PRECARIOUS PRESCRIPTIONS

PRECARIOUS PRESCRIPTIONS

Contested Histories of Race and Health in North America

LAURIE B. GREEN, JOHN MCKIERNAN-GONZÁLEZ,
AND MARTIN SUMMERS, EDITORS

UNIVERSITY OF MINNESOTA PRESS

Minneapolis
London

Portions of chapter 3 were previously published as "No License, Nor No Deplomer," in *Doctoring Freedom: The Politics of African American Medical Care in Slavery and Emancipation* (Chapel Hill: University of North Carolina Press, 2012), 114–38; copyright 2012 by the University of North Carolina Press; reprinted by permission of the publisher, www.uncpress.unc.edu. Chapter 8 was previously published as "Borders, Laborers, and Racialized Medicalization: Mexican Immigration and U.S. Public Health Practices in the Twentieth Century," *American Journal of Public Health* 101, no. 6 (June 2011): 1024–31.

Published by the University of Minnesota Press
111 Third Avenue South, Suite 290
Minneapolis, MN 55401-2520
http://www.upress.umn.edu

Library of Congress Cataloging-in-Publication Data

Precarious prescriptions : contested histories of race and health in North America / Laurie B. Green, John Mckiernan-González, and Martin Summers, editors.
    Includes bibliographical references and index.
    ISBN 978-0-8166-9046-6 (hc : alk. paper) — ISBN 978-0-8166-9047-3 (pb : alk. paper)
    1. African Americans—Health and hygiene. 2. Hispanic Americans—Health and hygiene. 3. Mexicans—Health and hygiene—United States. 4. Discrimination in medical care—North America. I. Green, Laurie B. (Laurie Beth), editor of compilation. II. Mckiernan-González, John Raymond, editor of compilation. III. Summers, Martin Anthony, editor of compilation.
    RA448.5.N4P74 2014
    362.1089'96073—dc23
                            2013028409

Printed in the United States of America on acid-free paper

The University of Minnesota is an equal-opportunity educator and employer.

20 19 18 17 16 15 14   10 9 8 7 6 5 4 3 2 1

Contents

Introduction

Making Race, Making Health

LAURIE B. GREEN, JOHN MCKIERNAN-GONZÁLEZ, AND MARTIN SUMMERS

IN 2009, the publication of *The Immortal Life of Henrietta Lacks* turned the attention of the American general reading public to a painful topic: the use and abuse of black bodies for scientific experimentation and medical education. Public reaction to science journalist Rebecca Skloot's account of the unauthorized acquisition of cancerous tissue from Henrietta Lacks, a working-class African American woman in Baltimore, and the subsequent revolution in cell culturing, placed the book on the bestseller list for an extraordinary number of weeks. This tale telescoped the complex relationship between ideas of racial difference and the hypervisibility and legal invisibility of African Americans in the development of biomedical thought and practice in the United States. The fact that the cells of Lacks's tumor were the first to reproduce ad infinitum, that this singular quality facilitated advancements in cell culturing technology, and that her cells went on to become the "standard laboratory workhorse" in almost all biomedical research for the next fifty years does little to obscure the larger dynamics that have characterized African Americans' relationship to the medical profession. Indeed, the case of Henrietta Lacks highlights these dynamics, which include the objectification and commodification of black bodies (in this case, black women's bodies), unethical and unauthorized medical research, black distrust of health care professionals, and persistent racial and socioeconomic disparities in health care access and quality.[1]

Stories of unauthorized dissections and medical experiments being conducted on black bodies have long circulated within African American communities and came to the fore in 1972 with revelations about the infamous Tuskegee Syphilis Study, in which the U.S. Public Health

Service between 1932 and 1972 observed approximately four hundred African American men with untreated syphilis. These histories gained broader recognition with science journalist Harriet A. Washington's 2006 publication *Medical Apartheid.* The Henrietta Lacks story now serves as a touchstone for what historians have been demonstrating for at least a generation now, that the Tuskegee study was hardly a unique episode given the role that race and racism have played in structuring the experiences African Americans have with biomedicine.[2]

Yet as unnerving as this story is, the encounters between the biomedical community and African Americans, and people of color more broadly, cannot be reduced to bromides of medical racism. This edited collection constructs a more complex portrait of the intertwined histories of race, medicine, and public health in the United States and its borderlands. In doing so, it extends lines of inquiry and analysis in terms of temporality, region, and race, ranging from Mexicans, Native Americans, African Americans, and government authorities in the nineteenth- and twentieth-century U.S.–Mexico borderlands; indigenous, Asian American, and Mexican American nurses and midwives in twentieth-century colonial Hawai'i and New Mexico; African American medical professionals, from Emancipation to the mid-twentieth century, in the South and nationally; and racialized groups, the mass media, and the state in the post–World War II era.

This diversity is not simply a matter of inclusion. By drawing them together in a single volume, we open new avenues for historical analysis. When taken together, the works of the scholars in this volume show that the dynamic interplay among categories of race, medicine, gender, and health were constitutive of social, cultural, and political processes far more broadly, and in more complicated and unpredictable ways, than we may have previously understood. We are not looking to present a model of medicalized racial formations but rather to encourage students and scholars in several fields to explore these relationships in order to better understand nation building, citizenship, poverty, health care, and the like.

THIS VOLUME emerged out of a conference held in November 2008 at the University of Texas at Austin, which brought together historians of medicine and of race from different generations and specialties, including most of the scholars whose studies appear in this volume.[3]

The conference aimed to advance a shared conversation among those concerned with the centrality of health and medicine to the history of race in the Americas and those whose work analyzes the significance of race in historical developments and conflicts over medical knowledge and practices. The papers at the conference also ranged across geographic boundaries and chronological lines. What excited us most were the ways in which discussions emerging out of the panels brought out in new ways the complexity of these intersecting histories. It was the historical contingency, more than the constancy of racism and medical authority, that came to the fore.

The chapters here illustrate how a bridging of the history of medicine and the history of race encourages an understanding of the relationship between race as a socially produced category of difference—its production and reproduction an act of racism itself—and race as a lived experience. In *Locating Medical History*, a 2004 volume edited by Frank Huisman and John Harley Warner assessing the state of the field of medical history, Susan M. Reverby and David Rosner made the observation that, although there had been important work in the history of medicine that took into account the centrality of gender, scholarship that looked at the history of medicine through the lens of race was lagging behind. They attributed this paucity to outmoded thinking about race, which was based more on a race relations model than a "race as discourse" paradigm. "The focus on the experience of particular people of color," they noted, "rather than the concept of race itself as an indicator of power relationships and an underlying assumption inherent in medical thinking, limited understandings of why race was critical in the history of health care."[4]

In the decade since Reverby and Rosner published their essay, and in the years directly preceding it, several scholars published works on the historic racialization of medicine, illness, and public health and the biomedical dimensions of racial formation in America. For scholars in race and ethnic studies, the history of medicine has provided a concrete way to connect the intellectual construction of racial difference, the material practices and policies that have emerged out of these constructions, and the lived experience of suffering and inequality. Their scholarship has presented a dynamic model for historians of medicine examining the ways in which people have been subjected to racist medical ideology, grappled with their health concerns, and engaged a medical and public health apparatus that has either excluded them altogether or included them on often unequal terms.

A much longer trajectory of scholarship in the history of race has informed this growing body of work within the history of medicine. For nearly half a century, scholars in the social sciences and humanities have illustrated how race is a historical, ideological process rather than a set of physical attributes or genetic traits. Whether articulated as racial formation, race making, or racialization, processes of producing racial categories and policing the boundaries between them occur in practically every realm of American life, including the law, public policy, the media, the academy, popular culture, and "the everyday."[5] As scholars have increasingly shown, race making also occurs in biomedicine, both in the impersonal realms of biotechnology and public health and in the more intimate domain of clinical practice.[6] Indeed, race making and medicalization—or, rather, race making through medicalization—is a dominant theme of this book. For the scholars assembled in this volume, medicalization means more than "the process whereby domains of life that were not previously so came under the aegis of medical practitioners and/or medical theories," as articulated by Ludmilla Jordanova in *Locating Medical History*.[7] Medicalization within a racial frame refers to the ways in which racial difference acquires the weight of truth through the production of biomedical knowledge and its deployment in therapeutic practice and public health policy. In this sense, race making takes the form of what historical sociologist Alondra Nelson has defined as "biomedical racialization."[8]

The chapters collected in this volume build on the scholarship of the past decade by starting from some basic premises: that assumptions about racial difference have been central to the development and evolution of categories within medical thought, that medical discourses and public health policies have been used in a variety of historical contexts to produce the normative citizen-subject, and that they have also been used to construct and police the raced, classed, gendered, and sexualized boundaries of national belonging. Some of the authors explore the ways in which medical knowledge and public health policy work to racialize certain groups—that is, to ascribe to people certain fixed biological qualities and traits that ostensibly determine temperament, capacity, and ability and that also allow social hierarchies to be explained as the natural results of these biological differences.

Other authors examine how racialized boundaries of citizenship, sovereignty, and national belonging are established, maintained, and, in some cases, undermined by professional medicine and vernacular healing cultures. And still others uncover the ways public health and professional medicine create social hierarchies that are based on racist assumptions of inferiority, backwardness, and difference.

Yet these studies also complicate these relationships in significant ways. They illustrate that the racialization of medical "problems" or the medicalization of racial differences have hardly been neat, coherent processes. Rather than assume their consistency and stability, for instance, several of the authors emphasize the multiple, often conflicting and competing narratives that are produced by, and in turn shape, these processes. To put it succinctly, acknowledging the existence of medical racism in America is only the starting point for our examinations of the relationship among medicine, race, and public health. The contributions here collectively tell a more complicated history of the relationship among medical knowledge, ideas of racial difference, health practices, and power.

Indeed, several of these scholars point to the complex nature of racialized groups' subjectivity, through an examination of contingency and intracommunity difference. In this sense, to borrow from medical historian Mary Fissell, this collection is a product of the cultural turn in the history of medicine, in which the focus of analysis "shift[s] from pattern to process, from understanding social categories as fairly static entities to analyzing how cultural categories work as ongoing sets of negotiations."[9] What Fissell calls "ongoing sets of negotiations" we address as the historically contingent processes that have shaped the making of race and the making of health in a variety of regions and among differently racialized groups in the United States, including within territories that were later incorporated as states.

Medicine and public health as arenas and practices of race making only partially convey the complex interplays among disease as a biological phenomenon, illness as a subjective experience, race as an ideological construct, and racism as a material practice.[10] It is critical that scholars approach the processes of racial formation and medicalization as dynamic projects that are constantly interacting and shaping one another. While medicine and public health are realms in which meanings of race are produced and contested, they also function as sites for the preservation of individual and collective well-being. What is lightly touched on in some of the chapters and more fully explored in others is the diverse ways in which racialized groups negotiate these arenas and practices and, in doing so, make demands on the health care profession or claims on the state to attend to their health needs.

Medical anthropologist Byron Good's challenge that scholars not reduce Western medicine to a form of biopolitical technology, an approach historians of medicine and race often pursue, based on their readings of Michel Foucault's work on this subject, is instructive in this regard. "Medical knowledge is not only a medium of perception, a 'gaze,' as one might take from Foucault," Good argues. "It is a medium of experience, a mode of engagement with the world. It is a dialogical medium, one of encounter, interpretation, conflict, and at times transformation."[11] Although Good was not referring specifically to race, his formulation provides an important conceptual framework for this volume. It suggests that studying the relationship between medicalization and racial formation cannot be limited to analyzing the state's construction and preservation of "normal" bodies. Rather, intellectual work on this front must attend to the full complexity of "biomedical racialization" *and* the pursuit of health as they are experienced and fought out within multiple arenas of everyday life.[12]

Over the past dozen years, a number of works have explored how people of color have engaged in this pursuit in the face of racially inflected and racist medical practices and public health policies.[13] However, making health, as a social and political practice, is itself a complicated undertaking that is marked by fracture and contestation as much as it is by solidarity. Indeed, the dialogical relationship that Good suggests characterizes the encounter between medical practitioners and sufferers might also be seen as a constitutive dynamic within marginalized communities if historians look closely enough.[14]

Even as they explore the ways in which marginalized groups engage and negotiate the professional- and state-generated discourses and practices that constitute them as objects of either exclusion or asymmetrical inclusion, several of the authors here also grapple with both the internal intricacies of the ways these groups respond and the contingencies that always accompany complex historical processes. In the process of making health, in other words, racialized groups do not always operate on some presupposed consensus of what best constitutes their collective interest; rather, negotiating the arenas of medicine and public health is bedeviled by differences along the lines of class, gender, sexuality, political persuasion, and immigrant status, and yet it can produce unanticipated and paradoxical alliances as well.

WHEN READ TOGETHER, the chapters assembled here speak to each other in significant ways, allowing readers to visit familiar themes of medical racism from new vantage points. Although the volume is organized chronologically, chapters that differ in region, temporality, or subject matter frequently intersect. For example, the collection is full of vivid case studies outlining how medical situations can become deeply ingrained in a given racial logic and policy frameworks connecting communities of color to the nation at large, giving assumptions about racial difference the ring of truth. Several contributors discuss historical contexts in which an officially sanctioned medical discourse portrayed people of color as threats to the state, even as the authors also recognize contradictions within these medical discourses. They also track the ways medical language moved across public health and medical institutions into other policy realms.

In "Making Crack Babies: Race Discourse and the Biologization of Behavior," Jason E. Glenn critically analyzes the 1980s firestorm unleashed by doctors' reports of a disturbing finding: Mothers addicted to crack cocaine were giving birth to babies with permanent neurological damage. Glenn argues that the medical spectacle of the "crack baby" offered a seductive storyline to a public that increasingly designated blacks as an urban underclass, "the offspring of poverty, joblessness, substance abuse, and criminal gang activity," which threatened America and was undeserving of public support. Glenn attributes the power of this story line to its links with other battlefront issues in the culture wars associated with the "Reagan Revolution," particularly the "War on Drugs." He asserts that public officials called for seemingly race-neutral policies to rescue "crack babies" by punishing the mothers and fathers who pushed crack cocaine into the veins of their unborn children. The "crack baby" epidemic provided a biological justification for draconian public policies such as mandatory sentencing laws for drug use, expanded policing, and the restructuring of welfare. As Glenn makes very clear, the only problem with the narrative is that medically, "crack babies" never existed; that is, there were no scientific studies linking maternal crack addiction to long-term damage to infant health. Drawing on copious evidence, he finds that "crack babies" provided a highly charged medical framework that became the basis for a harsher, more punitive set of public policies applied to African Americans.

Mark Allan Goldberg documents another instance in which an apparently extreme medical event provided government authorities the opportunity to engage in a particular political project, but in this case he addresses a real epidemic in the context of nation building in the Texas–Mexico borderlands. In "Curing the Nation with Cacti: Native Healing and State Building before the Texas Revolution," Goldberg highlights the ways that assumptions about racial difference were both pronounced and hidden in the Mexican government's attempt to combat cholera. In Texas in the 1830s, Mexican officials and American merchants sought ways to end their vulnerability and dependence on the goodwill of the Comanche, whom they perceived to be fundamentally different. However, when cholera threatened the stability of Mexican towns in the Comanche–Mexican–American borderlands, Mexican doctors ratified the use of peyote treatment regimens taken from "savage" ritual healing practices of Native Gulf Coast healers. Although many physicians relied on botanics and practiced various kinds of natural medicine, they considered health practices that grew from Native spirituality as unscientific, uncivilized, and unprogressive. Paradoxically, Mexican officials continued treating Indian nations as threats to the Mexican nation and yet, in the midst of the cholera crisis, happily prescribed peyote cactus button extracts to save the republic. Ritual peyote use by Natives confirmed their inherently savage nature even as Mexican peyote use provided succor in the times of cholera.

In Natalia Molina's chapter, "Borders, Laborers, and Racialized Medicalization: Mexican Immigration and U.S. Public Health Practices in the Twentieth Century," it is Mexican immigrants who constitute a menace, now that northern Mexico has been claimed as part of the United States. As with the history about which Goldberg writes, this menace is constructed and represented through racialized medical discourse, but in this case it is policed through immigration policy. Molina details three different points when the spectacle of medical interventions provided visual confirmation of the intimate threat "diseased" Mexican workers posed to American households: a 1916 typhus outbreak among

Mexican laborers in the Los Angeles area, medical inspections in the Bracero program in the 1940s, and private medical deportations of Mexicans and Latin Americans in the contemporary era. She demonstrates how disease, or merely the threat of it, marked Mexicans as "foreign," just as much as phenotype, native language, accent, or clothing. This association of their "foreignness" with their purportedly innate pathogenic capacity was forged at the same time that Mexican men and women provided the domestic service, custodial work, and farm labor needed to keep American families and homes fed, clean, and clothed. Moreover, the immigration policy and procedures that emerged reflected this contradiction. The medical inspections to which Mexican immigrants were subjected at the border were geared toward producing the "acceptable laborer," but they also stigmatized Mexicans as innate disease carriers. As Molina further demonstrates, the nature of the Mexican "threat" has changed. Whereas in the early twentieth century Mexican immigrants were viewed primarily as a threat to the nation's public health, in the current political climate undocumented Mexicans are seen as a threat to the nation's fiscal health.

As the chapters by Glenn, Goldberg, and Molina demonstrate, the articulation of racial difference through medical discourse and public health policy has a long history in the United States, a history that encompasses the experiences of, and relationships between, peoples before their incorporation into the American nation-state. Although at various moments medical events were exploited in order to demarcate the literal boundaries of the nation and the figurative boundaries of normative American-ness, the discourses and policies that emerged to confront these events were not without their own internal contradictions. Indeed, these contradictions bring into focus the illogic that was at the heart of the processes of medicalizing racial difference.

Several case studies show the myriad ways "Native," "local," and "traditional" healers interacted with Western biomedicine. In doing so, they point to the ways men and women in communities of color actively moved within and outside the formal structures of professional medicine and public health in order to establish their professional identities or intervene in medical crises in their communities.

Gretchen Long, in her chapter, "'I Studied and Practiced Medicine without Molestation': African American Doctors in the First Years of Freedom," traces how the growing status of allopathic medicine also affected African Americans who had practiced medicine during slavery and now sought to establish themselves as professional doctors. Focusing on two men who appealed their cases to the federal Freedmen's Bureau, which established offices throughout the former confederacy after the Civil War, Long finds that both faced racial injustice in their efforts to gain recognition. Her discussion of their attempts to exercise their full rights of citizenship might have ended at this point; however, Long surprises the reader with the information that the Freedman's Bureau did not treat their cases in similar ways. Influenced by the rising authority of allopathic medicine in Union Army hospitals, the bureau ascribed different values to the appeals of John Donalson, who had practiced herbal, Native American–influenced medicine in Austin, Texas, and Moses Camplin, who had learned the most modern of medical practices as an apprentice to his owner, a highly respected physician in Charleston, South Carolina. Most significantly, the differing values ascribed to their practices became bound up with race. The Freedmen's Bureau demanded a license for Camplin, but Donalson became "an African quack," ineligible for protection as a citizen. The chapter ultimately raises questions about the kind of freedom wrought by the Civil War, by asking what it meant to try to freely practice the craft of medicine under this new state definition of doctoring.

In "Complicating Colonial Narratives: Medical Encounters around the Salish Sea, 1854–1878," Jennifer Seltz further explores in the context of the Pacific Northwest how a tradition of cultural exchange in the area of health and healing gave way to more rigid racialized understandings of what constituted illness and the appropriate means of treating it. Eschewing the disappearing Indian narrative that has shaped much work on Native American history, Seltz considers the interaction among Indian agents, traders, farmers, and Native populations in a disease environment wrought by American political and commercial expansion into the Salish Sea area. She argues that the history of local healing exchanges between Native peoples and white settlers up until the late 1870s unsettles the assumption that a distinct Native healing tradition and a Western medical tradition existed in this area. However, as white Americans began to dominate the Puget Sound region, they increasingly constructed disease among Native peoples as "spatially and biologically separate" from themselves. These representations of a distinctive Native proclivity to disease, along with portrayals of indigenous healing as barbarous, worked to construct the narratives of Indians as a dying race and white American hegemony as inevitable. And yet far from behaving as a dying race with alien diseases and medical practices, Native people pressured the federal government to remember the medical obligations of its treaties. These protests, unsuccessful American efforts to curtail local healers' power, and settler attempts to dispossess Indian communities in the name of health, Seltz argues, reveal complex local histories that preceded and sometimes undercut sweeping claims about Native decline in the face of American expansion.

In "Professionalizing 'Local Girls': Nursing and U.S. Colonial Rule in Hawai'i, 1920–1948," Jean J. Kim examines dynamics of contestation over meanings of health and healing in the context of American imperial expansion. In Hawai'i, formal U.S. annexation in 1900 included the elaboration of a public health system that displaced indigenous male healers and placed medical care under the control of white physicians from the continent. In extending their authority over an urban and plantation workforce of native Hawaiians, contract laborers from Japan and other Pacific islands, colonial recruits from the Philippines, and others, health officials established a feminized, racially hierarchical nursing system based on white nurses and "local girls." "In Hawai'i, as in contemporary U.S. and British colonies," Kim asserts, "authorities sought to recruit indigenous and racialized women as nurses to secure colonial infrastructures by supplying needed labor, insulating white women from intimacy with colonial bodies, and supplying cultural brokering." On the U.S. continent in the early twentieth century, she argues, the increasing prevalence of white nurses professionally trained in allopathic medicine went hand in hand with the exclusion of black women from most nursing programs; however, in the imperial context "local girls" were racialized not by their exclusion but by their inclusion in the territorial public health system. This process cast Hawaiian nurses as an undifferentiated nonwhite group; however, the corps of "local girls" included Japanese American daughters of noncitizen laborers, who were in the majority, indigenous women, Filipinas, and others who were well beyond girlhood. Although they were taught that Western medicine and definitions of health and sanitation were superior, they nonetheless adapted and rejected different dimensions of American medical theories and nursing practices in ways that respected and preserved their communities' medical traditions.

Lena McQuade-Salzfass's chapter, "'An Indispensable Service': Midwives and Medical Officials after New Mexico Statehood," shifts our attention from biomedicine to the place of midwives in the transition to statehood for New Mexico. The change in status enfranchised close to 300,000 people, and many Americans felt threatened by the presence of a Nuevomexicano voting bloc presumed to be of mixed-race Indian–Spanish–Mexican descent. Birth practices, in particular, became the focus of these political anxieties. *Parteras*—Spanish-speaking community-based midwives in the United States—attended most births in New Mexico between World War I and World War II; to American authorities, they also represented tradition-bound practices and superstitions that needed to be eradicated in order to transform Mexican American women into American women. Despite these Americanizing priorities and the influx of federal funds through the landmark Maternal and Infancy Protection Act (Sheppard–Towner), the mostly white state health department employees of a Mexican American majority state were forced to recognize their inability to replace parteras across rural New Mexico. Public health officials in New Mexico instead tried to regulate parteras by hiring white nurses from outside New Mexico with little or no knowledge of Spanish to train and certify these parteras in their already established craft. Many parteras seized on the attempt to transform or displace them by actually pursuing licensing as an entryway into the professional health sector and an opportunity for geographic mobility. However, these nurses' public frustration with parteras' reluctance to conform helped authorize a Depression-era backlash against Mexican Americans in New Mexico, which, McQuade-Salzfass argues, meant that, "after New Mexico became a state, midwifery came to symbolize all that was different about New Mexico in the United States."

Another theme that bridges several chapters involves the complexity of claims by racialized citizen groups on the nation-state and its public health programs, in ways that complicate medical racism by defying predictable lines of contestation. John Mckiernan-González confronts such paradoxes in his chapter, "At the Nation's Edge: African American Migrants and Smallpox in the Late-Nineteenth-Century Mexican–American Borderlands." The hundreds of colonists he writes about responded to the dire conditions of the post-Reconstruction South by migrating to Mexico, at the behest of recruiters looking for laborers to work in the cotton fields of the powerful Compañia Agricola Tlahualilo. Ironically, three months later they appealed to the U.S. government for intervention, in protest of conditions that rivaled what they had left in Alabama. The State Department did take action, but only by casting its intervention as a medical mission to rescue American citizens who had been exposed to smallpox. Having become refugees, they were soon subjected to a high-profile U.S. Marine Hospital Service (USMHS) field trial to test potential smallpox serum vaccines. One could easily end this story with the tragic medical racism reflected in the USMHS's inoculations of African Americans with a potentially deadly serum. Mckiernan-González instead complicates this picture by tracing efforts by the refugees to leverage their status as research subjects to pressure the U.S. government into guaranteeing their safe passage back to their homes in the heart of the Deep South. Paradoxically, he argues, "The migrants' return is a compelling story of African American workers exploiting their role as commodities in an emerging laboratory-based American research economy, just as federal health officers exploited the migrants' high-profile illness while also laboring on behalf of the migrants' survival."

Fast-forwarding to the welfare state in the New Deal era, Verónica Martínez-Matsuda explores a different kind of encounter between the federal government and racialized agricultural laborers in the Texas borderlands. In "'A Transformation for Migrants': Mexican Farmworkers and Federal Health Reform during the New Deal Era," she analyzes Mexican American farm laborers' sojourns in New Deal resettlement camps established by the Farm Security Administration (FSA), most famously for white Dust Bowl refugees in California but actually in multiple states. Martínez-Matsuda refuses to be hemmed in by either of two opposite historical narratives: a hagiography of the FSA camps as utopias for migrant farmworker families or a critique of them as sites of exploitation that made laborers available for agribusiness. Although the chapter discusses the camps as projects of the most radical of New Deal agencies, intent on improving the lives of migrant families, she explores the complexity of Mexican Americans' approaches to their widely hailed modern medical programs. Again, one might have interpreted their responses in one of two ways: either a whole-hearted embrace based on migrants' desires to protect their children from malnutrition and tuberculosis or a rejection based on their attachments to longstanding modes of health care by midwives and healers. In fact, Martínez-Matsuda finds evidence of both reactions. Moreover, she concludes that even families who took full advantage of their status as medical subjects of the welfare state also resisted elements of another aspect of the FSA mission: to reshape them into model American citizens, "divested of the cultural and social attributes that defined their lives as ethnic Mexicans."

Moving into the 1960s, Laurie B. Green in "'Hunger in America' and the Power of Television: Poor People, Physicians, and the Mass Media in the War against Poverty" argues that the framing of disease within a racial (or a nonracialist) discourse does not necessarily function in a top-down manner, as the sole prerogative of either the state or medical professionals, nor as a reverse, bottom-up process in which racialized people determine their own narratives. In the embattled case of the "discovery of hunger in America," the mass media became part of the equation of power. As the ink was drying on the 1964 Civil Rights Act, activists in the Deep South began mounting protests to draw attention to worsening poverty. However, it was not until April 1967 that the federal government began to respond, after broadcast journalists, newspaper reporters, and photographers captured the shock of Robert Kennedy and other senators when they observed in Mississippi what they associated with World Hunger, including children with distended bellies. A subsequent report by human rights physicians challenged racist diagnoses of malnutrition that blamed black women for their children's hunger and instead laid blame on the federal government and southern congressmen. Green focuses on CBS's 1968 documentary "Hunger in America," which turned the tide of public concern by uncoupling hunger from blackness through a format that focused equally on Mexican Americans, Native Americans, poor whites, and blacks and foregrounded moving interviews with women and children. "In the historical context of the 1960s," she concludes, "there was no unified articulation of knowledge about malnutrition," and whether and how federal food policy would resolve the hunger crisis rested on who controlled the racial narrative of hunger.

Finally, one theme that emerges with particular clarity in the chapters by Martin Summers and Susan M. Reverby is the necessity of complicating the analytical categories of resistance and agency in histories of race, medicine, and public health. In "Diagnosing the Ailments of Black Citizenship: African American Physicians and the Politics of Mental Illness, 1895–1940," Summers examines how black physicians' approach to mental illness in the first half of the twentieth century was shaped by medical racism on one hand and by larger public health concerns on the other. In the post-Emancipation period, white physicians pointed to an increased incidence of insanity as evidence that African Americans were ill equipped to deal with freedom. Even as black physicians robustly disputed these racial degeneracy theories, they rarely addressed mental illness directly. In explaining the absence of a medical discourse on insanity within black medical professional circles, Summers argues that the profession's preoccupation with diseases that were an index of poverty and discrimination, such as tuberculosis, syphilis, and pellagra, enabled it to develop a critique of structural racism and inequality. When the profession did turn its attention to mental illness after World War I, it was mainly to address neurological injuries of African American veterans, which served as a testament for blacks' capacity for full citizenship. In the end, Summers maintains, although this imperative of citizenship was a necessary form of resistance to blacks' economic, social, and political marginalization, it also rendered invisible African Americans with functional mental illnesses in the eyes of black physicians. For Summers, the decisions that black physicians made—in a sense, their agency—is an important piece of the puzzle in understanding African Americans' continued skepticism of psychiatry as a legitimate resource for the preservation of mental health.

For Reverby, agency is also a useful analytical category, but one that must be complemented by historical contingency in order to develop a fuller understanding of historical phenomena. Counterpoised as they usually are against narratives of suffering and racism, narratives of agency and resistance can lead to an incomplete and impoverished rendering of history. Reverby develops this line of thinking in "Suffering and Resistance, Voice and Agency: Thoughts on History and the Tuskegee Syphilis Study." As she points out, voice and agency became the central analytic foci for historians trained in the 1970s who fought to create a new social history based on the premise that working-class people, women, and communities of color were not mere victims or followers but were actors who pushed back against structures of domination and who spoke for themselves. Immersed in the research of the events that occurred in Tuskegee, Reverby grappled with a key question: "Suffering and abuse are central to the story's core. In the face of what seems like a known story where suffering and death are the key to our outrage and endless pictures of 'abject' black men appear, what can we ask anew?" Through an examination of one of the men, often taken as paradigmatic of the suffering, she argues that an analytic frame of victimization and resistance is inadequate, even if it has added further dimension to the racist medical monsters trope that usually dominates accounts of the study. She goes further, asking how we separate out what happened from what is symbolically important. Reverby does not deny that race and racism were central to how the study at Tuskegee unfolded, but the totality of this sustained medical encounter between black rural Alabamans and the federal government—including motivations, decisions, and actions on all sides—cannot be fully understood by looking solely through those lenses.

Both Summers and Reverby challenge us to rethink the role of agency and resistance in historical examinations of the relationship among race, racism, medicine, and public health. Although Summers acknowledges the centrality of the concepts of resistance and agency to understanding how people of color have responded to racism, he also points to the ways in which resistance often fails to benefit everyone in marginalized communities. Reverby, on the other hand, impresses on us the importance of leavening our desire to see agency everywhere with a healthy dose of respect for historical contingency.

IT HAS BEEN more than fifty years since Charles Rosenberg's landmark study on cholera opened up new vistas for scholars who were interested in the intellectual, social, and cultural dimensions of sickness and health, and almost twenty-five years since Barbara Jeanne Fields's landmark article, "Slavery, Race and Ideology," encouraged scholars to view race as an historical, ideological process.[15] As a collection of essays by scholars who are working at the intersection of the histories of medicine and race, this volume seeks to open up new vistas as well. Thanks to the pioneering generation of scholars that made the social history of medicine a legitimate academic pursuit, the authors are able to investigate the subjective nature of disease and illness and the political dimension of medicine and public health without having to endure the charge that they are not giving due consideration to the objective and altruistic side of laboratory and clinical medicine. Thanks to an earlier generation of scholars who transformed our understanding of race from a natural division of humanity to, variously, a mode of representation, a logic of inclusion and exclusion, and one of the means by which group consciousness is formed and lived, the authors find it easier to locate the role of medicine in the production of racial discourses and the power relationships that flow from them. Far too often, the historical analysis of health and illness in American culture has been insulated from ongoing debates over the shape of citizenship and the nature of belonging in communities of color.

Yet an embrace of historical contingency—reflected in the terms that so often stand in as shorthand for this concept, such as *paradox, the unexpected,* and *messiness*—has also shaped the ways in which the contributors to this volume have approached their examination of the relationship between medicalization and racial formation. An example of this kind of contingency might be illustrated with a brief return to Henrietta Lacks. Paradoxically, even as the discriminatory, exploitative treatment she received emanated from larger social assumptions about racial difference and black inferiority, the harvesting of Lacks's cells reflected a fundamental belief in the biological sameness of African Americans and whites. This type of tension existed in scientific and medical thought going back to the Enlightenment and was most poignantly expressed in the use of enslaved African Americans for medical experimentation and demonstration.[16] By the time Lacks's tumor cells were excised in 1951, many people in mainstream scientific and academic circles openly challenged scientific claims about the radical difference associated with black bodies. Even as the fields of genetics and population studies continued to debate the utility of racial difference in explaining human variation, the idea that people of African descent were biologically inferior to, and naturally incompatible with, whites ceased to be one of the foundational pillars of post–World War II science and medicine. Many white Americans continued to believe in the racial distinctiveness of blood, emblematized by the American Red Cross policy of segregating white and "negro" blood in the early 1940s. However, the consensus among biologists, hematologists, physical anthropologists, physicians, and even many Red Cross officials was that this persistent belief amounted to nothing more than superstition.[17] And yet the very compatibility of Lacks's tumor cells, combined with her social location in the Jim Crow South, produced a scenario in which she, like countless other black and brown men and women, was enlisted in the cause of science without her knowledge and without compensation.

Even given the problematic nature of Lacks's conscription into the laboratory, it is undeniable that the research done with her cells, named HeLa according to standard laboratory protocol, has led to tremendous scientific progress, from the development of the polio vaccine to advances in virology. Within the medical and scientific communities, moreover, there are varied opinions with respect to the ethics of the original acquisition of the cells and whether or not Lacks's progeny should be beneficiaries of some of the profits generated by the commercialization of HeLa. For their part, Lacks's family had, and presumably continues to have, conflicted feelings about the research using her cells. These include anger at Johns Hopkins, where much of the early research was conducted, and bitterness toward the biotech companies that have profited handsomely from HeLa. Yet they also include pride in the knowledge that Lacks's cells (often personified as Henrietta herself by her family members) have contributed so much to scientific progress. Nonetheless, one of the points that unifies them is a recognition of the irony that Lacks's contribution has not materially affected their lives. As the experience of Henrietta Lacks and the ambivalence with which her family has come to understand it suggests, medical racism is an inadequate concept for understanding the role of ideas of racial difference in the complicated relationship among medical practitioners, public health officials, and sufferers and their social networks.

In the final chapter of this volume, Susan M. Reverby reflects on the history of the Tuskegee syphilis study and warns that by relying on familiar "binaries of suffering and resistance" among those subjected to medical racism—in this case poor African American men in Alabama—and paying less attention to historical contingencies and counternarratives of medical science and race, we may be sidestepping the very analysis we need to understand the tragedy. Indeed, many of us initially embarked on journeys to document the medical treatment, suffering, and voices of those targeted by racist medical knowledge and practice. Along the way, however, we confronted contradictions and paradoxes that muddied the waters, encouraging us to challenge static concepts of power that can so easily dominate studies of race and medicine. In taking up this challenge, we do not deny the millions of people of color who, like Henrietta Lacks and her family, have been the victims of deception and neglect at the hands of the medical profession and public health apparatus of the United States. Although it is imperative that we not forget the manifold instances of medical racism in American history, however, offering more nuanced analyses of historical contingency is critical to fully understanding how both race and health can be made and unmade in the biomedical arena.

NOTES

1 Rebecca Skloot, *The Immortal Life of Henrietta Lacks* (New York: Crown Publishers, 2010). On the visibility and legal invisibility of enslaved African Americans in biomedical practice, see Todd L. Savitt, "The Use of Blacks for Medical Experimentation and Demonstration in the Old South," *Journal of Southern History* 48 (1982): 331–48.

2 Harriet Washington, *Medical Apartheid: The Dark History of Medical Experimentation on Black Americans from Colonial Times to the Present* (New York: Random House, 2006). On Tuskegee see Susan M. Reverby, *Examining Tuskegee: The Infamous Syphilis Study and Its Legacy* (Chapel Hill: University of North Carolina Press, 2009); Susan M. Reverby, ed., *Tuskegee's Truths: Rethinking the Tuskegee Syphilis Study* (Chapel Hill: University of North Carolina Press, 2000); and James Jones, *Bad Blood: The Tuskegee Syphilis Experiment* (New York: Free Press, 1981).

3 Conference speakers included José Amador de Jesús, Nancy Bercaw, Lundy Braun, Laura Briggs, Jorge Canizares-Esguerra, Sherri Ann Charleston, Vanessa Northington Gamble, Mark Allan Goldberg, Pablo Gomez, Laurie B. Green, Judith Houck, Niklas Jensen, Richard Keller, Gretchen Long, Verónica Martínez-Matsuda, John Mckiernan-González, Lena McQuade-Salzfass, Jonathan Metzl, Natalia Molina, Thuy Linh Nguyen, David Oshinsky, Okezi Otovo, Leslie Reagan, Susan M. Reverby, Megan Seaholm, James Sidbury, Susan Smith, Martin Summers, Verónica Vallejo, and Jane Whalen.

4 Susan M. Reverby and David Rosner, "'Beyond the Great Doctors' Revisited: A Generation of the 'New' Social History of Medicine," in *Locating Medical History: The Stories and Their Meanings,* ed. Frank Huisman and John Harley Warner (Baltimore, Md.: Johns Hopkins University Press, 2004), 183.

5 Barbara Jeanne Fields, "Slavery, Race and Ideology in the United States of America," *New Left Review* 181 (1990): 95–118; Michael Omi and Howard Winant, *Racial Formation in the United States: From the 1960s to the 1990s,* 2nd ed. (New York: Routledge, 1994); and Thomas C. Holt, "Marking: Race, Race-making, and the Writing of History," *American*

Historical Review 100 (February 1995): 1–20. The literature on the social constructedness of race is vast, but representative works include David R. Roediger, *The Wages of Whiteness: Race and the Making of the American Working Class* (London: Verso, 1991); Neil Foley, *The White Scourge: Mexicans, Blacks, and Poor Whites in Texas Cotton Culture* (Berkeley: University of California Press, 1999); Melissa Nobles, *Shades of Citizenship: Race and the Census in Modern Politics* (Stanford, Calif.: Stanford University Press, 2000); Henry Yu, *Thinking Orientals: Migration, Contact, and Exoticism in Modern America* (New York: Oxford University Press, 2001); Mae Ngai, *Impossible Subjects: Illegal Aliens and the Making of Modern America* (Princeton, N.J.: Princeton University Press, 2005); Erika Marie Bsumek, *Indian-Made: Navajo Culture in the Marketplace, 1868–1940* (Lawrence: University Press of Kansas, 2008); Ariela J. Gross, *What Blood Won't Tell: A History of Race on Trial in America* (Cambridge, Mass.: Harvard University Press, 2008); and Peggy Pascoe, *What Comes Naturally: Miscegenation Law and the Making of Race in America* (New York: Oxford University Press, 2009).

6   On biotechnology and public health as sites of racial formation, see Keith Wailoo, *Drawing Blood: Technology and Disease Identity in Twentieth-Century America* (Baltimore, Md.: Johns Hopkins University Press, 1997); Wailoo, *Dying in the City of the Blues: Sickle Cell Anemia and the Politics of Race and Health* (Chapel Hill: University of North Carolina Press, 2001); Dorothy Roberts, *Fatal Invention: How Science, Politics, and Big Business Re-Create Race in the Twenty-First Century* (New York: New Press, 2011); Nayan Shah, *Contagious Divides: Epidemics and Race in San Francisco's Chinatown* (Berkeley: University of California Press, 2001); Alexandra Stern, *Eugenic Nation: Faults and Frontiers of Better Breeding in Modern America* (Berkeley: University of California Press, 2005); Natalia Molina, *Fit to Be Citizens? Public Health and Race in Los Angeles, 1879–1939* (Berkeley: University of California Press, 2006); and Samuel Kelton Roberts Jr., *Infectious Fear: Politics, Disease, and the Health Effects of Segregation* (Chapel Hill: University of North Carolina Press, 2009). We take the term *intimate domain* from historical anthropologist Ann Laura Stoler, "Tense and Tender Ties: The Politics of Comparison in North American History and (Post) Colonial Studies," *Journal of American History* 88 (December 2001): esp. 831, n4.

7   Ludmilla Jordanova, "The Social Construction of Medical Knowledge," in Huisman and Warner, *Locating Medical History*, 345. For a succinct critical discussion of the concept of medicalization, see the introduction to Cindy Patton, ed., *Rebirth of the Clinic: Places and Agents in Contemporary Health Care* (Minneapolis: University of Minnesota Press, 2010), xiv.

8   Alondra Nelson, *Body and Soul: The Black Panther Party and the Fight against Medical Discrimination* (Minneapolis: University of Minnesota Press, 2011), 25.

9 Mary Fissell, "Making Meaning from the Margins: The New Cultural History of Medicine," in *Locating Medical History*, 374.

10 The distinction between disease and illness has been an important analytical paradigm in the social history of medicine, and the scholars who observe it are too numerous to list here. For classic articulations of the distinction, see Arthur Kleinman, *The Illness Narratives: Suffering, Healing, and the Human Condition* (New York: Basic Books, 1988) and Charles Rosenberg, "Framing Disease: Illness, Society, and History," in *Explaining Epidemics and Other Studies in the History of Medicine* (Cambridge, England: Cambridge University Press, 1992), 305–18.

11 Byron Good, *Medicine, Rationality, and Experience: An Anthropological Perspective* (Cambridge, England: Cambridge University Press, 1994), 86. Also see Michel Foucault, *History of Sexuality: Volume 1: An Introduction*, trans. Robert Hurley (New York: Vintage Books, 1990); Foucault, *Birth of the Clinic: An Archaeology of Medical Perception*, trans. A. M. Sheridan Smith (New York: Vintage Books, 1994); Foucault, *Discipline and Punish: The Birth of the Prison*, trans. Alan Sheridan (New York: Vintage Books, 1995).

12 Excepting the racial dimension, this was, in fact, a line of argument developed by Foucault himself. See Foucault, *History of Sexuality: Volume 3: The Care of the Self*, trans. Robert Hurley (New York: Vintage Books, 1988); and Thomas Lemke, *Bio-politics: An Advanced Introduction* (New York: New York University Press, 2011), 50–52.

13 Important representative works include Jim Downs, *Sick from Freedom: African-American Illness and Suffering during the Civil War and Reconstruction* (New York: Oxford University Press, 2012); Gretchen Long, *Doctoring Freedom: The Politics of African American Medical Care in Slavery and Emancipation* (Chapel Hill: University of North Carolina Press, 2012); John Mckiernan-González, *Fevered Measures: Public Health and Race at the Texas–Mexico Border, 1848–1942* (Durham, N.C.: Duke University Press, 2012); Sharla M. Fett, *Working Cures: Healing, Health, and Power on Southern Slave Plantations* (Chapel Hill: University of North Carolina Press, 2002); Michelle T. Moran, *Colonizing Leprosy: Imperialism and the Politics of Public Health in the United States* (Chapel Hill: University of North Carolina Press, 2007); Nelson, *Body and Soul*; Wailoo, *Dying in the City of the Blues*.

14 For good examples of this kind of historical treatment, see Shah, *Contagious Divides*; Susan L. Smith, *Sick and Tired of Being Sick and Tired: Black Women's Health Activism in America, 1890–1950* (Philadelphia: University of Pennsylvania Press, 1995).

15 Charles E. Rosenberg, *The Cholera Years: The United States in 1832, 1849, and 1866* (Chicago: University of Chicago Press, 1962); Fields, "Slavery, Race and Ideology." See also Fields's essay, "Of Rogues and Geldings," *American Historical Review* 108 (December 2003): 1397–1405, which critiques scholars who have substituted what she perceives to be an

apolitical use of race as a category of analysis for critical exegeses on racism as a "crime against humanity."

16   Andrew S. Curran, *The Anatomy of Blackness: Science and Slavery in an Age of Enlightenment* (Baltimore, Md.: Johns Hopkins University Press, 2011); Savitt, "Use of Blacks."

17   Elazar Barkan, *The Retreat from Scientific Racism: Changing Concepts of Race in Britain and the United States between the World Wars* (New York: Cambridge University Press, 1993), esp. 279–339; Jenny Reardon, *Race to the Finish: Identity and Governance in an Age of Genomics* (Princeton, N.J.: Princeton University Press, 2005), esp. 1–44; Wailoo, *Drawing Blood*, 162–214; and Spencie Love, *One Blood: The Death and Resurrection of Charles R. Drew* (Chapel Hill: University of North Carolina Press, 1996), 183–214.

1

Curing the Nation with Cacti

Native Healing and State Building before the Texas Revolution

MARK ALLAN GOLDBERG

JUST TWELVE YEARS after Mexico declared independence from Spain, a cholera epidemic that had struck Europe, Asia, and North America made its way to Mexico. Cholera ravaged much of the nation, stretching from Chiapas in the south to Tamaulipas and Texas in the north. When it first appeared in New Orleans in late 1832, municipalities in Texas began to prepare for an imminent attack. The disease struck southern Mexico in the spring of 1833, and the federal and state governments sent preventive measures to city councils in the north to combat the disease. When the epidemic reappeared in Tamaulipas, state and municipal governments across the Texas–Mexico borderlands sent more measures, plus physician Pascual de Aranda's prescription. They later supplemented de Aranda's scrip with a different remedy, in which physician Ignacio Sendejas incorporated peyote, a plant associated with Native spirituality. Sendejas's cure became the state's preferred prescription.

Native health practices such as peyote healing made the Indians savage in the eyes of Mexicans.[1] Rooted in the Spanish colonial era, Mexicans based their notions of race partly on cultural practices. For Mexicans, Catholic customs were civilized and proper, and they considered anything beyond the Christian cultural realm uncivilized. For example, Indians in East Texas reportedly believed that "all internal maladies are caused by some witchcraft," a belief counter to Catholicism.[2] Mexicans recognized the power and skill of Native healers and continued treating Native healing arts as "superstitions" based on the spiritual character of Native healing. The Indians' use of chants, drums, and sucking to enact cures also appeared "heathen" to Mexican eyes.

These characterizations of Indian "savagery" shaped Indian relations and nation building in early national northern Mexico.

Centered on the U.S.–Mexico border, this is a story of state formation at the outer limits and meeting point of two nations and numerous Native communities. Through an analysis of different forms of healing during the 1833 cholera epidemic in the Texas–Mexico borderlands, this chapter examines the connections between medical practice and nineteenth-century state formation in Mexico and beyond.[3] Disease outbreaks brought everyday Native cultural practices to the forefront of elite Mexican visions of state formation, and the exchange of healing customs placed marginalized populations at the center of nation building. But the literature on state building often obscures the cultural elements of these instrumental political and economic processes.[4] In their national projects for the Mexican north, for example, Mexican state officials advocated individual land use and (limited) popular political representation, practices that were as cultural as they were political and economic. This study centers on the place of Native healing practices in nineteenth-century nation-building efforts. Centuries of tenuous yet interdependent relations set the stage for the exchange of peyote healing between Native peoples and Mexican officials. A focus on disease and healing helps depict Mexican nation building as a cultural negotiation as well as a political and economic one.

This study also uses the Mexican state's response to the 1833 cholera epidemic as a window into how health and healing shaped race making in the Texas–Mexico borderlands. As people constantly grappled with disease, the young Mexican nation grappled with colonizing a frontier region, securing its citizens against Indian raids, protecting claims to land, incorporating diverse peoples into the body politic, and now healing sick citizens in this moment of crisis. In the borderlands, Mexican officials were working to create "civilized" societies among "uncivilized," frontier peoples. Trying to build a nation on the margins, Mexico's elites promoted certain practices that they considered to be central to national progress, and they used culture to marginalize populations who, in their eyes, practiced "uncivilized," "savage" customs. For example, Native spiritual healing constituted improper medicine because it was not scientific. Mexican medical science, on the other hand, was not only proper but also modern and therefore constituted service to the young nation. However, the cholera epidemic forced Mexican doctors to draw from Native healers during the cholera epidemic. They stripped the peyote remedy from the taints of Indian spirituality and made it medical through scientific methods. Thus, Mexican authorities blurred the boundary between proper and improper national health practices when they adopted peyote healing as an integral component of modern public health. They relied on a practice that they had deemed savage and not Mexican. To understand how peyote found its way into Mexico's public health system in the Texas–Mexico borderlands, let us turn to cholera's arrival in Mexico.

THE 1833 CHOLERA EPIDEMIC IN TEXAS

Cholera did not only cause mortality rates to soar in the nineteenth century; it also caused much pain for those afflicted with the deadly disease. The disease produced dehydration, cramps, muscle spasms, and thirst. It caused uncontrollable vomiting, diarrhea, and sometimes bleeding.[5] Historian Christopher Hamlin argues that this horrible illness deeply affected not only the victims but also the communities in which they lived, before, during, and after an epidemic.[6] Cholera's appearance in southern Mexico in the fall of 1832 had such a ripple effect on the entire nation, igniting social and political activity across the young republic.

Once the federal government learned that cholera had invaded the republic through the southern state of Chiapas in February 1833, the news trickled down the political ladder from the national office to the *ayuntamientos,* or municipalities. The governor of the northern state of Coahuila y Texas responded with a list of thirteen preventive measures targeting dirty environments. Efforts at creating and maintaining clean public spaces even included regulations for households and targeted personal hygiene. For example, the *juntas de sanidad,* or Boards of Health, were in charge of "care of the streets, plazas and other passages of public use, and removing trash, rocks, . . . [and] other potentially harmful things," and people were told to "bathe and shower at least every Saturday."[7] For about a month, cholera spared Texas, even though the epidemic already had taken many lives in Louisiana to the east and farther south in Chiapas.

Later in the summer of 1833, cholera hit parts of northern Mexico.[8] The settlements in Coahuila, just south of Texas, promptly responded with public health initiatives. For example, the *ayuntamiento* of

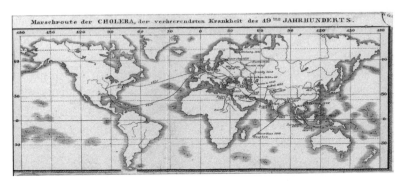

FIGURE 1.1. The global reach of the cholera epidemic. This is a portion of a larger map that shows diseases across the world in the early nineteenth century. It was published in German geographer Heinrich Berghaus's two-volume atlas *Physikalischer Atlas*. From *Planiglob zur Ubersicht der geographischen Verbreitung der vornehmsten Krankheiten*, by Heinrich Berghaus (Gotha, Germany: Justus Perthes, 1849). Courtesy of the David Rumsey Map Collection, www.davidrumsey.com.

Guerrero received twenty copies of a cholera prescription developed by Pascual de Aranda, a professor of medicine.[9] De Aranda first outlined a list of drinks that Indians at the Forlón Mission in Tamaulipas used to combat cholera earlier that summer, including vinegar and juices derived from lime, ashwood, and the *nejayote* plant. He used these liquids to concoct a plaster of "Lime whipped in Vinegar and Lemon juice" to apply to the stomach, legs, and joints. De Aranda then offered his own liquid mixture for patients to drink: a mixture of water, chamomile, laudanum, and citron syrup. The sick were also to apply a "hot brick to the plant of the feet, the brick wrapped in woolen cloth, or use bottles full of hot water, and friction all the body with the hand wrapped up in woolen cloth." For stomach cramps, de Aranda prescribed a stomach massage with whiskey and salt. Because of the difficulty acquiring medical supplies such as laudanum on the frontier, de Aranda noted that "in places where there is no means of obtaining the medicines mentioned in this curative method: first of all apply to the patient a strong infusion of mint, chamomile powder, and poppie, trying to get supplied at once of the medicaments already indicated."[10] De Aranda may have described such alternatives not only because certain medicines were rare in remote areas; he may have included plant cures because of the familiarity of these medical practices in the region. His inclusion of cactus and other local plants suggests that both physicians and the state government could support local healing practices.

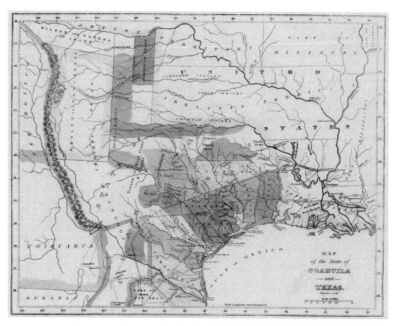

FIGURE 1.2. Map of the Texas–Mexico borderlands, 1833. From *Texas*, by Mary Austin Holley (Baltimore, Md.: Armstrong & Plaskitt, 1833). Courtesy of the Texas State Library and Archives Commission.

Cholera reached Texas in August. Settlers in Stephen F. Austin's colony felt the devastation, and Anglo Americans and African American slaves alike suffered.[11] By September, the people of San Antonio de Béxar had not yet felt the brunt of cholera. The *ayuntamiento* nevertheless prepared for a potential strike. Following the governor's orders, the municipality formed a *junta de sanidad*. The health board consisted of seventeen people, including "one *curandero* or *medio Medico*."[12] The inclusion of a *curandero* in the board of health indicated the popularity of the healers among the townspeople, another example of how local and state governments incorporated different healing methods in their battles with epidemic disease. The *junta* divided the town into five parts, and board members oversaw each section. As before, the Béxar *ayuntamiento* ordered the strict observation of public cleanliness and personal hygiene but followed with additional stipulations. If anyone got sick, heads of family had to report to *junta* leaders of their respective section and include details on symptoms. If the epidemic struck the city, members of the *ayuntamiento* were ordered to meet every three days and also to consult Alejandro Vidal, who was not a doctor but had medical knowledge. Because there were no physicians in the city, Vidal helped the city care for the poor, as he "offered his medical services . . . to the indigent free of charge."[13] A group of elites actually covered much of the cost of medicines and care for the city, and one resident and well-known politician, Erasmo Seguín, arranged to furnish the city with meat if cholera actually hit.[14] The last municipal preventive measure concerned the distribution of medicines. The Board of Health circulated information on three state-sanctioned prescriptions to citizens in each of the five sections of the city. The city ordered the *junta* to provide sufficient quantities of peyote to anyone who needed the medicine.[15] Thus, as the *ayuntamientos* were running out of viable options, Mexican physicians looked for less orthodox healing methods to stop the spread of disease.

DESPERATION FOSTERED CREATIVITY: PEYOTE AND CHOLERA

Mexican perceptions of their Native neighbors did not preclude doctors from appropriating Indian healing practices, as professional doctors could make any therapy "medical" through scientific testing. For professional doctors, medical practice could cut across cultural lines, but medical theory did not. The remedies Mexicans and Native peoples used were often the same; for example, both ingested plants as cures.[16] Doctors practiced "science," however, and Indian healers connected Native spirituality and healing. The exchange of peyote healing reveals both the ongoing traffic between science and Native health practices and the ongoing separation of Mexico from Native peoples. The peyote remedy for cholera carried political weight because the government of Coahuila y Texas promoted it as the most effective cure to the municipalities. Mexican officials promoted a cure from communities outside the nation to keep citizens alive inside the nation. The peyote cure traveled from the state of Nuevo León to Coahuila to Texas, undercutting the wide cultural gap that separated Native healing from Mexican medicine.

After independence, Mexicans had redefined Native savagery in national terms, questioning the fitness of Indians for Mexican society and, in turn, placing them outside the nation. When cholera ran rampant through Mexico in 1833, Native communities were excluded from the

Mexican government's public health program. Even if they were allies of the state, Native peoples who did not live in Mexican towns or settlements remained on the outside of the national public health project. However, the healing customs that made Native peoples heathen took on new meaning because the state found use for those practices since its health measures did not stem the epidemic tide. Learned from Indian customs, the use of peyote for healing revealed the state government's anxiety over the protection of its citizens. The cholera epidemic elicited a sense of crisis among federal, state, and municipal officials. Death rates soared, and the disease spread throughout much of the republic despite preventive efforts.

When the epidemic reappeared in the Texas–Mexico borderlands, the government supplemented its measures with Pascual de Aranda's prescription. Soon after, it introduced Ignacio Sendejas's remedy, which was similar to de Aranda's but incorporated peyote. Sendejas's method became the state's preferred prescription. Both physicians based their prescriptions on plant healing methods learned from the people of the Forlón Mission in Tamaulipas. They noted that the residents of Forlón successfully used juice derived from lime and *nejayote* and included the substances in their cures. Franciscans had established the mission in the Paso del Forlón in the Texas–Mexico borderlands in the early nineteenth century, targeting Indian nations who occupied the area.[17] Sendejas's knowledge of peyote may have originated at the Forlón, for its Native residents probably practiced a syncretic form of Catholicism that incorporated Native peyote rituals.

Because Mexican doctors drew a line between their scientific methods and lay healing, Ignacio Sendejas emphasized scientific theories to explain his inclusion of peyote, a plant associated with superstition, in his cholera remedy. He contended that the "abnormal flow of the digestive juices" produced deadly gases and caused cholera. He sought to break down those gases with a variety of chemicals and peyote:

One slice of peyote, one finger in width and two fingers in length, is allowed to boil [lightly] in one cup of water. The liquid is then strained. To this liquid is added as much purified slaked lime as will be held on a silver [coin]. It should then be [mixed well] and drunk. If the symptoms are not lessened within a half hour, the dose [can] be repeated.[18]

Sendejas believed that if the "development [of cholera] is arrested by a chemical substance which may have a diluent affinity, the terrible catastrophe can be prevented."[19] The doctor believed that the combination of lime and peyote was such a substance.

Unlike Sendejas, people used peyote for reasons other than science. For those who consumed the plant, the meanings surrounding peyote consumption depended on its purpose. Colonial documentation depicted various uses of peyote among Native peoples in areas ranging from East Texas to South Texas.[20] For example, Native peoples along the Rio Grande in the eighteenth century drank "peyote and [the juice of] other herbs which cause a disturbance of the senses producing visions and apparitions," enhancing their religious ceremonies.[21] Other Indians in the region organized lavish, community-wide feasts and occasionally invited people from neighboring villages to celebrate harvests, military victories, and changing seasons.[22] Anthropologist Rudolphe Troike claims that Texas Indians also used the hallucinogen before war to produce visions of their enemies' military tactics.[23] Though filtered through colonialist eyes, these descriptions suggest that many Indians believed in peyote's spiritual potency.

Spaniards had associated peyote consumption with irrational superstition and Native savagery, an idea that probably informed Ignacio Sendejas's perception of his remedy in 1833. From the moment that the Spaniards arrived in the sixteenth century, they defined Native spiritual cures as threats to the Catholic Church, and they targeted Indian healing.[24] But many Indians continued to look to the plant for healing therapy, which probably contributed to its survival into the nineteenth century. In the seventeenth century, moreover, people from all rungs of the social ladder sought out indigenous healers for various spiritual and medical needs, and they often consumed peyote.[25] Anthropologist Gonzalo Aguirre Beltrán argues that some Indian healers in the colonial era incorporated spiritual use of peyote into Catholicism as a way of maintaining Native rituals during the Mexican Inquisition.[26] And historian Omar Stewart contends that the development of missions in Texas helped spread knowledge of peyote, as people migrated with missionaries from areas in which peyote thrived to areas where it was less known.[27] Peyote was popular and survived attacks against it, even if the meanings of the practice changed over time and across cultures. Its historic and widespread use in the North for health purposes could explain Sendejas's familiarity with the cactus and its healing properties.[28] When Sendejas borrowed the cure, he gave it new meaning, arguing that the plant could counter the release of harmful digestive gases.

Grounding his remedy in medical science such as chemistry and physiology, Sendejas differentiated his remedy from other populations' forms of peyote healing. In his narrative, he addressed the character and potential popular reception of the plant cure, which revealed that he was conscious of the ways that his cure resembled folk cures. He referenced the plant's historic presence in Mexico and acknowledged its narcotic side effects. Perhaps he felt the need to do so because he was appropriating a plant associated with "superstitious" Indian beliefs that Native people often consumed specifically for hallucinations. Notions of gender also informed Sendejas's view of his prescription. Before he outlined his remedy, he wrote, "The following prescription has produced such admirable results, although at first it seems to be worthless and like one of those cures commonly known as [old women's remedies]."[29] Historically, female healers in Mexico incorporated peyote into their therapies. In the colonial era, Spaniards saw these women as a threat to Church authority because they garnered social power with their skills.[30] When Sendejas recorded his therapy, then, he worried that people might associate him with old women's "unscientific" cures. Therefore, he followed with a note that demonstrated the scientific efficacy of his method. "In order to dispel any apprehension, during the eight days that the epidemic has raged in [Monterrey]," Sendejas wrote, "over two hundred persons attacked by cholera have been cured with this prescription; and within the last seven days no one has died in the hospital, except . . . two patients."[31] Despite his declaration of peyote's curative power, however, Sendejas still felt the need to justify his use of the cactus. Perhaps he was aware of the discursive tension that arose from his reliance on a plant that Indians used for rituals. Through his self-conscious disclaimers about a cure associated with Native and "old women's" practices, Sendejas distanced himself, and Mexican men in general, from Native peoples and women. His narrative revealed the gender and racial hierarchies embedded in nineteenth-century Mexican scientific and medical practice.[32]

The state and the municipalities in the Texas–Mexico borderlands surely would not have promoted Sendejas's remedy if the physician had not proven its efficacy using scientific methods. Sendejas empha-sized the science of his prescription, stressing that its purpose followed nineteenth-century orthodox medicine. He distanced his method from the spiritual practices associated with peyote but maintained that the healing method he promoted was appropriate for a professional doc-tor. For Sendejas, Indians were "others" not because they used peyote as medicine but because they used it for spiritual therapies. Medical practitioners such as Sendejas and L. Rio de la Loza and R. Lucio (who experimented with tarantulas, which I discuss later) crossed cultural borders and searched for cures among those who stood outside the nation-state. Once they borrowed those practices, however, their mean-ings changed because they had to find ways to demonstrate that their use of Indian healing was scientific and untainted by Native peoples.

Several municipalities distributed the peyote remedy in their com-munities and praised its efficacy. In the fall of 1833, the peyote scrip circulated around the region. But it made it to only some of the frontier settlements. Political correspondence from September 1833 revealed that the Béxar *ayuntamiento* privileged the peyote cure over the other two that the state provided.[33] In October, officials reported that Béxar had escaped the epidemic.[34] The town of Goliad in South Texas and residents of Nacogdoches and several smaller settlements in East Texas also avoided the disease.[35] A few months after the end of the epidemic, the Goliad municipal council attributed the town's escape from cholera to the governor's measures, which included distribution of the peyote remedy.[36] Although several municipal officials claimed that the state-sanctioned measures saved many people from the ravages of cholera, the peyote remedy could not have been efficacious.[37] The politicians who penned the letters that praised the government's public health initiatives rarely questioned the governor's actions, at least in writing, and showed reverence to their superiors through correspondence. In the interest of their political careers, they had to praise the governor and attribute the escape from cholera to the actions of their superior. These political obligations obscure whether they truly believed that the peyote remedy was successful. For the most part, Mexican settlements in Texas escaped the ravages of cholera in 1833. The Anglo Americans in Austin's colony were the primary victims of the epidemic.

The disease resurfaced the next summer, causing much more dam-age in South Texas than before. This time, the *ayuntamientos* did not promote or report the use of peyote for cholera, despite the strength of the epidemic in South Texas. Perhaps cholera's strike was such a surprise that state officials did not have time to offer as much assistance as they did in 1833, especially considering that townspeople fled their homes so quickly. And the *ayuntamientos* themselves could not convene as often because of the migrations. The state-sanctioned appropriation of peyote was short-lived; Ignacio Sendejas's remedy served the victims of only the 1833 cholera epidemic.

MEDICAL PRACTICE, RACE, AND NATION IN NINETEENTH-CENTURY MEXICO

Ignacio Sendejas and the Mexican state's adoption of peyote held national implications because it occurred at a time when physicians and politicians were debating the role of medicine in the new nation. Before Mexican independence, elites throughout Spanish America began to adopt Enlightenment thinking that emphasized science and rationality to achieve progress and to apply methods of science to politics and society.[38] This approach to government influenced nation building after Mexican independence in 1821, and elites saw medicine as one way to bring about national progress. Professional medical practice was largely experimental, and doctors based what therapies worked and what did not work on experience. Lay healing was also empirical, but nineteenth-century physicians differentiated their work from that of other healers partly through their own dialogue with medical theories and practices from Europe.[39] In these physicians' eyes, their work was science because they considered such sciences as physiology and chemistry when treating illness. Plant healing itself bridged multiple medical worldviews because many healers used botanics. Yet the Indian version was often rooted in a spiritual tradition that many northern Mexican elites considered nonscientific and also a threat to Catholic values. For Mexican physicians, moreover, their contributions to science and to the medical profession were contributions to the Mexican nation.

In describing Native medicine and other Indian customs, many Mexicans tied their ideas about race to their visions for the emerging nation-state. Mexican officials defined the nation as a modern, capitalist state. They valued characteristics such as property ownership, education, and individualism, which they saw as crucial for the creation of a successful nation. These traits became associated with masculinity and Spanish ethnicity. Educated, property-owning men, then, had the ability to lead independent Mexico, whereas those without such qualities—women, Indians, slaves, and those without property—did not.[40] After Mexican independence, Indians became equal citizens before the law, and the state sought to incorporate Native peoples economically by privatizing lands that belonged to Indian communities and mission Indians.[41] Some Mexican elites thought Indians could adopt "national" ways of life if they rejected certain beliefs and practices, including Native spirituality. Still, many state officials pushed for their removal or for the seizure of Native lands.[42]

In the Texas–Mexico borderlands, however, Indians dictated the terms of their relationship with Mexican Texans, or Tejanos. Mexican state officials and businesspeople relied on Native peoples for military support and for trade goods, so they continued Spanish overtures toward Indians to uphold and develop peace treaties and to improve trade relations.[43] Struggles between Indians and settlers threatened stability, economic development, and the allure of the North for Anglo colonizers, whom the Mexican government considered essential to state formation in the region. Tejano officials, then, approved treaties and land grants for Indians, as all parties sought trade partners and military allies.[44] The use of peyote grew out of these longstanding interdependent relationships. Still, the Texas–Mexico borderlands was a place undergoing conquest, and Mexicans appropriated Native knowledge to serve the nation while denigrating their Indian allies' "savage" and "superstitious" ways.

Proper and improper medical practice constituted heathen Indianness for Mexican authorities. Mexican medicine was science; Native medicine was superstition. For example, Mexican official Juan Padilla reported on "superstitious" Native healing that he observed in East Texas, along the Texas–Louisiana, U.S.–Mexico border. Padilla commended Caddo Indians' "knowledge of many medicinal herbs which they use for wounds and other accidents with good results; although, in their method of cures," he continued, "there is always present superstition and excesses."[45] Padilla did approve of Caddo sedentary agricultural customs because they reflected Mexican visions of land use. But their spiritual healing practices and medical worldview made them suspect. In addition to plant healing, Mexican officials observed other Native healing rituals, constructing Native savagery through these observations. In the late 1820s, French scientist Jean Berlandier reported on healing traditions during his travels through Texas on a Mexican military expedition. Throughout his narrative, he distinguished between Indians and non-Indians based on cultural practices. Without identifying his subjects, for example, Berlandier wrote that the "crude medicine of the natives is limited to performance of a few superstitious ceremonies and the use of a few simple medications." These unnamed Indians called on medicine men "gifted with supernatural abilities" and plant knowledge.[46] Like Padilla, Berlandier recognized Native plant healing abilities but dismissed spiritual healing as superstition and unintelligence. In his critique, he described a hierarchy of knowledge that differentiated between Indian spiritual healing and European scientific medicine: "The natives are by no means of limited intelligence, though they are not gifted with that supernatural intelligence or genius that is the boast of both civilized worlds."[47] Like Berlandier, Mexican physicians contrasted Native healing with professional medicine, which many elite Mexicans saw as a symbol of Mexico's national civilized status.

Nineteenth-century Mexican doctors understood their medical practices as scientific and professional. In the 1830s, they organized a professional organization, the Academia de Medicina de Mégico (or Medical Academy of Mexico), to offer their "contributions to science, to support its theories, [and] make them known."[48] As part of this process of professionalization, physicians differentiated their healing practices from those of the masses. For example, a Doctor Schiede asked how the professional medical world could incorporate the "medicines known to the people of the countryside and unknown to doctors . . . [and] present these elements to the scientific domain."[49] Schiede suggested that science formed the boundary between physicians' work and that of most Mexicans living in the countryside. Mexican physicians were well aware of their limits and knew they could afford to learn more therapies. But for professional doctors, therapies gained legitimacy through scientific testing alone, using the "knowledge that makes up this [medical] science."[50]

Healing practices that doctors initially saw as "unscientific" could attain legitimacy in the profession. Although they did not always incorporate such cures as extensively as the Mexican government did during the cholera epidemic, doctors engaged what they deemed unconventional practices in the early nineteenth century. For example, Dr. L. Rio de la Loza and his colleague, R. Lucio, used tarantulas to create a concoction that caused sweats to combat illness.[51] They acquired the spiders from southern Mexico. They soaked them in alcohol for fifteen days and then prepared a solution with the liquid, ether, and cerate, which was a mixture of wax and resin. Rio de la Loza and Lucio used the cure on thirteen patients at the Hospital San Lazaro in Mexico City, mostly to treat leprosy, and recorded positive results in a Mexican medical journal. Patients produced abundant sweat for several days after taking the concoction, and their "clothes sometimes [got] completely soaked." The doctors further reported that the patient's pulse did not change much, and there were no digestive problems. They concluded that "from this animal product, some patients were cured, and if not, others obtained notable relief. The acquisition of the tarantulas has promoted the desire to improve the situation of the unfortunate [patients] attacked with this terrible disease with the most . . . efficacy, particularly in our nation."[52] The tarantula example demonstrates that doctors experimented with unfamiliar healing methods, and their work could make such practices scientific. Moreover, they did not limit their search for new therapies to moments of crisis.

Nineteenth-century Mexican doctors such as Lucio and Rio de la Loza understood their practice of medicine in broad terms, not limited to the local hospitals or communities in which they worked. In the introduction to the *Periódico de la Academia de Medicina de Mégico*, or *Journal of the Medical Academy of Mexico*, L. Blaquiere outlined the importance of the educated, elite class and of professional medicine in his definition of national progress.[53] For some Mexican physicians, plant healing would put Mexico on the global medical map, a source of national pride.[54] Doctors occasionally worked directly with the state, as Ignacio Sendejas did. And according to some physicians, refined public health institutions could bolster the national project, even though most Mexican cities and towns did not have developed public health infrastructures.[55] In general, doctors in Mexico struggled to control medical practice in the early national era. The availability of and people's preference for "unorthodox" medicine and lay healers strengthened physicians' determination to police the boundaries of the profession.[56] Thus, it is possible that the doctors' discussions about the different ways orthodox medicine served the nation were part of those efforts to control the medical profession. Still, in this medically pluralistic environment, their vision of the Mexican nation included modern scientific medicine and public health.[57]

This is the medical community to which Ignacio Sendejas belonged. Because many physicians viewed their therapies as the only legitimate ones, perhaps they thought Native healers, who did not belong to the profession, were not serving the nation through their medical practice. But Sendejas and others did not exclude Native peoples from their community solely on the basis of improper medicine; this was part of their larger exclusion from the modern Mexican nation. As we have seen with the Mexican representations of Indian healing, they understood medical practice in broader cultural terms, which included their ideas about legitimate science and also their views of proper religious practice and its role in healing. Professional physicians' and lay healers' therapies alike reflected their respective belief systems. Native versions of plant healing often were rooted in spiritual traditions that many non-Indian, northern Mexican elites considered unscientific and also savage, ideas that reflected widely accepted racial tropes. During the 1833 cholera epidemic in the Texas–Mexico borderlands, Ignacio Sendejas linked different forms of healing with the peyote remedy; however, he used the languages of science and race to fracture the tie that bound them together.

CONCLUSION

Ignacio Sendejas's appropriation of peyote during the 1833 cholera epidemic was a product of longstanding relations between the state and Native peoples in the Texas–Mexico borderlands. The exigencies of life in the borderlands required the different parties to develop economic and diplomatic relations to carry out their own political visions and to survive. Such mutual needs brought diverse groups together for cooperation, even in a violent context. These cross-cultural interactions and relationships set the stage for the Mexican–Native exchange of health practices during the cholera outbreak. Such cultural, political, and economic negotiations highlight the fluidity of power relations in the borderlands. Nevertheless, Ignacio Sendejas's and other Mexican officials' use of the peyote remedy reinforced Mexican nation-building and colonization projects, as the public health program allowed the government to fulfill its stated role as protector of the citizenry. The Mexican government's promotion of the doctor's remedy revealed contradictions in state officials' national imaginations. The state's use of the plant to heal Mexican citizens during the cholera epidemic meant that officials actually looked to cultures and people deemed threatening to the idea of a modern and progressive Mexico. The Mexican government's struggle to prevent the spread of cholera in the north forced physicians such as Ignacio Sendejas to engage therapeutic creativity and use peyote regardless of the image of the cactus in the eyes of Mexican officials. During these tumultuous times, Mexican elites embraced a plant that they had associated with so-called spiritual threats to society and had characterized as non-Mexican. Peyote allowed the state to carry out its main mission: the protection of Mexican citizens. A healing practice rooted "outside" the nation helped heal members of the national community. And the exclusion of Native communities from the state's public health agenda reinforced the boundary that placed Indians outside the polity.

The success of peyote for diverse patients in the region contradicted the racial theories that doctors applied when diagnosing illness. The cure defied the boundaries that medical theory established between human bodies of different racial backgrounds. A plant that historically cured Native peoples cured Texas residents in diverse ethnic communities in 1833. The efficacy of peyote certainly did not dismantle the scientific theories that "proved" human difference. And as the United States expanded into northern Mexico in the 1830s and 1840s, this science gained even more strength, central as it was to U.S. westward expansion. Anglo American scientists vaunted Anglo-Saxon racial superiority as U.S. Americans debated the future of an expanding nation that might force Anglos to rub elbows with racial inferiors. A new imperial power pushed into the region and faced its own health dilemmas. U.S. military surgeons also borrowed local healing practices to cure Anglo soldiers and to serve another national project. The contradictory process of cultural appropriation therefore shaped nation building for Mexico and the United States.

Unlike some other medicinal plants, such as purple coneflower (echinacea), Peruvian bark or cinchona (quinine), and ipecacuanha (an emetic), people continued to associate peyote with hallucinations, influencing racial ideologies and adding to the modern exclusion of

Native peoples, which may have prevented the full appropriation of peyote by Western medicine.[58] In the United States, peyote's hallucinogenic properties have made it difficult for some Native peoples to practice religious peyotism even under the American Indian Religious Freedom Act of 1978, which protected the use of peyote for religious purposes despite state and federal bans on hallucinogenic substances.[59] Because of peyote's effects, people continued to tie the plant to Native spirituality. The distance that those people created between approved botanics and peyote reinstated the exclusion of Native peyote healing from the parameters of modern medical science.

Tracing the role of Native healing in the making of a modern nation in Texas highlights the cultural contradictions of national expansion. Despite political officials' emphasis on proper and improper behaviors and healing practices in their national visions, officials crossed those boundaries to incorporate or reject aspects of local cultures during state formation. To serve the Mexican nation and further "civilization," doctors relied on "uncivilized" Native inhabitants and their cultural practices. Battles with sickness at the local level, which was an everyday concern, held national political significance, as people struggled with disease and state institutions worked to protect them. Moreover, ideas of nation and empire grew out of local interactions in addition to broader social and political visions. Emerging from existing cross-cultural relationships between Mexicans and Native peoples, the peyote exchange showed that nation building was a tangled negotiation in which populations and their everyday practices often excluded from the nation shaped the course of nation-state formation.

NOTES

The author thanks Laurie B. Green, Susan Johnson, John Mckiernan-González, Ron Numbers, James Schafer, Martin Summers, James Sweet, and the participants of the "Making Race, Making Health" conference for their comments and suggestions.

1   After Mexican independence, Mexicans in the Texas–Mexico borderlands used various ethnic labels that depended on the context. I use the term *Mexican* to refer to Mexican citizens, and I sometimes use *Tejano* (Mexican

Texan) when denoting the local character of Mexican national and ethnic identity. My use of ethnohistorical methods to recover Native history from European and Euro-American sources shapes the racial and ethnic terminology I use for Indigenous peoples. With an eye to the limitations of this method, I refer to Native peoples in the ways that the sources suggest they referred to themselves (e.g., Caddos and Xaranames). I mainly examine Native peoples in the aggregate, for example, when I explore Indian policy or Mexicans' perceptions of Indian peoples. In these cases, I use the terms *Native peoples* and *Indians* interchangeably.

2   Fray Juan Agustín de Morfi, *Excerpts from the Memorias for the History of the Province of Texas, Being a Translation of Those Parts of the Memorias Which Particularly Concern the Various Indians of the Province of Texas; Their Tribal Divisions, Characteristics, Customs, Traditions, Superstitions, and All Else of Interest Concerning Them*, trans. Frederick Chabot (San Antonio: Privately printed by the Naylor Printing Co., 1932), 26, 28.

3   For more on the connection between medicine and the nation in nineteenth-century Latin America, see Andrés Reséndez, *Changing National Identities at the Frontier: Texas and New Mexico, 1800–1850* (Cambridge: Cambridge University Press, 2005), 106–17; Steven Palmer, *From Popular Medicine to Medical Populism: Doctors, Healers, and Public Power in Costa Rica, 1800–1940* (Durham, N.C.: Duke University Press, 2003); Julyan G. Peard, *Race, Place, and Medicine: The Idea of the Tropics in Nineteenth-Century Brazilian Medicine* (Durham, N.C.: Duke University Press, 1999); Laura Cházaro, "Introducción. Historia, Medicina y Ciencia: Pasado y Presente de Sus Relaciones," in *Medicina, Ciencia y Sociedad en México, Siglo XIX,* ed. Laura Cházaro G. (Zamora, Mich.: El Colegio de Michoacán, 2002), 17–37; and David Sowell, "Contending Medical Ideologies and State Formation: The Nineteenth-Century Origins of Medical Pluralism in Contemporary Colombia," *Bulletin of the History of Medicine* 77, no. 4 (Winter 2003): 900–26.

4   Historians have used popular politics, the legal system, and local economies to show the local impacts on the national contours of state formation. See Reséndez, *Changing National Identities at the Frontier*; Patricia Nelson Limerick, *The Legacy of Conquest: The Unbroken Past of the American West* (New York: W. W. Norton, 1987); María E. Montoya, *Translating Property: The Maxwell Land Grant and the Conflict over Land in the American West, 1840–1990* (Berkeley: University of California Press, 2002); Raúl A. Ramos, *Beyond the Alamo: Forging Mexican Ethnicity in San Antonio, 1821–1861* (Chapel Hill: University of North Carolina Press, 2008); and Omar S. Valerio-Jiménez, "Indios Bárbaros, Divorcées, and Flocks of Vampires: Identity and Nation on the Río Grande, 1749–1894" (PhD diss., University of California, Los Angeles, 2001).

5   Christopher Hamlin, *Cholera: The Biography* (Oxford: Oxford University Press, 2009).

6   For more on the social, cultural, and political responses to cholera, see

Hamlin, *Cholera*, and Charles E. Rosenberg, *The Cholera Years: The United States in 1832, 1849, and 1866*, 2nd ed. (Chicago: University of Chicago Press, 1987).

7 *Ayuntamiento* of Béxar's proclamation, March 17, 1833, Béxar Archives (BA), Briscoe Center for American History (BCAH), University of Texas at Austin.

8 José Nicolás Elizondo to the *ayuntamiento* of Guerrero, July 19, 1833, Fondo Siglo XIX, Archivo General del Estado de Coahuila (AGEC) (hereafter cited as FSXIX).

9 Jesús Estrada to *ayuntamiento* of Guerrero, August 7, 1833, FSXIX.

10 Pascual de Aranda, "Curative Method for the Cholera Morbus," Vol. III: Bexar Archives, 1809–1836, Box 2R344, Medical History of Texas Collection, BCAH (hereafter cited as MHTC). Not my translation.

11 Miguel Arciniega to Superior Secretary of the Office of the Supreme Government of the State of Coahuila y Texas, August 26, 1833, Vol. IV: Nacogdoches Archives, 1804–1835, Box 2R344, MHTC; and J. Villasana Haggard, "Epidemic Cholera in Texas, 1833–1834," *Southwestern Historical Quarterly* 40, no. 3 (January 1937): 223–24.

12 In Spanish, *medio médico* translates to either "average healer" or "somewhat healer." Both translations deride the *curandero*'s medical skill and demonstrate the author's negative characterization of the healing style and the healer himself.

13 Report on the formation of a committee to combat cholera, September 9, 1833, BA.

14 List of contributors, September 8, 1833, BA; and Erasmo Seguín to *ayuntamiento* of Béxar, October 3, 1833, BA.

15 Miguel Arciniega to Béxar *ayuntamiento*, September 8, 1833, BA; Ficha 2417, Fondo Jefatura Política de Béjar, AGEC (hereafter cited as FJPB); and report on the formation of a committee to combat cholera, September 9, 1833, BA.

16 Doctor Schiede, "Observaciones sobre Objetos de Materia Medica," *Periódico de la Academia de Medicina de Mégico* 1 (1836): 11–15.

17 The Spanish targeted a number of Native communities, including Saracuayes, Truenos, Ximariguanes, and Mariguanes. See Fernando Ocaranza, "Fundacion de Nuevas Misiones Franciscanas en el Año de 1803," *The Americas* 11, no. 3 (January 1955): 453–55.

18 Ignacio Sendejas, "Metodo Curativo de la Colera Morbo, por el Ciudadano Ignacio Sendejas Boticario y Medico Encargado del Hospital, Seminario de Esta Ciudad, y Dado á Luz a Solicitud y Espensas de Algunos de Sus Amigos en Obsequio de la Humanidad Doliente," August 13, 1833, Box 2J140, Spanish Proclamations and Edicts, BCAH; and Box 2R344, Vol. V: Cholera in Texas, 1833-50, MHTC. Not my translation, except for bracketed words.

19 Ibid.

20 Fray Francisco Hidalgo to the Viceroy, November 4, 1716, in "Descriptions

of the Tejas or Asinai Indians, 1691–1722," trans. Mattie Austin Hatcher, *Southwest Historical Quarterly* 31, no. 1 (July 1927): 55–56.

21 Fray Antonio Olivares to the Viceroy, n.d., 1709, in Fray José Antonio Pichardo, *Pichardo's Treatise on the Limits of Louisiana and Texas: An Argumentative Historical Treatise with Reference to the Verification of the True Limits of the Provinces of Louisiana and Texas*, 2nd ed., ed. and trans. Charles Wilson Hackett (Freeport, N.Y.: Books for Libraries Press, 1971), 2:397.

22 Fray Vicente Santa María's narrative in Alejandro Prieto, *Historia, Geografía y Estadística del Estado de Tamaulipas*, 2nd ed. (Mexico City: M. Porrúa, 1975), 123–24.

23 Rudolph C. Troike, "The Origins of Plains Mescalism," *American Anthropologist* 64, no. 5 (October 1962): 950.

24 Gonzalo Aguirre Beltrán, *Medicina y Magia: El Proceso de Aculturación en la Estructura Colonial*, rev. ed. (Mexico City: Fondo de Cultura Económica, 1992), 135–54; Edward F. Anderson, *Peyote: The Divine Cactus*, 2nd ed. (Tucson: University of Arizona Press, 1996), 3–24; Richard E. Greenleaf, "Persistence of Native Values: The Inquisition and the Indians of Colonial Mexico," *The Americas* 50, no. 3 (January 1994): 351–76; and Omar C. Stewart, *Peyote Religion: A History* (Norman: University of Oklahoma Press, 1987), 17–30.

25 Amos Megged, "Magic, Popular Medicine and Gender in Seventeenth-Century Mexico: The Case of Isabel de Montoya," *Social History* 19, no. 2 (May 1994): 194–204.

26 Aguirre Beltrán, *Medicina y Magia*, 141–42.

27 Stewart, *Peyote Religion*, 26–27.

28 Sendejas was originally from Coahuila, and he practiced medicine and also sat on the municipal council in Saltillo. In the early 1830s, Sendejas went to Monterrey, Nuevo Leon, to oversee a seminary hospital. Lucas Mártinez Sánchez, "Juan Martín de Veramendi: El Texano que Murió en Moncolva. Año de 1833," copy from author.

29 Sendejas, "Metodo Curativo." Not my translation, except for the bracketed words. The English translation of the remedy translated the original Spanish words *remedios aquellos que llaman de viejas* into "household remedies." Although Sendejas probably was referring to household remedies when he wrote the prescription, I included the more literal translation, "old women's remedies," to demonstrate how gender shaped his description of his prescription.

30 Megged, "Magic, Popular Medicine and Gender," 194–204.

31 Sendejas, "Metodo Curativo." Not my translation.

32 For the racialization of female healers as superstitious in the antebellum U.S. context, see Sharla Fett, *Working Cures: Healing, Health, and Power on Southern Slave Plantations* (Chapel Hill: University of North Carolina Press, 2002), 45–47.

33 Manuel Jiménez report on formation of *junta de sanidad,* September 16, 1833, BA.

34 Miguel Arciniega to Governor of Coahuila y Tejas, October 9, 1833, BA.

35 José Miguel Aldrete to Miguel Arciniega, December 6, 1833, BA.

36 Ibid.

37 Medical research has shown that rehydration cures cholera. See David A. Sack, R. Bradley Sack, G. Balakrish Nair, and A. K. Siddique, "Cholera," *The Lancet* 363, no. 9404 (January 2004): 225–26.

38 David J. Weber, *Bárbaros: Spaniards and Their Savages in the Age of Enlightenment* (New Haven, Conn.: Yale University Press, 2005), 2–3; and Pamela Voekel, *Alone before God: The Religious Origins of Modernity in Mexico* (Durham, N.C.: Duke University Press, 2002), 171–89.

39 Cházaro, "Introducción," 21.

40 Nancy P. Appelbaum, Anne S. Macpherson, and Karin Alejandra Rosemblatt, "Introduction: Racial Nations," in *Race and Nation in Modern Latin America,* ed. Nancy P. Appelbaum, Anne S. Macpherson, and Karin Alejandra Rosemblatt (Chapel Hill: University of North Carolina Press, 2003), 4.

41 Weber, *Bárbaros,* 265.

42 Ibid., 275.

43 Juliana Barr, *Peace Came in the Form of a Woman: Indians and Spaniards in the Texas Borderlands* (Chapel Hill: University of North Carolina Press, 2007); James F. Brooks, *Captives and Cousins: Slavery, Kinship, and Community in the Southwest Borderlands* (Chapel Hill: University of North Carolina Press, 2002), 45–207; Pekka Hämäläinen, *The Comanche Empire* (New Haven, Conn.: Yale University Press, 2008), 18–180; Elizabeth A. H. John, *Storms Brewed in Other Men's Worlds: The Confrontation of Indians, Spanish, and French in the Southwest, 1540–1795,* 2nd ed. (Norman: University of Oklahoma Press, 1996); and David J. Weber, *The Spanish Frontier in North America* (New Haven, Conn.: Yale University Press, 1992), 204–35.

44 For more on Comanche–Tejano relations, see Ramos, *Beyond the Alamo,* 61–63; and Hämäläinen, *Comanche Empire,* 181–201. For more on Apache–Tejano relations, see José Francisco Ruíz, "Report of Observations and Additional Information about Indians Living in the Department of Texas by the Undersigned," in *Report on the Indian Tribes of Texas in 1828,* ed. John C. Ewers (New Haven, Conn.: Yale University Library, 1972), 6–7.

45 Juan Antonio Padilla, "Report on the Barbarous Indians of the Province of Texas," trans. Mattie Austin Hatcher, "Texas in 1820," *Southwestern Historical Quarterly* 23, no. 1 (July 1919): 48.

46 Jean Louis Berlandier, *The Indians of Texas in 1830,* ed. John C. Ewers (Washington, D.C.: Smithsonian Institution Press, 1969), 84–87. Quotes on 84.

47 Ibid., 55.
48 L. Blaquiere, "Prospecto," *Periódico de la Academia de Medicina de Mégico* 1 (1836): 7.
49 Schiede, "Observaciones sobre Objetos de Materia Medica," 11.
50 Carlos Gerard, "Concluye el Articulo sobre la Enfermedad en General," *Periódico de la Academia de Medicina de Mégico* 10 (1836): 304.
51 Doctors who used heroic therapies sought to restore the body's balance upset by an illness. The practice of sweating to return the body to its natural balance was a common heroic therapy in the nineteenth-century United States. See John Duffy, "Medical Practice in the Ante Bellum South," *Journal of Southern History* 25, no. 1 (February 1959): 55, 63; and John Harley Warner, "From Specificity to Universalism in Medical Therapeutics: Transformation in the 19th-Century United States," in *Sickness and Health in America: Readings in the History of Medicine and Public Health*, 3rd ed., ed. Judith Walzer Leavitt and Ronald L. Numbers, 87–101 (Madison: University of Wisconsin Press, 1997).
52 L. Rio de la Loza and R. Lucio, "Terapeutica. Apuntes sobre los Efectos de la Tarantula, Administrada al Interior," in *Periódico de la Sociedad Filoiátrica de México* (1844): 91–94. Quote on 94.
53 Blaquiere, "Prospecto," 4.
54 Schiede, "Observaciones sobre Objetos de Materia Medica," 11.
55 By comparison, the United States did not have a permanent public health department until 1866. For more on Mexican public health and the nation, see Manuel Robiedo, "Memoria del Año de 1844, Presentada al Consejo Superior de Salubridad por su Secretaria, y Leida en Session de 15 de Enero de 1845, que Presidió el Exmo. Sr. Gobernador del Departamento de México," *Periódico de la Sociedad Filoiátrica de México* (1844): 145–51. Quote on 146.
56 Luz María Hernández Sáenz, *Learning to Heal: The Medical Profession in Colonial Mexico, 1767–1831* (New York: Peter Lang, 1997), 227–63.
57 For more on medical pluralism and state formation in nineteenth-century Latin America, see Sowell, "Contending Medical Ideologies and State Formation," and Palmer, *From Popular Medicine to Medical Populism*, 1–154.
58 Saul Jarcho, *Quinine's Predecessor: Francesco Torti and the Early History of Cinchona* (Baltimore, Md.: Johns Hopkins University Press); and Michael A. Flannery, "From Rudbeckia to Echinacea: The Emergence of the Purple Cone Flower in Modern Therapeutics," *HerbalGram* 51 (2001): 28–33.
59 Steve Pavlik, "The U.S. Supreme Court Decision on Peyote in *Employment Division v. Smith*: A Case Study in the Suppression of Native American Religious Freedom," *Wicazo Sa Review* 8, no. 2 (Autumn 1992): 30–39.

2

Complicating Colonial Narratives

Medical Encounters around the Salish Sea, 1853–1878

JENNIFER SELTZ

SMALLPOX HAUNTED TRAVELERS around the Salish Sea in 1853. That summer a small group of people journeyed by canoe from Nisqually, on the southern end of the Sound, to Victoria, across the Straits of Juan de Fuca. This group probably included several men from Hawai'i, eastern Canada, and villages around the connected bays and waterways that Europeans called Puget Sound, as well as one Scot and, more unusually, one American. Most of these men were employees of the Hudson's Bay Company, still a regional power despite British relinquishment of claims to the territory south of the forty-ninth parallel five years earlier. The American, Theodore Winthrop, was a Yale-educated tourist from New England, thoroughly enjoying the rugged exoticism of his western travels, except for a mild case of smallpox he had recovered from while at an American army post on the Columbia River earlier that spring.[1] In fact, Winthrop was touring the Oregon country in the wake of a smallpox epidemic. Earlier that winter and spring, the disease had "spread with great virulence along the coast as far north as Cape Flattery" at the tip of the Olympic Peninsula.[2] William Tolmie, the Scottish Hudson's Bay Company official and physician who hosted Winthrop on his tour of the Sound, exchanged smallpox vaccinations for salmon and camas root with prominent local Native people at a village and crowded fishing site.[3] Several months later, another visiting American also discussed the recent wave of smallpox and Indian vaccinations as he took detailed notes on local fishing and farming techniques, vocabulary, population, and employment around Puget Sound. George Gibbs wrote of the "D'wamish" Indians, close to present-day Seattle, that "smallpox has as yet not been among them. Many of them it is said been vaccinated. Dr. Bigelow says that the vaccine matter from whites *does* take well."[4]

Both Winthrop and Gibbs made clear that these notes on smallpox and vaccine were details in a larger story of ailing and diminished regional Indian populations. In Gibbs's published writings on his travels as a government surveyor and scientist in the Northwest, the groups and individuals he met on this trip and later visits had all been "reduced" by sickness and by contact with whites.[5] Winthrop, a more romantic and less experienced observer, emphasized inevitable and collective demographic decline more strongly.[6]

Gibbs and Winthrop's preoccupations and the stories they told about smallpox and Indians are still familiar. In most surveys of North American history, the history of indigenous peoples, the moment at which their worlds start to change, begins with disease. Alfred Crosby's pioneering work on the devastating impact of introduced diseases such as smallpox, measles, and influenza on Indian peoples from the sixteenth through the nineteenth centuries established the centrality of epidemics to European conquest of the Americas.[7] Crosby's work set an enduring pattern and highlighted an ongoing and still unresolved debate. As an artifact of what came to be called contact, disease has mattered greatly in Native history and historiography. However, these histories of disease have often been implicitly framed around two related broad questions. First, how big were indigenous population numbers before European conquest? This question was part of a larger debate among historians, anthropologists, and archaeologists over the environmental history of the Americas and the environmental impacts of precontact populations. Second, how devastating were these diseases, and how much did their impacts cost Indian peoples the ability to mount a lasting resistance to colonialism? In other words, until very recently, the medical histories of Native peoples before the twentieth century and the ravages of colonial public health have been largely an argument about disease as a major factor in and reason for conquest.[8]

But as Theodore Winthrop and George Gibbs noted, almost in spite of themselves, new diseases reshaped the worlds of Natives and new-comers in more subtle ways. Among the people gathered at the village of Kowitchin who met the Hudson's Bay Company party, smallpox vaccine and vaccination had become trade items, integrated into long-standing social relationships and subsistence arrangements. For Gibbs and his naturalist and physician peers, Duwamish bodies' susceptibility to vaccination was another piece of evidence in long-running trans-atlantic debates about how and when smallpox vaccine worked. Both moments of exchange and discussion invoked larger questions about who bore responsibility for new diseases, how those responsible might compensate for the real and potential harm done by smallpox, and how illness separated and connected Indian and non-Indian bodies. Yet these large questions made sense only at smaller scales—the scales of daily life, of ongoing attempts to understand new circumstances. Recently, Paul Kelton, David Jones, and a number of scholars of First Nations medical history in Canada have tried to recapture some of the local contingencies of early epidemics.[9] As James Waldram, D. Ann Herring, and T. Kue Young point out, "The presence of new pathogens and the absence of immunity to them are insufficient as the sole explanation for epidemics in the Americas or elsewhere. Epidemics occur when the complex relationship between human populations and their social and physical environment is altered, disrupted, or conducive to the flourishing of micro-organisms."[10]

In the territory that became western Washington, nineteenth-century American boosters, observers, physicians, Indian agents, and settlers understood this dynamic, even as they trumpeted and amplified the myth of the automatically vanishing Indian. Native people were quick to remind them as well. Less than two years after the smallpox epidemic of 1853 and Winthrop and Gibbs's trips, indigenous people around Puget Sound signed treaties that, along with land cessions and the reservation of hunting and fishing rights, included the promise of "medicine and advice" from the U.S. government.[11] These treaties and the medical practices and debates they generated over the next twenty years connect questions about early epidemics and their local causes and effects with another key body of scholarship on Native health, which examines the goals, meanings, and consequences of colonial public health and medicine in the North American West, particularly in the first decades of the twentieth century.[12] However, the racial assumptions that underlay colonial medicine took time and effort to take root in the Pacific Northwest. In the quarter-century after George Gibbs and Theodore Winthrop's initial writings, arguments about who was responsible for Coast Salish people's diseases and care and to what extent those ailments differed from non-Indian people's sicknesses helped to constitute American authority in the region and to weaken it. Indians protested unfulfilled American medical obligations in the late 1860s and 1870s. At the same time, American agents tried, largely unsuccessfully, to curtail local healers' work and political and religious power. Settlers, manufacturing and reacting to smallpox and other disease scares, dispossessed Indian communities in the name of a newly racialized idea of local health. These episodes reveal interwoven patterns of exchange and tension between Indian and settler medical practices and theories. These complex local histories, in which Indian bodies only gradually and unevenly came to be seen as racially distinct and inherently less healthy than settler bodies, preceded and undercut sweeping claims about the inevitability of Native population decline in the face of American expansion.

Disease and imperial and national expansion were inarguably linked around the Salish Sea. By 1854, Native people along the Northwest Coast had endured at least two catastrophic smallpox epidemics, the first one probably beginning in the 1790s. Syphilis and tuberculosis were starting to become endemic. The arrival of dysentery, influenza, and other respiratory and gastrointestinal illnesses had come to mark the local calendar.[13] Although it probably never reached Puget Sound, malaria had decimated Indian groups from the lower Columbia to northern California in the early 1830s.[14] These illnesses, carried in the bodies of humans and mosquitoes, moved along trade and kin networks and through landscapes newly absorbed into and changed by the fur trade and its offshoots. Disease highlighted both the Puget Sound region's links to a commercial Pacific world and its place within a smaller geography defined by rivers, mountains, and coastlines as well as ties of kinship, trade, and violence. This Pacific world, linked by ships carrying the skins of beavers and otters, stretched from the Northwest Coast west to Hawai'i and Canton, south to the great harbors of California, Peru, and Chile, and north to the Russian posts in Alaska and across the Bering Strait in Siberia.[15] The local region extended south to the Columbia River, north across the Straits of Juan de Fuca from Vancouver Island to the Queen Charlotte Islands, and east through the passes of the Cascade Mountains to the Columbia Plateau.

Native and settler worlds mixed with and depended on each other. Around Nisqually, where Theodore Winthrop's canoe trip with William Tolmie began, Hudson's Bay tenants and newer American arrivals—known locally as King George men and Bostons, respectively—raised cattle and sheep imported from California. These livestock grazed on meadows first shaped by Indian burning or flooding for the growth of bracken, berries, and camas.[16] Medical knowledge and health practices,

like foodstuffs and agricultural techniques, also moved within neigh-
borhood networks, as King George men and local indigenous people
regularly exchanged domestic medical labor, remedies, and palliatives
for sprained ankles, broken bones, measles, and colds.[17]

Beyond these mundane exchanges, however, European and American
visitors had also been primed to see the Salish Sea as puzzling at least
since the publication of George Vancouver's journals at the end of the
eighteenth century, which represented the region simultaneously as a
landscape of death, an inviting Arcadia, and a populated place.[18] In
1792, Vancouver's expedition met Indians pockmarked by what he
recognized as smallpox; expedition ships also sailed by piles of skeletons.[19] In between describing a landscape of horror he named one
long sound for one of his lieutenants, praised its deep waters and calm
inlets, and compared its meadows with England's carefully created
aristocratic countryside.[20] Over the next fifty years, both English and
American visitors and settlers tried to explain how the region could
produce both beautiful (and potentially valuable) scenery and sickly
people. Indians' bad health might be evidence of both unproductive
land and poor prospects for non-Indian inhabitants.

American soldiers, explorers, and scientists tried to fit these contradictory impressions of the Northwest into familiar forms. Military
surgeons evaluated the climate of American posts in the Northwest,
wrote informal natural histories of each fort, and charted soldiers' illnesses. These assessments partly fit a template established by Congress
and the surgeon general in the early nineteenth century, itself consciously
based on sanitary records kept by the British military. The army's medical geographers were officially most interested in which local illnesses
might debilitate soldiers and how powerful these diseases might be—
how much they might affect the army's ability to pacify and occupy a
range of places, from west Florida to Oregon.[21]

These military assessments shifted unpredictably between what
we would now call standardized and subjective analyses of illness and
environment. They both rationalized and romanticized northwestern
bodies and northwestern places.[22] Physicians sorted the cases they
treated into categories defined partly by kind of disease or injury and
partly by which parts of the body were affected. Fevers came first. Next,
the sick soldier's body was divided up by system: respiratory, digestive,
"brain and nervous system," "fibrous and muscular tissues," "urinary

and genital organs." Wounds and abscesses—isolated injuries—also received their own categories. An 1853 medical topography of Fort Steilacoom began by situating the post within a grid, noting the post's latitude and longitude, its distance from Puget Sound, and its height above sea level.[23] After this quantitative beginning, J. M. Hader, the assistant surgeon at the fort, shifted rapidly into description and into a style that emphasized not the abstraction of cartographic measures but a ground-level and qualitative perspective. He could see the Cascades "by riding a few miles from the post." The local prairies were "beautiful and undulating," and nearby woodlands were also "most beautiful and park-like."[24] Haden clearly saw no contradiction between travelogue-style writing and precise medical recordkeeping. Describing the landscape of the fort—the trees that grew nearby, the amount and quality of water sources, the game and soil, the conditions of trails and waterways—provided proof that Haden had first-hand experience of Puget Sound, reassurance about American prospects, and information that allowed readers sensitive to common connections between marshy landscapes and fevers to draw their own conclusions.

Haden's initial assessment of Indian health in the region was both blunter and simpler than his observations on soldiers' health and the fort's setting. He claimed that "they seem to be passing away so rapidly before civilization, that but very few years will elapse before they are entirely extinct. Wherever the whites settle, they disappear as if there was something in civilization entirely incompatible with their existence."[25] But the rest of his discussion of Native health was at odds with this kind of formulaic thinking. Haden laid out specific examples of, and reasons for, Indian vulnerability to illness. Rather than just "something in civilization," he blamed Native peoples' mortality on individual diseases (measles, influenza, and dysentery), on unhealthy habits (scanty clothing and poor diet), on immoral behavior (prostitution and gambling), and on climate and atmosphere (damp winters and "offensive exhalations" in Indian villages).[26] Any regular reader of medical journals or domestic medicine manuals would have recognized at least individual parts of this litany of causes as common to unhealthy places and people—Indian and non-Indian—across the country.

Indians, Europeans, and Americans could also trade medical knowledge and practice and develop overlapping explanations for the devastations of epidemics in the region because on both theoretical and practical levels, all the people around Puget Sound in the first half of the nineteenth century shared some ideas of how individual bodies worked, what health and disease were, and the relation both bore to local environments. Euro-American and Native health cultures didn't parallel each other exactly. But the categories Indian people, King George men, and Bostons used to define well-being and illness, to make sense of bodily sensations, and to identify beneficial and harmful environments and substances were often mutually comprehensible. And at key moments, both Indians and non-Indians interpreted and took advantage of tensions and disagreements over disease theories and curing practices within the other group's culture.

Both Native and non-Native systems of understanding health focused on maintaining a balance between substances entering and exiting individual bodies, which were simultaneously dynamic and opaque, although they differed on what forces exactly needed to be balanced. Euro-American physicians saw bleeding and other therapies as a way to bring physical systems into balance. These practitioners diagnosed illness and tracked its progress by paying attention to how patients sweated, what their skin felt like, the speed and strength of their pulses, and the texture and color of their excrement. In the mid-nineteenth century, their diagnostic technologies were primarily their own senses and their own experience in observing the correlations between the insides and outsides of sick people's bodies (including their own), knowledge that was gained through access to both corpses and the living.[27]

Native healers also focused on balancing systems within the body and used their own expert sensory knowledge. As important, they knew their patients' bodies through access to spirit powers and diagnosed serious illness at times as the result of malignant objects entering victims' bodies.[28] Upper Skagit Indian Jackson Harvey remembered one diagnosis and eventual cure:

> The old man started to work, to sing and sing. He put his mouth on the girl's hip and pulled matter out of his mouth into the basin. He asked for another basin and poured matter in it. Once he drew the sickness out and showed it to us. It was like a worm, about as big as a gnat, and red from blood. It had been going all around in her body. The girl was all eaten up. Then the girl came through; she was healed. It took a long time for her to come back.[29]

Sick Americans, their anxious families, and their physicians would have recognized the healer's hard work, if not his songs, and the systemic illness that demanded a long recovery.

In both Indian and Euro-American society, less serious ailments, which were not necessarily the province of shamans or physicians, were also recognized by caregivers' readings of excretions, skin, pulse, and breath.[30] Remedies for minor sicknesses also focused on restoring bodily balance—whether by speeding harmful substances on their way or by slowing normal flows that had become dangerously accelerated. Both Indians and non-Indians drew on common stores of knowledge and medicines to bleed, sweat, and steam a range of illnesses out without calling in a doctor or shaman.[31] George Gibbs sorted northwestern Indians' health cultures into categories he understood, describing a range of practices and remedies in terms of regular and unorthodox practitioners and medicines designed to purge illness and infection from all the body's openings:

> Besides the regular practice of the tamahno-us men, who may be considered the faculty, the Indians used a number of plants as medicine, somewhat as herb doctors intrude their nostrums in the States. A decoction of the white-flowering or poisonous Kamas furnishes an emetic, and that of the cucumber vine . . . both an emetic and a cathartic. The root of a species of fern growing among the moss which covers the limbs of the maple and other trees in damp situations is chewed as an expectorant, and is made into a tea as a remedy for gonorrhea. Swellings produced by injuries they sometimes scarify. Sores that are slow in healing are cauterized, and they employ moxa [counter-irritants] by the application of coals of fire, and the powder left by worms under the bark of trees is also strewn to dry them up. This, and also potter's clay dried and powdered, is used for chancres. Suction by the mouth is employed as a topical remedy to alleviate pain, and this too is part of the practice of the tamahno-us doctors.[32]

Gibbs compared Indians' everyday remedies to quack medicines, but he still took the time to list them in some detail. Herb doctors—Indian or not—and their remedies were a fact of life, often a useful one. Inhabitants of the mid-nineteenth-century Oregon country, like other

Americans, drew on a catholic range of treatments for common medical problems. Despite the bitterness of contemporary medical practitioners' battles over professionalization and orthodox practitioners' attempts to draw a clear line between "regular" doctors and the herbalists, homeopaths, and others who claimed medical authority, many patients easily moved between the mercury- and opium-based medicines favored by orthodox physicians and homeopathic and botanical remedies.[33]

Gibbs and his contemporaries compared the theory and material culture of Indian and Euro-American medicine and found parallels and overlaps, but the everyday medical practices that melded both were also important grounds of cooperation and disagreement. For both Indians and newcomers, nursing care and the time spent following an illness through from inception to crisis to recovery or death mattered as much as any single kind of therapeutic treatment. Even in the case of the most dangerous illnesses and those clearly identified with newcomers in the Oregon country—smallpox, measles, sexually transmitted diseases, fevers, or influenza—daily domestic care could be as important as any treatment expert healers could provide.

Both Indian and non-Indian practitioners used expert training and techniques based on keeping the body's flows in equilibrium to figure out and deal with sickness in and on a person's body, but this tight focus by itself didn't provide enough information to diagnose and treat diverse ailments. To both kinds of experts, sickness made sense only within wider geographies. Illnesses took shape in dynamic environments, both geophysical and spiritual. For employees of the Hudson's Bay Company, homesickness, new climates, new diets, and new habits jarred foreigners' bodies into illness. For Native shamans, individual malice misdirected other-than-human powers into human bodies. In both cases, health began with perceptions of bodies as intersections for a range of processes that had to be connected and brought into balance. Both kinds of doctors worked directly on the body; both claimed special but not unlimited powers to expel or dissipate harmful substances from ailing bodies.[34] Both kinds of doctors did not spend all their time doctoring but had multiple roles in their respective communities. Moreover, both Native and non-Native healers maintained their position as experts only with difficulty. When people got sick and did not get better, both kinds of practitioners faced community suspicion and blame.[35]

The physicians who served—or failed to serve—groups who had

signed treaties with the United States in 1854 and 1855 bridged two worlds in other, more concrete ways, often annoying both Americans and Indians. Like other employees of the nineteenth-century Bureau of Indian Affairs, local agency doctors were often incompetent, alcoholic, or both.[36] Yet some physicians did work actively on behalf of and for indigenous people, and even when the local talent pool was thin, treaty signatories continued to press American officials to fulfill their medical obligations.[37] Within a few years of the treaty signings, agents around Puget Sound were explaining to the territorial superintendent of Indian affairs that "the want of a physician is very much felt among the Indians, and has been to them, of late, a source of great complaint. They urge that the terms of their treaty, in which they are promised the services of a physician, are not being fully complied with on our part."[38] By 1869, Indians around Puget Sound were irritated enough by the continuing absence of American doctors and medicines to take their concerns directly to Ely Parker, the newly appointed commissioner of Indian affairs. Four representatives of the Lummi and Nooksack Indians sent a letter pointing out the United States's failure to uphold its treaty obligations. Their first concern was the disappearance of annuities for land concessions, but their second was lack of medical attention. Whe-land-hur, Ge-le-whomist, Quima, Hump-Klalm, and Slow-el wrote,

> We were promised medicines and medical attendance for our sick, but we have only received two or three visits from a Physician in the past seven years. Many of our people die! for the want of medical assistance and help in time of sickness, which makes our heart sad, and fills us with sorrow! There is a Physician appointed for the Tulalip Reservation, but the remoteness of Tulalip from our reservation, prevent us from availing ourselves of his services in time of sickness and need.[39]

Three other groups of Indians, from Port Madison to the southern end of King County, made similar complaints to Parker over the next few weeks.[40] Puget Sound Indians also tried hard to exercise some control over agency physicians' appointments, lobbying superintendents for specific hires.[41] Less than two decades after the treaties' signing and the promise of medicines and physicians, how Native people dealt with sickness, as much as how and why they got sick, became a central area of conflict between Puget Sound Indians and Americans.

By the mid-1860s, American reservation agents and physicians commented more often and in tones of increasing frustration on what they saw as the problem of shamanism and associated indigenous healing practices. Earlier observers, such as George Gibbs, tended to see shamanism as a curiosity or a primitive parallel to an American or British doctor's practice. As the United States's official presence around Puget Sound increased, and as more outsiders entered the region, Americans began to draw sharper rhetorical lines between Native medicine, which they associated with violence, disorder, and superstition, and American medicine, which they linked to a largely theoretical but idealized civilizing process. Both during the wars that followed the hasty signings of the treaties and in the 1860s and 1870s, as reservation and agency boundaries and resources fluctuated (usually to no one's satisfaction), American officials struggled to establish both some sense of what was going on and some kind of authority on new reservations and at newly created agencies. In part because Americans could not always predict, let alone control, exactly when families would call on shamans' services, or what the consequences of shamans' activities would be, they mistrusted the practice.

Indian Bureau officials' specific reasons for objecting to shamanism varied, although almost all officials in western Washington identified the practice as a serious threat to the vexed American effort to turn Indians into recognizable Victorians. Many agents thought shamanism kept some Indians impoverished and unfairly enriched others. Agent W. B. Gosnell explained to the Washington superintendent of Indian affairs, in the midst of a hard winter in 1857 marked by near-starvation and widespread respiratory illness among Puget Sound Indians, that "the poor devils, when sick, will give the last rag they possess to obtain the mystic services of the 'tamanawas' man." Gosnell linked Native medical practices to gambling as a source of Indian destitution: Both were examples simultaneously of superstition and of profligacy, traits that widened the gulf between Indians and civilization.[42]

Agents also linked shamanism to other types of barbarity, pointing out that shamans' work both followed and led to intra-Indian violence, compromising agents' already tenuous ability to manage affairs on the new reservations. One employee just starting a job on the Skokomish reservation in 1861 reported, "On my arrival here I found difficulties existing between different families of Indians. It appears that a doctor had been shot by a relative of one of his late patients; the friends of both parties took it up, and several people were killed before I succeeded in quieting it down."[43] When "a disease similar to the hooping cough" killed a number of children near Fort Kitsap in the same difficult winter of 1857, agent G. A. Paige complained principally that local Indians had "with their usual superstition ascribed this sickness to the charms of their 'medicine men' which has had the effect of engendering feuds among the different families and bands."[44] Six years later at Neah Bay, James Swan simultaneously raised and dispelled fears of similar violence directed at non-Indian doctors and whites in general, noting,

> The superstitious Indians attribute the sickness and deaths of these chiefs, to the agency of some bad medicine or malign influence of the white men, and made open threat, that if [one chief died], they would retaliate on the whites. Happily their threats have not been obliged to be tested, nor do I with the intimate knowledge I have of their dispositions and intentions believe there is any danger even if John dies, of their attempting to execute this threat. . . . They also believe it is right to kill all the workers of bad spells who either as doctors or as [tamanawas] men cause the death of any members of the tribe or family. . . . They have no more hesitation or compunction in killing a white man than they have in killing one of their own sort.[45]

Swan, who unlike many agents had years of experience in the Northwest, was well aware of the intertwined histories of increased sickness, capitalist expansion, and settler colonialism on the western edge of the Olympic Peninsula. But he chose in his role as agent of the American state to focus on complex Makah political struggles and linked responses to illness only as an intrinsic cultural problem. By the mid-1860s, this kind of language, which made health practices essential to marking Indian people as fundamentally different from whites, was increasingly common and increasingly broad in its scope.

Within this new discourse, Indian houses as much as Indian bodies were at fault for poor health among Native peoples. Critiques of shamanism blended easily into increasingly vocal critiques of Indian domesticity, as agents and physicians gradually shifted their focus from

American responsibility for Native health to faulting Indian people for cultural deficits. Physicians consistently wanted to be able to make "Indians to live in homes which they should keep clean and free from smoke." They praised Indians for keeping their bodies clean, but thought they needed to learn to wash their clothes and the insides of their houses more often.[46] During a period when most American and British settlers in this area did their best to avoid hospitals and medical care outside domestic settings, Indian agents and doctors began advocating more centralized medical care not only as a way to keep local Indians minimally healthy but as a way to monitor Native populations, reform Indian domestic habits, and produce civilized Indians. By the 1860s, physicians began to fold all these goals into frequent pleas for money for hospitals. One agent wrote,

> With patients such as these, the physician must personally administer his prescriptions.—act as nurse—and see to the food they require; but unless he can have them collected in an Hospital, under his own eye, he cannot perform these duties, and consequently, but too often, finds his best efforts paralysed. Another suggestion I desire to offer, is, that dwellings constructed so as to exclude the weather, should be erected for these Indians; at present, their houses are neither wind- nor watertight.[47]

Physicians, agents, and superintendents argued for more than a decade, without much success, that government-funded hospitals would be the best way to ensure that "the strong concentrated medicines" of civilization would replace the "simple remedies and foolish sorcery called *timanimus*."[48]

Yet despite physicians' constant critiques of how Indians lived, dressed, ate, and traveled, they noted some Indians' good health at least as often as their sickliness. Immediately after Dr. Chalmers's long explanation of how much the Makahs at Neah Bay needed a hospital, he added that "this Tribe, is at present, physically, if not morally, far superior to their neighbours, and (considering the great number of children I see here) instead of decreasing in numbers, I should think they must be increasing."[49] Agency physicians and other employees were some of the most voluble commentators on Indian health and its connections to Puget Sound's climate and future in the two decades after the treaties were signed. Reservation doctors did not immediately or consistently see Native people as entirely different from other patients, either in bodily essence or behavior. These men evaluated Indian health using categories and standards that echoed those applied to American soldiers and to residents of cities with public health departments. Like Hudson's Bay Company employees earlier, but also like physicians used to competing with homeopathic and other unorthodox forms of treatments, doctors associated with reservations saw Indian compliance with their own diagnoses and prescriptions as a sign of civilization or good sense and reliance on other healers, especially shamans, as defiance and foolishness.

However, in a short time these doctors and officials also became more interested in separating Indian and white worlds, or in simultaneously minimizing the presence of Indians in an American Puget Sound and assimilating them into American habits, than in acknowledging any continued overlap and exchange between Indian and Euro-American health cultures. Agency doctors, like earlier military physicians and other observers, continued to pay close attention to Indian bodies, to how disease worked in Indian bodies, and to Indian habits, but their purpose was to justify, often unsuccessfully, a greater degree of intervention in Indians' lives rather than to come up with complex explanations for either sickness or health. When Byron Barlow became resident physician at the Puyallup reservation in March 1870 he attributed his patients' "rheumatism [and] bad colds with coughs and diarrhoea" to "exposure to the cold and dampness" and "squatting on the damp ground and passing the time in amusing themselves at cards and other games," while noting that "all in all they have been remarkably healthy." Physicians and agents, such as Barlow, who did not call for hospitals often focused on other methods of keeping Indians in place. Barlow went on to explain that "the great reason why there has been so little sickness this season is that the adults have been encouraged to labor regularly in the fields and to stay at home. This compensated employment has made them contented and kept them free from those dissatisfactions that in former years have told seriously on their health."[50] Barlow associated the decline of a more widely dispersed seasonal subsistence round and an increase in agricultural work on or near the reservation—in other words, Indian sedentism—with improved health.

Other American officials and settlers also shifted their discussions of the region's healthiness away from comparisons between Indians and non-Indians and assessments of emigrant health into efforts to define Indian sickness as spatially and biologically separate from American settlement. Twenty-three years after Theodore Winthrop and George Gibbs toured the Puget Sound country in the aftermath of a smallpox epidemic, other Americans and Canadians spent part of the fall blaming the travels of Native people for the spread of smallpox north and south on the West Coast.[51] Smallpox, no longer mostly the responsibility of newcomers to the region, had become Indians' fault, its contagion linked in newspapers and settler stories to Native mobility and Native houses.[52] Whereas agency physicians and other officials had bureaucratic investments in monitoring Indian sickness and in trying to garner resources to centralize Indian health care, other newcomers to the region had become less likely to depend on Indian labor or to see the fate of indigenous bodies as connected to settler prospects.

By the late 1870s, Puget Sound had become demographically American, and the region was firmly connected to the United States's postwar economic expansion. Over the next twenty years, a generation that renamed itself pioneers, struggling to hold on to power amid a flood of new arrivals, maneuvered to lay claim to the story of how Puget Sound had become American. As settlers appropriated and distorted local Indian identity as part of this struggle, they simultaneously worked to separate Indian and American spaces and bodies more clearly than ever before.[53] Drawing boundaries between American and Indian bodies also meant retelling the region's recent disease history and remapping geographies of illness to emphasize and naturalize the inevitability of Indian demographic decline and American increase. In these stories, Indian bodies were and would be inherently weaker and more vulnerable to disease, and Indian medical practice and medical epistemologies over the past seventy years had been simultaneously inflexible, persistent in the form of superstition, and entirely disrupted by new illnesses. As powerful as this version of Puget Sound's history eventually became, until the end of the nineteenth century it was both contested by Indian peoples and contradicted by a persistent, if reduced, mixed world of environmental and medical knowledge around the region.

NOTES

1 John H. Williams, ed., *The Canoe and the Saddle or Klalam and Klickitat by Theodore Winthrop* (Tacoma, Wash.: Franklin-Ward, 1913), 250–51.

2 *Annual Report of the Commissioner of Indian Affairs* (hereafter ARCIA) 1854, 447. For a broader discussion of the 1853 epidemic, see Robert Boyd, *The Coming of the Spirit of Pestilence: Introduced Infectious Disease and Population Decline among Northwest Coast Indians, 1774–1874* (Seattle: University of Washington Press, 1999), 165–71.

3 Williams, *The Canoe and the Saddle*, 275.

4 George Gibbs Notebooks of Scientific Observations of the Pacific Northwest, Western Americana Collection, Beinecke Rare Book and Manuscript Library, Yale University, New Haven, Conn.

5 George Gibbs, *Tribes of Western Washington and Northwestern Oregon* (Washington, D.C.: Government Printing Office, 1877), 173; Gibbs, "Report on the Indian Tribes of Washington Territory," in *Reports of Explorations and Surveys to Determine the Most Practicable Economical Route for a Railroad from the Mississippi River to the Pacific Ocean* (Washington, D.C.: Beverly Tucker, 1855–1860), 402, 428, 429.

6 Williams, *The Canoe and the Saddle*, 11, 28.

7 Alfred W. Crosby, "Virgin Soil Epidemics as a Factor in the Aboriginal Depopulation in America," *William and Mary Quarterly* 3rd ser., vol. 33 (1976): 289–99.

8 Key works include Noble David Cook, *Born to Die: Disease and New World Conquest, 1492–1650* (Cambridge, England: Cambridge University Press, 1999); Crosby, "Virgin Soil Epidemics"; and Henry F. Dobyns, *Their Number Become Thinned: Native American Population Dynamics in Eastern North America* (Knoxville: University of Tennessee Press, 1983).

9 Jody F. Decker, "Country Distempers: Deciphering Disease and Illness in Rupert's Land before 1870," in *Reading beyond Words: Contexts for Native History*, ed. Jennifer S. H. Brown and Elizabeth Vibert (Peterborough, Ont.: Broadview Press, 1996), 156–81; David S. Jones, "Virgin Soils Revisited," *William and Mary Quarterly* 3rd ser., vol. 60 (2003): 703–42; Paul Kelton, "Avoiding the Smallpox Spirits: Colonial Epidemics and Southeastern Indian Survival," *Ethnohistory* 51, no. 1 (Winter 2004): 45–71; and Kelton, *Epidemics and Enslavement: Biological Catastrophe in the Native Southeast* (Lincoln: University of Nebraska Press, 2007).

10 James B. Waldram, D. Ann Herring, and T. Kue Young, *Aboriginal Health in Canada: Historical, Cultural, and Epidemiological Perspectives* (Toronto: University of Toronto Press, 1995), 43. See also Mary-Ellen Kelm, *Colonizing Bodies: Aboriginal Health and Healing in British Columbia, 1900–1950* (Vancouver, B.C.: UBC Press, 1999).

11 Charles J. Kappler, ed., *Indian Affairs: Laws and Treaties,* vol. 2 (Washington, D.C.: Government Printing Office, 1904), 664, 672, 676.

12 See especially Kelm, *Colonizing Bodies,* and "Diagnosing the Discursive

Indian: Medicine, Gender, and the 'Dying Race,'" *Ethnohistory* 52, no. 2 (Spring 2005): 371–406.

13 George B. Roberts to Frances Fuller Victor, November 28, 1878, "Letters to Mrs. F. F. Victor," *Oregon Historical Quarterly* 63 (1962): 193–94.

14 Boyd, *The Coming of the Spirit of Pestilence*, 84–115; Sherburne Cook, "The Epidemic of 1830–33 in California and Oregon," *University of California Publications in American Archaeology and Ethnology* 43, no. 3 (1955): 303–26.

15 On disease and an eastern Pacific world, see David Igler, "Diseased Goods: Global Exchanges in the Eastern Pacific Basin, 1770–1850," *American Historical Review* 109, no. 3 (June 2004): 694–704, 714–19. The most comprehensive account of new illnesses in the Northwest is Boyd, *The Coming of the Spirit of Pestilence*. On British fur traders in the Pacific Northwest generally, see Richard Mackie, *Trading beyond the Mountains: The British Fur Trade on the Pacific, 1793–1843* (Vancouver, B.C.: UBC Press, 1997).

16 For similar processes elsewhere around Puget Sound, see Richard White, *Land Use, Environment, and Social Change: The Shaping of Island County, Washington* (Seattle: University of Washington Press, 1980), 14–34.

17 Joseph Heath, *Memoirs of Nisqually*, ed. Lucille McDonald (Fairfield, Wash.: Ye Galleon Press, 1979), 30, 48, 55, 72–73, 101, 127, 130–31.

18 For examples of nineteenth-century European and American newcomers comparing their impressions of the region's disease history with Vancouver's, see James G. Swan, *The Northwest Coast or, Three Years' Residence in Washington Territory* (1857; repr., Seattle: University of Washington Press, 1969), 211–12; and "Dr. John Scouler's Journal of a Voyage to N.W. America," *Oregon Historical Quarterly* 6 (1905): 198.

19 Edmond S. Meany, ed., *Vancouver's Discovery of Puget Sound* (New York: Macmillan, 1907), 98, 108, 123, 124–26.

20 For Vancouver's and other British explorers' views of Puget Sound as picturesque and pastoral, see Douglas Cole and Maria Tippett, "Pleasing Diversity and Sublime Desolation: The 18th-Century British Perception of the Northwest Coast," *Pacific Northwest Quarterly* 65, no. 1 (January 1974): 1–7.

21 Samuel Forry and Thomas Lawson, *A Statistical Report on the Sickness and Mortality in the Army of the United States, 1819–1839* (Washington, D.C.: J. Gideon, 1840), 325, 337.

22 For a longer discussion of shifts between personal and abstract styles of observation, see Linda Nash, "The Changing Experience of Nature: Historical Encounters with a Northwest River," *Journal of American History* 86, no. 4 (March 2000): 1605–10.

23 Assistant Surgeon J. M. Haden, "Medical Topography and Diseases of Fort Steilacoom," in U.S. Senate, *Report on the Sickness and Mortality in the Army of the United States*, 34th Congress, 1st and 2nd session, 1856, Senate Executive Document v. 18, no. 96, 478.

24 Ibid., 478.

25 Ibid., 480.

26 Ibid., 480–81.

27 On American physicians and anatomy, see Michael Sappol, *A Traffic of Dead Bodies: Anatomy and Embodied Social Identity in Nineteenth-Century America* (Princeton, N.J.: Princeton University Press, 2002). On diagnostic technique, see Steven M. Stowe, *Doctoring the South: Southern Physicians and Everyday Medicine in the Mid-Nineteenth Century* (Chapel Hill: University of North Carolina Press, 2004), 131–49; Conevery Bolton Valencius, *The Health of the Country: How American Settlers Understood Themselves and Their Land* (New York: Basic Books, 2002), 53–84; and John Harley Warner, *The Therapeutic Perspective: Medical Practice, Knowledge, and Identity in America, 1820–1885* (Cambridge, Mass.: Harvard University Press, 1986).

28 Boyd, *Coming of the Spirit of Pestilence,* 112; Myron Eells, *The Indians of Puget Sound* (Seattle: University of Washington Press, 1985), 411–16; William W. Elmendorf, *The Structure of Twana Culture* (1960; repr., Pullman: Washington State University Press, 1992), 481, 483, 506–7; Erna Gunther, "Klallam Ethnography," *University of Washington Publications in Anthropology* 1, no. 5 (January 1927): 297–99, 300; Alexandra Harmon, *Indians in the Making: Ethnic Relations and Indian Identities around Puget Sound* (Berkeley: University of California Press, 1998), 39; Herman Haeberlin and Erna Gunther, "The Indians of Puget Sound," *University of Washington Publications in Anthropology* 1, no. 5 (1927): 77–78; Marian W. Smith, *The Puyallup–Nisqually* (New York: Columbia University Press, 1940), 77–82, 87–90.

29 June McCormick Collins, *Valley of the Spirits: The Upper Skagit Indians of Western Washington* (Seattle: University of Washington Press, 1974), 200.

30 See Eells, *The Indians of Puget Sound,* 62.

31 See Swan, *The Northwest Coast,* 176–80; Collins, *Valley of the Spirits,* 208–9.

32 Gibbs, *Tribes of Western Washington,* 207–8.

33 For examples of domestic medicine in Washington Territory, see Swan, *The Northwest Coast,* 33–34, 176–80, 264–67.

34 Wayne P. Suttles, *Coast Salish and Western Washington Indians* (New York: Garland Publishing, 1974), 344.

35 See ARCIA 1861, 179; ARCIA 1865, 78; see also Coll Thrush, *Native Seattle: Histories from the Crossing-Over Place* (Seattle: University of Washington Press, 2008), 113: "Settler Joseph Crow . . . recalled the unsuccessful efforts of a Native doctor to heal patients in a house at Front and King Streets on the Lava Beds during a smallpox outbreak in 1864—after which the doctor, his skills now seen as useless, disappeared."

36 Truman Hack to W. B. Gosnell, October 9, 1857, *Records of Washington Territory Superintendent of Indian Affairs,* Microfilm A171, University

of Washington Libraries (hereafter WTSIA) Reel 23; M. T. Simmons to Nesmith, October 15, 1857, WTSIA Reel 17; E. C. Chirouse to Milroy, March 10, 1874, WTSIA Reel 26; ARCIA 1858, 222, 227.

37 G. A. Paige to Isaac Stevens, May 13, 1857, WTSIA Reel 20. In 1865 "the schoolboys of Tulalip Indian school" asked a visiting Washington, D.C. delegation for "if not a doctor, at least . . . the medicines required to help our poor health." See Appendix C, *Condition of the Indian Tribes* (Washington, D.C.: Government Printing Office, 1867), 18.

38 W. B. Gosnell to Nesmith, December 31, 1857, WTSIA Reel 23.

39 Whe-land-hur, Ge-le-whomist, Quima, Hump-Klalm, Slow-el, E. C. Finkboner, and Richard Romy to Commissioner of Indian Affairs, June 26, 1869, WTSIA Reel 14.

40 Iatab Wakletchow and Philip Seattle to Commissioner of Indian Affairs, July 5, 1869, and Chiefs of White River King County and Chiefs of Black River to Commissioner of Indian Affairs, July 6, 1869, WTSIA Reel 14.

41 Nesmith to R. C. Fay, April 21, 1857, WTSIA Reel 8.

42 W. B. Gosnell to Nesmith, December 31, 1857, WTSIA Reel 23.

43 G. A. Paige to W. B. Gosnell, June 30, 1861, WTSIA Reel 19. See also Brad Asher, *Beyond the Reservation: Indians, Settlers, and the Law in Washington Territory, 1853–1889* (Norman: University of Oklahoma Press, 1999), 160.

44 G. A. Paige to M. T. Simmons, December 31, 1857, WTSIA Reel 20.

45 J. Swan to Webster, March 31, 1863, WTSIA Reel 31.

46 L. Chalmers to H. Webster, July 30, 1862, WTSIA, Reel 31.

47 L. Chalmers to H. Webster, December 31, 1862, WTSIA Reel 31. See also Paget to Gosnell, July 30, 1861, WTSIA Reel 19; G. W. Weston to E. H. Milroy, October 1, 1873, WTSIA Reel 24.

48 R. H. Milroy to F. A. Walker, October 1, 1873, ARCIA 1873.

49 L. Chalmers to Henry Webster, December 31, 1862, WTSIA Reel 31.

50 Byron Barlow to Ross, April 31, 1870, WTSIA Reel 24.

51 Jennifer Seltz, "Epidemics, Indians, and Border-Making in the Nineteenth-Century Pacific Northwest," in *Bridging National Borders in North America: Transnational and Comparative Histories,* ed. Benjamin Johnson and Andrew Graybill (Durham, N.C.: Duke University Press, 2010), 91–92.

52 "Smallpox Prevalent in Victoria," *Washington Standard,* March 25, 1876, 2; "C.B. Hopkins Reports . . . ," *Washington Standard,* September 23, 1876, 3; "Citizens of Port Townsend . . . ," *Washington Standard,* September 30, 1876, 2; "Smallpox Scourge Still Exists in Victoria," *Washington Standard,* December 30, 1876, 2; Caroline Leighton, *Life at Puget Sound* (Boston: Lee and Shepard, 1884), 156.

53 Thrush, *Native Seattle,* 145–93; Harmon, *Indians in the Making,* 104–6, 148–49. For a broader discussion of this tendency, see Philip J. Deloria, *Playing Indian* (New Haven, Conn.: Yale University Press, 1998).

"I Studied and Practiced Medicine without Molestation"

African American Doctors in the First Years of Freedom

GRETCHEN LONG

IN THE EARLIEST YEARS OF FREEDOM, African Americans with hopes of becoming professional doctors faced a complex dilemma, perhaps more complex than most historians have recognized. Although many freedmen had practiced healing as slaves, by and large they had no formal medical education and no means of gaining one. In this respect, aspiring black doctors faced obstacles similar to those faced by African Americans trying to advance in education, land ownership, employment, and politics. In these areas, and in others, the end of slavery was followed by de facto and de jure racism that barred access to the professions and often to meaningful citizenship. Historians such as Vanessa Northington Gamble have rightly identified this racism as the key force in barring African American doctors, dentists, and nurses from the medical profession in the decades after emancipation.

In contrast to fields such as law and education, however, the medical field was also beset by complications that were distinct from racism. In the years immediately after the Civil War, not only the recently freed African Americans but American medicine itself stood at a critical juncture. In the decades before the Civil War, Americans had lived in a diverse medical landscape. Radically different types of health care, administered by many types of practitioners, and contradictory ideas about the nature of health and illness competed for patients and prestige. However, the Civil War brought about advances in medicine, especially in surgery and infection control. The Confederate and Union armies screened their doctors to ensure and regulate quality of care, favoring doctors of allopathic medicine. After the war, authorities held practitioners of other types of medicine in low esteem and barred herbalists, homeopaths, hydropaths, and the like from professional status.

The twin forces of racism and newly rigid professional standards worked powerfully in the lives of African American doctors and patients. Legacies of slavery and the vexed history of American medical practice challenged aspiring black doctors as they navigated the new terrain of both freedom and doctorhood.

Two African American healers—John Donalson of Austin, Texas and Moses Camplin of Charleston, South Carolina—appear sporadically in government records and correspondence in the early decades of emancipation. These documents throw light on the effect of changes in medicine on the ambitions of African American doctors. Their stories are remarkable in that we otherwise have few sources from this generation of black doctors, whose lives span both slavery and freedom. The experiences of these two doctors as they attempted to set up practice illustrate a number of struggles between authority, both medical and governmental, and free African Americans in the years immediately after the Civil War. They point to how the politics of race and the politics of medicine, both in periods of flux, intertwined in sites around the country. John Donalson and Moses Camplin tried, in the first years of freedom, to harness their new free status to a new professional status of physician. This coupling met with a tangle of success and failure and, for the historian, illustrates the intersection of a number of questions about racism on one hand and about the struggle over competing bodies of medical knowledge on the other.

Donalson and Camplin's stories survive because their letters and letters about them are preserved in the archives of the national office of the Freedmen's Bureau. Although health care was not part of the Bureau's original mandate, during Reconstruction some of its administrators in the various geographic districts took on limited responsibility for the medical care of former slaves.

Doctors working for the Freedmen's Bureau adhered to the medical methods of the Union army, eschewing the homeopathic and herbal medicine that had coexisted with allopathic medicine before the war. In the eyes of the Bureau, supporting the claim of a practitioner of alternative medicine would conflict with its assigned role of lifting the freedpeople out of superstition and into enlightened practices. This aspect of the Bureau's work proved important for John Donalson and Moses Camplin.[1]

Although both Donalson and Camplin called themselves doctors or physicians and, as far as the records show, were called and thought of as doctors by their communities, dissimilarities in the two men's training and background, their relationships with local black and white communities, their presentation to white authorities, and even their ambitions outweigh their shared vocation. However, Donalson and Camplin both realized that freedom changed their relationship both to the state and to local white authority, as well as to the claims they could make as doctors. Probably they were less aware of the effect that changing trends in the field of medicine would have on their careers.

Donalson and Camplin represent the first generation of black Americans to work out their adult citizenship in the context of emancipation. They were also the first generation of African American doctors who practiced medicine before the creation of black medical schools and in the beginning of more intense regulation of the medical profession by state and professional authorities. In the period after the Civil War, education and professional status became ever more tightly linked, and medical schools discriminated against African Americans. For Donalson, Camplin, and other African Americans who tried to make a living as physicians in the postwar South but whose names and stories have been lost to history, freedom ushered in a curtailment of their ability to practice medicine rather than the opportunity to prove themselves competent professional physicians. When faced with restrictions on their medical practices, Donalson and Camplin, in very different ways, mustered their literacy and their newfound political freedoms to make a case for themselves as doctors. However, their letters and surrounding documents reveal that the response of the federal government to each man's petition depended not just on each doctor's new status as a free citizen but also on changing trends in the American medical landscape.

JOHN DONALSON'S LETTERS TO THE
FREEDMEN'S BUREAU IN WASHINGTON

John Donalson of Austin, Texas had acted as healer to slaves and continued his practice with freedmen as his patients. He practiced the kind of medicine common in slave communities, relying on his knowledge of local plants with healing properties and on familiarity with the values, beliefs, and relationships within the slave community. It seems probable that Donalson, who listed his birthplace as Alabama on an 1880 census, had been a slave himself, although proof of his enslavement or of his manumission or freedom before 1865 is not evident in the records. In any case, Donalson's patients before the Civil War were almost certainly slaves and free blacks well integrated into slave culture.

Our earliest records of Donalson appear in 1866. During that year, a number of letters about him arrived in the national Freedmen's Bureau office in Washington. The letters came from Donalson himself, from local Freedmen's Bureau agents assigned to the Austin office, and from a group of newly free African Americans from the Austin area. In a letter to General Oliver O. Howard at the Freedmen's Bureau in Washington, Donalson sought redress against a number of parties in Austin, namely, various African American freedpeople, who he claimed had not paid him for medical services he had provided, and local Bureau agents who had refused to help him collect these debts. In a kind of stream-of-consciousness narrative, he recounted the history of his previous eighteen months, describing how local Freedmen's Bureau agents in Austin had undermined his practice in favor of one or more white doctors who had arrived on the scene.

In his letter, Donalson told of freedmen applying to the army in the spring of 1865 for help from white physicians and being told "get your Cold [colored] Drs." He claimed that Freedmen's Bureau agent A. Evans told him at that time to treat the freedmen and that "they will pay if they don['t] pay I will make them pay." When the white doctors later complained that Donalson "took all the custom [business] out of their hands," Donalson wrote, Evans refused to help him collect payments and "threw up the Name of Congering [conjuring]." The characterization of Donalson's medical practice as mere conjuring was a direct attack on his brand of medicine, which stood in stark contrast to that of the white doctors.[2]

Donalson's medical authority rested on self-compiled evidence and a claim to an organic, natural, and implicit connection to the people and land of central Texas—a claim that was less effectual during emancipation than it would have been before the war. Setting himself apart from standard white medical science—and perhaps unaware of the extent to which the Freedmen's Bureau was committed to standard medical science—Donalson claimed an authenticity specific to the climate and original people of Texas. He wrote, "I am not a Mineral Physician.

Professionally. I can use it but it not good in this Climate. I use rather herb. My father had Me Learned under an Indian phys when young. if any Man say that I ever Lost a case. he is vast mistaken."

Donalson was an astute observer of the changes in the medical options available to newly free African Americans, and this brief passage from his letter points to a number of aspects of the medical landscape for African Americans at this time. The arrival of emancipation brought with it the Freedmen's Bureau's oversight into areas of African American life that previously had been either strictly supervised by white owners or, in many cases, not supervised by white authority at all. Freed African Americans' medical care was a realm that fell between these two extremes. Masters had certainly been concerned about the health of their slaves; indeed, medical practice in a sense lay at the very crux of slave owners' abilities to maintain their slave workforce after the closing of the slave trade and of their claim that they were financially and emotionally invested in taking good care of their slaves. But practices such as Donalson's that used paradigms of healing foreign to white doctors may well have flourished during slavery, either ignored by slave masters or out of reach of white surveillance. Twentieth- and twenty-first-century historians of medicine and contemporary observers of enslaved healers throughout the South confirm the portrait that Donalson's letter paints of the changing nature of medical care in the nineteenth century, especially for African Americans.

Historian Sharla Fett argues that enslavement exposed African Americans to two parallel tracks of healing with separate ideas about health and sickness. White people controlled and supervised one system based on what Fett calls "soundness." The rubric underlying decisions about medical care, nutrition, and housing turned on understanding the bodies of slaves in relation to market value, labor, and reproductive potential. Treatments administered under this system by owners, doctors, and overseers tended to rely on the contents of a medicine chest. White owners decided when professional care was appropriate and what kind of physician would attend the slave. They paid the bills and granted or withheld consent for medical procedures. If the owner was a proponent of homeopathic medicine, he could call in a homeopath for his slaves. If he believed in a certain regimen of diet or exercise, he could order an overseer or nurse to provide it. The linking of medicine with the ownership of slaves' bodies, with financial concerns, and with racial hierarchy infused this breed of medicine with political meaning.[3]

Alongside this medicine, African American healers and families practiced a form of medical care in slave communities that Sharla Fett called "relational." Under this rubric, the goals of care were removed from the financial concerns of the slave owner. Enslaved healers, often women, attempted to make the patient comfortable and if necessary restore or retain proper relationships with other members of the community. Materials used for medicines tended to come from plants that were locally available and understood to be infused with healing power. Although Donalson's description of his own medical practice does not bring in all the elements of the relational care of slavery times as it is described by Fett, he clearly delineates between his own medical practice and that of the white doctor sent by the Freedmen's Bureau to look after the African Americans in Austin.

Donalson's distinction between the white doctor's "mineral medicine" and his use of "herb" gestures toward the divide that Fett describes. We can imagine that Donalson called the white doctor's medicine "mineral medicine" because of the medicines in the nineteenth-century doctor's medicine chest, such as calomel (mercurous chloride, a purgative), laudanum (tincture of opium, used as a pain-killer), and elixir of vitriol (ethylsulfuric acid, a tonic for stomach problems). Donalson was confident that his herbal remedies were more effective than mineral medicine and may even have been aware that some of the mineral medicines were dangerous, but the Freedmen's Bureau agents refused to take him seriously. They were fully committed to the kind of medical care administered by their white physician, a kind that was based on science, albeit faulty science.

Donalson's claim to rely on "rather herb" links his medicine to traditions of enslaved healers. His intriguing mention of his training, claiming to have been educated by "an Indian" at his father's direction, raises questions that archival evidence cannot answer. We know that in a census conducted fourteen years later Donalson described himself as an Alabama native, but we have no evidence of when he moved to Texas or where this training in Indian medicine took place. Historians describe relationships between Native Americans and African Americans in antebellum Texas as largely hostile.[4] In the 1850s, Texas saw its population (free Anglo and African American slave) rise dramatically alongside the flourishing of cotton plantations. These increases brought about conflict with Comanche communities who had established trade in Texas. It may have been during this period that Donalson and his father came in contact with Native American medical practice.[5] Of course, this conflict does not preclude the possibility that Donalson had received training from an Indian healer. Descriptions of Indian medicine in the Southwest stress native healers' reliance on herbs and spiritual forces.[6] This framework would certainly line up with archival evidence of Donalson's medical practice.

Donalson's claim that he could use "mineral medicine" if he liked, but found it wrong for the Texas climate, revealed an understanding of how and why the body heals that was distinct from the conceptual framework that was gaining ascendancy in medicine after the Civil War. He highlighted a key element of folk medicine and even of modern pharmacology—that the same substance, differently prepared or consumed by a patient with different ailments, or in a different environment, can have opposite effects. Donalson's letter stated, ominously, "I will send you apiece of this herb to test whether it is poison. Or No. as Sweet as honey. and as bitter as gall. Learn what that means."[7]

Donalson was affronted by the arrival in Austin of a white doctor who operated under the auspices of the Bureau and in a larger sense under a new wide umbrella of a "rational and methodical" approach to medicine, an approach that the Bureau was committed to establishing to the exclusion of all others. In contrast to this rational approach, Donalson often noted his own emotional reactions and those of the white Bureau agents he had had business with. He wrote, "Excuse a diranged Man—I attend day and Night. it got in the Ears of the whites they said to freedmen for dispite he's got no license; Nor no Deplomer. don't pay him youl Make that off of him." Donalson presents the white doctor hired by the Freedmen's Bureau as a competitor in the market for African American paying clients, but his complaints imply that he was not a competitor on a level playing field, as the agents had spread ridicule of Donalson's practice, perhaps destroying the trusting relationships he had formerly had with his patients.

It is unclear whether the white doctor to whom Donalson refers was providing treatment at a hospital or in an outpatient clinic. The leaders of the Freedmen's Bureau staffed hospitals and clinics with a combination of northern doctors recruited for the job and short-term southern white doctors.[8] Donalson's letter is silent on the exact nature of the white doctor's care or its medical setting; however, it is clear that he regarded it as "mineral medicine" and that the Freedmen's Bureau was actively promoting it over Donalson's herbal treatments.

In defense of his own medical expertise, Donalson offered testimony about his patients and the cures he had worked on them. According to Donalson, Austin had experienced an increased mortality rate since the local Freedmen's Bureau forced him to discontinue his practice. His letter gave a death tally among Austin residents. He wrote, "See how Many died since I quit Albert Brown &wife 2 Geo Rust 3 William Risher 4 Daniel Rust 5 Mrs. Niley Johnson 6 3 infants 9." Donalson wrote that he "showed Captain portor [sic] his reports. yesterday His Contanence fell." His letter continued to document Agent Evans's response, saying, "I ask him to read. He refused to read." In Donalson's view, having to show proof of cures was an imposition, but even after he had offered evidence about the rising mortality rate, white authorities still refused to take him seriously. As a result of the Bureau's interference, Donalson wrote, in order to continue his medical work, "I had to insure every Case. No Cure No pay."

Unfortunately for Donalson, he picked the wrong historical moment to launch a defense of herbal medicine or spiritual forces in healing. In the decades leading up to the Civil War, scientifically trained physicians fought back serious challenges from "irregulars" such as homeopaths, hydropaths, or the followers of Samuel Thomson, author of a popular book of herbal cures. Partly mindful of the chaotic state of standard American medical education and medical practice, American physicians undertook massive organizational and regulatory campaigns, attempting to arrive at and enforce uniform standards for medical education and licensing. Although a thorough overhaul of American medical schools did not occur until 1909, the regulatory movement was well afoot by the Civil War. During the war itself various regulatory bodies found new power, particularly in the North, where doctors in the Union army were held to unprecedented standards and inspectors worked to rid the army of irregular physicians. Banning homeopaths from joining the ranks of Union army surgeons or from gaining residencies at new hospitals in New York and Chicago was a victory for the regular physicians.[9] We hear a hint of this movement toward regulation in Donalson's complaint that the whites in Austin said to the freedmen, "he's got no license; Nor no Deplomer."

Donalson's first letter to General Howard detailing these complaints, according to the summary of that letter in the archives, was dated June 12, 1866. Howard's office apparently sent the letter on to Agent Evans in Austin, where it garnered a series of spirited reactions, attached to the summary. Before looking at those responses, however, let us turn to a letter from Moses Camplin that arrived in the Washington Bureau office the same year as Donalson's. Camplin's letter offers a look at a doctor who, although he was an African American and a former slave, practiced a kind of medicine very different from that of Donalson.

MOSES CAMPLIN'S LETTER TO THE FREEDMEN'S BUREAU IN WASHINGTON

In July 1866, Moses Camplin wrote to the Freedmen's Bureau about his struggles to practice medicine as a newly freed black man in Charleston, South Carolina. Camplin was enslaved until February 18, 1865, when Charleston fell to the Union army. The handwriting, language, syntax, and grammar of his tidily written and eloquent letter to the Freedmen's Bureau in 1866 serve as a testament to some significant education during his life as a slave. Camplin had worked for many years as assistant to a prominent white surgeon, and he set up his own medical practice two weeks after being freed.

Even before Camplin's letter to the Freedmen's Bureau, his name appears in at least one other Civil War–era document. A biography of Martin Delaney, an African American activist, writer, and Union army recruiter, described a meeting of "colored citizens of Charleston, South Carolina" who convened on March 29, 1865 to draft a resolution celebrating their freedom and honoring Union commanders and President Lincoln. Moses Camplin, enslaved until shortly before this date, was listed as the chairman of the colored citizens' committee.[10] Camplin's election as the chair one month after Charleston African Americans received their freedom shows his standing and respectability in the antebellum enslaved African American community and his investment in long-lasting and meaningful freedom for ex-slaves.

Like Donalson, Camplin sought assistance from the federal Freedmen's Bureau with his problem—namely, that local authorities were preventing him from continuing his practice of medicine. Donalson stated that he had learned medicine from a healer, and Camplin also had learned under a practitioner, but in his case his mentor was an allopathic physician, one of the foremost members of the medical establishment in his community. This difference proved crucial in Camplin's effort to gain the support of the Freedmen's Bureau in pursuit of his rights as a citizen and a professional. Camplin wrote that he had worked as a "servant" in the office of Dr. Thomas L. Ogier, "where," he stated, "I studied and practiced medicine without molestation." Camplin used the word "servant" as many antebellum whites did to refer to a slave who was property rather than a wage-earning servant. Camplin clarified his status in the letter's next sentence, which referred to February 18. He stated that it was "the 18the day of Febr'y 1865, when I received my freedom from the said Dr Ogier, and two weeks after I opened an office of my own."[11]

From these sentences in Camplin's letter, his allusions to his training with Ogier, and his initiative in opening up a practice of his own, readers begin to glimpse his life as a slave in Civil War–era Charleston. As a literate skilled slave in Charleston, Camplin was not the anomaly he might have been in other areas of the South. For generations, antebellum Charleston society and economy had fostered the development of an elite class of African Americans, both free blacks and skilled slaves, who had ties to white elite Charlestonians and who led lives vastly different from the majority of slaves in the rural South. Some urban slaves were hired out by owners for skilled work; others were essentially freelance agents who worked at a wide range of labor and provided their owners with a set payment weekly or monthly. These slaves had some freedom of mobility and a modicum of economic flexibility unheard of among slaves on South Carolina farms and plantations.

A central piece in understanding Camplin's life as a slave, his medical training, and the challenges he later faced as a free doctor is the position of his master and owner, Dr. Thomas Ogier, under whose supervision Camplin "studied and practiced medicine" in keeping with the medical traditions of the day. A prosperous urban physician, Ogier was wealthy, politically connected, and skilled in surgery; thus his influence extended through medical culture, political circles, and the urban slave-owning elite. By 1860, his household owned more than fifty slaves, and according to the 1860 census, he owned not only his own residence but another property that housed "slaves"—no number is given.[12] One of Ogier's sons was also a doctor, and the family's busy urban practice grew to include white families and their African American slaves.[13] Ogier presented case studies to the South Carolina medical community and published articles in journals such as the *American Journal of the Medical Sciences*. His articles reveal an interest in gynecology, innovative drug treatments for various diseases, and modern surgical technique as well as more abstract scientific questions such as the role of genetic heredity versus environment in transmission of conditions in families. Ogier also had an interest in medical education. In 1834, he coauthored a manual for "operative surgery" students. During the war Ogier was appointed as the chief division surgeon of the 1st Military District of South Carolina. Much of his time would have been spent organizing medical care for wounded and ill Confederate soldiers.[14]

If Camplin began working and studying medicine in Dr. Ogier's office in 1848, as his letter stated, then by February 1865, when Union soldiers marched into Charleston and Camplin set up his own practice, he had had almost twenty years of medical experience. In contrast to Donalson's letter, Camplin's presents a well-organized summary of the facts of his case. His voice is passionate in its plea for assistance from the Bureau but not hysterical or threatening. Just as the opening sentences of the letter give hints as to the kind of life Moses Camplin may have had as a slave, the appearance of the letter gestures toward the kind of orderly and law-abiding citizenship that Camplin imagined for African Americans.

While Camplin's letter grappled with an issue that encompassed his professional identity and livelihood as a physician, it also addressed more broadly the relationship between African Americans and municipal authority. He described his effort to open an office of his own, with a practice that would cater to African American patients. He wrote that shortly after opening his practice as a free man and "regular physician," he asked George Pelzer, a white Charleston doctor and city register, for "blank official Certificates so as to enable me to bury any that may die under my care."

According to Camplin, initially city register George Pelzer "readily complied with my request," then suddenly reversed his decision. After a year of Camplin's practicing medicine as a free man, the city register, under the direction of the white mayor, Peter C. Gaillard, refused to let him have death certificates, claiming that because he had not been to medical school and had no medical license, he was not legally authorized to certify death. Perhaps anticipating this maneuver by white authorities, two months after setting up his practice Camplin had tried to enroll in medical school at the South Carolina Medical College. Camplin wrote, "I called on Dr. Frost, Dean of the Medical College and brought to his notice my case—begging him if possible to let me have a medical License, for which, I would be willing to pay the highest price, but Dr Frost Said to me, the Medical College will not admit Colored men to its benefit, nor will the medical Board License any Colored person to practice medicine in the State of So. Ca."[15] Finally, Camplin wrote, "I called on the Mayor so as to have Some understanding with him relative to my case," but his visit was to no avail.

In his letter, Camplin pleaded with the Freedmen's Bureau to reverse the city authorities' decision and allow him to continue in practice as a regulated doctor and a free man. He noted that during the war two African American men, doctors Boseman and Becker, were physicians with the 54th Massachusetts Colored Regiment. He argued that because the United States recognized these black men as doctors and conferred that title on them in the Union army, then "South Carolina is obliged to do likewise." Camplin's writing of his letter demonstrated a faith, or at least a hope, that the power of the federal government could prevail against the racist policies of South Carolina. However, he held no illusions that doing so would be easy, for he added, "Were it in her power, she would have hung both Boseman, and Becker—long ago. South Carolina knows that no Colored man can possibly obtained [sic] a License to practice either Law, or medicine in any of these late Slaveholding States."[16] At the time of Camplin's letter, his inability to pronounce death and to interact professionally with the city coroner would "brake up my business entirely," he wrote.

Camplin's letter and the actions that led up to his writing to the Bureau—his initial request for and receipt of death certificates, his attempt to secure formal medical education and licensing, and his visit to the mayor—all reveal Camplin's ability and desire to work within the system of medical regulation and civil authority in place in Charleston at that time. His eagerness to join in these structures of power contrasts starkly with letters received later that year by the Bureau from and about herbalist John Donalson, who expressed no interest in qualifying for the "Deplomer" and whose behavior in some interchanges with Bureau agents was intemperate and emotional.

RESPONSES AND RESULTS

The attitude of the Bureau agents in Austin toward John Donalson, expressed both in their own reporting and in his, is revealing. Donalson's claim that the local agents were hostile to his sort of medicine was wholly borne out. However, the language used by agents Porter and Evans went beyond bias against herbal medicine and ventured into discourses of race. They equated the medical practices used by Donalson with ignorance, mental incompetence, and superstition. Not only was Donalson's kind of medical knowledge deemed ineffective; it was deemed ineffective because of the race of the practitioner. Their language brought in race explicitly, dismissing Donalson not only as a quack but as an African quack.

In his letter to the Bureau, Donalson complained that news of his treatments and hard work ("I attend day and Night") "got in the ears of the whites" in Austin and that they tried to steal his business, telling his patients that because he did not have a medical diploma he was not entitled to payment. When Austin locals learned of John Donalson's complaining letter to Washington, it provoked a flurry of accompanying correspondence from Austin Bureau agents and, on one occasion, a group of freedmen. Agent Evans wrote to the federal Bureau that "Serpent Dr John M. Donaldson [*sic*] is a non compusmentus freedman." (Evans apparently meant that Donalson was not *compos mentis*, of sound mind.) Furthermore, he wrote, Donalson "is known as a conjurer a believer in Witches, Hobgoblins and Ghosts." Evans wrote that he "put a quietus on his operations here In which act I am sustained by all the freemen of this place." Captain Porter, a subassistant commissioner who was appointed after Evans had left the post, had this comment about Donalson's activities in Austin: "His school of Medicine is a cross of the Botanical and African conjuring."[17]

Bureau agents' writings decried Donalson's beliefs in the supernatural and concluded that he was a "conceited simpleton practicing deception on the freedmen." Worse, his type of medical practice targeted those "colored people who were [inclined?] to be superstitious." Indeed, Evans wrote, "The better class of freedmen sustain me in my course with him." The concept of medicine, healing, and illness that Donalson represented, they believed, would hold freed people back from self-improvement and from joining the "better class" of African Americans who supported the Bureau and its activities. Agent Evans's "better class" of freedmen, whom Donalson accused of accepting bribes in return for their support, also weighed in on Donalson's complaint. In July 1866, the "Texas Lawyel Lege of Liberty" also wrote to the federal office of the Bureau in support of the agent Evans and against Donalson. The group of ex-slaves wrote that they were "glad to find that we have frinds in Washington." As to the conflict between Donalson and Evans, they said, "We will in shure you that it is not so for we is as well aquainted with our Agent as John Donalson. . . . Mr John Donalson we are well acquainted with him and do not wish to injure him but it is not strange to us that you has such a report given from the hand of him . . . for he is a pest. . . . He passes as a quack Doctor and we are sure his complainte is for his self." The Texas Lege of Liberty seemed ready to embrace the Bureau and a new, modern kind of medical practice. Their campaign was for new "mineral" medicine, overseen and advocated by the Bureau and white doctors instead of the herbal, essentialist medical structure that Donalson represented.[18]

Donalson may well have been owed thirty-five dollars by various freed people in Austin, as he claimed. Indeed, even the local agents who testified repeatedly to his mental instability and irrational medical methodology did admit that he had been "practicing medicine" and that he was regarded as a healer by freed people who were less advanced and modern than those in the Texas Lege of Liberty. His patients, though "superstitious" and backward, in contrast to the "better class" of citizens who had signed the petition, did in fact procure his services to cure illness of body and mind, whether the Bureau called such services "medical" or not. Donalson's patients sought him out after freedom to perform the same medical services he had provided under slavery. However, they quickly realized that with freedom came a different level of scrutiny and regulation of the medical marketplace by the government in the form of the Freedmen's Bureau, and that as a result they would not have to pay for the services they had received. As is clear from the correspondence, the Bureau, though trying to enforce contracts and payments in some areas of the society and economy, did not attempt to force freed people to pay for medical services they thought should be abandoned along with other benighted views that pervaded slave culture. One agent wrote of Donalson, "If he was able to conjure diseases out of his patients bodies, he ought to be able also to conjure his fees out their pockets, without the interference of the Bureau."[19]

In contrast to the Washington Bureau's simply sending Donalson's initial letter back to the agents in Austin for comment, the Freedmen's Bureau acted promptly on Moses Camplin's petition.

Shortly after writing his letter to the Freedmen's Bureau office, Camplin received good news in the form of General Order No. 1, issued by Major General R. K. Scott. Included in the General Order were the words, "Moses G. Camplin (Colored) will be permitted to practice medicine in this State, and to grant Certificates of Death of Patients."[20] The Freedmen's Bureau had been quick to recognize that Camplin was a qualified physician and to exert its authority over local officials in the defeated Confederate city. In Charleston, however, the white municipal authorities receiving this order were not content to leave the matter there. Rather, two weeks later the mayor of Charleston, Peter C. Gaillard, wrote to Scott's superior, objecting to Scott's order and explaining his reasons why Camplin should not be allowed to sign death certificates and thus practice medicine with city sanction. He acknowledged freely that Camplin was "well known in Charleston, having served many years in the office of one of our most respectable Physicians, in putting up prescriptions, and may be fully capable to prescribe, but has neither license nor diploma.... His certificate of death can not under our laws warrant burial any more than that of any other unprofessional man." Gaillard contended that it was not Camplin's "caste or color" that barred him from government-sanctioned medical practice but his lack of a diploma. He claimed that there was in fact one African American physician who had a diploma and to whom death certificates were freely given. Gaillard declined to identify this educated and regulated black physician by name and did not address the fact that no medical school in the state would accept Camplin as a student. If this black physician in fact existed, which is somewhat doubtful, he must have obtained his medical degree abroad, because by this time no American medical school had knowingly graduated a black doctor.[21]

Camplin's case gave Gaillard the opportunity to pursue a number of political and social projects at once. The first, and the one about which he was most straightforward, concerns the conflict between municipal and federal authority. Gaillard's language was quite explicit on this point as he protested "against the setting aside by military orders of an Ordinance of the City, the aim and object of which is the general good." Second, his objections on this legalistic point, along with his evocation of the possibly imaginary educated black doctor in Charleston, allowed him to claim that the central issue was one not of race but of public health and safety. The aim of the Charleston law, he wrote, was to "throw a shield of protection over the lives and persons of the whole community." Furthermore, he wrote, to "sustain the order of Genl Scott is to virtually remove this shield." Gaillard's tactic, to bar Camplin on grounds that were nominally other than race, foreshadows the tactics of the Jim Crow era, where poll taxes and literacy tests effectively barred African Americans from political participation without mentioning race.

Just as Camplin had anticipated Gaillard's tactics and attempted to enroll in a medical college, he likewise had anticipated the claim that he was barred from practice only because of his lack of formal medical education. In his initial letter to the Freedmen's Bureau, Camplin identified racism as the sole impetus behind Gaillard's actions. He named a specific white physician, Dr. Smythe, who practiced medicine in Charleston without a diploma.

No further correspondence between the Freedmen's Bureau and either Moses Camplin or Peter Gaillard is present in the archives, but other bits of information in the historical record give hints about the subsequent lives of Camplin and Donalson.

Neither man completely faded from the historical record after their efforts to establish themselves and their freedom in the 1860s. Their lives and records show that the entangled projects of freedom and medical professional identity were lifelong endeavors. After the flurry of letters to Washington about John Donalson's controversial practice, his public record is sparse but suggestive. He continued to clash with white authorities in Austin and was arrested for disturbing the peace in the spring of 1877. It is unclear whether he was ever able to make a postwar living from medicine. On the neatly written, close-ruled page of the 1880 census record, the letters "Dr," for "doctor," are written in above "John Donalson," actually crowding the name on the line above. His occupation is listed in a separate column as "laborer," possibly because the census taker ignored his medical practice. Given Donalson's attachment to his identity as a doctor fifteen years previous, he may well have insisted on this alteration in the census record, whether or not he was currently practicing medicine. In any case, he was able to eke out a small victory in the insertion of the title "Dr" in front of his name.[22]

Moses Camplin appears to have been able to continue his medical practice in spite of the controversy over death certificates. Either the Bureau ignored the mayor's letter and he was allowed to fill out death certificates, or he found a way around this predicament. When, serving in 1868 as president of the W. D. Middleton Class Union Society, he opened a bank account for the organization stipulating that the monies were for the "Charitable use of its own members," he listed his occupation as "physician" on the bank form.

Although no documents reveal why Camplin was able to continue to practice medicine whereas Donalson apparently was not, it is possible to see why the Freedmen's Bureau would have been willing to stand behind Camplin but not Donalson. Fortunately for Camplin, in terms of the tides of change sweeping the field of medicine during this period, he was well positioned to obtain the support of the federal government at the time of his petition. Although he had no diploma from a medical college, he had been trained by an eminent physician, surgeon, and researcher in the allopathic medicine favored by the federal government. On the other hand, Donalson had the deck stacked against him when he asked the federal government to support his efforts to continue in his practice of herbal medicine. Even discounting the racist attitudes of the local Bureau agents in Austin, the Freedmen's Bureau strove to offer modern, scientific medicine to the freedmen, and Donalson had little chance of changing their minds.

CONCLUSION

During these years, the entire medical profession was in a period of conflict and uproar over regulations and definitions about which types of doctors were bona fide physicians and which were quacks. The challenges that Donalson and Camplin faced show how changes in understandings of freedom and race, along with simultaneous turmoil in the field of medicine, shaped the ways in which black doctors were able to function as physicians. Despite the different outcomes of their appeals to the Freedmen's Bureau in Washington, however, their situations were similar in two important ways.

First, in the face of prevailing racial codes, the demands both men put to the Freedmen's Bureau show how relationships with the government were crucial to black doctors' ability to practice. Donalson and Camplin were particularly striking in their assertions that federal authority must and should take precedence over state or municipal government, and even over the local office of a federal agency. When Donalson's dealings with local Freedmen's Bureau agents went sour, he appealed to their superiors at the national level. Donalson's hope that the national-level Bureau would aid him in collecting unpaid debts owed by freedmen does seem naive, but it also demonstrates his apparent feeling of membership and investment in the U.S. government.

In his first year as a free man, Moses Camplin argued that to allow the law of a state or city to override federal authority was to relinquish the possibility of African Americans living as free citizens and professionals in the postwar South. Furthermore, he recognized the particular threat that black professionals posed to the white southern ideology. Far removed from agricultural and domestic labor, black physicians, particularly ones like him whose training was on a par with that of their white counterparts, by their very existence challenged and refuted a central tenet of proslavery thought: that African Americans were unable to grasp intellectual ideas such as those of biomedical science and were implicitly unable to comport themselves with the dispassionate composure required of professionals.

A second similarity between the situation of Donalson and that of Camplin concerns the end of slavery. A consideration of the medical licensing issue reveals the ironies and complexities involved in the relationship between slavery, freedom, and professional labor. Slavery robbed Camplin and probably Donalson of rights to their person and of wages for their labor and exposed them to sale and physical abuse. At the same time, the system of slavery did in a sense protect and shield their medical practices from the gaze and regulatory function of white-controlled government. Donalson, who presumably had charged fees for his medical services prior to 1866, remained unmolested by white authorities as long as his activities were confined within the underground economy of slave society. As long as Camplin was Ogier's "servant," his medical activities fell under the rubric of slave labor performed for his master, whether Camplin was driving the doctor's carriage, mixing prescriptions, or performing surgery. Slavery had masked the medical activities of both men, shielding them from white public jurisdiction before emancipation. During the years of early emancipation, before uniform licensing and regulation of physicians was instituted, Donalson found that by refusing to support his bill-collecting efforts, local Bureau agents in Austin could exclude his practice from the medical marketplace available in 1866 to Austin's African Americans. Camplin's experience reveals how Charleston city authorities, though lacking uniform criteria for medical education, did in fact license doctors by granting or withholding death certificates.

Despite these similarities and the centrality of racism to their professional struggles, the appeals to the Bureau by the two men met very different fates. The fact that Moses Camplin did succeed in building a career in medicine whereas John Donalson apparently did not may be owed in large part to the fact that the particular brand of medicine Camplin's master practiced was the brand favored by the government as a standard for the whole nation. The federal government, acting on its bias favoring "modern" medicine, intervened immediately on Camplin's behalf but referred Donalson's case back to the local agents in Austin—his adversaries.

Donalson and Camplin's experiences foreshadow a number of developments of the late nineteenth and twentieth centuries. Donalson's encounter with racist epithets spouted by agents of the federal government was echoed in the racial prejudice that raised barriers for aspiring medical professionals not only in the former Confederacy but in the North. The figure of the "African Conjurer" and the quack doctor plying his wares among the ignorant and superstitious plagued African American communities well into the twentieth century. Indeed, an uneducated and ignorant "doctor" doing more harm than good was a standard comic trope in minstrel shows and caricatures of African Americans. Donalson's failure to convince any white authorities of the validity of his herbal medicine crystallized alternative medicine's fall from respectability in the late nineteenth century. African American traditional healers, nurses, and midwives were left by the wayside in terms of professional status. Although herbal medicines and spiritualism would continue to be options available to American consumers, never again would those practitioners be able to claim parity with allopathic physicians in terms of state recognition.

Neither racism nor changes in medical practice can be called the single force that held African Americans back in their pursuit of medical careers after the Civil War. Rather, the two worked in tandem to narrow the path toward a medical career. Even for black doctors who, like Camplin, would probably have rejected herbal medicine, the path to recognition and respect from the dominant medical authorities was littered with obstacles during this period. As Camplin's experience made clear, the mark of slavery and presumed racial inferiority could trump twenty years of training under an eminent white doctor. As the nineteenth century waned, racially restrictive professional and graduate schools on one hand and nominally race-blind regulation on the other increasingly hemmed in aspiring black professionals. Throughout the first half of the twentieth century, African Americans who, like Camplin, sought medical training, particularly in fields such as surgery, found their paths blocked by admission policies at medical schools and by rules barring them from residencies at well-resourced white hospitals.

It is a piece of archival good luck that we have been able to examine these two men together. Finding one without the other might have denied us the opportunity to explore how various intellectual currents, in this case beliefs about medicine, influenced the ways in which white authorities understood and responded to racial difference. Their cases are not parallel and reveal different facets of the relationship between racial hierarchies and struggles over medical practice. Camplin's initial exclusion by local authorities and his subsequent victory at the hands of General Order No. 1 from the Freedmen's Bureau could be read as straightforward evidence of the Bureau's commitment to promoting African American men in their quest for professionalism. The Donalson case, in which the agents of the local and national Freedmen's Bureau disparaged him, reveals not only racism but also their powerful commitment to promoting one kind of medicine over another. The two men were united by race, by their faith that federal officials in Washington would right the wrongs inflicted on them, and by their memories and experiences during slavery. By 1866 and continuing to the end of their lives, however, their understandings of health, illness, and treatment formed a divide between them that allowed Camplin to practice medicine and relegated Donalson's professional identity to the margins of a census form.

Taken together, the letters by and about Camplin and Donalson remind us that African American participation in modern medical culture had roots both in legacies of slavery and in debates over appropriate practitioners in the mid-nineteenth century.

NOTES

Many thanks to Patricia Long for her tireless help and to Leslie Rowland, of the University of Maryland, for drawing my attention to these documents.

1 For more on the organization, limited success, and widespread failure of the Freedmen's Bureau's medical division, see Jim Downs, *Sick from Freedom: African American Illness and Suffering during the Civil War and Reconstruction* (New York: Oxford University Press, 2012).

2 "Dr. John Donalson to Gen Howard, Gen Gregry [*sic*], and Gen Kiddoo, 14 Dec. 1866," filed as "[D-105] 1866, Letters Received, ser. 15, Washington Hdqrs., RG 105" (see [A-3209]). Donalson's letter acknowledges receipt of a letter, dated September 12, 1866, from the three generals on December 13, 1866. This group, [A-3209], also includes earlier related letters and "endorsements"—notes written on the letters by the receiving clerk or another person—about related correspondence to the Endorsement of Capt. A. Evans, July 16, 1866, on a letter from Capt. A. Evans to Bvt. Col. Wm. H. Sinclair, July 16, 1866; Endorsement from Captain Bryon Porter (Freedmen's Bureau subassistant commissioner in Austin) from October 30, 1866; a letter from Capt. A. Evans to Bvt. Maj. Genrl. Kiddoo, July 30, 1866, filed as "[D-86] 1866, Letters Received, ser. 15, Washington Hdqrs., RG 105"; and a letter from A. Evans to Wm. C. Sinclaer, July 11, 1866. In [A-3275] are a letter from Mary Tomus and other freedmen to General Howard, July 26, 1866, and a letter from O. E. Pratt, Lieut. Col. and Lieut. Asst. Com. to Bvt. Col. Hmy. Sinclair (no date). Freedmen and Southern Society Project, University of Maryland, College Park. Bracketed numbers refer to the indexing system at the archive.

3 Sharla Fett, *Working Cures: Healing, Health, and Power on Southern Slave Plantations* (Chapel Hill: University of North Carolina Press, 2002), 15–20. One prominent slave owner expressing a preference for alternative medicine was James Henry Hammond, governor of South Carolina, who in 1840 directed his overseers that only homeopathy would be used on his plantation. After the war, however, allopathic medicine became almost exclusively the standard among white elites. See Gretchen Long, *Doctoring Freedom: The Politics of African American Medical Care in Slavery and Emancipation* (Chapel Hill: University of North Carolina Press, 2012), 29–30.

4 Randolph B. Campbell, *An Empire for Slavery: The Peculiar Institution in Texas, 1821–1865* (Baton Rouge: Louisiana State University Press, 1989), 58–60.

5 Pekka Hamalainen, *Comanche Empire,* The Lamar Series in Western History (New Haven, Conn.: Yale University Press, 2008), 305.

6 David Dary, *Frontier Medicine: From the Atlantic to the Pacific 1492–1941* (New York: Knopf, 2008), 13–17.

7 "Dr. John Donalson to Gen Howard, Gen Gregry [sic] and Gen Kiddoo, 14 Dec. 1866," [A-3209], Freedmen and Southern Society Project.

8 Downs, Sick from Freedom, 78–87.

9 John Duffy, From Humors to Medical Science, 2nd ed. (Urbana: University of Illinois Press, 1993), 150.

10 Frank A. Rollin, Life and Public Services of Martin R. Delaney, Sub-Assistant Commissioner, Bureau Relief of Refugees, Freedmen, and of Abandoned Lands, and the Late Major 104th U.S. Colored Troops (Boston: Lee and Shepard, 1868), 196–97.

11 "Moses G. Camplin to Brevet Maj. Gen'l, R. K. Scott 19 July 1866," [A-7054], Unregistered Letters Received, ser. 2923, South Carolina Assistant Commissioner, RG 107, [A-7054], Freedmen and Southern Society Project.

12 "Schedule 2: Slave Inhabitants in the District of Charleston, 14 June 1860," ancestry.com.

13 "Schedule 1: Free Inhabitants of the District of Charleston, June 1860," ancestry.com.

14 See, for example, T. L. Ogier, "Case of Induration and Enlargement of the Body of the Penis, with a New Method of Amputating That Organ," American Journal of the Medical Sciences (1836): 382–86; Ogier, "Hereditary Predisposition," Charleston Medical Journal Review 3 (1848); and Joseph I. Waring, "Charleston Medicine 1800–1860," Journal of the History of Medicine and Allied Sciences 31, no. 3 (1976): 336, footnote 47. For Ogier's military appointment, see Journal of the Senate of South Carolina: Being the Session of 1862. Electronic edition. South Carolina. General Assembly. Senate funding from the Institute of Museum and Library Services supported the electronic publication (http://docsouth.unc.edu).

15 "Moses G. Camplin to Brevet Maj. Gen'l R. K. Scott 19 July 1866," [A-7054], Freedmen and Southern Society Project.

16 Ibid.

17 Evans and Porter each wrote an endorsement on a summary of a letter from Donalson dated June 12, 1866. A. Evans, July 16, 1866 endorsement; Captain Bryon Porter, Sub Asst. Commr. endorsement Oct. 30, 1866 on letter from John Donalson of June 12, 1866, [A-3209], Freedmen and Southern Society Project.

18 "Mary Tomus and other freedmen to General Howard 26 July 1866," [M-94], [A-3275], Freedmen and Southern Society Project. In his letter of December 14, 1866, Donalson claimed that Evans bribed the members of the Lege to subscribe to the letter condemning Donalson's medical treatments.

19 Bryon Porter (Freedmen's Bureau subassistant commissioner in Austin), October 30, 1866 endorsement on summary of letter from John Donalson of June 12, 1866, [A-3209], Freedmen and Southern Society Project.

20 "Br. Maj Gen R. K. Scott to all whom it may Concern, 22 May 1866, vol.

11, p. 122, Letters Sent, ser. 2916, SC Asst. Comr. RG 105," [A-7054], Freedmen and Southern Society Project.

21   "Mayor P. C. Gaillard to Major General D. E. Sickles, 6 June 1866, and endorsements," filed as "[S-356], Letters Received, ser. 15, Washington Hdqrs. RG," [A-7054], Freedmen and Southern Society Project.

22   Arrest record, 1877, Austin History Center, Austin Public Library, Austin, Texas; U.S. Bureau of the Census, "Schedule 1: Inhabitants in the 1st Ward City of Austin, 3 June 1880, 6," ancestry.com. My own father's birth certificate from 1931 in Little Rock, Arkansas lists the occupation of his father, an African American college-educated, ordained Baptist minister, as "laborer." Donalson may have been listed as "laborer" almost automatically. Jerome Herbert Long birth certificate, in author's possession.

4

At the Nation's Edge

African American Migrants and Smallpox in the Late-Nineteenth-Century Mexican–American Borderlands

JOHN MCKIERNAN-GONZÁLEZ

ON JULY 23, 1895, secretary of state Edwin Uhl received a telegram from Torreon, Coahuila, stating that "one-hundred and fifty three negroes from [Tlahualilo] colony are here destitute. Surrounded by Mexican police to prevent them from entering town. Wire what to do. All are American citizens."[1] Secretary Uhl told the consul in Torreon to wait. Two days later, Uhl read a report that the group of "negroes [were] starving and almost in open rebellion to all authority. . . . I anticipate serious trouble."[2] Apparently, John McCaughan, a regionally prominent landowner, mine manager, and U.S. consul, had told the group of African Americans that they "must not be choice about the kind of work, nor particular as the amount of pay. They should scatter as much as possible. It will be impossible to find employment together, and by remaining in a body they only make it more difficult for aid and employment."[3]

McCaughan's prediction was wrong. By refusing to move as a body and continuing to articulate their collective demands, the migrants in Torreon catalyzed an executive branch decision on their behalf. On July 26, 1895 president Grover Cleveland ended the standoff: "War department will issue rations for one week. . . . If return to the colony is not practicable or consistent with humane considerations, let the consuls assure the railroad company that payment for the transportation of the sufferers to their homes will be strongly recommended."[4] The U.S. government now vouched for the costs of the railroad trip home to Alabama; however, the migrants had to find ways to guarantee food and shelter for their trip back home to Alabama.

This labor rebellion in northern Durango—led by black migrant families originally from Alabama, working on a cotton plantation in northern Mexico in 1895—forced the United States to go into Mexico and intervene on behalf of American citizens. The State Department seized on the presence of smallpox among the families to transform the politically volatile conflict between black American citizens and the powerful Compañía Agricola Tlahualilo into an American medical mission to protect American refugees from Mexico. Most histories of the Tlahualilo migration end their analysis of the migrants' situation with the declaration of a smallpox quarantine in Eagle Pass, Texas.[5] This chapter goes against the general grain of scholarship on race and medicine in the Progressive Era and argues that, in addition to treating labor migrants as medical threats, the medical mission and the subsequent U.S. Marine Hospital Service (USMHS) smallpox serum field trial strengthened the collective negotiating position of the migrants.

This chapter examines how black southerners in Mexico found their newfound status as the objects of an American medical mission useful to their demands to return home to Alabama. Moreover, they leveraged their status as objects of a federal smallpox serum field trial to guarantee their return against the wishes of white southern political authorities. The migrants' return is a compelling story of African American workers exploiting their role as commodities in an emerging laboratory-based American research economy, just as federal health officers exploited the migrants' high-profile illness while also laboring on behalf of the migrants' survival.

The 153-person collective in Torreon was part of a larger group of one hundred families (866 black men, women, and children, according to the railroad manifest) who left central Alabama in late January 1895 to work as sharecroppers in Mexico. Lured by promises given them by black emigration activist William Ellis and the Compañía Agricola Tlahualilo of racial democracy, higher shares, housing, and full rail passage to Mexico, they left Alabama by train expecting a familiar work setting in a foreign place. As diplomatic historian Fred Rippy argues, the Compañía Agricola Tlahualilo banked on the promise of skilled black southern labor, turning the migration into a "private venture conducted for the profit of a Mexican land company and a member of the Negro race." The Compañía's investors had already put a large amount of capital into building a sixty-mile-long private canal to irrigate a 17,000-acre dry lakebed and a private rail line connecting the tiny town of Mapimi with the Mexican International Railroad in Torreon.[6]

The appearance of the railroad in the iron-rich regions of the Mapimi basin led many Mexicans and foreign investors to believe the Great Mapimi Basin could become the next Mexican breadbasket. However, investors in the region's mines, farms, and plantations faced a common challenge: bringing in enough workers to match capital investment in a region that numbered maybe five thousand people in 1890.

Leaving kin and community for work outside the United States may have been a difficult decision for many of these families. However, the attraction of leaving the racial terror associated with Alabama after three years of an economic depression and two nationally infamous racially volatile gubernatorial and presidential elections is not so hard to imagine. The populist challenge to the Democratic Party in Alabama led to vitriolic and violent attacks on black and white men suspected of voting for the Populist Reuben Kolb over Democratic or Republican candidates.[7] Moreover, iron mines and steel mills in Alabama had begun to rely more heavily on the convict lease system for substantial numbers of their workers. In the aftermath of its sweeping victory in state elections in 1894, the Alabama Democratic Party moved to excise any claims black residents had on public office, public goods, public services, or public space. Because the majority of the migrants came of age during the twenty years after the Civil War, when African Americans openly voted in Alabama elections, these actions directly attacked their identities as citizens. The indifference to Alabama's political violence and coercive labor regimes must have made leaving industrializing urban Alabama for industrializing rural Mexico seem attractive.[8]

The general American indifference to recent events in Alabama made the migrants' ability to attract attention to their situation in Mexico even more striking. Migrant and coal miner Sam Claiborne set events in motion when he convinced the consul in Chihuahua that the migrants "found themselves in the worst form of bondage with [no] hope of ever securing liberty."[9] Migrant advocates presented the conditions as an issue for Americans in Mexico, a problem the American government ought to fix. Democratic president Grover Cleveland's directive to the State Department to guarantee passage to Alabama is a reminder of the success of this effort. The migrants' collective actions outside the nation's edge remind us of the importance, in historian Natalia Molina's words, of understanding how those "who are not citizens negotiate a sense of national identity, calibrating notions of citizenship and democracy in the process."[10] Although the migrants were citizens, collective actions against black southerners that preceded their decision to leave for Mexico in 1895 put the migrants on the margins of the American body politic. This is what makes their negotiations with the federal medical authority a window into the paradox of American medical citizenship: the simultaneous way sympathy and exclusion organize access to health care in the United States. Rather than focus on the dynamics of exclusion, the interpretation here argues that Camp Jenner was more a case of sympathy and exploitation, a twist on Beatrix Hoffman's succinct analysis of immigration and health care policy.[11] This chapter argues that these black southern migrants engaged a politics of entitlement to turn an American public health commitment to medical progress into an instrument of social membership and a vehicle for their return home.[12] In the process, this chapter calls attention to the obvious dependence of American medical authority on the tacit and active cooperation of their (detained) black migrant subjects.

FROM MIGRANTS TO REFUGEES: THE JOURNEY
FROM TORREON TO EAGLE PASS

A week after the standoff in Torreon, two hundred migrants stepped out of boxcars into the border town of Piedras Negras, Coahuila. Consul Jesse Sparks walked this group across the Rio Grande into Eagle Pass, Texas. The Associated Press remarked approvingly that Grover Cleveland, "regarding the case as one of the greatest emergencies involving the lives of American citizens," had guaranteed funds and rations in Eagle Pass.[13] Texas state health officer Jack Evans inspected the first group and "found them all healthy" but still placed them in abandoned boxcars under "quarantine with guards."[14] The call to quarantine the migrants ignored the absence of illness. Two days later, 170 more migrants arrived at Eagle Pass, and this time there were eight cases of smallpox. After repeated complaints by Eagle Pass customs collector William Fitch, state authorities moved the boxcars three miles north of Eagle Pass and assigned two armed guards to detain the migrants.[15]

When Fitch informed the secretary of the Treasury that there was "smallpox among negro refugees from Mexico," these five words added medical value to the existing federal investment in these black migrants. Smallpox structured the "commodity relationship" through which the

USMHS gained value from these black diasporic subjects; the USMHS provided food, shelter, nurses, and doctors partly to guarantee stable clinical conditions among the detained migrants for their field trial. In turn, the migrants used this visible public space to force the USMHS to confront southern state authorities to allow the migrants to return home.[16]

The actual practice of this Texas quarantine challenged most theories of quarantine. Fitch reported, "There are no guards to prevent the sick and well from intermingling and intercourse between the two camps is open." Furthermore, he cautioned, "if the negroes desired to escape there would have been no difficulty in their so doing, nor would their absence have been detected unless a large number escaped." People were willing to "mingle with these negroes when they were in town." Vendors treated the quarantined workers as a market opportunity. Eagle Pass residents openly ignored state dictums regarding the medical threat posed by the detained migrants, and this exasperated the local customs collector.[17] Some exploited the detainees' vulnerable status and ransacked their possessions, even though the city stationed four guards at the clearing. USMHS surgeon George Magruder blamed the "Mexicans and lower class of whites in the vicinity" for this outrage.[18] The theft confirmed Fitch's low opinion of the Texas State Health Office: "I do not believe the State Health Officer stationed at this place has a proper conception of the importance of isolation and precautionary measures."[19] For Fitch, the quarantine provided contact zones, not boundaries, between the town and the camp, between sick and well, and between black refugees and multiracial Eagle Pass.[20]

The USMHS representative was more anxious about smallpox treatment within the Texas quarantine. Magruder expressed shock at the extent to which the detainees made their own medical decisions: "Practically no attempt was made towards nursing or furnishing medical treatment to the sick, the management of each case is left to the individual fancy of the friends or relations and the burning of sage and drinking of yarb tea and other forms of negro medication were in progress at the time of my visit."[21] The trope "negro medication" registered his concern with the relative power and autonomy of the Tlahualilo migrants. The indifference of Texas state authorities provided the space for detainees to invert the relationship between state health officer and patient. Magruder considered the "fancy of friends and relations" to be a dangerous African American takeover of state-sanctioned medical spaces. He expected state medical authorities to provide food and water, tents, buildings, shelter, blankets, certified doctors, and nurses to attend to the smallpox patients. The modern American ideal embodied and promoted by the USMHS did not include black family members making the primary health care decisions and treatments in a state quarantine.[22] For Magruder, the Texas quarantine paralleled what historian Pekka Hammalainen and Samuel Truett call key characteristics of borderlands situations: "spatial mobility, situational identity, local contingency and the ambiguities of power."[23] This world turned upside down in the boxcar quarantine justified federal intervention.

Claiming that the threatened appearance of yellow fever in Galveston demanded his full attention, Texas state health officer Swearingen informed the USMHS that Texas was abdicating responsibility for the detainees.[24] Magruder took control of the detainees. The administrative transfer permitted the transformation of people ill with smallpox into subjects of a larger attempt to cure and prevent smallpox. At this point, the detainees became part of a larger history of American medical experimentation.

A COMMUNITY OF RESEARCHERS: THE USMHS, CAMP JENNER, AND THE PROMISE OF SERUM THERAPY

In the 1890s, American clinical researchers were making dramatic progress against the threats of germ-borne illnesses. The successful 1892 campaign to confine typhus to the Lower East Side in New York gave the USMHS leverage to demand more quarantine authority over ports across the United States. This authority became unilateral when Congress passed the 1893 National Quarantine Act.[25] Moreover, New York City's successful campaign against diphtheria made it clear, in city health officer Dr. Herman Bigg's words, that "disease is a removable evil," and consequently with the proper political will, "public health is purchasable."[26] For bacteriologists in the United States, antitoxin research was a promising way to develop cures and treatment for communicable diseases. News of diseased bodies crossing a distant and politically insignificant border provided a fortuitous chance to capitalize on the expanded USMHS mandate. When the USMHS assumed "charge of the negro colonists returning from Mexico," National

Hygienic Laboratory director J. J. Kinyoun and Surgeon General Walter Wyman called this situation "an opportunity not to be lost to put the serum therapy into effect."[27] Smallpox among a large number of detained migrants became a medical opportunity to demonstrate that the USMHS was in the international vanguard of serum therapy.

Magruder brought the detainees from the quarantine into a new space he named Camp Jenner, a place where the USMHS could combine their recently established authority over America's medical borders with innovative clinically based research.[28] The USMHS moved the detained migrants to a river bluff and meadow northwest of Eagle Pass, a locale effectively isolated by a creek over which they built a bridge to control the traffic between Camp Jenner and Eagle Pass.[29] USMHS staff separated men from women and children. Instead of one central camp, the USMHS built four smaller detention camps in the compound and assigned each colonist to one after thorough disinfection of their persons and their blankets. The USMHS increased rations, brought 140 tents from Waynesville, Georgia, and placed twenty armed guards around these camps. A two-hundred-bed tent hospital and a fourteen by twenty foot commissary addressed the immediate food and medical needs of the detainees. Nineteen additional people oversaw the detainees and maintained daily roll calls. Healthy people and smallpox survivors stayed in the camps, and those under treatment moved to the field hospital in Camp Jenner. The USMHS enhanced the material conditions and eliminated the general mobility of the Tlahualilo migrants, in return for their compliance as research subjects.

Until the post–World War II period, many doctors considered charity medical situations a reciprocal exchange between people needing medical services and doctors needing research opportunities.[30] But this exchange was also open to debate, for nineteenth-century doctors as distinguished as Sir William Osler considered clinical opportunities to have the potential to tear "the sacred cord binding doctor and patient."[31] Camp Jenner thus became a place where research principles challenged the imperative to help heal the sick. The detained migrants cooperated with the USMHS at the border because of their displacement, coerced detention, and hunger.[32] For the USMHS, the dependent status of the detainees opened up clinical research possibilities into a high-profile illness while proving the agency's ability to intervene in emergency epidemic situations to protect the nation's health. Although Magruder deplored the medical ambiguities of the Texas quarantine, the double status of Camp Jenner as a smallpox field trial and refugee camp with medical facilities undercut the research process and accepted medical principles.

In late February 1895, Kinyoun actively started applying diphtheria antitoxin methods to smallpox. Kinyoun and the USMHS wanted to demonstrate the general principle that serum application could induce a state of immunity. Kinyoun argued that USMHS Surgeon General George Miller Sternberg's observation that "the blood serum of an immune animal destroys the potency of vaccine lymph" meant that "[the filtered blood serum of an immune animal] could be used in the treatment of smallpox." Kinyoun and Sternberg believed the diphtheria model could work with other communicable diseases such as typhus and yellow fever.[33] In the introduction to his 1895 monograph on immunology, Sternberg made the following argument for smallpox serotherapy: "We infer that the blood and tissue juices of an individual who has recently suffered an attack of smallpox or scarlet fever contains an antitoxin which would neutralize the active poison of the disease in the circulation of another person immediately after infection. [This] can only be decided by experiment; but the experiment seems to me a legitimate one." The reasoning in this passage was important. Sternberg was confident that smallpox antitoxin could be obtained from vaccinated calves. The "practical application of bacteriological research" meant injecting smallpox antitoxin serum into human bodies as soon as possible.[34]

On his return from Germany, Kinyoun transferred diphtheria antitoxin production methods to smallpox.[35] Kinyoun told the public that "his special study of Roux's methods for the treatment of diphtheria by serum injection" was "one of the great discoveries in medicine, and has passed through the experimental stage and laid a new foundation for preventive medicine."[36] Kinyoun was hard at work establishing the same protocols for smallpox.[37] Public hospitals in New York City provided the first human trial of smallpox antitoxin therapy. Kinyoun prepared filtered smallpox serum in New York's vaccine farm on December 23, 1894.[38] Dr. Elliot, director of the New York City smallpox hospital, identified two "well developed" African American twenty-something male patients "with strong constitutions" in the early stages of the disease and injected fifteen milliliters of the serum into them.[39] The four-serum injection had no effect on one patient's bleeding, high fevers, pulse, respiration rate, or retention of water. The second patient survived but made his anger at the seven injections of vaccinated calf serum clear to Dr. Elliot.[40] The *New York Times* editorial board commented on the results, opining "that it was unwise to assume anything based on the improvement in one case" but expressed optimism for the potential of an "antitoxic serum which will reduce the severity of the disease at the early stages, and lower the mortality percentage for those who have failed to protect themselves by vaccination."[41] After a field trial in the Brooklyn Children's Hospital indicated a quicker recovery period among these children than other nonvaccinated people, Kinyoun knew he needed a larger field trial.[42]

The presence of smallpox among the Eagle Pass detainees sparked Wyman and Kinyoun's interest. They ordered rising young star Dr. Milton Rosenau, assistant director of the National Hygienic Laboratory, to Eagle Pass "with instructions to institute the treatment in a sufficient number of cases."[43] The promise of the antitoxin therapy gave Rosenau's trip west a heroic dimension. The *Houston Post* reported, "It is intimated that, aside from his going to supervise the sanitary precautions rendered necessary by the presence of a great number of refugees bound for Alabama from Mexico, Dr. Rosenau is especially designated to conduct scientific experiments in a new process of inoculating the smallpox virus."[44] Observers believed Rosenau was saving the migrants for science and for the welfare of the nation.

These national hopes for the medical experiment in vaccination complicated the relationship between the migrants and the USMHS. As the migrants fell under the control of the USMHS, antitoxin research transformed them from medical detainees to research subjects. Rosenau's arrival in Eagle Pass meant the end of open quarantine boundaries, commercial exchange between detained migrants and local residents, and, in general, migrant autonomy in the camps. Rosenau reported, "Discipline as strict as the circumstances seemed to demand was inaugurated; system and order soon followed the chaotic conditions which had prevailed."[45] Newspapers reported that Kinyoun was "manufacturing anti-toxine [*sic*] for diphtheria," and his partner Rosenau was "hard at work attending the negro colonists returning from Mexico."[46] The press made it clear that smallpox antitoxin was going to be part of the migrants' lives, grimly touching on the importance of black bodies to American clinical research efforts. Despite their previous defiance of the politically connected Compañía Tlahualilo and their skillful negotiations with the American State Department, the migrants' voices disappeared from the public record just as their bodies' actions grew increasingly well documented.

As a doctor with the USMHS, Rosenau had two working principles. The first was to treat people with smallpox to the best of his ability. The second was to test the smallpox antitoxin under field conditions. Camp Jenner was a field trial of the efficacy of serum vaccination before smallpox infection and, in a few cases, serum therapy after the onset of smallpox. In his report, Rosenau compared the clinical course of smallpox in people who received what he called a vaccination—that is, the smallpox serum antitoxin—to the course of smallpox among people denied a vaccination by authorities who under every other circumstance believed in vaccination.

The results of the field trial were very clear. The serum did not cure or prevent smallpox. There were 154 cases of smallpox in the camp. The USMHS treated 138 detainees from onset to recovery or death, 78 of whom survived discrete cases of smallpox, 35 of whom survived severe (or confluent) smallpox, and 25 of whom died. Doctors diagnose discrete cases when the pus blisters (pox) stay separate from each other; doctors diagnose confluent cases when the pox blisters expand into each other, creating wide and painful internal and external swaths of bleeding blisters. Both discrete and congruent cases of smallpox can be fatal; however, a person with discrete variola has a greater chance of survival.

A second list, "fatal cases by vaccination status," indicated that the serum field trial also meant observing the effects of unprevented and untreated smallpox infections on detained black migrants. Rosenau noted that the USMHS did not vaccinate fifty-five of the people they treated for smallpox. The USMHS did vaccinate approximately fifty different people before the onset of their smallpox. Moreover, some people received USMHS vaccinations after the onset of their infections. Most astoundingly, the USMHS "successfully vaccinated" fifty-five people who subsequently came down with smallpox. Ten of these "successfully vaccinated" people died of smallpox. In medical terms, a "successful" vaccination meant that the antitoxin provoked an immune response that looked similar to that of smallpox vaccination. The fifty-five cases of smallpox demonstrated that the immune response to the smallpox serum seemed to have little to do with smallpox infection. A successful

TABLE 4.1. Cases of smallpox, sorted by type (discrete, confluent, and fatal) and patient age, under U.S. Marine Hospital Service care at Camp Jenner

Patient Age	Number of Smallpox Cases			
	Discrete	Confluent	Fatal	Total
Under 10 years	30	2	3	35
Between 10 and 20 years	20	15	9	44
Between 20 and 30 years	18	13	6	37
Between 30 and 40 years	6	1	2	9
Over 40 years	4	4	5	13
Total	78	35	25	138

Note. In a discrete case of smallpox, the small and painful pus blisters (small pox) are independent. In a confluent case, the small blisters breach the tissue separating them, leading to severe internal and external bleeding. Both types can be fatal. Data from Milton Rosenau, "Report on the Camp Jenner Epidemic, Eagle Pass, Texas," *Annual Report of the Supervising Surgeon General* (Washington, D.C.: Government Printing Office, 1895), 234.

Vaccination Status	Number
Total cases with childhood vaccination	5
Total unvaccinated cases	21
Total successful vaccinations, take recorded	10
Total unsuccessful vaccinations No immune response to serum No immunity to smallpox	8
Total vaccinations, no take recorded No immune response to serum	9
Total	53

FIGURE 4.1. Fatal smallpox cases by vaccination status, Camp Jenner, 1895. From Milton Rosenau, "Report on the Camp Jenner Epidemic, Eagle Pass, Texas," in *Annual Report of the Supervising Surgeon General* (Washington, D.C.: Government Printing Office, 1895), 234.

vaccination take (a familiar immune response to the antitoxin serum) provided no guarantee against smallpox.

The list of fatal smallpox cases by vaccination status indicates a desire by Rosenau to compare the impact of smallpox serum vaccination with conventional smallpox therapy, because twenty-seven people received vaccinations and twenty-six people did not. Rosenau noted eight deaths among the people who did not show an immune response to the vaccination serum and ten among the people who did show an immune response to the USMHS vaccination. This did not prove that the successful serum vaccination mitigated the course of illness. However, Rosenau and Magruder believed that the smallpox serum could mitigate more severe cases of smallpox. Thus, they may have treated more severe cases among the detainees with whatever means they had available. Moreover, the vaccinated detainees were slightly older than the cohort average. The average age of the people who came down with smallpox in Camp Jenner was 20. The average age of people vaccinated against smallpox in Camp Jenner was 22.65, and the average age of people not vaccinated against smallpox in Camp Jenner was 16.5. Perceptions of the severity of the disease and the age of the patient with smallpox tilted Rosenau and Magruder's decision to use the serum. Rosenau clearly established some controls, but the controls did not rise to the double-blind ideal currently held for clinical trials.[47]

Did Rosenau use the severity of smallpox as the key calculus for use of the serum? This is impossible to know, because Rosenau probably would have been unable to predict who would come down with smallpox after receiving a vaccination. Instead, Rosenau held the black victims of smallpox and the Tlahualilo Company responsible for the serum's failure to mitigate the horrors of smallpox infection: "Smallpox is supposed to be a more fatal disease in the Negro. The epidemic had favorable soil on which to work on, viz: a number of pure-blooded, unvaccinated negroes with vitality depressed from bad and insufficient food, and exhausted from traveling on crowded freight cars."[48] Given that all the migrants shared the same miserable conditions in Tlahualilo and Eagle Pass, the claim that African Americans were more vulnerable to smallpox could not explain why some African Americans in Camp Jenner were able to survive their bout of smallpox. Nonetheless, Rosenau used full-throated racial metaphors to account for the divergence between the ambiguous clinical results in New York's Smallpox

Hospital and his dispiriting clinical observations in Camp Jenner. Camp Jenner marked the failure of the USMHS's smallpox antitoxin research endeavor. There was no double-blind clinical study or equal treatment of every patient in camp. The research at Camp Jenner did not result in the USMHS's conquest of smallpox. Instead, the Camp Jenner field trial and quarantine reflected mixed motives: to treat smallpox among American citizens, to contain smallpox among a large (racialized, stigmatized) population, and to test the smallpox antitoxin among a large cohort of people. Unsurprisingly, muddy medical intentions led to mixed outcomes. Camp Jenner ended up being a place where the USMHS kept American citizens "cooped up" until the State Department found a way to get the migrants back as a group to central Alabama.[49] In the fullest historical discussion of the camps in Eagle Pass, Karl Jacoby remarked that "Texas authorities responded to the potential passage of these sick migrants across their territory with what was to become an increasingly common tactic: recasting the U.S.–Mexico border as a medical boundary." Smallpox and quarantine mark the endpoint of inquiry rather than an opportunity to peer behind the medical terms of belonging in the United States.[50] As scholars shift to examine the tangled place of U.S. minorities in America's medical histories, the surprising actions by African American migrants while at the nation's edge make Camp Jenner a particularly fruitful place to emphasize contingency and complexity. For the migrants, Camp Jenner became the ground where they negotiated the conditions of their return to Alabama.

REFUGEES, DETAINEES, AND COLONISTS: MIGRANTS REWORK THE BOUNDARIES OF CITIZENSHIP

Leaving Camp Jenner was an endeavor in collective negotiation. The migrants refused to leave as individuals. The mayor of Birmingham and the governor of Alabama worked to prevent their return to their home state. The USMHS stopped funding the camp in mid-October. Rosenau left the detainees in the hands of USMHS surgeon Magruder, Texas state health officer Jack Evans, and the people in Eagle Pass, and he left on the Southern Pacific Railroad to help with bubonic plague in San Francisco. The majority of migrants stayed in Camp Jenner nearly a month and a half after Rosenau treated the last case of smallpox. Although that might have been their choice, every major city between Eagle Pass and Birmingham banned the entrance of the detained migrants, regardless of whether they had medical certification.[51] The perception that the migrants posed a medical threat to the New South overrode the USMHS guarantee that the detainees were free of smallpox. These decisions frustrated the State Department. As Sparks stated about Birmingham, "Every one of these negroes has a clean bill of health signed by Dr Magruder. No one permitted to get on the train without it. The action of this mayor is certainly arbitrary."[52] Despite these delays, Eagle Pass residents and the USMHS allowed the migrants to stay in Camp Jenner until the Southern Pacific Railroad could guarantee their trip home.

Concern with the condition of the migrants in Camp Jenner preceded Rosenau's departure; however, the migrants' situation in the camp provoked different forms of sympathy. In Eagle Pass, the county commissioners and the town agreed to continue feeding and clothing the migrants in the camps. The migrants' situation at the border had already struck a sense of sympathy and solidarity among African Americans in Texas. The *Houston Post* reported that President Abner of the Colored Baptist Association discussed "the condition of the colored people in Mexico. The president talked on the subject of these negroes abroad for about an hour, and their bad condition in Mexico."[53] According to a *Post* reporter in Luling, Texas, "The negroes all over this region are giving suppers and by other means raising money for the negro colonists quarantined at Eagle Pass."[54] Two months later, the *Post*'s coverage of the Foreign Mission of the Colored Baptists emphasized their successes in clothing and feeding the migrants, recognized support in Eagle Pass for the migrants' situation, and requested funds for food and winter clothing.[55] There seemed to be a subterranean thread of support for the migrants across black and some white communities in Texas.

The relative invisibility of individual white donations in the news coverage irked some in Texas's black communities. L. L. Campbell, editor of the black newspaper *Austin Herald*, penned a bristly response to calls by the Austin *Statesman* for black funds for the detainees in Camp Jenner: "Now do you mean to say that the Negroes are the only people who should be interested in this matter? It should concern every citizen. Let white men take steps to help these people. I am reliably told that white men led them there."[56] Campbell emphasized the shared American responsibility for the migrants' plight in Eagle Pass.

Other Americans openly rejected any shared connections with the

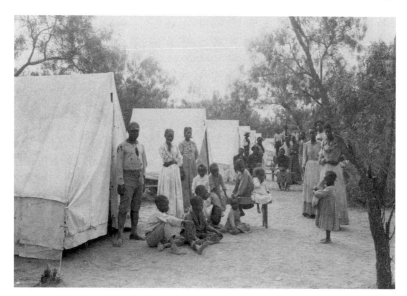

FIGURE 4.2. One of the designated tent compounds in Camp Jenner, 1895. From J. D. Whelpley, "Failure of Negro Colonization in Mexico," *Frank Leslie's Weekly*, October 31, 1895, p. 286. Collection no. 4289, M. J. Rosenau Papers, Southern Historical Collection, Wilson Library, University of North Carolina at Chapel Hill.

experiences of the migrants in Texas. The *San Antonio Express* editorial board argued that the migrants' inability to achieve settler status in Mexico justified American intervention, for "even though the colonists forfeited their citizenship by leaving the United States to settle in Mexico, the burden of American responsibility should be extended to rescue the colonists of Tlahualilo from their attempt to establish an independent existence."[57] In this vision of an American political community, it was the responsibility of federal authorities to free the freedmen and their adult children of their delusions of independence and self-ownership. This was an expression of sympathy for the migrants, as long as they accepted their position at the margins of American society. Many used their editorial space to reject potential attempts to express sympathy for the migrants. As the *Birmingham Age Herald* noted, "The press both North and South charged with more triumph than pity, declare negroes as colonists are and always have been a failure, which is the equivalent that a negro is incapable of self-government."[58] This was a mandate for racial domination, easily confirmed by the spectacle of Camp Jenner.

Southern authorities considered the migrants to be a political threat and used the language of medicine to justify their exclusion. Mayor

Vanhoose repeatedly banned the appearance of "diseased colonists" in Tuscaloosa and threatened to expel the migrants after their return.[59] The mayor of Birmingham declared that he would refuse to allow any train with Tlahualilo migrants aboard to stop at the train station.[60] The Tlahualilo migrants' successful appropriation of federal authority prompted local public quarantines against healthy ex-detainees by prominent partisans of the New South's racial order.

Yet the Camp Jenner detainees used federal medical authority to defy southern political borders. The migrants refused to leave Camp Jenner until the USMHS guaranteed their return to Alabama.[61] Camp Jenner provided the physical space to help the migrants force the USMHS to advocate on their behalf. They demanded that USMHS surgeon Magruder certify that they were free of smallpox.[62] They refused to accept local employment, perhaps for fear of being left isolated on another unfamiliar plantation, this time in Texas.[63] Their fears proved to be warranted. Despite the USMHS promise to guarantee their return home, the state of Alabama allowed women and children who arrived in Birmingham to detrain but transferred the adult men to the Campion mines in Blunt County, Alabama, 100 miles away from Tuscaloosa, where they were forced to work.[64] These miner conscripts were fortunate because within a week, they had made their way back to Tuscaloosa.[65] In other cases, Southern Pacific employees stopped their trains in the woods between Tuscaloosa and Birmingham, allowing the migrants off the train and permitting the rest of the train to stop in Birmingham.[66] Ultimately, the migrants outlasted the Compañia Tlahualilo, the state of Texas, the USMHS, and the governor of Alabama and made their way home.

Camp Jenner raised visible boundaries around the Tlahualilo migrants, symbolically separating these four hundred people from the rest of the United States. Historians have focused on Camp Jenner as a medical border, a final medical tragedy to the difficult odyssey of these African American migrants.[67] However, the migrants' own actions disrupt this conventional narrative. Their position as highly visible wards of the USMHS forced the American federal state to move them through San Antonio, Houston, New Orleans, and Birmingham, against the express wishes of powerful white southern political authorities. On October 17, the migrants formed a committee composed of Reverend Charles Cook, Reverend G. W. Smith, Henry Wilson, Thomas Means, and Reverend T. P. Phillips to express "the heartfelt gratitude of the refugees to the people of Eagle Pass for their many charitable deeds towards the unfortunate returning colonists." They also expressed appreciation to Magruder for the "masterly manner Camp Jenner was conducted and to Dr. Evans for his unsparing labors on behalf of the colonists." Finally, they thanked consul Sparks for his efforts in helping them "out of bondage in Mexico." Samuel Parnell made this very clear when he sent Sparks a telegram from Tuscaloosa expressing "all of the dew respects for you kind and pernevolent aid and asistern of aiding us to our Homes you have did a great thing for the poore colored colney that went to Mexico and I truly thank you."[68] Magruder, Texas state health officer Jack Evans, and Sparks were the people who helped them meet their key demands on federal authority. Sparks helped force the confrontation between the first group of migrants and consul McCaughan in Torreon. He was also the key liaison in the negotiations between the Southern Pacific Railroad and the Tlahualilo migrants. Magruder emerged in importance in mid-October to defend their right to return home, especially when he sought to ensure that the USMHS passport enabled passage through the hometown quarantines awaiting the migrants. Finally, Evans and the neighbors in Eagle Pass never registered a complaint about the presence of Camp Jenner in Eagle Pass. Instead, they treated the migrants like new residents and, after mid-September, helped provide food and local employment. Parnell's telegram spoke to the importance the migrants placed on their return home and a willingness to recognize that the people who detained them met their key demand.

Movements and negotiations across stark medical boundaries—the actions of Camp Jenner's many communities—better illustrate the complex intersection of race and disease status in a nation with a growing research economy. Camp Jenner did more than define the conditions for life stripped of political and social rights.[69] Rather, the migrants turned Camp Jenner into a site of ongoing negotiation where national authorities wrestled with American citizens over basic questions of illness, citizenship, and national identity. The migrants and their medical authorities turned a meadow north of Eagle Pass into a border space that was also central to national medical institutions, a political situation that linked medical exploitation and community assertion, a place both in the margin and in the mainstream.[70] Black southern migrants in Mexico made Camp Jenner the nation's edge.[71]

NOTES

I acknowledge the work of Martin Summers, Laurie B. Green, Laura Briggs, and Sarah Deutsch. These issues are covered in far more depth in my book *Fevered Measures: Public Health and Race at the Texas–Mexico Border, 1848–1942* (Durham, N.C.: Duke University Press, 2012).

1   Consul Jesse Sparks, "Fifteen cases of contagious disease. Surrounded by Mexican police to prevent entry into town, July 21, 1895," *Failure of Scheme to Colonize Negroes in Mexico,* House Document 169, 54th Congress, 13.

2   Sparks, "Negroes almost in open rebellion, July 23, 1895," *Failure of Scheme,* 13.

3   Consul John McCaughan, "Erroneous belief consular officers offer financial relief (July 19, 1895)," *Failure of Scheme,* 17. For McCaughan's prominent career as an industrialist in Torreon, see John Mason Hart, *Empire and Revolution: The Americans in Mexico since the Civil War* (Berkeley: University of California Press, 2002), 201–5.

4   Grover Cleveland, "If return to the colony is not practicable (July 26, 1895)," *Failure of Scheme,* 13.

5   Karl Jacoby calls the migrants' detention "an early medicalization of the Mexican border." His analysis is the first public connection of the black migrants to the general scholarship on the history of Mexican migration to the United States. Jacoby, "Between North and South: The Alternative Borderlands of William Ellis and the African American Colony of 1895," in *Continental Crossroads: Remapping U.S.–Mexico Borderlands History,* ed. Samuel Truett and Elliott Young, 209–39 (Durham, N.C.: Duke University Press, 2004).

6   J. Fred Rippy, "A Negro Colonization Project in Mexico," *Journal of Negro History* 6, no. 1 (1921): 66–73, esp. 67; William K. Meyers, "Politics, Vested Rights and Economic Growth in Porfirian Mexico: The Company Tlahualilo in the Comarca Lagunera," *The Hispanic American Historical Review* 57, no. 3 (1977): 435.

7   Michael Fitzgerald, *Urban Emancipation: Popular Politics in Reconstruction Mobile* (Baton Rouge: Louisiana State University Press, 2002); Fitzgerald, *The Union League Movement in the Deep South* (Baton Rouge: Louisiana State University Press, 1989).

8   For scholarship that examines organized white violence and the persistence of black political participation and property ownership, see W. E. B. Du Bois, *Black Reconstruction in America, 1860–1880* (1935; repr., New York: Free Press, 1992); C. Vann Woodward, *The Strange Career of Jim Crow* (New York: Oxford University Press, 1955); Jane Dailey, Glenda Gilmore, and Bryant Simon, eds., *Jumpin' Jim Crow: Southern Politics from the Civil War to Civil Rights* (Princeton, N.J.: Princeton University Press, 2000); and Douglas Blackmon, *Slavery by Another Name: The*

Re-Enslavement of Black Americans from the Civil War to World War II (New York: Anchor Press, 2009).

9   "Mr. Burke to Mr. Uhl, May 28, 1895" (received June 4, 1895), 54th Cong., 1st sess., H.R. Doc. No. 169, Enclosure No. 12, p. 2.

10   Natalia Molina, *Fit to Be Citizens: Public Health and Race in Los Angeles, 1879–1939* (Berkeley: University of California Press, 2008), 3. For Angel Island, Ellis Island, and the El Paso border, see Anna Pegler Gordon, *In Sight of America: Photography and Immigration Policy* (Berkeley: University of California Press, 2009). See also Amy Fairchild, *Science at the Borders: Immigrant Medical Inspection and the Creation of the Modern Industrial Labor Force* (Baltimore, Md.: Johns Hopkins University Press, 2003). For the impact of state heteronormativity on communities of color, see Alexandra Minna Stern, *Eugenic Nation: Frontiers and Faultlines of Better Breeding in Modern America* (Berkeley: University of California Press, 2005); and Nayan Shah, *Contagious Divides: Epidemics and Race in San Francisco's Chinatown* (Berkeley: University of California Press, 2001).

11   Beatrix Hoffman, "Sympathy and Exclusion: Access to Health Care for Undocumented Immigrants in the United States," in *A Death Retold: Jesica Santillan, the Bungled Transplant, and Paradoxes of Medical Citizenship*, Keith Wailoo, Julie Livingston, and Peter Guarnaccia, eds. (Chapel Hill: University of North Carolina Press, 2006), 238–41.

12   This argument challenges the periodization for the shift in the politics of race in public health from regulation to entitlement as sketched out in Shah, *Contagious Divides*, 6–7. For two key examples of this periodization in the United States, see Barbara Guttman Rosenkrantz, *Public Health and the State: Changing Views in Massachusetts, 1842–1936* (Cambridge, Mass.: Harvard University Press, 1972), 178–84; and Alondra Nelson, *Body and Soul: The Black Panther Party and the Struggle against Medical Discrimination* (Minneapolis: University of Minnesota Press, 2011), 5–11. There is an ongoing tension between entitlement and exclusion around medicine, a tension that can be seen in slave medicine and colonial medical practices. In this case, the Tlahualilo migrants were able to engage a politics of entitlement in an age of open exclusion.

13   "Deluded Colonists," *Los Angeles Times,* July 30, 1895, 3.

14   "Will Feed the Negroes," *Houston Post,* July 28, 1895, 2.

15   "Collector William Fitch to Surgeon General Wyman, August 4, 1895," Box 150, Entry 11.1, Correspondence with Southern Quarantine Camps, Record Group 90, United States Marine Hospital Service, National Archives, Washington, D.C.

16   William Fitch, "Smallpox among Negro Refugees from Mexico," *Weekly Abstract of Sanitary Reports* 10, no. 31 (August 3, 1895), 619–20; Keith Wailoo, *Dying in the City of the Blues: Sickle Cell Anemia and the Politics of Race and Health* (Chapel Hill: University of North Carolina Press, 2001), 7–9.

17   Fitch, "Smallpox among Negro Refugees from Mexico," 619–20.

18 George Magruder, "August 4, 1895," 1, Box 150, Entry 11.1, Correspondence
    with Southern Quarantine Camps, Record Group 90, United States Marine
    Hospital Service, National Archives.

19 William Fitch, "Report, August 4, 1895," 4, Box 150, Entry 11.1,
    Correspondence with Southern Quarantine Camps, Record Group 90,
    United States Marine Hospital Service, National Archives.

20 On contact zones, see Mary Louise Pratt, *Imperial Eyes: Travel Writing
    and Transculturation* (New York: Routledge, 1992), 6.

21 George Magruder, "August 4, 1895," Box 150, Entry 11.1, Correspondence
    with Southern Quarantine Camps, Record Group 90, United States Marine
    Hospital Service, National Archives.

22 Sharla Fett, *Working Cures: Healing, Health, and Power on Southern
    Slave Plantations* (Chapel Hill: University of North Carolina Press, 2002),
    61–82, esp. 72 and 74; Bernard Vogel, *American Indian Medicine* (Norman:
    University of Oklahoma Press, 1970); Todd Savitt, "Black Health on the
    Plantation: Masters, Slaves and Physicians," in *Sickness and Health in
    America: Readings in the History of Medicine and Public Health,* 3rd ed.,
    ed. Judith W. Leavitt and Ronald Numbers, 351–68 (Madison: University
    of Wisconsin Press, 1997).

23 Pekka Hammalainen and Samuel Truett, "On Borderlands," *Journal of
    American History* 98, no. 2 (September 2011): 338.

24 Milton Rosenau, "Report on the Camp Jenner Epidemic, Eagle Pass,
    Texas," *Annual Report of the Supervising Surgeon General* (Washington,
    D.C.: Government Printing Office, 1895); "Telegram, R. M. Swearingen
    to Surgeon General Walter Wyman, August 10, 1895," in ibid., 234.

25 Howard Markel, *Quarantine! East European Jewish Immigrants and
    the New York City Epidemics of 1892* (Baltimore, Md.: Johns Hopkins
    University Press, 1997), 166–80.

26 Evelynn Hammonds, *Childhood's Deadly Scourge: The Campaign to
    Control Diphtheria in New York City* (Baltimore, Md.: Johns Hopkins
    University Press, 2002), 221.

27 J. J. Kinyoun, "The Application of Serotherapy," in *Annual Report of the
    Supervising Surgeon General of the United States Marine Hospital Service*
    (Washington, D.C.: Government Printing Office, 1897), 779.

28 See Markel, *Quarantine!,* 40–58, and Lucy Salyer, *Laws Like Tigers:
    Chinese Immigrants and the Shaping of American Immigration Law* (Chapel
    Hill: University of North Carolina Press, 1995), 37–68.

29 George Magruder, "Smallpox at Eagle Pass, Texas among Negro Colonists
    Returning from Mexico," in *Annual Report of the Supervising Surgeon
    General* (Washington, D.C.: Government Printing Office, 1895), 370–73.

30 Susan Lederer, *Subjected to Science: Human Experimentation in America
    before World War II* (Baltimore, Md.: Johns Hopkins University Press,
    1995), 2–8.

31 Ibid., 1, 2, 22–25. Magruder and Rosenau fit Harriet Washington's trans-

historical portrait of "overachieving adepts with sterling reputations, impressive credentials, and social skill sufficient to secure positions of great responsibility." See Harriet Washington, *Medical Apartheid: The Dark History of Medical Experimentation on Black Americans from Colonial Times to the Present* (New York: Doubleday, 2008), 13.

32   The World Health Organization currently prohibits medical research in refugee camps.

33   Kinyoun, "Application of Serotherapy," 767, 772–73.

34   George Miller Sternberg, *Immunity, Protective Inoculation and Serotherapy* (New York: William and Wood, 1895), v, iv.

35   "Surgeon Kinyoun at Koch's Laboratory," *Philadelphia Inquirer*, January 18, 1891, 3.

36   "Roux's Diphtheria Treatment. Dr. Kinyoun to Introduce It in This Country," *Daily Charlotte Observer*, October 20, 1894, 2.

37   Sternberg, *Immunity*, v.

38   "J. J. Kinyoun: Smallpox Serum Remedy Tested," *New York Times*, January 23, 1895, 4.

39   Kinyoun, "Application of Serotherapy," 775. Contemporary sources reveal no first name for Dr. Elliot.

40   "J. J. Kinyoun: Smallpox Serum Remedy Tested," 4.

41   Ibid.

42   Kinyoun, "Application of Serotherapy," 779.

43   Ibid.; "Help for the Prodigals," *The State* (Columbia, South Carolina), August 9, 1895, 1.

44   *New Orleans Picayune*, "A Government Scientist Sent to Texas on an Important Mission." Reprinted in the *Houston Post*, August 7, 1895, 4.

45   "Milton Rosenau to Walter Wyman, August 14, 1895," Box 150, Entry 11.1, Correspondence with Southern Quarantine Camps, Record Group 90, United States Marine Hospital Service, National Archives.

46   "Mr. Eccles Brings News of His Trip," *Daily Charlotte Observer*, August 25, 1895, 1.

47   Lederer, *Subjected to Science*, 1–25, esp. 20–25. Also John Harley Warner, *The Therapeutic Perspective: Medical Practice, Knowledge, and Identity in America* (Princeton, N.J.: Princeton University Press, 1997), 235–50.

48   Milton Rosenau, "Smallpox—some peculiarities of the Camp Jenner epidemic—a clinical study of 137 cases," in *Annual Report of the Supervising Surgeon General of the United States Marine Hospital Service for the Fiscal Year 1896* (Washington, D.C.: Government Printing Office, 1896), 234–44.

49   "Negroes Who Have Been Cooped Up in Camp Jenner to Be Sent Back to Alabama," *Dallas Morning News*, September 23, 1895, 1.

50   Jacoby, "Between North and South," 224; Donald Hopkins called Camp Jenner "an unusual importation of cases." See Hopkins, *The Greatest Killer: Smallpox in History, with a New Introduction* (Chicago: University of

Chicago Press, 2002), 324. Historians and public health officers treat the emerging research economy separately from smallpox interventions. See T. R. Bender and J. M. Michael, "Fighting Smallpox on the Texas Border: An Episode from the Public Health Service's Proud Past," *Public Health Reports* 99, no. 6 (1984): 579–82; and James Colgrove, *State of Immunity: The Politics of Vaccination in 20th Century America* (Berkeley: University of California Press, 2006). Michael Willrich, *Pox: An American History* (New York: Basic Books, 2011), 65–68, 112, 179, 194, treats Rosenau and Magruder as antagonists; their commitment to research in the field linked the two.

51 "Birmingham Quarantine against Negro Colonists," *Houston Post,* October 15, 1895, 2.

52 Jesse Sparks, "Birmingham to Prevent Negroes En-Route from Entering City, October 3, 1895," United States Consulate, the State Department, *Despatches from United State Consuls in Piedras Negras, 1876–1906* (Washington, D.C.: National Archives, 1963), reel 1.

53 "Church Meeting," *Houston Post,* July 26, 1895, 2.

54 "Negroes Giving Suppers," *Houston Post,* August 17, 1895.

55 "Foreign Mission of Colored Baptists of Texas in Session," *Houston Post,* October 16, 1895, 1.

56 L. L. Campbell, "The Statesman Calls for Colored Help," *Austin Herald,* August 3, 1895, 2.

57 "The Negro as a Pioneer," *San Antonio Express,* July 28, 1895, 4.

58 J. T. Harris, "The Mexican Failure," *Birmingham Age Herald,* August 24, 1895, 3.

59 Birmingham State Herald, "Homeward Bound," reprinted in *Tuscaloosa Times,* October 16, 1895, 1.

60 "Birmingham Quarantine against Negro Colonists," *Houston Post,* October 15, 1895, 2.

61 L. L. Campbell, "Negro Colonists: Trying to Secure Homes for the Unfortunate," *Austin Herald,* August 18, 1895, 3.

62 George Magruder, "Report on the Establishment and Administration of Camp Jenner, Eagle Pass, TX," *Weekly Abstract of Sanitary Reports* 10, no. 45 (October 25, 1895): 957–59.

63 Sparks, "Birmingham to Prevent Negroes En-Route from Entering City."

64 Birmingham News, "Ungrateful Are the Negroes Brought Back to Alabama," reprinted in *Tuscaloosa Times,* October 8, 1895.

65 Birmingham State Herald, "Homeward Bound," reprinted in *Tuscaloosa Times,* October 16, 1895, 1.

66 Newspaper, Eagle Pass Guide, "Clippings from the Eagle Pass Guide Newspaper, November 3, 1895," United States Consulate, the State Department, *Despatches from United State Consuls in Piedras Negras, 1876–1906* (Washington, D.C.: National Archives, 1963), reel 1.

67 Ibid.

68 Ibid.

69 Giorgio Agamben, *Sovereign Power and Bare Life* (Stanford, Calif.: Stanford University Press, 1998). Agamben argues that extreme conditions in spaces such as labor camps and immigrant detention zones define the exercise of sovereignty, where the state demonstrates its ability to operate outside its own scrutiny. For this argument for the Mexican borderlands, see Gilberto Rosas, "The Thickening Borderlands: Diffused Exceptionality and 'Immigrant' Social Struggles during the 'War on Terror,'" *Cultural Dynamics* 18 (2006): 335–49.

70 John Nieto Phillips, "From Margin to Mainstream: The Brave New World of Borderlands History," *Journal of American History* 98, no. 2 (September 2011): 338.

71 Susan M. Reverby, *Examining Tuskegee: The Infamous Study and Its Legacy* (Chapel Hill: University of North Carolina Press, 2009), 56–71.

5

Diagnosing the Ailments of Black Citizenship

African American Physicians and the Politics of Mental Illness, 1895–1940

MARTIN SUMMERS

MENTAL HEALTH EXPERTS in the United States have long recognized that, as a group, African Americans underuse mental health services. This lack of use has resulted in an underrepresentation of African Americans in outpatient services and their overrepresentation in inpatient services, especially public hospitals. This is largely because the failure to seek and receive outpatient care often means that one's condition is more severe by the time there is any medical intervention. Mental health professionals point to both structural and cultural factors to explain this lack of voluntary engagement with the mental health care system. These include a lack of mental health resources in African American communities, the perception on the part of blacks that psychiatry is Eurocentrically biased, and blacks' historical mistrust of the medical profession. Additionally, experts argue that mental distress is often understood within a religious framework and that African Americans respond to it as an opportunity to "renew one's commitment to a religious or spiritual system of belief." Finally, psychiatric care is eschewed by blacks, according to many professionals, because of the stigma associated with mental illness and the belief that mental distress can be overcome through "self-reliance and determination."[1] All these factors have contributed to the lack of a tradition of seeking psychotherapy in the African American community. Although these are all compelling reasons, few scholars have attempted to put them in a larger historical context.[2]

This chapter is an attempt to historicize what has become something of an axiom in the thinking of mental health care professionals.

Although it does not deny the important influence that issues of access and culture have played in blacks' underuse of mental health services, it seeks to deepen our understanding of this contemporary phenomenon, mainly by examining the historical role of black physicians in shaping African Americans' relationship to psychiatry. From its formation in the late nineteenth century to roughly the middle of the twentieth, the black medical profession largely neglected to address problems of mental illness in the African American community. To be sure, some black physicians were interested in diseases and disorders associated with the mind and the nervous system, and they explored and advocated for the various disciplines that emerged to address these diseases and disorders, such as neurology, psychoanalysis, psychobiology, and even eugenics. However, this interest did not translate into collective efforts—at either the institutional or organizational level—to promote mental health among African Americans until the mid-twentieth century. Even as psychiatry gained medical authority in the early twentieth century through its incorporation of laboratory- and clinic-based knowledge and its liberation from the asylum, it was much slower to obtain legitimacy in the black medical profession and larger African American community.

Several factors contributed to the black medical profession's somewhat detached relationship to mental illness and psychiatry. Many were external to the profession itself. Racism in American medicine, including the practical exclusion of African Americans from the American Medical Association (AMA) and the American Psychiatric Association (APA) and the obstacles that African American physicians had to face in pursuing specialties, made it difficult for any black physician who might be interested in devoting his or her career to tackling the problem of mental disease. The absence of psychopathic hospitals to serve the black community, the limited number of state hospitals dedicated to the care of mentally ill blacks, the discriminatory hiring practices of hospitals that admitted black patients, and the inability of most African Americans to afford private treatment surely made psychiatry a not particularly remunerative specialty for black physicians before World War II.

But as we will see, along with these external barriers to the development of a robust black psychiatric community in the early twentieth century, internal rationales inhibited the black medical profession from engaging psychiatry in a way that encouraged ordinary African Americans to see it as a potential asset as opposed to something alien and stigmatizing. These internal rationales were shaped by the tenuous relationship that African Americans had to the nation-state as citizens. In the formative years of the black medical profession, black physicians used their medical authority to draw attention to diseases for which there were clear somatic origins that could be identified as the consequences of segregation and economic discrimination. Diseases that were the result of deficient nutrition, unsanitary homes, and poorly serviced neighborhoods provided black physicians, nurses, and public health experts with the ammunition to take aim at structural racism and inequality. The indeterminacy of the causes of mental illnesses gave them less purchase in the black medical profession's battle on behalf of the collective health of the race. Indeed, when the profession did turn its attention to mental illness and transform that attention into institutional substance, it was mainly to address neurological injuries of African American veterans. The focus on damage to the nervous system certainly gave physicians a greater degree of certainty regarding the etiology, or cause, of mental illness; perhaps equally important was the status of those who suffered from these injuries. In much the same way that somatic diseases allowed black physicians to point to the lack of full citizenship rights for African Americans, mental illness among black soldiers was a testament to the race's capacity for citizenship. In other words, somatic diseases and mental diseases held differential value when it came to conceptualizing health and illness as indexes of African American social membership in the United States.[3] Ultimately, the lack of full citizenship rights shaped the ways that the black medical profession approached mental illness in the first few decades of the twentieth century and consequently contributed to the marginalization of African Americans with functional mental illnesses and personality disorders and of psychotherapy as a legitimate therapeutic practice.

THE IDEOLOGICAL CONTEXT OF BLACK MEDICAL PROFESSIONALIZATION

Even though there have been black folk and professional healers in what is today known as the United States since the colonial period, the beginning of the black medical profession might be located in 1895. It was in the fall of that year that physicians Robert Fulton Boyd and Miles Vandahurst Lynk, in Atlanta for the Cotton States and International Exposition, arranged a meeting with ten other doctors to explore the possibility of forming a professional medical organization for people of African descent. In the near half-century since its founding, very few black physicians had gained membership in the AMA, largely because of the racial exclusion policies of the AMA's constituent local and state medical societies. As early as the 1880s, African American doctors had begun forming their own local and state medical societies for networking opportunities, camaraderie, and the exchange of knowledge, but it was not until 1895 that they formed the National Medical Association (NMA).[4]

The NMA was founded just as a school of thought on the condition and prospects of the post-Emancipation "Negro" was maturing. Proponents of racial degeneracy theory—which included physicians, social scientists, popular writers, and politicians—claimed that emancipation had an overall deleterious effect on African Americans. Loosed from the "civilizing" institution of slavery and constitutionally incapable of caring for themselves, African Americans were physically and mentally deteriorating as a race. This degeneration took the form of an atavistic reversion to the "savagery" of their ancestral past, purportedly evident in the increase of criminal activity and sexual assault by African Americans. It could also be seen in the increasing morbidity and mortality rates among blacks. These proponents of racial degeneracy pointed to the growing incidence of diseases such as tuberculosis and syphilis as well as insanity as evidence that African Americans were on the verge of racial extinction.[5]

In addition to serving as a vehicle for the professionalization of black physicians, then, the NMA early on assumed responsibility for defending the race against reactionary racial degeneracy rhetoric. One of the main ways it did this was through the pages of the *Journal of the National Medical Association*. From the beginning of its publication in 1909, the *JNMA* regularly included editorials, feature articles, and transcripts of presidential addresses that refuted the claims of racial degeneracy theorists. They did so by challenging the objectivity of racial degeneration studies and emphasizing the socioeconomic, rather than racial, causes of high morbidity and mortality among the black population. Nonetheless, they acknowledged escalating illness and death rates

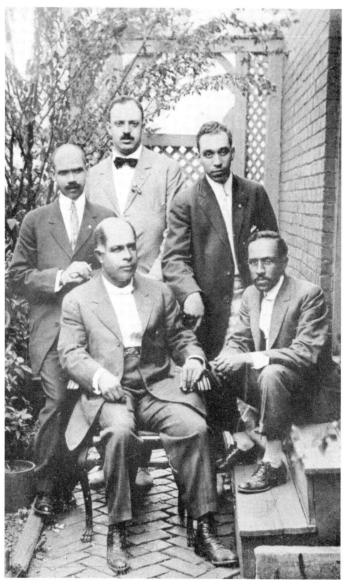

FIGURE 5.1. Editorial staff of the *Journal of the National Medical Association*. Courtesy of General Research and Reference Division, Schomburg Center for Research in Black Culture, the New York Public Library, Astor, Lenox, and Tilden Foundations.

by stressing the need for more black professional health care workers and, in a classic middle-class reform posture, by exhorting working-class blacks to make their home environments more sanitary, improve their personal hygiene, and eschew folk healing practices.[6]

Clear indication that the black medical profession was not as interested in mental illness is the fact that neither individual physicians nor the NMA as a whole went to great lengths to refute the insanity component of racial degeneracy theory. Within a quarter century after emancipation, many white physicians had begun to comment on the upward trend in insanity rates among African Americans. They argued that freedpeople and their descendants were ill equipped to handle the strain of modernity and, consequently, suffered from mental alienation. J. F. Miller, the white superintendent of North Carolina's public asylum for African Americans, expressed this idea in a speech before the Southern Medico-Psychological Association in 1896: "In his ignorance of the laws of his being, the functions of citizenship and the responsibilities and duties which freedom imposed, demands were made upon the negro which his intellectual parts were unable to discharge. In his former condition none of these things disturbed his mind."[7] In other words, the salubrious environment of slavery gave way to the stress-filled landscape of freedom, generating a higher incidence of insanity in a morally and biologically underdeveloped people.

Many white physicians and psychiatrists in the 1910s and 1920s continued to regurgitate the same arguments that were advanced by medical experts in the post-Emancipation period.[8] This is not particularly surprising, given that these physicians and psychiatrists existed in a cultural environment that was saturated with images and narratives of the atavistic "negro." What is interesting to note is that, despite having matured by the World War I era, the black medical profession largely failed to engage with these reactionary ideas about insanity among African Americans. In the post-Emancipation period, there was little institutional or organizational infrastructure for black physicians to develop a counterdiscourse of mental illness in the black community. This was not the case in the 1910s and 1920s. Why, then, did black physicians ignore the white medical establishment's framing of black insanity even as they vigorously challenged other aspects of racial degeneracy discourse, particularly with respect to tuberculosis and other infectious diseases?

This is not to say that mental illness was never a topic of discussion among black physicians and other professionals. Articles either directly or indirectly dealing with mental disorders occasionally appeared in the *JNMA* throughout the first decade of its publication. Neurasthenia and pellagra-induced dementia received some coverage in the journal. Contributors to the journal also occasionally invoked the problem of insanity more as a rhetorical move to criticize racial degeneracy theory than as a general accounting of mental health issues in the black community. For instance, one editorial raised the issue of mental illness in its refutation of racial degeneracy theory. Rather than directly addressing theorists' claims of increased rates of insanity among blacks, however, the editorial turned the tables and suggested that it was the paternalism of racial conservatives that was tantamount to mental illness. Pointing out the tendency of racial degeneracy proponents to preface their claims with assurances that they had blacks' best interests at heart, the editorial trenchantly remarked that "the contention of the white man that because he owned the Negro in slavery he understands him in freedom constitutes the real 'Dementia Americana.'"[9]

However, these occasional references to mental illness paled in comparison to the numerous articles in mainstream (white) medical and psychiatric journals that attributed increasing rates of insanity in the black community to emancipation and exposure to "civilization." This reluctance to engage in a larger professional discussion of mental illness had its corollary in the absence of any sophisticated organizational or institutional efforts to address the presence of mental illness in the black community in the 1910s and early 1920s. There were several reasons for this. One factor that contributed to this lack of interest in mental illness was the relationship (or, rather, nonrelationship) between the professionalization of black physicians and the emergence of psychiatry as a science-based discipline.

THE POLITICAL AND IDEOLOGICAL CONTEXT OF BLACK PSYCHIATRIC PROFESSIONALIZATION

Even in the mainstream medical profession, mental illness did not occupy a central place in physicians' sense of their responsibility for the prevention and curing of disease. In part, this was caused by the lack of consensus among physicians about the etiology, classification, and treatment of mental illness. In part, it was caused by the professional antagonism between institutional psychiatry and a more science-based psychiatry that emerged in the late nineteenth century. Moreover, this nonconsensus and the split between institutional and scientific psychiatry were related.

Over much of the nineteenth century, psychiatry as a field was limited to the asylum, and its practitioners were asylum superintendents. They understood mental disease to have a physiological or somatic basis even though they could not draw direct correlations between symptoms or abnormal behavior and actual brain lesions. Superintendents grouped asylum inmates according to their behaviors rather than their diseases, and they used moral management as the main therapeutic regimen. Moral management was organized around the principle of removing the insane from their existing environment, placing them in a tranquil and ordered setting, and treating them through a regularized routine that included labor, rest, and a nutritious diet. Institutional psychiatry was as much custodial as it was curative and characterized more by the management of patients than the systematic apprehension of mental disease itself.[10]

By the 1870s, advances in the understanding of brain anatomy and the central nervous system set the stage for a new generation of specialists to challenge the hegemony of institutional psychiatry. Neurologists did not depart from the somatic understanding of mental illness; rather, they localized the physiological origins of mental illness to damage to the nervous system. Influenced by a European model of scientific and clinic-based medicine, neurologists claimed greater medical expertise in the study and treatment of insanity. They criticized institutional psychiatrists for being "isolated from medicine" and more concerned with the administration of asylums. Institutional psychiatrists defended their management of asylums and reinforced the necessity of interacting with actual patients in order to fully understand mental illness. Nonetheless, advocates for a more scientific psychiatry eventually prevailed. Despite their resistance to efforts to elevate scientific and clinic-based medicine in the profession, asylum superintendents found their outdated conceptions of psychiatry displaced by a new consensus. Throughout the 1890s, the main professional society, the Association of the Medical Superintendents of American Institutions for the Insane, increasingly expanded its membership beyond institutional psychiatrists to include assistant physicians of asylums, many of whom were sympathetic to neurology. The association eventually changed its name to the American Medico-Psychological Association.[11]

Several historians have noted that the shift to a scientific psychiatry contributed to an expansion of the boundaries of the profession "outward into the community." The locus of the treatment of mental illness began its slow migration from an institutional environment to noninstitutional settings such as the psychiatrist's private office, the psychopathic hospital, and the outpatient clinic. This shift ultimately meant the "implicit abandonment of institutionalized patients," those with chronic mental illness, those who could not afford private treatment, and those who had no access to outpatient clinics.[12] The development of a scientific psychiatry also eventually laid the groundwork for what historian Elizabeth Lunbeck calls the "psychiatry of everyday life"—that is, the transformation "from a psychiatry of insanity to a psychiatry that took the whole of the human endeavor for its subject."[13] Even though neurologists were not embedded in institutions and, indeed, framed the asylum as inimical to the study and treatment of mental illness, it was this very institutional network that moved the field of psychiatry onto more scientific terrain.

What did the absence of an institutional infrastructure and network mean for the black medical profession in particular and for the black community in general? And how did this shape the contours of black thought about mental illness and mental health at both the professional and popular levels? After the Civil War, mentally ill African Americans who were institutionalized found themselves in segregated wards. Some states, including Virginia and North Carolina, established public asylums exclusively for African Americans. Very few asylums in the South had black physicians on staff, and none had black superintendents. Indeed, the first black superintendent of a mental institution was not appointed until 1926.[14] Outside these mental hospitals, there were limited psychiatric facilities in general hospitals that served African American communities. Before the opening of U.S. Veterans' Hospital No. 91 in Tuskegee, Alabama in 1923, apparently none of the approximately two hundred black-controlled or segregated hospitals and sanitariums in the country had neurology or psychiatric departments or neurologists or psychiatrists on staff.[15] Frederick Douglass Memorial Hospital in Philadelphia appears to have been the only black hospital that provided the services of a neurologist, although French-born white American Alfred Gordon was not on the hospital's staff.[16] Thus, black physicians were rarely in positions to really work with mentally ill populations. Certainly, the limited educational opportunities available to African American physicians interested in mental illness impeded the development of a black psychiatric profession worthy of note before the 1920s. Most African American physicians received their medical education at either Howard University Medical School or Meharry Medical College, neither of which had formal programs in psychiatry until after World War II. As southern medical schools, Howard and Meharry were not unusual in this regard; southern medical schools in general did not begin offering training in psychiatry until the late 1920s.[17] Howard was ahead of Meharry in training students in neurology and psychiatry, probably because of its proximity to the federal mental hospital, Saint Elizabeths. One of the hospital's staff members, Dr. Benjamin Karpman, began offering courses in dynamic psychiatry at Howard in the mid-1920s and supervised or mentored a number of the school's graduates who went on to do their clinical rotations or pursue research at Saint Elizabeths. One of those graduates, Dr. Ernest Y. Williams, ended up establishing a psychiatric service at Freedmen's Hospital, Howard's teaching hospital, in 1939. Along with Justin Hope, Williams also served as an assistant professor of psychiatry and neurology at Howard's medical school in the early 1940s. In contrast, Meharry did not set up a psychiatry department until 1961, although faculty members did offer courses in psychiatry as early as the 1930s.[18]

Even for African American medical students who received some instruction in psychiatry and neurology, the opportunities to pursue either as a specialty were severely restricted. Internships at hospitals with clinical training programs were rare for African Americans, and residencies were practically nonexistent. White hospitals routinely excluded African Americans from their residency programs, and there were few black-controlled or segregated hospitals with sufficient resources to support residencies. Even the few black hospitals that did offer residencies by the late 1930s did so in the fields of surgery, pediatrics, obstetrics, gynecology, pathology, and radiology. In the main, however, there were only about two dozen African American specialists in any field of medicine in the entire country by the end of the 1930s. The numbers of black specialists continued to be depressed into the postwar period as a result of new policies adopted by medical specialty boards, which required that prospective members finish a three-year residency at a hospital that had the imprimatur of the AMA.[19]

The exclusion of African American physicians from medical specialties was animated by run-of-the-mill white racism that became buttressed by professional consensus after the release of the Flexner report in 1910. Largely responsible for the standardization of medical education in North America, the Flexner report led to the closure of many sectarian medical schools and medical schools that catered to African Americans and women. The author of the report, Abraham Flexner, recognized the importance of training black health care professionals but argued that they should perform mainly a public health function. In other words, black physicians and nurses were necessary to serve as barriers between blacks, who were a "potential source of infection and contagion," and white society.[20]

Although black health professionals were loath to agree with the motivations behind such characterizations of their responsibility, they did recognize their public health obligations. Shortly after the *JNMA* began publication in 1909, Dr. John A. Kenney, medical director of the hospital at Tuskegee Institute, a black college, and the journal's managing editor, wrote an article that captured the urgency of the public health role of black physicians. In it, he engaged the larger debate of racial degeneracy. "In many places, without quibbling over such academic questions as whether the Negro is dying as rapidly as some other people, or whether there is some racial inherency productive of its high mortality, or whether it is due to environment," Kenney argued, "the race is realizing that its death-rate is high[,] that certain diseases are taking more than their fair toll of human life from its ranks, and many of these diseases are preventable."[21] From an objective standpoint, this was true. Black morbidity and mortality rates were higher than those of whites. Whereas racial degeneracy theorists and many white health professionals pointed to these higher rates as evidence of racial inferiority, black physicians and health activists stressed socioeconomic causes.[22] In assessing the overall health of the race, the black medical and public health establishment put an emphasis on somatic diseases, especially diseases spread by infection, such as tuberculosis and syphilis; those that were the result of vitamin deficiency, such as pellagra; and those that were caused and exacerbated by the environment, such as pulmonary diseases. They did this not only because these diseases posed a significant threat to black communities. The focus on somatic diseases also allowed black physicians and health activists to expose the physical trauma of racism. These same people believed that the masses of blacks were, to a certain extent, responsible for the unhealthy environments in which they lived and urged them to adopt middle-class values of thrift, industry, sobriety, and self-control. Yet they also exploited high morbidity and mortality rates in order to make, as historian Susan Smith argues, "political claims on the state."[23]

In other words, black health professionals argued that the collective unhealthiness of the race was fundamentally connected to their lack of full citizenship rights. The political valence of the black public health discourse was clearly expressed in Dr. A. M. Brown's 1914 presidential address before the NMA. After running off a list of problems with the individual and collective hygiene of African Americans that would have resonated well with racial degeneracy theorists, Brown went on to criticize Jim Crow and call for the leveraging of federal resources. "It is then proper . . . to direct energy toward the removal of all causes over which he [the Negro] has no control," Brown declared,

> and to which his civic life is amenable, namely the disregard for his domestic environments, his insanitary homes, his lack of sewer hygiene, his poverty, his low wages, his destitution, his privation, his lack of employment, his ignored rights in railway stations, in depots, and his poor accommodations with regard to street railway and railway privileges. It is time for the profession to appeal in the Negro's behalf to the national government for the protection of this class of humanity in the form of conservation funds.[24]

The black medical and public health profession focused on somatic diseases because they could make direct linkages between environment, behavior, and etiology. They could then use those linkages to argue for better economic opportunities, an amelioration of segregated environments (if not an end to segregation altogether), and the investment of resources into a black public health infrastructure.

The indeterminacy around the causes of mental illness meant that it was not as politically freighted as diseases such as tuberculosis, syphilis, and pellagra. Because of the lack of consensus on how mental disorders originated and evolved in individuals, the specter of mental illness did not allow black health activists to make demands for better-paying jobs, improved sanitation, better housing, and so forth.

In this regard, it is significant that the first concerted effort among African American physicians to provide systematic care for mentally ill blacks was propelled by the massive problem of "war neuroses" experienced by veterans in the years after World War I.[25] Damage to the nervous system gave physicians a clear etiological provenance that they could associate with mental illness. Moreover, the fact that these "war neuroses" were evidence of African Americans' sacrifice for a country that did not fully recognize them as citizens gave the existence of mental illness in the black community the same potential political purchase that tuberculosis or pellagra held.

Opened in 1923, U.S. Veterans' Hospital No. 91 in Tuskegee was dedicated to the treatment of black veterans. In its initial projected allocation of bed space and staff positions, the U.S. Veterans Bureau made an important statement that the treatment of mental disorders would be considered as important as the treatment of infectious diseases. The six hundred beds were to be equally divided between veterans suffering from neurological disorders and those who had contracted tuberculosis. Of the twenty physician positions, ten were reserved for neuropsychiatric specialists.[26] Despite the initial reluctance of the U.S. Veterans Bureau and the adamant opposition of the local white community, the Tuskegee hospital very early on was staffed and supervised by black physicians, nurses, and administrators.[27] Historian Anne C. Rose argues that the actual clinical treatment of mentally ill veterans became secondary to the importance of demonstrating the race's ability to run a sophisticated treatment facility. According to Rose, very little attention was paid to the etiological, classificatory, and therapeutic specificity of mental disease.[28] There may be some truth to this, but it is also clear that the establishment of the veterans' hospital at Tuskegee accelerated psychiatric specialization in the black medical profession and consequently increased the legitimacy of the discipline.

Indeed, shortly after U.S. Veterans' Hospital No. 91 opened its doors, the *JNMA* was touting the opportunities it presented to black physicians to break into the "hitherto impenetrable field of neuropsychiatry."[29] Some in the NMA understood the neurological disorders that were the result of combat stress to potentially have an important influence on the ways black physicians approached mental illness more generally. For instance, John A. Kenney argued that mental illness was not limited to returning veterans who were confined to institutions. "The World War with its disastrous sequelae has served as nothing else to bring out the importance of this subject, not alone to physicians serving disabled soldiers in Government Hospitals, but to the general practitioner who is often called upon to diagnose, if not to treat, some of the unfortunate victims of that terrible ordeal," he wrote.[30]

The watershed nature of the establishment of U.S. Veterans' Hospital No. 91 is also reflected in the pages of the *JNMA* in another way. Before the mid-1920s, few articles by specialists appeared in the journal. Most of the articles directly or indirectly addressing mental illness were by general practitioners who addressed insanity in vague, occasionally moralistic language. The few specialist articles were penned largely by Alfred Gordon or another white neurologist associated with Douglass Memorial Hospital in Philadelphia, Dr. R. Wellesley Bailey. Gordon and Bailey tended toward a discussion of mental illness that was based on a hereditarian understanding of etiology and that advanced a combination of eugenics and a modernized moral treatment regimen as the most preferable form of intervention.[31] By the early 1930s, readers of the *JNMA* were encountering articles on mental illness more frequently. Moreover, they were encountering articles written by psychiatrists who were quite eclectic in their understandings of the origins, development, treatment, and prevention of mental illness. One might read a synthesis of the research on neurosyphilis or clinical studies that focused on the psychical origins of insanity and the efficacy of occupational therapy and psychotherapy.[32]

Beginning in 1933, the *JNMA* included a regular department dealing with mental illness. Edited by Dr. Alan P. Smith, the Department of Neuropsychiatry included abstracts of research and clinical studies, information on professional organizational meetings, and notices of postgraduate clinics, courses, and fellowships. Smith, a graduate of the University of Iowa's College of Medicine, was the first African American to become a member of the APA. Another of Smith's colleagues, Dr. Prince P. Barker, was also an APA fellow and a certified member of the Board of Psychiatry and Neurology.[33] The latter half of the 1930s witnessed the publication of far more articles on insanity than had ever appeared in the journal. With the very few exceptions of those written by neurologists and psychiatrists treating acute cases in general hospitals, most contributions came from psychiatrists working with institutionalized populations, and topics ranged from the persistent question of the hereditary nature of insanity to the therapeutic innovations of insulin shock therapy and the anticonvulsant drug dilantin sodium.

African American medical professionals were beginning to more fully incorporate a scientific-based psychiatry into their understanding of what constituted health threats for blacks. Just as Kenney suggested in 1924, Smith, Barker, and others reminded their fellow physicians that the interdependence of the mind and the body, of the psychical and the somatic, made mental health indispensable to the overall health of the race. Some acknowledged that psychiatry had to be demystified, or as Barker put it, be given "more of a 'down-to-the-earth' feel," but there was no denying the cognate relationship between the principles of psychiatry and medicine. "Psychiatry must continue to emphasize the environmental, social and psychologic implications of disease but there is a decided current movement in psychiatry to avail itself in increasing measure of the biological perspective of medicine," an editorial in the *JNMA* asserted. "Psychiatry as a specialty is founded on medicine."[34] In effect, psychiatry was increasingly being considered as important as any other specialty in addressing the health needs of African Americans.

But even as psychiatry was beginning to be mainstreamed within the black medical profession, there was little integration of the specialty into everyday medical practice, despite the many pronouncements of its most enthusiastic promoters. For instance, there was little interaction between these early black psychiatrists and noninstitutionalized people who may have been experiencing mental distress. Few black psychiatrists were engaged in psychotherapy as a form of treatment for neurotic disorders or as a method of preventing psychoses in the black community. This was not the result of the school of psychiatric thought to which they adhered. Many, if not most, of them were committed to dynamic psychiatry, or the approach that understood mental illness to be as much a product of the interaction between the person and the environment as it was a result of brain lesions.[35] In its emphasis on the emotional, psychological, and social dimensions of mental disease—and, indeed, on the importance of recognizing the cumulative effect of life experiences on the ability of an individual to socially adapt to his or her environment—dynamic psychiatry encouraged early intervention as the proper mechanism for treating and preventing mental illness. As was the case with the emergence of neurology in the late nineteenth century, the ascendancy of dynamic psychiatry furthered the movement of mainstream psychiatric practice from large, impersonal institutions with increasingly elderly and chronically ill populations to outpatient clinics, psychopathic hospitals, and private offices.[36]

This was not the case with African American psychiatrists. Given that private psychotherapy required a certain level of disposable income, it is not surprising that few black psychiatrists would have been able to cultivate a large enough clientele to make private practice financially viable.[37] But there was very little work done to establish outpatient clinics or facilities within existing hospitals that would handle acute psychotic cases. Indeed, in 1937 Smith lamented the lack of a mental health infrastructure that could serve the African American community. "There is an urgent need," he wrote, "for facilities for the development of a Negro Mental Health Program to adequately study and treat inadequate personalities who present an abundance of overlooked and still correctible disturbance of emotional balance, abnormalities in conduct and social relationships and maladjustments in school and work." Even though Smith was on the staff of the Tuskegee veterans' hospital, he argued for the importance of establishing psychopathic hospitals and child guidance centers, the latter of which were especially needed to address the social adjustment of black youth in urban environments.[38]

Two years after Smith's article appeared, the historically black North Carolina college, St. Augustine's, hosted a meeting of the Committee for the Development of Psychopathic Hospitals and Other Mental Hygiene Resources for Negroes. Shaped by the principles of social psychiatry, the committee called for the development of mental health training centers. These centers, initially proposed to be located at Howard and Meharry, would train psychiatrists, psychiatric nurses, psychiatric social workers, and clinical psychologists to work in psychopathic hospitals and outpatient clinics. The NMA endorsed the idea in an editorial penned by John A. Kenney in 1940. Recognizing the "utter scarcity of Negro psychiatrists to participate in the prevention and treatment of disease," Kenney strenuously argued that a social psychiatry approach was needed to reduce the high number of mentally ill African Americans within custodial institutions. Like his colleagues during the formative years of the NMA, Kenney placed an emphasis on the federal government's responsibility in addressing the health needs of the black community. "We hope the authorities will see that the establishment of such a training center will make possible the preparation of such personnel as will be necessary for the prosecution of a nation-wide program among Negroes for the prevention, early recognition, and control of mental disease in this group," Kenney declared. "Once such a program has become effective, we may expect a much smaller load of Negro patients in the traditional hospitals for the insane, of Negroes in jails, on the chain gang, and of Negro delinquents erroneously incarcerated in reformitories [sic]." The teaching centers never materialized, at least not in the way that the committee envisioned it.[39] Still, Kenney's attempt to make political claims on the state suggests that by the 1940s the black medical profession had elevated mental illness and mental health to the same level that an earlier generation of black physicians had reserved for somatic diseases.

This did not translate into the development of a robust mental health infrastructure in African American communities, however. Few hospitals that served primarily African American patients had mental hygiene clinics, and community mental hygiene clinics were scarce in African American neighborhoods in the 1940s. New York City had the lion's share of those that did exist, with Harlem Hospital establishing a mental hygiene clinic in 1943 and two Jewish American psychiatrists, Hilde Mosse and Frederic Wertham, founding Lafargue Mental Hygiene Clinic in Harlem in 1946. These two clinics joined black psychologists Kenneth and Mamie Clark's Northside Child Guidance Center, which had been operating since the mid-1930s.[40] St. Louis's Homer G. Phillips Hospital and John A. Andrew Memorial Hospital in Tuskegee also opened mental hygiene clinics before the end of World War II. Freedmen's Hospital opened a psychiatric service in 1939 and a child guidance center in 1941, yet it did not have sufficient resources to support psychiatry clinical clerkships for Howard University medical students as late as the end of that decade.[41] This dearth of black psychiatrists continued into the 1960s. In the middle of that decade, black psychiatrists made up only 5 percent of all black health care professionals. Although African Americans only made up 1.6 percent of psychiatrists in the United States, this percentage did not differ substantially from the percentage of African Americans in the physician profession (2 percent). Nonetheless, the author of a study on race and

to address mental illness. The black psychiatric profession was born, one might argue, out of black physicians' engagement with the neuropathic problems encountered at U.S. Veterans' Hospital No. 91. With the establishment of that federal facility and the maturation of black psychiatrists who worked there, the problem of mental illness—and the promise of mental health—attained greater visibility in the black medical profession as a whole.[45]

This newfound commitment to addressing mental illness focused more on forms of mental disease that were somatic in origin and that were responsive to somatic therapies. There was little attention given—at least at the institutional level—to mental diseases that were psychical in nature. Nor was much energy spent on working with noninstitutionalized populations or using psychotherapy as an ameliorative agent for functional disorders. The point of this chapter is not to cast blame but rather to explain why the black medical profession did not engage racial degeneracy discourses of black insanity or the larger issue of mental health in the black community until the 1930s. To be sure, the ravaging effects of infectious diseases demanded the attention of the black medical profession in the early twentieth century. As I have tried to show, however, the professional formation of black physicians, the internal debates in the field of psychiatry, and the tangible political and economic objectives attached to black public health activism conspired to prevent the development of a robust black psychiatric profession that would have made mental illness more intelligible at the popular level and that would have made the mentally distressed individual subject to more progressive and humane medical intervention.

The absence of a robust black psychiatric profession before World War II prevented the development of a "psychiatry of everyday life" in the African American community, in which psychiatry was applicable to "everyone, not only the patently insane."[46] Of course, economics and culture played important roles in inhibiting this development. The prohibitive costs of psychotherapy precluded most African Americans from seeking it as a form of treatment from private psychiatrists. Moreover, through the first half of the twentieth century, the majority of African Americans resided in the South, parts of which were particularly resistant to psychiatry due to the confluence of traditionalism, skepticism of science, and evangelical Christianity.[47] But we should not take for granted that this was an inevitable outcome, a product of the interaction between structure and culture with little room for agency. In the process of attending to the health care needs of their communities, black physicians made decisions with respect to the problem of mental illness among African Americans in the first half of the twentieth century, decisions that, along with other factors, continue to shape African Americans' relationship to psychiatry.

NOTES

I thank Jim Downs, Dennis Doyle, Laurie B. Green, and John Mckiernan-González for their helpful comments on various drafts of this chapter. I also thank Adebukola Oni for her research assistance.

1   See the 1999 report by the Office of the U.S. Surgeon General for an overview. *Mental Health: A Report of the Surgeon General* (1999), http://www.surgeongeneral.gov/library/mentalhealth/home.html, quotes on 82, 87. Also see Robin D. Stone, "Mind over Matter: A Conversation about African American Mental Health," *The Crisis* 111 (November–December 2004): 32–35; Billy Jones, "Current Mental Health Issues Affecting Black Americans," in *Black Psychiatrists and American Psychiatry*, ed. Jeanne Spurlock, 205–15 (Washington, D.C.: American Psychiatric Association, 1999); Lloyd C. Elam, "Development of the Department of Psychiatry at Meharry Medical College," in Spurlock, *Black Psychiatrists and American Psychiatry, 67–75.*

2   One of the few scholars to have done so is Anne C. Rose, although her study focuses on the South as a region rather than solely on African Americans. See Rose, *Psychology and Selfhood in the Segregated South* (Chapel Hill: University of North Carolina Press, 2009). See also several of the essays in Spurlock, *Black Psychiatrists and American Psychiatry.*

3   On social membership, see Natalia Molina, *Fit to Be Citizens? Public Health and Race in Los Angeles, 1879–1939* (Berkeley: University of California Press, 2006), 3.

4   Herbert M. Morais, *The History of the Afro-American in Medicine* (Cornwells Heights, Pa.: Publishers Agency, 1978), 66–68; Michael Byrd and Linda Cayton, *An American Health Dilemma: A Medical History of African Americans and the Problem of Race* (New York: Routledge, 2002), 2:113–14.

5   For a few examples, see J. F. Miller, "The Effects of Emancipation upon the Mental and Physical Health of the Negro of the South," *North Carolina Medical Journal* 38 (November 20, 1896): 285–94; J. Allison Hodges, "The Effect of Freedom upon the Physical and Psychological Development

of the Negro," *Richmond Journal of Practice* 14 (June 1900): 161–71; Frederick Hoffman, "Race Traits and Tendencies of the American Negro," *Publications of the American Economic Association* 1st series, XI (August 1896). For general discussion see George M. Fredrickson, *The Black Image in the White Mind: The Debate on Afro-American Character and Destiny, 1817–1914* (1971; repr., Hanover, N.H.: Wesleyan University Press, 1987); Susan L. Smith, *Sick and Tired of Being Sick and Tired: Black Women's Health Activism, 1890–1950* (Philadelphia: University of Pennsylvania Press, 1995), 8–10. Expectations that African Americans would become extinct increased in the immediate years after the Civil War. See Jim Downs, *Sick from Freedom: African-American Illness and Suffering during the Civil War and Reconstruction* (New York: Oxford University Press, 2012).

6   For a good example that combines a number of these approaches, see "An Impending Crises [*sic*]," *JNMA* 1 (October–December 1909): 232–36.

7   Miller, "Effects of Emancipation," 289.

8   For two examples, see W. M. Bevis, "Psychological Traits of the Southern Negro with Observations as to Some of His Psychoses," *American Journal of Insanity* 78 (July 1921): 69–78; Mary O'Malley, "Psychoses in the Colored Race: A Study in Comparative Psychiatry," *American Journal of Psychiatry* 71 (October 1914): 309–37.

9   "Ethnology," *JNMA* 4 (October–December 1912): 354.

10 Gerald N. Grob, *Mental Illness and American Society, 1875–1940* (Princeton, N.J.: Princeton University Press, 1983), 32–46.

11 Ibid., 51–69; Albert Deutsch, *The Mentally Ill in America: A History of Their Care and Treatment from Colonial Times,* 2nd ed. (New York: Columbia University Press, 1946), 276–77; Jacques M. Quen, "Asylum Psychiatry, Neurology, Social Work, and Mental Hygiene: An Exploratory Study in Interprofessional History," *Journal of the History of the Behavioral Sciences* 13 (1977): 3–11.

12 Grob, *Mental Illness and American Society,* quotes on 46 and 71. Also see Quen, "Asylum Psychiatry," esp. 7–10.

13 Elizabeth Lunbeck, *The Psychiatric Persuasion: Knowledge, Gender, and Power in Modern America* (Princeton, N.J.: Princeton University Press, 1994), 46–77.

14 "The Dawn of a Better Day," *JNMA* 17 (October–December 1925): 209–10; "Opening of State Hospital for the Colored Insane in West Virginia," *JNMA* 18 (July–September 1926): 136.

15 See Vanessa Northington Gamble, *Making a Place for Ourselves: The Black Hospital Movement, 1920–1945* (New York: Oxford University Press, 1995), 42, for figures on black hospitals in the United States.

16 Gordon was on the Jefferson Medical College's faculty, and his articles on the hereditary nature of neurosis and psychosis regularly appeared in the *JNMA* in the 1920s.

17 Rose, *Psychology and Selfhood,* 28.

18 Charles Prudhomme and David F. Musto, "Historical Perspectives on

Mental Health and Racism in the United States," in *Racism and Mental Health: Essays*, ed. Charles V. Willie, Bernard M. Kramer, and Bertram S. Brown (Pittsburgh, Pa.: University of Pittsburgh Press, 1973), 42–43; Jeanne Spurlock, "Early and Contemporary Pioneers," in Spurlock, *Black Psychiatrists and American Psychiatry*, 5–7; *Annual Report College of Medicine Howard University, 1941–1942*, 8, in Howardiana Collection, Moorland–Spingarn Research Center, Howard University, Washington, D.C.; Elam, "Development of the Department of Psychiatry," 70, 73; James Summerville, *Educating Black Doctors: A History of Meharry Medical College* (Tuscaloosa: University of Alabama Press, 1983), 146.

19 Thomas J. Ward Jr., *Black Physicians in the Jim Crow South* (Fayetteville: University of Arkansas Press, 2003), 60, 72–74. There were exceptions. For the biography of Liberian-born Solomon Fuller, who did postgraduate work with psychiatric luminaries Emile Kraepelin and Alois Alzheimer at the University of Munich, see Morais, *History of the Afro-American in Medicine*, 104–5.

20 Abraham Flexner, *Medical Education in the United States and Canada: A Report to the Carnegie Foundation for the Advancement of Teaching* (1910; repr., New York: Arno Press, 1972), 180.

21 John A. Kenney, "Health Problems of the Negroes," *JNMA* 3 (April–June 1911): 127; Byrd and Cayton, *American Health Dilemma*, 178–79.

22 Smith, *Sick and Tired*, 10–11; Samuel K. Roberts Jr., *Infectious Fear: Politics, Disease, and the Health Effects of Segregation* (Chapel Hill: University of North Carolina Press, 2009), 47–55.

23 Smith, *Sick and Tired*, 34.

24 A. M. Brown, "The Profession and Conservation of Negro Health," *JNMA* 6 (October–December 1914): 200.

25 DeHaven Hinkson, "Problems in the Rehabilitation of Victims of War," *JNMA* 14 (October–December 1922): 229–31.

26 L. B. Rogers to National Medical Association, June 2, 1923, reprinted in *JNMA* 15 (July–September 1923): 204.

27 For in-depth discussions of the Tuskegee controversy, see Gamble, *Making a Place for Ourselves*, 70–104; Raymond Wolters, *The New Negro on Campus: Black College Rebellions of the 1920s* (Princeton, N.J.: Princeton University Press, 1975), 137–91.

28 Rose, *Psychology and Selfhood*, 18–19.

29 "Dawn of a Better Day," 210.

30 Kenney, "Review of Francis M. Barnes Jr., *An Introduction to the Study of Mental Disorders*," *JNMA* 16 (January–March 1924): 75.

31 For examples, see Gordon, "Mental Abnormalities and the Problem of Eugenics," *JNMA* 15 (January–March 1923): 5–10; and Bailey, "Mental Hygiene: Its Necessity and Socio-Economic Importance," *JNMA* 17 (January–March 1925): 1–5.

32 George C. Branche, "Syphilis of the Brain and Cord," *JNMA* 21 (April–June 1929): 52–57; Alan P. Smith, "Mental Hygiene and the American Negro,"

JNMA 23 (January–March 1931): 1–10; Prince P. Barker, "Neuropsychiatry in the Practice of Medicine and Surgery," *JNMA* 23 (July–September 1931): 109–16.

33   "Department of Neuropsychiatry," *JNMA* 25 (November 1933): 192–94; "Dr. Alan P. Smith Elected to Membership in the American Psychiatric Association," *JNMA* 22 (October–December 1930): 205; "Who's Who— Dr. Prince P. Barker," *JNMA* 32 (November 1940): 138. This increasing attention to mental disease in the interwar period contrasts somewhat to the mainstream (white) medical profession, where mental illness was very early on understood within a biomedical framework, even if those who made its treatment their professional purpose were somewhat marginalized within the AMA. Nervous and mental diseases were subjects within the AMA's Section on Medical Jurisprudence as early as 1887 and received their own section in 1900. See Grob, *Mental Illness and American Society,* 265–87; Morris Fishbein, *A History of the American Medical Association, 1847 to 1947* (Philadelphia: W. B. Saunders Company, 1947), 1095, 1149–50.

34   Smith, "Mental Hygiene and the American Negro," 1; Barker, "Psychiatry and General Medicine," *JNMA* 32 (September 1940): 222; "Psychiatry and Medicine," *JNMA* 27 (February 1935): 28–29.

35   Lunbeck, *Psychiatric Persuasion,* 118–19; Nathan G. Hale Jr., *The Rise and Crisis of Psychoanalysis in the United States: Freud and the Americans, 1917–1985* (New York: Oxford University Press, 1995), 157–66. Dynamic psychiatry was an expansive category, including Freudian psychoanalysis and Adolf Meyer's psychobiology, which relied less on the unconscious as an etiological factor. There were probably more psychobiologists than psychoanalysts in the ranks of black psychiatrists in the mid-twentieth century. As Prince Barker pointed out in a 1940 article, "Psychobiology is taught in the leading medical schools and is doubtlessly America's major contribution to psychiatry, competing with and in many instances supplementing or supplanting Freudian Theory." See Barker, "Psychiatry and General Medicine," 222–23.

36   Grob, *Mental Illness and American Society,* 286–87. Also see Hale, *Rise and Crisis of Psychoanalysis,* 158–59.

37   This obstacle persisted into the postwar period. See Harold Rosen and Jerome D. Frank, "Negroes in Psychotherapy," *American Journal of Psychiatry* 119 (November 1962): 456–60.

38   Smith, "The Availability of Facilities for Negroes Suffering from Mental and Nervous Diseases," *Journal of Negro Education* 6 (July 1937): 450–54, quote on 453.

39   "The Proposed Development of Teaching Centers for Negro Personnel in Psychiatry," *JNMA* 32 (January 1940): 34. The conference did directly lead to the founding of a mental hygiene society at U.S. Veterans' Hospital No. 91. See C. P. Prudhomme, "A Mental Hygiene Society Organized at Tuskegee," *JNMA* 33 (January 1941): 34–35.

40   "Two New Clinics Planned: Harlem Hospital to Have Tumor and Mental

Hygiene Services," *New York Times,* May 26, 1943, 20; Dennis Doyle, "'Where the Need Is Greatest': Social Psychiatry and Race-Blind Universalism in Harlem's Lafargue Clinic, 1946–1958," *Bulletin of the History of Medicine* 83 (Winter 2009): 746–74; Gerald Markowitz and David Rosner, *Children, Race, and Power: Kenneth and Mamie Clark's Northside Center* (Charlottesville: University of Virginia Press, 1996).

41 "Mental Hygienists Hold N.Y. Confab," *The Chicago Defender,* natl. ed., February 20, 1943, 6; "Guidance Clinics Aid 900 Children Yearly," *Washington Post,* January 29, 1941, 5; "Howard Dean Hails Interne Acceptance," *Washington Post,* October 17, 1948, M21.

42 Joseph H. Douglass, "Racial Integration in the Psychiatric Field," *JNMA* 57 (January 1965): 1–7. Douglass's conclusions were not race-specific. They were based on the ideal ratio of one psychiatrist for every 2,000 people.

43 Rosen and Frank, "Negroes in Psychotherapy"; Jonathan Metzl, *The Protest Psychosis: How Schizophrenia Became a Black Disease* (Boston: Beacon Press, 2009).

44 I take the ideas of the differential visibility and the commodification of diseases from Keith Wailoo, *Dying in the City of the Blues: Sickle Cell Anemia and the Politics of Race and Health* (Chapel Hill: University of North Carolina Press, 2001). On commodification, Wailoo writes, "To call attention to disease as 'commodity' is merely to emphasize its place in a network of exchange relationships, where—much like any object—the *disease concept* and the *illness experience* acquired value and could leverage resources, money, or social concessions" (9). "Landscapes of prevailing diseases" is quoted on 55.

45 The black medical profession continued to vigorously take on the issue of mental illness in the wake of World War II. See Ellen Dwyer, "Psychiatry and Race during World War II," *Journal of the History of Medicine and Allied Sciences* 61 (April 2006): 117–43.

46 Lunbeck, *Psychiatric Persuasion,* 307.

47 Rose, *Psychology and Selfhood,* 20–32, 69–81.

"An Indispensable Service"

Midwives and Medical Officials after New Mexico Statehood

LENA MCQUADE-SALZFASS

"ABOUT 800 MIDWIVES deliver babies in New Mexico," reported state director of maternal and child health Hester Curtis in the late 1930s.[1] She continued her assessment of the primarily Spanish-speaking Nuevomexicana midwives of New Mexico, explaining that their "chief qualifications seem to be extreme age, poor eyesight and a large stock of superstitions with which to meet emergencies."[2] In conclusion, Curtis lamented that because of the rural nature of the state, "time-honored folkways," and the lack of readily available medical facilities, it was "unrealistic to suppose" that the public health department could "eliminate" New Mexico's midwives. Hester Curtis echoed the sentiments of many early twentieth-century medical professionals in her disparaging appraisal of midwives as second-rate health workers. Read more closely, however, her account also reveals the specific ways midwifery in New Mexico was deeply intertwined with constructions of the state's racial difference and the legacies of colonialism that shaped public health.

Delfina Cordova, a practicing midwife in Gallina, New Mexico who "never lost a mother" in her thirty years of active health service to the women and families in her rural community, challenged the notion that midwives provided substandard care. She asserted, "Women who had their babies at home were better off and recuperated sooner and more completely than those who went to the hospital or to the doctor in town."[3] Cordova argued that New Mexican midwives were successful because they attended women in their own homes, remained flexible about payment, and provided services in Spanish and within a more familiar cultural framework, all of which facilitated better birth outcomes. Refuting the charge that midwifery was a symbol of New

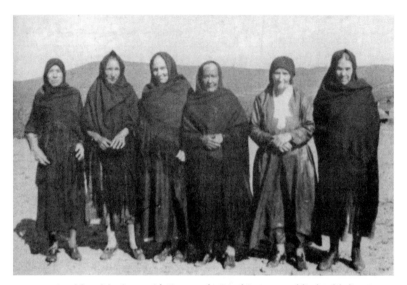

FIGURE 6.1. New Mexican midwives as depicted in state public health literature. *New Mexico Health Officer,* December 1938, p. 47. New Mexico Supreme Court Law Library State Agency Collection. Courtesy New Mexico State Records Center and Archives, Accession No. 1998-027.

Mexico's ongoing backwardness, Cordova and other New Mexican midwives insisted that the public health department recognize their crucial health care work. The divergent perspectives of Hester Curtis and Delfina Cordova highlight the politicization of midwifery and the contested process of making meaning about birth attendants in New Mexico in the first half of the twentieth century.

In 1912, New Mexico joined the nation as its forty-seventh state and ushered in a new era of political enfranchisement for the state's majority Nuevomexicano population. Although statehood extended the full legal privileges of citizenship to New Mexicans, most Americans considered Nuevomexicanos to be of a presumed Indian–Spanish–Mexican descent as well as inferior and illegitimate members of an imagined white nation. As nationally circulating newspapers described it, Nuevomexicanos constituted a "mongrel population too ignorant and lazy to assume the privileges of full citizenship."[4] In the politically and socially fraught post-statehood period, *parteras*—or Spanish-speaking midwives—played a key discursive role in the production of New Mexico as a racially distinct and suspect political space.[5] The 1919 formation of the state public health department marked the initial campaign to manage and modernize the health practices of New Mexicans. The attempt to regulate and replace parteras through midwifery laws and birth education classes was crucial to this project. The public health department implicitly relied on the irreplaceable labor of local midwives, while public health campaigns publicly perpetuated racialized depictions of Nuevomexicana midwives as anachronistic, "superstitious," "folk" healers—relics of New Mexico's cultural past that had to be "eliminated" with state incorporation. Coming out of increased interactions between state-sanctioned public health workers and community-based health care practitioners, state public health workers marshaled the long-established practice of parteras as evidence of the racial distance between Nuevomexicano communities and emerging medical norms in the United States.

In the United States, the medicalization of childbirth involved shifting pregnancy and childbirth to hospitals under obstetric authority. By the early twentieth century, pregnant women and their families who had access increasingly sought out the option to give birth in hospitals. After a sustained campaign by American physicians to situate labor and delivery within their professional domain, coupled with public policies regulating and prohibiting lay reproductive techniques, middle-class women increasingly opted for obstetricians over midwives, effectively pushing midwives out of practice.[6] This was the case in spaces throughout the nation where women were excluded from mainstream medical care on the basis of racial segregation, poverty, geography, immigrant status, and lack of English language fluency. In marginalized communities, women continued to serve as and rely on midwives to meet basic reproductive health care needs.[7] Noting this stratification of birth services in the first half of the twentieth century, historian Susan Smith argued that "American midwifery did not disappear—it was racialized."[8]

Expanding Smith's framework, this chapter turns our attention to midwifery in New Mexico, where more than 900 Nuevomexicana parteras delivered an estimated 40 percent of state citizens throughout the late 1920s and more than 27 percent of births by the end of the 1930s.[9] The history of midwifery in New Mexico stands out from that in other states because of New Mexico's specific geopolitical relationship with the nation, including the imperial and colonial dynamics of incorporation, the numerical majority of enfranchised Mexican American (and, later, Native American) citizens after statehood, and the legal designation of both Spanish and English as official state languages.[10] Because of the formal enfranchisement of Mexican Americans through statehood, the mostly Anglo public health authorities in New Mexico used the work of parteras to symbolize a key racial difference between New Mexico and the United States and to justify their own labors educating and disciplining these "Mexican" midwives. This chapter argues that after New Mexico became a state, midwifery came to symbolize all that was different about New Mexico in the United States.

COLONIAL CONTEXTS FOR NEW MEXICAN REPRODUCTIVE HEALTH

The history of New Mexico's imperial acquisition from Mexico by the United States in 1848, followed by a protracted period of colonial relations between the New Mexico territory and the federal government (1850–1912), shaped the contours of public health care in this region. After the Mexican–American War (1846–1848), the Treaty of Guadalupe Hidalgo stipulated that Mexican inhabitants of the newly conquered U.S. Southwest could remain in the territory and become U.S. federal citizens. Federal citizenship in the United States entitled New Mexicans to the protections of the Constitution but, importantly, did not extend the political rights (including the right to elect their own officials and to self-representation at the federal level) conferred only through citizenship in a recognized state. Over the next sixty-two years, Congress, backed by public sentiment, rejected New Mexico's bids for statehood no less than fifteen times, leaving the territory and its inhabitants in a subordinated position of provisional inclusion within the nation. As Albert Beveridge, influential senator and chair of the Senate Committee on Territories, surmised, New Mexico "had a savage and alien population."[11] He deemed that New Mexicans were incapable of self-rule, necessitating that "we govern our territories without their consent."[12]

Legal historian Laura Gómez aptly characterized the relationship between territorial New Mexico and the United States as that of a "contiguous colony" wherein a Mexican population was conquered in the U.S. war with Mexico and subsequently denied the right of self-governance for more than three generations. The New Mexico territory was an important piece of the mainland westward expansion that would be incorporated as a state once the region was sufficiently "Americanized," or once Euro-American settlers gained a stronger foothold in politics and the economy, including the practice of medicine and public health. The always contentious colonizing process of superimposing Euro-American ideals and institutions onto existing Native and Nuevomexicano communities had its roots in the territorial period and continued after statehood was granted in 1912.

During this period, health maintenance and medical practices became key arenas for colonial impositions, resistances, and negotiations. Vaccination of children in New Mexico provided a key example of national publicity and community assertion. In 1905, the *New York Times* featured a full-page article on New Mexico titled "Most Un-American Part of the United States." As proof of the danger of considering New Mexico part of the nation, Gilson Willets singled out the "un-American attitude of the Mexicans of New Mexico towards the public menace called smallpox." "Not one Mexican in a hundred among the poorer classes" believed that their family could avoid smallpox, the author erroneously concluded, "so they do nothing to stamp it out."[13] According to this account, the absence of vaccination among Nuevomexicanos served as evidence of unfitness, lack of drive, and even the contaminating hazard of New Mexicans. Vaccination against smallpox, a European disease introduced to Indian peoples in the Americas during the Spanish conquest, first began in New Mexico in 1808 but dropped off because of a lack of funding during the Mexican and American territorial periods, leaving many poor families no other option but to suffer or die. Moreover, observers blamed inadequate health provisions on "Mexicans of the poorer classes" and used them as proof of the need to "wait until this most un-American part of our country is Americanized" before extending statehood.[14] As U.S. territorial subjects, Nuevomexicanos were not given access to the vaccine but then were also publicly blamed for their resulting infections. This continued after statehood in 1912, leading one Nuevomexicano community in Rio Arriba to implement their own measures to protect their community's health. After the vaccination of a few children in 1923, community members cast back to health knowledge developed during Spanish and Mexican rule and "inoculated everybody from those first treated."[15] In the absence of adequate public health services, the people themselves manufactured and administered their own vaccines. Even after statehood was granted, state and federal officials continued to ignore the health care needs of Nuevomexicanos, forcing many poor and rural communities to take health matters into their own hands. Colonial relationships in territorial New Mexico worked through and reinforced ideologies of racial hierarchy and white supremacy, imbricated with heteropatriarchal norms of gender and sexuality. During the territorial period, federal legislators continuously denied New Mexico's petitions for statehood well after it had met all the numerical and "native-born" population requirements for admission as a state. To cite one example, both Idaho and Wyoming, rural western territories with smaller populations, were both granted statehood two decades before New Mexico.[16] Undergirding these federal rejections of New Mexican statehood was an ideology of racially exclusive national reproduction, one that valued only births to white, "fit" parents. The births and lives of Nuevomexicanos and Native Americans in the territory of New Mexico literally did not count toward the Euro-American body politic of the nation envisioned by the Congress. Congressional representatives characterized the Spanish-speaking people of New Mexico as a "mongrel" race comprising a "mixture" of Spanish, Mexican, Indian, African, and European parentage and thus unfit for self-governance.[17] These officials associated Nuevomexicanos with mongrelization—or fantasies of animalistic and unregulated sexuality and reproduction. In the minds of congressmen John C. Box and Thomas A. Jenkins, because Mexicans themselves were a product of "racial mixing" they were especially likely to further intermingle with whites and African Americans, making "the blood of all three races flow back and forth between them in a distressing process of mongrelization."[18] Federally authorized debates about New Mexico's fitness for national belonging hinged on constructed notions of New Mexicans as racially problematic sexual and reproductive subjects. Nuevomexicanos vigorously refuted these dominant perceptions of their racial inferiority and inability to manage their own well-being. In one example, some leading Nuevomexicanos joined Euro-American statehood boosters in advancing a gendered counterlogic, one that depicted the Spanish-speaking people of the territory as the direct descendants of "pure" and "noble" Spanish women, heirs themselves to a colonial heritage.[19] Scholars have pointed out that claims of "pure" Spanish lineages in New Mexico are historically inaccurate, do not account for the *mestizaje* in the territory, and rely on problematic notions of white supremacy that privilege Spanish and European descent above Native and African ancestry. This counterdiscourse of proper European reproduction can also be understood as an attempt to legitimize Nuevomexicanos as valid citizen subjects within the terms of the nation-state. These racialized struggles over reproductive self-competence and citizenship formed the context in which public health developed in the state.

The sixty-two-year period New Mexico spent as a federal territory of the United States left an indelible mark on the health care infrastructure and on the bodies and well-being of the inhabitants of this region. The late development of a state public health department in 1919 and subsequently the state's ineligibility to participate in federally funded health projects stand out as clear consequences of New Mexico's colonial relationship to the nation. Without an established public health department, New Mexico was ineligible to receive grants from the Federal Children's Bureau in 1918 and under the National Rural Health Act of 1919.[20] In a largely rural state with the highest infant mortality rate in the United States, these continuing forms of national exclusion had tangible negative consequences. Even though New Mexico enriched the nation through its vast addition of territory, natural resources, labor power, and the facilitation of transcontinental railroads, the majority of Nuevomexicanos did not benefit from this transfer of wealth, nor were they eligible for the same federal funds enjoyed by other American citizens in states with existing public health departments.

Once New Mexico became a state, Nuevomexicanos played an important role in the development of public health. In the years preceding the state public health bill, several health crises garnered much public attention. First, the army turned away a number of New Mexicans attempting to enlist during World War I, ostensibly because they had tuberculosis. In 1918, a deadly influenza epidemic swept through the state, killing thousands, including the youngest son of the governor, Octaviano Larrazolo. As one health official remembered, at this point, "the people's demand [for public health] was unmistakable."[21] Governor Larrazolo oversaw the establishment of a state department of health in 1919, and he appointed a local leading Hispana, Adelina Otero-Warren, as chair of the state board of health from 1919 to 1922. As Ann Massmann explains, Otero-Warren's "position as chair of this committee is particularly noteworthy because it was an otherwise all-male, public health doctor–dominated board."[22] Following Otero-Warren, Hispanas consistently held one of the five appointed positions on the state board of health from 1933 through the 1950s.[23]

Although Nuevomexicanos were instrumental in establishing and monitoring the state public health department, this representation did not carry over into the logic or staffing of this state agency. From 1919 through the 1950s, of the more than one hundred employees who served as Public Health Department directors, division directors, and district health officers, all had Euro-American surnames. It was not until 1953 that Alex Armijo became the first Spanish-surnamed director of a department, division, or district of public health in New Mexico.[24] For twenty-four years, in a state where Nuevomexicanos made up more than half the population, the state health department never gave state administrative medical authority to a Mexican American. This gross underrepresentation marked public health in New Mexico as a Euro-American dominated space and continued to make the colonial notion that Nuevomexicanos were unfit to manage their health part of the continuing dynamic of public health in twentieth-century New Mexico.

Some of the first steps of the newly established public health department involved "Americanizing" birth practices and medical licensing in New Mexico. As historical sociologist Elena Gutiérrez argues in *Fertile Matters,* discursive and material control over reproduction and women's bodies "served as a crucial tool of colonization and social repression of entire communities."[25] Women's ability to give birth is politically charged in part because reproductive capacity represents the potential to produce future citizens or territorial subjects. Beyond giving birth to the nation's future generations, reproductive capacity is also linked to the transmission of social and cultural identities through child rearing and family maintenance.[26] Therefore, nation-states closely monitor and regulate women's reproductive capacities to uphold heteronormative patriarchal standards of domesticity, in addition to the inheritance of wealth, notions of racial purity, and images of national unity.[27] In the post-statehood era in New Mexico, the public health department moved to monitor and standardize birth practices. Women's bodies, their function before and after delivery, and the work of birth attendants came under direct public health jurisdiction and scrutiny. The public health department was particularly interested in parteras and their practices, especially the degree to which these midwives diverged from embodied white, middle-class, and professional norms.

INDISPENSABILITY OF PARTERAS IN NEW MEXICO

Writing at a time when midwifery was still nationally controversial, bilingual nurses and lifelong residents of northern New Mexico Mary Marquez and Consuelo Pacheco concluded, "Tribute should be paid to her, for it was the partera who, at a particular period in New Mexico's development, provided an indispensable service to the Spanish-American population."[28] Parteras in New Mexico played a vital role in the region's reproductive health, serving primarily rural, economically impoverished Nuevomexicanas and their families who often had no other access to physicians or hospitals well into the twentieth century. In addition to facilitating the physiological aspects of labor, delivery, and postpartum care, parteras also attended to the psychological, spiritual, religious, and cultural dimensions of giving birth.[29] Parteras' skills as community health workers combined with their accessibility helps to explain why Hispanos continued to prefer parteras to medical or hospital delivery through World War II.

The lifework of two different parteras, Virginia Perea Sánchez from San Mateo and Susana Archuleta from Santa Fe, exemplify the multidimensional roles parteras undertook as community health workers. Responsible for delivering hundreds of babies in her west New Mexico town of San Mateo, Sánchez is remembered for her work not only in assisting laboring women but also in addressing the unmet health needs of her predominantly Hispano community. "To this day," reflected San Mateo resident Abe Peña, "I think of Doña Virginia Perea Sánchez as my surrogate mother, someone who was there when I breathed life and gave that first cry."[30] Peña recalled that the Civilian Conservation Corps brought the first doctor to San Mateo in the 1930s but that the agency denied the doctor's services to the surrounding community unless it was an emergency. Peña continued, "But Doña Virginia was always there, and in many ways she was more than a doctor to us."[31] Peña's recollection points to his assessment of the relative merits of parteras, who were committed to addressing a range of community health needs. In her role as a midwife and healer, Sánchez helped deliver babies and created social health networks essential for survival in the face of poverty and racist exclusion from mainstream medical care. Likewise, Santa Fe midwife Susana Archuleta elaborated on her expansive understanding of community health:

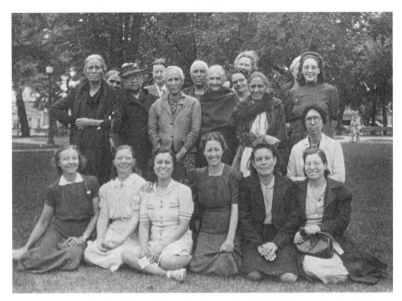

FIGURE 6.2. Midwife Club members, Las Vegas, New Mexico, ca. 1941. Fran Leeper Buss Oral History Collection, Schlesinger Library, Radcliffe Institute, Harvard University, W382248-1.

The midwife was a friend of the family. She made herself that way. We knew when the husbands were unemployed, and we had a lot of deliveries that we were never paid for. Or sometimes people would give us a string of *chile* or they would butcher a calf for us. That was money. But there we'd be, money or not.[32]

In this example, Archuleta explains that as a midwife in the 1940s she was also aware of the larger economic and social circumstances of the families of the women who she delivered. Given that they accepted various forms of payment or performed deliveries for free, Archuleta highlights that being a partera was principally about providing midwifery services regardless of monetary gain. Her emphasis that a midwife "made herself" a friend of the family implies that parteras did more than deliver babies but also were consciously and actively part of the larger social fabric that facilitated the overall health and welfare of their communities.

In their practice, parteras went beyond the biomedical model of diagnosing disease and focused instead on the larger social context in which women experienced pregnancy and labor. Parteras were fluent in Spanish (usually the first language of their patients) and often shared religious, spiritual, and even, at times, familial ties with the women they assisted. For example, parteras evoked Roman Catholic saints such as San Ramón to ease delivery and protect the mother and infant. One partera, Jesusita Aragón, hung a painting of Nuestra Señora de Guadalupe above her delivery bed in her home.[33] Some parteras maintained lifelong connections with the babies they delivered, at times even serving as the *madrina*, or godmother. In contrast, some Euro-American doctors in New Mexico were unable to speak Spanish, which was a major limitation in the officially bilingual state of New Mexico. As Dr. Johnson, a monolingual English-speaking physician performing deliveries at the Medical Center in Cuba, New Mexico, put it, "I know these women like to talk to someone in Spanish, and I don't understand Spanish."[34] Clearly, many factors contributed to the preference for parteras.[35]

In New Mexico, parteras were widespread throughout the state and continued to deliver more than a quarter of the babies until the 1940s. The actual percentage of statewide partera-assisted deliveries may have been even higher because not all parteras or the families they assisted went through official state channels to document births. This high percentage of midwife deliveries highlights the importance and autonomy of parteras in the Hispano-majority regions of central and northern New Mexico. State vital statistics from 1929 through 1941 indicate that midwives were active in all thirty-one New Mexico counties, although their rate of delivery varied based on the demographics of the population. The predominantly Euro-American regions in the southeastern part of the state bordering Texas had the lowest percentages of midwife-assisted births, whereas the counties with Hispano majorities along the Rio Grande and the Sangre de Cristo Mountains in the central and northern parts of the state had midwife delivery rates above 50 percent.[36] A 1930s federal study of the Spanish-speaking villages in northern New Mexico further documents the existence of active parteras in almost all of the thirty-two villages surveyed.[37] Parteras' extensive work was particularly evident in the Hispano region of northern New Mexico, including Guadalupe, Mora, Sandoval, San Miguel, and Taos counties, where parteras and family members made up for the lack of doctors and nurses, assisting at 70 percent or more of all births into the 1940s.[38] As recently as the 1960s, San Miguel and

Mora counties, which are primarily Hispano, had partera delivery rates of 29 and 21 percent, respectively.[39]

A closer snapshot of birth practitioners in Valencia County, New Mexico provides additional evidence of the indispensability of parteras to Hispano communities. In 1928, patients with Spanish surnames represented just over one-half of recorded births. Records indicate that there were no doctors present for these Nuevomexicano births. Instead, parteras delivered 83 percent of these babies, with family members and neighbors delivering the remaining 17 percent. In contrast, doctors delivered 88 percent of the babies to women with Euro-American surnames.[40] These birth statistics reveal a strong association between licensed physicians and Euro-American births as well as between parteras and Mexican American births. These statistics illustrate the racial dimension of medical access to licensed physicians and, perhaps, a strong preference among Nuevomexicanos for the skills of parteras.

To fully grasp the indispensability of parteras, it is also necessary to historicize the absence of public health and private medicine in many early twentieth-century New Mexican communities. In 1922, by its own admission, the New Mexico public health department estimated that only 35 percent of the state population was receiving even "moderately adequate" health services.[41] Almost a decade later, the public health department was reaching only an additional 5 percent of the population. In large part, these dismal health service statistics stemmed from chronic underfunding of public health in the state and a subsequent absence of sufficient health personnel. During the first few years after its establishment in 1919, the New Mexico public health department funded only four visiting nurses for a state over one-and-a-half times the size of New England. Additional federal funding, made available through the Social Security Act in 1936, raised the number of county public health nurses to forty-two; this still meant some counties in New Mexico had only one public health nurse.

In addition to the shortage of public health services, many New Mexicans also had very limited access to physicians, who charged for their services and usually practiced in regions with higher population densities. A national comparative study of health factors in 1940 found that the U.S. average ratio of physicians to citizens was 1 to 748, whereas in New Mexico this ratio was 1 to 1,211.[42] New Mexico was a large, predominantly rural state crisscrossed by deserts and mountain ranges, raising serious transportation issues for rural residents. Many New Mexican families lived more than one hundred miles from the nearest doctor or hospital, further reducing access to modern medical care.

Even if geography and the scarcity of physicians could be addressed, the costs of private medical care at birth were prohibitive for the many New Mexicans who lived in poverty and at subsistence levels. For example, in 1937 the per capita savings for the United States was $156, whereas in New Mexico it was only $26.[43] Typically, doctors in New Mexico charged $30 for maternity care in a hospital—more than the total annual saving of the average New Mexican. In contrast, some parteras charged only $4 to $10 for deliveries and also accepted other forms of payment. According to a 1941 Work Projects Administration oral history, parteras "never charged for their services, but left it to the patient's family to give what they thought their services were worth."[44] Some families gave parteras corn, beans, chili, goats, or grain. If a family could not pay, "the father of the child helped the partera's husband with his planting or gathered his crops for him; or sometimes the women would go in the fall and plaster the partera's house. All tried to pay, for they never knew how often they would need her."[45] Some doctors in New Mexico refused to treat rural Hispana women. The federal 1935 Tewa Basin Study on the lives and health of rural Hispanos in northern New Mexico recorded, "Doctors will not make the trip out [to Hispano villages] unless sure of pay," and, the study concluded, "the people are, of course, unable to pay."[46] In the face of this exclusion from medical care, the work of parteras truly was indispensable for many economically impoverished Nuevomexicanos.

Not all Nuevomexicanos relied on parteras; some notable exceptions illustrate how socioeconomic class further complicated the use of birth attendants in New Mexico. It is possible that modern birth practices served as part of a larger constellation of identity construction through which some Nuevomexicanos could further their elite status. For example, when Cleofas Jaramillo, the daughter of a wealthy Hispano family, became pregnant in 1908, her husband "engaged the most noted obstetrical specialist" for the birth, requiring the couple to travel out of the state to Denver, Colorado.[47] Though quite unusual, this example demonstrates that class status might grant access to health care unavailable to most Nuevomexicanos.

For most Nuevomexicanos, however, a preference for parteras

coupled with significant structural and institutional barriers that compromised access to hospital and physician health care made midwifery indispensable well into the twentieth century. In this respect, New Mexico resembled other regions of the country where racialized marginalization in medicine extended the period during which midwives were both actively sought for their skills and crucial in their provision of care, as also documented among African Americans in the South and Japanese Americans on the West Coast and in Hawai'i.[48] Scholars of race and midwifery have noted that the presence of practicing midwives in communities of color and immigrant neighborhoods throughout the twentieth century often signaled a complicated combination of race-based exclusions from mainstream medicine and pregnant women's inclination toward birth attendants who shared linguistic, cultural, and religious worldviews.[49] The indispensability of parteras in New Mexico indicated both the inequitable distribution of private and public health among the state's rural and economically impoverished Nuevomexicano communities and a preference for the extensive community health work provided by parteras.

MIDWIFERY LAWS AND SHIFTING ACCOUNTABILITY

In the first half of the twentieth century, New Mexico passed a series of midwifery laws that required parteras to register with the public health department, attend birth education classes, and restrict the scope of their practice. These midwifery laws looked very similar to other efforts across the country, but the distinct historical situation of New Mexico turned midwife licensing into a form of colonial incorporation after statehood. First, the very existence of these laws in New Mexico indicates that the public health department was aware not only of the extensive work of parteras but also of their own inability to replace the critical labor of these health care practitioners. In essence, midwifery laws and education requirements in New Mexico were a mechanism for the public health department to appropriate the work of parteras and dismiss their extensive empirical knowledge and autonomy. Second, midwifery licensing laws placed reproductive health care practices under the purview of the state public health department. This was an attempt to shift parteras' accountability away from the communities where they worked and toward the state institution charged with monitoring and credentialing their practices. Finally, these laws transformed midwifery in New Mexico by outlawing specific reproductive health techniques and prohibiting certain women from practicing midwifery. Consequently, through institutionalizing mechanisms to ensure partera compliance, these laws rendered certain birth practices and practitioners illegal. In this way, midwifery was a microcosm of a larger process of colonization where the health practices of the formerly territorial subjects of New Mexico were appropriated, scrutinized, and regulated to meet Euro-American and middle-class health norms.

Within three years of its establishment, the New Mexico public health department promulgated the state's first laws governing the practice of midwifery. Initially issued in 1922 and updated in 1937, these regulations dictated the parameters of legal midwifery practice. Before state-organized health programs, parteras practiced their skills based on the demands of their local communities, and community members held parteras accountable by requesting the services of those who most met their needs. As Ramon Del Castillo explained in his life history of Diana Velazquez, a *curandera* and partera from Texas, "Velazquez earned her 'credentials' when she proved her healing skills to the community. . . . Her reputation flourishes as a result of actual work accomplished, in contrast to traditional Western practices, where one must certify theoretical competence before being allowed to practice."[50] The 1922 midwife laws shifted existing systems of health accountability, entitling only the public health department, not communities, pregnant women, and their families, to determine the adequacy of birth practitioners.

The 1922 public health midwife regulations defined midwifery as conducting or managing any "form or stage of parturient labor" by a person "not duly licensed by the laws of the State of New Mexico to practice medicine."[51] It is important to note that this law was the first to establish labor and delivery as a medical event in New Mexico. Oral histories with Mexican Americans in New Mexico reveal alternative conceptions of childbirth as a time when "the whole family would rally around" and "render an opinion" on how they thought the birth was progressing.[52] The midwife regulations of 1922 legally medicalized childbirth, entitling only those licensed to practice medicine or certified as midwives to manage births.

In constructing the legal parameters for acceptable reproductive practices, this law also created a new category of "illegal" birth practitioners. Under the heading "Midwife Prosecuted," a 1929 publication of the New Mexico public health department reported, "Upon the request by the State Bureau of Health a midwife operating in Sierra County was prosecuted last week, in the District Court at Hillsboro, for failure to report births that she attended."[53] Although the outcome of this particular trial was not recorded, it should be noted that this midwife faced prosecution because of her failure to report births, not necessarily because of her work delivering infants. The threat of prosecution affected the work of traditional birth attendants and healers in New Mexico. For example, lifelong *curandera* Gregorita Rodriguez from Cerro Gordo outside of Santa Fe explained, "The people still came to me for treatment. I hesitated to treat them without the proper papers, but I did not know how I would ever be licensed" because she had previously been rejected for certification by a local hospital on the grounds that she was "too old."[54] Gregorita continued, "I had been warned that I needed a license to protect myself in a world where that was important."[55] Public health midwifery laws were intended to protect the public from potential harm from unregulated practitioners, but when applied in New Mexico these laws also transformed Nuevomexicanas with extensive community support and a wide repertoire of healing practices into illegal subjects.

Mirroring other midwifery laws throughout the nation, New Mexico's 1922 midwifery law demarcated professional medical boundaries by institutionalizing a hierarchy of practitioners. Because there were simply too many people in New Mexico who chose not to or could not access doctors and hospitals, parteras remained a crucial part of health maintenance in the state. Their vital presence forced New Mexico's public health department to focus most of its policy efforts on incorporating parteras into the state health care system. Additionally, parteras were vocal advocates of their long-established craft, and because they were members of the Mexican American majority in the state, their existence and critical work on behalf of Nuevomexicano communities granted them a degree of negotiating power. The relative incorporation of parteras and other informally trained health practitioners challenged the racial boundaries around medicine in New Mexico.

Some medical professionals resented this challenge. The New Mexico midwife laws of 1922 appropriated the work of midwives, allowing the state to continue benefiting from their crucial services but also institutionalizing new legal parameters that ensured a familiar American racial hierarchy in reproductive health services. For example, in the midwife's pledge, parteras had to promise not to conduct any internal exams nor "pass fingers or instruments" into a woman's birth canal under any circumstances.[56] Demarcating the body's interior as the sole province of doctors limited the work of parteras and constructed a professional hierarchy relegating midwives to lower status positions in consolidating health fields. It also made the necessary and routine practices of many parteras illegal. Ostensibly this law was designed to reduce maternal infections, but in an era before antibiotics, medical professionals too were often unable to prevent and cure bacterial infections. For the most part, public health midwifery laws divested Nuevomexicanas of their autonomy as reproductive health care workers and invalidated their knowledge and training about birth and reproductive matters even while relying on their labor to address the shortage of state and federally funded public health services. Conversely, these laws also transferred legal and institutional authority about birth to primarily Euro-American male doctors and secondarily to Euro-American female public health nurses who had access to medical and public health education and credentialing.

Midwifery laws in New Mexico were part of a larger trend after statehood that brought the formerly territorial subjects of New Mexico into subordinate positions in an emerging national health care hierarchy. In this new era, parteras had to be granted permission to practice midwifery by the public health department rather than by their community, and their right to practice could be withheld or revoked. At the same time, these laws created a new space of illegality for parteras who refused or were unable to comply with new regulations. Statehood incorporation followed by midwifery laws created a limited and more scrutinized realm in which parteras practiced. As public health oversight of midwifery accelerated in the decades before World War II, parteras were often evoked as evidence of the foreign and racially distinct space of New Mexico. With the promulgation of midwifery laws, the public health department increasingly attempted to bring New Mexico's pregnancy and birth practices in line with national norms through midwifery education policies.

MIDWIFERY EDUCATION AND THE PRODUCTION
OF NEW MEXICAN "FOREIGNNESS"

Early public health efforts to address what officials saw as the inevitable problem of midwifery in New Mexico included raising funds
and attracting qualified public health nurses to educate and certify
midwives in the state. In describing public health work, health officials often perpetuated the notion that New Mexico was an exotic,
foreign space greatly in need of Americanization. "You may wonder
why any nurse would choose to work in a state [New Mexico] with
so few facilities," Dorothy Anderson, director of child hygiene and
public health nursing in New Mexico said to policymakers and public
health officials at a national conference for maternal and infant health
care in 1926.[57] She continued, explaining, "Her efforts are worthwhile
because of the great need for the work and the fact that even the most
ignorant try to follow her directions, even though in doing it they may
have to give up some age-old superstition."[58] In this national address,
Anderson depicted New Mexico as a region where white, female nurses
endowed with the "pioneer spirit" performed "greatly needed" work
educating "the most ignorant" New Mexicans who clung to "age-old
superstitions" and "believe[d] in their medicine women rather than in
modern methods."[59] In the context of New Mexico, descriptors such
as "superstitions" evoked the indigenous and Catholic health practices of Nuevomexicanos and racialized people of Spanish Mexican
descent. Typical of public depictions of New Mexico in the 1920s and
1930s, Anderson's statement contributed to the larger discourse that
produced New Mexico as an anomalous space within the nation, one
that needed reproductive health intervention to be brought within
national norms.

Public health midwifery education in New Mexico became financially feasible with the support of key pieces of federal legislation,
most importantly the Maternal and Infant Protection Act of 1921 (also
known as the Sheppard–Towner Act) and the Title V funds appropriated through the Social Security Act in 1936. At first, state-sponsored
midwifery education was conducted by a handful of public health nurses
who traveled the state educating midwives through ten elementary
classes that highlighted hygiene and compliance with public health regulations. In addition, the public health department began certifying lay

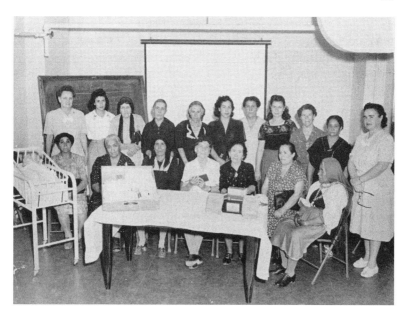

FIGURE 6.3. Midwife classes, Albuquerque, New Mexico, ca. 1945. Fran Leeper Buss Oral History Collection, Schlesinger Library, Radcliffe Institute, Harvard University, W382244-1.

midwives who had successfully completed training and had undergone an annual physical examination. In the late 1930s and increasingly as doctors and nurses left the state for World War II, midwifery education programs expanded through the work of public health nurse midwife consultants, midwife institutes, and the establishment of midwifery demonstration sites. Running through all these midwifery education programs were contestations and at times collaborations over what constituted acceptable knowledge and practice regarding birth. In this way, parteras turned midwife education into a contested site for negotiating New Mexico's and New Mexicans' belonging within the nation.

Teresa McGowan, one of the first Sheppard–Towner field nurses employed in New Mexico, exemplifies the experiences of many early public health nurses in the state. McGowan, a white woman originally from Idaho, was hired by the New Mexico pubic health department in 1923 to work for several months educating midwives in rural communities "far from doctors and trained nurses" in Doña Ana County, along the New Mexico–Mexico border.[60] Like most public health nurses working in New Mexico, McGowan was young, not yet married, and raised and trained outside the state of New Mexico. Although the records do not indicate whether McGowan herself was fluent in Spanish, many public health employees and doctors working in New Mexico did not speak the language of their patients. Furthermore, the training some public health nurses received did not adequately prepare them for the poverty they encountered in New Mexico. For example, McGowan routinely carried a "complete set of demonstration material" including clean bedding, clothing, and equipment. However, McGowan quickly discovered that she was ill equipped to address the reality in which parteras worked without access to consumer goods because "it is usually impossible for them [midwives] to buy even the least expensive articles." Working through these obstacles, McGowan trained and certified twenty-six midwives during her three-month educational tour of southern New Mexico.

Before Teresa McGowan left New Mexico, her public health supervisor commented on her work, noting, "They [midwives] have improved from women with no knowledge of the first principles of proper procedure to ones of utmost carefulness in their methods and practices."[61] Coded into this praise of McGowan's capacities as a midwife instructor was the reciprocal trope of parteras as "women with no knowledge," or, in Anderson's words, the "most ignorant." These particular assessments of New Mexican midwives, reiterated throughout the documents of the public health department, encapsulate the ways medical knowledge was a site for the continued negotiation of colonial relationships and racial construction in the state. Early public health descriptions of parteras, many of whom had decades of regionally and culturally specific experience delivering babies, as "ignorant" at best and "superstitious" or actively harmful at worst invalidated their skills and knowledge because they were not recognizable to the public health department.

Despite early public health distrust in the work of parteras, the department was forced to recognize that "midwives will be with us for many years to come."[62] In explaining this continuing necessity for midwives in New Mexico, public health officials "constantly" stated, "New Mexico's problems are different!"[63] With congressional appropriation of funding to the state from the Social Security Act and the U.S. Children's Bureau in 1936, New Mexico was able to expand its programs aimed at promoting the health of mothers and babies. With increased funding, the public health department strengthened its efforts to train and certify midwives by hiring a nurse–midwife consultant, Frances Fell, who was a public health nurse with additional training in midwifery. Her job was to instruct parteras through a series of ten classes "emphasizing the importance of cleanliness, non-interference, recognition of abnormal conditions, use of silver nitrate [to prevent infant blindness], and filling out the birth certificate."[64] By the early 1940s, especially with the shortage of physicians leaving the state for the armed services during World War II, the public health department increasingly relied on parteras who had a combination of training from public health nurse–midwives, other local parteras, and their own direct experience. In 1942 the public health department explained, "Realizing the important position the midwife usually holds in her community, many women have been reached through instructions of midwives in classes and institutes."[65]

The presence of parteras in public health midwifery education is evidence of a complicated response to the difficulties and rewards created by the public health department. Many parteras took the opportunity to learn more about pregnancy, labor, and delivery through public health programs. Besides limited attendance in grade school, midwifery classes were often the only formal education outlets available to parteras. For example, after a ten-lesson course in midwifery offered in San Miguel County in the early 1920s, seven parteras passed an examination and earned midwifery certificates. News of this class and certification spread to the neighboring communities of Trementina and Los Vijiles, where groups of fifteen and ten women, respectively, requested public health training and midwifery certification.[66] Another partera, Jesusita Aragón, participated in the two-week public health–sponsored midwifery institute in Las Vegas, New Mexico. At this midwifery institute, Aragón remembered there were "about thirty to forty-five women from different places Los Lunas, Santa Rosa, Wagon Mound, and only me from Trujillo."[67] Aragón explained, "The class had many interesting things. I didn't like to miss the meetings nor the movies."[68] However, Aragón, who first learned midwifery from her grandmother and had been delivering babies since she was fourteen, also indicated that she had already learned many of the things being taught at the public health class. She noted that her grandmother had taught her to wear her apron "years ago," as well as many other techniques and skills to assist women through pregnancy, during birth, and postpartum.[69] Aragón's experiences indicate how parteras drew on many different sources of training and education to continue meeting the reproductive needs of women in their communities.

In August 1945, the New Mexico department of public health promulgated the nation's first Nurse–Midwife Regulations, which issued state licenses for the practice of nurse–midwifery.[70] To obtain this license, an applicant had to be a registered nurse in New Mexico who had successfully completed a course of training from a recognized school of midwifery. Although this licensure opened up an important avenue for future nurse–midwives, parteras, regardless of their direct experience, lacked the formal training required for this professional license. Despite their exclusion from midwifery licensing, parteras continued to practice in New Mexico well into the second half of the twentieth century, although their numbers declined from an estimated 800 in 1945 to fewer than 100 by 1965. As this history illuminates, midwifery laws and education were never designed to legitimate and advance parteras as professional health care workers. Rather, these laws helped contain their practices until further medical and public health infrastructure could be developed in the state. These policies reveal much about the consolidation of racialized and gendered health hierarchies in early twentieth-century New Mexico and the centrality of reproduction to demarcating national belonging. Today, New Mexico leads the nation with the highest percentage of midwife-attended births in the nation. Behind this contemporary resurgence in midwifery is a long history of parteras who provided an indispensable service.

NOTES

1 Hester B. Curtis, "Division of Maternal and Child Health," *State of New Mexico Department of Public Health Tenth Biennial Report* (1937–1938): 47.

2 There is a rich body of scholarship and much debate about the racial and ethnic identity labels for the Spanish-speaking people of mixed Native, Spanish, Mexican, and African descent in New Mexico. Reflecting the complexity of racial and ethnic designation in New Mexico, I use several different terms when identifying Spanish-speaking and Spanish-surnamed people in New Mexico. In this chapter, I use *Nuevomexicano/a* to designate people of Native, Spanish, Mexican, and African ancestry who lived in the U.S. territory and later the state of New Mexico, because this was a common self-referent. I also use the term *Hispano/a* to designate Nuevomexicanos in the period after statehood was granted in 1912. In using this term, I follow Gabriel Melendez's assertion that "*Hispanoamericano* and its diminutive *Hispano,* connoted a transnational solidarity among and between *Mexicanos* on both sides of the Bravo, much like the present day use of *latinoamericano* or *latino.*" Additionally, following the legal and historical scholarship of Laura Gómez, at times I use *Mexican American* to foreground the racialized experience of New Mexicans of Mexican origin. Finally, at times I use *Spanish American* because this was the official, public designation of the Spanish-surnamed people of New Mexico starting in the 1920s and is used throughout the public health archival material. Selected sources on this debate include Laura Gómez, *Manifest Destinies: The Making of the Mexican American Race* (New York: New York University Press, 2007); Phillip B. Gonzales, "The Political Construction of Latino Nomenclatures in Twentieth Century New Mexico," *Journal of the Southwest* 35, no. 2 (1993): 158–85; Charles Montgomery, *The Spanish Redemption: Heritage, Power and Loss on New Mexico's Upper Rio Grande* (Berkeley: University of California Press, 2002); Gabriel A. Meléndez, *So All Is Not Lost: The Poetics of Print in Nuevomexicano Communities, 1834–1958* (Albuquerque: University of New Mexico Press, 1997); John M. Nieto-Phillips, *The Language of the Blood: The Making of Spanish-American Identity in New Mexico, 1880s–1930s* (Albuquerque: University of New Mexico Press, 2004); and Clara E. Rodríguez, *Changing Race: Latinos, the Census, and the History of Ethnicity in the United States* (New York: New York University Press, 2000).

3 "Birth-Delivery," August 16, 1961, Anne M. Smith Collection, 1961–1965, Fray Angélico Chavez Library, Santa Fe, New Mexico (hereafter cited as AMS MSS).

4 Nieto-Phillips, *Language of the Blood,* 91.

5 Many New Mexican parteras were fluent in both Spanish and English.

6 For an overview of histories of midwifery and obstetrics in the United

States, see William Ray Arney, *Power and the Profession of Obstetrics* (Chicago: University of Chicago Press, 1982); Judith Walzer Leavitt, *Brought to Bed: Childbearing in America, 1750–1950* (New York: Oxford University Press, 1988); Judy Barrett Litoff, *American Midwives, 1860 to the Present* (Westport, Conn.: Greenwood Press, 1978); and Richard W. Wertz and Dorothy C. Wertz, *Lying-In: A History of Childbirth in America* (New Haven, Conn.: Yale University Press, 1989).

7 Charlotte G. Borst, *Catching Babies: The Professionalization of Childbirth, 1870–1920* (Cambridge, Mass.: Harvard University Press, 1995); Gertrude Jacinta Fraser, *African American Midwifery in the South: Dialogues of Birth, Race, and Memory* (Cambridge, Mass.: Harvard University Press, 1998); and Susan L. Smith, *Japanese American Midwives: Culture, Community, and Health Politics, 1880–1950* (Chicago: University of Illinois Press, 2005).

8 Smith, *Japanese American Midwives*, 42.

9 *New Mexico Health Officer* (1937–1938): 28.

10 Selected histories of parteras in New Mexico include Fran Leeper Buss, *La Partera: Story of a Midwife* (Ann Arbor: University of Michigan Press, 2000); and Felina Mychelle Ortiz, "History of Midwifery in New Mexico: Partnership between Curandera-Parteras and the New Mexico Department of Health," *Journal of Midwifery & Women's Health* 50 (2005): 411–17. Pueblo Indians in New Mexico were denied the right to vote under Article VII, Section 1 of the Constitution of New Mexico. Miguel Trujillo Sr. of Isleta Pueblo successfully sued the state of New Mexico for the right to vote. Joe S. Sando, *Pueblo Nations: Eight Centuries of Pueblo Indian History* (Santa Fe, N.M.: Clear Light Publishers, 1992).

11 David Holtby, *Forty-Seventh Star: New Mexico's Struggle for Statehood* (Norman: University of Oklahoma Press, 2012), 42.

12 Ibid.

13 Gilson Willets, "Most Un-American Part of the United States," *New York Times*, August 20, 1905.

14 Ibid.

15 Myrtle Greenfield, *A History of Public Health in New Mexico* (Albuquerque: University of New Mexico Press, 1962), 11.

16 For more about the New Mexico statehood debate see Robert Larson, *New Mexico's Quest for Statehood, 1846–1912* (Albuquerque: University of New Mexico Press, 1968); and Holtby, *Forty-Seventh Star*, 2012.

17 Pablo Mitchell, *Coyote Nation: Sexuality, Race, and Conquest in Modernizing New Mexico, 1880–1920* (Chicago: University of Chicago Press, 2005), 17.

18 Gregory Rodriguez, *Mongrels, Bastards, Orphans, and Vagabonds: Mexican Immigration and the Future of Race in America* (New York: Vintage Books, 2007), 166.

19 Nieto-Phillips, *Language of the Blood*, 75.

20 Greenfield, *History of Public Health in New Mexico*, 14.

21 Ibid., 18.

22 Ann Massmann, "Adelina 'Nina' Otero-Warren: A Spanish–American Cultural Broker," *Journal of the Southwest* (Winter 2000): 891.

23 These women included Mrs. David Chavez Jr. (1933–1936), Mrs. Tobias Espinosa (1937–1939), Mrs. Elizabeth Gonzales (1940–1951), and Mrs. Amalia Sanchez (1952–1955). Greenfield, *A History of Public Health in New Mexico,* Appendix G.

24 For a list of public health administrators, 1919–1955, see Greenfield, *History of Public Health in New Mexico,* Appendix G.

25 Elena R. Gutiérrez, *Fertile Matters: The Politics of Mexican-Origin Women's Reproduction* (Austin: University of Texas Press, 2008), 3.

26 George Sanchez, "'Go After the Women': Americanization and the Mexican Immigrant Woman, 1915–1929," *Stanford Center for Chicano Research Working Paper Series* 6 (1984).

27 Rickie Solinger, *Pregnancy and Power: A Short History of Reproductive Politics in America* (New York: New York University Press, 2005).

28 Mary N. Marquez and Consuelo Pacheco, "Midwifery Lore in New Mexico," *American Journal of Nursing* 64 (1964): 81–84.

29 Nasario García, "Curanderismo: Folk Healing," in *Old Las Vegas: Hispanic Memories from the New Mexico Meadowlands* (Lubbock: Texas Tech University Press, 2005), 112–29.

30 Abe Peña, *Memories of Cíbola: Stories from New Mexico Villages* (Albuquerque: University of New Mexico Press, 1997), 46.

31 Ibid.

32 Nan Elsasser, ed., *Las Mujeres: Conversations from a Hispanic Community* (New York: Feminist Press, 1980), 39.

33 Buss, *La Partera,* 11.

34 "Hospitals Available for Delivery," August 17, 1961, AMS MSS.

35 Sarah Deutsch, *No Separate Refuge: Culture, Class, and Gender on an Anglo-Hispanic Frontier in the American Southwest, 1880–1940* (New York: Oxford University Press, 1987), 48.

36 "New Mexico: Summary of Vital Statistics," *New Mexico Health Officer* (1942).

37 Marta Weigle, ed., *Hispanic Villages of Northern New Mexico: A Reprint of Volume II of the 1935 Tewa Basin Study, with Supplementary Materials* (Santa Fe, N.M.: Jene Lyon, 1975), 67.

38 "New Mexico: Summary of Vital Statistics," 17, 24, 29, 31, 35.

39 Anne M. Smith, "Interview with Miss Anne Fox, Nurse–Midwife Consultant," August 16, 1961, AMS MSS.

40 Daphne Arnaiz-DeLeon, archives and historical services director at the New Mexico State Records and Archives Center (SRAC) in Santa Fe, graciously compiled a database containing extracted information from all the birth certificates filed in Valencia County (the only county with available birth records at the SRAC) during the years 1928–1930. Because the original birth certificates have restricted viewing access, this database was the only

way for me to analyze the birth attendants. In the 1920s, Valencia County included all its current territory plus what is today known as Cibola County. It was located near the west-central part of New Mexico below Albuquerque and extending west toward the Arizona border. I used my judgment to distinguish Spanish and Euro-American surnames. Valencia County also included the Pueblos of Acoma and Laguna, but Native American births were not recorded by the public health department until 1943. From the available data it is impossible to more accurately identify racial and ethnic status.

41 Greenfield, *History of Public Health in New Mexico*, 26.

42 Gerhard Hirschfeld and Carl W. Strow, "Comparative Health Factors among the States in 1940," *American Sociological Review* 11 (1946): 42–52.

43 "Twenty-Five Years of Public Health in New Mexico," *New Mexico Health Officer* 12, nos. 3 and 4 (1944): 62.

44 "Parteras 'Midwife,'" February 25, 1941, Work Projects Administration New Mexico Collection, Center for Southwest Research, University of New Mexico, Albuquerque.

45 Ibid.

46 Weigle, *Hispanic Villages of Northern New Mexico*, 67.

47 Cleofas Jaramillo, *Romance of a Little Village Girl* (Albuquerque: University of New Mexico Press, 2000), 96.

48 Fraser, *African American Midwifery*; and Smith, *Japanese American Midwives*.

49 Sheryl Nestle, *Obstructed Labour: Race and Gender in the Re-Emergence of Midwifery* (Vancouver, B.C.: UBC Press, 2006).

50 Ramon Del Castillo, "The Life History of Diana Velazquez: *La Curandera Total*," in *La Gente: Hispano History and Life in Colorado*, ed. Vincent C. De Baca (Denver: Colorado Historical Society, 1998), 229.

51 State of New Mexico Bureau of Public Health, *Regulations Governing the Practice of Midwifery*, sec. 10, ch. 145 (November 20, 1922), 1.

52 Eremita García-Griego de Lucero, "I'm Going to Have a Baby / Voy a tener un niño," in *Comadres: Hispanic Women of the Río Puerco Valley*, ed. Nasario García (Albuquerque: University of New Mexico Press, 1997), 177.

53 *New Mexico Health Officer's Weekly Bulletin*, February 1929. University of New Mexico, Health Historical Collection, Albuquerque, NM (hereafter cited as HHC, UNM).

54 Edith Powers, *Singing for My Echo: Memories of Gregorita Rodriguez, a Native Healer of Santa Fe* (Santa Fe, N.M.: Cota Editions, 1987), 73–75.

55 Ibid., 73.

56 State of New Mexico Bureau of Public Health, *Regulations Governing the Practice of Midwifery*, 3.

57 Dorothy R. Anderson, "Why New Mexico Nurses Cooperate in Maternity and Infancy Work," *American Journal of Public Health* 16 (1926): 473–75.

58 Ibid.

59 Ibid.

60 *New Mexico Health Officer's Weekly Bulletin*, January 13, 1923, HHC, UNM.

61 *New Mexico Health Officer's Weekly Bulletin*, September 22, 1923, HHC, UNM.

62 *Bureau of Public Health 5th Annual Report* (1927–1928): 2.

63 *New Mexico Health Officer Annual Report* (1941): 17.

64 *New Mexico Health Officer Tenth Biennial Report* (1937–1938): 47–48.

65 *New Mexico Health Officer Annual Report* (1942): 29.

66 Louise Wills, "Instruction of Midwives in San Miguel County," *Southwestern Medicine* 6 (1922): 276–79.

67 Buss, *La Partera*, 52.

68 Ibid.

69 Ibid.

70 *New Mexico Health Officer Annual Report* (1947): 43. State of New Mexico Department of Public Health, "Nurse–Midwife Regulations for New Mexico," August 4, 1945, Authorizing Act Chapter 39, Laws of 1937.

7

Professionalizing "Local Girls"

Nursing and U.S. Colonial Rule in Hawai'i, 1920–1948

JEAN J. KIM

MULTIPLE AND WIDELY CIRCULATING representations of "local girls," or indigenous Hawaiian, Asian, and mixed-race women working in Hawai'i as nurses in the first half of the twentieth century, bear haunting resonances with the racialization of black nurses working domestically on the U.S. continent and with nonwhite nurses working across a wide range of contemporary British and U.S. colonial possessions. In 1924, *The Queen's Hospital Bulletin* described the emergence of local girls in Honolulu through "a nurses' training school" engaged in "developing Island girls with character to give cheerfully a much needed service to the community."[1] In 1949 Brigid Maxwell, in her overview of the British colonial nursing service, wrote that throughout Britain's colonies "the Colonial Office hopes to train more and more local girls" who would learn their profession from British metropolitan supervisors in Africa, Asia, and the Pacific.[2] In disparate colonial regimes, local girls, like African American women entering the nursing profession in the U.S. South at the turn of the century, were racialized through nurses' training programs. Before World War II, a health administrator in Hawai'i observed that "local girls cannot compete with the experience of mainland *haole* girls," or white women, and that "Japanese don't make good executives," extending a prevalent stereotype and rationale used to limit advancement of African American women in nursing to Asian American women in Hawai'i, a U.S. settler colony.[3] Geographically disparate yet overlapping constructions of nurses such as these suggest a continuity between domestic U.S. racialization and colonial racial exigencies as they were articulated in medicine and raise further questions about the origin, geographic expanse, colonial genealogy, and racial power of the category "local girl."

This chapter situates the racial and imperial paradigms that produced the category of local girls in the 1920s in the contexts of the U.S. metropole and contemporary developments in African, Asian, and Pacific colonies, where governing transitions placed an emphasis on improving colonial welfare by recruiting nonwhite indigenous and racialized professionals. By the 1920s, when the children of plantation labor migrants in Hawai'i entered the nursing profession, Warwick Anderson suggests that in the Philippines and elsewhere, colonial modalities underwent a liberal shift characterized by changes in the ethos of empire, the embrace of allopathic medicine by Western-educated indigenous elites, and the incomplete sanitary citizenship of minorities whose full inclusion in colonial states was often challenged on health grounds.[4] As part of a profession that was underscored by imperial aims, Asian, Hawaiian, and mixed-race local nurses were poised to reproduce, incorporate, and resist colonial medical epistemologies as brokers of colonial biomedicine and indigenous and ethnic ideas about health and healing.[5] In Hawai'i, local girls became important to territorial public health measures because they possessed clinically relevant cultural affiliations with a polyglot colonial labor force; however, their professionalization underscored their racial difference and subordinate status, even as supervisors celebrated their assimilation. Furthermore, their participation in health care did little to change developing patterns of Filipino and Hawaiian marginalization in public health.[6]

The continuities and discontinuities between the colonial and domestic construction of white and nonwhite women in nursing signal nuanced colonial taxonomies grounded in paradigmatically shared material and managerial experiences of colonialism and racial exclusion in Asia, Africa, the Pacific, and the United States, and they demonstrate the production of racial categories through the practice and professional structure of biomedicine.

INSULAR AND CONTINENTAL CONVERGENCES
OVER SUGAR AND SOVEREIGNTY

The racial paradigms and structural foundations of U.S. colonialism in Hawai'i, like the gendered and racial hierarchy of nursing, radiated from developments on both the U.S. continent and across contemporary empires operating in the Pacific. Medical technologies, tropical agriculture, ideas about the human body and personhood, labor regimes, and migrants circulated practically and paradigmatically between the Americas, Africa, and Europe, to Asia and the Pacific, especially in the nineteenth century, creating unique cultural, practical, and ideological ties.[7] Asian contract workers became the predominant source of labor for sugar cultivation on plantations that spread from the Americas to Oceania, Asia, and South Africa to meet increased European demand for tropical products in the wake of the abolition of slavery. In the Pacific, British, French, German, and U.S. plantation interests looked to each other for models of labor management, settler colonialism, and imperial rule. In these exchanges, the United States both led and followed its European counterparts. Gerald Horne argues that U.S. nationals provided aggressive models of indigenous land expropriation and racial dominance that shaped wider patterns of imperialism in the Pacific.[8]

In Hawai'i, U.S. investors began their experiment in commercial sugar cultivation using Hawaiian labor in 1835, and by the end of the century the industry transformed Hawai'i's economy, politics, and demographics. U.S. continental developments such as settlement of the West Coast; the Civil War, which disrupted southern sugar production; and the 1875 Reciprocity Treaty, which ensured favorable sugar prices, fueled commercial expropriations of Hawaiian land, racialized labor recruitment, and prompted a coup against Hawai'i's reigning monarch in 1893. Sanford Dole, son of U.S. Protestant missionaries, declared Hawai'i a republic in 1894 and sought U.S. annexation. As the Spanish–American War expanded into the Philippines in 1898, Congress passed the Newlands Resolution, which annexed Hawai'i over opposition from domestic sugar producers and anti-imperialists. In 1900 Hawai'i gained territorial status, which required the abolition of contract labor, Chinese immigration exclusion, and a ban on Asian naturalization as U.S. citizens.

As racially exclusive laws and social etiquette solidified segregation and African American subordination on the U.S. continent, novel racial and imperial triangulations and proximities took shape in new U.S. insular colonies. After the Gentlemen's Agreement between the United States and Japan in 1907 cut off planters' supply of male labor migrants from Japan and its territories, colonial labor migration from the Philippines supplied the sugar industry's continuous demands. Other nations from which planters and the Hawaiian Bureau of Immigration recruited laborers and settlers between 1854 and 1905 included China, the Azores, Germany, Korea, Okinawa, Russia, Fiji, the Gilbert Islands, Scandinavia, and Puerto Rico.[9] White settlers, Asian labor migrants ineligible for naturalization, the racialized children of Asian labor migrants born locally into U.S. citizenship, predominantly male Filipino colonial migrant laborers, Pacific Islanders recruited to work in Hawai'i from the mid-nineteenth century onward, and indigenous Hawaiians were positioned unevenly in colonial institutions, citizenship status, and access to health care. The professionalization of nurses in the 1920s reflected and deepened many of the imperial asymmetries of Hawai'i's multiracial population under U.S. colonial rule.

PROFESSIONAL STRATIFICATIONS AND THE APORIA
OF EMPIRE IN U.S. NURSING HISTORY

Sociologists and historians have written extensively about the gendered, class, and racial dynamics of the U.S. continental profession of nursing, but they have generally overlooked its imperial genealogy, which is important for locating Asian women in the field and framing the local girl as both colonial construct and racial subject.[10] Beginning in 1870, white reformers transformed nursing from a category of servitude into a skilled occupation through professionalization activities including recruitment of women from higher socioeconomic backgrounds, establishment of training schools and alumni organizations, universal educational standards, and legislation to regulate the credentialing of nurses. In the resulting hierarchy, white graduate nurses from racially exclusive hospital training programs relied on the assistance of untrained practical nurses and nurse's aides, who were poor or working class and often women of color.[11] In 1910 and 1920, leaders in the profession were overwhelmingly white and supportive of racially exclusive training programs.[12]

Based on analyses of the racialization of professional nursing, Evelyn Nakano Glenn has paralleled the experiences of African American women in the U.S. South, Japanese women in northern California and Hawai'i, and Mexican women in the Southwest, respectively, on the basis of their restricted citizenship and regional racial binaries.[13] Joan Manley, on the other hand, categorizes Asian and white nurses together because of their predominance as registered nurses working

above black and Latino women, a development that took shape after
the Civil Rights Act of 1964 formally removed racial barriers against
black women in nurses' training programs and hospital employment
but failed to create opportunities for their advancement because of the
availability of Asian colonial and other immigrant nurses to fill shortages of trained staff.[14]

In their interpretations of these professional incommensurabilities
between women of color, both Glenn and Manley overlook the productive role of colonial subjection and imperial inequalities in both
transnational labor migration and Asian women's professionalization
as nurses, a status that offered women unique opportunities and constraints. Missing from Glenn's account of nursing in Hawai'i are native
Hawaiians and the dynamics of U.S. imperialism, which structured racial
minority status through unequal categories of citizenship, indigeneity,
and colonial migration. A consideration of the imperial dynamics of
nursing is necessary for understanding how women of color were articulated into the field across the United States and its colonies.

Although the colonial history of U.S. nursing is plainly evident in
primary source material produced by prominent leaders in the field, its
authors have ignored the power dynamics of their tutelary professional
roles abroad.[15] Academics, on the other hand, have largely underappre-
ciated the significance of colonial expansion to the profession. Darlene
Clark Hine has importantly cited the years from 1890 to 1925 as critical
to the racialization of nursing because this period saw rapid expansion
of the profession at the same time that Jim Crow segregation became
institutionalized in the United States.[16] Equally worthy of note, however, is that in addition to marking the rise of racial segregation and
the expansion of nursing, the years from 1890 to 1925 also marked a
formative period in U.S. overseas imperial expansion.

New U.S. colonies and imperial projects constituted arenas for the
professionalization of nursing as leaders in the field exported training models abroad that were still evolving on the U.S. continent. M.
Adelaide Nutting, known for becoming the first professor of nursing
in the United States, remarked in her 1923 survey of American nursing
schools that in addition to establishing 1,300 programs between 1900
and 1920, U.S. nurses had also "built up" schools "in the Philippines,
in Hawaii, in Porto Rico, and in Cuba." She also remarked that "75
trained nurses" were employed "in far Alaska" to spread U.S.-based

models of nurses' education.[17] By the turn of the century, the military further propelled nurses throughout new U.S. possessions. Edith Aynes, a career army nurse, traces nursing in the U.S. military to the inception of U.S. settler struggles for independence from England in 1775. In 1818, the U.S. Army formed a Medical Department that employed 3,000 nurses during the Civil War. Nurses later gained permanent recognition and official status in the military during the Spanish–American War, which initiated the movement of white civilian and army nurses to the Philippines for work with the Red Cross.[18] Additional U.S. nurses became the first directors of training schools for Filipino women in 1907.[19] White nurses also traveled to Hawai'i for work or as a stopping point en route to Japan or China to establish hospital-based nurses' training programs. Despite their overwhelming overrepresentation in the profession between 1910 and 1950, white nurses were in constant demand in Hawai'i to assume managerial roles.[20]

One of the few historians to examine the colonial functions of U.S. nursing is Catherine Ceniza Choy. In the Philippines, Choy argues, white nurses played an important leadership role in empire while upholding and interpreting their work complementarily according to established imperial narratives. White nurses attempted to recruit Filipino women of the higher classes as a putatively benevolent policy, but they did so on the basis of racialized ideas about Filipino uncleanliness and backwardness that bridged older imperial racial binaries with newer American colonial science. Choy argues that nurses' training programs ultimately prepared Filipino women to meet the needs of U.S. imperial authority and, later, prepared Filipino nurses to relieve professional shortages in the U.S. metropole.[21] This colonial structure created what Choy calls an "empire of care" in which "nurses from countries with comparatively higher nursing shortages" migrated to serve "primarily highly developed countries such as the United States, Canada, and the United Kingdom."[22]

Unique partnerships between nursing, imperial expansion, and colonialism were also prevalent throughout British colonies in Africa and Asia, where "local girls" appeared. Lavinia Dock and Nutting describe British and American nurses traveling around the world to establish professional nursing in Canada, Australia, New Zealand, Africa, India, Japan, China, Korea, Cuba, Puerto Rico, and the Philippines.[23] In these locations U.S. nursing educators, like their British counterparts, shared what Brigid Maxwell described as an ambition "to penetrate to the oddest corners of the earth" as they trained nonwhite women and constructed colonial whiteness as hygienic and scientifically grounded.[24] Applicants to the British Colonial Nursing Service, who were required to possess "first-class physique and health," brought indigenous women, described by Maxwell as "girls," in small numbers from Hong Kong and Africa to the British metropole for further hospital training.[25]

In Hawai'i, as in contemporary U.S. and British colonies, authorities sought to recruit indigenous and racialized women as nurses to secure colonial infrastructures by supplying needed labor, insulating white women from intimacy with colonial bodies, and supplying cultural brokering. By feminizing nursing and recruiting educated women to assume lower professional roles, U.S. nurses in the Philippines and Hawai'i and British nurses across most of Africa restructured professional health care and marginalized indigenous medicine and male health care providers in the process.

NURSING THE EMPIRE: COLONIAL GENEALOGIES OF NURSING

Asian American women's entrance into nursing in Hawai'i in the 1920s grew from roots in nineteenth-century missionary domesticity, imperial constructions of Hawaiian women, and shifting legitimations of U.S. imperialism. Federal public health officers in Hawai'i, a U.S. territory, institutionally linked Hawaiian epidemiology to health surveillance on the U.S. continent. Ira Hiscock, professor of public health at Yale University, described Hawai'i as "the first Pacific outpost of America's health defense," where public health conditions were "of extreme importance to the rest of the United States and to the Army and Navy forces."[26] Among existing threats to this outpost's health security were the islands' cultural, geographic, and epidemiological proximity to Asia. In the face of these racialized risks, ethnic assimilation and population-wide adherence to territorial public health and hygiene mandates carried implications not only for the welfare of Hawai'i as a U.S. possession but also for the health status of the U.S. continent and for the stability of military projection in the Pacific region.

Because infections deadly to Europeans were not a part of Hawai'i's indigenous disease ecology in the eighteenth and nineteenth centuries, modern developments in immunology, sanitation, and bacteriology that enabled European colonialism across tropical Asia and Africa were not vital to white survival and settlement in Hawai'i. However, public health advancements were still significant for U.S. imperialism in Hawai'i because they facilitated the discursive conceptualization of differences between sovereign healthy whites and vulnerable Hawaiians before annexation. Later, in the postannexation context of closer epidemiological ties between Hawai'i and the U.S. continent, nursing in Hawai'i, like public health and medicine, was poised to buttress the imperial objectives of increasing workers' productivity, protecting the health of white colonists and military personnel, reproducing healthy citizen families in the 1920s, and producing narratives of indigenous and immigrant bodies that justified imperial interventions and the hegemony of Western medicine and institutions. Dynamic imperial objectives appeared in diverse public health policies, from nineteenth-century vaccination campaigns, leprosy segregation, racial quarantines and sanitary fires, and twentieth-century antituberculosis and infant and maternal hygiene work.[27]

Advances in U.S. imperialism over Hawai'i and the institutionalization of Western medicine, which included feminized indigenous and nonwhite nursing, went hand in hand by the start of the twentieth century when white settler physicians largely monopolized authority over the human body as the Board of Health officially outlawed the practice of indigenous Hawaiian medicine.[28] Over the course of the nineteenth century, white settlers considered Hawaiians to be a "dying race," and philanthropists concerned with preserving the Hawaiian population—which fell from an estimated 300,000 to 1 million in 1778 to 40,000 in 1900—placed special responsibility for Hawaiian health on Hawaiian women.[29] Starting in 1820, American missionary wives often complained about the poor domestic skills of Hawaiian women and their deficiencies as nurses. Missionary men and women also claimed urgency in teaching native women appropriate domestic habits and nutritional principles in order to reverse trends of high infectious disease mortality.[30] Walter Murray Gibson implored Hawaiian women in 1880 to "learn to become nurses," and to take "a place by the sickbed" so that "the Hawaiian nation may be given to hope for its perpetuation."[31] These pointed admonitions to Hawaiians absolved foreigners for bringing novel infectious diseases to Hawai'i and for playing a role in introducing malnutrition to Hawaiians through land dispossession and disruptions of Hawaiian settlement patterns and agriculture.

In the last quarter of the nineteenth century, white doctors drove a small group of chiefly Hawaiian men trained in Western medicine out of the local profession and condemned traditional Hawaiian healers known as *kahuna lapa-au,* leaving informally trained Hawaiian women, formally trained white American women, and Franciscan sisters to provide nursing care under their direction at custodial institutions such as Hawai'i's settlement at Molokai for people suffering from Hansen's disease, or leprosy, and at the Queen's Hospital, founded by Queen Emma Rooke and King Kamehameha IV in 1859 to serve native Hawaiians.[32] Nursing then entered native Hawaiian school curricula in gendered ways that became institutionalized through hospital-based training programs. Starting in the 1890s, young Hawaiian girls took "hospital practice" classes at the Kamehameha School for Girls, and they could enroll at the Kauikeolani Children's Hospital's nursing school from 1910 to 1917.[33] In 1903, the Trustees of Queen's Hospital supported nurses' training but did not open a school until 1916 because supervisory white nurses from the East Coast were expensive to employ, turned over at a high rate, and exhibited disciplinary problems such as the tendency to strike.[34] The Queen's Hospital program affiliated with and then absorbed the Kauikeolani training school in 1928.

The initial 1911 grant for the Queen's Hospital school stipulated a preference for recruiting native Hawaiian women, or students with some "aboriginal blood." This indigenous preference was later deleted without the knowledge of its benefactor, Honolulu businessman M. S. Grinbaum. However, the school's first recruits in 1912 were Hawaiian, and its first graduate in 1917, Annie Kamanoka, was Hawaiian.[35] Predominantly white Punahou Academy and predominantly Japanese McKinley High School were not initial recruitment sites, indicating the indigenous target of such programs and their direction against reversing the putative extinction of the Hawaiian race, which settlers institutionally advanced but culturally disavowed by faulting a presumably endogenous Hawaiian incapacity for sovereignty.[36]

The operation and ethos of the nurses' training school at Queen's Hospital, like its continental counterparts, melded gentility with military discipline. Applicants were required to secure references, exhibit good health, remain free from physical blemishes or deformity, display cheerful and kindly dispositions, and have good eyesight and teeth. They were also expected to embody high moral ideals and to lead by example in maintaining good hygiene through regular practices of brushing their teeth, drinking milk, and wearing shoes.[37] Supervision was constant and rigidly hierarchical. Nurses wore uniforms, worked twelve hours per day, and were obliged to work extra hours to make up for any time away from work due to illness. Women were also subjected to daily physical inspections for neatness and proper attire.[38] Head mistresses and administrators were carefully selected from the U.S. continent.[39]

As standards for training increased under the heavy influence of U.S. continental professionalization patterns, and as a diverse working class increasingly came under public health surveillance, Hawaiian women diminished within the profession. Half of the first graduating class of the Queen's Hospital's training school in 1919 was Hawaiian. When the Territorial Board of Nursing accredited the school in 1921, it struggled to attract pupils and graduated only five women in 1924.[40] Over the course of the 1920s, however, local women began to consider nursing a viable career choice. When admission standards rose to require a high school diploma along the lines of U.S. continental programs in 1929, the school graduated a large of class of twenty-six.[41] However, when the University of Hawai'i contributed public health nursing courses to the program, it graduated only eighteen women.[42] When completion of at least one year of university education became a nursing school prerequisite "to secure young women with more matured minds" along the lines of "the best schools of nursing" in the United States, according to Dorothea Hunt, president of the graduating class of 1933, the size and diversity of the student body plummeted.[43] Only five women graduated, two of whom were Japanese American, one Portuguese, and two white.[44] In contrast, the 1929 graduating class included five Hawaiians, six Japanese, two Koreans, four Chinese, and one woman each of the following ethnicities: Portuguese, Russian, Spanish, "Anglo-Saxon," Australian, and "white."[45] The trend of decreasing Hawaiian and increasing local, especially Japanese American, presence in nursing continued with higher educational requirements. By 1936, the training school's course of study extended to four years. When it closed in 1968, 67 percent of the school's 1,283 graduates were Japanese American, indicating their majority status among trainees over the ensuing years.[46]

Local girls in nursing were primarily the daughters of immigrants, and they supplied an answer to the problems of white graduate nursing turnover and colonial efforts to secure public health as a prerequisite to continued imperial ties with the United States.[47] The term *local girls* described an obvious gendered dimension of the nursing profession, and the *local* designation further signaled race, generation, and geography. For nurses of Asian descent, whose parents were ineligible for naturalization as U.S. citizens, *local* referred both to nativity in the islands and the U.S. citizenship they gained from it. Because of the greater numbers of Japanese women than women of other ethnicities in the territory, "local girls" were often Japanese American. Even though some local girls would be considered white in the United States, local girls maintained ethnic and class ties that excluded them from mainstream *haole* society. The term *girls* further designated these women's lower professional status in relation to white women who worked as supervisors. Graduates of the Queen's Hospital training school were referred to as "girls," even though they could be up to thirty-eight years of age.[48] All local girls were fortuitously positioned to take up professionalizing opportunities initially established for training Hawaiian and part-Hawaiian women as U.S. colonial health objectives expanded.

As Glenn notes, white nurses who were trained on the U.S. continent and employed in Hawai'i were skeptical of the professional capacities of local nurses.[49] However, the expansion of public health nursing and new infant and maternal health programs organized by the Territorial Board of Health gave new importance to reaching heterogeneous racialized plantation and urban working-class populations with hygiene and health surveillance programs. This objective opened the doors to Asian American and other local women in nursing because cultural knowledge became a key to implementing professional principles in this area.[50] Public health nursing, first introduced to Honolulu under the private charity auspices of the Panama settlement in 1906, moved nurses beyond the confines of the hospital and, according to Olive MacLean, required cultural insider status with Hawai'i's multiethnic population.[51] Local girls were able to bridge gaps between territorial public health policies necessary for U.S. imperial governance and the needs of racialized migrant laborers who were beginning to form settler communities in the territory.

In Hawai'i's colonial, racial, and gendered economy, women of diverse ethnic backgrounds, especially the daughters of immigrants, pursued nursing because of a range of constraints including racial barriers to other fields, lack of financial resources to pursue training in professions such as teaching, and patriarchal subordination within families to brothers, whose education parents prioritized. Other women chose the field because it held value for them as a means of improving the welfare of their communities. Despite choosing nursing because of class and racial barriers, Janet Song, a graduate of the Queen's training school in 1925, described public health nursing as valuable to communities and noted the clinical significance of cultural intimacy between nurses and patients "of the same nationality," who could communicate freely.[52] Across ethnic lines, local nurses were able to use multiple linguistic resources, including pidgin and community acquaintances who could translate. In contrast, white graduate nurses were often unable to form close ties with local communities because they continually moved through an unstable and unpredictable revolving door as they relocated or married white professional and managerial men from the plantations.[53] In contrast, some local girls worked and lived in the camps and continued to work after marriage because they could not afford to retire as wives.

Despite the homogenizing connotation of the *local girl* label, epidemiological differences between ethnic groups and disparities in public health inclusion were prevalent. These differences stemmed from the varying degrees of family formation, citizenship, local nativity, and colonial subject status of each ethnic group. First-generation Asian labor migrants remained aliens because they were unable to naturalize as U.S. citizens until the federal repeal of this ban between 1943 and 1952. However, Japanese, Okinawans, and Koreans were able to access local sexual reproduction at a high rate through marriage and family formation with co-ethnic women who migrated to Hawai'i as brides between 1907 and 1923. U.S. colonial subjects who came to Hawai'i as laborers from the Philippines were "nationals" when they first arrived from 1906 to 1934, after which they became "aliens" with the promise of eventual Philippine liberation from U.S. imperial governance under the Tydings–McDuffie Act. Native Hawaiians and white settlers were U.S. citizens, but this status was imperially imposed on the former group. Additionally, the Hawai'i-born children of Asian labor migrants carried U.S. citizenship but continued to face racial discrimination and restricted social and class mobility, especially through World War II. Filipino labor migrants, as a predominantly male population, had less access to family formation with co-ethnic women than did Japanese,

Okinawan, and Korean migrants. As a consequence, Filipinos had less access to citizenship through birthplace nativity in Hawai'i. In 1931, among 30,333 single Filipino men living on plantations, only 0.2 percent possessed U.S. citizenship, compared with 49.4 percent of single Japanese men.[54] Their lesser degree of family formation and citizenship through birth in Hawai'i translated additionally into their lower access to territorial and plantation health programs that focused increasingly on family welfare.

To planters, the racialized citizenship of Japanese Americans prompted improved housing, recreation, and welfare services that benefited families rather than single men as part of attempts to reproduce this generation as plantation labor in the 1920s and 1930s. New territorial health resources also focused on families, women, and children as the colonial state expanded to catalogue vital statistics, regulate sexual reproduction, and promote hygienic assimilation across the territory's entire population, including within nonwhite settler communities for the first time since U.S. annexation. The relative ethnic exclusion of Filipinos from public health services reflected their simultaneous status as labor migrants and U.S. colonial subjects. Private and public institutional exclusion, rather than inclusion, operated as the primary means of regulating their exposure to illness, rate of reproductive sexuality, and demands on the state. During the Depression, the sugar industry reported repatriating 7,300 Filipinos because of disability, their large or "extra large" families, incarceration in a public institution, or unemployment.[55] Because they were U.S. colonial subjects facing exclusion and deportation rather than medical rehabilitation and care, the relative shortage of co-ethnic Filipino nurses in Hawai'i, who came from U.S. colonial training programs in the Philippines rather than the territory, was consistent with the broader marginalization of Filipinos in public health provisions. As local girls expanded public health services to racialized communities, they did so within the existing parameters of territorial health inequalities and exclusions.

CULTURAL POLITICS OF EMPIRE

Although their status as nurses was partly an artifact of indigenous exclusion from Hawai'i's public health infrastructure, local girls both advanced and challenged racialized U.S. colonial myths and recognized

existing health disparities as brokers of biomedicine. In national publications, they symbolized successful Americanization and thereby mo-
bilized support for continued U.S. colonization of Hawai'i. As medically trained practitioners, however, they simultaneously extended and
resisted clinical epistemologies that suggested the incomplete hygienic
citizenship and the racialized pathology of ethnic minorities. In 1927,
The Queen's Hospital Bulletin reached U.S. readers with illustrations
of the nursing school's progress in photographs that showed student
nurses wearing their nursing uniforms and, elsewhere, their "native
garb" to illustrate the normative power of the profession juxtaposed
against the polyglot background of Hawai'i's population. A caption
below one photo described "Some of Our American Student Nurses in
their Former Native Costumes," indicating a teleology in which women's
colorful cultural attire along with their ethnic and racial specificity, all
located temporally in the past, has been superseded by the uniformity
of purpose and values represented in other photos of student nurses in
their plain, modern, white professional outfits.[56]

Although women who worked as nurses in Hawai'i exhibited much
more complex cultural allegiances as they negotiated their citizenship in
a settler colony, nursing was a field where assimilation was on display
in gendered and racial terms. Local girls circulated discursively as visible symbols of the tutelary transformation of heterogeneous "Native"
girls' culture and physical appearance to conform with U.S. models.
Nursing schools also normalized women into middle-class habits that
permitted them to venture into new social and cultural arenas while
their status as local girls underscored their difference from whites, from
fully mature women, and from graduate nurses. The students' living
quarters contained formal dining and sitting areas. Milk was served
at meals, and students were trained in how to properly set a mealtime
table along with proper methods for making beds and cleaning house
according to white middle-class standards. Although their labor was
exploited in the hospital through compulsory night duty requirements
that taught them little and laboratory assignments meant to save on the
costs of hiring regular technicians, in their accommodations students
were provided with linens and access to a tennis court and swimming
pool.[57] In this assimilationist context, which coincided with an aggressive Americanization campaign in schools and other public institutions, nursing school pupils also learned about each other's cultures by

exchanging ethnic foods, forming interethnic friendships, and protecting each other from the harsh supervision that dormitory life afforded.

A second area where local nurses brokered colonial constructs was in their interpretation of the relationship between culturally specific beliefs about health and illness and biomedical explanations. Colonies became extraordinarily productive sites for generating knowledge about nutrition and the impact of food components on physiological function and efficiency. In the 1930s, a compelling narrative emerged on plantations and in the territory that reduced a broad range of health problems, including infant mortality and tuberculosis, to faulty dietary choices based on Hawai'i residents' overreliance on the dietary staple of white rice. In the literature on a local pediatric dental condition that was implicated in the morbidity and mortality of Hawaiians, Filipinos, Japanese, and other East Asians in particular, this faulty diet was known as the "oriental" diet.[58] As part of an epistemological apparatus to explain high rates of Hawaiian morbidity and mortality without implicating imperial economic, land, and social policies, this new emphasis on "oriental" diets as the cause of poor Hawaiian health outcomes sanitized U.S. imperial sovereignty in the territory. Researchers advocated native Hawaiian diets for Hawaiians and plantation workers of all backgrounds but in ways that appropriated Hawaiian staples to support U.S. imperial land usage and class inequalities. Some local nurses resisted this and other hegemonic claims of allopathic medicine in addition to mainstream white American claims of monopoly over scientific knowledge of the human body.

Even as they actively facilitated education in balanced diets and infant and child care and provided advice alongside white nurses and doctors in birth control and sexual sterilization, women who worked as local nurses did not necessarily internalize the broader political claims and assumptions of contemporary colonial narratives on the pathological status of "oriental" diets or the broader cultural dichotomies implied by the organization of healthy and unhealthy behaviors along racial and ethnic lines. Betty Sora, a registered nurse and the daughter of a plantation family who married a plantation worker, resisted the cultural coding of all matters of health and the contention that Hawai'i's nonwhite communities held beliefs about health that were either radically different from or inferior to those of white Americans. In a 1982 interview conducted by Ruth Smith as part of a history of public health nursing on the island of Kauai from 1920 to 1955, Sora used the strategies of scientific translation, contextualization, and correction to refute the categorical juxtaposition of Japanese or other ethnic healing beliefs against putatively more rational *haole* practices.[59] Sora maintained a pluralistic understanding of the legitimacy of a wide range of beliefs about health, and she repeatedly rejected their exoticization.

When Smith good-naturedly invited Sora to respond with benign amusement at her anecdote of Japanese waitresses admonishing Smith for taking her son out in public before he was thirty days old, Sora translated this belief into scientific terms to inform Smith that the Japanese prohibition against leaving the house for thirty-three days "has something to do with the six weeks, you know post-partum, you know it takes that long for the uterus to go down to its normal size and shape then."[60] She not only volunteered a scientific basis for this belief but considered the thirty-three-day rule to be a conservative estimate of how long women's bodies needed for full return to their physiological state before pregnancy. Sora also remained steadfastly sympathetic to multiethnic health practices in her explanation of why Filipino women wanted to drink warm water after deliveries. She simply stated that they must have been told that drinking warm water after delivery reduced cramps, whereas cold water was damaging. By doing so, she indicated that all women are given advice during childbirth and that following recommendations, even in the absence of a detailed rationale, is common in such circumstances. She also explained that a Japanese custom of not washing one's hair for thirty-three days after delivery was a measure to prevent catching a cold. She then added matter-of-factly, "Now of course you have driers, so you can dry your hair right away."[61] This comment normalized the underlying logic of this practice, while Sora acceded that technological innovations had since rendered it obsolete.

Like Sora, other local girls supported multiple health care systems and beliefs. Irene Cabral reported her regular use of herbal and alternative treatments.[62] Other local girls reported their empirical belief in Japanese birthing proscriptions that Smith assumed were transient. When Smith asked Tsugie Kadota when the Japanese belief that babies should not be taken out in public until thirty days after birth disappeared, Kadota surprised her by stating that her own postpartum recovery was especially difficult after she violated this rule by waiting only one week.[63] Peggy Nishimitsu attributed her failing eyesight to her violation of the prohibition against reading during the one-month postpartum period.[64] When Smith told Nellie Hiyane her story of being chastised by Japanese waitresses for taking her newborn son outdoors too early, Hiyane interjected by stating that there were many more handicapped and disfigured children at that time, implying that precautions Japanese mothers took with their newborns were shaped by their awareness and anxieties about the prevalence of these occurrences.[65]

In her answers to Smith's questions about ethnic food ways, Sora contradicted paternalistic stereotypes about ethnic dietary deficiency when she described Filipino men as good cooks with good diets. The most problematic feature of Filipino diets she cited was their low meat content, which she speculated to be responsible for causing anemia. Other local girls also refused the essentialist implications of Smith's dietary questions. Rather than cite ethnicity as the most relevant determinant of nutrition, Miyoko Ednaco emphasized economic rather than cultural constraints. She explained that diets were dictated by economy, accessibility, and availability. People ate to their satisfaction whatever "filled you up" based on what they could afford.[66] She did admit, however, that her family "didn't eat good" because they could not afford milk or meat, but this did not prevent them from being healthy.[67] Hiyane communicated that past efforts to Westernize ethnic diets were unnecessary on health grounds.[68] Nishimitsu described nutrition in the past as superior because people kept vegetable gardens and did not eat candy and junk foods, which she identified as unhealthy.[69] None of these women cited the occurrence of excessive white rice consumption by any ethnic group.

When asked about rates of patient compliance with medical and nursing instructions, local girls were sympathetic toward patients' rejection of medical proscriptions. Some had resisted medical surveillance and compulsory health interventions first-hand. Cabral disclosed that when she was a child, a white visiting nurse threatened to take her and her siblings away from their mother after they were identified as underweight.[70] Nishimitsu, who was also identified as underweight, was forced to take cod liver oil supplements in school that she attempted to avoid by carrying rocks in her pockets during school weigh-ins.[71] Local girls' unique outlook on biomedicine was shaped in part by their simultaneous experience as the subjects and agents of normalizing and racializing colonial medicine.

Sora explained noncompliance as a rational response to unnecessary instructions. She stated that mothers who did not need prenatal classes were put into them, even though they read on their own and were motivated to learn outside the class setting. She also noted that Filipino mothers, who were not brought into these classes, should have been involved, recognizing that needs were uneven between ethnic groups and that outreach efforts were not always rational.[72] By noting public health programs' failure to adequately serve Filipino mothers, Sora also referenced an important inequality that was reproduced by territorial medicine. As U.S. colonial subjects insufficiently incorporated into the field of nursing, Hawaiians and Filipinos also faced the highest rates of infant and maternal mortality and tuberculosis infection through the 1930s, indicating the reflexivity between poor health, exclusion from professional health care, and exploitation as indigenous and migrant U.S. colonial subjects.[73]

CONCLUSION

Everywhere U.S. sovereignty extended, so did nursing, allowing women the unique opportunity for professional development, travel, adventure, and dedication in serving a national mission through their skill and learning. Although historians and sociologists have criticized the material exploitation inherent in nurses' training programs, the gendered dimensions of nursing that facilitated that exploitation, and the racial grounds that ensured the hierarchical exclusion of women of color in the most highly skilled areas of the profession, these authors have largely not considered the ways white women participated in imperial projects that involved the training and normalization of indigenous and Asian women in U.S. colonies and the complex colonial inequalities such practices entrenched. As African American women were excluded from nursing on the U.S. continent, quite a different set of principles guided the colonial incorporation of nonwhite women in Hawai'i under the U.S. models of professionalization that nursing supervisors and hospital programs adopted.

In Hawai'i, the "local girl" had multiple colonial roots, emerging at the nexus of U.S. imperial expansion in the Pacific and imperatives to sanitize and epidemiologically rehabilitate the colony as a bridge between the U.S. continent and other island colonies. White women attempted to export metropolitan gendered models of female nursing abroad, and they also picked up in colonies their largely unsuccessful efforts to recruit middle-class women into the profession. From the Philippines, these colonial trajectories later brought U.S. colonial women of color to the U.S. metropole to fill nursing positions in a way that interfered with African American women's own efforts to advance in the field, especially after 1965. In Hawai'i, the incorporation of indigenous Hawaiian and later racialized Asian women born locally into U.S. citizenship into the profession supported shifting U.S. imperial labor and reproductive interests as Hawai'i became a U.S. territory and a U.S. military outpost in the Pacific.

The early professional feminization of nursing in Hawai'i excluded Hawaiian men from healing roles, and later rigid educational requirements for nurses' training increasingly excluded Hawaiian women. However, these imperial nursing programs allowed local girls at times to provide professional care that improved the lives of local communities, even as the institutions through which they worked reproduced existing indigenous and interethnic health inequalities, such as the relative exclusion of Filipinos and Hawaiians from health services. The story of American nursing is one of class, gender, and racial subordination and segregation, but it is also a story of imperial expansion involving the recruitment of indigenous and Asian colonial and migrant women in subordinate roles. Within Hawai'i's settler colonial infrastructure, local girls both reproduced and challenged the racializing impulses of colonial biomedicine.

NOTES

Research and writing for this chapter were supported by the Center for the Comparative Study of Race and Ethnicity at Stanford University and the U.S. Studies Center at the University of Sydney.

1 *The Queen's Hospital Bulletin* 1, no. 1 (June 1924): 2.

2 Brigid Maxwell, "Colonial Nurse," *American Journal of Nursing* 49, no. 7 (July 1949): 455.

3 Evelyn Nakano Glenn, "From Servitude to Service Work: Historical Continuities in the Racial Distribution of Paid Reproductive Labor," *Signs* 18, no. 1 (Autumn 1992): 27; Darlene Clark Hine, *Black Women in White: Racial Conflict and Cooperation in the Nursing Profession, 1890–1950* (Bloomington: Indiana University Press, 1989), 99; Susan Smith, *Japanese American Midwives: Culture, Community, and Health Politics, 1880–1950* (Urbana: University of Illinois Press, 2005), 112.

4 Warwick Anderson, *Colonial Pathologies: American Tropical Medicine, Race, and Imperialism in the Philippines* (Durham, N.C.: Duke University Press, 2006), 4.

5 Conversations with Martin Summers and John Mckiernan-González have helped frame these ideas.

6 David Scott similarly argues that dependency and underdevelopment persisted after the late colonial extension of liberal rights in British colonies. "Colonial Governmentality," *Social Text* 43 (Autumn 1995): 213–15.

7 Lisa Lowe, "The Intimacies of Four Continents," in *Haunted by Empire: Geographies of Intimacy in North American History,* ed. Ann Laura Stoler (Durham, N.C.: Duke University Press, 2006), 193; Moon-ho Jung, *Coolies and Cane: Race, Labor, and Sugar in the Age of Emancipation* (Baltimore, Md.: Johns Hopkins University Press, 2006).

8 Gerald Horne, *The White Pacific: U.S. Imperialism and Black Slavery in the South Seas after the Civil War* (Honolulu: University of Hawai'i Press, 2007), 2–3.

9 Ralph Kuykendall, *The Hawaiian Kingdom, Volume III: 1874–1893, The Kalakaua Dynasty* (Honolulu: University of Hawaii Press, 1967), 122–35.

10 Ann Game and Rosemary Pringle, *Gender at Work* (Sydney: George Allen and Unwin, 1983), 99–100; Joan E. Manley, "Sex-Segregated Work in the System of Professions: The Development and Stratification of Nursing," *Sociological Quarterly* 36, no. 2 (Spring 1995): 301.

11 Glenn, "From Servitude to Service Work," 23–25, 27.

12 Hine, *Black Women in White,* 99–101; Evelyn L. Barbee, "Racism in U.S. Nursing," *Medical Anthropology Quarterly* 7, no. 4 (December 1993): 357; Manley, "Sex-Segregated Work," 304.

13 Glenn, "From Servitude to Service Work," 9–10.

14 Manley, "Sex-Segregated Work," 307.

15 M. Adelaide Nutting and Lavinia L. Dock, *A History of Nursing: The*

Evolution of Nursing Systems from Earliest Times to the Present, 4 vols. (New York: G. P. Putnam's Sons, 1907–1912), 3: 116–236; M. Adelaide Nutting, "Thirty Years of Progress in Nursing," *American Journal of Nursing* 23, no. 12 (September 1923): 1030.

16 Hine, *Black Women in White,* 99–101.

17 Nutting, "Thirty Years of Progress," 1028.

18 Edith A. Aynes, "Army Nursing," *American Journal of Nursing* 40, no. 5 (May 1940): 539; Nutting and Dock, *A History of Nursing,* 4:308; Catherine Ceniza Choy, *Empire of Care: Nursing and Migration in Filipino American History* (Durham, N.C.: Duke University Press, 2003), 23.

19 Nutting and Dock, *History of Nursing,* 4:308; Choy, *Empire of Care,* 23.

20 Eileen Tamura, *Americanization, Acculturation, and Ethnic Identity: The Nisei Generation in Hawaii* (Urbana: University of Illinois Press, 1994), 232–33.

21 Choy, *Empire of Care,* 10, 41–42.

22 Ibid., 2.

23 Nutting and Dock, *A History of Nursing,* 4:122–322.

24 Maxwell, "Colonial Nurse," 455.

25 Ibid.

26 Ira V. Hiscock, *A Survey of Public Health Activities in Honolulu, Hawaii, Including Official and Voluntary Agencies, under the Auspices of the Chamber of Commerce of Honolulu; and a Brief Survey of the Major Health Problems of the Territory, Made with the Aid of the Kauai, Maui, and Hilo Chambers of Commerce* (New Haven, Conn.: Committee on Administrative Practice, Public Health, 1935), 12.

27 See Michelle Moran, *Colonizing Leprosy: Imperialism and the Politics of Public Health in the United States* (Chapel Hill: University of North Carolina Press, 2007); and James Mohr, *Plague and Fire: Battling Black Death and the Burning of Chinatown in 1900* (New York: Oxford University Press, 2005).

28 Bradley E. Hope and Janette Harbottle Hope, "Native Hawaiian Health in Hawaii: Historical Highlights," *Californian Journal of Health Promotion* 1 (2003): 4.

29 Kuykendall, *The Hawaiian Kingdom,* 122.

30 Francis John Halford collates missionary perspectives in *9 Doctors and God* (Honolulu: University of Hawai'i Press, 1954), 53, 180.

31 Frances R. Hegglund Lewis, *Nursing in Hawaii* (Node, Wyo.: Germann-Kilmer, 1969), 40–43.

32 Ibid., 44–45, 56, 58.

33 Ibid., 58, 61. Robert W. Shingle considered the nursing school a modern hospital feature. "Report of the President," *Queen's Hospital Annual Report* (1915): 5–6.

34 Ruby LoRaine Carlson, "A Case Study of Queen's Hospital School of Nursing, 1916–1968" (PhD diss., University of Hawai'i at Manoa, 1999), 21.

35 Hegglund Lewis, *Nursing in Hawaii,* 11.

36 Carlson, "A Case Study of Queen's Hospital," 22.

37 Ibid., 23–24.

38 Pat Loui, "Queen's Nursing School Caps 50th Class," *Honolulu Star Bulletin and Advertiser,* May 1963.

39 Paul Withington complained about high U.S. nurses' turnover. "Report of Resident Physician," *Queen's Hospital Annual Report* (1920): 15.

40 *The Queen's Hospital Bulletin* 5, no. 3 (August 1924): 1.

41 *The Queen's Hospital Bulletin* 9, no. 4 (September–October 1932): 8–9.

42 *The Queen's Hospital Bulletin* 11, nos. 1–12 (1935): 7–9; and Carlson, "A Case Study of Queen's Hospital," 58–63.

43 Dorothea Hunt, "Yesterday, Today and Tomorrow," *The Queen's Hospital Bulletin* 10, nos. 1–3 (September 1933): 3.

44 *The Queen's Hospital Bulletin* 7, nos. 7–12 (July 1936): 4–13.

45 Mary Hayashi, "Senior Class History," *The Queen's Hospital Bulletin* 5, nos. 9–10 (March–April 1929): 2.

46 Carlson, "A Case Study of Queen's Hospital," v, 68, 70.

47 Glenn, "From Servitude to Service Work," 27.

48 "The Queen's Hospital Training School," *The Queen's Hospital Bulletin* 5, no. 1 (June 1928): 6.

49 Glenn, "From Servitude to Service Work," 26.

50 Hegglund Lewis, *Nursing in Hawaii,* 8.

51 Olive MacLean, "Nursing in Hawaii," *American Journal of Nursing* 39, no. 10 (October 1939): 1083.

52 *The Queen's Hospital Bulletin* 2, no. 2 (July 1, 1925): 4.

53 Lela M. Goodell, "Plantation Medicine in Hawaii from 1840 to 1964: A Patient's Perspective," *Hawaii Medical Journal* 54 (November 1995): 789.

54 Hawaii Sugar Planters' Association, *Census of Hawaiian Sugar Plantations* (Honolulu: Hawaiian Sugar Planters' Association, 1931).

55 John Butler, "The HSPA and the Labor Problem in Hawaii," presented before the Senate on April 13, 1933 by J. K. Butler, May 29, 1933, H. S. P. A. Archives, KSC Box 23, Folder 28, 7. Margaret Catton estimates that the Social Service Bureau helped repatriate 1,748 Filipinos in *Social Service in Hawaii* (Palo Alto, Calif.: Pacific Book Publishers, 1959), 54.

56 *The Queen's Hospital Bulletin* 3, no. 11 (April 1927): 1.

57 Agnes Collins, "Report of the Superintendent of Nurses," *Queen's Hospital Annual Report* (1916): 21–23.

58 Jean J. Kim, "Experimental Encounters: Filipino and Hawaiian Bodies in the Imperial Invention of Odontoclasia, 1928–1946," in *Alternative Contact: Indigeneity, Globalism, and American Studies,* ed. Paul Lai and Lindsey Claire Smith, 117–40 (Baltimore, Md.: Johns Hopkins University Press, 2011).

59 Betty F. Y. Sora, interview by Ruth Smith, Grove Farm Oral History Project, "Public Health Services and Family Health on Kauai, 1920–1955,"

February 16, 1982, typed transcript, Grove Farm Homestead Museum, Kauai.

60 Ibid., 7.

61 Ibid., 6.

62 Irene Cabral, interview by Ruth Smith, Grove Farm Oral History Project, "Public Health Services and Family Health on Kauai, 1920–1955," February 26, 1982, typed transcript, Grove Farm Homestead Museum, Kauai, 28.

63 Tsugie Kadota, interview by Ruth Smith, Grove Farm Oral History Project, "Public Health Services and Family Health on Kauai, 1920–1955," February 26, 1982, typed transcript, Grove Farm Homestead Museum, Kauai, 17–18.

64 Peggy Nishimitsu, interview by Ruth Smith, Grove Farm Oral History Project, "Public Health Services and Family Health on Kauai, 1920–1955," May 14, 1982, typed transcript, Grove Farm Homestead Museum, Kauai, 12.

65 Nellie Hiyane, interview by Ruth Smith, Grove Farm Oral History Project, "Public Health Services and Family Health on Kauai, 1920–1955," February 16, 1982, typed transcript, Grove Farm Homestead Museum, Kauai, 23.

66 Miyoko Ednaco, interview by Ruth Smith, Grove Farm Oral History Project, "Public Health Services and Family Health on Kauai, 1920–1955," June 6, 1982, typed transcript, Grove Farm Homestead Museum, Kauai, 20.

67 Ibid., 20.

68 Hiyane, interview by Ruth Smith, 34.

69 Nishimitsu, interview by Ruth Smith, 11.

70 Cabral, interview by Ruth Smith, 25.

71 Nishimitsu, interview by Ruth Smith, 5.

72 Sora, interview by Ruth Smith, 8.

73 Hawaiians and Filipinos were disproportionately affected by tuberculosis. L. L. Sexton, "Report of the Anti-Tuberculosis Bureau," *Board of Health Annual Report* (Honolulu, 1910): 159; and F. E. Trotter, "Report of the President and Executive Officer Board of Health," *Board of Health Annual Report* (Honolulu, 1933): 5.

8

Borders, Laborers, and Racialized Medicalization

Mexican Immigration and U.S. Public Health Practices in the Twentieth Century

NATALIA MOLINA

THROUGHOUT THE TWENTIETH CENTURY, U.S. public health and immigration policies intersected with and informed one another in the country's response to Mexican immigration. Three historical episodes illustrate how perceived racial differences influenced disease diagnosis: a 1916 typhus outbreak, the midcentury Bracero Program, and medical deportations that are taking place today. Disease, or just the threat of it, marked Mexicans as foreign, just as much as phenotype, native language, accent, or clothing. A focus on race rendered other factors and structures, such as poor working conditions or structural inequalities in health care, invisible. This attitude had long-term effects on immigration policy and on how Mexicans were received in the United States.

U.S. immigration policy was fairly open until the end of the nineteenth century because immigrant labor was needed to help build and settle the expanding country. Federal restrictions on immigration did not appear until 1891, when Congress passed the first comprehensive immigration law. The law allowed immigrants to be barred from the United States for various reasons, ranging from being convicted of a crime to being considered likely to become a public charge, but many involved standards of fitness. Anyone considered "feebleminded," "insane," or likely to spread a "dangerous and loathsome contagious disease" was barred from the United States. An immigrant who was allowed entry into the United States but later fell ill and became a public charge (or even was thought likely to become a public charge) faced the possibility of deportation.[1] In the early twentieth century, as public health as a field and profession became more established, it increasingly influenced immigration policy.

At the same time that U.S. immigration and public health policies were becoming more interwoven, Mexican immigration to the United States began to increase. From 1900 to 1930, the Mexican population in the United States more than doubled every ten years. By 1930, an estimated 1.5 million Mexicans and Mexican Americans lived in the United States.[2] Most Mexicans arrived as low-paid laborers who worked mainly in industries such as agriculture and railroad building. Nativists denounced Mexican immigrants as unable to assimilate, less intelligent than white Americans, and "for the most part, Indian"[3] and therefore racially inferior. Increasingly, these stereotypes took the form of negative medicalized representations, giving rise to significant ramifications for immigration policy and securing the nation's borders. Public health standards based on perceived racial difference influenced both the treatment and perceptions of Mexican immigrants, not just at the time they crossed the border but long after they settled in the United States.

MEDICALIZED BORDERS IN THE NATION'S INTERNAL BORDERLANDS

Medicalized representations of Mexicans in the United States can be traced back to when what is now the U.S. Southwest was still a part of Mexico. The ideology of Manifest Destiny gained popularity during the Mexican–American War (1846–1848) and provided justification for U.S. expansionism. Dedicated believers in Manifest Destiny were compelled to portray white Americans as superior to Mexicans and Native Americans. Expansionists argued that after the U.S. takeover, Mexicans and Native Americans would eventually disappear in the Southwest because these peoples were not as biologically fit as Americans.[4]

Mexican immigration to the United States increased in the second decade of the twentieth century, driven by the need for laborers, particularly in the Southwest's burgeoning agricultural industry. The demand for laborers was conveniently met by refugees fleeing the ravages of the Mexican Revolution. Mexicans were ideal migrant laborers: sojourner men who traveled to secure work but would eventually return home. Such workers needed no capital or social investment; they needed little more than a willing employer and transient housing.

Although immigration laws did not severely restrict Mexican immigration at this time, public health standards helped shape attitudes and regulations directed at this new laboring class. As Amy Fairchild found in a study of the nation's borders, medical inspectors indoctrinated incoming immigrants by demonstrating to them the social and industrial norms they needed to succeed as workers in the United States.[5] Thus, far from excluding workers, health inspectors could shape immigrants into an acceptable laboring class. In the borderlands, however, such practices could also stigmatize Mexicans.

Before the enactment of restrictive laws such as the 1917 Immigration Act, which imposed a head tax and literacy test, medical screenings already regulated Mexican immigration. Mexicans underwent intrusive, humiliating, and harmful baths and physical examinations at the hands of the U.S. Public Health Service (USPHS) at the U.S.–Mexico border beginning in 1916. The rationale was the belief that Mexicans were bringing disease into the United States.[6] Thus, public health policies helped secure the U.S.–Mexico border and mark Mexicans as outsiders even before the advent of more focused gatekeeping institutions, such as the border patrol, created in 1924.

The connections between public health policies and the development of long-lasting representations of Mexicans as disease carriers are demonstrated by the response to a 1916 typhus outbreak in Los Angeles County. The disease spread from person to person, spurring the creation of local policies derived from the premise that all Mexicans spread disease. The typhus cases in Los Angeles preceded a quarantine on the U.S.–Mexico border in Texas the next year, also spurred by a handful of cases. Nonetheless, as Alexandra Stern, writing about the Texas quarantine, argues, these practices "fostered scientific and popular prejudices about the biological inferiority of Mexicans."[7] These medically driven policies had far-reaching social and political effects.

When a Mexican laborer at a Southern Pacific Railroad camp near Palmdale (twenty miles north of Los Angeles) came down with typhus in June 1916, health officials were alarmed. Typhus is an infectious disease caused by rickettsia (a bacterialike microorganism) and transmitted to humans through lice and tick bites.[8] Although not contagious, in the right conditions (overcrowding, lack of facilities for bathing and washing clothes, poor sanitation), typhus can rapidly become an epidemic.[9] Ultimately, twenty-six people contracted the disease (including twenty-two Mexican railroad workers) over a five-month period from June to October 1916. The outbreak killed five people, all of them Mexican.[10]

Public health officials at the county, state, and national levels soon became involved. County measures to contain the outbreak involved hygiene, sanitation, and education campaigns, all aimed exclusively at Mexicans. Howard D. King of New Orleans warned, "Every individual hailing from Mexico should be regarded as potentially pathogenic."[11] The stigma of the typhus outbreaks marked every area where Mexicans lived as needing inspection. In thirty railroad camps in California, health officials were particularly aggressive; they used cyanide gas to destroy lice, ticks, and other pests.[12]

The California State Board of Health pressured railroad employers to play a role in containing the typhus outbreak. Officials drew up an eight-point list of regulations, printed in both English and Spanish, and labor recruiters distributed the list to the various railroad camps. The regulations applied to every man, woman, and child living in the camps, not just to laborers. All the regulations focused on improving personal hygiene; not one addressed the inferior living conditions in the camps.

Mexican laborers expressed frustration over the attention paid to their individual actions, with no mention of structural problems in the camps, such as a dearth of toilets and bathing facilities. This frustration is clear in a formal letter of complaint sent to the Mexican consul in Los Angeles by a group of Mexicans who lived in a desert camp about 140 miles east of the city. The men, angry over the crudeness and impracticality of the antityphus procedures and the overt racism of the regulations, submitted their complaint just two weeks after the state board issued the regulations:

> Dear Sir:
>
> Due to the difficult circumstances we find ourselves in this for-eign country, we look to you asking for help in this case. We are enclosing a copy of the severe law that the railroad line has imposed on us Mexicans who work on the track, which we do not see as a just thing, but only offensive and humiliating. When we crossed the border into this country, the health inspector inspected us. If the railroad line needs or wants to take such precautions it is not necessary that they treat us in this manner. For this, they would need health inspectors who assisted every individual with medical care and give us 2 rooms to live, one to sleep in and one to cook in, and also to pay a fair wage to obtain a change of clothes and a bar of soap. This wage they set is not

enough for the nourishment of one person. Health comes from this and these precautions are the basis for achieving sanitation. Health we have. What we need is liberty and the opportunity to achieve it. We need a bathroom in each section of camp and that the toilets that are now next to the sleeping quarters be moved. Many times their bad smell has prevented us from even eating our simple meal. Furthermore, we can disclose many other details which compromise our good health and personal hygiene[.] With no further ado, we remain yours, graciously and devotedly, your attentive and faithful servants. We thank you in advance for what you may be able to do for us.

> Felipe Vaiz,
> José Martinez,
> Felipe Martinez,
> Adolfo Robles,
> Alejandro Gómez,
> Alberto Esquivel.[13]

Drawing on an alternative epistemology, the men explained that their living conditions resulted from systemic inequality, not from ingrained cultural habit. Unlike the state and county officials who crafted reports that avoided charging the railroad companies with any responsibility for the presence of disease and dirt in the camps, the workers did not hesitate to assign blame where it belonged. Health officials focused their efforts to stem the typhus outbreaks on remedying Mexicans' "unclean habits," but the letter writers pointed out the obvious: The unsanitary living conditions that so disturbed health officials were created and maintained by the railroad employers. By failing to treat typhus as a threat to the public at large, officials constructed the disease as uniquely Mexican. This preference for making race the organizing principle for understanding typhus also transformed Mexicans from unfortunate victims of a serious disease into active transmitters of deadly germs, thus adding a medicalized dimension to existing nativism. Armored by their presumed scientific objectivity, health officials gave wide circulation to constructed categories of Mexicans as unclean, ignorant of basic hygiene practices, and unwitting hosts for communicable diseases. These images were embedded in medical and media narratives and in public policy.

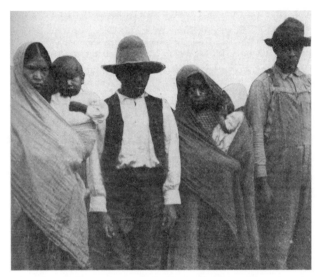

FIGURE 8.1. This photograph of Mexican families appeared on the cover of the *California State Board of Health Monthly Bulletin,* October 1916, to illustrate the dangers of Mexican immigration.

Visual depictions of Mexicans linked them with disease. In October 1916, for example, the cover of the *California State Board of Health Monthly Bulletin* was emblazoned with a photograph of Mexican men, women, and children who lived in the railroad camps. The caption, "The type of people who are bringing typhus and other diseases into California from Mexico," ensured that not even the most naive reader could miss the point.[14] Used in this way, the word *type* reduced all Mexican immigrants to a static archetype. Race, not symptoms, became shorthand for *disease carrier.*[15]

Although the potential typhus epidemic was contained, it spurred widespread changes in immigration inspection procedures. General inspections at the border increased, even for laborers who crossed daily. The Los Angeles County Health Department received assurances that in the future, disinfections at the El Paso border would be performed by USPHS staff. Indeed, the USPHS planned to establish multiple inspection stations along the Texas border, in El Paso, Eagle Pass, Laredo, and Brownsville—a move county officials applauded.[16] Mandatory inspections continued into the late 1920s, further demonstrating the extent to which Mexican immigrants and disease had become conflated.[17]

BRACERO PROGRAM AND HEALTH

The idea that Mexicans were likely to spread disease continued to shape immigration policies in the decades that followed, notably in the Bracero Program. In 1942, the United States and Mexico collaborated in creating this guest worker arrangement, which operated until 1964. The Bracero Program brought four million Mexican men to the United States to work in agriculture and other industries such as railroads to fill World War II labor shortages. The physically rigorous nature of the work the U.S. government was recruiting workers for necessitated assurances that they would be productive and that they posed no public health threat.

This recruitment took place in the wake of deportation programs carried out just a few years earlier. During the Great Depression, everyday citizens and government officials alike scapegoated Mexican immigrants as both drains on the U.S. economy and cultural outsiders. These attitudes led to deportations (voluntary and involuntary) that sent an estimated 1.6 million Mexicans back to their homeland. Although the majority of deportations had ended by 1935, Mexicans who sought medical care at public institutions still risked deportation. The coexistence of the deportations and guest worker program illustrates the pliability of a racial logic that could view Mexicans as liabilities and resources simultaneously.[18]

Scholars have informed our understanding of the Bracero Program by looking at the complexity of the government policy and administration that drove the program.[19] More recently, researchers have shown how the workers themselves exhibited agency as they negotiated this program and how the program affected not just them but also their families, bringing a much-needed gender analysis to this area of study.[20] These recent scholarly works, along with other sources, such as newspaper articles and previously untapped oral interviews, combine to support the conclusion that health policies that were central to the Bracero Program continued to regard Mexicans as health threats rather than critically examining systemic inequalities created and maintained by the Bracero Program. These policies, overseen and sanctioned by the federal government, signaled a new era in medical racial profiling, thus offering a new framework for disciplining labor.

Braceros were recruited in Mexico and underwent health screenings in both Mexico and the United States. In Mexico, personnel from the USPHS, along with the War Manpower Commission and the Farm Security Administration, oversaw the contracting of workers, in collaboration with Mexican officials. Mexicans seeking to participate in the program were required to pass a physical examination by both U.S. and Mexican public health doctors in accordance with U.S. immigration policies and railroad company regulations. U.S. public health officials used standards developed by the U.S. military for conducting medical screenings. Officials required every prospective bracero to undergo a physical examination, with chest x-rays to check for tuberculosis, serological tests to check for venereal disease, psychological profiling, and a chemical bath. They tested applicants to see whether they were capable of the arduous labor expected of them, checking their hands for calluses and their bodies for scars. Inspectors could interpret fresh scars as evidence of injury or pain, thus potentially disqualifying the applicant.[21]

Mexicans found the examinations tiring and humiliating. In her research, historian Ana Rosas found that men could wait anywhere between six and ten hours to be examined. Physicians directed the men into an examination room that held as many as forty men at a time, where they had to undress and undergo an examination the doctors conducted in English.[22] Scholar Barbara Driscoll notes that recruits complained to Mexican officials that USPHS officials were harassing them.[23] Applicants who passed this examination and were accepted to the program found that their trials were not over: They underwent yet another compulsory physical examination when they arrived in the U.S. bracero camps.[24]

Mexican men did their best to retain their dignity through this process. Historian Deborah Cohen interviewed men applying to the Bracero Program and found that Mexican men recast parts of the exams in a positive light. The men wanted to be seen as strong, healthy, and hardworking, so they willingly extended their calloused hands to inspectors as evidence of these qualities. This image was important to them not just as potential participants in the Bracero Program but as male breadwinners for their family and as part of their own sense of masculinity. Applicants also recalled trying to subvert the x-ray examination by drinking large quantities of milk beforehand. They did this not because they had something to hide but because they feared the physicians might find some small imperfection that could be used to disqualify them from the program.[25]

Despite the perception that Mexicans posed a public health threat, the War Manpower Commission, created during World War II to balance the labor needs of agriculture, industry, and the armed forces, was not always willing to fully fund the USPHS physicians' work. When the USPHS moved from its original location in Mexico City to San Luis Potosi, the employees asked to take the x-ray equipment with them. The War Manpower Commission denied permission, on the premise that x-rays were too costly. In 1945, however, a railroad company in eastern Florida complained that a bracero in its employ had an active case of tuberculosis. After this complaint, the USPHS received permission to move the x-ray equipment to its new office, although the head of the War Manpower Commission refused to purchase any more medical equipment.[26]

In the United States, contracted workers underwent a second inspection at USPHS processing centers that duplicated the procedures they experienced in Mexico. USPHS centers in and around El Paso, Texas, the largest port of entry into the United States from Mexico, processed many of the braceros. Often the braceros were transported in cattle cars.[27] Personnel routinely processed 800 to 1,600 braceros at a time and in some cases more than 3,100.[28] Carlos Cordella, a processing employee, described how braceros were asked to strip and then were sprayed with a white powder on their hair, face, and "lower area," a procedure that embarrassed them. Some tolerated the situation with humor, declaring, "I guess we're gringos now."[29]

Many other problems arose in the U.S. inspections. Pedro Ortega reported that U.S. doctors sold the x-ray films of men who had passed the physical exam to braceros who worried about passing. He also reported that doctors occasionally gave penicillin to braceros with the goal of keeping them in good health for six months, the length of their contract.[30]

Although health standards were ostensibly important selection criteria, once braceros were hired, the employers did not adhere to the same standards in providing safe working and living conditions. According to a report from California's State Senate Fact Finding Committee on Labor and Welfare, inadequate health and accident insurance and employee housing ranked among the laborers' most frequent complaints.[31]

In one case in Santa Barbara, California, in 1963, the U.S. Department of Labor was called into a work camp to conduct a special investigation after receiving reports that "wretched conditions existed in the camps." The laborers charged that they had been threatened with return to Mexico if they filed any complaints. Braceros with health problems claimed that they received "unsympathetic treatment from camp doctors." They also complained that they were not given enough to eat and were often served spoiled meat and that their wages were not paid in full.[32] It is striking that concerns about access to health care and the standard of living persisted throughout the Bracero Program's twenty-two-year existence. It is also striking that these concerns involved a government program, carried out by the very same government that was enacting laws and policies dedicated to eradicating the diseases that were spawned by the conditions in which the workers were forced to live.

In its final years, the Bracero Program faced a congressional opponent in representative Edward Roybal. Representative Roybal began his career as a public educator with the California Tuberculosis Association and is remembered for his many years of fighting for the rights of his constituents in East Los Angeles, first as a council member and then as a member of Congress for more than three decades. Representative Roybal publicly denounced the substandard living conditions in the bracero camps and the poor health of the workers and argued against renewing the Bracero Program.[33]

Thus, although the Bracero Program ostensibly upheld strict health standards, in practice it stigmatized Mexicans as bearers of disease while ignoring the systemic conditions that gave rise to disease. Even when investigations repeatedly brought to light problems in the camps, government officials did not rush to ameliorate the problems. Conditions found in the bracero camps were reminiscent of those found in railroad camps fifty years earlier, but change would have required dealing with widespread systemic problems and would have threatened the very existence of the Bracero Program.

MEDICAL DEPORTATIONS

The consistent representation of Mexicans as disease carriers unworthy of social membership in U.S. society led to the conclusion that they were unworthy recipients of publicly funded health care. This philosophy is exemplified by the frightening modern-day practice of patient deportation by hospitals. Some hospitals, without prompting from the federal government, are taking it upon themselves to return patients to their home countries if they are undocumented, without insurance, and in need of long-term care. This occurs because, by law, hospitals that accept Medicare are required to secure continuing care before discharging Medicare patients. Except in California and New York, Medicare does not pay for long-term care for undocumented patients, so hospitals undertake a large financial burden when they accept such patients.

Hospital administrators who deport patients do not necessarily secure health care in the patients' home country. One attorney whose practice specializes in these cases objected, "If somebody has a serious illness and needs continuing care, a hospital can't simply discharge them onto the street, much less put them onto a plane."[34] These hospital-initiated deportations shine a light on how deportations are being performed today outside the purview of Homeland Security.

In today's climate, in which many view Latino immigrants as an economic, cultural, and social threat, it is not surprising that Latino immigrants are often the targets of medical deportations. Although the deportation of immigrants by hospitals originated not to regulate immigration from Latin America but rather as a response to the perceived burden of patients from other countries who are unable to pay for their care, these deportations are nonetheless undergirded by the same racial logic that led to public health screenings during the 1916 typhus outbreak and the Bracero Program, in which immigrant Mexicans were consistently characterized as a problem for or threat to U.S. society. In addition, these deportations are connected to other contemporary medical practices and acts that stigmatize Mexicans, such as the passage of California Proposition 187 in 1994, which sought to withhold public services from undocumented immigrants.[35] Anthropologist Leo Chavez provides a fascinating look at the contemporary categorization of Latinos as threats through medical discourse in his examination of immigrants as organ transplant recipients.[36] Similarly, anthropologist Jonathan Inda examines how immigrants are constructed as incapable of governing themselves through his research on changes in immigration and welfare policy, such as the Personal Responsibility and Work Opportunity Reconciliation Act of 1996.[37]

Hospital deportations suggest that little has changed in the workplace for immigrants since the early twentieth century. Low-wage, low-skilled immigrants routinely perform the most dangerous jobs, yet they are not provided health care as part of their employment and earn too little to purchase their own health insurance. According to a recent special issue of the *American Journal of Industrial Medicine* on occupational health disparities, "Immigrant Latino workers have fatal traumatic injury rates that are one-third higher than U.S. workers overall. Hispanic workers also experience high rates of nonfatal, lost-work injuries and prolonged recover times. Studies show that such workers commonly work in the more dangerous jobs, receive little training, and are exploited by employers."[38]

Focusing on the cost of providing long-term care to injured immigrants reinforces the image of Latinos as a threat and potential burden, obviating examination of the systemic inequalities that place Latinos in this position. Journalist Deborah Sontag has documented cases of deportations resulting from what she calls a "collision of two deeply flawed American systems, immigration and health care." She writes about Luis Alberto Jimenez, an undocumented Guatemalan immigrant who was working as a gardener in Florida when he became the victim of a drunk driver in an auto accident. Uninsured, Jimenez owed hospital and rehabilitation bills of $1.5 million. The hospital, Martin Memorial, obtained a court order and "forcibly returned him to his home country," according to a hospital administrator, although an appeal was pending. The hospital did not notify Jimenez's family of the deportation.[39] In Phoenix, Arizona, as a Mexican patient lay in a coma, hospital personnel, without the family's permission, took her fingerprints to begin deportation proceedings.[40]

Not all deported immigrants are undocumented. Some hospitals routinely return both documented and undocumented immigrants simply because they are uninsured. A Tucson, Arizona hospital attempted to send a sick baby, born in the United States to an undocumented Mexican couple, to the parents' home country. The process was stopped only after legal intervention.[41]

Because these deportations are not part of an official government program, no official statistics exist on how many immigrants have been affected, but the increasing prevalence of examples suggests a trend. St. Joseph's Hospital in Phoenix, which has a large Mexican immigrant population, has reported deporting ninety-six immigrants. Since 2007, ten immigrants have been returned to Honduras from Chicago, Illinois hospitals. In San Diego, California, the Mexican consulate reported eighty-seven medical cases, most of which ended in deportation. The Guatemalan foreign ministry listed fifty-three deportations by U.S. hospitals from 2003 to 2008.[42]

In addition, medicalized repatriation programs have been privatized as companies have developed to provide the services usually undertaken by federal immigration authorities. One such company is MexCare, located in San Diego, which bills itself as "an alternative choice for the care of the unfunded Latin American national." MexCare works with "any hospital seeking to defray un-reimbursed medical expenses" to transport patients to their home country. MexCare emphasizes that it only transports patients when they have received the authorization of the patient or family.[43] By contrast, Steven Larson, an expert on migrant health and an emergency room physician, considers repatriation a "death sentence" in some cases. "I've seen patients bundled onto the plane and out of the country, and once that person is out of sight, he's out of mind."[44]

MexCare is also vague about the hospitals it has collaborated with, thereby raising some doubt about the transparency of its practices. Although its Web site includes a testimonial section, it does not mention the source of the testimonials. One such anonymous quote reads, "Our hospital has used MexCare several times. They help us provide care to our unfunded Latin American patients. They do it all, from start to finish. We are very pleased with their service."[45] Because MexCare is a private company performing a function usually reserved for the federal government, it is difficult or impossible to independently verify the legality or morality of its practices.

Although transnational patient dumping is a recent phenomenon, it nonetheless follows patterns established throughout the twentieth century in which medical discourse is used to distinguish desirable and undesirable members of society. The emergence of private companies such as MexCare is symptomatic of a neoliberal era in which private companies take over activities once performed by public entities. The seeming ease with which a private company can transport a patient in critical condition from Chicago to Honduras is also a feature of the era of globalization. Yet the same racial logic that gave rise to harmful policies and practices in the typhus epidemic and Bracero Program continues to affect Mexicans and other Latin American immigrants.

CONCLUSIONS

How a problem is defined shapes the solution. Negative representations of Mexicans as disease carriers and health burdens shaped the programs, policies, and practices of immigration and health agencies. Many documented cases illustrate the medicalization of the Mexican immigrant historically. The reaction to typhus outbreaks in the early twentieth century and the development of health policy standards in the Bracero Program revolved around representations of Mexicans as a threat to public health. Race served as an interpretive framework for explaining the typhus outbreaks and for developing a double screening policy for braceros entering the United States and thus precluded any need to ameliorate the living conditions of workers once they had settled in the United States. Such reasoning, firmly established, obviated a deeper investigation into the systemic inequality that fostered the inferior health and living conditions of Mexican laborers. Because medical discourse has the power to naturalize racial categories, it has also in some cases naturalized societal inequalities.

The fact that medical discourse had a demonstrable influence on perceptions and consequently on the treatment of Mexican immigrants does not mean that all programs failed to implement changes that improved the public's overall health and welfare. To the contrary, public health agencies and practitioners have carried out many genuinely successful efforts, from reducing infant mortality rates to maintaining pure water supplies. Nonetheless, the power of public health discourse to affect perceptions of race and to contribute to inequalities continues in the twenty-first century.

Latino immigrants who face deportation by U.S. hospitals today, like their counterparts before them, are perceived as unworthy of U.S. aid. Hospital deportations continue to obscure the global structure of inequality: People immigrate to developed nations in search of work, the destination countries benefit from the cheap labor without providing the necessities of a sustainable community, and then the immigrants become scapegoats for the problems that inevitably arise. The situation today did not arise spontaneously but rather flows from the long history of negative representations of Mexicans as outsiders who are unfit to be citizens.

NOTES

I thank the audiences to whom I presented versions of this article for their helpful comments: American Public Health Association; Making Race, Making Health Conference, University of Texas, Austin; and the Department of Chicano–Latino Studies, University of California, Irvine. I also thank Anne-Emanuelle Birn, Ian Fusselman, Meg Wesling, and the anonymous journal reviewers for their helpful comments.

1   Allan Kraut, *Silent Travelers: Germs, Genes, and the "Immigrant Menace"* (New York: Basic Books, 1994).

2   Mark Reisler, *By the Sweat of Their Brow: Mexican Immigrant Labor in the United States, 1900–1940* (Westport, Conn.: Greenwood, 1976), 56.

3   U.S. Congress, House Committee on Immigration and Naturalization, Hearings before the Committee on Immigration and Naturalization, House of Representatives, 70th Congress, First Session, February 21–April 5, 1928 (Washington, D.C.: Government Printing Office, 1928), 60.

4   For more on Manifest Destiny, see Reginald Horsman, *Race and Manifest Destiny: The Origins of American Racial Anglo-Saxonism* (Cambridge, Mass.: Harvard University Press, 1981).

5   Amy Fairchild, *Science at the Borders: Immigrant Medical Inspection and the Shaping of the Modern Industrial Labor Force* (Baltimore, Md.: Johns Hopkins University Press, 2003).

6   Alexandra Minna Stern, *Eugenic Nation: Faults and Frontiers of Better Breeding in Modern America* (Berkeley: University of California Press, 2005), 57.

7   Ibid., 59.

8   Typhus symptoms can include high fever, headaches, chills, and severe muscular pain, followed by the appearance of a rash. The disease is serious and can be fatal for the very young, the elderly, and those already in poor health. See "Epidemic Louse-Borne Typhus," http://www.who.int/mediacentre/factsheets/fs162/en/index.html.

9   The World Health Organization notes, "Louse-borne Typhus is the only rickettsial disease which can cause explosive epidemics in humans." Ibid.

10 In addition to the twenty-two Mexican railroad workers, one person in the city of Los Angeles contracted typhus, two people in the county (but not from the railroad camps) were affected, and no details are available about the one remaining case. There were also outbreaks in areas outside the county: seven cases in Banning (Riverside County), one in Livermore (Alameda County), one in Bakersfield (Kern County), and three in Tulare (Tulare County). *California State Board of Health Monthly Bulletin* (Sacramento: State Board of Health), June–December 1916.

11 H. D. King, "Frequency of Tuberculosis among Negro Laundresses," *Journal of Outdoor Life* 11 (1914): 275. King also wrote about the problems of

miscegenation; see King, "Miscegenation: An Old Social Problem," *New Orleans Medical and Surgical Journal* 66 (1914).

12   Los Angeles County Health Department, "Quarterly Health Report, 7/1–9/30/16," Records, Los Angeles County Department of Health Services Library, Main Office, Los Angeles (DHS). Delousing procedures at this time typically involved routine baths, laundering clothes, and cleaning living quarters. Use of cyanide gas was not common because of the effects chemical gases could have on the central nervous system. In Prussia, however, the military used hydrocyanic acid to fumigate Gypsy dwellings and railway carriages. The key ingredient was sodium cyanide, and the substance also contained sulfuric acid and water. See Paul J. Weindling, *Epidemics and Genocide in Eastern Europe* (Oxford: Oxford University Press, 2000), esp. chapter 4, "The First World War and Combating Lice."

13   F. Vaiz et al. to Mexican consul, October 17, 1916, *Foreign Consulate Records for Los Angeles, Archives Secretaria de Relaciones Exteriores* (Secretary of Foreign Relations), Mexico City.

14   *California State Board of Health Monthly Bulletin,* October 1916, cover.

15   Vicente Rafael, "White Love: Surveillance and National Resistance in the U.S. Colonization of the Philippines," in *Cultures of United States Imperialism,* ed. A. Kaplan and D. Pease (Durham, N.C.: Duke University Press, 1993), 185–218. Rafael argues that these types of photographs flatten out identity, causing individuals to be seen merely as racial types.

16   "Quarterly Health Report, 7/1–9/30/16," 5.

17   Howard Markel and Alexandra Minna Stern, "Which Face? Whose Nation? Immigration, Public Health, and the Construction of Disease at America's Ports and Borders, 1891–1928," *American Behavioral Scientist* 42, no. 9 (1999): 1314–31; John Mckiernan-González, "Fevered Measures: Race, Contagious Disease and Community Formation on the Texas–Mexico Border, 1880–1923" (PhD diss., University of Michigan, 2002); Alexandra Minna Stern, "Buildings, Boundaries, and Blood: Medicalization and Nation- Building on the U.S.–Mexican Border, 1910–1930," *Hispanic American Historical Review* 79, no. 1 (1999): 41–81.

18   Natalia Molina, *Fit to Be Citizens? Public Health and Race in Los Angeles, 1879–1939* (Berkeley: University of California Press, 2006), 141.

19   Kitty Calavita, *Inside the State: The Bracero Program, Immigration, and the I.N.S.* (New York: Routledge, 1992).

20   Ana E. Rosas, "Flexible Families: Bracero Families' Lives across Cultures, Communities, and Countries, 1942–1964" (PhD diss., University of Southern California, 2006); Debra Cohen, "Masculine Sweat, Stoop-Labor Modernity: Gender, Race, and Nation in Mid-Twentieth Century Mexico and the U.S." (PhD diss., University of Chicago, 2001).

21   Barbara A. Driscoll, *The Tracks North: The Railroad Bracero Program of World War II* (Austin: Center for Mexican American Studies, University of Texas at Austin, 1999), 55, 73, 91; Cohen, "Masculine Sweat, Stoop-Labor Modernity," 267.

22   Rosas, "Flexible Families," 67.

23 Driscoll, *Tracks North*, 93.

24 Rosas, "Flexible Families," 197.

25 Cohen, "Masculine Sweat, Stoop-Labor Modernity," 267–68, 71–74, 87–89.

26 Driscoll, *Tracks North*, 93–94.

27 Julius Lowenberg, Bracero History Archive, http://braceroarchive.org/items/show/68.

28 S. Sánchez, oral interview, Bracero History Archive.

29 C. Corella, oral interview, Bracero History Archive.

30 P. Ortega, oral interview, Bracero History Archive.

31 Ruben Salazar, "Braceros Cast in Complex Role," *Los Angeles Times*, November 26, 1962, 3, 30.

32 Ruben Salazar, "U.S. Probe of Bracero Complaints Scheduled: Charges of 'Special Nature' on 'Wretched Conditions' Cited; Full Report Promised," *Los Angeles Times*, November 14, 1963, 30.

33 "Bracero Plan to Be Opposed by Rep. Roybal," *Los Angeles Times*, January 10, 1963, 10.

34 Deborah Sontag, "Deported by U.S. Hospitals," *New York Times*, August 3, 2008, A1.

35 California Proposition 187 was approved via referendum by California voters in 1994 to prevent undocumented immigrants from receiving public benefits or services, including health care and education. Legal challenges prevented it from being implemented. Ostensibly, Proposition 187 was directed at all undocumented immigrants, but in California's political and cultural climate, it was understood that the proposition's primary target was Mexicans. P. Hondagneu-Sotelo, "Women and Children First: New Directions in Anti-Immigrant Politics," *Socialist Review* 25, no. 1 (1995): 169–90.

36 Leo R. Chavez, *The Latino Threat: Constructing Immigrants, Citizens, and the Nation* (Stanford, Calif.: Stanford University Press, 2008).

37 Jonathan X. Inda, *Targeting Immigrants: Government, Technology, and Ethics* (Malden, Mass.: Blackwell, 2006).

38 H. Solis, "Foreword to Disparities Special Issue," *American Journal of Industrial Medicine* 53, no. 2 (2010): 81.

39 Sontag, "Deported by U.S. Hospitals." See also Sontag, "Jury Rules for Hospital That Deported Patient," *New York Times*, July 28, 2009; Sontag, "Deported in Coma, Saved Back in U.S.," *New York Times*, November 9, 2008, A1.

40 "Mexicano Es Deportada en Estado Vegetativo" [Mexican is deported in vegetative state], *La Opinion*, March 12, 2008, http://www.proquest.com.ezproxy.lib.utexas.edu.

41 Sontag, "Deported by U.S. Hospitals."

42 Ibid.

43 MexCare, http://mexcare.com.

44 Sontag, "Deported by U.S. Hospitals."

45 MexCare, http://mexcare.com.

9

"A Transformation for Migrants"

Mexican Farmworkers and Federal Health Reform during the New Deal Era

VERÓNICA MARTÍNEZ-MATSUDA

IN 1946, the *Texas Spectator*, a periodical known for muckraking journalism, reprinted a story from the *Washington Post* titled "Camps Aid to Valley Workers: Projects at Robstown Are Transformation for Migrants." The account, written by Agnes E. Meyer, described the tragic case of a pregnant migrant woman whose experiences, Meyer claimed, "[exemplified] the contrast in health conditions as well as in the whole tenor of life between the camp and the Mexican quarter of Robstown," a town located just west of Corpus Christi. The story reported as follows:

> She could have had her baby delivered without charge through the camp arrangements with the local physicians. But this poor creature had more confidence in the mid-wives to which she had always been accustomed. She slipped out of camp when she felt the baby coming, to an old hag who acts not only as midwife but as *curandera* or curer of all ills, natural [and] supernatural. As the woman's placenta would not separate from the uterus, the midwife pulled at it until she had turned it inside out. When the distracted husband summoned help, rigor mortis had already set in but the midwife still had the bloody mess in her hands.[1]

Meyer's report carefully contrasted what she presented as the superstitious, supernatural, and unconventional practices of the curandera, or healer, to the more modern, sanitary, and professional services of the camp physicians. After offering some insight into the curandera's healing rituals and dual home and work environment, Meyer concluded, "No wonder Robstown has a staggering infant and maternity death rate." In contrast, Meyer gushed, "The camps where housing is clean and medical facilities first-rate have conquered even the all-prevalent intestinal afflictions to a point where not a single infant has succumbed to them." In juxtaposing migrants' tragic medical choices against the triumph of the Farm Security Administration's (FSA) modern health services, Meyer presented the problem of "curing" Mexicans as cultural and not simply based on their lack of resources.[2] The larger tragedy here resulted from Mexicans choosing medical services that resulted in the death of their babies when, in their established labor camps across the country, the FSA presented an option that ended infant mortality. Beginning in 1938, until the camp program was terminated in 1947, the FSA offered migrants subsidized medical care through a series of agricultural workers' health plans administered in the federal labor camps. The guarantee of a healthier life such services offered, according to people such as Meyer, left little to be debated about the advantages or disadvantages of curanderas or doctors. If Mexican migrants were to secure a healthy future, they had to transform their cultural practices and embrace the camps' professional practitioners and modern medicine.

Camp evidence suggests that many families did indeed seek and even fight to protect their families' wellness by using the FSA's health resources. In July 1941, for example, Atilano and Matilde Suárez signed a statement addressed to President Franklin Roosevelt titled "A Petition for a Chance to Live," along with 155 residents of the Weslaco, Texas, labor camp.[3] The petition contested a recent notice of eviction for families who had exceeded the "one-year occupancy rule" aimed at discouraging permanent residency. At the time they signed the petition, the Suárezes had a newborn son and a daughter who was only about a year and a half old.[4] In their appeal, the petitioners stressed the importance of remaining in the labor camp to secure their family's health and well-being.

Migrants' seemingly contradictory responses to federal intervention in their domestic, cultural, and medical affairs reveal the struggle they encountered within their households, community, and in daily interactions with government officials and public health representatives over the best way to address their health needs and concerns. In negotiating the camps' medical program, migrants acted on a calculated choice to have the government care for them in an effort to improve their families' prospects for a healthier future. Their varied choices also challenged federal officials to extend their definition of migrant citizen-ship (in both juridical and cultural terms) and concurrently exposed an inherent paradox in the camp's medical program. That these two stories could coexist demonstrates the contradictory reality surround-ing the FSA's social reform efforts. Ultimately, the FSA contributed to both improved migrant health and racialized discourses concerning Mexican farmworking families' cultural practices that further encoded their status as second-class citizens.

The FSA's contradictory approach to health reform for migrant laborers yields several crucial lessons about the role of the welfare state that reemerged most concretely during the "War on Poverty" in the 1960s. The FSA's idealistic labor camp program provided migrant farmworkers critical care to combat the alarming rates of disease, malnourishment, infant mortality, and economic poverty that affected their families. In an unprecedented manner, the agency took migrants' health conditions seriously, they defended migrants' right to govern-ment attention, and they applied significant federal funds to aid migrant farmworkers' everyday lives. This extraordinary level of federal com-mitment and responsibility to care for the nation's farmworkers was truly promising.

In the process of conducting this effort, however, the FSA's medical program reflected, deepened, and even produced problematic cultural biases that further exploited and racialized different poor and working-class groups across the United States. In Texas, as this chapter will show, the FSA celebrated the rationality and modernity of Anglo culture over the ignorance and backwardness of Mexican culture to promote and help affirm the medical program's contributions to social reform. As they struggled to receive medical attention and sanitary housing on their own terms, Mexican migrants unmasked these contradictions rooted in the FSA's programing efforts and fought to keep the FSA's commitment to improved health working in their favor.

This chapter begins by explaining the broader historical and socio-economic setting from which the labor camp program emerged to high-light the logic behind the government and medical authorities' concern for migrants' health on one hand and migrants' desires to protect their families on the other. I argue that federal officials' needs to maintain support for the camp program led them to remain flexible in the way they promoted their medical objectives among local communities and agricultural employers. FSA agents argued that migrants' improved health was central to their cultural reform while also affecting both the spread of contagions and their efficiency as workers. The alarming portrayal of Mexican families in need of curing was advanced alongside the claim of producing stronger bodies that were critical to industrial farming. As World War II got under way, the FSA's ability to address migrants' needs was stymied by conservative political attacks against "sociological experimentation," leaving the gains Mexicans encountered through the camp's medical program vulnerable to termination.[5]

The chapter shifts next to showing how, in the process of advancing their medicalized project, FSA officials pathologized Mexicans' domestic and cultural practices as unhealthy, harmful, and degenerative. This discourse allowed the agency to carry out a valuable program of health education (aimed primarily at farmworking women), but it also promoted racialized views of Mexican culture and poverty as it reinforced normative American standards of health and hygiene. Ironically, this strategy allowed the FSA to allocate medical resources to families very much in need of them, even as it established an official discourse of Mexican migrants as unable to care for themselves. Such policies, I argue, foreshadowed the kind of struggles that arose again in the 1960s as Americans debated social theories explaining the "culture of poverty," especially, the interplay between cultural ignorance, poverty, race, and disease.[6] Laurie B. Green's chapter in this volume insightfully analyzes the scope of these struggles in relation to America's fight against hunger.

As Mexican migrants mediated their engagement with health authorities and state-generated medical ideologies and practices, they forced a discussion of their human and civil rights to the forefront of national debate. Beyond demonstrating their own desire and determination to improve their lives, Mexican migrants' willingness to participate in the camps' social programs advanced their claims to national belonging. This was especially powerful in Texas, where the majority of labor camp inhabitants were American-born, legal citizens. In light of the narrative of invisibility, exclusion, and marginalization that had long characterized Mexican Americans' experiences as farmworkers and U.S. citizens, the political consciousness and promise imbued in their daily actions remains one of the camp program's most important legacies.

THE FEDERAL MIGRATORY LABOR CAMP PROGRAM

Although the radicalism of a predominantly Mexican and Filipino workforce brought the matter of farmworkers' domestic conditions to the government's attention during strikes in the early 1930s, it was a simultaneous change in the ethnoracial composition of California's agricultural labor force that finally resulted in the formation of a labor camp program. Between 1935 and 1938, more than 300,000 Dust Bowl migrants, most of whom were white, arrived in California in search of work. The "Okie exodus," depicted in John Steinbeck's influential novel *The Grapes of Wrath* (1939), encouraged widespread debate over the issue of government intervention, especially for families abased by the economic crisis of the Great Depression. Steinbeck's idyllic and romanticized depiction of "Weedpatch Camp," a place where the Joad family found hot showers, indoor privies, free medical care, and regular recreational activities, was intended to show Americans the promise of the federal camps in addressing migrants' socioeconomic needs.[7]

The first labor camp was built in 1935, and by 1942 there were ninety-five permanent and mobile camps in service across the nation, with accommodations for an estimated 19,464 families, or 83,695 individuals.[8] Most of the labor camps were located in seven states: California, Oregon, Washington, Idaho, Arizona, Texas, and Florida. Texas had the second largest concentration of permanent labor camps, after California. At this time, camp inhabitants included Japanese Americans (many of whom were transferred from World War II U.S. internment camps to the FSA camps to work as farm laborers), Mexican Americans, African Americans, and increasingly after 1942, imported foreign-born workers, primarily from Mexico, Jamaica, and the Bahamas. White Dust Bowl migrants had not entirely disappeared from the camps' population, but their numbers had dwindled as many found employment in better-paying wartime industries.

In establishing a national camp program, the FSA (and its predecessor, the Resettlement Administration) demonstrated great initiative in fighting rural poverty. In its early stages, the camp program was led by one of President Franklin Roosevelt's "Brain Trust" leaders, Rexford Tugwell, an agricultural economist well known for his left-leaning politics. Tugwell was also advised in the creation of the program by people such as Carey McWilliams, who had long advocated for measures to protect farmworkers against the abuses of corporate agriculture in California. Those first working on the camp program were, in great part, idealistic people who had a genuine interest in providing migrant families the necessary resources—including sanitary housing, regular employment, improved education, and a healthy diet—to combat the causes of their destitution. According to Michael Grey, an expert on New Deal medicine, "the rigor with which the FSA pursued its mandate established its reputation as one of the most socially conscious of all New Deal programs."[9]

It was this same idealism and concern for the broader socioeconomic conditions affecting migrant families (beyond the Dust Bowl refugees) that placed the FSA under constant attack from powerful growers and their organizations, such as the Associated Farmers and American Farm Bureau. The FSA was regularly fighting for the federal funding and political backing needed to stay active. As a result, it never realized any effort to transform the systemic abuses inherent in standard farm labor practices. Instead of altering the deeper sources of farmworkers' poverty and directly challenging the conditions in capitalist agriculture that created such problems in the first place, the FSA increasingly focused its attention on reforming migrant families.

Consequently, the great paradox in the FSA's labor camp program lies in the fact that it emerged from a sincere and strong commitment to aid migratory workers, but in the process of doing so, it reinforced culturally biased notions that racialized struggling farmworkers. Ironically, this often resulted from the same efforts to draw public attention to migrants' socioeconomic plight. It was this same visibility, and more specifically the degraded nature by which some migrants were made visible, that helped perpetuate existing discourses blaming them for their condition. Considering Mexican migrants' experiences in Texas within this framework reveals a more complex narrative, where health became the terrain on which broader struggles around race and labor were waged.

The curandera story opening this chapter must be understood within this contradictory framework to fully grasp the complicated nature of Mexican migrants' encounters with the FSA. Meyer's article first appeared in the *Washington Post* on April 22, 1946, less than one month after President Harry S. Truman signed the Farmers Home Administration Act, abolishing the FSA.[10] Although termination of the camp program did not arrive until one year later (on July 31, 1947), it was already clear, as Meyer herself warned, that "one of the only serious efforts ever put forth to help ease the plight of the Latin American migrant worker [was] headed for the ash can."[11] Because her report could help drum up support for the camp program, it is possible that the FSA recruited Meyer to publish her findings. Meyer was undoubtedly influenced by Joseph Cowen, the FSA's regional director, and Dr. Lee Janice, the FSA's field medical officer, who accompanied her on her tour of the South Texas camps and surrounding communities. Whether Meyer's account was published in an attempt to save the program, out of a benevolent concern for Mexican migrants' welfare, or both, the outcome was the same. The report contributed to a broader discourse stemming from the FSA that indicted Mexican migrants' cultural practices as primitive in relation to the virtues of modern hygiene, nutrition, childrearing, and social responsibility available in the federal camps. It was through this process of delimiting Mexican migrants' health awareness and medical choices that the FSA became an agent fueling Mexican farmworkers' racialization.

THE CAMPS AS A "PUBLIC BARRIER TO THE SPREAD OF DISEASE"

Although some criticized the FSA for engaging in matters that appeared well beyond their domain, FSA officials contended that medical care provisions, including preventive health services and health education, were central to their overall objective of rehabilitation, or socioeconomic uplift, among rural families. To support their claims, the FSA used national surveys conducted by the U.S. Public Health Service and other medical organizations to highlight migrants' health deficiencies in relation to those of nontransients. In the border area of Hidalgo County, Texas, where Mexican migrant families made up a significant portion of the general population, studies found that tuberculosis rates were approximately eight times as high as the national median in the 1930s, "averaging nearly 400 cases per 1,000 residents compared with 51 cases per 1,000 nationally." In general, migrants' mortality rate from tuberculosis was almost 200 times higher than among the total U.S. population. Diseases induced by malnourishment and an unbalanced diet were also more prevalent among Mexican migrants. According to a 1931 report on the health and nutrition of Mexicans living in Texas, "from 1924 through 1935, there were [a total of] 7,550 deaths from pellagra in the state, an average of 755 per year [and] a death rate three times greater than that for the United States as a whole." Pellagra is a disease brought on by a niacin (a type of vitamin B) deficiency, which causes harm to the body's digestive system, skin, and nerves. A child suffering from pellagra ordinarily appears malnourished and has severe skin lesions and swelling on his or her face, hands, and feet. Doctors who analyzed the pellagra problem in Texas linked their disturbing findings directly to the existing farm labor system, particularly its reliance on a migratory workforce.[12]

FSA officials insisted that migrant farmworkers carried various contagions when they traveled through different communities, creating a serious health hazard and burden to more than just themselves. To make this claim clear, Baird Snyder, FSA chief engineer, requested that his team of sanitary and public health engineers collect "additional data on pathogenic disease along the streams of migration, with special emphasis on those loci at which [the FSA had] erected these public barriers [the migrant camps] to the spread of disease." According to Snyder, this particular enterprise would allow the FSA to "evaluate, as time wears on, the actual public health value of a migratory camp against pathogenic disease." Snyder was confident that over time the FSA would prove that the federal migrant camps were "worth to the public health alone all that they cost."[13]

The engineers' preliminary findings in Texas demonstrated how closely pathogenic diseases and agricultural labor migration were tied together. As Karl Buster, District 5 engineer, noted,

> The geographical lines of incidence of typhoid closely follow the geographical lines of migration of casual farm labor. . . . disease does follow the lines of communication. Typhus fever has been followed across the state from the western portion to the eastern portion. The dreadful influenza epidemic followed transportation lines through the state. Dysentery and typhoid epidemics follow the cotton pickers in their migration to new fields. We know the line of migration of cotton pickers originates in the southern portion of the state and extends north through the central and eastern portion, thence northwest and terminating in the area around Lubbock.[14]

Snyder recognized the great value this information had both for the FSA and public health studies throughout the country. The proof of widespread disease among migrant workers, particularly among Mexicans "originating in the southern portion of the state," allowed the FSA to argue that the construction of the camps would be an asset to local communities, not a social and economic liability, as many contended. To garner support for the establishment of the camp program in South Texas, for instance, Ernest Wilson, FSA field supervisor, told the Kiwanis Club in Sinton, "Children will go to your schools free of communicable diseases and with clean bodies." Moreover, "workers having better living conditions and medical care will be able to render a much better service to the farmers for whom they work."[15] Although the FSA may have been genuinely interested in improving migrants' health and socioeconomic status by providing sanitary housing, clean water, toilets, and a steady diet, they still claimed communities needed protection against the menace of migrants' poor health. There was some truth to this claim, given the communicable nature of tuberculosis and other diseases Mexican migrants suffered from, but this public discourse had damaging consequences.

By drawing on American middle-class public health ideologies that pathologized Mexican migrants' sociocultural customs and beliefs as menacing to their families' and communities' well-being, FSA officials drew on familiar narratives that linked cultural deficiency to race and citizenship. As historians Nayan Shah and Natalia Molina have convincingly argued, by the early twentieth century, health and hygiene became increasingly accepted as fundamental characteristics of American identity. Health specialists commonly claimed that unless people could learn to adopt good "modern" health practices and maintain a higher standard of living, they were a threat not simply to their own health and prosperity but also to that of the nation. Those unable or unwilling to meet the nation's developing health standards were not "fit" for social membership.[16] As the FSA and public health officials worked to "clean up," transform, and modernize Mexican migrants' bodies and daily cultural practices, they claimed to restore their civic virtue and demonstrate Mexican migrants' worthiness for citizenship to the rest of the nation. With the onset of World War II and increased attacks on the New Deal's liberal programing, the FSA's concerns in this regard expanded to reveal how Mexican migrants' healthy bodies (both foreign and American born) were essential to agricultural production and the war effort. In Texas, FSA camp administrators argued that Mexican migrants posed a serious health threat to themselves, their families, and the communities in which they traveled, primarily because they were ignorant of the factors that contributed to disease and illness. Their "unhealthy" cultural practices, domestic behavior, and medical choices made their ability to act as responsible citizens questionable. Demonstrating this opinion, the Council of Women for Home Missions, an organization actively involved in several of the FSA camps, reported in 1938 that one of the factors contributing to high infant mortality rates among Mexican migrant families was the "ignorance of the mother." To support their claim, the organization included the following story in their report:

> When the Martinez twins came, the mother was rushed to the hospital in an effort to save her life and that of her children. In ten days the mother was back in camp [a non-FSA facility]. A few more days and she was in the cotton fields again, the mites cuddled in a box at her side. In six weeks all that was left to her was a memory and two nameless graves in a field.[17]

As a final remark, the authors exclaimed, "Sometimes the struggle is longer but the end is too often inevitable," meaning that such conditions regularly resulted in tragedy if not eliminated.

Although the Council of Women for Home Missions also pointed to the unsanitary environment, constant moving, and insufficient wages as matters that likewise "spelled tragedy for the [migrant] baby," by attributing the infants' "inevitable" death to the mother's poor judgment, they affirmed that socioeconomic conditions were not entirely to blame for Mexican migrants' detrimental health status. Such claims were representative of the movement in public health reform and social welfare under way in the United States around this time. In general, the 1920s and 1930s saw a significant shift away from focusing on the environment and privation (i.e., external conditions and poverty) as the causes for disease toward faulting individuals (particularly mothers) and cultural behavior. To improve immigrants' prospects for living a healthy life, reformers believed that mothers had to be taught the science of home management, involving nutritious cooking, domestic sanitation, and hygienic care of children.[18]

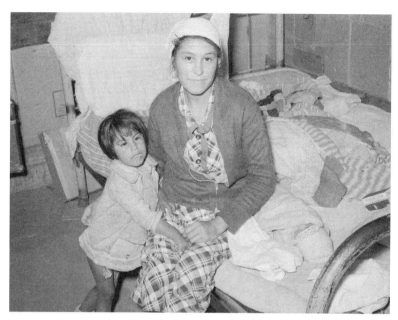

FIGURE 9.1. A Mexican mother in her home after giving birth. Crystal City, Texas (March 1939). Photograph by Russell Lee; courtesy of the FSA/OWI Photographic Collection, LOC, LC-USF34-032352-D.

Several photographs taken by the FSA's documentary division demonstrate the extent to which Mexican migrants' domestic realm remained a focal point for the agency's health reform and cultural redevelopment efforts in the late 1930s. For example, Russell Lee's images of Mexican farmworkers' living conditions in Crystal City, Texas, taken in 1939, included the following photograph and accompanying caption:

> Mexican Mother and Child in Home. This Woman Had Given Birth to Baby on Bed While She Had an Advanced Case of Gonorrhea. The Baby at Time Picture was Taken was Ten Days Old. The Baby Slept in the Same Bed with the Mother and She was Caring for Both It and the Small Child by Her Side.

In a series of similar photographs, Lee observed that Mexicans were unaware of the health risks they posed to their families and communities and thus were partially responsible for the social and health-related problems in their lives—as if having an infant in a mother's bed was bad, or peculiar to Mexican Americans. Photographs by chroniclers such as Lee, however, concealed, even as they highlighted, the structural poverty and racial inequality affecting Mexican migrants in order to draw the viewer's attention (through the explicit caption) to what they portrayed as the subject's lack of health awareness. Unlike the FSA's more iconic imagery of the Dust Bowl migrants, which worked to depict white migrants as victims of their social circumstances and featured their poverty as an object of sympathy, the ethnic Mexican migrants in Lee's images were faulted for their condition.[19] The national dispersal of these representations had dangerous implications for pathologizing Mexicans' domestic practices and racializing what was fundamentally a structural problem. Still, the images justified the FSA's intervention in matters of preventive health education and sociocultural reform. The photographs of diseased Mexican bodies called for action that reassured viewers (mainly middle-class Americans) that their concerns and fears surrounding Mexicans' ignorance would be met.

CLEANING UP THE "DIRTY RIVAS"

In 1941, Joseph N. Cowen, camp manager for the federal labor camp in Sinton, Texas, reported his findings on whether migrant families received any permanent educational values from residence in the FSA camps. To show that migrant families were learning important standards and codes of behavior that would influence their lives, Cowen included the following transcript from a conversation he had with one of the Mexican American migrants residing at the camp:

> COWEN: Emilio, do you think that your people learn very much, get any permanent good or education from living in these camps? That is, do you think they change their habits any?
> EMILIO: Well . . . when the dirty Rivas first came here, they were called the Dirty Rivas. We had them clean up. Now, the Dirty Rivas is the Clean Rivas.[20]

Cowen's decision to use Emilio's humorous response as an affirmation of the positive impact the labor camp program was having on "[Emilio's] people" reveals the transformation public officials hoped would take place inside the camps. That the camps served as a site in which the practice of "cleaning up" the "Dirty Rivas" occurred underscores the dramatic role the FSA played in shaping Mexican migrants' domestic lives. By identifying Mexican migrants' "habits" (i.e., their transgressive cultural practices) as the source of their deficiency, the FSA promoted discourses that pathologized Mexican migrants' poor health in racial terms.

As the transcript also suggests, however, FSA agents did not engage in this effort alone; Mexican migrants were willing, and often eager, to "clean up." Although some may have found the camps' medical program patronizing and even culturally offensive, Mexican migrant families recognized that the camps' resources presented a valuable opportunity to combat the health dangers posed by their unsanitary living conditions, lack of medical attention, and poverty. For many, as the Weslaco camp petitioners made clear, the camp's medical program offered "a chance to live." In their willingness to grapple with the FSA's medical project, Mexican migrants demonstrated that they were not merely objects of the FSA's reform efforts but engaged those efforts on their own terms.

A study of the workshops, lessons, and committees facilitated by the labor camps' home management supervisors (HMSs) best illustrates the degree to which federal officials hoped to impose new practices of domestic behavior, institute new standards for proper medical care, and transform migrants' cultural and traditional values to better meet the notion of good health and citizenship the FSA desired. These forms of health education were carried out in each of the camps nationwide, meaning that the FSA did not exclusively target Mexican farmworkers in their efforts. Even so, Mexican migrants' experiences best illuminate how the camps' workshops created a contested space where they were pressured to adopt modern and dominant American standards of health, hygiene, diet, and personal care. Arguably, FSA officials assumed that all migrants inhabiting the camps were ignorant of such standards regardless of their ethnoracial identity. But in Texas, where Mexican American families made up the majority of the camp population, the HMS and camp nurses reinforced racial ideologies that defined Mexican Americans as non-Americans. By maintaining beliefs about their culture as deficient, they failed to incorporate Mexican migrants' knowledge about nutrition and health care into their lessons.

Not unlike earlier progressive reformers, the HMS believed that migrant women, particularly those who were mothers, had the ability to change their families' traditional practices by instituting the changes toward "better health" the FSA promoted. In this sense, migrant women (and, to a lesser extent, the adolescent girls) were key mediators in negotiating the pressures associated with the FSA's medical program and critical actors in shaping the government's health measures in a way that could meet their families' needs. Migrant women attended lessons and engaged in discussions on numerous topics, including "Questions about Your Teeth," "Typhoid and the Fly," "Home, Hygiene and Care of the Sick," "Keep[ing] Fitness with the Right Foods," and "Diets to Fit the Family Income." In these classes, they were taught how to make soaps, shampoos, and toothpaste, to can foods and make budgeted grocery lists, to prepare recipes for "a well balanced diet," and to keep dangerous pests and disease carriers out of their homes.[21]

To further inculcate the ideas introduced in the home management workshops, camp officials encouraged migrant women to participate in various "women's committees" responsible for maintaining and instituting appropriate measures of health and sanitation in the federal camp. In this regard, migrant women acquired some authority to facilitate and regulate the adoption of guidelines and recommendations promoted by the FSA's health program. In Texas, the women who made up such committees were primarily Anglo, not because of any apparent racial bias by the HMS but because they were the more permanent residents with family incomes supported by year-round agricultural employment. Mexican families did not live in the camps' "labor homes" but rather inhabited the "temporary shelters" for shorter-term residents. Located closer to the camps' administrative center, these shelters subjected Mexican families to more regular supervision in their adoption of the camp policies, including appropriate health standards. In the Crystal City camp, for instance, an "Inspection Committee" accompanied the camp nurse, Miss Chandler, in making a weekly examination of the more temporary residents' living environment. In an ironic outcome, the camp section or district having the cleanest shelters, comfort stations, and shared grounds received one bar of soap for each family in that section.[22]

In addition to holding lessons on matters of hygiene, nutrition, and childcare, both nurses and the HMS frequently instructed the camps' migrant women on matters related to sex education, family planning, and birth control. Information on such topics as "Preparation for Pregnancy," "The Question of Sexual Relations," "Step by Step in Sex Education," "Preparing for Marriage," and "Feeding the Child for Health" were distributed to women (in both English and Spanish) as part of this effort. Although such lessons probably provided useful information about syphilis, gonorrhea, and other sexually transmitted diseases, they also presumed that Mexican women did not know about sex. To ensure that migrant mothers were following the right measures in caring for their pregnancies, the FSA required that they attend regular prenatal and postpartum clinics and carefully monitored their attendance. At the Crystal City camp, for example, Miss Chandler frequently publicized a list of names expected at the "baby clinic" in the camp newspaper.[23] When migrant mothers failed to adhere to the program's expectations, the camp nurse or the "women's committee" paid the family a visit at their shelter home. According to the FSA, "constant supervision" by the nurses and doctors was necessary for a "well baby."[24]

The most coercive measure the FSA practiced over expectant mothers in the labor camps was the insistence that a physician be present when migrant women gave birth. According to Michael Grey, this demand "represented an unusually explicit government effort to monitor and modify medical practice for that period."[25] The FSA's medical program, however, reflected broader public health measures seeking to transform obstetric care into a practice exclusive to licensed physicians, or (at the very least) to professionally trained midwives. As Lena McQuade-Salzfass's revealing study on reproductive health in New Mexico argues, this battle was not simply cultural. Such measures commonly promoted racial pathologies around women's birth choices that ignored their poverty. In 1940, studies found that 71 percent of nonwhite women in the United States were still delivering their babies with the help of a midwife, suggesting that it was a familiar and acceptable choice for their working-class milieu.[26] But the tragic case involving the Mexican woman from Robstown underscored for FSA officials, as it was meant to do for sympathetic readers, why only physician-attended births were a responsible choice. To train ethnic Mexican farmworkers to trust and use the camps' modern medical services, the FSA aimed to convince them that such practices guaranteed better health outcomes.

MIGRANTS' ENCOUNTERS WITH FEDERAL HEALTH REFORM

As camp residents, the Robstown woman and her husband understood the choice they were making by "slipping out" to acquire the birthing services of a midwife and healer, or partera. Even though the FSA taught migrant women about the benefits of delivering their babies with doctors in modern medical facilities, and despite the fact that the FSA's health plan, the Agricultural Workers Health Association, would have covered all costs associated with the birth, the couple decided to pay $35 for the services of the partera. Given the circumstances, why did they make such a costly decision? Although it is impossible to know for sure what influenced their choice, a few important possibilities are worth considering. One explanation is that a language barrier might have existed between the medical staff and the migrant woman and her family. By the early 1940s, federal officials were aware that this was a serious matter affecting migrants' willingness to participate in the medical program, particularly in regions such as South Texas, where a majority of the migrants were Spanish speakers. For this reason, R. C. Williams, the FSA's chief medical officer, noted that "a working knowledge of Spanish as spoken by the average Mexican [was] important for the camp nurses." "Should they not have a working knowledge of Mexican-Spanish [at the time of employment]," he suggested that they be "required to begin a study of this language at once."[27] FSA officials reasoned that if the medical staff spoke some Spanish, they would seem more "sympathetic to Mexican migrants," making migrants more likely to trust in their health services than those they traditionally relied on.[28]

Another reason could have been that the Robstown woman preferred the assistance of a female, Mexican partera, whose birthing practices were probably more familiar and comforting than a male physician and clinic, where parturition was treated solely as a medical (not holistic) practice. Unlike the male physician, parteras customarily provided both emotional and physical care, including abdominal massages and various herbal tea remedies before and after delivery. In most cases, parteras also allowed the woman's relatives to assist in the birth, possibly explaining the presence of the so-called "distracted husband" in Meyer's account, and engaged in traditional rituals such as saving the placenta and umbilical cord for special treatment according to custom. It appears that these are not things Meyer understood or cared to acknowledge, which calls to question the extent to which she accurately depicted the couple's experience when she recorded her version of the story.

Although any or all of these factors may have influenced the Robstown couple's decision, what is most suggestive of their choice to deliver their baby as they preferred, and not as federal officials saw fit, is that it demonstrates how migrants found ways to challenge the pressure to conform to the customs and standards federal officials imposed. In other words, it shows that although migrants may have chosen to participate in the camps' medical and social welfare reforms in exchange for housing and other amenities, they continued to practice their own approaches to family management and health care based on their personal convictions. In this way, their actions subverted FSA medical discourses that highlighted the cultural (versus structural) sources behind their vulnerable condition. Racialized depictions such as Meyer's discredited the medical knowledge and skill Mexican midwives maintained in order to link superstitious "old hags" and senseless Mexican families in a narrative of tragic outcomes. By subverting, altering, or even evading the FSA's reform measures, however, migrant families questioned to what extent a visit to the doctor would truly improve their status as Mexican farmworkers.

Mexican families were willing to manage the cultural racism imbued in the FSA's practices to bring about more lasting improvements to their conditions. They participated in the program because they recognized that federal attention to their plight was valuable—even if, paradoxically, it perpetuated negative perceptions of Mexican families' domestic lives. Although camp documents make it difficult to evaluate to what extent migrant families appreciated the services the FSA's health program provided, their engagement suggests that many recognized it provided a valuable service, source of relief, and the potential for improved living. Given the high rate of disease, malnutrition, and infant mortality, it is not surprising that many families did appreciate the practical lessons in health and hygiene, medical attention, financial assistance, and even female camaraderie that the camps' program afforded. Although some migrants may have resented the health program's paternalistic approach, they also understood that these services allowed them to better balance their work in the fields with their work and responsibilities at home.

This was the sentiment several Mexican American families expressed in November 1941 when they requested permission to leave some of their family members in camp as the "head of family" migrated to West Texas for cotton picking. In their plea to extend their stay, the Robstown, Texas migrants cited reasons of health conditions, economic subsistence, educational factors, and general domestic safety as evidence of why they desired to stay in camp. Henry C. Daniels, the camp's manager, supported their request, assuring leading FSA officials that it would not "be a question of turning away eligible farm workers [for residence] so that these women and children can remain in the community."[29] Even though FSA supervisors acknowledged "Latin-American families' particular need for sanitary housing and steady schooling," they ultimately reiterated that the labor camps should remain temporary shelter communities.[30] Despite losing the case, the Robstown families successfully pressured the FSA to evaluate their commitment to safeguarding migrants' health and in this way demonstrated a critical agency in shaping the medical program. They also exposed the FSA's depiction of Mexican families as having to be coerced into the camps' health care system as false. This appeal showed how some migrants were actually trying to pressure the federal government into granting extended aid.

Migrants' diverse responses to the FSA's health program suggest the important negotiation involved in deciding how best to use the services available to them. Although these decisions often involved significant mediation between migrant families and FSA officials, they were also settled among migrant families themselves, further demonstrating the internal complexities in migrants' encounters with the FSA. Oral histories with former camp residents sometimes reveal a humorous interpretation of their experiences. The telling of amusing stories, particularly among migrant families and communities, connotes an important understanding of themselves as outsmarting camp officials and the FSA's reform objectives. The accounts describe migrants as anything but ignorant in their cultural practices. Instead, such narratives show how Mexican migrants were willing to engage the FSA and play along with the program's expectations for their own benefit.

Mr. Herón Ramirez, for instance, remembered that his mother was fairly receptive to the ideas and lessons promoted by the HMS at the McAllen, Texas camp. About matters related to cooking and nutrition, he exclaimed,

> When it came to the food, we experimented! My family would eat spinach and artichoke, and roast turkey and things we had never had before because they told mom it was good for us. If the nurse or those lessons told you it was good for your brain and that sort of thing, we ate it.[31]

Ms. Ramirez was eager to treat her family to a healthful diet that did not represent Mexican food choices because she trusted it was good for them. The story, as Mr. Ramirez described it, showed a Mexican household enthusiastic about the FSA's recommendations and willing to try them. Even so, Mr. Ramirez's discussion of the camps' surplus commodities suggested that his family still found ways to push the boundaries of expected engagement with the medical program. Though not as nutritious, Mr. Ramirez remembered fondly the cookies his mother made with the camp's food supply. He stated, "You know those peanut-butter cookies, the ones with the fork marks on top? Ooh, my mother made the best ones!" The cookies were a regular favorite among Mr. Ramirez and his siblings.

The family's use of commodities that were less favored further demonstrates how they negotiated the programs' acculturation efforts. For example, describing his family's regular weekend trips to visit relatives in neighboring Starr County, Ramirez amusingly recalled,

> We'd go see grandma and grandpa and the house where we were born and raised. My mother would take powdered milk and eggs [supplied through the camp program] that nobody liked to eat, and give them to grandpa so that he could mix it with the slop to feed his pigs.

Such accounts, though lighthearted, express the important ways migrants embraced the FSA's health reform project while adapting the resources it offered to serve as they saw fit. The Ramirez family's use of the FSA's food distribution presumably went beyond what program officials intended, but for this migrant family, it still served as a source of sustenance that aided their condition. In this way, we see again that migrant families were mindful agents negotiating and molding the FSA's medical program to attend to their needs.

Migrant children, not unlike their parents, also weighed the pressure FSA officials exerted to comply with the medical program against the rewards it promised to deliver. Alcario Samudio, who resided at the Weslaco, Texas camp, remembered lining up one day to have his tonsils removed at the camp clinic. As he described it,

> There was this one day that there was a whole line over there [by the clinic], and I went to check why that line was there. I thought they were giving something away. But no, they were taking tonsils out! And they were gonna give free ice cream and comic books,

so my brother and I both got in line. There was a whole line of kids! We had no problem.[32]

In a similar manner, Mr. Samudio stated that the nurse would sometimes line everyone up to give them shots "for this and that," and he would think "Ah, what the hell, I might as well do it!" The memory of such experiences, though seemingly carefree, offers a valuable insight into the way migrants made daily decisions that determined their willingness to participate in the camps' health project.

In choosing to reside in one of the federal camps, migrants were conscious of the pressure to adhere to the FSA's medical standards and health education programming. Upon entering the camp, for instance, each family was required to pass a thorough health examination at the medical clinic and take a series of vaccinations, primarily for typhoid, smallpox, diphtheria, and whooping cough. During peak season, it was not uncommon for the camp nurse and doctor to conduct more than a hundred medical examinations in one week.[33] The program's health administrators subjected incoming residents to medical screenings in order to identify any illness "likely to endanger the health of other camp occupants, or chronic conditions likely to render the applicants ineligible for camp residence."[34] Even after residing in the camp for a period of time, migrants were expected to have regular examinations and keep up with the required immunizations. A report on the Robstown camp concluded that "these precautions kept some of the most backward migrants from using the labor centers," resulting in "a phenomenal health record for young and old alike in a countryside haunted by tuberculosis and intestinal diseases."[35] Presumably, those considered "backward" were migrants who were unwilling to undergo the camps' medical treatment or had conditions beyond the FSA's ability to care for.

That the FSA's medical program chose not to concentrate its efforts on those migrants with serious medical conditions illustrates how it functioned mostly as a preventive measure that attempted to control the spread of communicable diseases or illnesses among migrants, especially as they traveled throughout the country. By the early 1940s, congressional investigations, political attacks, and budgetary cuts pressured the FSA to reformulate its health objectives to better reflect the nation's wartime agenda. To do so, the agency had to prove that their foremost concern was not to promote the social welfare, physical well-being, or more general rehabilitation of migrant families but to erase any obstacles to farm labor production. Therefore, the Migrant Medical Program existed in the camps not simply to keep migrants healthy but, more importantly, to keep them working.

Exemplifying this concern, *The Dawson County Courier* exclaimed in a story published on October 30, 1941 that the medical service was given at the Lamesa, Texas, camp "to improve the health and therefore increase the working days of farm laborers in the area."[36] On a similar note, in a 1944 speech before the annual convention of the American Public Health Association, Dr. Frederick D. Mott, acting chief medical officer for the FSA, proudly announced that "the FSA camps had only a 1.5 percent loss of available man-days due to illness-related absenteeism," a figure that compared quite favorably with the "national average for industrial workers [which was at] about 3.7 percent."[37] According to Mott, this fact reflected the "effectiveness of the volume of services" delivered through the Migrant Medical Program.

CONCLUSION

Although the FSA may have identified migrants inhabiting the camps primarily as workers and sought to improve their overall condition so as to ensure their labor potential, the measures they used had implications that were far more profound and far-reaching. The FSA's medical program set an important standard for direct federal intervention in matters of medical care, social welfare, and cultural reform. It also provided farmworkers with unprecedented services to stay healthy, including sanitary housing, regular immunizations, health education, and a steady and nutritious diet. For Mexican migrants in Texas these resources were critical to combating the dire health and poor domestic conditions they faced as a result of their unstable employment and their second-class status as racial minorities in the United States. Mexican migrants took advantage of the FSA's idealistic effort to foster stronger workers and better citizens because they recognized it could significantly improve their lives. The gains they could acquire with the federal government's intervention outweighed the costs associated with the FSA's pathologizing discourses that advanced cultural-racist logic portraying Mexicans as careless, backward, and menacing.

As Mexican migrants resided in the camps, participated in the project's social programs, and took advantage of the services the FSA offered (sometimes even advocating for them), they exercised a sense of national belonging that made them invested in and a part of a government that historically excluded and marginalized them. New Deal legislation securing workers' rights, such as the National Industrial Recovery Act (1933) and the Social Security Act (1935), specifically barred farmworkers from federal protection. Mexicans were also distinctly targeted during the Great Depression by local community agencies that labeled them nonresidents and unworthy burdens on public relief rolls. The treatment of Mexicans as outsiders, undeserving of federal labor protections and civic resources, contributed to government-sponsored deportation campaigns between 1929 and 1935 where an estimated 1.6 million Mexicans left the United States. Approximately 60 percent of those deported were U.S. citizens.[38] The FSA's labor camp program therefore offered an exceptional opportunity to renew Mexican working-class families' faith in the state. By allowing the government to care for them, Mexican migrants advocated for the human and civil rights frequently denied to them and challenged the parameters of federal responsibility to poor Americans.

Despite their investment in the FSA's efforts, Mexican American farmworkers' ability to bargain for improved conditions weakened with the introduction of the Bracero Program in 1942, which turned FSA attention to the recruitment of foreign-born farmworkers. In the Southwest—with the exception of Texas, which had been excluded by the Mexican government from participating in the program until 1947 because of rampant labor abuse and discrimination against Mexicans in the state—the FSA used the majority of its labor camp facilities to house the guestworkers they imported. Initially, the agency tried to balance its care for both Mexican American migrant families and Mexican braceros. For instance, until 1946, when the FSA was terminated, access to medical attention continued to be available for all farmworkers (even foreign contract workers) under the Agricultural Workers Health Associations the FSA established. But increasingly, as braceros arrived in larger numbers, the camps were stripped of most of the social programming aimed at improving Mexican American migrant families' lives. Such actions demonstrated one of the perpetual problems plaguing the FSA's efforts. Despite its benevolent intentions to improve Mexican Americans' socioeconomic status, they paradoxically contributed to the forces inducing their poverty and poor health. By introducing labor competition that undermined Mexican American farmworkers' ability to have stable employment, earn fair wages, and demand sanitary housing, the FSA made Mexican Americans' efforts to secure a brighter future that much harder.

The complexity of Mexican migrants' encounters with the FSA's health reform measures reveals the value of analyzing the intersections of citizenship and the medicalization of race, gender, and work in more complicated terms. Mexican families left remarkable evidence, given their status as migrant laborers, documenting their engagement with the FSA. Their diverse expressions concerning the role of the Migrant Medical Program in their lives remind us that those who relied on the FSA's medical services and participated in its education efforts, even if at times reluctantly, did so out of a calculated effort to secure their families' well-being. The negotiation they partook in was critical to framing the FSA's efforts on their terms and to challenging the FSA's practices consigning their cultural identity to something primitive in need of "curing." Their responses illuminate how Mexican American migrants claimed the right to receive medical attention and sanitary housing—to be entitled to the protections of American citizenship—without being divested of the cultural and social attributes that defined their lives as Mexicans. As migrants and racialized others, the families who participated in the camp program set an important precedent in defining the role of the welfare state. Although the struggle to negotiate the boundaries of federal intervention in social welfare and public health would reemerge most concretely in the 1960s, it is not too bold to argue that underserved families, especially migrants, continue to challenge this realm of federal responsibility even today.

NOTES

Thank you to Laurie B. Green, John Mckiernan-González, and the anonymous reviewers who offered helpful suggestions for improving this chapter. Members of the Industrial and Labor Relations School women's writing group and the Society for the Humanities de Bary writing group on "Spaces of Permeability and Alternative Infrastructures" also provided invaluable feedback.

1   Agnes Meyer, "Camps Aid to Valley Workers: Projects at Robstown Are Transformation for Migrants," *Texas Spectator,* May 5, 1946, 3. The original articles appeared in the *Washington Post* (April 22–23, 1946) as part of a series Meyer conducted on wartime America focusing on selected southern states.

2   I use the term *Mexican* in this chapter to keep with contemporary usage but also because citizenship status was rarely specified in camp records. Where it is possible, I am careful to differentiate between citizens and noncitizens and between foreign- and U.S.-born people by using the terms *Mexican American* and *Mexican national.*

3   "A Petition and Explanation of Reason for Stay of Execution on Certain Orders of this U.S.D.A. Camp of Recent Date," July 2, 1941, box 486, folder "RP-TX-35-912-135 Complaints Weslaco Migratory Labor Camp," Record Group (RG) 96, FSA, National Archives and Records Administration (NARA).

4   Bertha Suárez, interview by author, Weslaco, Texas, February 29, 2008.

5   Sidney Baldwin, *Poverty and Politics: The Rise and Decline of the Farm Security Administration* (Chapel Hill: University of North Carolina Press, 1968), 325, 353–54.

6   Oscar Lewis, *Five Families: Mexican Case Studies in the Culture of Poverty* (New York: Basic Books, 1959).

7   John Steinbeck, *The Grapes of Wrath* (New York: The Viking Press, 1939) and *The Harvest Gypsies: On the Road to the Grapes of Wrath* (*The San Francisco News,* 1936); Brian Cannon, "Keep on-a-Goin': Life and Social Interaction in a New Deal Farm Labor Camp," *Agricultural History* 70, no. 1 (Winter 1996), 1.

8   U.S. Congress, House of Representatives, Committee on Agriculture to Investigate the Activities of the Farm Security Administration, *Hearings, Pursuant to H. Res. 119,* Part 3 (1944), 1164–67; "FSA Migratory Camp Population Reports and Employment and Earnings of Families Living in FSA Camps," box 19, folder "AD 124 All Regs. 183 Migratory Labor Social Security Tables on Interstate Migrants 1937," RG 96, FSA, NARA. After the FSA became involved in the recruitment of foreign farmworkers in 1942, the number of camps continued to fluctuate depending on regional need. In August 1945, for example, the federal government managed camps at 191 sites in twenty-six states (47 were permanent, and 144 were mobile). Wayne David Rasmussen, "A History of the Emergency

Farm Labor Supply Program, 1943–1947," Agricultural Monograph No. 13, U.S. Department of Agriculture Bureau of Agricultural Economics (Washington, D.C.: Government Printing Office, 1951), 180.

9   Michael R. Grey, *New Deal Medicine: The Rural Health Programs of the Farm Security Administration* (Baltimore, Md.: Johns Hopkins University Press, 1999), 3.

10 Baldwin, *Poverty and Politics,* 401.

11 Meyer, "A Look at Labor Camps," *Texas Spectator,* June 30, 1947, 6,7, 11.

12 Grey, *New Deal Medicine,* 27–28; Carey McWilliams, *Ill Fares the Land: Migrants and Migratory Labor in the United States* (Boston: Little, Brown, 1942), 173, 177, 243, 286.

13 Baird Snyder, FSA chief engineer, to Karl Buster, FSA District 5 engineer, November 6, 1939, box 10, folder "AD 124 R-8 Migratory Camps Medical Care," RG 96, Farmers Home Administration (FHA), NARA.

14 Karl Buster to Baird Snyder, November 22, 1939, box 10, folder "AD 124 R-8 Migratory Camps Medical Care," RG 96, FHA, NARA.

15 "Migratory Labor Camp Near Completion," *The Weslaco News,* Weslaco, Texas, December 7, 1939.

16 Natalia Molina, *Fit to Be Citizens? Public Health and Race in Los Angeles, 1879–1939* (Berkeley: University of California Press, 2006), 2; Nayan Shah, *Contagious Divides: Epidemics and Race in San Francisco's Chinatown* (Berkeley: University of California Press, 2001), 12.

17 Adela J. Ballard, "The Mexican Migrant," as cited in *They Starve That We May Eat: Migrants of the Crops,* compiled by Edith E. Lowry (New York: Council of Women for Home Missions and Missionary Education Movement, 1938), 36.

18 Richard A. Meckel, *Save the Babies: American Public Health Reform and the Prevention of Infant Mortality 1850–1929* (Baltimore, Md.: Johns Hopkins University Press, 1990), 99, 121.

19 On Dust Bowl migrant imagery, see Wendy Kozol, "Madonnas of the Fields: Photography, Gender, and 1930s Farm Relief," *Genders* 2 (Summer 1988): 1–23.

20 Monthly Narrative Report (MNR), Sinton, Texas, August 1, 1941, RG 96, FSA, NARA, Southwest Region, Fort Worth, Texas.

21 MNR, Harlingen, Texas FSA Camp, April 1942, box 486, folder "RP-TX-36-183-01 Monthly Narrative Report of Home Management—Sept. 1941," RG 96, FSA, NARA.

22 Genevieve Rhodes, HMS, MNR, Crystal City, Texas FSA Camp, November 1941, box 488, folder "RP-TX-38-183 1941 Crystal City Mig. Camp, Camp Population Report," RG 96, FSA, NARA.

23 *Spotlight,* Crystal City, Texas camp newspaper, September 12, 1941, p. 6, box 17, folder "RP-M-163-1941 Newspapers and Magazines," RG 96, FHA, NARA.

24 *Migrant Mike,* Yuma, Arizona camp newspaper, November 28, 1941, box

97, folder "RP-AZ-11 (000-900) Yuma Migratory Labor Camp," RG 96, FSA, NARA.

25　Grey, *New Deal Medicine*, 86.

26　Charlotte Borst, *Catching Babies: The Professionalization of Childbirth, 1870–1920* (Cambridge, Mass.: Harvard University Press, 1995), 157.

27　R. C. Williams, FSA chief medical officer, to C. M. Evans, FSA regional director, "Suggestions with Reference to the Medical Care Program for the Migratory Labor Camps," March 26, 1940, box 10, folder "AD 124 R-8 Migratory Camps Medical Care," RG 96, FHA, NARA.

28　Dr. W. W. Alexander, FSA administrator, to R. C. Williams, FSA chief medical officer, May 7, 1940, box 10, folder "AD 124 R-8 Migratory Camps Medical Care," RG 96, FHA, NARA.

29　Henry C. Daniels, Robstown camp manager, to W. A. Canon, FSA assistant regional director, November 7, 1941, Robstown Files, RG 96, FSA, NARA Southwest Region, Fort Worth, Texas.

30　W. A. Canon, FSA assistant regional director, to Henry C. Daniels, Robstown camp manager, November 28, 1941, Robstown Files, RG 96, FSA, NARA Southwest Region, Fort Worth, Texas.

31　Mr. Herón Ramirez, interview by author, Pharr, Texas, July 18, 2008.

32　Alcario Samudio, phone interview by author, May 13, 2008.

33　Owen H. Eichblatt, camp manager, MNR, Princeton, Texas, FSA Camp, May 1942, box 488, folder "RP-TX-38-183-01 Monthly Narrative Report," RG 96, FSA, NARA.

34　As cited in Grey, *New Deal Medicine*, 94.

35　Meyer, "Life on the Rio Grande: A 1946 Model," *Washington Post*, April 22, 1946, Pro Quest Historical Newspapers.

36　"Report on Lamesa Farm Workers Community Historic District, 1991," 13, Lamesa File, Texas Historical Commission, Austin, Texas.

37　Grey, *New Deal Medicine*, 205; Frederick D. Mott and Milton I. Roemer, *Rural Health and Medical Care* (New York: McGraw-Hill, 1948), 429.

38　Natalia Molina, "Borders, Laborers, and Racialized Medicalization: Mexican Immigration and US Public Health Practices in the 20th Century," *American Journal of Public Health* 101, no. 6 (June 2011): 1024–31.

10

"Hunger in America" and the Power of Television

Poor People, Physicians, and the Mass Media in the War against Poverty

LAURIE B. GREEN

IN THE MOST RIVETING SCENE of the 1968 CBS documentary "Hunger in America," prominent white pediatrician Raymond Wheeler asks black fourteen-year-old Charles, who is seated beside his younger brother and sister in their grim, dimly lit home in Hale County, Alabama, what he has for lunch at school. "Nothing," responds Charles shyly, as the camera zooms in. He has told Wheeler that he has peas for breakfast, but only sometimes. His school provides subsidized lunches, but Charles says he doesn't have the twenty-five cents to pay. "Well, what do you do while the other children are eating?" queries Wheeler. "Just sit there." "Where do you sit?" "I sit where all the children be seated," Charles tells him. "How do you feel toward the other children who are eating when you don't have anything?" "Be ashamed," Charles admits, now in a near whisper. "Why are you ashamed?" "Because I don't have any money," the boy says. A voice-over by famous CBS broadcaster Charles Kuralt earlier reported that Charles's family couldn't afford food stamps, which were not free but had to be purchased monthly. Wheeler, examining Charles's younger brother and sister before turning to the boy, has told us that such children "get up hungry, go to bed hungry, and never know anything else in between." The resulting malnutrition impairs children's physical and mental development, he asserts, "and they never catch up. Malnutrition impairs their performance for life."[1]

For most people who watched "Hunger in America," Charles and his siblings represented the most vulnerable faces of hunger in the United States, which in 1967 had been "discovered" in the Mississippi Delta by Robert F. Kennedy and other senators. Kennedy and the rest of the

committee had reported their shock at finding conditions they associated with world hunger—that is, hunger in poor nations.[2] Produced
by Martin Carr and associate produced by Peter Davis, the show aired
on May 21, 1968, as part of the network's *CBS Reports* documentary
series.[3] Besides the Hale County segment, three others featured Mexican
Americans in San Antonio, whites in Loudoun County, Virginia, and
Navajos in Tuba City, Arizona. Television allowed viewers to imagine
these malnourished children as individuals and to see beyond the immediate crisis to the potential for permanent developmental damage
and psychological scarring. Viewers could identify with the children's
suffering; by helping them, one could secure hope for their future.

So, too, did another medical sequence stir powerful responses,
this one occurring a few minutes into the documentary and filmed in
an emergency pediatric ward in San Antonio. The camera focuses on
a doctor's attempt to resuscitate an infant, who unexpectedly died as
this footage was being shot. We hear Kuralt's voice-over: "Hunger is
easy to recognize when it looks like this." He continues, "This baby is
dying of starvation. He was an American. Now he is dead." This is not
an intimate scene that stirs compassion and hope. It establishes that
hunger is a tragedy striking American citizens. These two stunning
scenes, opposite in many ways, melded the shame felt by the individual child with the shame of the American public for its government's
inaction.

"Hunger in America" captured more attention than any other salvo
in the fiercely contested political battle over hunger that erupted in the
late 1960s. It also provoked more response than had any television
documentary to date. CBS News president Richard Salant reported to
his colleagues that 300 callers had phoned the night the show aired,
many to inquire about how to send money to the people in the program, and that callers had kept two secretaries busy the entire next
day.[4] The broadcast also prompted a hail of criticism from southern
congressmen, the secretary of agriculture, and citizens who accused CBS
of fabricating the existence of starvation. "Hunger in America" swept
all the major television awards, even as CBS contended with a Federal
Communications Commission (FCC) hearing and Federal Bureau of
Investigation (FBI) inquiry.

Eleven months earlier, in June 1967, the publication of *Hungry
Children* by Wheeler and five other physicians who toured Mississippi

after the "discovery of hunger" had cemented their harrowing findings about actual starvation to a critique of the federal government for allowing southern officials to obstruct food distribution. *Hungry Children* had provoked fierce rebuttals to Wheeler's charge that Mississippi officials were trying to "eliminate the Negro Mississippian." The shift from this politicized epidemiological report to "Hunger in America" warrants special attention. Pediatricians serve as interlocutors in three of the segments. In contrast to *Hungry Children,* their presence in the documentary foregrounds their medical professionalism and heartfelt concern for the infants and children they examine. Contemporaries identified the broadcast, not the medical report, as the turning point in bringing public awareness to hunger and malnutrition in the wealthiest country in the world.[5]

Through the medium of television, "Hunger in America" galvanized public concern by uncoupling the crisis from Mississippi's infamous relations of race and power and reassigning it to the quartet of subjects presented in the program. This view beyond Mississippi also unhinged hunger and malnutrition from blackness. Paradoxically, audiences responded favorably to "Hunger in America," even though a competing racial discourse painted the face of American poverty black and, most commonly, female and explained it as the result of cultural characteristics rather than political and economic factors. At least temporarily and for a large portion of the audience, the broadcast deracialized the crisis of hunger and malnutrition by establishing a sympathetic portrayal of deserving women, infants, and children from multiple groups.

Whether they lauded "Hunger in America" or denounced it, contemporaries referred to the "power of television" to explain its impact and suggested that the broadcast illustrated television's unfulfilled social potential. Somewhat awed CBS executives claimed that the documentary had elevated the network's stature and advanced the struggle against poverty—even more so than Edward Murrow's 1960 *CBS Reports* documentary about migrant workers, "Harvest of Shame." Opponents, meanwhile, scrambled to contain what they too perceived as the "power of television."[6]

Television had a unique capacity to involve audiences in what was unfolding on screen through its specific production and reception practices.[7] "Hunger in America" presented "the reality" of hunger through a carefully crafted visual narrative that conveyed authenticity and objectivity. It shocked viewers. What they thought they knew—that starvation and malnutrition existed in poor countries but not America—was not true after all.

Television's transformation of medical exposé into a portrayal of suffering that inspired activism forms the focus of this chapter. It shows that in the 1960s, there was no unified articulation of knowledge about malnutrition. Hunger and malnutrition were unstable social, political, and medical categories reformulated in particular historical milieus. Race was central to the larger political context in which understandings of hunger and malnutrition developed, a context that was further mediated by the technologies of mass culture.[8]

Few scholars of the postwar civil rights and antipoverty movements explore whether, and if so, how, it matters that the rise of these movements coincided with the ascent of television broadcasting. Conversely, most scholarship on medicine and visual culture has looked at images associated with scientific research or public health campaigns but not social movements. Television historians who have analyzed "Hunger in America" focus more on its political message as one of a series of "muckraking" broadcasts.[9]

Here, I explore television in the context of an intense struggle in the late 1960s over who got to control the meanings and ramifications of hunger, which was tightly bound up with gendered ideas about race. "Hunger in America" transformed contested medical knowledge into a compelling human drama that eluded familiar, negative images of blackness to which poverty had been staked. More than any other scene, the one in which Raymond Wheeler interviewed Charles drew sympathy, at a historical moment when black teenagers were frequently depicted as threats to society. The chapter analyzes this 1968 documentary in order to explore why the power of television allowed its producers to create a visual narrative that remobilized medical knowledge and represented to many a watershed in the politics of hunger.

PROTESTING STARVATION, 1967–1968

Neither conflict nor violence nor suffering would have been new to television watchers in May 1968. The months leading up to the broadcast convulsed with uprisings in Czechoslovakia and France that threatened to overturn the existing order. In the United States, antiwar protest intensified as the nightly news broadcast footage from Vietnam and from the unloading of body bags at home. Perhaps most pertinently for the shaping of "Hunger in America," images of peaceful civil rights demonstrators being brutalized by white supremacists had been partially superseded by images in which blacks themselves appeared threatening, whether in the visage of Black Power militancy or urban uprisings in Harlem, Watts, Newark, Detroit, and elsewhere.

The historical context preceding "Hunger in America" also included groundbreaking civil rights and antipoverty legislation. In summer 1964, president Lyndon Johnson had signed the hard-fought Civil Rights Act, the Equal Opportunity Act—a central component of which was the War on Poverty—and the Food Stamp Act. The Food Stamp Act formalized and expanded a pilot program initiated by President John Kennedy in 1961 and was administered by the U.S. Department of Agriculture (USDA).[10] In theory and sometimes in practice, the program allowed families to buy more nutritious food than they received through the existing surplus commodities program, in which the government helped farmers keep prices high by purchasing and distributing agricultural products such as flour and cheese.

Antipoverty and racial justice protests by poor people had drawn public attention to worsening hunger and malnutrition, despite the War on Poverty program. The replacement of surplus commodities with food stamps, which the poorest families could not afford, and the fact that nonrepresentative local boards determined eligibility, helped precipitate the hunger crisis. In winter 1966, former black farm laborers in the Mississippi Delta, displaced by mechanization or evicted for striking for a minimum wage, occupied a deserted air force base in Greenville to publicize their plight and pressure the federal government to intervene. To be sure, their demands included more than food, but their public statement began, "We are here because we are hungry and cold and we have no jobs. Our children can't be taught in school because they are hungry."[11]

Outside Mississippi, protesters challenging poverty and racial justice confronted similar conditions. In 1967, black community activists in Memphis began battling infant mortality and childhood malnutrition as part of a broader agenda of black self-determination. In March 1968, this crisis became bound up with the historic strike of Memphis sanitation workers, who earned such low wages that they qualified for food stamps.[12] Also in March, tenant farmers and laborers working with the Southern Rural Research Project in Selma, Alabama made national headlines when they traveled to Washington, D.C. to testify in federal court about county officials' rejection of both the surplus commodities and food stamp programs. They perceived this denial as a response to the Voting Rights Act. The farmers and Southern Rural Research Project attorney Don Jelinek had also helped the CBS film crew locate interviewees for "Hunger in America."[13]

A different intervention in Mississippi in 1967 precipitated what became known as the official "discovery of hunger in America." During a public hearing on the War on Poverty in Jackson on April 10—one of ten inquiries by the Senate Subcommittee on Manpower, Employment, and Poverty across the U.S.—nationally known local activists Fannie Lou Hamer and Unita Blackwell, and National Association for the Advancement of Colored People Legal Defense and Educational Fund attorney Marian Wright (later Edelman), testified about the growing crisis. All linked their statements to the historical context of civil rights and the collapse of the plantation system. Blackwell described a situation in one county where parents had to trade on school lunches and integration: They could send their children to an integrated school, where subsidized lunches cost thirty cents, or an all-black school, where they cost fifteen cents. Wright appealed to the senators "to go and just look at the empty cupboards in the Delta and the number of people who are going around begging just to feed their children. . . . Starvation is a major, major problem now." This hearing received extensive media coverage, in part because of senator Robert F. Kennedy's rising popularity. The reportage before the hearing had focused on political fights over the War on Poverty; afterwards hunger and starvation took center stage.[14]

Kennedy and committee chairman Joseph Clark's legendary tour of the Delta the next day became the touchstone for attention to hunger in the United States. Reports, photographs, and TV footage recorded the senators' shock when, as CBS reporter Daniel Schorr put it, they "visited squalid shacks, talked to poor Negroes earning $6 a day for cotton chopping and many earning nothing, saw children with distended bellies." Schorr reported that after returning to Washington, committee members sprang into action, meeting with Secretary of Agriculture Orville Freeman and writing to President Johnson to request emergency

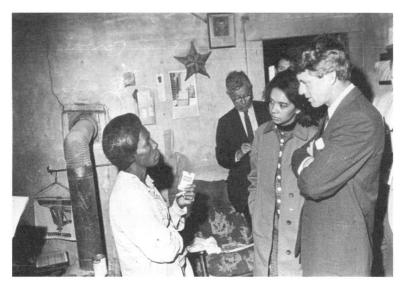

FIGURE 10.1. Unidentified woman speaking in her home with Marian Wright and Robert F. Kennedy, with Daniel Schorr in the background, during the senators' tour in the Mississippi Delta, April 11, 1967. AP Images.

food. However, much coverage obscured the complex ways in which Hamer, Blackwell, and Edelman had connected hunger to the political economy of racism.[15]

MEDICAL REFRAMING OF HUNGER

At a June 16, 1967, press conference, the doctors who had taken their own tour of six Mississippi counties injected the weight of scientific evidence into the "discovery of hunger" and criticized Congress for adding to the disaster by refusing to make food stamps available at no cost. Their revelations fanned the flames of a political fight that had erupted after the senators' tour over whether starvation actually existed. Although reported sympathetically in the national press, the doctors' revelations triggered attacks on their objectivity from within the South, thereby situating medicine as a contested field. Race was at the heart of this conflict over objectivity and the question of who had access to the truth.[16]

In fact, these doctors had never extracted science from the historical and political context, nor had Leslie Dunbar, who initiated the investigation as director of the Marshall Field Foundation. Dunbar had previously directed the Southern Regional Council (SRC), a research and activist civil rights organization, and in his tenure at the Field Foundation he had supported projects pertaining to children, poverty, and racial justice.[17] Raymond Wheeler, based in Charlotte, North Carolina, chaired the SRC's executive board. Yale pediatrics professor Milton Senn had researched malnutrition for the World Health Organization and surveyed child health in preschools run by Friends of the Children of Mississippi, which received funding from the Field Foundation. Dr. Cyril Walwyn, medical advisor to Friends of the Children of Mississippi and the team's sole black physician, had provided health care for poor African Americans first at Tuskegee and then at the Afro-American Hospital in Yazoo City, Mississippi. Dr. Joseph Brenner, a Massachusetts Institute of Technology professor and clinician, had recently hosted an international conference on malnutrition, learning, and behavior. Alan Mermann, a Yale professor of pediatrics who practiced privately and in a school system, had conducted a study on school health in Lowndes County, Alabama. Harvard child psychiatrist and Field Foundation board member Robert Coles had worked with rural families in Mississippi and Appalachia and with East Coast migrant farmworkers and recently published *Children of Crisis: A Study of Courage and Fear*. He and Brenner had been medical activists during the civil rights movement. These physicians visited six counties to examine "the health and living conditions of a representative group of Negro children enrolled in a pre-school program sponsored by the Friends of the Children of Mississippi."[18]

The SRC published the group's report, which included Mermann and Coles's observations on Alabama and Appalachia, and Wheeler's individual report, as *Hungry Children*. The publication combined epidemiology, first-person narrative, and political critique. An initial section asserted that infants can be damaged before they are born if mothers cannot secure prenatal care. All infants and young children must have basic nutritional and medical needs met in order to thrive, yet the families they visited had no means to provide them. A second section described living conditions they observed: contaminated water, potentially disease-bearing mosquitos, and the absence of electricity, window screens, and medical care. The core section of the report detailed the horrible physiological consequences of chronic malnutrition. A typical sentence reads,

> What we saw clinically—the result of this condition of chronic hunger and malnutrition—was as follows: wasting of muscles; enlarged hearts; edematous legs and in some cases the presence of abdominal edema (so-called "swollen" or "bloated" belly); spontaneous bleeding of the mouth or nose or evidence of internal hemorrhage; osteoporosis—a weakening of the bone structure— and, as a consequence, fractures unrelated to injury or accident; fatigue, exhaustion, and weakness.[19]

Lastly, the doctors made recommendations about adequate food distribution and the creation of local medical and dental institutions.

Clinical language dominated *Hungry Children,* but political criticism in a rights-based language framed the text. The doctors expressed shock that such conditions existed in the United States, given the nation's vast "technological and scientific resources."[20] More pointed commentary followed: "Welfare and food programs (including the commodity food program) are in the hands of people who use them selectively, politically, and with obvious racial considerations in mind." Food, they argued, is a human right; its denial constitutes a violation of rights. They insisted that their aim was not to "quibble over words"; what they observed, however, could not be summed up as "malnutrition." "They are suffering from hunger and disease, and directly or indirectly they are dying from them—which is exactly what 'starvation' means."[21]

Wheeler's appended report elicited sharp condemnations from white southerners, who reversed blame and assigned it to African Americans themselves. "Frequently throughout the Mississippi Delta," he wrote, "we heard charges of an unwritten but generally accepted policy on the part of those who control the state to eliminate the Negro Mississippian either by driving him out of the state or starving him to death."[22] He had thought such a charge "beyond belief" but now found it credible. These words probably struck a moral chord with northern readers but threw down the gauntlet to southern politicians. Wheeler received hate mail attacking the doctors as liars, "damn Yankees," or dupes of civil rights groups. Writers accused him of fabricating evidence but, ironically, blamed women who bore "illegitimate babies" as the cause of what hunger did exist. Wheeler received more hate mail a month later after he testified before the Senate subcommittee.[23]

The televised hearings on July 11–12 enacted a public drama involving the six doctors, a photographer, federal and state officials, and poor people from Virginia, New Mexico, Arkansas, South Dakota, and South Carolina. Mississippi senator James Eastland declared himself a friend of blacks who would leave Mississippi if they moved away. Eastland's Senate colleague John Stennis accused the doctors of purposely misleading the public: "I think it is an unintentional libel and slander of the grossest sort to come here at this high level of testimony, with a national television audience, and try to put a libel like that." Likewise, they challenged photographs documenting child malnutrition in Mississippi as fabrications. In response to these accusations, Wheeler, speaking emotionally as a native southerner, held the state's politicians responsible for the wretchedness of the region's poor. Such men had obstructed all "courageous and noble leadership when all of us had nothing to lose but the misery and desolation which surrounds all of our lives."[24]

Stennis and Eastland then introduced Dr. A. L. Gray, director of the Mississippi State Board of Health, who had been charged by that state's governor with investigating public health to determine whether children were "starving to death." The report is stunning. Based on findings of five physicians in four counties, it detailed visits to county health and welfare departments, clinics, Head Start programs, and private homes. At each juncture, the committee asserts that there were no known cases of starvation, yet they conclude that "in many localities sanitary conditions are below the acceptable minimum and there are varying degrees of under nutrition, malnutrition and anemia, as there are in other parts of the nation."[25]

The presentation of dueling medical reports and interventions by leading politicians signaled that the battle for adequate food for the poorest Americans would be a hard-fought one.

INVESTIGATIONS AND PUBLICATIONS

As southern congressmen led by powerful House Agricultural Appropriations Subcommittee chairman Jamie Whitten, also a Mississippian, used political muscle to block the expansion and restructuring of food programs, government and nongovernment investigators worked to determine whether hunger (a subjective experience) and malnutrition (a medical condition) existed beyond Mississippi. Such evidence would signal a national crisis rather than an exceptional one. CBS's investigation commenced after the release of *Hungry Children*. Peter Davis recalls that the germ for the documentary originated with Robert Kennedy's suggestion to CBS News executive producer Don Hewitt.[26] Robert Coles had a similar idea, which he pursued with former CBS News president Fred Friendly. Coles also wrote to Leslie Dunbar that reporters at the doctors' press conference "thought a good, serious documentary would be terribly helpful to our cause."[27]

Two other investigations also commenced. The Committee on School Lunch Participation, a coalition of the nation's five largest women's groups, conducted a nationwide survey of local school lunch programs. Meanwhile, the Citizens' Board of Inquiry into Hunger and Malnutrition in the United States, headed by Leslie Dunbar and Morehouse College president emeritus Benjamin Mays, held hearings in Kentucky, West Virginia, Virginia, South Carolina, Texas, and Alabama. It also conducted field trips on Indian reservations, in migrant camps in Florida, Kentucky, Mississippi, and the rural counties around San Antonio, and in the cities of Boston, Washington, D.C., and New York.

The publications produced by these investigations spurred political action. In April 1968, a month before "Hunger in America," school lunch committee chairwoman Jean Fairfax announced the release of *Their Daily Bread*, which criticized the USDA for allowing states to control how they financed the state contribution to the program, including passing off costs to its recipients. Immediately after the release, agriculture secretary Freeman pledged his support for federal guidelines, and the Senate—missing from its numbers senators away for the Easter holiday—overturned its agriculture committee's rejection of a school lunch bill and approved a pilot program to provide lunches to preschoolers.[28]

Whereas *Their Daily Bread* assessed the status of a key food program, the Citizens' Board's ninety-six-page report, *Hunger, U.S.A.*, spelled out the full parameters of the crisis. It incorporated medical evidence and arguments elaborated in *Hungry Children* but encompassed forty-eight states. Moreover, it combined physicians' analysis with personal testimony about hunger and its consequences for families, reports from multiple public health and food industry experts, evidence

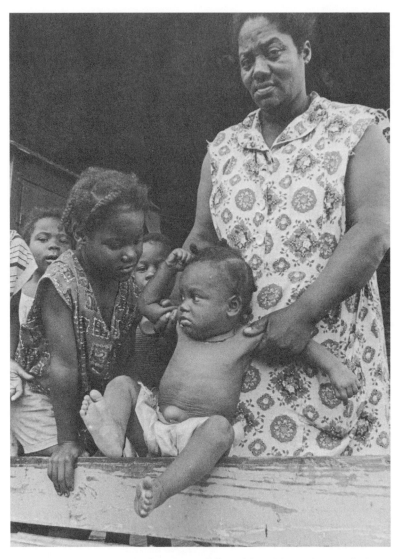

FIGURES 10.2 AND 10.3. At the request of the Southern Regional Council, photo-journalist Al Clayton took these and other pictures documenting severe malnutrition among children in Mississippi. These photographs were circulated at the July 1967 Senate Subcommittee hearings and published in 1969 in *Still Hungry in America*, by Robert Coles, photos by Clayton, World Publishing Co. Courtesy of Al Clayton.

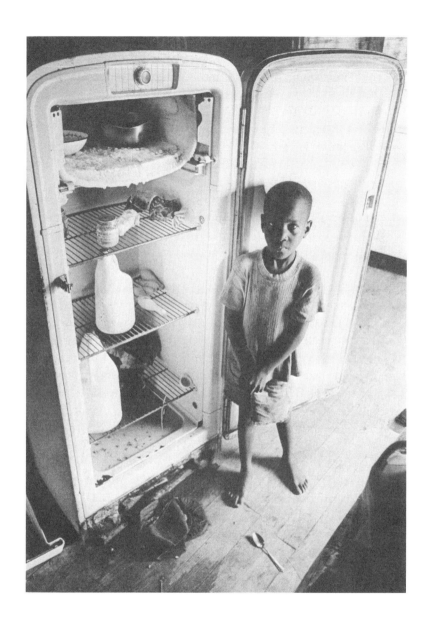

about the efficacy of federal programs, and charges that agricultural policy supported growers rather than poor people.[29] It became the most influential publication on hunger and malnutrition of this era.

These publications provided fodder for the Poor People's Campaign, initiated by Dr. Martin Luther King Jr. but carried out by his Southern Christian Leadership Conference after his assassination on April 4, 1968. Beginning in early May, the campaign brought to the capitol caravans of African Americans, Mexican Americans, Puerto Ricans, Native Americans, and poor whites.[30]

What has gone unnoticed in scholarly studies of the campaign is the increasing significance of hunger. An advance contingent, the Committee of 100, first addressed the hunger crisis at the end of April in a statement to the Secretary of Agriculture. Beginning on May 23, two days after the broadcast of "Hunger in America," poor people themselves testified before the Senate Subcommittee on Employment, Manpower, and Poverty. And on June 12, hundreds of demonstrators converged at the Agriculture Department building to demand changes in food programs.[31]

When CBS News producers conceived of "Hunger in America," they could not have anticipated that the broadcast date would coincide with the Poor People's Campaign. Initially, they projected an air date at Thanksgiving time, but instead, it aired just as protesters intensified demands for an overhaul of federal food programs and, simultaneously, as much of the media coverage began turning negative. Sympathetic journalists highlighted the egregious conditions that participants endured at home. In such constructions, race denoted poverty and vulnerability. But others began using racially coded language and ominous images associated with Black Power and urban rebellions. This coverage overrode the diversity of the campaign by casting participants as black, disorganized, and threatening, often portraying black women as welfare cheats and black men as social menaces.[32]

TRANSFORMATION OF MEDICAL ACTIVISM INTO DOCUMENTARY TELEVISION

Through the prism of late-1960s' network documentary television, the politics of hunger struck a different chord from its coverage in print media, published reports, and even nightly news shows. Ironically, part of what made "Hunger in America" so effective was that documentary producers borrowed conventions and technologies from cinema and from television news and entertainment programming. The "reality" of hunger in the documentary represented not the raw footage of a rolling camera but the craftsmanship of camera operators, editors, writers, and directors who pieced together a seamless and powerful audiovisual narrative. In other words, the "real" of television news programs was not the same as the natural.[33]

The genealogy of the very name of the documentary reflects the yearlong struggle over who controlled the narrative of hunger. CBS initially named the project "Starvation in America." After the face-off at the July 1967 hearings, they changed it to "Starving Americans," then to "Starvation—American Style" in December and "Hunger: American Style" in January 1968. Two months before the broadcast, CBS executives settled on "Hunger in America," a statement of fact and shift to a subjective experience that might elicit emotional responses. The broadcast had not abandoned medicine and politics but incorporated them into a moving drama.[34]

Television news audiences had probably seen images of hunger in war-torn Biafra or among the poor in India, but for most this would have been their first witnessing (through television) of the visage of hunger in the United States. Searing scenes depict the sensory and psychological experiences of hunger and malnutrition, the physiological impact of starvation, the impact on the future for children unable to learn, and the gross inadequacy and uneven implementation of USDA food programs. Bold graphics show that of ten million hungry Americans, only half were served by federal food programs. The four-part structure took the problem out of Mississippi, but unlike *Hunger, U.S.A.,* it spotlighted sites in the South and Southwest, perhaps to strike a chord among northern and midwestern viewers.[35]

"Hunger in America" features multiple characters and layers of narration. Most memorably, it incorporates extensive footage of children and mothers describing their problems. As the omniscient narrator, Charles Kuralt gazes straight at the camera, appearing to speak directly to viewers and connect them to the "real world." In a significant innovation, each part also features a guest narrator, three of them pediatricians. The fourth, Father Ralph Ruiz, who ministered in the barrio, draws out the subjective experience of hunger. Ruiz speaks with a youth who attends school without lunch and a pregnant Mexican American woman who cannot afford the nutritious food that her doctor advises she eat. Dr. Stephen Granger, along with a nurse, visits a white family in Loudoun County whose children exhibit the same signs of severe malnutrition as do those in each of the other sequences, yet the parents refuse government assistance. In a wrenching scene at the Indian hospital in Tuba City, Dr. Jean Van Duzen shows David Culhane, the principal reporter, infants with kwashiorkor and marasmus, the deadliest forms of malnutrition. Finally, Dr. Raymond Wheeler, introduced as a member of the Field Foundation team, shows us the environment in which Hale County's poorest residents live and takes us into Charles's home—little more than a shack. The doctors demonstrate that they are not outsiders rehearsing a political argument but are acquainted with and concerned about these families.

Narrative tension builds throughout "Hunger in America," from the opening sequence that cuts from the recently opened HemisFair exposition to San Antonio's west side barrio and emergency pediatric hospital ward, to Kuralt's final charge that USDA policies threatened the survival and well-being of fellow Americans. Television documentary producers took cues from Hollywood and television dramas. They presented compelling stories with central characters and a narrative arc revolving around characters' confrontation with and possible resolution of a problem, often one involving an imbalance of power.[36] Narrative tension also unfolded within each segment. In the San Antonio section, for example, compelling interviews with mothers and youth precede Culhane's interview with Bexar County commissioner A. J. Ploch, who declares himself unconcerned with whether food-deprived children can learn in school because every society has to have "Indians and chiefs." In Hale County, a pregnant woman speaks about giving birth to babies who died because of her prenatal malnutrition, the hospital's refusal to admit her because of her lack of funds, and racist welfare officials who have denied her assistance. We learn that when she gives birth shortly after being filmed, she loses this baby as well.

As a whole the program, broadcast in May 1968, substituted visual narratives of chronically hungry mothers, infants, and children for images of protests that in fact had occurred in each site. In San Antonio, Father Ruiz's Inner City Apostolate and the Chicano movement had garnered national attention. Native American activists from Tuba City had gone to the capital with the Poor People's Campaign. Hale County,

Alabama was located in one of the most hotly contested regions of the civil rights movement. And in wealthy Loudoun County, struggles over school desegregation and poverty resources had shaped the political landscape. The program's effectiveness revolved around its distance from such conflicts, yet this very success placed it squarely back into the conflicts that had remained off-screen.[37]

Paradoxically, the program's geographic and social diversity unsettled ubiquitous images of poverty that attached it to race, even as it paired each location with a specific racialized population. Specifically, it uncoupled hunger from blackness. "Hunger in America" contained references to histories of racial discrimination, such as Kuralt's opening comment in the Hale County segment ("It has never been easy to be a Negro in Alabama") or the opening scenes that cut from Anglo tourists enjoying HemisFair to San Antonio's west side, home to "400,000 Mexican Americans, half the city's population." However, it placed the onus not on the race of the malnourished but on government priorities, racist practices, and historical material changes such as the replacement of tenant farmers with mechanized cotton pickers.

The shared sense of intimacy constructed by the broadcast illuminates how the "power of television" could shift racial meanings more than medical reports. As framed in "Hunger in America," the interviewees appear to share a universal humanity instead of a racially marked one. Poor women and children seem to look beyond the interviewer and into the eyes of the viewer, who had the impression of peering directly into their lives. The camera does not merely pan the interior spaces of homes; it dwells on them, through darkened but warm lighting. The camera zooms in so closely on the children that the viewer can look into their eyes, observe their expressions, nearly touch sores on their faces, almost bat away the flies they are too lethargic to notice. Through the television screen, viewers could feel that they were at once in the room with them and safely in their own homes.

The interviewees, in part, become the objects of this gaze, yet the slow-paced conversations, unlike the clipped sound bites of the nightly news, also allow the interviewees to become subjects, personalities within the documentary. The CBS team had made this on-screen interaction possible by paying extensive visits to the families. *New York Times* television critic Jack Gould asserted the day after the show aired, "The graphic portrayal of youngsters permanently handicapped by malnutrition and the disheartening death rate among neglected citizens in many ways was more vivid than the TV scenes of the poverty march on Washington." If Gould's assessment was true, the documentary had managed to at least temporarily displace racist images of demonstrators in the capitol with compelling portraits of women and children living in circumstances like those presented in testimony to the Senate Subcommittee.[38]

This reciprocal construction of intimacy hinges on alternative images of both race and gender. The producers spotlighted poor but functional nuclear families, easily recognizable and indeed normative for TV watchers, given the propensity of producers to feature nuclear families in entertainment programs. These meanings were never straightforward. The families in "Hunger in America" have not stepped out of suburban sitcoms, and yet that dissonance influenced the construction and reception of the documentary. The families in "Hunger in America" confront real problems that must be resolved through massive societal changes.[39]

Apparently, then, the families portrayed in "Hunger in America" would have been "normal" but for circumstances created by historical ruptures and government negligence, even callousness. Nearly all the interviewees are women and children, but there is an off-screen husband and father in every household who gains a presence through interviewers' questions and wives' references to them as hardworking yet unable to earn enough to sufficiently house, clothe, and feed their families, or unemployed because of disability or another fault not their own. These are not the iconic black female-headed households so reviled today, nor the emasculating black women of Daniel Moynihan's 1965 "culture of poverty" thesis, who had generated a "tangle of pathology" that had ensnared their families. Significantly, at a time when the "population bomb" had captured attention as a problem looming over not only poorer countries but the United States, "Hunger in America" drew attention to malnourished mothers whose babies died days after birth or suffered severe physical and mental developmental problems.[40] Neither mothers nor fathers are to blame here. They needed to rely on government programs, but their dependency did not follow from purported cultural defects. In contrast, during the Loudoun County segment the unsettling expression of derision toward welfare recipients by a father with severely malnourished children marks him as different. Race stands out most sharply in this case; poor and white stand in for ignorance, even cultural inferiority, perhaps implicitly the cause of his children's malnutrition.

The documentary's projection of an American narrative of hunger, counterposed to world hunger, elicited indignation at the exclusion of American citizens from the "American dream." In this respect, "Hunger in America" resembled the documentary journalism and photography of the New Deal, most notably John Steinbeck's portrayal of dust bowl refugees in *The Grapes of Wrath*.[41] However, whereas Steinbeck spotlighted white farm families whom he depicted as temporarily down on their luck, "Hunger in America" concentrated on blacks, Mexicans, Native Americans, and poor whites who had long endured poverty but now faced more dire circumstances. It focused on starvation, an absolute, not poverty in general. By stressing malnutrition as a collective concern of all Americans toward their own fellow citizens, they unhinged it from derogatory connotations of blackness, a transition that had become a precondition for government action. The documentary then asked audiences to critically assess the actions (or inaction) of their government—not poor people.

Audiences experience television differently from how they listen to radio or watch movies. Media studies scholar Lynn Spigel argues that television did not so much wrap viewers up in an imaginary world and isolate them from the real one, as with cinema, as transport them into a constructed real world as seen through the television screen. Most made that journey in living rooms with family members or friends.[42] These social viewing practices fueled responses. CBS News president Richard Salant wrote his colleagues, "And contrary to what I think I have always seen in the New York ratings in the 10 to 11 P.M. period, on both Arbitron and Nielsen the last quarter hour got a higher rating than the first quarter hour."[43] Viewers had called others to watch the show. During and after the broadcast many had walked to their telephones, or to find pen and paper, perhaps while talking to others. CBS's telephones began ringing before the show was over.

These responses bespoke the emergence of an attentive national public that bore witness to this crisis and, for some viewers, became spontaneously involved in its solution. By deciding to send money or even join the antipoverty movement, viewers stepped outside the world of television and the channels of government. They established one-to-one contact with Charles and other subjects of the film, with whom they simultaneously identified and dis-identified.[44]

"Hunger in America" also triggered directly political responses. Senator Jacob Javits told Congress that his office had been swamped with mail, which was also true of other congressmen. He also requested a copy of the broadcast to show before the Senate Subcommittee on Manpower, Employment, and Poverty hearing on hunger the next week. Agriculture secretary Freeman announced the day after the broadcast that he would start implementing surplus food programs over objections by county officials. However, Freeman also called a press conference to denounce the broadcast and call for equal airtime to defend his office against charges made by the documentary.[45]

More intense conflict erupted in the House of Representatives. As chair of the House Appropriations Subcommittee on Agriculture, Jamie Whitten initiated a months-long investigation using agents on loan from the FBI to pursue every person in the documentary and determine whether the producers had invented stories or misrepresented normal situations as starvation. And Henry B. Gonzalez, the first Mexican American member of Congress, furious at the show's juxtaposition of the infant fatality at Robert B. Green Hospital in San Antonio to the HemisFair exposition, which he had promoted, attacked the film as deceptive. He demanded an investigation by the FCC to judge whether its producers had adhered to the Fairness Doctrine. That Gonzalez, long a champion of labor and civil rights, found himself on the same side of the fence as A. J. Ploch compels a return to the more complex interaction between the documentary itself and the historical and political context surrounding it. If "Hunger in America" sparked both accolades and attacks, they arose from television's power to carve out a narrative that reflected the larger tumultuous period of antipoverty and racial justice movements but did not reproduce it.[46]

CONCLUSION

One of the most prominent crusaders against hunger in the United States, Dr. Jean Mayer, a French-born Harvard nutritionist who served on the Citizens' Board and, beginning in 1969, as a special advisor on hunger to President Nixon, called CBS News in 1971 at the time of the FCC hearing on the broadcast. He wanted to let Salant and other executives know that he was "writing the newspapers as well as the White House to say that 'Hunger in America' was a watershed broadcast and that ten million people now have food stamps that they wouldn't have if it were not for 'Hunger in America.'"[47] To ascribe this much power to this one production and hence remove it from the larger fabric of this era was strategic. Nonetheless, it is no small point that Mayer as a premier nutritionist who had gained national recognition for his important work in the crusade to end hunger and malnutrition would make this claim.

Beginning in spring 1967, physicians such as Mayer, Wheeler, and Coles had presented themselves on a national stage as medical authorities who alone—unlike southern politicians—could make determinations about starvation. Their civil rights–inflected conclusions had drawn a political backlash from southern officials, who themselves claimed to be the unbiased evaluators of their citizens' well-being and addressed hunger in racist terms.

Television quite literally framed their concerns differently, however. "Hunger in America" brought together three articulations of medical knowledge. First, interviewees spoke directly to the camera, and hence the audience, about their subjective experiences. The riveting close-up with Charles powerfully conveyed the physical and psychological suffering resulting from hunger and malnutrition. The same is true of scenes in which pregnant mothers describe their inability to purchase the nutritious food that would ensure their babies' survival. Issues of health, medicine, and politics are packed into these scenes, but their emotional power comes from the framing of these interviews.

Second, the producers incorporated harshly lighted scenes of infants dying of malnutrition in hospital wards. These images spoke a thousand words. Doctors at the San Antonio hospital and the Indian public hospital dealt repeatedly with infant mortality, but it appalled TV audiences. By juxtaposing these scenes to those of the close-up interviews with women and children, the narrative emphasized the full range of the tragedy, from infant mortality to the physical and mental stunting of children.

Finally, the innovative use of a level of narration in which physicians became key characters as interlocutors between local people and a national audience proved greatly effective. These were not the talking heads that present-day watchers of TV documentaries might expect. The doctors converse with members of hungry families about whom they evidently care a great deal. Kuralt introduces Raymond Wheeler, for example, as one of the doctors who investigated hunger for the Field Foundation. However, in the scene with Charles he has his back to the camera, which films over his shoulder, zooming in on the youth. The conventions of television allowed the producers to shape these medical moments such that they destabilized threatening connotations of blackness on which the politics of hunger hinged in the historical context of the late 1960s. Significantly, the producers spotlighted four locales, none of them Mississippi but also none of them in northern cities that had erupted in race riots. They presented hungry children as American citizens and as members of nuclear families, making the latter status evident when it was not visually apparent. These elements steered the narrative away from blackness as a stand-in for the *cause* of malnutrition and from stereotypes such as the licentious black mother, the lazy father, the urban rioter, or the welfare cheat. Charles's expression of pain could make sense only in this context. As a television documentary, "Hunger in America" was both of this world and outside it, confined to a carefully constructed visual narrative far from the protests in Washington and from the medical exposé in *Hungry Children*. In this way, it contributed to the struggle over the future of millions of hungry Americans.

NOTES

Many thanks to the Institute for Advanced Study for providing the support I needed to develop this project and to my colleagues there, especially Daniela Caglioti, Steven Pierce, and Andrew Rotter, and to Martin Summers and John Mckiernan-González for their invaluable insights in the editing of this chapter.

1   "CBS Reports 'Hunger in America' as Broadcast over the CBS Television Network, Tuesday, May 21, 1968, 10:00–11:00 P.M., EDT" (New York: Columbia Broadcasting System, 1968); Martin Carr and Peter Davis, "Hunger in America," 16mm, *CBS Reports* (New York: CBS, May 21, 1968). All quotations and summaries of the documentary are from the transcript or broadcast.
2   The post–World War II concept of world hunger was tied to the formation of the United Nations International Children's Emergency Fund (UNICEF). UNICEF initially addressed child malnutrition in war-ravaged Europe but shifted to "backward" countries in Asia, Latin America, and Africa.

Gertrude Samuels, "The Child's Name Is Today," *New York Times,* June 1, 1952, SM16.

3   Carr had won an Emmy for "Gauguin in Tahiti." Davis went on to win multiple awards for the *CBS Reports* documentary "The Selling of the Pentagon" (1971) and the film documentary *Hearts and Minds* (1974).

4   Richard Salant to Lou Dorfsman, May 23, 1968, Walter Cronkite Papers, Box 2M647, Hunger in America BB Folder, Dolph Briscoe Center for American History, University of Texas at Austin.

5   Southern Regional Council (SRC), *Hungry Children* (Atlanta, Ga.: SRC, 1967).

6   *New York Times* critic Jack Gould stated, "The power of television to rock the status quo has been brilliantly demonstrated in the case of the Columbia Broadcasting System's documentary entitled 'Hunger in America,'" in "Hunger Is Not for Quibbling," June 23, 1968. Agriculture secretary Freeman wrote CBS president Frank Stanton, "Television is too powerful to be allowed to subject the American public to shocking inaccuracies for the sake of eliciting emotional responses." Charles Kuralt Collection, Folder 154, Southern Historical Society, University of North Carolina–Chapel Hill.

7   Marita Sturken and Lisa Cartwright, *Practices of Looking: An Introduction to Visual Culture,* 2nd ed. (New York: Oxford University Press, 2009), 135–36, 230.

8   On hunger as a historical category see Nick Cullather, *The Hungry World: America's Cold War Battle against Poverty in Asia* (Cambridge, Mass.: Harvard University Press, 2010), and James Vernon, *Hunger: A Modern History* (Cambridge, Mass.: Harvard University Press, 2007).

9   David Serlin, *Imagining Illness: Public Health and Visual Culture* (Minneapolis: University of Minnesota Press, 2010); Leslie J. Reagan, Nancy Tomes, and Paula A. Treichler, eds., *Medicine's Moving Pictures: Medicine, Health, and Bodies in American Film and Television* (Rochester, N.Y.: University of Rochester Press, 2007); Bert Hansen, *Picturing Medical Progress from Pasteur to Polio: A History of Mass Media Images and Popular Attitudes in America* (New Brunswick, N.J.: Rutgers University Press, 2009); Chad Raphael, *Investigated Reporting: Muckrakers, Regulators, and the Struggle over Television Documentary* (Urbana: University of Illinois Press, 2005), esp. 33–61.

10 Legislative History of the Food Stamp Program, http://www.fns.usda.gov/snap/rules/Legislation/.

11 James C. Cobb, *The Most Southern Place on Earth: The Mississippi Delta and the Roots of Regional Identity* (New York: Oxford University Press, 1992), 269–70; John Dittmer, *Local People: The Struggle for Civil Rights in Mississippi* (Urbana: University of Illinois Press, 1994), 366–68; Mark Newman, *Divine Agitators: The Delta Ministry and Civil Rights in Mississippi* (Athens: University of Georgia Press, 2004), chapter 6. Quote is from Cobb, 269.

12   Laurie B. Green, "Saving Babies in Memphis: The Politics of Race, Health
     and Hunger during the War on Poverty," in *The War on Poverty: A New
     Grassroots History, 1964–1980,* ed. Annelise Orleck and Lisa Hazirjian,
     133–58 (Athens: University of Georgia Press, 2011). These activists teamed
     up with pediatricians at St. Jude Children's Research Hospital.

13   Don Jelinek, telephone interview by author, March 11, 2011, Berkeley,
     Calif.; Peter Davis, interview by author, Cambridge, Mass., November 29,
     2010; Bernadette Carey Washington, "Food Stamp Program Is Protested,"
     Washington Post, March 25, 1968; Roy Reid, "Suit Today Will Seek to
     Force Freeman to Feed the Starving," *New York Times,* March 25, 1968.

14   *Examination of the War on Poverty. Hearings before the United States Senate
     Committee on Labor and Public Welfare, Subcommittee on Employment,
     Manpower, and Poverty, Ninetieth Congress, First Session, on Apr. 10,
     1967* (Washington, D.C.: Government Printing Office, 1967), 582, 585,
     592–94, 647–57. Quote is on 655; clippings about the Jackson hearing
     in Scrapbook, Joseph S. Clark Papers, Historical Society of Pennsylvania,
     Philadelphia.

15   *Subcommittee Hearings, April 10, 1967,* 3; Clark Scrapbook; Daniel Schorr
     Papers, Box 60, Folder 2, Manuscripts Division, Library of Congress,
     Washington, D.C.; Nick Kotz, *Let Them Eat Promises: The Politics of
     Hunger in America* (Garden City, N.Y.: Doubleday, 1971), 1–6.

16   Nan Robertson, "Severe Hunger Found in Mississippi," *New York Times,*
     July 17, 1967, 14; SRC, *Hungry Children.*

17   Kotz, *Let Them Eat Promises;* and Leslie Dunbar Papers, Finding Aid,
     Manuscript, Archives, and Rare Book Library, Emory University, Atlanta,
     Georgia.

18   *Hunger and Malnutrition in America Hearings before the United States
     Senate Committee on Labor and Public Welfare, Subcommittee on
     Employment, Manpower, and Poverty, Ninetieth Congress, First Session, on
     July 11, 12, 1967* (Washington, D.C.: Government Printing Office, 1967),
     5, 8, 11–12, 13–14, 19, 20–21, 24–25; SRC, *Hungry Children.* Quotation
     is on 2. Friends of the Children of Mississippi was founded after the Office
     of Economic Opportunity gave in to pressure to shut down the Head Start
     program there, ii. Little, Brown published *Children of Crisis* in 1967.

19   SRC, *Hungry Children,* 6–7.

20   Ibid., 11.

21   Ibid., 6–7.

22   Ibid., 27.

23   Raymond Wheeler Papers, Series 1, Folder 38, Southern Historical
     Collection, University of North Carolina–Chapel Hill.

24   *Hunger and Malnutrition in America Hearings.* Quotations on 64, 65, 104.

25   Ibid.; "Observations on the Health Status of Indigent Families in Leflore,
     Humphreys, Washington and Bolivar Counties," 232.

26   Peter Davis interview; Peter Edelman note, June 22, [1967], Robert F.
     Kennedy Papers, Box 58, Folder: Hunger, Notes, John F. Kennedy

Presidential Library and Archives, National Archives and Records Administration, Boston.

27 Robert Coles to Leslie Dunbar, June 23, 1967, Box 2, Folder: Les Dunbar, 1966–1975, Robert Coles Papers, Southern Historical Collection, Wilson Library, University of North Carolina at Chapel Hill.

28 Committee on School Lunch Participation, *Their Daily Bread* (Atlanta, Ga.: McNelley–Rudd Printing Service, 1968), 3–4. See also Susan Levine, *School Lunch Politics: The Surprising History of America's Favorite Welfare Program* (Princeton, N.J.: Princeton University Press, 2008); John W. Finney, "Senate Approves Pilot Lunch Plan," *New York Times,* April 18, 1968; "School Lunch Extension Voted by Senate, 38–14," *Washington Post,* April 18, 1968.

29 Citizens' Board of Inquiry into Hunger and Malnutrition in the United States, *Hunger, U.S.A.* (Boston: Beacon Press, 1968), 2, 3, 7, 9, 13, and chapter 2, "Documenting the Extent of Hunger and Malnutrition in the United States," 16–38.

30 Taylor Branch, *At Canaan's Edge: America in the King Years, 1965–68* (New York: Simon & Schuster, 2006); Adam Fairclough, *To Redeem the Soul of America: The Southern Christian Leadership Conference and Martin Luther King, Jr.* (Athens: University of Georgia Press, 1987); Amy Nathan Wright, "Civil Rights 'Unfinished Business': Poverty, Race, and the 1968 Poor People's Campaign" (PhD diss., University of Texas at Austin, 2007); Gerald McKnight, *The Last Crusade: Martin Luther King, Jr., the FBI, and the Poor People's Campaign* (Boulder, Colo.: Westview, 1998).

31 Earl Caldwell, "Campaign of Poor Begins in Capital," *New York Times,* April 30, 1968; Vincent J. Burke and Jack Nelson, "Poor Present Series of Demands upon Nation," *Los Angeles Times,* April 30, 1968, 8; *Hunger and Malnutrition in the United States: Hearings before the Subcommittee on Employment, Manpower, and Poverty of the Committee on Labor and Public Welfare on S. Res. 281 to Establish a Select Committee on Nutrition and Human Needs, 90th Cong., 2nd sess., May 23, 29, June 12, 14, 1968* (Washington, D.C.: Government Printing Office, 1968); "Poor Post Agriculture Vigil: Marchers List Demands, Get Permit for June 19 Rally," *Washington Post,* June 13, 1968.

32 Robert C. Maynard, "They Are Born Hungry," *Washington Post,* May 19, 1968, B1; Paul Valentine, articles in *Washington Post,* June 8, June 16, June 9, and June 11, 1968; and Jean M. White, "Leadership Crisis Perils Poor March," *Washington Post,* June 9, 1968; Richard Lentz, *Symbols, the News Magazines, and Martin Luther King* (Baton Rouge: Louisiana State University Press, 1990), 308–37.

33 Michael Curtin, *Redeeming the Wasteland: Television Documentary and Cold War Politics* (New Brunswick, N.J.: Rutgers University Press, 1995), 188–89; Sturken and Cartwright, *Practices of Looking,* 230.

34 Bud Benjamin to Bill Leonard, June 30, 1967, Hunger in America— Investigation folder; Martin Carr to Benjamin, July 14, 1967, Hunger in

America—Investigation folder; Leonard to Richard Salant, December 1, 1967, Starvation in America folder; Benjamin to Ernest Silverman, January 5, 1968, Starvation in America folder; and Bud Benjamin to Messrs. Salant, Leonard, Hewitt, Carr, and Silver, March 26, 1968, Hunger in America BB folder, all in Cronkite Papers, Box 2M647.

35 Peter Davis interview.

36 Curtin, *Redeeming the Wasteland,* 177–82.

37 Douglas Watson, "Low Wages Are Blamed for Poverty in Loudoun," *Washington Post,* February 3, 1968, E16; Maurine McLaughlin, "Void Freedom-of-Choice School Plan in Loudoun County, Court Is Urged," *Washington Post,* April 26, 1967, B1.

38 Davis interview; Carr discusses harrowing sights in home visits in memo to Benjamin, August 30, 1967, Cronkite Papers, Box 2M647, Hunger in America—Investigation folder; Jack Gould, "TV: Hunger Amid Plenty, 'C.B.S. Reports' Examines Recurring Picture of Starvation across U.S.," *New York Times,* May 22, 1968, 95.

39 Curtin, *Redeeming the Wasteland,* 189, 191.

40 Paul R. Ehrlich's 1968 *Population Bomb* (New York: Ballantine, 1968) helped shift attention from poor countries to the United States. On black women as "population bomb" see Rickie Solinger, *Wake Up Little Susie: Single Pregnancy and Race before Roe v. Wade* (New York: Routledge, 1992).

41 John Steinbeck, *The Grapes of Wrath* (New York: Viking, 1939).

42 Lynn Spigel, *Make Room for TV: Television and the Family Ideal in Postwar America* (Chicago: University of Chicago Press, 1992), esp. chapter 4; Sturken and Cartwright, *Practices of Looking,* 49, 94.

43 Richard Salant to Lou Dorfsman, May 23, 1968, Cronkite Papers, Box 2M647, Hunger in America BB folder.

44 Interview with Ralph Ruiz by author, San Antonio, Texas, August 7, 2010.

45 Louise G. Colon to Mike Silver, May 22, 1968, in Kuralt Papers, Folder 153; Tom McGowan, "Personnel Quizzed at Hospital," *San Antonio Light,* October 9, 1968, clipping in Cronkite Papers, Box 2M647, Hunger in America BB folder; "Pupils to Get Free Books in Loudoun," *Washington Post,* June 5, 1968, B3; Salant to Dorfsman, May 23, 1968, Cronkite Papers, Box 2M647, Hunger in America—BB folder; Ben A. Franklin, "Freeman Asks Equal Time to Rebut C.B.S. Film," *New York Times,* May 28, 1968.

46 Subcommittee on Department of Agriculture and Related Agencies Appropriations, *Department of Agriculture Appropriations for 1970: Hearing before a Subcommittee of the Committee on Appropriations,* 91st Cong., 1st sess., March 17, 1969 (Washington, D.C.: Government Printing Office, 1969), 51; Congress. House. Congressman Henry B. Gonzalez of Texas, 90th Congress, 2nd Session, *Congressional Record* (September 23, 1968), 27811.

47 Salant to Benjamin, Klinger, Leonard, Wolff, Davis, March 22, 1971, Cronkite Papers, Box 2M647, Hunger folder.

11

Making Crack Babies

Race Discourse and the Biologization of Behavior

JASON E. GLENN

ALTHOUGH RECENT MEDICAL RESEARCH has discredited the concept of the crack baby,[1] as a narrative of urban behavioral degeneracy it played a pivotal role in the creation of a post–civil rights reconception of race. The revelation that there was no sound empirical evidence supporting the classification of developmentally challenged newborns as "crack babies" is now more than ten years old. However devoid of empirical evidence, it was nevertheless a story of such powerful cultural resonance that it heavily contributed to the demonization of the poor urban underclasses: Americans who experience systemic poverty and joblessness and whose existence has never been captured by national unemployment statistics. This demonization in turn provided political support for increased law enforcement surveillance, an end to the Aid to Families with Dependent Children program, racially disparate extreme mandatory minimum sentencing legislation, and the continued support for a criminal justice approach to addressing substance abuse that by all accounts has failed to achieve its goals.[2]

This chapter explores the role that the intensified war on drugs played in redefining race in America in the aftermath of the civil rights movement. In post-1960s America, discourses on race have become obscured in nebulous discourses of crime, personal responsibility, illegal immigration, and most recently, terrorism. Such discourses have a tremendous amount of political currency and are often used to galvanize public support for policies that increase the power and authority of the state. In turn, the state uses its increased power to police racialized bodies in order to demonstrate the need for its increased authority.

To understand the emergence of crack babies we must deconstruct its wide cultural resonance. Crack babies shared four parents that made them perfect cultural symbols of the wretchedness of the urban underclasses of the 1980s: poverty, joblessness, substance abuse, and criminal gang activity. They were the outcomes of everything perceived wrong with America.

The looming crisis of crack babies, couched in a discourse of health, can best be understood as what Stephen Toulmin describes as a "scientific mythology": dramatic representations of how the world works that stimulate our emotions, validate our hopes, make sense of our fears, and lend both cosmic and scientific sanction to our order of living.[3] Crack babies performed the cultural work of taking all the nebulous white, middle-class, and post–civil rights movement guilt of the 1970s and alleviating that guilt by providing new justifications for categorizing the urban poor as undeserving and degenerate.

This chapter investigates the role that the crack baby narrative played in redefining the racial antithesis against which American identity is constructed. The crack baby narrative helped policymakers come to a new consensus as to how newly coded racial discourses of behavioral pathology and personal irresponsibility could be used to manufacture consent for neoliberal economic policies and dismantle the New Deal state.

RACE AND HEALTH

The histories of the production of biomedical knowledge and discourses of race are strongly intertwined. The conceptual revolution that led to the birth of the biological sciences in the nineteenth century and the transformation of medicine into a clinical practice backed by laboratory and clinical experimentation also led to the creation of the biological categories of race. As Michel Foucault argues, the production of biological knowledge became thinkable when "Man" became a formal object of investigation in the West. "Man's" history, language, society, economic organization, and most notably his biology all became areas of specialized study.[4] It is the production of biological knowledge that allows the rise of the "bio-power" of the state: "an explosion of numerous and diverse techniques for achieving the subjugations of bodies and the control of populations."[5]

The concept of "race" and the emergence of the concept of "Man" were birthed out of the lay-humanist revolution in the fifteenth century, initiated as a way to valorize the hopelessly fallen status of laypersons in the cosmogony of Latin Christianity of medieval Europe.[6] This intellectual break shifted the concept of humans as hopelessly irredeemable spiritual beings to "Man": a political being redeemed by his rationality (or irredeemable in his lack thereof, as in the case of *indíos* and *negros*).[7] The peculiar characteristic of this concept "Man," Sylvia Wynter argues, is that for the first time in human history this local, culture-specific conception of what it means to be human was overrepresented in the West as if it were an objective, general understanding of the entire human species.[8] It was the humanists' assumptions of the uniformity of human existence, yet defining that uniformity in their own culture-specific terms, that led to both a huge intellectual rupture and fallacy. On one hand, believing in the uniformity of human existence led them to also insist that the cosmos and natural world were likewise uniform. This insistence enabled epistemic shifts in astronomy and physics that led to the birth of the natural sciences by making the idea of "laws of nature" thinkable.

On the other hand, that same assumption about the uniformity of human existence led Europeans to interpret the peoples they encountered during the exploratory voyages of the Portuguese and the Spanish as lacking the rationality and civic organization of political "Man."[9] This fundamental lack became symbolically mapped onto their physiognomies, which led to the intellectual fallacy of racial categorization. Within this new human taxonomy, *indíos* and *negros* (defined as irrational, pagan, idolatrous barbarians) were legitimately exploitable and enslavable.[10]

Similarly, in the nineteenth century the reconceptualization of "Man" as biological being led to two divergent intellectual trajectories. On one hand, the epistemic rupture of the Darwinian revolution insisted on a uniformity of biological existence that enabled the birth of the biological sciences. On the other hand, the reconceptualization of "Man" as biological being enabled the social hierarchies that emerged during Europe's enslavement of Africans and colonial expansion to be scientifically verified in the nineteenth century in new discourses of biological determinism and natural selection.

This biopolitical organization of knowledge, based on a Darwinian understanding of humans as purely biological beings, was widely challenged during the global anticolonial and human rights struggles of the mid-twentieth century, of which the American civil rights movement was a part. Because, as Michael Omi and Howard Winant argue, the hard, fixed color line that emerged in the racial formation of the United States served the pivotal role in defining America as a white, free nation,[11] and the challenges waged against the color line left the United States with something akin to an identity crisis. In response, by the late 1960s there was a backlash—a retreat from racial justice in both the academy and in public policy[12]—that amounted to a counterreformation of race relations. If the old discourses of biological determinism (social Darwinism, eugenics, and racial science) had been abandoned, a new biology of behavior emerged in the discourse of sociobiology by the late 1960s.[13] As Stephen Jay Gould pointed out, this "new biological determinism" should be understood as the result of "contemporary social and political forces": a revival of racism expressed as frustration with the failure of costly social welfare programs aimed at reducing crime and poverty.[14]

In the ashes of this identity crisis, the biology of behavior movement gave birth to new categories of inclusion and exclusion that could once again ground American identity. Between the late 1960s and the 1980s, the previous conception of genetically selected humanness as symbolized by white, free citizens was transformed to behaviorally selected humanness (where one's behavior is recognized as a better proxy for his or her genetic selectedness than skin color), now symbolized by the middle, upper, and investor classes of suburban America, of which whites were the archetype but not the rule. At the same time, the conception of genetically dys-selected humanness as symbolized by black Americans was transformed to be symbolized by the poor and underclasses of the urban inner cities, of which blacks were the archetype but were increasingly joined by Latinos. The crack baby narrative helped solidify this racial transformation by providing concrete links to the discourses of sociobiology and the biologization of behavior.

The use of behavior and social or socioeconomic status as proxies to indicate biological fitness or genetic selectedness was certainly not new and is reminiscent of social Darwinism and the eugenics movement. Until approximately the 1930s, the main thrust of university scholarship used a social Darwinist frame to define black Americans as innately inferior. After World War II and all the stigma then attached to social Darwinism and eugenics, this type of scholarship was largely dismissed as biased pseudoscience. However, by the 1980s a new corpus of biological knowledge emerged to reassert such claims. With the "breaking" of the genetic code and the development of a new biology of behavior in the fields of sociobiology and evolutionary psychology, these biomedical knowledges tended to minimize environmental and cultural models of social behavior in favor of revised genetic theories hailed as finally truly scientific. Such analyses offered a rebuttal to new work in the social and behavioral sciences that, as a result of the social uprisings of the period and the entrance of previously excluded scholars who challenged the status quo of the traditional disciplines, analyzed urban conditions as the results of poverty, discrimination, and social injustice.

In this historical context we can understand the emergence of crack baby narratives. The resonance they had with the American public and the enthusiasm with which they were received resulted from the cultural work that such narratives performed, defining for Americans a refined category of behavioral dys-selectedness against which to define optimal being. Crack mothers, "crack whores," crack-dealing fathers, and crack babies symbolized the worst in degraded behavioral wretchedness. Dealing with them would not necessitate millions of dollars in spending on social programs but instead a dramatically amped-up war on drugs and a drastic expansion of the U.S. prison system. Crack babies, in particular, played a central role because of their intersection with many different culture war discourses that were politically hot during this time: crime, poverty, drug abuse, welfare, personal responsibility, and reproductive rights. Because crack babies were at the same time helpless, innocent, and wretched because of their supposed attenuated brain development, political drug warriors couched their crusade against inner-city minorities in a discourse of benevolence: as a mission to protect the innocent and prevent future crack babies from being born. These narratives played a central role in redefining a normative American identity in which race was reified through a biologization of behavior.

MAKING CRACK BABIES

The birth of the crack baby is situated within the broader cultural preoccupation with crack cocaine use in the United States from the mid-1980s through the early 1990s. This cultural preoccupation carried with it the perception that crack cocaine was the most addictive drug ever introduced in the United States (it was not), that its use was concentrated among inner-city black Americans (it was not), and that its sale and distribution were responsible for an explosion of gang violence and the deterioration of American cities (a correlation, yes, but not the cause).[15] Together, these perceptions, as expounded on in national media coverage, created the idea that the nation was facing a crack epidemic.[16] A brief introduction to the roots of that perception will help ground an analysis of the crack baby phenomenon.

Conception: The Crack "Epidemic"

In September 1986, in a speech from the White House, Ronald Reagan, joined by wife Nancy, informed the nation that "drugs are menacing our society. They're threatening our values and undercutting our institutions. They're killing our children." Prompted by the media attention surrounding the sudden cocaine-related death of college basketball star Len Bias in June of that year, Reagan exclaimed that "today there's a new epidemic: smokable cocaine, otherwise known as crack. It is an explosively destructive and often lethal substance which is crushing its users. It is an uncontrolled fire." Shortly after the president's warning, Mrs. Reagan chimed in, exclaiming, "Today there's a drug and alcohol abuse epidemic in this country, and no one is safe from it—not you, not me, and certainly not our children, because this epidemic has their names written on it." For all the hard work they had done in their first five years in office, the First Lady pointed out that there were "dark" forces working against the future of America's children: "Our job is never easy because drug criminals are ingenious. They work everyday to plot a new and better way to steal our children's lives. . . . For every door that we close, they open a new door to death."[17]

Reagan made a special request of media organizations near the end of this speech: "You have a special opportunity with your enormous influence to send alarm signals across the nation." It was a call to help fight the War on Drugs by covering it from a perspective sympathetic to Reagan's drug policies. Accordingly, the White House instructed the Drug Enforcement Agency (DEA) to allow ABC News to accompany them on "crack house" raids. As the head of the New York office of the DEA reported, "Crack is the hottest combat-reporting story to come along since the end of the Vietnam War."[18] In 1986, more than a thousand crack stories appeared in the press, with more than four hundred reports on NBC alone. *Time* and *Newsweek* made crack cocaine a cover story ten times between 1986 and 1992.[19] Such coverage was instrumental in producing the perception that crack use was an epidemic.

Shortly after his address, Reagan declared October Crack Cocaine Awareness Month, alluding to the death of Len Bias as an example of how cocaine, "long masquerading as glamorous and relatively harmless," was indeed "a killer."[20] To drive home the threat, Reagan continued: "Tragically, it is sold to and used by even 11- and 12-year olds. To mothers and fathers, boys and girls at this age are children. To a cocaine dealer, they are just another market."[21] If the language used here seems extreme, it paled in comparison to the doomsday discourse that accompanied the birth of the crack baby.

Birth of the Crack Baby

In a July 30, 1989 article for the *Washington Post*, Charles Krauthammer warned that "the inner-city crack epidemic is now giving birth to the newest horror: a bio-underclass, a generation of physically damaged cocaine babies whose biological inferiority is stamped at birth."[22] Krauthammer, quoting the American Enterprise Institute's Douglas Besharov,[23] further explained that "this is not stuff that Head Start can fix. . . . This is permanent brain damage. Whether it is 5 percent or 15 percent of the black community, it is there." Krauthammer likened cocaine-exposed children to "a race of (sub)human drones." Their future, he stated, "is closed to them from day one. Theirs will be a life of certain suffering, of probable deviance, of permanent inferiority. At best, a menial life of severe deprivations" that would exhaust the resources of our educational system, fill the prisons to overflowing, and completely drain the coffers of social welfare. Krauthammer concluded that "the dead babies may be the lucky ones."[24] In August of that same year the *Washington Post* allowed Besharov to pen his own editorial that detailed the criminally negligent behavior of "crack-crazed" mothers.[25] By 1987, many of the thousands of media stories about this drug focused on the "epidemic" of crack babies.[26]

Ira Chasnoff gave birth to the frenzy in September 1985 with an article in the *New England Journal of Medicine (NEJM)* in which he suggested that "prenatal cocaine exposure could have a devastating effect on infants."[27] In December 1986 the *NEJM* followed up on Chasnoff's article with a special report on the medical complications of cocaine abuse. The report argued that the use of crack, described as "almost pure cocaine" (an egregious mistake in pharmacological analysis), could contribute to "spontaneous abortions." It further warned that infants exposed to crack were "at risk for higher rates of congenital malformations, perinatal mortality, and neurobehavioral impairments."[28] By 1987 the topic had generated so much interest that *Neurotoxicology and Teratology* published a special edition focusing on the developmental effects of addiction, particularly cocaine. Among the findings, researchers reported that an infant born to a woman using cocaine typically had a lower birth weight, length, head circumference, and Apgar score[29] and an abnormal heart rate accompanied by tremors and hypertonicity.[30] Another study in the series found that drug-using mothers were much more likely to abuse or neglect their infants, and such children stood a greater chance of being placed in foster care.[31]

Popular news sources ran with this information. A few days after Chasnoff's first article, CBS aired a story about an eighteen-month-old crack-exposed infant and explained to viewers that the baby would grow up to have "an IQ of perhaps 50" and be "barely able to dress herself."[32] In the September 15, 1986 edition of *Time*, crack was named "issue of the year."[33] An article in *Sober Times* proclaimed that "cocaine ingested by a pregnant woman can cause premature birth or cerebral strokes in the unborn child. It is unsafe at any dosage," the authors warned, quoting Henry Wasiewski of Hershey Medical Center, "even just one hit of cocaine may be enough to cause defects or death."[34] By the November elections of 1986 this media frenzy made being "tough on drugs" resonate strongly with voters.[35] The drug issue was rated the most important problem facing America in polls taken between 1986 and 1992.[36]

When George Bush became president, he also held a prime-time press conference—the first of his presidency—to emphasize the continued threat posed by drugs. Holding up a small bag of crack, Bush asserted, "Our most serious problem today is cocaine, and in particular, crack." No one was safe, he admonished: "When hundreds of thousands of babies are born each year to mothers who use drugs—premature babies born desperately sick—then even the most defenseless among us are at risk."[37] Bush reinforced this dire warning with a crack baby photo-op the next day by visiting a hospital room for babies abandoned by drug-addicted mothers, where he scooped up "Little Edward" to give Americans a glimpse of an "authentic" crack baby.[38]

A 1989 *Washington Post* article by Marcia Greene painted an alarming scenario of the mothers of crack babies. As she described, "Parents seeking the next crack fix have abandoned their young children in the streets and in hospitals. They have sold food stamps and their children's clothes for drug money. A few even have sold their children as prostitutes."[39] Lending further credence to the crack baby narrative, a 1990 front-page *New York Times* article proclaimed,

> Parents and researchers say a majority of children exposed to significant amounts of drugs in the womb appear to have suffered brain damage that cuts into their ability to make friends, know right from wrong, understand cause and effect, control their impulses, gain insight, concentrate on tasks, and feel and return love. . . . As adults, they may never be able to hold jobs or control anger.[40]

By 1991, the president of Boston University went so far as to lament the expenditure of so many health care dollars on "crack babies who won't ever achieve the intellectual development to have consciousness of God."[41] Judy Howard, a pediatrician at the University of California at Los Angeles, regularly gave interviews warning of the horrors of crack babies, telling *Newsweek* that in crack babies, the part of their brains that "makes us human beings, capable of discussion or reflection" had been "wiped out."[42] More drastic language was applied to the supposed havoc that crack babies would wreak on the world as they grew older. A September 17, 1989 *Washington Post* article warned of "A Time Bomb in Cocaine Babies," and a September 15, 1990 article in the *St. Louis Post-Dispatch* declared a "Disaster in Making: Crack Babies Start to Grow Up."

Most pertinent about the crack baby story is that its structure specifically frames the behavior of the mothers and the biological condition of the infants as antithetical to basic human nature. Crack-addicted mothers were inhuman in their neglect of caring for their unborn babies, a supposed violation of the most basic of human instincts. Crack babies were inhuman by outcome of that neglect, their hypothesized deficiencies in mental, emotional, and developmental capacity physical evidence of their degeneration. In this era of biologized behavior, the pathological irresponsibility of urban, jobless, crack-using or crack-dealing parents had been biologically stamped into the next generation.

REVELATION OF THE MISDIAGNOSIS

What is striking about these assertions is not only the horrific picture they paint but that there seem to have been no sound or verified scientific studies to support such claims. As explained in a meta-analysis of earlier research studies on the impact of cocaine use during pregnancy on infants and young children that appeared in a March 2001 issue of *Journal of the American Medical Association (JAMA)*, the very idea of a "crack baby" has no scientific standing:

> Among children aged 6 years or younger, there is no convincing evidence that prenatal cocaine exposure is associated with developmental toxic effects that are different in severity, scope, or kind from the sequelae of multiple other risk factors. Many findings once thought to be specific effects of *in utero* cocaine exposure are correlated with other factors, including prenatal exposure to tobacco, marijuana, or alcohol, and the quality of the child's environment.[43]

The article cites serious methodological flaws in the bulk of the research conducted studying the impact of prenatal cocaine exposure, including the failure to distinguish cocaine exposure from other drugs, a lack of control groups to consider basic factors such as malnourishment and a lack of prenatal health care, and a general lack of understanding of normal infant behavior. However, it would be a mistake to explain the reporting of this "scientific mythology" simply as a matter of the naiveté of lay reporters unable to distinguish between sound and unsound scientific practice. As Gideon Koren and others explained in a 1989 study, journal editors systematically rejected articles whose results tended to nullify the crack baby hypothesis, even when they used more sound research methods.[44] According to the authors,

> Our analysis revealed that the likelihood of a [nullifying] study being selected for presentation was negligible, whereas a positive

study was likely to be accepted in 57% of cases. It is generally assumed that studies are selected for presentation or publication based on objective scientific criteria. In selecting criteria for this assessment we tried to identify those elements in an abstract that reviewers are likely to use. The data indicated that negative abstracts were similar to or better than positive abstracts. In particular negative abstracts tended to verify cocaine use more frequently, which is probably the most important independent variable in such studies.[45]

As this study illustrates, stories verifying the existence of crack babies had an irresistible radiance with medically trained audiences, journal editors, and reviewers throughout the late 1980s. The persistence of the crack baby story, despite nullifying evidence, and the zeal with which policymakers latched on to the issue, suggests Americans were enthralled by the crack baby narrative. This confirmation of black urban behavioral pathology captivated and fed the American consciousness. Here, the interface between biomedical research (compromised by the biomedical gaze that sought to biologize a social condition caused by urban poverty and neglect), the corporate agenda of news organizations, media representations, and policymakers seeking to capitalize on the fear generated in those representations, all combined to create the phenomenon of the crack baby. At a micro level, these forces produced a chain of events in which mostly black and Latina lower-class women who consumed crack cocaine during pregnancy were demonized and singled out for special prosecution from the courts.[46] Taking a broader view, the crisis of crack babies helped create support for a drastically more aggressive War on Drugs, which changed the face of American policing, transformed the United States into an incarceration state, and created the prison industrial complex.

CRACK BABIES AND PUBLIC POLICY

With the intense media focus, Congress held fourteen hearings on crack babies and prenatal drug exposure between 1986 and 1992. Such legislative attention led to the enactment of a number of laws that resulted in numerous criminal convictions for prenatal drug use. Hospitals, especially emergency rooms, began testing expectant women for cocaine, often secretly, and reporting positive tests to police. Many women were jailed, and tens of thousands of children were put into foster care.[47] By 1995, thirteen states required doctors to report drug use by pregnant women or positive drug tests in newborns to law enforcement. There were also nine states that specifically defined drug use during pregnancy as child abuse, addressed by any means from mandatory treatment to a criminal investigation and the possible removal of the child.

By 1995 between two hundred and three hundred women were prosecuted for using drugs while pregnant, almost all of them for cocaine.[48] In a throwback to the eugenics movement, government programs began pushing long-lasting hormonal birth control implants or injections on poor urban women and welfare recipients,[49] and private organizations started offering "crack mothers" money to buy more drugs in exchange for being sterilized.[50] The bulk of these policies were enacted between 1988 and 1991, when the prenatal cocaine exposure media hysteria peaked. Such policies have perpetuated the historical pattern of treating the procreation of black Americans as the cause of urban poverty and crime.[51] However, these arguments had been thoroughly discredited[52] after the release of the Moynihan report in 1965, which described the conditions in urban ghettos as the result of a "tangle of pathology" in the black family while negating the impact of racial oppression and systemic discrimination.[53] Boosted by the new discourses of sociobiology and the biology of behavior, the personal irresponsibility of "crack mothers" provided new grounds for pathologizing the urban poor.

WHITE HOUSE RESPONSE

Seizing on such horrific reports, Donald Ian MacDonald, director of the Office of National Drug Control Strategy, alerted U.S. attorney general Edwin Meese to the crisis of illegal drug use during pregnancy on June 17, 1988. MacDonald cited two examples of hospitals in Miami and Philadelphia where 20 percent of pregnant women had tested positive for illegal drugs. MacDonald further referenced the oft-cited crack baby symptoms of premature birth and physical and behavioral abnormalities "that have been reported as a result of cocaine use by the mother. Among the most distressing," MacDonald warned, "are the effects on the baby's brain," and he supplied for Meese a photocopy of one study citing such birth defects.[54] The article, "Brain Lesions in Cocaine and Methamphetamine Exposed Neonates," like the ones mentioned earlier, controlled for cocaine use as opposed to methamphetamine but did not control for other factors, such as alcohol and tobacco use, malnutrition, and access to prenatal care. However, the picture painted was particularly dire, finding that neonatal strokes were common in 35 percent of the infants born to drug-addicted mothers.[55]

MacDonald also sent a memo to Reagan's communications director on the necessity of maintaining a high profile on the drug war. "Recent poll numbers," he pointed out, "show that our best issue, as far as Presidential approval and Republican/Democrat differential, is the drug issue. We have about a 20 point spread, while our other issues on peace, economy, etc., have only a two-to-three point difference. With that in mind," MacDonald concluded, "our efforts should be focused on building the foundation that has already been laid by the President and First Lady."[56] MacDonald was acknowledging that the political future of Republicans depended on sustaining public fears about drugs. To further that goal, MacDonald requested Reagan's presence at a White House luncheon to thank media chief executives for their "extraordinary" coverage of the drug problem in the wake of Reagan's call for media organizations to address this issue.[57] This cooperation from media outlets helped maintain fear about the lurking specter of drugs and, most importantly, the inner-city, criminalized segments of the population associated with drugs in the American consciousness.

"FOCUS ON THE USER" CRUSADE

To lay the intellectual groundwork for the next phase of the drug war, MacDonald authored a position paper proposing a strategy to keep the nation's attention focused on the drug issue as a continuing crisis. The paper, titled "Focus on the User," served as the conceptual foundation for the religious zeal of a crusade that characterized all subsequent federal drug policy. It began with MacDonald reiterating the success of the public health and public awareness "Just Say No" campaign. However, MacDonald explained that the number of remaining users was far too high. For such users, "education and prevention efforts are less likely to be successful."[58] Pointing to earlier remarks by Reagan, when he argued that "we will insist [drug users] take responsibility for their own actions,"[59] MacDonald suggested that "user accountability" be the theme of the new era of the drug war. Drawing on the discourses of personal responsibility, substance abuse was specifically framed as an issue of individual bad behavior. This framing found particular resonance in the Reagan era's retreat from social justice in almost all areas, including workers' rights, social welfare, and racial and sex discrimination in the workplace and in higher education.

The first task necessary for such a change in attitude, MacDonald argued, was to overcome the "erroneous perception of the drug user as powerless" and instead acknowledge that "nearly all drug use starts with a willful act" and "most illegal drug users can choose to stop."[60] This strategy, attacking the idea of powerlessness, was a total negation of the consensus in the substance abuse medical literature, which recognizes high relapse rates in addiction treatment that fails to treat the mental health disorders from which most chronic addicts suffer.[61] By categorizing addiction as a failure of personal responsibility, MacDonald took the problem out of the realm of health policy and placed it in the realm of criminal justice.

"Previous demand reduction policies," MacDonald continued, have "suggested compassion for the drug user, including ample opportunities to stop drug use and . . . receive medical treatment." In a sly twist, MacDonald then made it seem as if his new "user accountability" crusade was actually a different form of empathy. "The emphasis on compassion is as it should be," MacDonald argued reassuringly, but "unfortunately, individuals have great difficulty in changing established behavior, especially when the reinforcing power of drugs tends to override health considerations and the psychological effects of the drugs themselves often conceal the real consequences from the user." Therefore, "solid accountability for stopping one's own drug use can be an effective stimulus to help individuals overcome drug-using behavior."

MacDonald's new frame of personal responsibility fit perfectly with concurrent conservative discourses used to dismantle the New Deal policies of the state. In this respect, a penal approach rather than a treatment one "made sense" while it allowed MacDonald to maintain that he had the user's well-being in mind. "A sound policy must," MacDonald asserted, "administer compassion with a firm hand if it is not to 'enable' the very behavior which it seeks to avoid." MacDonald concluded that individuals who continued to ignore the perils of drug use should face swift and certain sanctions. The goal was not to punish the users "but to cause them to stop their destructive behavior and to prevent other individuals from ever starting."[62] With these words, MacDonald set the White House on a course to launch an urban military drug crusade in a manner in which policymakers could feel as if they were acting compassionately.

MacDonald subsequently circulated memos to all White House offices informing them of the new "Focus on the User" crusade with instructions to tailor their programs and public addresses accordingly. It was this "crusade" that solidified the hysteria surrounding crack cocaine and crack babies into the American consciousness. Its conceptual foundation of "user accountability" was part of a larger racialized discourse of "personal responsibility" that has characterized much public policy debate over the past three decades. Far from being neutral, the discourse on personal responsibility has often been a thinly veiled condemnation of the black lower classes, particularly related to the perception that welfare primarily benefits blacks who lack a suitable work ethic.[63]

The most significant policies to emanate from the drug hysteria were the Omnibus Drug Abuse Acts of 1986 and 1988. Enacted on October 27, the Omnibus Anti-Drug Abuse Act of 1986 was a blueprint for the new drug control strategy that emphasized punishment and incarceration over treatment and educational awareness. It authorized $1.7 billion in new war funding, adding to the previous drug control budget of $2.2 billion. It increased mandatory sentencing for sales and possession, eliminated probation or parole for certain sellers and repeat offenders, and instituted an automatic sentence of death for any murder committed by a person involved in the drug enterprise. The bill established a "good faith" exception to the evidence exclusionary rule, where evidence illegally seized by officers would no longer be excluded from a criminal case. Officers needed only to testify that they conducted illegal searches in good faith and that in time, a proper search warrant would have been granted.

Treatment and prevention took a back seat to enforcement, new prison construction, and interdiction. The law established the block grant program to which state and local law enforcement agencies could apply for use in fighting the drug war but made the distribution of funding—even for projects not related to law enforcement—contingent on states passing similar legislation. States that favored a more tempered approach had no choice but to join the crusade. The law declared drugs a threat to national security, made large-scale trafficking violations federal offenses, and allocated $278 million for the Department of Defense to militarize its interdiction efforts along the southern border.

The 1988 bill represented the legislative height of the "Focus on the User" crusade, as demonstrated by the billions of new dollars allocated for law enforcement agencies. Subtitle A, dubbed the User Accountability Act, stipulated that any person convicted of a drug offense be deemed ineligible for federal benefits—including federally subsidized student loans, Social Security, and Medicare—and authorized the withholding of federal highway funds to any state that did not revoke the driver's licenses of drug offenders. It even directed the attorney general to study the feasibility of prosecuting federal drug-related offenders without affording them constitutional rights.[64]

The bill provided $1.5 billion in block grants for law enforcement in addition to more than $300 million for hiring new federal officers. It allocated $200 million for new prison construction and $600 million in international aid as conditional grants for source countries to eradicate drug crops.[65]

The law also set a distinction between crack and powder cocaine, establishing the 100-to-1 ratio of mandatory minimum sentencing for cocaine offenses. Under this rubric, possession of 5+ grams of crack carried a mandatory five-year minimum; 50+ grams carried a ten-year mandatory sentence. It took 500 grams or more of powder cocaine to receive the same five-year sentence, or 5,000 grams for the mandatory ten-year sentence, even though powder cocaine is the manufacturing base of crack.[66] The overwhelming majority of those prosecuted for crack cocaine offenses are black. Despite the fact that a 1995 U.S. Sentencing Commission report found this statute was egregiously racially discriminatory,[67] so strongly was crack cocaine associated with the social pariah of the black, urban, criminal gang member that there was no congressional, judicial, or executive branch support for correcting the racial bias in the law until 2007.[68]

Most importantly, the bill streamlined the process for asset forfeiture, allowing the proceeds from confiscated assets to go directly to the operating budgets of law enforcement agencies, and lifted restrictions on the amount they could collect in forfeitures. It turned the drug war into a cash cow as every car, boat, house, bundle of cash, and tract of property seized during a drug arrest went directly into the coffers of state and local police agencies. This meant higher salaries and millions worth of new vehicles and equipment. This development eventually led to a $500-billion-per-year profit motive for sustaining the drug war,[69] creating powerful, financially vested interest groups whose financial futures depend on maintaining the war.

By the late 1980s, the War on Drugs became the main contributor to the largest exponential growth of prison inmates in U.S. history. In the forty years since the War on Drugs began, the U.S. jail and prison population has grown to eleven times its size in 1971, from about 200,000 inmates to more than 2.3 million. This period also saw a total transformation of inmate demographics. Up until the beginning of the War on Drugs, whites made up the majority of the U.S. prison population, commensurate with their percentage of the general population. Since the War on Drugs began in the aftermath of the civil rights movements, blacks now make up 49 percent of all prison inmates, with Latino/as making up another 27 percent. By 1989–90, twenty-three states had a racial disparity in drug arrest rates of more than five blacks to every one nonblack.[70] Although blacks account for only 13 percent of monthly drug users, according to annual National Institute on Drug Abuse surveys, they make up 35 percent of all arrests for drug possession, 55 percent of all convictions for possession, and 74 percent of all prison sentences for possession.[71]

Before 1970, drug offenders made up roughly 16 percent of the prison population.[72] Of the 2.3 million people now incarcerated, roughly 60 percent are drug-related convictions. Of drug offenders, 45 percent are for charges related to crack. Of those convicted for crack, 88.3 percent of them are black.[73] Mandatory sentencing is also a huge factor: The California "three strikes" law, which requires life in prison for third-time offenders, has sentenced more people for drug possession than for all violent offenses combined, and it has sentenced twice as many marijuana users to life sentences as murderers, rapists, and kidnappers combined.[74]

To put this in perspective, a prison system that had consistently been 75 percent white with around 200,000 inmates is now 75 percent black and Latino, with more than 2.3 million inmates.[75] What is to be made of the fact that this drastic transformation took place at a time when the United States was, at least in name and on paper, struggling to put behind it the era when blacks functioned in the American consciousness as the antithesis of what it meant to be American, to be human? This period represents a time when the nation's antiblack discourse was refocused into a nebulous anti-crime rhetoric that focused on urban behaviors. Such rhetoric was reinforced by deindustrialization and its disproportionate impact on blacks, a rising income inequality between the upper and working classes, a prevailing discourse of racialized welfare stereotypes, an increased policing of reproductive behaviors of the racialized female body, and dramatized media and political responses to the burgeoning trend of crack use.[76]

The War on Drugs was a nuanced way to refocus racial attitudes in an ambiguous, post–civil rights discourse of "being tough on crime" and "taking back our streets." After more than a decade of relaxed attitudes toward drug use, it was an indication that the social upheaval of the 1960s and 1970s was over. It was time for America to get back to conservative family values. As the 1970s drew to a close, the United States was passing more than two decades of crisis. An era of violent protests, race riots, Vietnam, political assassinations, Watergate, and a recession had sapped the progressive, transformative energy out of the country. Americans seemed to want to put the traumas of the previous decades behind them. The decisive election of Ronald Reagan was perceived as a mandate for change,[77] and it brought with it the promise that the traumatic, countercultural fighting of the previous era could be laid to rest.

On the whole, the 1980s was a counterreformation period in American thought and politics, when conservatives sought to reverse the transformations brought about with the civil rights and countercultural movements of the 1960s and 1970s. It was a movement whose ideological foundations were laid with the 1964 presidential campaign of Barry Goldwater,[78] gained momentum under Nixon, and finally came to fruition under the Reagan and Bush presidencies.

The crack baby narrative served as key evidence demonstrating the need for this counterreformation, now grounded in the new discourses of behavioral biology. It demonstrated for Americans the dysfunctionality and irresponsibility of black American families. It affirmed that Americans were right to despise the inner cities and criminalize their inhabitants. It proved that black men were heartless, drug-dealing thugs and that black women were lazy welfare queens who used the state's money to get high rather than take care of their children. The overwhelming popularity of the Reagan presidency demonstrates the extent to which this movement resonated with the American middle class. In this sense, the exponential growth in the prison population—focused primarily on blacks and Latinos and beginning right after the civil rights movement and the height of the Black Power and Nationalist movements—was an American cultural response to correct the social up-heavals of the previous decades. The narrative of the crack baby helped focus these feelings into a new socially acceptable enemy: crack users.

A SOLUTION TO THE AMERICAN IDENTITY CRISIS

The crack baby phenomenon illustrates how stories, regardless of their empirical grounding, can nevertheless be major motivators of historical events. In this case, the narrative of the crack baby—at least temporarily, but long enough to have wide-reaching effects—became constructed in scientific journals and news articles as fact. Americans found the narrative so enthralling because it solved the post-1960s American identity crisis. It did so by reinscribing race in a discourse of behavioral biology that regrounded American identity against the savages of the urban jungle.

As Charles Rosenberg argues, "ideas always have a structural role."[79] To fully comprehend the religious zeal of the antidrug crusade, and the powerful manner in which the narrative of the minority, hedonistic, and criminal-minded addict resonates with the American consciousness, we need to understand how these narratives function to inscribe inner-city drug users into a liminal space of alterity. It is through the inscription of certain groups into spaces of liminal alterity—the space of conceptual Otherness—that a society defines itself, produces its sense of well-being, and motivates collective behavior.[80] It is by the omnipresent threat posed by liminal groups that states legitimate their claims for power and authority, and by the persecution of liminal groups that individuals within a society come to realize themselves as fully human.[81]

In this history the interplay between media representations, scientific research, and policymakers gave birth to the crack baby phenomenon and subsequently constructed drug use as a racial problem. As a discourse of racial behavioral degeneracy, it helped foster the political climate in which incarceration and the death penalty took the place of segregation and lynching.[82] As a discourse to reaffirm for us who is, and who is not, civilized, the crack baby narrative functioned as a mechanism by which the urban poor were sacrificed in a ritual of justice and retribution that functioned to create identity-affirming cohesion for the rest of American society while granting ever more power to the state. The crack baby narrative facilitated the development of a new American political consensus for using newly coded discourses of race to galvanize the political support to dismantle the public welfare and social justice reforms enacted since the Great Depression and the civil rights movement.

NOTES

1 Deborah Frank, Marilyn Augustyn, Wanda Knight, Tripler Pell, and Barry Zuckerman, "Growth, Development, and Behavior in Early Childhood Following Prenatal Cocaine Exposure: A Systematic Review," *Journal of the American Medical Association* 285 (March 28, 2001): 1613.

2 David Boyum and Peter Reuter, *An Analytic Assessment of US Drug Policy* (Washington, D.C.: AEI Press, 2005).

3 Stephen Toulmin, "Contemporary Scientific Mythology," in *Metaphysical Beliefs*, ed. Alasdair MacIntyre (London: SCM Press, 1957), 13–78.

4 Michel Foucault, *The Order of Things: An Archaeology of the Human Sciences* (1970; repr., New York: Vintage, 1994).

5 Michel Foucault, *History of Sexuality, Vol. 1: An Introduction* (1978; repr., New York: Vintage, 1990), 140.

6 Sylvia Wynter, "Unsettling the Coloniality of Being/Power/Truth/Freedom: Towards the Human, after Man, Its Over-representation—An Argument," *New Centennial Review* 3, no. 3 (Fall 2003): 257–337.

7 Sylvia Wynter, "New Seville and the Conversion Experience of Bartolomé de Las Casas, Part One," *Jamaica Journal* 17, no. 2 (1984): 26.

8 Wynter, "Unsettling the Coloniality of Being/Power/Truth/Freedom."

9 Sylvia Wynter, "1492: A New World View," in *Race, Discourse, and the Origin of the Americas: A New World View*, ed. Vera Hyatt and Rex Nettleford, 5–57 (Washington, D.C.: Smithsonian, 1995).

10 Sylvia Wynter, "New Seville and the Conversion Experience of Bartolomé de Las Casas, Part One," 25–32; and "New Seville and the Conversion Experience of Bartolomé de Las Casas, Part Two," *Jamaica Journal* 17, no. 3 (1984): 46–55.

11 Michael Omi and Howard Winant, *Racial Formation in the United States: From the 1960s to the 1990s* (New York: Routledge, 1994).

12 Stephen Steinberg, *Turning Back: The Retreat from Racial Justice in American Thought and Policy* (Boston: Beacon, 1995).

13 Howard Kaye, *The Social Meaning of Modern Biology: From Social Darwinism to Sociobiology* (1986; repr., New Haven, Conn.: Yale University Press, 1997).

14 Stephen Jay Gould, *Ever Since Darwin: Reflections in Natural History* (New York: Norton, 1979), 201, 237–39.

15 Caroline Acker, *Creating the American Junkie: Addiction Research in the Classic Era of Narcotic Control* (Baltimore, Md.: Johns Hopkins University Press, 2002).

16 Steven Belenko, *Crack and the Evolution of Anti-Drug Policy* (Westport, Conn.: Greenwood, 1993).

17 Ronald Reagan, "Address to the Nation on the Campaign against Drug Abuse," September 14, 1986, http://www.reagan.utexas.edu/resource/speeches/1986/091486a.htm.

18 Alexander Cockburn and Jeffrey St. Clair, *Whiteout: The CIA, Drugs and the Press* (London: Verso, 1998), 74.

19 U.S. Sentencing Commission, *Special Report to the Congress: Cocaine and Federal Sentencing Policy* (Washington, D.C.: Government Printing Office, 1995), 122.

20 Office of the Press Secretary for Ronald Reagan, Press Release, "Crack/Cocaine Awareness Month 1986," October 31, 1986, in the files of Richard L. Williams, folder "Crack Cocaine," box OA 19050, Reagan Presidential Library, Simi Valley, California.

21 Ibid.

22 Charles Krauthammer, "Children of Cocaine," *Washington Post*, July 30, 1989, C7.

23 Besharov coined the term "bio-underclass."

24 Krauthammer, "Children of Cocaine."

25 Douglas Besharov, "Crack Babies: The Worst Threat Is Mom Herself," *Washington Post*, August 6, 1989.

26 Mariah Blake, "'Crack Babies' Talk Back: Young Writers Take Aim at a Media Myth Built on Wobbly, Outdated Science," *Boston Phoenix*, September 17, 2004, 32.

27 Ira Chasnoff, William Burns, S. Schnoll, and Kayreen Burns, "Cocaine Use in Pregnancy," *NEJM* 313 (1985): 666–69.

28 Special report, "Medical Complications of Cocaine Use," *NEJM* 315, no. 23 (1986): 1495–1500.

29 Lynn Ryan, Saundra Ehrlich, and Loretta Finnegan, "Cocaine Abuse in Pregnancy: Effects on the Fetus and Newborn," *Neurotoxicology and Teratology* 9 (1987): 295–99.

30 Enrique Ostrea, Paul Kresbach, David Knapp, and Kenneth Simkowski, "Abnormal Heart Rate Tracings and Serum Creatine Phosphokinase in Addicted Neonates," *Neurotoxicology and Teratology* 9 (1987): 305–9.

31 Diane Regan, Saundra Ehrlich, and Loretta Finnegan, "Infants of Drug Addicts: At Risk for Child Abuse, Neglect, and Placement in Foster Care," *Neurotoxicology and Teratology* 9 (1987): 315–19.

32 Blake, "'Crack Babies' Talk Back," 32.

33 Roger Rosenblatt, "Special Report. The Enemy Within: A Nation Wrestles with the Dark and Dangerous Recesses of Its Soul," *Time*, September 15, 1986.

34 Emanuel Peluso and Lucy Peluso, "Motherhood & Drugs," *Sober Times* (April 1989): 42.

35 Craig Reinarman and Harry Levine, "Crack in Context: Politics and Media in the Making of a Drug Scare," *Contemporary Drug Problems* 16, no. 4 (Winter 1989): 535–78.

36 Eva Bertram, *Drug War Politics: The Price of Denial* (Berkeley: University of California Press, 1996), 138.

37 Craig Reinarman and Harry Levine, *Crack in America: Demon Drugs and Social Justice* (Berkeley: University of California Press, 1997), 22; George Bush, "Address to the Nation on the National Drug Control Strategy," September 5, 1989, George Bush Presidential Library. http://bushlibrary .tamu.edu/research/papers/1989/89090502.html.

38 Craig Malisow, "Deal of a Lifetime: Drug Addicts Can Get Hard Cash to Be Sterilized or Go on Birth Control," *Houston Press*, February 27, 2003.

39 Marcia Greene, "Abuse, Neglect Rising in D.C.; Drugs Ravage Home Life," *Washington Post*, September 10, 1989, A1.

40 Sandra Blakeslee, "Adopting Drug Babies: A Special Report; Child-Rearing Is Stormy When Drugs Cloud Birth," *New York Times*, May 19, 1990, 1.

41 Katherine Grieder, "Crackpot Ideas," *Mother Jones*, July/August, 1995.

42 Ibid.

43 Frank et al., "Growth, Development, and Behavior in Early Childhood Following Prenatal Cocaine Exposure: A Systematic Review," 1613.

44 G. Koren, K. Graham, H. Shear, and T. Einarson, "Bias against the Null Hypothesis: The Reproductive Hazards of Cocaine," *The Lancet* 2, no. 8677 (December 16, 1989), 1440–42.

45 Ibid., 1441.

46 Belenko, *Crack and the Evolution of Anti-Drug Policy.*

47 Blake, "'Crack Babies' Talk Back."

48 Grieder, "Crackpot Ideas," 5.

49 Dorothy Roberts, *Killing the Black Body: Race, Reproduction, and the Meaning of Liberty* (New York: Pantheon, 1997).

50 Craig Malisow, "Deal of a Lifetime."

51 Roberts, *Killing the Black Body.*

52 William Ryan, *Blaming the Victim* (New York: Vintage, 1971).

53 Daniel Moynihan, *The Negro Family: The Case for National Action* (Washington, D.C.: Office of Policy Planning and Research, U.S. Department of Labor, 1965).

54 Memorandum, Donald Ian MacDonald to Attorney General, "Drug-Free Pregnancy," June 17, 1988, files of Donald Ian MacDonald, folder "National Drug Enforcement Policy Board, 7 of 9," box OA 19364, Reagan Presidential Library.

55 Suzanne Dixon and Raul Bejar, "Brain Lesions in Cocaine and Methamphetamine Exposed Neonates," *Pediatric Research* 23 (April 1988): 405A.

56 Macdonald to Thomas Griscom, "Memorandum on Drug Initiative," April 14, 1987, files of Donald Ian MacDonald, folder "Crusade for a Drug Free America, 1 of 4," box OA 19322, 1.

57 MacDonald, "Schedule Proposal Request," February 3, 1988, files of Donald Ian MacDonald, folder "West Wing Correspondence Drug Policy 9/87–11/88, 3 of 4," box OA 16758.

58 MacDonald, "Working Paper: Focus on the User," February 12, 1988, files of Donald Ian MacDonald, folder "Crusade for a Drug Free America, 1 of 4," box OA 19322, 1.

59 Ronald Reagan, "Remarks Announcing the Campaign against Drug Abuse and a Question-and-Answer Session with Reporters," August 4, 1986, http://www.reagan.utexas.edu/resource/speeches/1986/080486b.htm.

60 MacDonald, "Working Paper: Focus on the User," 2.

61 Jason E. Glenn and Helen Wu, "Sobriety," in *Encyclopedia of Substance Abuse Prevention, Treatment, and Recovery,* ed. Gary Fisher and Nancy Roget (Los Angeles: Sage, 2008).

62 MacDonald, "Working Paper: Focus on the User," 3–4.

63 Martin Gilens, *Why Americans Hate Welfare: Race, Media, and the Politics of Antipoverty Policy* (Chicago: University of Chicago Press, 1999).

64 Comprehensive Anti-Drugs Act of 1988, H.R. 4842, 100th Congress, http://thomas.loc.gov/.

65 Pub. L. 100-690, Nov. 18, 1988, 102 Stat. 4181.

66 U.S. Sentencing Commission, *Cocaine and Federal Sentencing Policy* (Washington, D.C.: Government Printing Office, 1995), iii.

67 Ibid.

68 James Morone, "Enemies of the People: The Moral Dimension to Public Health," *Journal of Health Politics, Policy and Law* 22, no. 4 (August 1997): 993–1020.

69 James Bovard, "Seizure Fever: The War on Property Rights," *The Freeman* 46, no. 1 (January 1996): 6–13; Dan Baum, *Smoke and Mirrors: The War on Drugs and the Politics of Failure* (Boston: Little, Brown, 1996), 254.

70 Kenneth Meier, *Politics of Sin: Drugs, Alcohol, and Public Policy* (Armonk, N.Y.: M. E. Sharpe, 1994), 119–21.

71 F. Butterfield, "More Blacks in Their 20s Have Trouble with the Law," *New York Times,* November 5, 1995, A18.

72 *Sourcebook of Criminal Justice Statistics Online,* http://www.albany.edu/sourcebook/pdf/t654.pdf.

73 U.S. Sentencing Commission, *Cocaine and Federal Sentencing Policy,* xi.

74 Jerome Skolnick, "Tough Guys," *American Prospect* 8, no. 30 (February 1997): 86–91.

75 Patrick Langan, *Race of Prisoners Admitted to State and Federal Institutions, 1926–1986* (Washington, D.C.: U.S. Department of Justice, Office of Justice Programs, Bureau of Justice Statistics, 1991); *Correctional Populations in the United States* (Washington, D.C.: U.S. Department of Justice, Office of Justice Programs, Bureau of Justice Statistics, 1995).

76 Steinberg, *Turning Back;* Jennifer Eberhardt, Phillip Goff, Valerie Purdie, and Paul Davies, "Seeing Black: Race, Crime and Visual Processing," *Journal of Personality and Social Psychology* 87, no. 6 (2004): 876–93; William Julius Wilson, *When Work Disappears: The World of the New Urban Poor* (New York: Vintage, 1997); William Julius Wilson, *The Bridge over the Racial Divide: Rising Inequality and Coalition Politics* (Berkeley: University of California Press, 1999); Ange-Marie Hancock, *The Politics of Disgust: The Public Identity of the Welfare Queen* (New York: NYU Press, 2004); and Belenko, *Crack and the Evolution of Anti-Drug Policy.*

77 Norman Amaker, *Civil Rights and the Reagan Administration* (Washington, D.C.: Urban Institute Press, 1988), 3.

78 Rick Perlstein, *Before the Storm: Barry Goldwater and the Unmaking of the American Consensus* (New York: Hill and Wang, 2001).

79 Charles Rosenberg, *Explaining Epidemics and Other Studies in the History of Medicine* (Cambridge: Cambridge University Press, 1992), 6.

80 Asmarom Legesse, *Gada: Three Approaches to the Study of an African Society* (New York: Free Press, 1973), 114–15; Michael Taussig, *Mimesis and Alterity: A Particular History of the Senses* (New York: Routledge, 1993), 129; Victor Turner, *The Ritual Process: Structure and Anti-Structure* (Chicago: Aldine, 1969), 128.

81 Legesse, *Gada,* 115; Turner, *The Ritual Process,* 110–11.

82 Charles Ogletree and Austin Sarat, eds., *From Lynch Mobs to the Killing State: Race and the Death Penalty in America* (New York: NYU Press, 2006).

12

Suffering and Resistance, Voice and Agency

Thoughts on History and the Tuskegee Syphilis Study

SUSAN M. REVERBY

VOICE AND AGENCY became the central analytic foci for my generation as we fought to create a new social history and to make concerns of race, gender, class, and sexuality crucial to the historical enterprise. Two quick anecdotes of my own travels through graduate school illustrate this. When I was first in graduate school in the late 1960s, I took a European intellectual history course at New York University with renowned scholar Frank Manuel. In the middle of some lecture on an obscure French revolutionary thinker, I raised my hand and asked, "Professor Manuel, who believed these ideas and did anything with them?" Manuel raised himself up, peered down at me through his glasses past the other one hundred students in the class, and said, "That, my dear, is the wrong question."

In 1973 (after a several-year dropout from graduate school), I considered going back and went to speak to Herbert Gutman, one of the leaders of what was then called the New Labor History. Gutman was working on his magisterial book *The Black Family in Slavery and Freedom*, which would become the historical answer to the seemingly scurrilous Moynihan report. After I explained my interests, I politely asked him what he was doing. Unfurling the almost Talmudic looking scrolls of paper that surrounded him, he showed me plantation records of slave names and long genealogical connections. "There," he said, triumphantly pointing, "Mary was named after her great-grandmother." I panicked. I had no idea what he was trying to tell me and why it mattered.

Now, many decades later, I can happily say I survived to become deeply focused on the questions of voice and agency and to understand what Gutman was trying to tell me about agency through naming practices. I learned to have an answer to Manuel's response that I was asking the wrong question about whose voice I should worry about, even if he must be turning his in grave to know I have a professorial chair in the "history of ideas." I thought I knew finally how to think about this: searching for voice among those assumed not to have one while documenting suffering to consider the multiple forms that agency might take, from a full-scale revolt, to the naming of a child, to survival itself.

Yet in the place where the answers seemed to have created an extensive industry in African American history, the limitations of this approach must be assessed. For as American studies scholar Jeffrey Ferguson argues, "The broad and diverse discourse on African Americans has yielded many books, but only two basic stories: those of suffering and resistance." Ferguson goes on to claim that these stories provide "no sure answers" about the meaning of suffering and resistance while limiting our analytic insights.[1] For he wants us to consider that "resistance serves more of a rhetorical deal-closer than an analytical concept, more of an answer that ends or suspends the conversation than a problem that opens it up to new territory."[2]

To attempt to step up to Ferguson's critique of this historiographic binary and often sophisticated "racial melodramas," I am going to focus on some of my thinking that comes from completing two (and too) long book projects on what has come to be called the infamous Tuskegee syphilis study and was more formally known as a study of "Untreated Syphilis in the Male Negro."[3] I will use two examples from this work to meditate about the tropes historians use and the analysis we do and need to do in the history of medicine or health care and race.[4]

If anything has been paradigmatic of the relationship of African Americans to the American health care system in the twentieth century, it has to be this Study. To summarize, the crucial facts seem clear at first: In a forty-year study (1932–1972) white government doctors from the U.S. Public Health Service (PHS) found approximately 400 African American men presumed to all have late-stage, and therefore not infectious, syphilis in and around Tuskegee in Macon County, Alabama. After some initial treatment was given and then stopped, the PHS provided aspirins and iron tonics, implying through deception that these were to cure the men's "bad blood." PHS doctors also told nearly 200 controls—men without the disease—that they were being cared

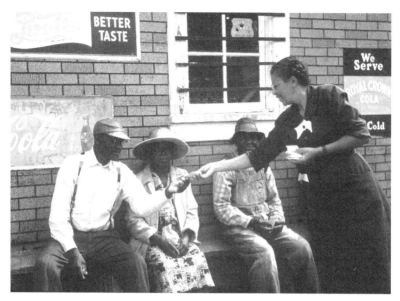

FIGURE 12.1. Nurse Eunice Rivers Laurie handed out a packet of aspirins and vitamins to a man in the study in Tuskegee. Source: National Archives.

for with the same simple medications. The only permission asked for was the right to autopsy the bodies after the men had died in exchange for payment for a decent burial. Doctors and a nurse connected to the county health department, the venerable black educational institution Tuskegee Institute (now Tuskegee University), and the Tuskegee Veterans Administration Hospital provided assistance and did the x-rays, tests, and autopsies. Given the complexity of syphilis, many of the men survived their disease and others were felled by it. Those still infectious could have passed it on to wives or sexual partners, and through them to children.

The Study went on not for one year but for forty, through the Depression, World War II, the Cold War, and into the civil rights era and beyond, as a changing number of administrators, epidemiologists, doctors, and nurses made it possible. It began at a time when there was "modern treatment" for syphilis in the form of heavy metals and malarial fever therapy and continued into what is usually considered the curative penicillin era of the post–World War II years. The PHS did what it could all those years to keep the men from treatment, even though some made it to treatment and many may not have been helped even if they had been given penicillin because their organ damage was too extensive.

Since 1972, the Study's cultural malleability has gained it a central position in the American pantheon of experimental monstrosities and racial injustices. When the Study ended, the stories began. The knots that tie racism to experimentation, a fearful disease to the black male body, sexuality to the state, and gender and class to claims of racial collaboration give the stories their cultural staying power and their deep place in collective memories. Poems, music, movies, documentaries, books, articles, institutional review board training sessions, bioethics texts, a federal apology in 1997 at the White House, and endless whispering keep the story of the Study alive. New events renew and reinvigorate its telling, however mythic, from Barack Obama's former minister Jeremiah Wright's "God Damn America" sermon to its use by right-wing politicians to frighten black voters and gain opposition to government-sponsored stem cell research during election referendums in Missouri and Michigan.

The Study has become a site of collective memory and a contentious ground for a civic—rather than a civil—war battlefield. As its story gets repeated, its truths pass between different communities as fictions become facts and rumors become truths.[5] Often just the word *Tuskegee* is uttered in the context of racial injustice, and its meaning is implied or assumed to be known. Suffering and abuse are central to the story's core. In the face of what seems like a known story where suffering and death are the key to our outrage and endless pictures of "abject" black men appear, what can we ask anew?

The key voice from the men in the Study and its prime example of the suffering endured comes from the late Herman Shaw, who died in 1999 at the age of ninety-seven. A farmer and textile mill worker, Herman Shaw, with his grace, charm, and eighth-grade education, emerged out of what is often seen as "600AfricanAmericanilliteratesharecroppers," as if the men were one word, one group, with just one story. Shaw gave testimony about the Study at Ted Kennedy's Senate experimentation hearings in 1973, is visible in the documentaries made in the 1990s, and served as spokesman for the men at the federal apology at the White House in 1997. Shaw's story of what happened to him is emblematic of how the suffering of the men in the Study is recounted. His powerful tale—of going to receive appropriate drugs at a rapid treatment center

for syphilis in Birmingham in the late 1940s and being sent home—
stands as a key moment in the Study's horrific tellings.

As Shaw related many times, and especially at the Kennedy hearings
in the Senate in 1973, which also became dramatized in the fictional
play and movie on the Study, *Miss Evers' Boys,*

> In the late 1940's—I do not remember the exact date—they sent
> me to Birmingham. . . . I saw a nurse roaming through the
> crowd. . . . She said that she had been looking for a man that was
> not supposed to be here and his name is Herman Shaw. Naturally
> I stood up. She said come here. She said, "what are you doing
> here?" I said, "I do not know, they sent me here." They got me a
> bus and sent me back home.[6]

With his story, Herman Shaw becomes almost a twentieth-century medical runaway slave who tries to escape but gets caught and returned to
enslavement to the Study. This dramatic moment of resistance and defeat
links the Study to the horrors of slavery and the deadly toll of racism.

In all the interviews and writing about the Study, however, no one
seems to have asked Mr. Shaw who sent him to the rapid treatment
center and why? So focused on the horror of his coming close to treatment, on his suffering and being denied it at the last moment, the questions that are not asked are, How did he get there in the first place?
Was it merely a mistake? Was the "they" who sent him to Birmingham
someone from the study in Tuskegee or some other family member or
health professional?

I tried to ask him some about this in 1998, when he was ninety-six
years old.[7] By then, the story was confounded with so many other events
in his life that it was impossible to even separate when he learned what.
He talked about the "state conscripting him to Birmingham," but I was
not clear what this meant. He did say, "The only remorse I have about
it is in [19]47 the rumors came out that they were treating us for bad
blood; and they had found the medicine that alleviated the pain and
withheld it and didn't give it to us." But there was no way to tell when
he found out about penicillin, what he knew and when.

In the context of the efforts to keep the men from treatment, Mr.
Shaw's denial of care is taken as one more tragic or horrific example
of the PHS's deadly callousness. It may indeed be that he was sent back

home because the center in Birmingham had a list of the names of the men in the Study, as his statement implies.

However, there is another possible explanation if we want to escape a focus on suffering and consider more fully historical contingency. At least in Birmingham during the mass campaign, the drugs were being given only to those with early cases of syphilis. The state health officials stated this clearly in their 1940s news accounts: "Unfortunately, some inferred that all cases of syphilis were eligible for penicillin treatment, when actually its use was limited to early cases. This inaccuracy was never completely corrected. Many chronic cases demanded penicillin treatment of practicing physicians and public clinics and were not always satisfied as to the reasons for its refusal."[8] Was Mr. Shaw then sent back home because he was in the study or because it was presumed that he was not an early case?

Mr. Shaw's story becomes even more complicated once the medical records are used that became available just a few years ago. Mr. Shaw was originally a control switched into the syphilitic category after 1945 when his tests turned positive. There is no way to know whether he had been positive before and just did not register on an earlier blood test or whether this was a new infection. It is possible that he should have been treated in Birmingham because he could have been in the early stage and infectious. But if he was not and it was known he was in the Study, his being turned away could have been because of the stage of his disease. The irony is that even though he was turned away in Birmingham, Mr. Shaw actually was given penicillin in the 1950s.

Herman Shaw's story gives us another clue as to what might have happened to others: Some did get to doctors more often than the focus on the Depression years makes us think. In 1953 and 1956, Mr. Shaw was hospitalized for a total of twenty days for pneumonia. The treatment was penicillin every three hours for nine of those twenty days. His status in the Study did not affect his care. Did this make a difference in his syphilitic illness? We will never know.[9]

Others, the now available medical records show, actually were treated in Birmingham at the rapid treatment center or at the local health department.[10] "May 1951 Penicillin 5,000,000 units R.T.C.," report the records in one man's case while his wife was treated at the Macon County Health Department. Another forty-nine-year-old man in the Study had a similar experience: Both he and his wife were treated at the same time in 1949 at the rapid treatment center in Birmingham. Still another man, who died from a stroke, not syphilis, remained a syphilitic in the Study even though he too had penicillin in 1949 in Birmingham, supposedly twenty-seven years after his first infection.[11] It is not clear why some men who were clearly in latency also were treated. Mr. Shaw remembers being turned away, and there is no reason to doubt him. What about these other men, and why were they not turned away?

What do we do with our story based on suffering and the inability to escape when we examine these experiences? Do I count this as a form of agency, however unintended? Or when it comes to medicine, might we want to consider the role of uncertainty and historical contingency?[12] I do not think we can consider Mr. Shaw an agent of his own life in this aspect of the Study because he did not choose to get pneumonia, nor resist being sent back from Birmingham. Yet his escape through getting pneumonia is not really resistance either. So what terms do we use to understand this, and what are its consequences for how we tell the story of the Study? Might the concept of historical contingency be of more use to us here?

There is more at stake here in trying to understand this than a seemingly arcane debate between historians about analytic categories and tropes. Because Tuskegee has become such a powerful metaphor for racism, government perfidiousness, and medical deceit, it should be no surprise that there has also developed what one scholar labels the counternarratives that question the suffering by focusing primarily on the science.[13]

These counternarratives refocused attention on the medical uncertainties among syphilologists and the questions over heavy metal therapies and penicillin for late latent syphilis. Were the medical scientific decisions so dreadful, those writing the counternarratives asked? Was the "discourse of horror," as anthropologist Richard Shweder labeled the narrative of the Study, used to justify modern "research regulation" unfair once more of the facts were known? Oncologist Dr. Robert W. White asked whether there should even have been an apology.[14]

Shorn of the liberal rhetoric that had underlain historians' work on the Study nearly twenty years earlier, the new critics found the debates in the medical literature about the type and duration of efficacious treatment, how common nontreatment was, and whether the provision of penicillin would have made a difference. These new narratives took the uncertainty and subthemes of earlier histories and brought them to the front of analysis.[15] Using this analysis, they argued for a different kind of historical judgment. Their conclusions supported an earlier review of studies on cardiovascular syphilis treatment that concluded that "the therapeutic efficacy of penicillin in the treatment of cardiovascular syphilis is not established" because of the lack of controlled trials even though a wide range of dosages of the drug were being used.[16]

The counternarratives hoped to make a similar point: The symbolic "Tuskegee" is wrong because the *real* Study was not so horrific or out of character for the times for both whites and blacks. The oft-quoted belief that 60 to 70 percent of those with tertiary syphilis did not die from it was used to counter the sense of the public narrative that hundreds of the men died because of the PHS's malfeasance.

Racism is labeled a "presentist" worry, whereas the medical science gets elevated and shorn of its racial assumptions. "Efficacy" of the drugs—both the heavy metals and penicillin—became a central concern rather than the attempts to withhold treatment.[17] The medical belief that latent syphilis would not kill everyone and acceptance of the claims of the PHS that the contagious were treated serves the arguments that the study was not so terrible. These counternarratives argued that most of the men either died early, before penicillin, or might not have been helped by it and that the danger to their lives was not borne out by the epidemiological evidence.

Rather than denouncing these counternarratives as confused, overtly racist, or efforts to protect scientific research, we need to consider their arguments.[18] This has to be done by appeals to what we can know about what happened rather than the "truths" that have prevailed, however useful they are to current political considerations.[19]

We will probably never know from the incomplete men's records and reports whether the PHS's assertion that they made the men sicker and that the syphilitics died earlier until the antibiotic era is really true for everyone in the Study. The conflicts on the autopsies, the lack of records on those who dropped out, the ways in which controls were switched to syphilitics, and the evidence that some of the syphilitics who probably never had the disease in the first place should have been the controls muddy the data. It is impossible to know whether the penicillin would have changed the health outcomes of those still alive in the antibiotic era and whether those decades out from their initial

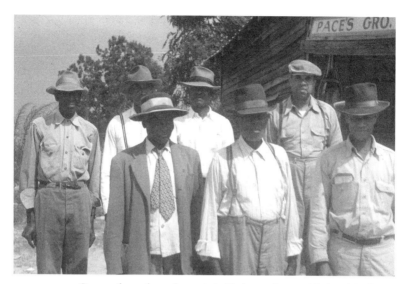

FIGURE 12.2. Group of men from the study in Tuskegee. Source: National Archives.

infections would have been helped. But even a syphilis study that used white patients at Stanford in 1948 and withheld treatment concluded, "Should penicillin prove effective, all arguments against the routine treatment of latent syphilis should vanish."[20] By the mid-1950s, penicillin became routine in medical practice even with those in latency. And in the 1970s, when the Study became more public, anyone still alive and willing to be treated was given penicillin.

Tuskegee's symbolic power works, however, because of revulsion over the idea that the PHS deceived the men and their families, watched for years as they died whether from syphilis or not, and then carved up their bodies at autopsies. These are the images that float through cultural consciousness. It cannot be forgotten that the men were treated as a public health problem to be watched. Even if only one man was harmed at the time (and we know it was more), or only one man passed the disease on to his wife and children, it would matter. The men were treated as a population, rather than individuals, without their knowing, and the deception that went on so long will haunt Tuskegee forever.

Although the reigning medical belief before penicillin was that "if the patient has had syphilis for 25 years without clinical disease, he is to be congratulated not treated," even a leading syphilologist who defended the Study in the 1970s wrote, "I followed the advice, with exceptions, of course."[21] The historical fact is that the men were not given a choice, and they were intentionally lied to because the PHS doctors thought they were doing little harm to those who were expected to get little attention. If the men became "exceptions," it was not because the PHS wanted it this way. If we see them as individuals and understand that the situation in Alabama changed over the forty years, we can then see how some managed to get to treatment. Our focus becomes the men and their families, not just the intentions of the PHS. Their voice matters, and their suffering takes on a different kind of more nuanced meaning, even if we would be hard-pressed to label it resistance.

The counternarratives bring up what their authors' claim are "medical facts" of this deeply flawed study, as if the science can be separated from its political context, as if the history does not form a kind of testifying, and as if the facts are easy to know. These "medical facts" as they were defined in the Study were suffused with racial concepts and rested on beliefs about racial difference. Above all in this study, race mattered, and it made the science. Whether it is morals or methods, or racism and medical science, these counternarratives are a way to separate out concerns about the ways science can create race and perpetuate racism, whether it is done overtly or in more subtle ways. This segregation of race and science cannot be done because they co-create one another.

We cannot look at the Study as if the symbolic Tuskegee does not exist. The symbolism informs how we understand the facts, what questions we ask, what explanations we offer. In turn, as with any historical event that becomes mythic, examination of the facts often does little to undermine a powerful and useful story. There is a truth to what actually happened, and trying to understand it does matter. In this sense, the counternarratives should be read, their facts measured, and the arguments considered, if for no other reason than to understand why they are being made. But our task also must be what historian Walter Johnson argues for the historiography of slavery: "focusing attention on the present life of the past, on what elements of the past are drawn upon at any given moment in history and the power structured processes through which they are selected and enforced."[22]

What are the lessons here as we struggle to find new tropes to explain the complexity of voice and agency and the limits of using suffering and resistance as the historical skeletons on which to build our analysis? Let me be very clear. We still need to document the suffering (even if we refuse it as melodrama), to search for the voices of those who have been unheard, to be sophisticated about what we think is agency, and to be concerned with the multiple forms of resistance.[23] However, we must also be very aware of historical contingency, of the uncertainty in medicine that allows racial assumptions to fill in the lacunae in analysis and practice, and be cognizant of the ways historical accounts provide for political and personal metaphors. We cannot be limited by the binaries of suffering and resistance as we search for a way to understand a more complex past.

NOTES

1   Jeffrey B. Ferguson, "Race and the Rhetoric of Resistance," *Raritan* 28 (Summer 2008): 4.

2   Ibid., 8.

3   On race and melodrama, see ibid. and Linda Williams, *Playing the Race Card: Melodramas of Black and White from Uncle Tom to O.J. Simpson* (Princeton, N.J.: Princeton University Press, 2001). On the study, see Susan M. Reverby, ed., *Tuskegee's Truths: Rethinking the Tuskegee Syphilis Study* (Chapel Hill: University of North Carolina Press, 2000) and *Examining Tuskegee: The Infamous Syphilis Study and Its Legacy* (Chapel Hill: University of North Carolina Press, 2009).

4   As a caveat, I am of course well aware that *race* does not mean *black* any more than *gender* means *women*. But because my work has been on African Americans and medicine and on this study, my focus will be on African Americans. Parts of the discussion of the study appear in *Examining Tuskegee*.

5   Susan M. Reverby, "More Than Fact and Fiction: Cultural Memory and the Tuskegee Syphilis Study," *Hastings Center Report* 31 (September–October 2001): 22–28.

6   "Testimony by Four Survivors," in Reverby, *Tuskegee's Truths*, 144.

7   Interview with Herman Shaw, Tallassee, Alabama, November 9, 1998.

8   George A. Denison and W. H. Y. Smith, "Mass Venereal Disease Control in an Urban Area," *Southern Medical Journal* 39 (March 1946): 197. This argument is more fully developed by Robert W. White, "Misrepresentations of the Tuskegee Study of Untreated Syphilis," *Journal of the National Medical Association* 97 (April 2005): 564–81.

9   Record 478, Box 32, Tuskegee Syphilis Study Medical Files, Tuskegee Syphilis Study Administrative Records, 1930–80, Centers for Disease Control Papers, National Archives and Records Administration—Southeast

Region, Morrow, Georgia. In 1958, Dr. Bunch, on fluoroscope, wrote that Shaw suffered from "syphilitic aortitis." But Bunch often made this diagnosis because a man was in the Study. Mr. Shaw died in 1999, but the cause was not given.

10 For more analysis of the records see Reverby, *Examining Tuskegee,* and Tywanna Whorley, "The Tuskegee Syphilis Study: Access and Control over Controversial Records," in *Political Pressure and the Archival Record,* ed. Margaret Procter, Michael G. Cook, and Caroline Williams, 109–18 (Chicago: Society of American Archivists, 2005). I am grateful, as we all should be, to Tywanna Whorley, whose Freedom of Information Act filing made the opening of the medical records possible.

11 Record A12S, Box 1; Record 540, Box 36; Record 534, Box 35, Tuskegee Syphilis Study Medical Files.

12 I am following here some of the analysis of Walter Johnson, "On Agency," *Journal of Social History* 37 (Fall 2003): 113–24. As Johnson writes about slavery, "any form of activity is not resistance" (116).

13 The term is Richard Shweder's; see "Tuskegee Re-Examined," *Spiked* online, January 8, 2004, http://www.spiked-online.com/Articles/0000000CA34A.htm.

14 Thomas Benedek, "The 'Tuskegee Study' of Syphilis: An Analysis of Moral Versus Methodologic Aspects," in Reverby, *Tuskegee's Truths,* 213–35. The article was first published in 1978. The other major counternarratives are Thomas Benedek and Jonathan Erlen, "The Scientific Environment of the Tuskegee Study of Syphilis, 1920–1960," *Perspectives in Biology and Medicine* 43 (Autumn 1999): 1–30; Robert W. White, "Unraveling the Tuskegee Study of Untreated Syphilis," *Archives of Internal Medicine* 160 (March 13, 2000): 585–98; and Shweder, "Tuskegee Re-Examined." Shweder's article was then picked up by *Arts and Letters Daily* and widely circulated on the Web. Robert White has also written numerous other articles on the study, including critiques of my work, particularly in the *Journal of the National Medical Association.*

15 In 1973, the federal investigating committee made an effort to scour the medical literature on treatment for late latent syphilis and concluded that the men should have been treated, especially after penicillin became widely available.

16 R. K. St. John, "Treatment of Cardiovascular Syphilis," *Journal of the American Venereal Disease Association* 3 (December 1976): 149.

17 See H. Jack Geiger to the American Public Health Association's "Spirit of 1848" e-mail subscription list, "Re: Shweder Article on Tuskegee," January 24, 2004, http://www.spiritof1848@yahoogroups.com. See also Reverby, "More Than Fact and Fiction" and Reverby, "'Misrepresentations of the Tuskegee Study'—Distortion of Analysis and Facts," *Journal of the National Medical Association* 97 (August 2005): 1180–81.

18 Both Robert White's and Richard Shweder's articles were debated on

the American Public Health Association's "Spirit of 1848" e-mail subscription list when they appeared; see http://www.spiritof1848-subscribe @yahoogroups.com.

19 White has been dogged in his efforts to get the facts about the study out. Although we have disagreed in and out of print, I do appreciate his efforts to counter much of the mythology.

20 Reverby, "More Than Fact and Fiction," 27.

21 R. H. Kampmeier, "The Tuskegee Study of Untreated Syphilis," in Reverby, *Tuskegee's Truths,* 200.

22 Johnson, "On Agency," 118.

23 On race and melodrama see Ferguson, "Race and the Rhetoric of Resistance," and Williams, *Playing the Race Card.*

Contributors

Jason E. Glenn is assistant professor of history of science and medicine at the Institute for the Medical Humanities, University of Texas Medical Branch at Galveston.

Mark Allan Goldberg is assistant professor of history at the University of Houston.

Laurie B. Green is associate professor of history at the University of Texas at Austin. She is the author of *Battling the Plantation Mentality: Memphis and the Black Freedom Struggle*, which won the 2008 Philip A. Taft Labor History Book Award, and the coeditor, with Thomas C. Holt, of *The New Encyclopedia of Southern Culture*, vol. 24, *Race*.

Jean J. Kim is an independent historian; she earned her PhD in history from Cornell University.

Gretchen Long is associate professor of history at Williams College. She is the author of *Doctoring Freedom: The Politics of African American Medical Care in Slavery and Emancipation*.

Verónica Martínez-Matsuda is assistant professor of labor relations, law, and history at Cornell University's School of Industrial and Labor Relations.

John Mckiernan-González is assistant professor of history at Texas State University. He is the author of *Fevered Measures: Public Health and Race at the Texas–Mexico Border, 1848–1942*.

Lena McQuade-Salzfass is assistant professor of women's and gender studies and directs the career minor in women's health at Sonoma State University.

Natalia Molina is associate professor of history and urban studies at the University of California, San Diego. Her work sits at the intersections of race, culture, and citizenship. She is the author of *Fit to Be Citizens? Public Health and Race in Los Angeles, 1879–1939.*

Susan M. Reverby is McLean Professor in the History of Ideas and professor of women's and gender studies at Wellesley College. She is the author of several books, including most recently *Examining Tuskegee: The Infamous Syphilis Study and Its Legacy.*

Jennifer Seltz is assistant professor of history at Western Washington University.

Martin Summers is associate professor of history and African and African diaspora studies at Boston College. He is the author of *Manliness and Its Discontents: The Black Middle Class and the Transformation of Masculinity, 1900–1930.*

Index

Academia de Medicina de Mégico (Medical Academy of Mexico), 13, 14

Africa, 143–45, 148–50

African American physicians: during Civil War, 54; criticism of, as "conjurer" in post–Civil War period, 46, 55–57, 61; detached relationship of, to mental illness and psychiatry, xxi, 91–110; Euro-American physicians compared with, in nineteenth century, 46–50; exclusion of, from medical specialties, 100–101; Flexner report on, 101; focus of, on somatic diseases, 93, 101–2, 108; and Freedmen's Bureau, xv–xvi, 44–62, 64n18; herbal medicine practiced by, 47–50, 55, 59, 61; and hunger in the South, 218; medical schools for, 45, 100–101; professionalization of, 93–97; and professionalization of Euro-American physicians, 43–45, 50, 62; psychiatric professionalization of, 97–110, 112n19, 113n35; public health role of, 101–2; racism against, 43, 45, 51–58, 60–62, 92, 94, 100–101; and slaves' medical care, xvi, 43, 45–46, 47, 48, 60; in South Carolina, xvi, 44, 51–54, 57–62;

statistics on, 107–8; in Texas, xvi, 44, 45–51, 55–62

African Americans: in antebellum Texas, 48–49; citizenship of, xxi, 102; and crack baby narrative, xiii–xiv, 240, 247, 248; diseases of, xxi, 94, 96, 101–2, 108, 262–71; and hunger in the South, xx, 213, 215–22, 229, 232; lack of full citizenship rights for, 102; and Lacks cancer study, vii, viii, xxiii–xxiv; living conditions of, 96, 102; mental health services underused by, xxi, 91–92, 109–10; mental illness among, xxi, 91, 96, 103–4; and midwives, 128; as migrants in Mexico during late-nineteenth century, xviii–xix, 67–70; military service by, xxi, 93, 103–4, 108–9; morbidity and mortality rates of, 50, 94, 101, 102, 111n5; Moynihan report on the black family, 228, 248, 261; negative stereotypes of, 222, 224, 228, 232, 253–54; in nursing, xvii, 143, 146–47, 160, 161; poverty and hunger of, in 1960s, xx, 213–22, 226; in prison population, 253, 255; public policies against, in Reagan era, xiii–xiv, 237, 247–55; return of Tlahualilo migrants from Eagle

277

CONIECTANEA BIBLICA • NEW TESTAMENT SERIES 24

SAMUEL BYRSKOG

Jesus the Only Teacher

Didactic Authority and Transmission
in Ancient Israel, Ancient Judaism
and the Matthean Community

Almqvist & Wiksell International, Stockholm
1994

Abstract

Byrskog, S. 1994. Jesus the Only Teacher. Didactic Authority and Transmission in Ancient Israel, Ancient Judaism and the Matthean Community. Coniectanea Biblica. New Testament Series 24. 501 pp. Monograph. Dissertation Lund University. ISBN 91-22-01590-6.

Keywords

Bible, New Testament, Matthew, Gospels, Old Testament, Isaiah, Sirach, Dead Sea scrolls, Rabbinic literature, Teacher, Pupil, Disciple, Scribe, Prophet, Tradition, Transmission, Gospel tradition, Jesus tradition, Jesus, the Righteous Teacher, Ben Sira, Rabbi, School, Authority, Narrative, Teaching, Biography, Orality, Literacy.

Printed in Sweden by Graphic Systems, Malmö   ISBN 91-22-01590-6

Per Angela, Franca
Mia moglie e amica

Contents

Part One

Didactic Authority and Transmission in Ancient Israel and Ancient Judaism

Ch. 1. Didactic Authority and the Settings of Transmission

Ch. 2. Didactic Authority and the Motives of Transmission

Ch. 3. Didactic Authority and the Process of Transmission

Part Two

Jesus as Teacher and Transmission in the Matthean Community

Ch. 4. Jesus as Teacher and the Setting of Transmission

Introduction

1. The Purpose of the Study

When circumstances forced some early Christian theologians to define and defend their faith, it seemed important to claim that Jesus was the only teacher. Although the terminological evidence is sometimes meagre, the concept is clearly present in several Christian writings from the second century and on. It was taken from the NT, especially from Matt 23:8 containing the important phrase "for one is your teacher" (εἷς γάρ ἐστιν ὑμῶν ὁ διδάσκαλος).[1]

Among the early apostolic fathers, Ignatius of Antioch is of most interest.[2] In the letters composed some time during the first decades of the second century C.E., he reveals an interest in Jesus as teacher. Both passages using διδάσκαλος for Jesus put a particular emphasis on Jesus as the *only* teacher. Eph. 15:1 discusses the coherence between teaching and action and puts forth Jesus as the example: "There is then one teacher (εἷς οὖν διδάσκαλος) who spoke and it came to pass, and what he has done even in silence is worthy of the Father." Magn. 9:1 points out that just as the Jews came to a new hope, also the Christians endure so that they may be found disciples of Jesus Christ "our only teacher" (τοῦ μόνου διδασκάλου ἡμῶν). Even the prophets were disciples in the spirit and looked forward to Jesus as teacher (Magn. 9:2).

Among the church fathers, Clement of Alexandria (c. 150–215 C.E.) is perhaps most significant.[3] In his view, the tradition is truly preserved by those who adhere in speaking and hearing to no one else but the one teacher. "For one is the teacher (εἷς γάρ ὁ διδάσκαλος) both of him who speaks and of him who hears" (Strom. I 12:3). The Christian brotherhood exists on the basis of having only one teacher (Strom. V 98:1f). This teacher is Jesus, and no one else. Not even the angels will stand the test as teachers of all philosophers and of the first generation of men (Strom. VI 57:3–5). God's first begotten Son, through whom God created all things and whom all the prophets call the Wisdom, is "the teacher of all created beings" (ὁ τῶν γενητῶν

---

[1] NORMANN, *Christos Didaskalos,* 28.
[2] For discussion, see NORMANN, *Christos Didaskalos,* 83–91; BAUER/PAULSEN, *Briefe des Ignatius,* 40, 53f; SCHOEDEL, *Ignatius,* 77f, 123–125.
[3] For discussion, see FASCHER, *TLZ* 79 (1954) 338f; *idem,* Logos-Christos, 193–207; NORMANN, *Christos Didaskalos,* 153–177.

ἁπάντων διδάσκαλος).[1] Accordingly Strom. VI 58:2 refers to what was rightly said, namely "do not call each other teacher on earth" (μὴ εἴπητε ἑαυτοῖς διδάσκαλον ἐπὶ τῆς γῆς). E. Fascher goes as far as to call Clement's christological discussion "eine Fuge zum Thema Mt 23:8."[2] And certainly, Clement's writings—especially the Stromateis—contain several further passages which may appear as allusions to or direct quotations of Matt 23:8.[3]

What was of interest to some ancient Christians is of interest also to modern exegetes. But the subject of Jesus as the only teacher has aroused only a modest interest among NT scholars. While several studies dealing with Jesus as teacher in the NT exist,[4] only few scholars make a point out of the fact that Jesus appears even as the *only* teacher. This investigation deals with the subject in one limited part of early Christianity—the Matthean community. *The purpose of this study is to investigate the relationship between the understanding of Jesus as the only teacher and the transmission of the Jesus tradition in the Matthean community.* I will explain this purpose further. An account and evaluation of the scholarly discussion on this subject will first help us to clarify the problems involved.

2. The Scholarly Discussion

The various studies dealing with Matt 23:8–10 separately discuss of course the notion of Jesus as the only teacher. However, this passage is *in itself* not the main focus of the present investigation.[5] Comments made by different scholars suggest that the concept is broader and vital to the whole question concerning the transmission of the Jesus tradition in early Christianity.[6]

G. Kittel argued in his book *Die Probleme des palästinischen Spätjudentums und das Urchristentum* from 1926 for the need to study the laws of transmission within a comparative perspective.[7] Among the peculiarities of the transmission reflected in the NT, he brought special attention to the constant focus on Jesus:

"Was im Rabbinat völlig, auch in Ansätzen, fehlt, ist die bewusste Beschränkung des Traditionsstoffes auf e i n e Person, auf den e i n e n Mann ... Jeder, auch der grösste

---

1   Strom. VI 58:1.
2   Logos-Christos, 205.
3   Cf. e.g. Paed. I 17:3; I 25:2; Strom. II 9:4; II 14:3; II 24:3; IV 162:5.
4   See RIESNER, *Lehrer,* 74–79, 505–507. His bibliography contains many other works related to the same subject.
5   I will discuss certain aspects of these verses below pp. 207f, 284–290, 299–302.
6   I will concentrate on some major contributions only. For a survey of research about the transmission of the Jesus tradition, see RIESNER, *Lehrer,* 1–79, including information concerning the study by several early—partly neglected—scholars.
7   *Probleme des palästinischen Spätjudentums,* 62–70.

und verehrteste Schriftgelehrte, steht für seine Schüler i n der Reihe, und seine Isolierung, seine Herausnahme aus der Traditionskette, ist völlig undenkbar. Für den Jesusjünger ist alle Lehre und Tradition aller anderen Autoritäten verschwunden. Die Reihe, die Traditionskette hat aufgehört zu existieren. Wert, tradiert zu werden, ist nur noch das Wort und die Geschichte des Einen."[1]

In a footnote probably aimed to modify the emerging form-critical approach to the gospels, Kittel adds: "Die I s o l i e r u n g der Jesustradition ist das Konstitutivum des Evangeliums; sie aber hat nie, auch in keinem Stadium der palästinischen Traditionsbildung, gefehlt."[2]

Kittel's basic observation is obvious. No one would deny the difference between the focus on Jesus in the gospels and the appearence of many teachers side by side in the rabbinic writings. But Kittel wrote his book at a time when the form-critical approach to tradition and transmission was beginning its advance among NT scholars.[3] The footnote shows that he believed the focus on Jesus to be more challenging than it might appear at first sight. It implies that the unique position of Jesus in the young Christian communities was a driving force which effected careful attention to the transmission of the Jesus tradition from early on. In the following decades, scholars were to use Kittel's observation in basically two directions.

The first direction is best seen in the classical studies by R. Bultmann and M. Dibelius.[4] Bultmann's *Die Geschichte der synoptischen Tradition* from 1921 was enlarged and published again in 1931. Bultmann partly acknowledges Kittel's observation. When he discusses some early collections of traditions, he refers to Kittel's study and points out that we sometimes find the Jesus tradition in an isolated form at a secondary stage of transmission, without the voices of several authorities.[5] This isolated form of the early collections prepared the creation of the gospels. But as is well known, Bultmann locates the process of isolating the Jesus tradition within the various activities of the Christian—Palestinian or Hellenistic[6]—communities. He does not pay sufficient attention to Kittel's footnote pointing out that the isolation of the Jesus tradition was present already from the beginning. According to Bultmann, it was essentially the needs of the communities that motivated and guided the transmission. Faith in the resurrected Christ intimately correlated with these motives of transmission emerging in various life settings. The resurrection faith did not include an interest in Jesus' his-

---

[1]   *Probleme des palästinischen Spätjudentums,* 69.

[2]   *Probleme des palästinischen Spätjudentums,* 69 n. 3.

[3]   For early surveys of the antecedents to form criticism, see FASCHER, *Methode,* 4–51; EASTON, *Gospel,* 1–27.

[4]   K.L. SCHMIDT, *Rahmen,* was the third form-critical pioneer. But his study from 1919 was never revised to comment on Kittel's view, and it does not, as far as I can see, discuss how the focus on Jesus related to the transmission of the Jesus tradition.

[5]   *Geschichte der synoptischen Tradition,* 393f.—BULTMANN, *ibid.,* 42 n. 1, refers to the same section of Kittel's study.

[6]   Cf. e.g. *Geschichte der synoptischen Tradition,* 254.

tory for its own sake. Rather, since it effected a levelling of any distinction between the earthly and the resurrected one,[1] the focus on Jesus generated the incorporation of a number of new sayings with various origin into the Jesus tradition.[2] It was the needs of the communities together with the resurrection faith that caused the isolation of the Jesus tradition. To seek for one specific factor or interest independent of these motives is futile, since "ein geistiger Besitz objektiviert sich auch ohne spezielle Zwecke."[3]

The enlarged edition of Dibelius' *Die Formgeschichte des Evangeliums* from 1919 was published in 1933. Although he does not refer to Kittel, he clearly recognizes the distinctive focus on Jesus within early Christian tradition and transmission. In comparing the paradigms with the halakhic stories of the rabbinic literature, Dibelius specifically points out that the characteristic feature in the transmission of the paradigms is that they concern decisions depending on the authority of one man only, not on the voices of several persons from different times.[4] And in a different context, he stresses that the appreciation of the tradition, the authenticity and the authority were driving forces in the collection of some Jesus-sayings.[5] But nevertheless, Dibelius also subordinates these forces of transmission to the needs and activities of the Christian communities. Interest in the past tradition was not a sufficient motive of transmission for people directing their primary attention and hopes towards the future.[6] The transmission of the Jesus tradition was essentially motivated by and had its life setting within the general—and in Dibelius discussion rather abstract—activity of preaching.[7] This is especially true of the paradigms and the paraenetic material.[8] "Der Prediger ist es, der zugleich überliefert und erzählt."[9]

It remains unclear if Bultmann and Dibelius would at all have been able to conceive settings and motives of transmission independent of the common activities of the Christian communities. Bultmann was apparently not satisfied with Dibelius' emphasis on the preaching as the sole life setting.[10] He added various other settings: "Apologetik und Polemik wie Gemeindebildung und Disziplin sind ebenso in Rechnung zu setzen und daneben

---

1   *Geschichte der synoptischen Tradition*, 135, 373, 395f.
2   *Geschichte der synoptischen Tradition*, 106, 132–136, 156, 220.
3   *Geschichte der synoptischen Tradition*, 393.
4   *Formgeschichte*, 142.
5   *Formgeschichte*, 243.
6   *Formgeschichte*, 10, *passim*.
7   *Formgeschichte*, 8–34, *passim*. Dibelius uses "Predigt" both as general category for all activities by which the early Church communicated its message and doctrines and as a more specific category for the sermon itself. For some critique of this inconsistency, see STENDAHL, *School of Matthew*, 13–19.
8   *Formgeschichte*, 66, 239, 262–264.
9   *Formgeschichte*, 66.
10 *Geschichte der synoptischen Tradition*, 42, 64.

schriftgelehrte Arbeit."[1] But his additions were activities in which the Jesus tradition was used for a certain purpose. Transmission was not performed for its own sake. Dibelius occasionally spoke of early Christian teachers.[2] But it seems that he primarily thought of the teachers as persons using the Jesus tradition in paraenesis. And this was for Dibelius also the setting of transmission. If Bultmann and Dibelius should have conceived separate settings and motives of transmission at all, they would probably have hastened to integrate them into other activities of the Christian communities. The focus on Jesus did not motivate the transmission. The common activities constituted the settings of transmission and the needs of the community created the focus on Jesus.

Scholars objected to the approach taken by Bultmann and Dibelius already after the first edition of their books.[3] Others have accordingly used Kittel's observation to imply more specific settings and motives of transmission. B. Gerhardsson initiated in his dissertation *Memory and Manuscript* from 1961—with a second edition from 1964—modern scholarship to a more concrete picture of tradition and transmission.[4] While aiming to enlighten scholars about the technical side of early Christian transmission through a study of rabbinic Judaism first of all, he is aware of the distinctive features of the Jesus tradition. To mention one such feature, there is a repeated stress in several of Gerhardsson's studies on Jesus as the *only* teacher. He mentions it in reference to Kittel's study already in his dissertation and relates it to Jesus' statement in Matt 23:10.[5] Within the specific setting of Christian work on "the word of the Lord," the understanding of Jesus as the only teacher functioned to motivate transmission and to further the isolation of the Jesus tradition.

Gerhardsson has elaborated his observation in several studies, most extensively in *Tradition and Transmission in Early Christianity* from 1964, *The Origins of the Gospel Traditions* from 1979 and "Der Weg der Evangelientradition" from 1983,[6] the two latter based on previous lectures. The subject relates in Gerhardsson's view to three aspects of the Jesus tradition.[7]

---

[1]   *Geschichte der synoptischen Tradition,* 64.

[2]   *Formgeschichte,* 66, 241.

[3]   Cf. e.g. FASCHER, *Methode,* 52–144, 186–234; KOEHLER, *Problem;* EASTON, *Gospel,* 59–81; TAYLOR, *Formation,* 11–19, *passim,* knowing also of Bultmann's 2nd ed. of his book, which he describes as merely "a restatement of the argument with additional matter and comments on subsequent developments" (*ibid.,* 15).

[4]   Cf. also RIESENFELD, *SE* 1 (1959) 43–65, though his observations were "mainly based on considerations issuing from recent studies carried out in Uppsala" (*ibid.,* 51), namely on Gerhardsson's preparations for his dissertation (*ibid.,* 51 n. 1).

[5]   *Memory,* 332f.

[6]   *Tradition and Transmission,* 40–44; *idem, Origins of the Gospel Traditions,* 47–49, 51, 67f; *idem,* Weg der Evangelientradition, 79–82, 91–93. Cf. also *idem,* Gospel Tradition, 536.

[7]   Cf. Weg der Evangelientradition, 82.

First, there is a formal isolation of the tradition. The Jesus tradition occurs explicitly only in the gospels. We hardly ever find actual quotations of the Jesus tradition in the framework of proclamation, teaching and admonition visible in the NT outside of the gospels. The Jesus tradition has apparently not arisen and been preserved in the general life settings of the Christian communities. Second, there is an isolation in content. The Jesus tradition concerns only Jesus. Not even John the Baptist plays any role independent of Jesus. This exclusive focus on Jesus suggests a strong motive of transmission. Third, other early Christian authorities did not enrich the Jesus tradition under their own names. This does not mean that there were no interpretative adaptations. Early Christians may in good faith even have added certain new creations to the Jesus tradition. But the absence of their names in connection with the adaptations and additions suggests that what is quoted in the gospels is what was felt to be Jesus tradition.

R. Riesner developed Gerhardsson's approach in his dissertation *Jesus als Lehrer* from 1981—with a third expanded edition from 1988. Gerhardsson had mentioned more popular settings of transmission than the rabbinic colleges. Riesner places Jesus' didactic role as the originator of the gospel tradition within the perspective of educational measures and transmission techniques that are earlier and more general than the ones emerging in the rabbinic Judaism of the tannaitic and amoraic periods. In Riesner's work, the concept of Jesus as the only teacher plays a significant role as the specific feature of the Jesus tradition on several occasions.[1] Riesner first brings attention to it when he discusses motives of transmission unrelated to the general needs of the communities.[2] He connects it closely with a biographical and historical interest in Jesus.[3] Just as there was, to be sure, an interest in the Jesus tradition for certain practical purposes, there were also motives of transmission independent of the needs of the Christian communities, person-oriented motives of transmission relevant already before Easter.[4] Riesner uses Kittel's observation primarily to argue for the genuine origin and authentic wording of the Jesus-sayings. The consistent focus on Jesus makes it unlikely that the young Christian communities attributed sayings from other authorities to Jesus, and it makes probable that they preserved even sayings without immediate social relevance. The understanding of Jesus as the only teacher constituted from the very beginning "ein außerordentliches Tradierungsmotiv."[5]

Both Gerhardsson and Riesner clearly acknowledge that the common ac-

---

[1] *Lehrer,* 37–40, 54, 57, 264, 351f, 417–419, 500. Cf. also *idem,* Jesus as Teacher and Preacher, 208.

[2] *Lehrer,* 37–40.

[3] *Lehrer,* 29–32, 35–37.

[4] *Lehrer,* 351f.

[5] *Lehrer,* 352.

tivities of the Christian communities produced an active interest in the Jesus tradition.[1] Gerhardsson stated early that the traditions were "marked by the use which was made of them in the many-sided activity of the young Church."[2] The transmission was not entirely "passive," as W.H. Kelber later described Gerhardsson's approach.[3] But unlike Bultmann and Dibelius, Gerhardsson introduced the important distinction between transmission as a *deliberate act* within a special setting on one hand, and the *use* of the traditions within various activities on the other: "it is one thing to state that traditions have been *marked* by the milieu through which they passed; another to claim that they simply were *created* in this secondary milieu."[4] This view, which Riesner later adopted, relates to the concept of Jesus as the only teacher. The isolation of the Jesus tradition is inconceivable if we do not assume the existence of separate settings of transmission.[5] The common activities did not constitute the primary settings of transmission and the needs of the community did not create the focus on Jesus. Rather, it was the focus on Jesus that was the driving force from the beginning, furthering separate settings and preservative acts of transmission.

The presentation of these different views suffice to indicate the importance of the subject and the problems involved. Kittel, Bultmann, Dibelius, Gerhardsson and Riesner point clearly to the significant connection between the concept of Jesus as the only teacher and the transmission of the Jesus tradition. It is true that others have occasionally made more or less casual remarks about the fact that rabbinic Judaism in distinction to early Christianity contains teaching from a large number of different individuals.[6] But to this date, no one has devoted a separate study to the subject. A detailed inquiry into this phenomenon holds promise to reveal factors essential for a fuller understanding of transmission in early Christianity. But the five scholars have also different opinions about the issue at stake. Their disagreements indicate the specific problems at hand.

---

[1] Cf. e.g. GERHARDSSON, *Memory,* 330f; *idem,* Weg der Evangelientradition, 85–87; RIESNER, *Lehrer,* 35, 55–60.

[2] *Tradition and Transmission,* 43.

[3] *The Oral and the Written Gospel,* 8–14.—GERHARDSSON, Gospel Tradition, 520–527, gives a critique of Kelber's account and points out himself that "not even the most 'academic' halachists among the Rabbis were completely uninfluenced by the social life around them" (*ibid.,* 527). See further below pp. 338f, 341, 348f, 397, 400f.

[4] GERHARDSSON, *Tradition and Transmission,* 43.

[5] RIESNER, *Lehrer,* 57.

[6] Among more recent scholars, cf. e.g. WIEFEL, *NovT* 11 (1969) 116; NEUSNER, *Development,* 2, 187, 190f; *idem, Rabbinic Traditions* III, 33, 85, 90; STANTON, *Jesus of Nazareth,* 128f; MUSSNER, Beschränkung auf einen einzigen Lehrer, 34, 36; CHILTON, Targumic Transmission, 39; MUSSNER, *Tractate on the Jews,* 233–235; P.S. ALEXANDER, Rabbinic Biography, 41; MUSSNER, *TBer* 13 (1985) 169f; *idem, Kraft der Wurzel,* 110; *idem,* Die Stellung zum Judentum, 211, 224; CHILTON, *Profiles of a Rabbi,* 120.

3. The Basic Problems of the Study

I will approach the problems of this study from the perspective of some general definitions and assumptions. The present study concerns tradition and transmission, *traditum* and *traditio*. The two cannot be separated from each other. There is no tradition without transmission, and there is no transmission without tradition. But although there are over-lappings between the two, *I will use "tradition" for the transmitted material and "transmission" for the transmitting process.*[1]

This study will concentrate on tradition as that which comes from the past, with the sociologist E. Shils as "anything which is transmitted or handed down from the past to the present."[2] The tradition does not necessarily have to speak explicitly about the past; it does not have to be embraced by a large number of people; it does not have to span over generations. It even happens that a teacher deliberately formulates sayings to serve as traditions from the beginning. In such cases, a tradition is at hand as soon as a saying is received by the first pupil(s) in accordance with the teacher's intention. But I rarely discuss such situations here. The important thing is that those who transmit at a certain time understand the material as older than themselves. Further, a tradition is the object of transmission. Transmission involves, among other things, communication between two partners. But in distinction to general forms of communication, transmission is always of something that existed already before the situation arises.[3] I thus adopt a broad and general definition which focuses on the *temporal aspect of tradition and transmission.*

Tradition and transmission may in turn take many forms. Gerhardsson provides a model which makes it possible to discuss the complicated phenomenon of tradition in an analytical manner. He proposes a basic distinction between "inner" and "outer" tradition, and within the latter category between verbal, behavioural, institutional and material tradition.[4] The "inner" tradition externalizes itself in words, practices, fellowship and inanimate objects. This phenomenological model serves as a general basis for my approach to the various forms of tradition. I will focus primarily on *the verbal aspects of the "outer" tradition.* The study deals first of all with transmitted words of and about significant persons. But as Gerhardsson points out,[5] the different aspects of tradition usually interact. The words of tradition do not normally remain isolated from the rest of life. The genuine

---

[1] For the use of this terminology, see D.A. KNIGHT, *Rediscovering,* 5–20; *idem, ABD* 6 (1992) 634.

[2] *Tradition,* 12.

[3] Cf. ANDERSEN, Oral Tradition, 25f.

[4] Gospel Tradition, 500–504.

[5] Gospel Tradition, 503.

transmitters are personally involved in the vital content of the tradition—in the "inner" tradition. They are not only mechanically handing on the tradition. It affects their *behaviour*. They also often belong to a fellowship—an emerging *institution*—which centres on the shared belief in the "inner" tradition. In the ideal case, the transmission takes place within a social setting held together by a motivating engagement. In order to understand the transmission process, it becomes necessary to pay attention to the interactions that appear within—and also around—the transmitting group. For the purposes of this study, *transmission includes the preservative and elaborative work with the verbal tradition that takes place within the interactions of a group motivated by a common interest in the vital content of the tradition.*[1]

These definitions clarify the general approach to tradition and transmission in this study. There are also some basic assumptions *pertinent to the Jesus tradition.* These assumptions emerge from the scholarly debate. All five scholars mentioned above agree on one important point: within a comparative perspective, the constant focus on Jesus was *the* characteristic feature of the Jesus tradition. Jesus—his person, ministry, death and resurrection—constituted the factual content of the tradition. This does not mean that the OT was unimportant. On the contrary, the OT exhibited its authoritative influence and interacted with the focus on Jesus during the various stages of transmission. But it means that the vital centre of the Jesus tradition was not an impersonal object. "The heart of Early Christianity was a Jesus Christ-centered relation to God."[2] A basic assumption in this study is consequently that *transmission of material concerning words and deeds of an esteemed person exhibits features that are not as evident in the transmission of material concerned with impersonal matters.* My task is to find those features.

Kittel, Bultmann and Dibelius did not relate the issue to the presentation of Jesus as teacher. Gerhardsson and Riesner think of it in connection with the characterization of Jesus as the only teacher in Matt 23:8–10. They have both shown that Jesus' own activity as teacher constituted an important condition for the *origin* of the Jesus tradition. They also think—more implicitly—that the *continued* process of transmission was marked by the understanding of Jesus as teacher. Another basic assumption of my study is that *the understanding of Jesus as teacher was particularly important for the transmission of the Jesus tradition.* It is not as evident that the material attributed to persons understood in totally different terms is transmitted in the same way. I will, therefore, focus especially on transmission of material from and about a teacher.

---

[1] I will not deal with the material tradition externalizing itself in inanimate objects. The sources do not provide sufficient information concerning the function of such objects in early Christianity.

[2] GERHARDSSON, Gospel Tradition, 508.

The relation between the understanding of a person as teacher and the transmission is confirmed from a quick look at the Pauline literature and tradition. Paul himself had a group of co-workers around him.[1] Although H. Conzelmann's hypothesis, that Paul was the leader of a wisdom school in Ephesus,[2] is difficult to ascertain from the available evidence,[3] it is likely that Paul did educate his closest associates. In spite of this, he never refers to himself as the "teacher" (διδάσκαλος) of his co-workers.[4] And he never calls the co-workers "disciples" (μαθηταί). This may be a coincidence. But it is nevertheless striking to notice that the didactic label appears in the Pastorals.[5] 1 Tim 2:7; 2 Tim 1:11 refer to Paul as teacher.[6] Paul is now a teacher with a doctrine. 2 Tim 3:10 praises Timothy for observing closely the doctrine of Paul, and 2 Tim 4:3 blames other people for accumulating for themselves teachers to suit their own desires, instead of keeping to the only sound doctrine. When Paul's teaching became a tradition to be transmitted, the didactic label explicitly came to the surface.[7]

The review of the scholarly discussion, the definition of tradition and transmission and the two assumptions show that the purpose of this study is connected with three basic issues. First, there is the question of the setting of transmission. No one would deny that transmission, generally speaking, may take place in a number of various settings. But Gerhardsson and Riesner have pointed out that there existed in antiquity didactic settings in which transmission was a deliberate and specific act. There was a kind of "programmatic transmission." This is most plain in rabbinic Judaism. There is also some evidence suggesting that trained teachers were responsible for the transmission of the Jesus tradition.[8] It is necessary here to go one step further and ask *if there were situations in which the authority of a person considered in some way to be a teacher—whether alive or not—constituted the*

---

1   E.E. ELLIS, *NTS* 17 (1970–71) 437–452; HOLMBERG, *Paul and Power,* 58–72; OLLROG, *Paulus und seine Mitarbeiter.*
2   *NTS* 12 (1965–66) 231–244; *idem,* Schule des Paulus, 85–96. Conzelmann is followed by e.g. PEARSON, Hellenistic-Jewish Wisdom Speculation, 43–66 (with some critical remarks); LEVISON, Rhetoric, 37; STUHLMACHER, Christusbild, 159f. The dissertation by H. LUDWIG, *Der Verfasser des Kolosserbriefes.* Ein Schüler des Paulus. University of Göttingen 1974, developing Conzelmann's hypothesis further, was not available to me.
3   For criticism of Conzelmann, see OLLROG, *Paulus und seine Mitarbeiter,* 114–118; P. MÜLLER, *Paulusschule,* 270f. Cf. also LÜHRMANN, *ZTK* 67 (1970) 450–452.
4   Cf. OLLROG, *Paulus und seine Mitarbeiter,* 114 n. 24.—When Paul uses διδαχή (Rom 6:17; 16:17; 1 Cor 14:6) or διδάσκειν (1 Cor 4:17), he thinks of his activity in the Christian communities, not among his own co-workers.
5   I assume that the Pastorals are post-Pauline.
6   Cf. also Acts 13:1.
7   Cf. MEADE, *Pseudonymity,* 126: "... in the Pastorals, Paul is not *a* teacher or one who teaches, but *the* teacher."
8   ZIMMERMANN, *Die urchristlichen Lehrer.* Cf. also SCHÜRMANN, Lehrende, 429f.

essential identity marker for the settings of transmission.

Second, there is the question of the motives of transmission. Why did people find it important to transmit teaching? What was their "internal" drive? I am here interested in motives relating to a specific person—in conceptions that the transmitters had about a certain teacher.[1] We may call them "person-oriented motives of transmission." As already said, I assume that a basic understanding of Jesus as teacher is evidence of an essential willingness to transmit the Jesus tradition. It is, however, possible to differentiate this motive in different ways. Bultmann and Dibelius, on one hand, tended to exclude an interest in the history and the life of Jesus. What was of importance, it seems, was the teaching in itself, which the evangelists framed with biographical notices. And the teaching was not always attached to Jesus' own person. Sayings of foreign origin often entered into the Jesus tradition. Various needs and practical considerations of the Christian communities were decisive. Riesner, on the other hand, speaks explicitly of a historical and a biographical interest within the transmission process. There were motives independent of the general needs and considerations of the communities. They were, so to say, "non-practical." As is evident, the issue concerns the transmitters' interest in relating the Jesus-sayings to the episodal material.[2] I will differentiate three basic motives of transmission depending on how closely the transmitters related the transmitted teaching to a specific teacher: (1) a motive in which the teaching was an entity independent of the life and the status of the teacher, (2) a motive in which the teaching was integrated within the life of a specific teacher and (3) a motive in which the teaching was integrated within a process that enhanced the teacher to an exclusive status of authority by means of validating labels. I will speak of didactic, didactic-biographical and didactic-labelling motives of transmission.[3] It is necessary to ask *to what extent the didactic-biographical and didactic-labelling motives of transmission, exhibiting an interest in the life and status of Jesus as teacher, interacted with the purely didactic motives focusing on the teaching itself.*

The third issue concerns the actual process of transmission. How did the setting determined by didactic authority and the person-oriented motives of transmission correlate with the transmission process? Only those procedu-

---

[1] Also MANSON, *Sayings of Jesus,* 9f, includes a personal interest in Jesus himself among the motives for preserving and collecting the sayings of Jesus.

[2] BOMAN, *Jesus-Überlieferung,* 35, stated: "Die Volkskunde lehrt uns, daß, wenn eine Überlieferung von einer geschichtlichen Person entsteht, diese Überlieferung eine zusammenhängende Erzälung bildet, weil die Person und nicht die Einzeltaten im Zentrum stehen." In my view, Boman never proved his assertion. But he rightly saw that the focus on Jesus in the gospel tradition challenged the form-critical isolation of Jesus-sayings from the episodal material.

[3] I understand "didactic" as a characteristic applicable to various components present in a teaching situation: to the person speaking or acting (teacher), to the communicated and transmitted material (teaching) and to the recipients and transmitters (pupils).

res and techniques are of interest which reveal a significant "personal specificity," i.e. where the setting and conceptions about the individual teacher
correlated with the discernable objects and acts of transmission. The issue
has several different aspects. An area of disagreement is the extent to which
the verbal tradition was *identified* as *Jesus* tradition. Bultmann and Dibelius
could conceive a variety of sayings that became utterances of Jesus. The focus on Jesus functioned apparently to attract sayings of different origins.
Gerhardsson and Riesner think that, in general, the focus on Jesus prevented other sayings from entering into the body of Jesus traditions. Another area of interest concerns the *means* of transmission. In a study aimed
as an alternative to both Bultmann's and Gerhardsson's approaches, Kelber
sets up a strict dichotomy between oral and written means of transmission.[1]
He shows convincingly that the means of transmission affects the hermeneutical process through which the traditions are conveyed, and yet, we
need to pose the question if the understanding of Jesus as the only teacher
and the person-oriented motives of transmission allow for the strict dichotomy. Finally, the process of transmission concerns the *preservation and
elaboration* of the tradition. While Bultmann and—even more—Dibelius
did not exclude the notion that the young communities preserved sayings
from Jesus, they stressed that the communities created new ones. Riesner
emphasizes the preservative aspects of transmission. Gerhardsson repeatedly points to the intricate interplay between the preserved tradition and the
interpretative adaptations, between fixed and flexible characteristics of the
tradition. It is necessary to ask *how these three areas in the process of transmission—the identification of traditions, the means of transmission, the
preservation and elaboration of traditions—correlated with the setting and
the person-oriented motives of transmission.* Only in this way can we determine how and to what extent the understanding of Jesus as the only teacher
was *the* essential factor in the transmission of the Jesus tradition.

As we go along, I will define the problems further. These are only the
basic problems related to my task. They are broad and span over large
fields in the whole of the NT. To make the topic workable, I will concentrate on a limited—though still rather vast—range of material.

4. The Basic Material of the Study

In selecting the basic material, I have used five criteria which are essential
for a study of the problems at hand:

1. The material should concern the activities of a person described in
some way as a *teacher*.

---

1   *The Oral and the Written Gospel.*

2. The material should state a *name* or a *significant title* of the teacher. This does not mean that the exact identity of the teacher must be evident in all cases. What is important is that a possibility exists to identify a tradition by reference to the teacher.

3. The material should portray a teacher accorded an *authoritative status*.

4. The material should indicate the existence of one or several *pupils* of the teacher.

5. The material should permit the *possibility to study* the relationship between the teacher and the pupil(s) as the setting for *actual transmission* of teaching given by the teacher.

A gospel must serve as the basic material. The gospels often refer to Jesus as teacher. Other explicit referents of the term διδάσκαλος appear only on three occasions (Luke 2:46; 3:12; John 3:10). In striking contrast, the remaining writings of the NT mostly use the term διδάσκαλος for Christian teachers,[1] once for Jewish teachers (Rom 2:20). With the exception of the Pastorals, which, as we saw, are concerned with Paul as teacher, the writings outside of the gospels do not constitute transmission literature in which traditions are explicitly related to a specific teacher. But the gospels present teaching as coming from Jesus.

It is impossible to treat all four gospels in one study. To make analytical work possible, I will deal only with Matthew's gospel narrative.[2] The concept of Jesus as the only teacher occurs most clearly here. P.-G. Müller points also to the relation between Matthew's general picture of Jesus as the only teacher and the transmission of the Jesus tradition in the Matthean community.[3] To be sure, Matthew was to some extent a creative interpreter of tradition.[4] But regardless of whether he always recorded existing traditions or not,[5] the picture he gave of Jesus as teacher indicates that he thought

---

[1] Acts 13:1; 1 Cor 12:28, 29; Eph 4:11; 1 Tim 2:7; 2 Tim 1:11; Jas 3:1. Cf. also 2 Tim 4:3; Heb 5:12. For discussion and further literature, see ZIMMERMANN, *Die urchristlichen Lehrer,* 92–140, 194–213.

[2] I will use "Matthew" somewhat variously, sometimes for the *written composition*—the narrative with its implied author—itself and sometimes for the *unknown person* behind the major parts of the canonical gospel. In the former case, I will write in the present tense, in the latter case, in the past tense. I will use a similar procedure in regard to other books carrying the name of certain persons, e.g. the later prophets in the OT. Expressions such as "the gospel of," "the narrative of" or "the book of" will be used only when it is necessary to clarify further which of the referents that is intended.

[3] *Traditionsprozeß,* 157–161.

[4] Cf. STANTON, *Gospel,* 326–345.

[5] For the view that Matthew is a liturgical midrash on Mark, see GOULDER, *Midrash and Lection,* 28–69, 137–52, *passim.* For criticism of Goulder's hypothesis, see MORRIS, Jewish Lectionaries, 129–156; STANTON, *ANRW* II 25:3 (1985) 1938f; FRANCE, *Matthew: Evangelist and Teacher,* 116f. For criticism of his use of the term "midrash," see FRANCE, Jewish Historiography, 99–127; *idem, Matthew: Evangelist and Teacher,* 202–205 (with lit.). Cf. also the review of Goulder's book by GERHARDSSON, *SEÅ* 45 (1980) 147–149.—For the view that Matthew is a midrash on or a midrashic embellishment of Mark and Q, see GUNDRY, *Matthew,* 623–640, *passim.* For criticism—some-

of his story not only as a literary fiction,[1] but also as a presentation of traditions from and about Jesus—as report.[2] It is a story, but it is in large measure "story as report." Matthew's story intends to tell about something which happened in the past. It exhibits a "diachronic" dimension of conveying traditions from and about Jesus.

In order to provide a comparative perspective, I have selected relevant material from Matthew's sociocultural background and environment—the sociocultural situation. The reconstruction of such a situation requires that we avoid restricting the comparative frame to the ideas and practices emerging from only one block of ancient material. The risk of making onesided or anachronistic assumptions about the Matthean process of transmission is limited when we include a broad range of material related to Matthew's sociocultural situation, aiming for a view which surveys the phenomena of transmission without strictly chronological and genetic classifications.

I have, however, restricted myself to material from ancient Israel and ancient Judaism. I have not included a comparison with Greco-Roman material. It is of course true that the Hellenistic world was the civilization of the "paideia."[3] And as the culture of the "paideia" influenced large aspects of life in antiquity,[4] Hellenistic schools certainly contributed to the development of educational institutions and practices among the Jews.[5] M. Hengel has repeatedly pointed to the influence of Hellenism on the Jewish culture,[6] though distinctions between the two do seem to exist.[7] This affects our view of the common separation between Hellenistic and Palestinian Christianity.[8] Nevertheless, not only would an account of these didactic fea-

---

what apologetic—of Gundry, see PAYNE, Midrash and History, 177–215.

[1] Cf. the opposite emphasis by FRANKEMÖLLE, *Jahwebund,* 351.

[2] Cf. BORING, *Continuing Voice,* 256.

[3] So e.g. MARROU, *History of Education,* 95–101.

[4] Already JAEGER, *Paideia* I, 6, stated long ago: "Und in der Form der Paideia, der 'Kultur', haben die Griechen endlich ihre geistige Gesamtschöpfung als Erbe an die übrigen Völker des Altertums weitergegeben."

[5] HENGEL, *Judaism and Hellenism* I, 70–78; RIESNER, *Lehrer,* 179–182; HENGEL/MARKSCHIES, *'Hellenization' of Judea,* 19-29. For the same phenomenon reflected in the rabbinic literature, see DAUBE, *HUCA* 22 (1949) 239–262; LIEBERMAN, *Hellenism,* 47-82; GERHARDSSON, *Memory,* 27, 50f, 56f, 88f, 91f, 109, 124–126; FISCHEL, Studies in Cynicism, 372–411; *idem, Rabbinic Literature, passim;* COHEN, *PAAJR* 48 (1981) 57–85. Cf. also the more general discussions by e.g. S. STEIN, *JJS* 8 (1957) 13–44; SHIMOFF, *JSJ* 18 (1987) 168–187; M. LUZ, *JSJ* 20 (1989) 49–60; P.S. ALEXANDER, Quid Athenis et Hierosolymis?, 101–124.

[6] *Judaism and Hellenism* I–II, idem, *Jews, Greeks and Barbarians;* HENGEL/MARKSCHIES, *'Hellenization' of Judea.* Hengel has developed his view in several articles.

[7] For a critique of Hengel's position, see the reviews by FELDMAN, *JBL* 96 (1977) 371–382; *idem, HUCA* 57 (1986) 83–111; *idem, JSJ* 22 (1991) 142–144.

[8] MARSHALL, *NTS* 19 (1972–73) 271–287. Cf. already LARSSON, *SEÅ* 28–29 (1963–64) 81–110.

tures in the Greco-Roman material by far exceed the limits of my investigation. What is more important, this material does not, as far as I can judge, contain to any larger degree situations that meet the fifth criterion mentioned above.[1] A survey by D.E. Aune even concludes that it provides "very little" information about important aspects of oral tradition and transmission.[2] It is furthermore difficult to avoid the impression, which forms the opinion of a majority of scholars,[3] that the main author of the narrative was most at home in Jewish-Christian circles.[4] All the arguments for a Jewish-Christian author also account for the view that the writings from ancient Israel and ancient Judaism reflect Matthew's *primary* sociocultural situation.[5] And as R.A. Culpepper points out, "the basic stimulus to teach and preserve tradition through disciples already had a long history in Judaism."[6]

5. The Basic Methods of the Study

In order to use the material for the problems of this study, I need to place them within the analytical boundaries of some basic methods. There are essentially two methodological issues involved, one pertaining to the understanding of sociocultural phenomena and one to the use of texts for reconstructing conceptions and practices.

---

[1] Epicuros (c. 341–270 B.C.E.) and his school constitute perhaps an exception. Epicureanism developed into a cult of the teacher and the adherence to this one teacher led to (careful) transmission of Epicuros' teaching. Already the Epicurean specialist DEWITT, *Epicuros,* 3, stated: "His handbooks of doctrine were carried about like breviaries; his sayings were esteemed as if oracles and committed to memory as if Articles of Faith." For further discussion of the transmission, cf. e.g. RENGSTORF, *TDNT* IV, 424f; CULPEPPER, *School,* 101–121; MALHERBE, Self-Definition, 47f (with lit.); BALCH, *Forum* 7:3–4 (1993) 197–199 (with lit.).

[2] Prolegomena, 98.

[3] Cf. the list given by DAVIES/ALLISON, *Matthew* I, 10f.

[4] WONG, *Interkulturelle Theologie,* 2–27, gives a recent survey of the most important contributions. For arguments in favour of a Jewish-Christian author, see e.g. DAVIES/ALLISON, *Matthew* I, 7–58; U. LUZ, *Matthäus* I, 62–65. For critical reviews of the literature arguing for Gentile-Christian authorship, see STANTON, *ANRW* II 25:3 (1985) 1916–1919; FRANCE, *Matthew: Evangelist and Teacher,* 102–108.—It seems that even NEPPER-CHRISTENSEN, *Matthæusevangeliet,* 18–23, now thinks of the gospel as written by a Jewish-Christian author for a Jewish-Christian context, a view which he earlier, in *idem, Matthäusevangelium,* tried to refute.

[5] It is not necessary for the purposes of this study to discuss further the authorship, date and location for the creation of Matthew's narrative. In addition to the Jewish-Christian setting, I only assume that Matthew created his narrative on the basis of—and thus later than—a version of Mark's narrative and that he was both a creative individual and a representative of a community, which in itself may have consisted of several interrelated groups. For Matthew as an exponent of his community, see U. LUZ, *Matthäus* I, 59-61.

[6] *School,* 188. Cf. also RIESNER, *Lehrer,* 179: "Die jüdische Schule wurde nicht erst vom Hellenismus ins Leben gerufen."

The setting, the motives and the process of the Matthean transmission constitute phenomena occurring within a sociocultural situation. They are not literary fictions of a text. All five scholars referred to in the previous account of the scholarly discussion agree that the phenomena partly gain their significance within a comparative perspective. W. Goldschmidt, an anthropologist, stresses the fact that each society operates within the field of cultural continuity.[1] "Every social system has a past and is directed to the future."[2] *The phenomena of transmission occurring within the Matthean community must be seen within a field of continuity relating to the past and to the future of their sociocultural situation.* For the purpose of this study, there are four aspects of the comparative method that need separate comment.

First, the comparative perspective aims towards *a holistic view of the phenomena.* This holistic approach suggests that the phenomena cannot be studied apart from their location in the broader framework of the sociocultural—and literary—situation. It is of course necessary to focus on certain items of special interest: the setting, the motives and the process of transmission. But the ideas and practices attain their primary meaning and significance within the context of their own configurational whole.[3] This implies that before any comparison can take place, we need to perceive the phenomena transmission within their own immediate situation.[4]

Second, the patterns of tradition and transmission emerge as the description of *how ideas and practices manifestly function among persons who understand themselves as adherents of a teacher.* The comparison does not focus on the views and practices of the "historical" teacher. Those features are of interest only when the teacher understands himself as a pupil of a previous teacher. This approach does not mean that I neglect theoretical statements about transmission. It will sometimes even be necessary to focus on those statements specifically. They occur mostly in the rabbinic literature and usually reflect views of persons involved in transmission. The functional approach merely means that I concentrate on those who perform transmission, not that I neglect their ideas.

Third, the comparative material should serve as the basis for a *sociocultural reconstruction.* The comparison is not strictly interpretative, in the sense that phenomena are interpreted through an implicit assumption of genetic relationships to other phenomena with similar causes. Nor is it merely illustrative, serving only to show that similar phenomena existed elsewhere. The aim of my study is to see the Matthean transmission within the context of its sociocultural background and environment, manifested in ancient Is-

---

[1] *Comparative Functionalism,* 53–56.
[2] *Comparative Functionalism,* 53.
[3] See HULTKRANTZ, *Metodvägar,* 112–118.
[4] TALMON, The "Comparative Method," 320–356.

rael and ancient Judaism. This means, to be more precise, that I make the phenomenological comparison by reconstructing the broad sociocultural situation.[1] When this reconstruction emerges from a sufficiently broad range of material, it is possible to avoid moulding my understanding of the Matthean transmission into pre-conceived schemata based on meta-theoretical presentations reflecting my own cultural matrix.[2] Through the reconstruction, the setting, the motives and the process of the Matthean transmission are explainable in terms of their own sociocultural situation. The patterns of the Matthean transmission emerge out of a comparison with patterns inherent in the sociocultural situation itself.

Fourth, the comparison seeks both for *contrasts and similarities.* The review of the scholarly debate shows the tendency to approach the phenomena exclusively through contrastive comparison. It is, however, a valid historical—and theological—task also to point out the similarities. This study assumes that the specific contours of the Matthean transmission best emerge when the comparison includes an account of the similarities within its basic contrastive perspective.

We reach the phenomena of transmission through the study of various texts. The material consists of texts from literary productions, and to some extent from inscriptions. A text textualizes a real world, and at the same time creates its own world by its textualization. For the purpose of this investigation, it is necessary to make the step (back) from the text as a literary fiction to the extra-fictional level—to the sociocultural situation. *The text serves as an "index" to the sociocultural situation of real persons.*[3] After all, the textual world and the real world both depend on language embedded in a common social system.[4] Of course, I will try to avoid making the "referential fallacy." It is not certain—it is even unlikely—that each and every item in a text refers to extra-textual circumstances. Some features are primarily "mirrors" reflecting the self-contained textual world. But some are also "windows" transparent for the world outside of the text. As will be e-

---

[1] D.P. WRIGHT, *Disposal of Impurity,* 8, speaks of "historical reconstruction" as the attempt to "deduce cultural connections between cultures by examining phenomenological similarities." I will study comparable phenomena in various social contexts within one—allegedly very broad—field of cultural continuity. Cf. HULTKRANTZ, *Metodvägar,* 88f, 96–99, describing the study of religious phenomena within different regions of one culture.

[2] MALINA, *New Testament World,* 10, rightly states: "If commentators, historians, and ordinary Bible readers derive meaning from the New Testament, the question we might put to them is whether such meaning comes from *their* cultural story or the cultural story of the people who produced the texts." Cf. also *idem, Christian Origins,* 5–12; KELBER, *Semeia* 39 (1987) 121–126; MALINA/ROHRBAUGH, *Commentary,* 1–14; ROBBINS, *Jesus the Teacher,* xxi.

[3] So KINGSBURY, *NTS* 34 (1988) 459, though he rarely asks for sociocultural phenomena. But cf. *idem, Matthew as Story,* 147–160; *idem,* Analysis of a Conversation, 259–269.

[4] MALINA/ROHRBAUGH, *Commentary,* 15.

specially evident in the treatment of Matthew, I am here thinking of broad and essential features visible in the narrative of the story.[1]

My basic approach to the texts is *"user-oriented"* in the sense that *the texts are testimonies about their ancient users.* The users of interest in this study are persons who transmitted traditions. The transmitters were not only authors and not only readers/hearers of texts. They were both. When they composed a text, they normally depended on other traditional texts which they had read/heard. And the text they themselves produced was often a means through which they expressed their own interpretation of the traditional texts and of their own situation.

I will regard the transmitters' use of texts as reflections of *conceptions* that they cherished. The focus will in these cases be on the transmitters as persons who encoded their conceptions in the signs of a text which they composed through interaction between the reception of earlier traditions and the creation of new material.[2] This makes it necessary to combine form- and redaction-critical approaches with the methods of the new literary criticism. The integration of methods will become especially evident in my treatment of Matthew's narrative. Certainly, the recent discussion of narrative structures in the gospels, as well as in other genres of texts,[3] stresses the risk of making an "intentional fallacy" and consequently pays more attention to the texts' semantic autonomy than to the real author's intentions. But as D.B. Howell points out in his analysis of Matthew's narrative rhetoric, the position that totally ignores the role of the author is to be avoided.[4] The author uses communicative conventions which to some extent condition the response of the readers/hearers.[5] In its modest applications,

---

[1]   The term "narrative" is used variously by scholars. FUNK, *Poetics,* 2f, lists three main references of the term. I will follow GENETTE, *Narrative Discourse,* 27, according to whom "story" (French "histoire") is the content—the signified—and "narrative" (French "récit") is the means—the signifier. I do not distinguish sharply between narrative and narrative text. CHATMAN, *Story and Discourse,* 19, uses the term "discourse" to describe "the means by which the content is communicated."—GENETTE, *ibid.,* 27; *idem, Narrative Discourse Revisited,* 13–15, uses also "narrating" (French "narration") for the real or fictive situation which produces the narrative. I will occasionally, in chapter 6, discuss the real act of "narrativizing" the existence.

[2]   My treatment of Sirach is an exception. As it seems, the hebrew Sirach is to a large extent a composition from the teacher himself. I will therefore assume that the transmitters' conception about Ben Sira emerged primarily as they read/heard his own writing.

[3]   For a brief survey of this trend in NT studies, see BYRSKOG, *Nya testamentet och forskningen,* 18f (with lit.).—For commentaries and monographs on Matthew using narrative criticism, see R.A. EDWARDS, *Matthew's Story;* KINGSBURY, *Matthew;* D.R. BAUER, *Structure;* KINGSBURY, *Matthew as Story;* R.H. SMITH, *Matthew;* W.G. THOMPSON, *Matthew's Story;* WEAVER, *Missionary Discourse;* HOWELL, *Inclusive Story;* HEIL, *Death and Resurrection;* M. DAVIES, *Matthew.* There are also numerous articles.

[4]   *Inclusive Story,* 44–50. Cf. the positive remark on this in the review by U. LUZ, *TLZ* 117 (1992) 189, who himself combines form- and redaction-critical approaches with narrative criticism in his commentary on Matthew.

[5]   E.D. HIRSCH, *Validity,* 1–23, tried to refute the notion of a text's semantic

the new literary criticism develops form and redaction criticism and helps us to see also the intentions and conceptions of the author.

I will also regard the transmitters' use of texts as reflections of *practices* that they performed within the transmission process. Here the focus will be on the transmitters as persons who worked on the texts. The text is not only a reflection of conceptions. It is also a testimony of how the work of transmission proceeded. Since the transmitters used texts in a constant interchange between traditional material and their own creativity, the common distinction between tradition and transmission on one hand, and redaction and text composition on the other, becomes somewhat fluid. The redactors were also transmitters and the texts they produced reflect the transmission. This is even more so if we assume that ancient, written texts essentially were part of an oral currency where the composition itself often entailed transmission,[1] though without necessarily being fused with other activities in the communities.

The methods serve to locate the specific problems at hand within an adequate analytical perspective. They should not pose a limit to the range of issues that can be brought into discussion. And no one-dimensional method would do justice to the complexity of all the material. Further methodological considerations will therefore occur as I bring individual problems and material into the discussion.

6. On the Content of the Book

The book falls into two separate parts: the reconstruction of the sociocultural situation of transmission and the analysis of transmission in the Matthean community. I have chosen to allow each part to stand for itself. This is in accordance with the aim to provide a holistic perspective. It means that the reader of the first part of the book will find discussions of phenomena that do not always correspond to phenomena within the Matthean situation but are important for providing the holistic view.

In order to facilitate comparison, I have—as far as possible—structured each part similarly in regard to chapters and sections. The out-line of the book corresponds to the basic problems mentioned above. First, I will ask about settings of transmission determined by the authority of a person considered in some way to be a teacher. What is important is the perspective of the transmitters themselves. The question is whether the transmitters in any

---

autonomy already before it entered into the studies of biblical scholars.

[1] Cf. KELBER, *The Oral and the Written Gospel,* 43 n. 224.—HENAUT, *Oral Tradition,* argues the thesis that the written gospel text has textualized the oral tradition beyond recognition. But since Henaut acknowledges that orality and literacy do not represent two incompatible media (*ibid.,* 94–99, *passim*), his conclusion is, as far as I can see, not mandatory even from his own presuppositions.

sense were familiar and associated with such settings. Second, I will study the person-oriented motives of transmission. The issue of interest is the function of the transmitters' understanding of the teacher for motivating transmission. Third, I come to the actual process of transmission. Here the correlation between the settings and motives of transmission on one hand, and the transmission process on the other, will be studied.

The presentation of the results differs in the two parts. The first part is more synthetic and the second more analytic. An analytical manner of presentation needs no defence here. The synthetic presentation in the first part is due to the vast amount of relevant material from different places and times. The various writings from ancient Israel and ancient Judaism are each, in a sense, independent compositions in need of separate treatment. Each book in the OT stands for itself and is often the object of separate studies; the recent discussion about the Dead Sea scrolls—published and un-published—points to an increasing need to treat each of these documents in its own right; and there is now an awareness of the fact that even the rabbinic literature, in which an idiosyncratic teaching has always been difficult to distinguish from a generally accepted teaching, consists of various pieces of writings with their own integrity. An analytical presentation, arranged around the chronological order of each piece of material, would by far exceed the limits of this—already rather lengthy—book. It would also make it more difficult for the reader to focus on the specific phenomena of interest. I have therefore presented each item as part of a body of material larger than the individual writing. And these bodies of material are in turn, once they have been defined in chapter one, arranged around the primary issues and the emerging hypotheses.

Part One

Didactic Authority and Transmission in Ancient Israel and Ancient Judaism

Chapter 1

Didactic Authority
and the Settings of Transmission

1. Introductory Remarks

Various texts from ancient Israel and ancient Judaism maintain that settings characterized by didactic features occurred in a number of different situations. Not all of these situations involved transmission of traditions related to a specific teacher.[1] Training—whether in the home or in more organized forms—served different purposes: basic education of boys and girls was in early times given within the family;[2] a trade had to be learnt;[3] military training was necessary;[4] the son of the king was given special education for his future office;[5] the different duties of the priest probably required organized training.[6] These situations are not my concern here. For the purposes of this study, *only those settings are of interest in which—as we will see more clearly in the following chapters—the pupils by various means acknowledged the authority of a certain teacher and in which this acknowledgement related to a process of transmission.*

The material is not restricted to the appearance of certain significant terms and expressions only. Since the teacher-pupil relationship expresses itself first of all as an interaction between the two partners, I will look further than to the didactic terms only. For instance, the term "prophet" (נביא) is normally used for persons performing a number of various activities.[7] And certain texts speak of the prophet as a man of God (איש [ה]אלהים),[8] seer

---

[1] See e.g. excursus 1 below.

[2] For the family as the setting of education, see RIESNER, *Lehrer,* 102–118 (with lit.).

[3] Cf. 1 Chr 25:8.

[4] Cf. Judg 3:2; 2 Sam 22:35; Isa 2:4; Mic 4:3; Pss 18:35; 144:1; 1 Chr 5:18. Cf. also Judg 8:20; 2 Sam 2:14; Cant 3:8.

[5] Cf. 2 Kgs 10:1, 5f; 1 Chr 27:32.

[6] Other didactic settings are of course conceivable. I will discuss the existence of elementary and scribal schools in ancient Israel below excursus 2. Neither in such schools was the transmission of traditions related to one specific teacher the primary characteristic of the pupils' activity.

[7] Jörg JEREMIAS, *THAT* II, 8f. Cf. already FASCHER, *ΠΡΟΦΗΤΗΣ,* 148f.

[8] Cf. e.g. 1 Kgs 20:28; 2 Kgs 4:40, 42; 6:6. The expression is used 29 times for Elisha.

(ראה)[1] or visionary (חזה).[2] This variety of terms and expressions shows that
the activities of the prophets seemed to be other than purely didactic ones.
As it happens, only the false prophet is explicitly called "teacher" (מורה) in
the OT (Isa 9:14).[3] However, the terminological evidence in no way
exhausts the evidence. Various texts speak of individuals or groups understanding certain persons as authoritative teachers from whom specific teaching can be received.

There are two steps involved in this chapter. First, I will refer to some
texts implying that the ancient transmitters might have conceived a teacher-
pupil relationship *within the material they used*. I am not concerned to
prove the historicity of the teacher-pupil relationship here. It is sufficient,
as a first step, to show that people, among whom there were transmitters,
might have written and read/heard texts depicting interactions between a
teacher and pupils. Second, I will ask if these brief accounts about a teacher-
pupil relationship in any sense corresponded to *the actual existence* of
schools. The two steps represent the search for the existence of two related
sociocultural phenomena: *accounts about the teacher-pupil relationship and
manifestations of the relationship in social settings*.

2. The Teacher-Pupil Relationship

I think here of "the teacher-pupil relationship" as *an interaction seen from
the perspective of the ancient transmitters as users of texts*. Of interest are
configurations of a teacher producing a body of instructions which is received by the pupil(s).

2.1. Elijah and Elisha

1 Kgs 19:19–21; 2 Kgs 2:1–18 depict Elijah's relation to Elisha.[4] 1 Kgs
19:19–21 pictures the initial interaction between the two. Just as Moses ap-
points Joshua as his successor (Num 27:18–23),[5] Elijah choses Elisha to take

---

[1]   Cf. e.g. 1 Sam 9:9.

[2]   Cf. e.g. 2 Sam 24:11; Amos 7:12. Cf. further RENDTORFF, *TDNT* VI, 809f; Jörg
JEREMIAS, *THAT* II, 9f; KOCH, *Prophets* I, 15f. The different expressions are discussed
as role labels by PETERSEN, *Roles*, 35–88. For a summarizing discussion of the prophetic titles, see WILSON, *Prophecy*, 136–141 (with lit.).

[3]   Cf. also Hab 2:18.

[4]   For discussion of the material concerning Elijah and Elisha, see WILSON, *Prophecy*, 192–212 (with lit.). For the Elisha material, cf. also STIPP, *Elischa*. For Elisha as the
follower of Elijah, cf. SCHÄFER-LICHTENBERGER, *ZAW* 101 (1989) 210–222.

[5]   Cf. also the crossing of Jordan by both Joshua and Elisha (Josh 3; 2 Kgs 2:6–14).
For the (intended) similarities between the two persons, cf. CARROLL, *VT* 19 (1969)
413; HOBBS, *2 Kings*, 19; SCHÄFER-LICHTENBERGER, *ZAW* 101 (1989) 198–222.

up his ministry. Elijah transfers his powers—his identity and status[1]—by casting the mantle over Elisha (1 Kgs 19:19).[2] Elisha, in turn, acknowledges his willingness to follow after (הלך אחרי) Elijah (1 Kgs 19:20f). Following also means serving (שרת) Elijah (1 Kgs 19:21).[3] These expressions are not technical terms for discipleship here,[4] but they do indicate the beginning of a fellowship which prepares Elisha to become the legitimate successor of Elijah.

B. Lang points to the didactic character of the interaction between Elijah and Elisha. The text implies, according to Lang, "that the head of the school brings the candidate into the ranks of the pupils by throwing his coat over him."[5] While there is no evidence that Elijah brings Elisha into a larger body of pupils within a school, the text does suggest that Elisha enters into contact with a specific master.

2 Kgs 2:1–18 confirms the didactic implications to some extent.[6] When Elijah rises into heaven in a chariot (2 Kgs 2:12), Elisha cries "my father" (אבי). No doubt, the term "father" spelled authority to the ancient Israelites.[7] Since the father is a teacher in the OT,[8] and since the term "father" is also used for other persons acting as teachers or advisers (Gen 45:8),[9] Elisha's exclamation may convey a didactic connotation. It is his own teacher that is taken away.

Ancient Jewish texts strengthen the didactic understanding of the relationship between Elijah and Elisha. Sir 48:8, 12; Bell. 4:460 depict Elisha as the legitimate successor of Elijah. Various texts also imply a didactic interpretation of the relationship between the two. Josephus pictures Elisha as the disciple (μαθητής) of Elijah, both in his account of 1 Kgs 19:19–21 (Ant. 8:354), where Elisha is also Elijah's servant (διάκονος), and

---

[1]   Cf. VIBERG, *Symbols of Law,* 134: "The mantle is a well-known symbol for the identity and status of the person who is wearing it." Viberg does not, however, discuss the act of Elijah. But cf. STACEY, *Prophetic Drama,* 85f.

[2]   Cf. also 2 Kgs 2:8, 13f and the comments by GUNKEL, *ExpTim* 41 (1929–30) 185; DEVRIES, *1 Kings,* 239.

[3]   Cf. also 2 Kgs 3:11.

[4]   A. SCHULZ, *Nachfolgen,* 19. Cf. also LARSSON, *Vorbild,* 30; G. KITTEL, *TDNT* I, 213.

[5]   *Monotheism,* 95.

[6]   A. SCHMITT, *Entrückung,* 47–139, gives a detailed treatment of 2 Kgs 2:1–18. For the prophetic succession in this passage and its relation to the concept of the Mosaic prophet (Deut 18:15–18), cf. CARROLL, *VT* 19 (1969) 400–415; SCHÄFER-LICHTENBERGER, *ZAW* 101 (1989) 213–220.

[7]   RINGGREN, *TWAT* I, 8.

[8]   Cf. e.g. Exod 10:2; 12:26f; 13:8, 14; Deut 4:9f; 6:7, 20f; 11:18f; 32:7, 46; Josh 4:21f; Judg 6:13; Pss 44:2; 78:3–6.

[9]   Cf. also Judg 17:10; 18:19. DE VAUX, *Israel,* 49, mentions also 2 Kgs 2:12 in this connection. LANG, *Schule,* 192–195, argues that the many references to a father teaching his son in Proverbs (1:8, 10, 15; 2:1; 3:1, 11, 21; 4:1–4, 10, 20; 5:1, 7, 20, etc.) should be understood exclusively in the sense of the teacher instructing his pupil. Similarly e.g. DÜRR, *Erziehungswesen,* 107; RÜGER, *Oral Tradition,* 112. Differently e.g. HERNER, *Erziehung,* 58f; DE VAUX, *ibid.,* 49; LIPIŃSKI, *Scribes,* 162.

of 2 Kgs 2:1–18 (Ant. 9:28).[1] Tg. Neb. 2 Kgs 2:12 changes Elisha's cry "my father" to "(my) teacher" (רבי). And the rabbinic literature refers quite frequently to Elijah and Elisha as examples of the relationship between teacher and pupil.[2]

2.2. Elisha and the Sons of the Prophets

Elisha is associated with the sons of the prophets. The expression "sons of (the) prophets" (בני [ה]נביאים) occurs in 1 Kgs 20:35; 2 Kgs 2:3, 5, 15; 4:1, 38 (*bis*); 5:22; 6:1; 9:1; Amos 7:14 (בן נביא). Only 1 Kgs 20:35; Amos 7:14 use the expression without any connection to Elisha.[3]

Although these "sons" never call Elisha "father,"[4] he appears as their leader (2 Kgs 2:15; 4:1, 38; 9:1). 2 Kgs 4:38; 6:1 indicate perhaps a didactic relationship. In both texts the sons of the prophets sit in front of (ישבים לפני) Elisha—an early form of a yeshivah.[5] This is the only common activity of the group mentioned. The preposition לפני points here to a gathering of a more formal kind.[6] Such a gathering implies that a respectful attitude—as the one between a teacher and his pupils—is involved.[7] The references to a place of meeting suggest perhaps that the sons of the prophets are gathered for instruction by Elisha.[8]

Also Samuel appears as the leader (אב, נציב) of a group (חבל, להקה) of prophets (1 Sam 10:5–12; 19:20). They seem to have a common dwelling-place (נוית, נויח) where they live together (1 Sam 19:18–23). However, Samuel is not an actual teacher of a group of attentive pupils. The term נציב has no didactic connotations. The peculiar place called נויח, נוית is not a school house. It is probably related to נוה, "meadow," "dwelling-place."[9] The group of prophets is throughout ecstatic (1 Sam 10:5–10; 19:20–24). It is not accurate to connect them with the group around Elisha. They are never called "sons of the prophets."[10]

---

1   Cf. also Ant. 9:33.—RENGSTORF, *TDNT* IV, 428f, claims that Elisha was not a disciple but merely a servant of Elijah. This distinction would seem strange at least to Josephus. He refers to Elisha as "both disciple and servant" (καὶ μαθητὴς καὶ διάκονος) of Elijah (Ant. 8:354). On Josephus, see further HENGEL, *Charismatic Leader,* 16–18; WILKINS, *Concept of Disciple,* 111–116.

2   b. Ber. 7b; b. Sanh. 68a; Mek. on 12:1; 13:19 (Lauterbach I, 14:152; 177:101). For further references, cf. HENGEL, *Charismatic Leader,* 17 n. 4.

3   For summarizing discussion, see WILSON, *Prophecy,* 140f (with lit.); HOBBS, *2 Kings,* 25–27.

4   But cf. 2 Kgs 6:21; 13:14 and the discussion by WILLIAMS, *JBL* 85 (1966) 345–347; PHILLIPS, *Father,* 188; A. SCHMITT, *Entrückung,* 111–114.

5   I.e. a place where pupils sit in front of their teacher. Cf. GEVARYAHU, *ASTI* 12 (1983) 7.

6   Cf. Ezek 8:1; 14:1; 20:1; 33:31.

7   GÖRG, *TWAT* III, 1018f.

8   Josephus develops the didactic implications. Ant. 9:106, in the account of 2 Kgs 9:1, calls the sons of the prophets the disciples (μαθηταί) of Elisha. Ant. 9:68 also refers to the elders sitting with Elisha in his house (2 Kgs 6:32) as disciples.

9   MCCARTER, *1 Samuel,* 328f.

10   WILSON, *Prophecy,* 141, points to the differences between the two groups. For

2.3. Isaiah and His Disciples

Certain texts in Isaiah give the impression that Isaiah of Jerusalem is a teacher in some regard.[1] Scholars have proposed that Isaiah actually belonged to the upper-class aristocracy of the city and enjoyed some education in wisdom circles.[2] J. Fichtner even speaks of him as a converted scribe.[3] Whatever Isaiah's own social and professional location may have been, certain texts suggest that he is a teacher. They present the prophets as teachers in a general fashion.[4] To be sure, 30:20 probably refers to Yahweh—not the prophets—as teacher. But 9:14 depicts false prophets as false teachers.[5] And 28:7–9 speaks of drunken priests and prophets who chastise Isaiah for teaching (יורה) knowledge.[6]

8:16 provides the most explicit claim for the existence of supportive groups around the later prophets. It appears within 6:1–9:6, the so-called memoirs of Isaiah. Although these memoirs, if accepted as a unit at all,[7] are to some extent composite,[8] most scholars see no obstacle in regarding 8:16 as reflecting a genuine event in Isaiah's prophetic career. But whatever the historicity,[9] the central section (7:1–8:18)[10] of the memoirs now appears within the political context of the Syro-Ephraimite war circa 735–732 B.C.E (7:1).[11] Isaiah's warnings to king Ahaz (c. 735–715 B.C.E.) about

---

discussion of Samuel's prophetic role in the Samuel traditions, see WILSON, *ibid.,* 169–184 (with lit.). Cf. also MOMMER, *Samuel.*

[1]   I will use the expressions "Isaiah of Jerusalem," or "First Isaiah," and "Second Isaiah" for the major individual behind or within parts of Isa 1–39 and 40–55 respectively. I will use "Third Isaiah" for the major individual(s) behind or within the oldest material in Isa 56–66, without deciding if Third Isaiah actually was a single individual or not.

[2]   For surveys of the discussion, see VERMEYLEN, Proto-Isaïe, 39–58; E.W. DAVIES, *Prophecy and Ethics,* 29–36; VON LIPS, *Weisheitliche Traditionen,* 70–72.

[3]   *TLZ* 74 (1949) 75–80.—GEVARYAHU, *JBQ* 18 (1989–90) 64, claims that Isaiah was a "סופר and the leader of a circle of young intelligentsia called יודעי ספר 'literate ones'." But Gevaryahu is too bold in his briefly substantiated conclusions.

[4]   Only rather late material (37:2; 38:1; 39:3) call Isaiah "prophet" (נביא). 8:3 says that he married a "prophetess" (נביאה), though, as JEPSEN, *ZAW* 72 (1960) 267f, points out, this observation should be treated with caution. However, for Isaiah's prophetic characteristics in general, cf. EATON, *VT* 9 (1959) 145–147.

[5]   Many commentators regard 9:14 as a late gloss. But cf. OSWALT, *Isaiah,* 253f n. 2.

[6]   It is questionable if Isa 28:10 (13) pictures Isaiah as a teacher of children. Cf. DRIVER, 'Another Little Drink', 53–57; GÖRG, *BN* 29 (1985) 12–16.

[7]   Cf. IRVINE, *ZAW* 104 (1992) 216–231.

[8]   Cf. W. DIETRICH, *Jesaja,* 62–87; KAISER, *Isaiah 1–12,* 114–117; WERNER, *BZ* 29 (1985) 1–30; KAISER, *TRE* 16 (1987) 645–647; REVENTLOW, *BN* 38–39 (1987) 64–66; HØGENHAVEN, *Gott und Volk,* 77–80.

[9]   In a recent attempt to prove that Ahaz conducted a neutralist course strongly supported by Isaiah, IRVINE, *Isaiah,* 75–109, minimizes the historical accuracy of the elements in the texts implying Ahaz' submission to Tiglath-pileser III.

[10]   LESCOW, *ZAW* 85 (1973) 315.

[11]   Cf. 2 Kgs 16:5–9; 2 Chr 28:5–21.

the consequences of an alliance with Tiglath-pileser III (c. 745–727 B.C.E.) are ignored and the prophet withdraws. Isaiah moves to the periphery of the establishment and appears in dissonant opposition to the official policy.[1]

At this time of crisis, a testimony is to be bound and a torah sealed.[2] This activity takes place "among my disciples" (בלמדי). Since there is no adversative at the beginning of 8:16 to signal a new subject, some interpreters understand the verse as a continuation of the preceding statements from Yahweh.[3] The three other instances using forms of למד (50:4 [*bis*]; 54:13) describe Yahweh as teacher. He appears as a teacher also elsewhere in Isaiah (2:3; 28:26; 30:20; 48:17; 51:4).[4] According to this understanding of 8:16, both verbs are imperatives.[5] However, the decisive argument against this interpretation is that it obstructs a uniform reading/hearing of the first person pronouns in 8:17f. The simple waw links the prophet speaking in the first person in 8:17f with the one speaking in 8:16. In addition, it is not impossible that the children in 8:18 refers to the disciples,[6] and not (only) Isaiah's physical children (7:3; 8:3)

Textcritically בלמדי is uncertain. The versions render the expression variously. Most MSS of the LXX read "in order not to learn" (τοῦ μὴ μαθεῖν). Tg. Neb. Isa 8:16 reads "they do not wish to learn" (לא צבן דיילפון). Scholars have accordingly exceeded in conjectures about the original reading,[7] or omitted it altogether.[8] But such a procedure is unnecessary.[9] The condensed language in 8:16 could easily have created different interpretations when the original situation no longer provided any clear reference of meaning.[10]

The transmitters might in 8:16 have conceived persons who receive specific torah from Isaiah. It is Isaiah who binds and seals. The two verbs, חתום

---

[1] Cf. CARROLL, *Prophecy,* 140f; WILSON, *Prophecy,* 272f.

[2] I will use "torah" as a collective designation for teaching and sacred tradition. I will use "the Torah" only when that which is codified in sacred Scripture is in view.

[3] So e.g. BOEHMER, *ARW* 33 (1936) 171f; SCHEDL, *Rufer des Heils,* 242; W. DIETRICH, *Jesaja,* 96 n. 41; ERLANDSSON, *Jesaja,* 27; REVENTLOW, *BN* 38–39 (1987) 66f.

[4] The context of Isa 30:20 points to a singular reference to Yahweh as teacher. For further discussion of Yahweh as teacher in Isaiah, see SCHAWE, *Gott als Lehrer,* 63–69, 134–137.

[5] The term צור may be an imperative or an infinitive absolute. The counterpart is vocalized as an imperative in the BHS (חתום). It may also, with a different vocalization, be understood as an infinitive absolute (חתם).

[6] So e.g. D. JONES, *ZAW* 67 (1955) 237; EATON, *VT* 9 (1959) 148; LINDBLOM, *Prophecy,* 160f; GEVARYAHU, *JBQ* 18 (1989–90) 67.

[7] For surveys of different proposals, see WIDENGREN, *Literary and Psychological Aspects,* 69f n. 4; D. JONES, *ZAW* 67 (1955) 232f; WHITLEY, *ZAW* 90 (1978) 29; IRVINE, *Isaiah,* 207f.

[8] FOHRER, *Studien,* 142.

[9] Many commentators accept בלמדי as original. So e.g. WILDBERGER, *Jesaja* I, 343; CLEMENTS, *Isaiah 1–39,* 100; KAISER, *Isaiah 1–12,* 196 n. 9; WATTS, *Isaiah* I, 122; OSWALT, *Isaiah,* 230.

[10] D. JONES, *ZAW* 67 (1955) 233 n. 34.

and צוּר, are probably absolute infinitives.[1] An imperative interpretation would either suggest that Isaiah utters a prayer to Yahweh or a command to an anonymous person. But in the following verse Isaiah speaks of Yahweh in the third person, not in direct prayer, and no other person capable of performing Isaiah's command is present. The waw at the beginning of 8:17 links the two verses and shows that the verbs in 8:16 are infinitives replacing finite verbs in the first person. As Isaiah waits and hopes (8:17), he himself binds and seals (8:16).[2]

The object of sealing is torah (תורה).[3] This suggests that the people around the prophet are pupils receiving divine instruction through the prophet. Also prophets, not only priests, are imparters of torah.[4] This contradicts in no way the idea that torah comes from Yahweh.[5] The instruction of the prophet conveys divine torah in Isaiah: 1:10 calls an oracle of the prophet "torah of our God"; 30:9f parallels the people's refusal to listen to Yahweh's torah with disrespect for the seers and prophets. It is therefore probable that the expression "to seal torah" (חתום תורה) in 8:16 means that Isaianic disciples receive divine instruction from Isaiah. They are Isaiah's pupils.

Perhaps Isa 1–39 maintains the existence of prophetic disciples on two further occasions. First, after the singular address in 8:11, a specific group of people is in 8:12–15 admonished together with Isaiah to judge the situation differently than the rest of the people. These persons may be identical with the disciples in 8:16.[6] It is not impossible to read/hear the pericope within the same historical situation as 8:16.[7] Second, 30:8 might imply that Isaiah has a group of close associates.[8] Isaiah is commanded to perform an act of writing "with them" (אתם). It is impossible to state with certainty that this indicates the involvement of attentive followers.[9] The preposition with the suffix can also be rendered "before them." But the possibility of interpreting it as a reference to Isaiah's disciples should at least be recognized.

Two texts in Isa 40–55 also deserve attention. First, there is the plural address in 40:1f.[10] Someone commands a group, not an individual, to pro-

---

[1]   So e.g. DUHM, *Jesaia,* 62; A. KLOSTERMANN, *Schulwesen,* 10; FOHRER, *Studien,* 140 n. 30; WILDBERGER, *Jesaja* I, 342f; KAISER, *Isaiah 1–12,* 194f n. 1; WATTS, *Isaiah* I, 122; HØGENHAVEN, *Gott und Volk,* 97.
[2]   RIGNELL, *ST* 10 (1956) 47, understands the two verbs in 8:16 as infinitive constructs being subordinated in an adverbial manner to the finite verbs in 8:17.
[3]   For the significance of the testimony, see below pp. 160f.
[4]   Cf. ÖSTBORN, *Tōrā,* 127–168.
[5]   Cf. JENSEN, *Use of tôrâ,* 18–27, 58–121.
[6]   WILDBERGER, *Jesaja* I, 345; LESCOW, *ZAW* 85 (1973) 325f; WATTS, *Isaiah* I, 119; HØGENHAVEN, *Gott und Volk,* 96f. Cf. also KAISER, *Isaiah 1–12,* 190f.
[7]   WILDBERGER, *Jesaja* I, 336.
[8]   Cf. GEVARYAHU, *JBQ* 18 (1989–90) 67.
[9]   The BHS advises deletion of אתם.
[10]   Cf. EATON, *VT* 9 (1959) 152; D. MICHEL, *TRE* 8 (1981) 520f; BLENKINSOPP, *Prophecy,* 210f, 214; WILSON, Community of the Second Isaiah, 54.

claim the end of the exile to Jerusalem.[1] Although there is no evidence to
ascertain the identity of this group,[2] the text does present the giving of the
task in the form of an address to several individuals. Second, 52:8 mentions
a number of watchmen (צֹפִים) rejoicing together with the individual herald.
The prophets often use the image of the watchman (צפה, שֹׁמֵר)[3] in reference
to their own activity (Isa 21:6–10; 62:6; Jer 6:17; Ezek 3:17; 33:2, 6f; Hab
2:1).[4] It suggests here that Second Isaiah is associated with a group of prophetic disciples.

> Scholars sometimes connect the twofold reference to disciples (לִמּוּדִים) in 50:4—part
> of the third servant song—with 8:16 in order to show that Second Isaiah understands
> himself, or is understood, as continuing the activity of the group gathered around
> Isaiah of Jerusalem.[5] However, even if we accept the MT as it stands,[6] we can draw
> no conclusion in this direction. First, the text does not picture the ones who are taught
> as Isaiah's disciples. Rather, as in 54:13, they are taught by Yahweh.[7] Second, in the
> third servant song (50:4–9[–11]),[8] the speaker may be someone who in the second
> song (49:3)[9] and elsewhere (41:8f; 44:1f, 21) is called "Israel."[10] The surrounding
> context speaks of Yahweh as teacher (51:4). And just as 51:7 mentions Israel as ha-
> ving Yahweh's teaching (תּוֹרָה), so 50:4 depicts the speaker as one who hears "as
> those who are taught." Isa 40–55 applies the concept of hearing on Israel also else-
> where, sometimes in connection with mentioning servant(s) (42:18–20, 23, 43:8–10,
> 12; 48:8a).[11] At the most, we might assume that knowledge of 8:16 and some kind of
> educational process caused the rather uncommon adjectival form of לִמֻּד[12] in 50:4.[13]

2.4. Jeremiah and His Followers

Jeremiah also appears as a teacher. It is not impossible that Baruch initiated
such an understanding of the prophet. A number of factors point to Ba-

---

[1]   Cf. also Isa 35:3f.
[2]   P.-E. BONNARD, *Second Isaïe*, 85.
[3]   The term צפה is most frequent.
[4]   Cf. also Isa 56:10; Hos 9:8; Mic 7:4.
[5]   J.L. MCKENZIE, *Second Isaiah*, 116f. Cf. also e.g. EATON, *VT* 9 (1959) 152f;
LINDBLOM, *Prophecy,* 161; G.A.F. KNIGHT, *Servant Theology,* 144; WILKINS, *Concept of Disciple,* 50.
[6]   Cf. the different proposals listed by HAAG, *Gottesknecht,* 171f. Cf. also MEREN-
DINO, *ZAW* 97 (1985) 349–352.
[7]   JENNI, *THAT* I, 875; SCHAWE, *Gott als Lehrer,* 135–137; KAPELRUD, *TWAT*
IV, 581.
[8]   The term עבד occurs here only in 50:10, by some scholars regarded as a later comment on 50:4–9.
[9]   There is not sufficient indication for deletion of יִשְׂרָאֵל.
[10] Cf. also 45:4; 48:20.
[11] Cf. also 35:5. For further arguments to this end, see METTINGER, *Servant Songs,*
33f.
[12] Outside of Isa 8:16; 50:4 (*bis*); 54:13, it occurs only in Jer 2:24; 13:23.
[13] So already A. KLOSTERMANN, *Schulwesen,* 19–22; RIESSLER, *TQ* 91 (1909)
606f; DÜRR, *Erziehungswesen,* 110. The affinities in this verse to wisdom teaching and
Egyptian education have been listed by RIESNER, *Lehrer,* 159f.

ruch's own prominent social position and educated skill.[1] It is especially revealing that a seal impression which is probably Baruch's own has been found in an archive containing some bullae of royal officers.[2] In any event, on the basis of the scribal features of Jeremiah's ministry visible in the texts,[3] we may assume that ancient transmitters conceived the prophet partly as a teacher. Jeremiah is both expected and able to write (29:1; 30:2; 36:2; 51:60).[4] And the scribes are connected, though in a polemical context, with the wise men as the ones responsible for Yahweh's instruction (8:8).[5] Since priests appear together with wise men and are assigned a teaching responsibility (2:8; 18:18),[6] Jeremiah's priestly background could be a further indication of his didactic activity,[7] perhaps located near the temple.[8]

The book of Jeremiah also indicates that the prophets have groups of followers. Jeremiah is not entirely alone.[9] Among several persons of scribal profession associated in some way with Jeremiah, Baruch, the son of Neriah, is the most important one (32:12f, 16; 36:4–32; 43:3, 6; 45:1–5). The texts maintain that he is closely attached to Jeremiah: he is involved in Jeremiah's personal affairs (32:12f; 16); when Jeremiah is instructed to write, it is in fact Baruch who writes (36:2–4, 28–32); Baruch is summoned to read a scroll in place of Jeremiah (36:5f); Baruch is together with Jeremiah made responsible for the prophecies and even liable to persecution (36:18f); he accompanies Jeremiah to Egypt (43:6). While details might have been added at different times,[10] and while the accounts depict a rather narrow part of Jeremiah's career,[11] the fact that several independent texts

---

[1]   MALLAU, *TRE* 5 (1980) 269 (with lit.). Cf. also LUNDBOM, *JSOT* 36 (1986) 107. The article by H.M.I. GEVARYAHU, Baruch ben Neriah the Scribe (Hebrew), in: *Zer Ligevurot.* FS Z. Shazar. Jerusalem 1973, 209–238, was not available to me.

[2]   AVIGAD, *IEJ* 28 (1978) 52–56.—From the same unknown place in Judah is also the seal of Jerahmeel, the king's son (Jer 36:26), published by Avigad in the same article. As far as I can judge, the identification is in both cases certain. For discussion, cf. also AVIGAD, *Hebrew Bullae,* 27–29, 128; *idem,* Contribution of Hebrew Seals, 199–102; SHANKS, *BARev* 13:5 (1987) 58–65; AVIGAD, Hebrew Seals, 11f.

[3]   Cf. LUNDBOM, *JSOT* 36 (1986) 107f.

[4]   Cf. also the images employed in e.g. 17:1, 13; 22:30; 31:33.

[5]   WEINFELD, *Deuteronomy,* 162. For broader discussion of this verse, see MC-KANE, *Prophets,* 102–112, and the critical comments by WHYBRAY, *Intellectual Tradition,* 22–24.

[6]   Cf. CODY, *Priesthood,* 119.

[7]   For the priests as teachers in the OT, cf. also e.g. Lev 10:10f; 14:57; Deut 17:9–11; 24:8; 31:9–13; 33:10; 2 Kgs 17:27; Ezek 7:26; 22:26; 44:23f; Hos 4:6; Mic 3:11; Zeph 3:4; Hag 2:10–13; Mal 2:7–9; 2 Chr 15:3; 17:7–9; 19:8–10; 35:3. Also Ezra was a priest (Ezra 7: 1–5, 11f; Neh 8:2, 9). For Ben Sira, see STADELMANN, *Ben Sira,* 12–26, 40–176; OLYAN, *HTR* 80 (1987) 261–286, and below pp. 46f.

[8]   Cf. 7:2; 19:14; 26:2, 7, 10; 28:1, 5; 35:2, 4.

[9]   VAN DER PLOEG, *RB* 54 (1947) 36, thinks of Jeremiah "comme un homme solitaire."

[10]   Cf. CARROLL, *Jeremiah,* 44f, 61.

[11]   Cf. MALLAU, *TRE* 5 (1980) 269f.

mention Baruch is noteworthy. This observation leads G. Wanke to the conclusion that Baruch was in fact closely associated with Jeremiah.[1] It is not only fiction. Whatever the exact historicity of the accounts, the texts themselves picture Baruch as the faithful follower of Jeremiah.

Other persons related to scribal families also appear. Seraiah, son of Neriah and thus a brother of Baruch, is presented as some kind of royal chief quartermaster at the court of Zedekiah (51:59). It is not certain that he actually was a scribe. The impression of his name found on a seal does not—like the seal of his brother—include the scribal title.[2] At any rate, the texts portray his close relation to Jeremiah. He is entrusted with a written oracle from the prophet (51:59–64). We may also notice Jeremiah's close association with the eminent scribal family of Shaphan.[3] Three of Shaphan's sons come to Jeremiah's aid:[4] Ahikam rescues Jeremiah in the face of a mortal threat (26:24); Elasah is one of the persons delivering Jeremiah's letter to the exiles (29:3); Gemariah allows his chamber in the temple court to be used for the reading of the scroll dictated by Jeremiah to Baruch (36:10),[5] and together with other officials, he protects Jeremiah and Baruch (36:12–19) and urges king Jehoiakim not to destroy the scroll (36:25).[6] Even Shaphan's grandchildren support Jeremiah (36:11, 13; 40:5f).

Certain texts might imply that Jeremiah's own family also is interested in the prophet. Although there is no statement claiming that Jeremiah serves as a priest himself, we do find that Jeremiah is the son of Hilkiah,[7] who is a member of the priestly family at Anathoth (1:1). We also come across other influential relatives.[8] With the possible exception of 11:18–12:6,[9] no text maintains that Jeremiah is openly hostile to these men. R.R. Wilson may go beyond the evidence when he regards them as Jeremiah's actual support group,[10] but the texts do picture them as keenly interested in the message and ministry of Jeremiah.

---

[1]　*Baruchschrift,* 147. Cf. also MALLAU, *TRE* 5 (1980) 271.

[2]　AVIGAD, *IEJ* 28 (1978) 56; *idem, ErIsr* 14 (1978) 86f.

[3]　Cf. MUILENBURG, Baruch the Scribe, 235f; METTINGER, *Officials,* 31–34; WILSON, *Prophecy,* 247f.

[4]　Perhaps Ezek 8:11 indicates a fourth son, Jaazaniah. His conduct, however, is rather different and the passage may be secondary. Cf. ZIMMERLI, *Ezekiel* I, 241.

[5]　There is not sufficient evidence to distinguish between two Gemariahs, one in 36:10 and another in 36:12, 25. See DEARMAN, *JBL* 109 (1990) 406 n. 8.

[6]　A seal impression probably identifying Gemariah has been found in the city of David. See SHILOH, *Excavations,* 20, 61, pl. 35:3. Cf. also *idem,* City of David, 461f; *idem, IEJ* 36 (1986) 33f; SHILOH/TARLER, *BA* 49 (1986) 204f. As the impression of Seraiah, it does not contain the scribal title. Cf. AVIGAD, *Hebrew Bullae,* 129 n. 164.

[7]　Cf. 2 Kgs 22:4–14; 23:4, 24. The identification of Jeremiah's father as the high priest of Josiah is however uncertain.

[8]　Cf. 32:6–15 (the uncle Shallum and the cousin Hanamel); 35:4 (the cousin Maaseiah); 21:1; 29:25f; 37:3 (the priest Zephaniah, son of Maaseiah).

[9]　Cf. HOLLADAY, *Jeremiah* I, 370f.

[10]　*Prophecy,* 233–235.

2.5. Ezekiel and His Followers

Two features make Ezekiel appear as a teacher. First, the image of the watchman (צֹפֶה) is used to describe the office of the prophet (3:17; 33:2, 6f). The didactic connotation of the image in Ezekiel emerges from its constant relation to הִזְהִיר, usually rendered "to enlighten" or "to warn."[1] This term is part of the Hebrew didactic terminology.[2] With one exception (Dan 12:3), the hiphil carries a didactic connotation in the OT (Exod 18:20; 2 Kgs 6:10; 2 Chr 19:10). Ezekiel is not only a watchman of warning, but also of teaching and interpretation. Second, Ezekiel's priestly background (1:3) might imply a teaching activity. The priests are in Ezekiel held—both positively and negatively—responsible for the instruction (תּוֹרָה) of the people (7:26; 22:26; 44:23f). 22:26 uses הוֹדִיעַ for priestly instruction, and this is the term that 16:2; 43:11 employ for Ezekiel's address to the people. Although this feature does not necessarily suggest the teaching of certain doctrines, it allows for the assumption that Ezekiel performed some kind of priestly teaching.[3]

The book of Ezekiel occasionally speaks of people attentively gathered around the prophet. The texts describe the elders of the people (8:1; 14:1; 20:1) and the people themselves (33:31) as assembled in a formal gathering, sometimes in the prophet's own house.[4] They sit in front of (יֹשְׁבִים לְפָנַי) Ezekiel, just as the sons of the prophets sat in front of their master Elisha (2 Kgs 4:38; 6:1).[5] Some of Ezekiel's activity appears to be addressed to larger audiences.[6] But there is also indication of a more limited activity, restricted to his own house and directed to a group of attentive listeners gathered in front of him.[7]

23:45 provides perhaps a reference to a Zadokite support group.[8] Certain righteous men (אֲנָשִׁים צַדִּיקִם) occur as judges of the sinful sisters—the people of Israel and Judah. The Zadokites receive a positive evaluation in Ezekiel.[9] The priestly character of the book of Ezekiel points in the same direction.[10]

---

[1] SIMIAN-YOFRE, Wächter, Lehrer oder Interpret?, 151–162.
[2] Cf. ZUCK, *BSac* 121 (1964) 229f.
[3] Cf. CODY, *Priesthood,* 118f.—ZIMMERLI, *Ezekiel* I, 71, understands Ezek 18, 33:1–20 as pieces of didactic instruction given by Ezekiel, and thus as further indications of Ezekiel's role as teacher.
[4] Cf. also 3:24 and GEVARYAHU, *ASTI* 12 (1983) 7.
[5] In 2 Kgs 6:32 the elders sit with (יֹשְׁבִים אֵת) Elisha in his house.
[6] Cf. Ezek 11:25. For the symbolic acts of Ezekiel as a kind of street theatre, see LANG, Street Theater, 297–316.
[7] Cf. ZIMMERLI, *TRE* 10 (1982) 769.
[8] WILSON, *Prophecy,* 285.
[9] Cf. e.g. 40:46; 43:19; 44:15f; 48:11.
[10] Cf. ZIMMERLI, *Studien* II, 169; *idem, Ezekiel* I, 52; *idem, Ezekiel* II, 552.

2.6. Jesus ben Sira and His "Sons"

Sirach reflects in its Greek translation[1] to some extent the Hebrew text[2] written by a person commonly called Jesus b. Sira,[3] active in Jerusalem[4] during the early decades of the second century B.C.E. To the ancient readers/hearers of the text, Ben Sira must have emerged as a devout scholar of wisdom. Even the first known reader/hearer of his words expresses this view (Prol. 7–11). Partly in reference to himself, Ben Sira also praises the wisdom that the scribe acquires through intensive professional study (38:24–39:5). The frequent use of wisdom terminology and wisdom concepts places Ben Sira within broad streams of sapiential influences, Jewish and extra-Jewish.[5] The scribe is now an intellectual, a scholar.[6]

Ben Sira's scholarly devotion is combined with his teaching activity.[7] The scribe is also a teacher (39:8) and Ben Sira says about himself that his knowledge became so vast and overflowing that he shared his education and teaching with all those who were seeking wisdom (24:30–34).[8] The hymn closing the book describes Ben Sira's own striving for wisdom and invites those untrained to the house of education, to Ben Sira's yeshivah (51:23, 29).[9]

Perhaps the attentive reader/hearer would connect Ben Sira's teaching

---

[1] For discussion of the relationship between the Greek and the Hebrew, see B.G. WRIGHT, *No Small Difference.*

[2] For discussion of the Hebrew text, see DI LELLA, *Hebrew Text;* RÜGER, *Text und Textform.*

[3] The name varies in different passages. Cf. Prol. 7; Sir 50:27; 51:30. For discussion, see Rudolf SMEND, *Weisheit des Jesus Sirach erklärt,* xivf; SKEHAN/DI LELLA, *Wisdom of Ben Sira,* 3f; MACK, Sirach, 66. I will use the expression "Ben Sira."

[4] 24:10f states that wisdom has found its permanent dwelling-place in Zion/Jerusalem. The Greek of 50:27 inserts the explanatory gloss ὁ Ἱεροσολυμίτης.

[5] For a list of Ben Sira's wisdom terminology and pericopes, see MARBÖCK, *Weisheit im Wandel,* 13–16. For Ben Sira's relation to Jewish and extra-Jewish thinking, cf. the different positions taken by e.g. PAUTREL, *RSR* 51 (1963) 535–549; MARBÖCK, *ibid.,* 160–173; MIDDENDORP, *Stellung Jesu Ben Siras, passim;* HENGEL, *Judaism and Hellenism* I, 138–153, 157–162; *idem, JSJ* 5 (1974) 83–87; JACOB, Wisdom and Religion, 248–253; HENGEL, *Jews, Greeks and Barbarians,* 121–123; GOLDSTEIN, Jewish Acceptance and Rejection, 72–75; KAISER, Gottesgewißheit, 77f; *idem, VF* 27 (1982) 79–85; J.T. SANDERS, *Ben Sira and Demotic Wisdom, passim;* MACK, *Wisdom,* 78–80, 91f, 111–137, 166; LEE, *Form of Sirach 44–50,* 243–245; MACK/MURPHY, Wisdom Literature, 374f; SKEHAN/DI LELLA, *Wisdom of Ben Sira,* 40–50, and the discussion below pp. 85–87. The view of older scholars is rehearsed by PAUTREL, *ibid.,* 535–537.

[6] For a survey of the discussion about the scribes, see SCHNABEL, *Law and Wisdom,* 63–69. Cf. also e.g. FISHBANE, *Biblical Interpretation,* 23–37; BAR-ILAN, Writing in Ancient Israel, 21–24; LIPIŃSKI, Scribes, 157–164; SALDARINI, *Pharisees, Scribes and Sadducees,* 241–276; ORTON, *Understanding Scribe;* GAMMIE/PERDUE (eds.), *Sage in Israel;* VON LIPS, *Weisheitliche Traditionen,* 63–65.

[7] LANG, *Monotheism,* 152, wrongly speaks of Ben Sira as "a private scholar."

[8] Cf. LÖHR, *Bildung aus dem Glauben,* 46.

[9] For the school of Ben Sira, see below pp. 67–69.

activity with a priestly profession. We have observed numerous OT references implying the didactic functions of the priests.[1] There are even sporadic statements about contacts between wisdom circles and priests (Jer 18:18). During the post-exilic period, the temple may have taken over educational responsibilities earlier related to the court.[2] H. Stadelmann and S.M. Olyan have argued that Ben Sira regarded himself as a priest.[3] Although the question has been the object of much debate and no explicit evidence can be given,[4] we should notice that Ben Sira is well informed about the priestly functions and supports the temple, the priesthood and the cult.[5] Perhaps some of the lyric forms used in the book derive from cultic settings.[6]

It is possible to regard major parts of Sirach as composed for didactic purposes. Prol. 12–14 describes the book as directed towards those who strive for education and wisdom. Although Ben Sira's scholarly activity appears partly as an exegetical search in the Scriptures[7] and as an attempt to comprehend the meshalim,[8] popular education is a key-concept throughout the book.[9] The use of Sirach at Masada might suggest that it was early the object of deliberate study, and perhaps memorized.[10] This would be of no surprise in view of the didactic, catechetical and mnemonic forms it contains.[11] We could also mention the repetitions (2:7–18), the pedagogical questions (10:19–29; 36:8) and the acrosticon (51:13–30).[12]

Sirach also speaks of pupils. The recipients of Ben Sira's teaching are repeatedly addressed "(my) son" (בני/τέκνον), "sons" (בנים/τέκνα).[13] To be sure, this designation may suggest that the recipients of the teaching are

---

1   Cf. above p. 43 n. 7.

2   Cf. excursus 2 below.

3   STADELMANN, *Ben Sira,* 12–26, 40–176; OLYAN, *HTR* 80 (1987) 261–286.

4   The variant ὁ ἱερεὺς ὁ σολυμείτης in 50:27 is secondary.

5   Cf. 7:9f, 29–31 (14:11[G]); 24:10f, 15; 35:6–11(G32:8–13); 38:11; 45:6–26; 46:16; 47:2; 49:1; 50:1–24. For a survey of the discussion about the relations between cult and wisdom, see VON LIPS, *Weisheitliche Traditionen,* 46–51.

6   Cf. BAUMGARTNER, *ZAW* 34 (1914) 169–186.

7   Cf. 2:16; 3:21; 32(G35):15 (דורש תורה/ὁ ζητῶν νόμον); 39:1.—The use of דרש to denote exegetical study of the Scriptures is prominent at Qumran and probably present also here. Cf. SCHIFFMAN, *Halakhah at Qumran,* 55f, and below p. 74. For discussion of its significance in Sirach, see STADELMANN, *Ben Sira,* 252–255.

8   Cf. 1:25; 3:29 (13:26[G]); 20:20; 38:33–39:3; 47:15, 17. For emphases on the scribe's task to understand meshalim in Sirach, see BICKERMAN, *Jews,* 168; ORTON, *Understanding Scribe,* 67f.

9   Cf. (Prol. 3, 12, 29) Sir 1:27; 4:17, 24; 6:18; 8:8; 16:25; 18:14, etc.

10   So MIDDENDORP, *Stellung Jesu Ben Siras,* 32f, 98f.

11   STADELMANN, *Ben Sira,* 308.

12   Does the Hebrew text of 51:29 indicate that cantillation was practised in the yeshivah of Ben Sira? Cf. the translation of the text below p. 67.

13   Cf. 2:1; 3:1; 3:17; 4:1, 20; 6:18, 23(G), 32; 10:28; 11:10; 14:11; 16:24(G); 18:15; 21:1; 23:7; 31(G34):22; 37:27; 38:9, 16; 40:28; 41:14. In 39:13(G) they are addressed as υἱοὶ ὅσιοι.

young men starting their pursuit of wisdom. But it is also the traditional manner in wisdom literature for calling the students to attention.[1] Ben Sira's ethical admonitions further convey the impression that the teaching is directed to persons able to take moral responsibility. 7:15 even indicates that they can be active in practical occupations. Stadelmann locates them in the upper middle-class of Jerusalem.[2]

2.7. The Righteous Teacher and the Qumran Community

The Dead Sea scrolls often use different forms of מורה to refer to some kind of teacher: the Damascus Document uses מורה (20:28), מורה צדק (1:11; 20:32), יוריהם (20:1) יוריהם (3:8), יורה הצדק (6:11) and יורה היחיד (20:14); the commentary on Habakkuk mentions a certain מורה הצדק(ה) (1:13; 2:2; 5:10; 7:4; 8:3; 9:9f; 11:5); 1QpMic 8–10:6 gives the orthographic variation מורי הצדק;[3] 4QpIsaᶜ (4Q163) 21:6 uses מורה; 4QpHosᵇ (4Q167) 5–6:2 refers to מוריהם; 4QpPsᵃ 3:15, 19; 4:27 read, most likely, מורה הצדק; the same expression appears in 4QpPsᵇ 1:4 and probably in 4QpPsᵇ 2:2.

Although these instances refer to a teacher, not all of them concern the human teacher appearing in the history of the community, the Righteous Teacher.[4] 4QpIsᶜ (4Q163) 21:6; 4QpHosᵇ (4Q167) 5–6:2 occur in contexts too fragmentary to give the term a clear referent. The context of CD 3:8 gives the impression that "their teacher" refers to God. Also CD 2:12; 3:13f; 6:3; 7:4; 20:4 picture God as revealer and instructor. Other documents indicate that the members of the community regard God as teacher and understand themselves as God's disciples.[5] I will discuss CD 6:11 below,[6] but we should note already here that this passage hardly provides a direct reference to the Righteous Teacher. The rest of the instances, however, probably refer to the Righteous Teacher.[7]

---

1   For Proverbs, see above p. 37 n. 9. For the Dead Sea scrolls, see below p. 52. This designation is also common in other wisdom writings.

2   *Ben Sira,* 27–39.

3   For this form of מורה, see G. JEREMIAS, *Lehrer der Gerechtigkeit,* 147 n. 3.

4   I prefer to translate מורה הצדק with "the Righteous Teacher" instead of "the Teacher of Righteousness." For arguments, see below pp. 119–122.

5   For God as teacher, cf. e.g. 1QH 2:17; 4:27f; 6:9; 7:10, 26f; 10:4–7, 14; 11:4; 12:33; 1QS 4:22; 10:13; 11:17f; 1QSb 3:23; 11QPsᵃ 19:2f; 24:9. The Temple scroll presents God as the sole legislator, though this document may be of pre-Qumranic origin. For the members of the community as God's disciples, cf. 1QH 2:39; 7:10, 14(?); 8:36; 1QM 10:10.—Some scholars think of CD 3:8 as a reference to Moses as teacher. This is unlikely.

6   See pp. 126f, 129f.

7   I. RABINOWITZ, *VT* 8 (1958), 393f, thinks that the term denotes a guide. But guidance becomes effective by virtue of the teaching (CD 1:11). And outside of the scrolls, the meaning of the term favoured by Rabinowitz is, as far as I know, not the primary one. It is questionable if מורה is the Semitic counterpart of καθηγητής in Matt 23:10. See

A.-M. Denis, J. Murphy-O'Connor and others believe that also CD 20:28 is a reference to God as teacher.[1] I regard it as unlikely. God is nowhere else called מורה, only יוריהם (CD 3:8). And it is not possible to claim that the teacher (מורה) and God (אל) are parallel in CD 20:28. The people listen to the teacher but confess before God. Of importance is, as I will explain later,[2] that CD 20:28 probably parallels CD 20:32, which explicitly speaks of מורה צדק. This observation leads even P.R. Davies, who in his own work on the Damascus Document often builds on Murphy-O'Connor, to regard a reference to God as teacher in CD 20:28 as "improbable."[3]

The didactic understanding of the Righteous Teacher emerges not only from the use of מורה, but also from the depiction of him as a wise scribe. Although the term חכמה is not common in the scrolls, wisdom teaching is important for the community. The scrolls use other semantically related terms (השכיל, הבין, הודיע, הורה, ירה, למד).[4] Sometimes these terms refer to God, who as teacher gives revelation (of wisdom) to members of the community;[5] sometimes we find similar designations for a community functionary or different functionaries assigned a didactic task.[6]

These general wisdom features make it natural to estimate the person giving the group its internal identity in similar categories. The Righteous Teacher appears as an eminent scribe.[7] A commentary on Psalm 45:2 in 4QpPsᵃ 4:27 applies the term סופר, "scribe," to מורה הצדק.[8] 4QpPsᵃ 1:19

---

[1]   DENIS, *Thèmes de connaissance,* 176; MURPHY-O'CONNOR, *RB* 79 (1972) 559 n. 50. Cf. also e.g. KNIBB, *Qumran Community,* 76; CALLAWAY, *History of the Qumran Community,* 114; *idem, RevQ* 14 (1990) 641.

[2]   See below pp. 189f.

[3]   *Damascus Covenant,* 195. Davies' pre-Qumranic dating of the Damascus Document causes him to regard וישמעו לקול מורה (20:28) as an addition to the pre-Qumranic conclusion of the Admonitions (CD 1–8, 19–20).

[4]   For wisdom and wisdom teaching at Qumran, see LIPSCOMB/SANDERS, Wisdom at Qumran, 277–285; ROMANIUK, *RevQ* 9 (1978) 429–435. Cf. also LÜHRMANN, *ZAW* 80 (1968) 90–97; KÜCHLER, *Frühjüdische Weisheitstraditionen,* 88–109; J.A. DAVIS, *Wisdom and Spirit,* 29–44; SCHNABEL, *Law and Wisdom,* 190–226; SANDELIN, *Wisdom as Nourisher,* 54–70; VON LIPS, *Weisheitliche Traditionen,* 130f; NEWSOM, Sage, 373–382; MENZIES, *Early Christian Pneumatology,* 84–87. The dissertations by J.E. WORRELL, *Concepts of Wisdom in the Dead Sea Scrolls.* Claremont Graduate School 1968, and S.J. TANZER, *The Sages at Qumran.* Wisdom in the "Hodayot." Harvard University 1986, were not available to me.

[5]   For references, cf. above p. 48 n. 5.

[6]   For the Maskil (משכיל), cf. CD 12:21; 13:22; 1QS 1:1(?); 3:13; 9:12–20; 4Q298 1:1. For the teaching function of the guardian (פקיד, מבקר), cf. CD 13:6–8; 1QS 6:14f; 4Q266 line 16. I do not need to discuss the relationship between the different designations.

[7]   ORTON, *Understanding Scribe,* 124–130.

[8]   ORTON, *Understanding Scribe,* 124, claims that the term סופר "is not used of the Essene leader in the extant scrolls." Unfortunately Orton has not noticed the present passage. It would have given support to his general thesis. NIEHR, *TWAT* V, 929; KARRER, *ZNW* 83 (1992) 15, state that the term does not occur at all in the scrolls. To be sure, 4QpPsᵃ 4:27 is somewhat corrupt, but the presence of סופר is most likely since the begining of Ps 45:2b (לשוני עם), which contains סופר, is explicitly referred to at the end of the previous line.

probably calls the Teacher מליץ דעת, "interpreter of knowledge." The scribal assessment of the Teacher emerges also through the use of מחוקק, "sceptre," and דורש התורה, "interpreter of the Torah," in CD 6:2–11, if we take them as references to the Teacher.[1] As regards מחוקק, it is noteworthy that Sir 10:5 translates this term with γραμματεύς and—even more—that the tannaitic midrashim and the targumim, with only one exception (Judg 5:14), understand all OT passages using the term (Gen 49:10; Num 21:18; Deut 33:21; Isa 33:22; Pss 60:9; 108:9) as references to scribal torah teaching.[2] As regards דורש התורה, we should notice that Ezra, the scribe, according to Ezra 7:10 regards it as his task to interpret—search out—the Torah of Yahweh (לדרוש את תורת יהוה).[3]

The didactic assessment of the Righteous Teacher might relate to the depiction of him as priest. 2 Chr 15:3 (כהן מורה) and the hiphil of ירה, which is frequently used to denote directions delivered by priests (Lev 10:11; 14:57; Deut 17:10f; 24:8; 33:10; Ezek 44:23), indicate that the very term מורה may be read/heard against priestly connotations in the OT.[4] 4QpPsa 3:15; 4QpPsb 1:4f connect positively מורה הצדק and (ה)כוהן.[5] 1QpHab 2:8 calls an important person within the community הכוהן.[6] 4QpPsa 2:18 refers to such a person with בכוהן.[7]

> There is some indication for understanding the Teacher as being of Zadokite lineage, though the scrolls never say this explicitly.[8] First, the identity of a certain Zadok points in this direction. The name Zadok appears by itself three times. 3Q15 11:3, 6 refer to the tomb of Zadok. CD 5:5 mentions Zadok in a statement about the sealed book of the torah which was kept in the ark and not revealed until the coming of Zadok. Scholars give different suggestions concerning the identity of Zadok in CD 5:5.[9] Y. Yadin and—more explicitly—B.Z. Wacholder, on one hand, identify him with the Teacher.[10] J.C. Vanderkam and J. Maier, on the other hand, dispute any futuristic

---

1   See below pp. 126f.

2   For references, see VERMES, *Scripture and Tradition,* 51–55. Cf. also O. BETZ, *Offenbarung und Schriftforschung,* 27–35; G. JEREMIAS, *Lehrer der Gerechtigkeit,* 272f; ORTON, *Understanding Scribe,* 54f, 127; FISHBANE, Scribalism, 453 n. 24.—The meaning of מחוקק in 4QGenFlor (4Q252) 5:2 is different.

3   Cf. also Sir 32(G35):15.

4   Cf. also Mic 3:11.

5   4QpPsb 1:5 is somewhat corrupt and does not have the definite article in front of כוהן.

6   1QpHab 2:2 mentions the Teacher explicitly.

7   Cf. also the expression "the last priest" (כוהן האחרון) in 4QpHosb (4Q167) 2:3. But it is uncertain if the expression refers to the Teacher. The impression given is rather opposite to the one given in 4QpPsa 2:17–19.

8   DIMANT, Qumran Sectarian Literature, 545f n. 292; J.M. BAUMGARTEN, *ANRW* II 19:1 (1979) 233–236, are critical to the assumption that the Teacher actually was a Zadokite.

9   For surveys of different proposals, see WERNBERG-MØLLER, *VT* 3 (1953) 314f; VANDERKAM, *RevQ* 11 (1984) 561–564; J. MAIER, *RevQ* 15 (1991) 234–237.

10   YADIN (ed.), *Temple Scroll* I, 395; WACHOLDER, *Dawn of Qumran,* 99–140; YADIN, *Temple Scroll,* 228; WACHOLDER, *RevQ* 12 (1986) 351–368. Cf. also J.M.

connotations in CD 5:2–5 and interpret the passage as referring to the priest of David[1] or the beginning of the Zadokite high priest office.[2] Perhaps a middle way is appropriate. An allusion to David's priest clearly appears.[3] CD 5:2–5 relates Zadok to David and identifies the sealed book locked up in the ark with Deuteronomy or perhaps the whole Pentateuch.[4] But the OT connects Zadok only indirectly with the bringing of the ark from the Philistines to Kiriath-jearim (1 Sam 6:21–7:2), and later to Jerusalem (2 Sam 6:1–19; 1 Chr 13:1–16:42).[5] A future allusion to the appearance of the Teacher is therefore possible.[6] Although it is difficult to identify the sealed book of the torah with the Temple scroll, it seems clear that a certain Zadok should bring important teaching to the community. If this interpretation is correct, is is possible to associate the Teacher with the Zadokite priesthood. Second, a number of times there is a strong emphasis on the sons of Zadok (בני צדוק). They occur as a leading group in the community (1QS 5:2, 9; 1QSa 1:2, 24; 2:3; 1QSb 3:22; 4QFlor 1:17).[7] The expression "sons of Zadok" might have been coined on the basis of Ezek 44:15 (CD 3:21–4:4) and is perhaps historically related to a struggle against the illegitimate Hasmonean priesthood.[8] If my interpretation of CD 5:2–5 contains some truth, this expression connects the "sons" both with the Teacher and the Zadokite priesthood. It is noteworthy that the expression בני צדוק is not entirely fixed. Also בני צדק occurs (1QS 3:20, 22). A variant of 1QS 9:14 from cave four (4QS[e]) contains בני הצדק instead of בני צדוק.[9] These variations suggest that the leading group is sometimes associated with the Zadokite priesthood and sometimes with the Righteous Teacher.[10] Third, it is possible to regard the Teacher as a high priest. There are not only texts using the absolute הכוהן for the wicked priest (1QpHab 8:8, 16; 9:9; 11:4, 12; 12:2, 8; 4QpPs[a] 4:8[?]). 4QpPs[a] 3:15 uses it for the Teacher.[11] H. Stegemann has tried to demonstrate that the term always denotes the high priest in the pesharim.[12] Although the correctness and usefulness of Stegemann's analysis is uncertain today,[13] 1QpHab 11:4–8 might imply that the Teacher performs high-priestly functions on the day of Atonement as it is celebrated at Qumran.

In view of the strong didactic identity given to the Righteous Teacher in the scrolls, it is obvious that the members of the community should appear as his pupils. True, the published scrolls do not speak about disciples or pupils of the Righteous Teacher. The Qumranites are presented as disciples of

---

BAUMGARTEN, *ANRW* II 19:1 (1979) 235f.

[1] VANDERKAM, *RevQ* 11 (1984) 561–570.

[2] J. MAIER, *RevQ* 15 (1991) 231–241.

[3] Cf. 2 Sam 8:17; 15:24f, 27, 29, etc.

[4] Cf. STEGEMANN, Origins of the Temple Scroll, 245 n. 70.

[5] But cf. 2 Sam 15:24f, 29.

[6] J. MAIER, *RevQ* 15 (1990) 240f, ventures some possible polemical intentions of the historical depiction.

[7] For the superior status of the sons of Zadok, see LIVER, *RevQ* 6 (1967) 4–7.

[8] So SCHWARTZ, Priestly View of Descent, 159f.—LIVER, *RevQ* 6 (1967) 24–30, tries to reduce the anti-Hasmonean background.

[9] For this fragment, see MILIK, *RB* 67 (1960) 414.

[10] Cf. J.M. BAUMGARTEN, Recent Qumran Discoveries, 152.

[11] Cf. also 1QpHab 2:8; 4QpPs[a] 2:18.

[12] *Entstehung der Qumrangemeinde,* 102 nn. 328, 329.

[13] See WISE, *RevQ* 14 (1990) 587–602. Cf. also J.J. COLLINS, Origin, 165–167; SIEVERS, *The Hasmoneans,* 76.

God (CD 20:4),[1] sometimes in clear allusion to Isa 50:4 (1QH 7:10, 14[?]; 8:36).[2] They form a brotherhood (CD 6:20–7:3; 1QS 6:10, 22; 1QSa 1:18), with all the members on the same level as disciples of God.[3] However, we also gain the impression that they are attached to the teaching believed to have originated with the Teacher.[4] Perhaps they are addressed as his "sons" (בנים), as may be indicated if we read/hear CD 2:14 as an utterance from the Teacher.[5] In addition, if they are eager to know the divine mysteries, they must listen to the Teacher to whom special revelation has been given (1QpHab 2:2f; 7:4–8). He has come to lead them on the way of God (CD 1:11). They are to listen to his teaching for their own salvation (CD 6:7–10; 20:27–34; 1QpHab 2:2; 8:1–3; 1QpMic 8–10:6f; 4QpPs[a] 1:19).

> Early Qumran scholars often understood the phrase "their faith in the Righteous Tea-cher" (אמנתם במורה הצדק) in 1QpHab 8:2f as salvific faith in the person of the Tea-cher, with allusions to the Pauline concept of faith in (πίστις ἐν) Jesus Christ.[6] But the expression probably refers to faith in the teaching of the Teacher. The commentary on Habbakkuk uses the hiphil of אמן on three occasions (2:4, 6, 14). The object, in-dicated with ב, is nowhere a person. It is always an impersonal object representing the will of God.[7]

2.8. The Rabbis and Their Pupils

The rabbinic literature pictures the rabbis as scholars. They devote them-selves entirely to the study of different aspects of torah. This is their basic and primary task.

Perhaps the clearest testimony of this uniform view of the rabbis is the absence of a variety of labels attributed to them. The term מורה occurs oc-

---

1 Cf. also 1QH 2:39; 1QM 10:10.

2 Cf. the allusion (במעני לשן) in reference to the Teacher in 4QpPs[a] 4:27 .

3 Cf. KAPELRUD, *TWAT* IV, 581f.

4 Cf. ZUMSTEIN, *Relation du maître et du disciple,* 67–69; 77–80; FISHBANE, Mikra at Qumran, 361f.

5 So LEMAIRE, L'enseignement essénien, 196. Cf. also 4Q525 1:12.—In 1QH 5:24 the "I" claims to be surrounded by a specific group of individuals who are called "those joined to my assembly" (נצמדי סודי) and "men of my council" (אנשי [עצ]תי) or perhaps "men of my covenant" (אנשי [ברי]תי). 1QH 5:23 mentions more generally "my friends" (רעי), "those who entered my covenant" (באי בריתי), "all those who have come together around me" (כול נועדי) and "those who ate my bread" ([או]כלי לחמי). But these expres-sions do not depict a specifically didactic relationship.

6 For surveys of the discussion, see G. JEREMIAS, *Lehrer der Gerechtigkeit,* 142f; H. BRAUN, *Qumran und das Neue Testament* I, 169f.

7 For further discussion, see G. JEREMIAS, *Lehrer der Gerechtigkeit,* 142–146; Jürgen BECKER, *Heil Gottes,* 176–180. Cf. also the similar conclusions by e.g. W.D. DAVIES, *Setting of the Sermon on the Mount,* 217–219; H. BRAUN, *Qumran und das Neue Testament* II, 171f; THYEN, *Sün-denvergebung,* 85; ZIESLER, *Meaning of Righteousness,* 103; FISHBANE, Scribalism, 451.

casionally,[1] but it is rare.[2] The label "father" (אב) is more common.[3] It often appears in relation to the name of early scholars.[4] But its frequency as a designation for early masters should be compared with a developing tendency to avoid it for the rabbis.[5] Nowhere is it used to address a rabbi.[6] A baraita in b. Ber. 16b even pictures a sporadic attempt to restrict its use to Abraham, Isaac and Jacob only. The targumim, though merely of indirect value here, replace אבי with רבוני/רבי or מרי when it occurs as an address to Saul (Tg. Neb. 1 Sam 24:12), Elijah (Tg. Neb. 2 Kgs 2:12), Naaman (Tg. Neb. 2 Kgs 5:13) and Elisha (Tg. Neb. 2 Kgs 6:21; 13:14). As it seems, only one label becomes, with some variations, prominent in rabbinic writings: "Rabbi" (רבי), "Rab" (רב) or "Rabban" (רבן). And it functions to a large extent merely as a title for the qualifed scholar.

The scholarly devotion is not an end in itself. It is an integral part of the teaching activity. Numerous texts present the rabbis as teachers studying and transmitting torah together with a group of pupils. The well-known statement attributed to the early sage Joshua b. Peraḥiah (c. 104–78 B.C.E.)—together with Nittai of Arbela (c. 110 B.C.E.) one of the five pairs (זוגות)—in m. ʾAbot 1:6 is characteristic:

עשה לך רב	Set up for yourself a teacher
וקנה לך חבר	and get yourself a companion.[7]

Study is not a private matter.[8] Advanced study generally takes place under the guidance of a recognized teacher and in close association with fellow-students.[9] The primary term used for a rabbinic disciple, תלמיד, mostly refers to a person who wants to learn torah.[10] We find a teacher and a group of learning pupils. The texts picture a setting that is didactic and collegiate.

Excursus 1: *Joshua as the Pupil of Moses*

Joshua appears in some Jewish writings as the pupil of Moses. We find this both in

---

[1] Cf. e.g. b. Ketub. 23a, 79a; y. Šabb. 11b; y. Šeqal. 47c, 51a.

[2] DALMAN, *Worte Jesu*, 276; G. JEREMIAS, *Lehrer der Gerechtigkeit*, 316.

[3] Cf. KOHLER, *JQR* 13 (1901) 567–580; STRACK/BILLERBECK, *Kommentar* I, 918f; DALMAN, *Worte Jesu*, 278f; BONSIRVEN, *Judaïsme Palestinien* I, 274f; SCHRENK, *TDNT* V, 977f; SCHÜRER, *History* II, 327; RIESNER, *Lehrer*, 109f.

[4] Best known is perhaps Abba Saul, designated thus already in m. Peʾa 8:5; m. Kil. 2:3; m. Šabb. 23:3; m. Šeqal. 4:2; m. Beṣa 3:8; m. ʾAbot 2:8; m. Mid. 2:5; 5:4, etc.

[5] Cf. already KOHLER, *JQR* 13 (1901) 580.

[6] Its occurrence in b. Mak. 24a is secondary. Cf. STRACK/BILLERBECK, *Kommentar* I, 919.—Sifre on Deut 6:7 is not relevant here. Cf. Joachim JEREMIAS, *Abba*, 44 n. 64.

[7] Cf. also m. ʾAbot 1:16; ʾAbot R. Nat. A 8.

[8] Cf. ABERBACH, Relations Between Master and Disciple, 7f.

[9] Cf. e.g. m. ʾAbot 6:5; b. Ber. 63b; b. Šabb. 63a; 147b; b. Taʿan. 7a, 8a; b. Ketub. 111a; b. Mak. 10a; ʾAbot R. Nat. A 12, 14; Sifre on Deut 31:14; Gen. Rab. 69:2; Qoh. Rab. on 7:7.

[10] RENGSTORF, *TDNT* IV, 431f.

Josephus' (Ant. 6:84)[1] and in the rabbinic writings (Sifre on Num 27:18, 23; Sifre on Deut 31:14; Sifre Zuṭ. on 27:18f; Deut. Rab. 11:10).[2] Although it is impossible to determine the historicity of the relationship between Moses and Joshua,[3] the later Jewish texts picture it to some extent in the same way as the OT itself.[4]

The terminology in the OT is noteworthy.[5] It is as נער, "a young boy," that Joshua follows Moses (Exod 33:11). This is exactly the term used for a follower of Elijah (1 Kgs 18:43). Gehazi is also regularly called the נער of Elisha (2 Kgs 4:12, 25; 5:20; 8:4).[6] Furthermore, Joshua repeatedly occurs as the משרת, "servant," of Moses (Exod 24:13; 33:11; Num 11:28; Josh 1:1).[7] The same root (שרת) describes Elisha's service to Elijah (1 Kgs 19:21). A followers of Elisha may also occasionally be called משרת (2 Kgs 4:43; 6:15).[8]

Joshua is with Moses in intimate places, as Moses climbs the mountain (Exod 24:13; 32:17) or enters the tent (Exod 33:11; Num 11:28; Deut 31:14). According to Exod 17:14, Joshua is even entrusted with a memorial (זכרון)[9] to be recited to others.[10] Filled with spirit (Num 27:18) of wisdom (Deut 34:9), he finally takes over the office from Moses (Num 27:12–23; Deut 1:38; 31:7f, 23; 34:9). He has been prepared for his task, before he is publicly appointed at the express command of Yahweh (Num 27:15–21).[11]

Some texts picture Moses as a servant of Yahweh.[12] Although this expresses a status of honour, it also implies that the words of Moses receive their importance through his dependence on Yahweh. Joshua therefore occasionally introduces his utterances with reference to what Yahweh himself, not Moses, said (Josh 24:2).

But the book of Joshua also conveys the impression that Joshua continues to be bound both to Moses' person and teaching after the death of the master. Joshua occurs in a typological relation to Moses.[13] Although the texts do not picture him as a second Moses, they portray a figure like Moses:[14] just as the people obeyed Moses, they now obey Joshua (Josh 1:17); just as Moses (Exod 19:10), Joshua makes the people consecrate themselves before an important event (Josh 3:5; 7:13); just as Moses (Deut

---

1   Cf. also Ant. 3:49 and the discussion by FELDMAN, *HTR* 82 (1989) 351–376.

2   Cf. also m. Abot 1:1; Mek. on 12:1 (Lauterbach I, 14:151) and the discussion by LOHSE, *Ordination*, 25–27.

3   For surveys of the discussion concerning the "historical Joshua," see SOGGIN, *Joshua*, 14–18; DONNER, *Geschichte*, 127f.

4   RIESNER, *Lehrer*, 278f. Differently RENGSTORF, *TDNT* IV, 427f.

5   For Joshua as the follower of Moses in the Pentateuch, see SCHÄFER-LICHTEN-BERGER, *ZAW* 101 (1989) 206–210.

6   CD 8:20f maintains this understanding of Gehazi.

7   Sir 46:1 maintains this understanding of Joshua.

8   Cf. WESTERMANN, *THAT* II, 1020.

9   On the force of זכרון, see CHILDS, *Memory*, 66–70; SCHOTTROFF, *'Gedenken'*, 299–328, esp. 305.

10   Cf. GANDZ, *PAAJR* 7 (1935–36) 6–8.

11   The public appointment at the command of Yahweh is a feature emphasized by RENGSTORF, *TDNT* IV, 427f, to the extent that Joshua cannot be understood as a disciple of Moses.

12   Exod 4:10; 14:31; Num 11:11; 12:7f; Josh 1:1f, 7, 13, 15, 8:31, etc.; 1 Kgs 8:53, 56; 2 Kgs 18:12; 21:8. For the use of this designation for Moses in the Dtr, see RIESE-NER, *Der Stamm* עבד, 186–191.

13   CHILDS, *Introduction*, 245.

14   RENDTORFF, *Old Testament*, 165.

9:25–29), Joshua intercedes for sinful Israel (Josh 7:6–9); just as Moses (Deut 31:1–33:29), Joshua gives his last will before his death (Josh 23:1–24:28). Moses' own teaching reaches also a normative status. It is essential for Joshua to follow the teaching of Moses exactly (Josh 1:7, 13; 4:10; 8:30–35; 11:15, etc.). Joshua depends on the law of Moses which assumes a decisive position. It is not to be separated from Joshua's mouth but meditated upon and obeyed (Josh 1:8). Joshua speaks of the book of the law from Moses as the guide for the people of Israel (Josh 23:6). Obedience or disobedience to this law determines their success or failure.

It seems quite certain, however, that the relationship between Joshua and Moses depicted in the OT did not constitute an *actual* setting of transmission. *This relationship is of little value in a phenomenological comparison of tradition and transmission.*

3. The Schools

Various people, among whom there were the ancient transmitters, wrote and read/heard several texts from ancient Israel and ancient Judaism as accounts about a teacher-pupil relationship. I have not yet discussed if the persons writing and reading/hearing these brief accounts actually identified themselves as pupils within the didactic interaction depicted in the texts. The expression "ancient transmitters" is still vague and without clear historical contours. We must now go outside of the textual world itself. The next question is if these didactic accounts corresponded to the manifest existence of schools.

I will speak of a "school" when the pupil appears *within a larger group of people basing its identity on the authority of a specific teacher.* I am not primarily interested in educational settings defining the institutional framework *apart* from the teacher.

It is not possible to relate each and every text speaking of a teacher-pupil relationship to a discussion about schools. And a detailed inquiry into the historicity of each account respectively would at any rate hardly yield much result. Evidence—and also space—allows only for a more general discussion.

3.1. The Schools of the Ancient Prophets

Settings of elementary and scribal education did normally not imply the undisputable authority of a single teacher in ancient Israel.[1] The person in charge of higher education was probably highly esteemed,[2] but he still re-

---

[1] For the existence of elementary and scribal schools in ancient Israel, see excursus 2 below.

[2] LEMAIRE, *Écoles*, 54–57, makes a distinction beween teachers in charge of higher education and of local elementary education. While the former were highly respected, the latter were not. For a similar phenomenon in Greek education, see NILSSON, *Schule*, 53; MARROU, *History*, 145–147. For later Jewish education, see RIESNER, *Lehrer*, 185f.

mained nothing more than one teacher among many, and he could be replaced.[1] The goal of education was merely to provide knowledge and skill.[2] Certainly, the teachers could carry out their task with authority and refined methods of persuasion.[3] But the teacher is usually anonymous in the present texts. The teaching was essentially *independent* of the teacher himself.

A pupil of a prophetic teacher could not separate teacher and teaching to the same degree. A. Lemaire concludes his account of the schools during the time of the monarchy by pointing to the distinctive feature of the prophetic school and stressing that the prophets conveyed their teaching through deep personal involvement.[4]

However, the possibility that prophetic disciples formed a kind of school has for a long time been a matter of debate.[5] Scandinavian scholars recognized the importance of the prophetic disciples early. In 1926 S. Mowinckel brought attention to such a group around Isaiah.[6] J. Lindblom later agreed and assumed "that as a rule the classical prophets were surrounded by a circle of disciples who had attached themselves to the great prophetic personalities, regarding them as their teachers and masters."[7] These groups were, according to Lindblom, the continuation of the sons of the prophets, though with the difference that they now "occupied themselves with other and more important matters,"[8] i.e. the transmission of the prophetic traditions.[9] Other scholars remain sceptical. R.E. Clements has repeatedly pointed to the meagre evidence. The general existence of such disciples has

---

1   Cf. the plurality of teachers mentioned in Prov 5:13.
2   DEMSKY, *EncJud* VI, 385.
3   CRENSHAW, Wisdom and Authority, 10–29.
4   *Écoles,* 70f: "A la différence des écoles royales et sacerdotales, dont l'enseignement, surtout celui de l'école sacerdotale, devait être assez fixe et stéréotypé, impersonnel, l'enseignement prophétique était probablement très personnalisé, la personnalité propre de chacun des prophètes jouant un rôle considérable. C'est pourquoi, alors que la tradition biblique n'a conservé le nom d'aucun des maîtres de l'école royale ou de l'école sacerdotale, elle nous a transmis ceux des grands prophètes quitte à ce que leurs disciples, tels le deutéro-Esaïe, restent dans l'anonymat."
5   I do not need to discuss the social location of prophecy, such as its relation to the cult. For a summary of this debate, see WILSON, *Prophecy,* 8–10; TUCKER, Prophecy, 348–354.
6   *Jesaja-disiplene.* Cf., as early as in 1925, *idem, Profeten Jesaja,* 19.
7   *Prophecy,* 161.
8   *Prophecy,* 161.
9   I. Engnell was Mowinckel's main Scandinavian discussion partner. In spite of disagreements, Engnell also accepted the importance of the prophetic disciples. Cf. e.g. ENGNELL, *Gamla Testamentet* I, 41; *idem, SEÅ* 12 (1948) 114f; *idem, SBU* I, 1557f; *idem, Essays,* 143 n. 45, 168, 266. See also his articles on individual prophets in *SBU* I–II.—Among NT scholars, MEADE, *Pseudonymity,* 17–43; RIESNER, *Lehrer,* 283–288; SATO, *Q und Prophetie,* 317–336, have brought attention to these groups as an analogy for understanding the transmission of the Jesus tradition. More than Riesner, Meade and Sato point to the creative—not only preservative—activity of these groups. MEADE, *ibid.,* 9–11, 26f, 32, 38 n. 74, is sceptical about the value of regarding these groups as schools, but he assumes a more static definition of a school than necessary.

not been proven, in his view, and the almost total silence about them and their activities in the prophetic books counsels further caution.[1] It is not possible, according to Clements, to locate the transmission of the prophetic traditions within settings of prophetic schools.

Several scholars claim today that the writings attributed to prophets reflect more or less extensive work within prophetic schools. In particular, modern scholars use the label of a school to explain (parts of) the formation of Amos, Hosea, Isaiah and Ezekiel.

Some find explicit traces of the school of *Amos*. Not only was Amos, according to this view, a learned man who himself enjoyed some education in wisdom circles.[2] Lindblom refers to Amos 3:13 as evidence for the existence of disciples around the prophet.[3] Amos summons the addressees—the alleged disciples—to hear and attest against the house of Jacob how Yahweh punishes Israel's crimes (3:14f). But the context hardly allows for Lindblom's interpretation. The addressees are perhaps the same as those referred to in 3:9. These non-Israelites are to see Israel's guilt in a similar manner as the persons addressed in 3:13 are to hear the announcement of punishment.[4] The effect might be purely rhetoric.[5] Lindblom also refers to Amos 7:10 which mentions Amaziah's accusation of conspiracy against Amos. Lindblom comments: "A conspiracy presupposes more than one man."[6] But this observation does not allow any conclusion about the existence of disciples. I. Engnell uses Amos 7:14f to show that Amos was a prophet's son after his call, a member of a prophetic guild. But Engnell admits himself that in and of itself "this interpretation is not absolutely mandatory."[7]

Although there are no explicit statements in Amos that the prophet functioned like a teacher surrounded by a number of pupils forming a kind of school, scholars use the tradition and redaction history behind the book as an argument in this direction.[8] Not many modern interpreters argue that the present book as a whole goes back to Amos himself.[9]

H.W. Wolff, in particular, considers the composite character of the book as best explained by reference to a school of Amos.[10] He finds six redactional layers alto-

---

[1]   *Old Testament Study*, 78. Cf. also e.g. *idem, Prophecy*, 28, 45–47; *idem, Deliverance*, 69f; *idem, Isaiah 1–39*, 100; *idem, VT* 30 (1980) 436; *idem*, Ezekiel tradition, 119–136; *idem, Int* 36 (1982) 119; *idem, JSOT* 31 (1985) 96, 113 n. 22; *idem*, Chronology of Redaction, 283–294; *idem*, Prophet and his Editors, 212.

[2]   Cf. KOCH *et al., Amos* I, 4; *idem, Prophets* I, 38, 49; LANG, *Monotheism*, 98f. For Amos' relation to wisdom, see WOLFF, *Amos' geistige Heimat;* TERRIEN, Amos and Wisdom, 448–455.

[3]   *Prophecy*, 161.

[4]   WOLFF, *Joel and Amos*, 200.

[5]   MAYS, *Amos*, 68f; RUDOLPH, *Joel – Amos – Obadja – Jona*, 163, 165.

[6]   *Prophecy*, 161.

[7]   *Essays*, 133.

[8]   BIRKELAND, *Traditionswesen*, 67–69; ENGNELL, *SBU* I, 66f, stress the oral element behind the book of Amos.

[9]   But cf. R. GORDIS, *HTR* 33 (1940) 239–251; BOTTERWECK, *BZ* 2 (1958) 176–189.

[10]   *Joel and Amos*, 108–111. Cf. also LINDBLOM, *Prophecy*, 239–242; WILLI-PLEIN, *Vorformen*, 59.—RUDOLPH, *Joel – Amos – Obadja – Jona*, 98, 102, 264 n. 4, is critical of Wolff's hypothesis in this regard but still speaks of Amos' "Freundeskreis"

gether.[1] Three of these derive from the eighth century and three from the following centuries, down to the post-exilic period. The first redactional activity during the eighth century took place, according to Wolff, in the old school of Amos. Wolff assigns the activity of this school chronologically to 760–730 B.C.E. and geographically to Judah, perhaps Beer-sheba.[2]

There are no explicit references indicating that *Hosea* had pupils. Nevertheless, H.S. Nyberg presupposed as early as in 1934 the existence of certain persons as the initial carriers of the oral tradition behind the MT.[3] In the sphere of Nyberg's influence, others also recognized existence of such persons.[4] A large number of more recent scholars presuppose a faithful group of followers, who received and transmitted the message of Hosea.[5]

Wolff again receives the credit for trying to give the group clear historical contours. In an influential article from 1956, he placed Hosea within the context of pre-Deuteronomic and prophetic-levitical groups in the northern kingdom.[6] At the end of his essay,[7] and more explicitly in his commentary,[8] Wolff calls members of this group "experts in the transmission of Hosea's words."[9] They formed the school of Hosea. Wolff argues for three large transmission complexes behind the present book, supplemented by later Deuteronomic and Judaic redactions.[10] The first complex (Hos 1–3) contains portions of the prophet's own *memorabilia* (2:4–17; 3:1–5),[11] with additional biographical notes composed by a disciple (1:2–6, 8f; 2:1–3, 18–25). The second section (Hos 4–11) spans over a longer time of Hosea's activity. The nucleus of the tradition consists of several kerygmatic units which contain sketches of scenes that someone within the circle of disciples wrote down soon after their actual occurrence. Some of the sketches reflect Hosea's public preaching (4:1–9:9; 10:9–15); others were originally addressed to the inner circle around the prophet (9:10–10:8; 11:1–11). The

---

(*ibid.*, 100) and assumes "daß es in Juda einen Kreis von Menschen gab, denen seine Verkündigung und sein Geschick am Herzen lag" (*ibid.*, 252).

[1] *Joel and Amos*, 106–113.

[2] Cf. Amos 5:5; 8:14.—WOLFF, *Joel and Amos*, 110, 239, 332, considers Beer-sheba to be an ancient cultic meeting place for pilgrims. Thus, "the school of Amos ... made contact with pilgrims to Beer-sheba from the northern kingdom and discussed with them the words of the master" (*ibid.*, 110).

[3] *ZAW* 52 (1934) 241–254; *idem, Studien.*

[4] E.g. BIRKELAND, *Traditionswesen*, 63; ENGNELL, *SBU* I, 983f; LINDBLOM, *Prophecy*, 244f.—E.M. GOOD, *SEÅ* 31 (1966) 21–63, speaks occasionally of "disciples" (*ibid.*, 29) and "intelligent people" involved in the process of transmission (*ibid.*, 23, 55), but he remains sceptical as to whether we can talk about Hosea as the master of a school (*ibid.*, 62 n. 69). Cf. also HALDAR, *Cult Prophets*, 156.—For a recent assessment of Nyberg's contribution, cf. NISSINEN, *Prophetie*, 2–16, 41–43.

[5] E.g. EISSFELDT, *Old Testament*, 391; WILLI-PLEIN, *Vorformen*, 221, 243f, 247, 251f; ANDERSEN/FREEDMAN, *Hosea*, 52f, 58; WILSON, *Prophecy*, 230; RUPPERT, Beobachtungen, 176; BLENKINSOPP, *Prophecy*, 100; Jörg JEREMIAS, *Hosea*, 18f; EMMERSON, *Hosea*, 5; YEE, *Composition*, 128; RIESNER, *Lehrer*, 285; SATO, *Q und Prophetie*, 319, 326f.—STUART, *Hosea – Jonah*, 10, 12, reflects on this group merely as an audience of Hosea's oracles.

[6] *TLZ* 81 (1956) 83–94.

[7] *TLZ* 81 (1956) 94 n. 71.

[8] *Hosea*, xxiif, xxix–xxxii, 75.

[9] *Hosea*, 75.

[10] Exilic or post-exilic additions—perhaps from the Dtr—occur in 1:1; 14:10.

[11] For the definition of the *memorabile*, see WOLFF, *Hosea*, 57f.

third transmission complex (Hos 12–14) builds partly on three similar sketches depicting scenes from the public (12:8ff; 13:9ff) and from within the group of Hosea's followers (14:2–9).

Some texts in *Isaiah* maintain, as we have seen, the existence of prophetic disciples. According to Mowinckel, these disciples functioned as transmitters preserving and elaborating the tradition.[1] Their consciousness of being themselves inspired prophets stimulated and carried a creative activity within a group of dominating personalities and "less distinguished men."[2] Members of this prophetic school performed more or less extensive work in Isaiah, Micah, Zephaniah, Nahum, Habakkuk, Deuteronomy 32, the Decalogue (Exod 20:2–17; Deut 5:6–21) and the Deuteronomic body of regulations. Although Mowinckel went beyond what evidence can justify,[3] he did bring attention to the importance of prophetic disciples in the process of transmission. More recent scholars have also tried to explain the tradition and redaction history of Isaiah by assuming the existence of an Isaianic school.[4]

It has become rather customary to speak of Second Isaiah as a disciple of Isaiah of Jerusalem.[5] Despite disagreements concerning the structure and composition of Isa 40–55,[6] scholars often assume that several oracles stem from a single individual.[7] His anonymity[8] does not conceal that his activity coincided with the Persian king Cyrus (c. 559–529 B.C.E.).[9] Since the text presupposes the situation of the exile, Second Isaiah was probably one of the exiles. To be sure, there is no explicit evidence that he was a disciple. But nevertheless, some interpreters maintain that he was acquainted with the earlier Isaiah tradition and that he was active within a group of descendants from the incipient Isaianic school.

Even if we accept B. Duhm's famous separation of Isa 56–66 from the rest of Isaiah,[10] we face notable disagreements among recent scholars as to whether these chapters come from one author or represent a collection of texts from many different

---

1   *Jesaja-disiplene*, 11f. Cf. also *idem, Tradition*, 67–71.

2   *Tradition*, 68.

3   MOWINCKEL, *Jesaja-disiplene*, 13, mentions himself that there are no explicit connections between Isaiah and the writings carrying the names of other prophets.

4   Cf. e.g. D. JONES, *ZAW* 67 (1955) 226–246; EATON, *VT* 9 (1959) 138–157; *idem*, Isaiah tradition 58–76; SCHREINER, Buch jesajanischer Schule, 143–162; GEVARYAHU, *JBQ* 18 (1989–90) 62–68.

5   E.g. MOWINCKEL, *Jesaja-disiplene*, 15; *idem, Tradition*, 69; D. JONES, *ZAW* 67 (1955) 237, 245f; EATON, *VT* 9 (1959) 151–156; ENGNELL, *SBU* I, 1145f; J.L. MCKENZIE, *Second Isaiah*, xxi–xxiii; ENGNELL, *Essays*, 266; RIESNER, *Lehrer*, 286; SATO, *Q und Prophetie*, 335.

6   For surveys of research, see SCHOORS, *God Your Saviour*, 1–31; MELUGIN, *Formation*, 1–7; RICHTER, Hauptlinien, 116–122; WHYBRAY, *Second Isaiah*, 20–42. Cf. also KRATZ, *Kyros*.

7   The servant songs (42:1–4[–9]; 49:1–6[–12]; 50:4–9[–11]; 52:13–53:12) present a special problem. For surveys of interpretation, see NORTH, *Suffering Servant*, 6–116; HAAG, *Gottesknecht*; JEPPESEN, Herrens lidende tjener, 113–126.

8   Scholars usually regard Isa 40:1–8(–11) as reflective of the prophet's commission. However, the opening apostrophe (40:1f) addresses a plurality, and the "I" commanded to cry out (40:6) is not unambiguously the prophet. If the servant of Yahweh is identified with the prophet, further statements about the call, commission, suffering, and death of the prophet could be adduced. But this also remains uncertain.

9   Cf. Isa 41:2f, 25; 44:28; 45:1, 13; 46:11; 48:14f. For an analysis, see LAATO, *Servant*, 166–195.

10   *Jesaia*, xiiif, xviiif.

hands.[1] In any event, there are indeed several similarities between Isa 56–66 and Isa 40–55.[2] While some scholars would explain this feature by reference to common authorship,[3] a great number of other scholars are convinced that some of the material in Isa 56–66 comes from one or several disciples of Second Isaiah.[4]

P.D. Hanson has tried to identify the group behind Isa 56–66.[5] As O. Plöger,[6] he discovers a conflict between a prophetic-visionary group and a hierocratic party in control of the re-established cult and the political community. While the hierocratic party relied on Ezek 40–48 in the restoration of the community, the visionaries adhered to and applied the promises of Isa 40–55. Out of this social matrix, there arose polemical and apocalyptic ideas among the visionaries. And within this setting, Isa 56–66 took shape, according to Hanson. The continuous struggle of the dissident visionaries, the followers of Second Isaiah, is further reflected in Zech 9–14.

We have seen that also *Ezekiel* contains accounts about prophetic followers. Although the present book appears to be rather uniform and coherent, a majority of modern scholars discover a growing process.[7] One cannot explain the apparent unity by reference to a single author, whether Ezekiel himself[8] or an anonymous author during the post-exilic period.[9] The coherence is, according to this view, the result of a unified tradition and redaction history.

The detailed studies by W. Zimmerli have strongly influenced the complicated discussion of these issues.[10] Several scholars have accepted the existence and importance of Ezekiel's followers.[11] But Zimmerli thinks of their activity as a specific interpretative activity. Instead of perceiving the growth as the addition of independent glosses, Zimmerli thinks of a process of continuous exegesis on a kernel element. He calls it "Fortschreibung." To some extent, Ezekiel himself initiated this process. The tumultuous years of the exile brought new experiences which caused an updating of

---

[1]   For surveys of research on Isaiah 56–66, see PAURITSCH, *Gemeinde*, 1–6, 8–30; VERMEYLEN, *Isaïe* II, 451–454; SEKINE, *Tritojesajanische Sammlung*, 3–23; KOENEN, *Ethik*, 1–7; STECK, *Tritojesaja*, 3–9.

[2]   See below pp. 145f.

[3]   E.g. MAASS, "Tritojesaja?," 153–163.

[4]   E.g. ELLIGER, *Einheit des Tritojesaia*, 125; *idem, ZAW* 49 (1931) 138 n. 1; *idem, Deuterojesaja in seinem Verhältnis, passim;* BIRKELAND, *Traditionswesen*, 39; MOWINCKEL, *Tradition*, 69; ZIMMERLI, *Gottes Offenbarung*, 233; EISSFELDT, *Old Testament*, 342f; SCHREINER, *Buch jesajanischer Schule*, 146; WESTERMANN, *Isaiah 40–66*, 27f, 299, 307; P.-E. BONNARD, *Second Isaïe*, 316f; P.D. HANSON, *Dawn of Apocalyptic*, 32–208; CARROLL, *Prophecy*, 152; BLENKINSOPP, *Prophecy*, 217, 245; KOCH, *Prophets* II, 153.

[5]   *Dawn of Apocalyptic.*

[6]   *Theokratie und Eschatologie.*

[7]   Cf. the indications of such a process listed by EICHRODT, *Ezekiel*, 20; Rudolf SMEND, *Entstehung*, 165f. For surveys of research into the tradition and redaction history of Ezekiel, see LANG, *Ezechiel*, 1–17; ZIMMERLI, *TRE* 10 (1982) 767–769; *idem, Ezekiel* II, xi–xviii. Cf. also POHLMANN, *Ezekielstudien.*

[8]   *Contra* GREENBERG, *Ezekiel 1–20*, 3–27.

[9]   *Contra* Joachim BECKER, Erwägungen zur ezechielischen Frage, 137–149; *idem,* Ez 8–11, 136–150.

[10]   *Ezekiel* I, 68–74; *idem*, Phänomen der "Fortschreibung," 174–191.

[11]   Cf. e.g. HOWIE, *Date and Composition*, 85–99; ENGNELL, *SBU* I, 947; LINDBLOM, *Prophecy*, 266; WEVERS, *Ezekiel*, 22–30; EICHRODT, *Ezekiel*, 41f; BLENKINSOPP, *Prophecy*, 194f; WILSON, *Prophecy*, 285f; RENDTORFF, *Old Testament*, 209; BROWNLEE, *Ezekiel 1–19*, xxxvi.

earlier material. But depending on Mowinckel, Zimmerli thinks that a school of Ezekiel was the primary location of the interpretative activity. During Ezekiel's own life and after his death, the school was responsible for the continuous exegesis of older units and for the process that led to the coherent impression of the present book.

The assumptions concerning the schools sometimes go beyond what evidence can prove. This is partly true of Wolff's attempt to define the schools of Amos and Hosea. In particular, the contours of the group around Hosea are not as clear as Wolff claims.[1] There are two problematic points. First, it is difficult to say with sufficient certainty that a group of disciples—an incipient school—constituted the original addressee of Hos 9:10–10:8; 11:1–11; 14:2–9. As is well known, any attempt to penetrate down to the "historical Hosea" is fraught with immeasurable difficulties.[2] The text is, if not corrupt,[3] at several instances problematic. And while Hosea certainly directs Yahweh's word to different groups, it is impossible to tell whether the notations about the addressees reflect an authentic situation or not. No episodal scenario occurs. In addition, there are no signs that the addressees formed a close fellowship.[4] These considerations also undermine the certainty of Wolff's claim that some texts represent sketches from the original hearers.[5] Second, the levitical character of the group is difficult to prove. Since the many connections between Hosea and Deuteronomy cannot be denied,[6] and since some of these connections may be genuine,[7] it is reasonable to assume that Hosea was acquainted with pre-Deuteronomic traditions. But it is not as obvious that Hosea was related to the Levites. Not only is their history shrouded in darkness.[8] In particular, there is no reason to assume that Hosea's acquaintance with cultic matters and Israel's old traditions necessarily implied contacts with the Levites.[9] Hosea could also have attained

---

1   For various reactions to Wolff's hypothesis, cf. e.g. GUNNEWEG, *Tradition,* 102; RENDTORFF, *ZTK* 59 (1962) 150–152; RUDOLPH, *Hosea,* 23; STECK, *Israel,* 197, 199–201; CODY, *Priesthood,* 123f; VON RAD, *Theology* II, 139; VAN DER WOUDE, Prophets, 47; BLENKINSOPP, *Prophecy,* 99f.

2   Cf. the extreme scepticism of ENGNELL, *SBU* I, 983; E.M. GOOD, *SEÅ* 31 (1966) 62 n. 69.

3   Instead of speaking of a corrupt text, some scholars refer to the peculiarities of the northern dialect. Cf. e.g. RUDOLPH, *Hosea,* 20–22; MAYS, *Hosea,* 5; VAN DER WOUDE, Prophets, 43f; STUART, *Hosea – Jonah,* 13.

4   The following addressees of Yahweh's word through Hosea appears: Israel, sometimes indicated with "Ephraim" or simply "you" (2:3, 4; 4:1, 15; 5:1, 8; 6:4; 9:1, 5, 7; 10:12–15; 11:8; 12:10; 13:4, 9–11); the priests (4:4f; 5:1); the royalty (5:1); Samaria (8:5); Judah (6:4, 11). At the beginning of the book, Yahweh speaks directly to Hosea (1:2; 3:1).

5   Cf. the scepticism of WILLI-PLEIN, *Vorformen,* 247.

6   The substantial links between the two books are listed by WEINFELD, *Deuteronomy,* 366–370. Cf. also recently ZOBEL, *Prophetie,* 17–22, 35–49, 51–87, 96f, 99f.

7   WILSON, *Prophecy,* 227f.

8   Cf. CODY, *Priesthood, passim.* For a summarizing account of the history of the Levites, see DE VAUX, *Israel,* 361–366.

9   RENDTORFF, *ZTK* 59 (1962) 151f; RUDOLPH, *Hosea,* 23; VAN DER WOUDE,

this knowledge elsewhere.[1]

Hanson also overstates his case, in my opinion. It is true that to a large extent Isa 56–66 fits well into the picture given by Hanson. The polemical thrust of many oracles is obvious: the social criticism launches accusations against the decline in righteous behaviour towards fellow countrymen (56:1a; 57:1, 12; 58:2; 59:4, 9, 14; 64:5) and looks forward to its restoration (58:8; 60:17, 21; 61:3, 10f; 62:1f);[2] the criticism is linked with polemic against false attitude to fasting (58:1–5), failure to keep the sabbath (58:13), dietary offences (65:4; 66:17), immorality and idolatry (57:3–10, 13; 65:1–7) and general sinfulness (59:1–15); harsh judgement is pronounced against the ones responsible for the situation (56:9–12). The result might have been that the visionaries were thrown out of the community (66:5). However, it seems that Hanson overstates the polarization between the two groups.[3] Eschatological dreams occur also in texts of priestly background (Ezek 38–48; Zech 1:7–6:8). Second Isaiah and his disciples may even have been influenced by the Ezekiel tradition.[4] And it is far from evident that the visionary group was entirely opposed to the cult. Focusing on Isa 56–66 only,[5] we may question if 66:1–4 actually implies that the group rejected sacrifices. This would indeed be unique in the history of Israelite religion. It is possible that the reaction was against the attempt to make the temple an indispensible precondition for worship and against acts reflecting a syncretic and illegitimate cult.[6]

It is also peculiar—and perhaps significant—that the group which is faithful to Yahweh and cast out of the community are the ones who tremble at the word of Yahweh (Isa 66:2, 5). This manner of speaking is almost identical with the description of the group that supported Ezra's mission (Ezra 9:4; 10:3).[7] Since also Ezra was critical of prevailing practices within the post-exilic community, it is not certain that Isa 66:2, 5 depict an entirely different kind of group.[8] The scribal character of some of Third Isaiah's exegesis, noted independently of this manner of speaking,[9] becomes interesting from this perspective.

Prophets, 47.

[1]   RUDOLPH, *Hosea,* 23.—GUNNEWEG, *Tradition,* 102, thinks Hosea belonged to a group of cult prophets.

[2]   Cf. also Yahweh's own righteousness in 56:1b; 59:16f; 63:1.

[3]   Cf. ACKROYD, *Int* 30 (1976) 412–415; CARROLL, *JSOT* 14 (1979) 3–35.

[4]   See below pp. 185f.

[5]   For a critique of Hanson's treatment of Zech 9–14, see REDDITT, *CBQ* 51 (1989) 631–642.

[6]   For a survey of different interpretations of these verses, see SEKINE, *Tritojesajanische Sammlung,* 45f.

[7]   Cf. BLENKINSOPP, *Prophecy,* 250.—Isa 66:2 uses חרד על and Isa 66:5 אל חרד. Ezra 9:4; 10:3 use חרד ב. In Ezra 10:3 the object of trembling is not Yahweh's word but his commandment (מצוה). Elsewhere in the OT, the participial form of חרד occurs only in 1 Sam 4:13.

[8]   *Contra* SEKINE, *Tritojesajanische Sammlung,* 59f.

[9]   D. MICHEL, *TViat* 10 (1965–66) 213–230.

The difficulties we face in determining the identity of the prophetic schools more closely are due to the meagre explicit evidence forcing a circular way of reasoning. Scholars argue that the redactional character of the prophetic books implies the existence of schools preserving and elaborating the traditions of each prophet respectively. Although this kind of reasoning is sometimes unavoidable in sociocultural reconstructions made on the basis of texts providing only fragmentary information about the issue at hand, its presence should provoke the necessary caution. Nevertheless, if elementary and scribal schools existed in ancient Israel from early on,[1] it is not inconceivable that the brief accounts about a teacher-pupil relationship present in some prophetic texts actually were manifest in the form of schools. We have seen that some texts speak of gatherings in front of the prophet in rather formal terms. *The possibility that the transmitters of the prophetic teaching thought of themselves as members of a school identifying itself by reference to a certain prophet should not be rejected altogether.* In chapter three, I will explore further if the growth of the prophetic traditions corresponds to such a view.

Excursus 2: *Elementary and Scribal Schools in Ancient Israel*

Ever since A. Klostermann's study *Schulwesen im alten Israel* from 1908, scholars have often assumed that elementary and scribal schools existed in Israel from the pre-exilic period and onwards.[2] Klostermann based his conclusions mainly on texts such as Isa 28:9–13; 50:4–9; Prov 22:17–21.[3] Although they may provide—at the most—some indirect support,[4] other data are also present.

The OT gives further information.[5] There are references to persons capable of reading and writing,[6] and also of counting.[7] These references occur at various places in

---

[1] See excursus 2 below.

[2] For literature on schools and education in ancient Israel, see LEMAIRE, *Écoles,* 93 n. 70. Cf. also GOLKA, *VT* 33 (1983) 257–270; N. LOHFINK, *KatBl* 108 (1983) 86–97; LEMAIRE, *VT* 34 (1984) 270–281; N. LOHFINK, *BK* 39 (1984) 90–98; CRENSHAW, *JBL* 104 (1985) 601–615; LANG, *Wisdom,* 7–12; SHUPAK, *RB* 94 (1987) 98–119; HARAN, Literacy, 81–95; LIPIŃSKI, Scribes, 161–164; PUECH, Écoles, 189–203; LEMAIRE, Sage, 165–181; *idem, ABD* 2 (1992) 305–312.—The recent interest in this subject among NT scholars appears in the (partial) treatment given by RIESNER, *Lehrer,* 153–163, 278–288, 507f; SATO, *Q und Prophetie,* 314–342; WILKINS, *Concept of Disciple,* 43–91; VON LIPS, *Weisheitliche Traditionen,* 31.

[3] *Schulwesen,* 19–40.

[4] After the publication of Klostermann's essay, it has been recognized that Prov 22:17–21 is part of a larger collection perhaps showing indication of dependency on the Egyptian instruction of Amen-em-Opet. Parallels to this collection, which extends to Prov 24:22, have also been found in the oriental Sayings of Ahikar. For a summarizing discussion and literature, see EISSFELDT, *Old Testament,* 52 n. 64, 474f. For a more recent (and positive) assessment of the connections with Amen-em-Opet, see RÖMHELD, *Wege der Weisheit.*

[5] LEMAIRE, *Écoles,* 34–45, summarizes the biblical evidence.

[6] Not all persons were literate (Isa 29:12). I cannot here discuss if the literacy was restricted to specific groups or more wide-spread. Arguments for the wide diffusion of literacy are given by e.g. RIESNER, *Lehrer,* 112–115; DEMSKY, Extent of Literacy, 349–

the OT.[1] The conclusion of G. von Rad reflects a wide-spread assumption: "In Israel ... writing was known. But writing has to be taught. Handwriting, however, was never taught without accompanying material. It follows from this that there must have been schools of different types in Israel."[2]

The emergence of a royal administration during the pre-exilic period created the need for educated officals,[3] also scribes. If we think of the scribes as a professional class of wise men,[4] we may assume a connection between the need for officials and the production of wisdom literature. The wisdom motifs in the OT—especially in Proverbs—then constitute indications for the existence of scribal schools.[5]

Extra-biblical data support the biblical indications. Some scholars think that the epigraphical findings at places such as Arad, Aroër, Gezer, ʿIzbet Ṣarṭah, Qadesh-Barnéa, Kuntilat-Ajrud and Lakish indicate the existence of elementary schools.[6] And a comparison with neighbouring cultures reveals the wide-spread existence of educational institutions at this time. The strong influence from Egypt during the early monarchy makes it probable that schools of similar kinds existed also in pre-exilic Israel.[7]

Although recent scholars have not rejected the possibility that elementary and scribal schools existed at an early time in ancient Israel, there is also a growing awareness of the fact that the evidence is meagre. Only the cumulative combination of different pieces of evidence carries sufficient weight. A. Lemaire's rather extensive argumentation, published in 1981,[8] for the early existence of schools in ancient Israel provoked further debate. R.N. Whybray's criticism, published even before Lemaire's study,[9] against the assumption that there were professional wisdom schools in ancient Israel has been reinforced and developed by F.W. Golka in regard to the elementary education.[10] Golka does not deny that there are numerous references to schools in neighbouring cultures. He stresses rather that the absence of such references in the OT then

---

353; MILLARD, Evidence for Writing, 301–312; DEMSKY, Writing, 10–16 (with lit.). Arguments for the limited diffusion of literacy are given by e.g. HARAN, Literacy, 81–95; PUECH, Écoles, 189–203.

7   HERNER, Erziehung, 61–63.

1   E.g. Deut 6:9; 11:20; 17:18f; 24:1, 3; 27:8; Judg 8:14; Isa 8:1; 10:19; 29:11; 30:8; 34:16; 50:1; Jer 3:8; 25:13; 29:1–32; 30:2; 32:12; 36:2–32; 45:1; 51:60f; Ezek 2:9f; 24:2; 37:16, 20; 43:11; Hab 2:2; Job 31:35–37. The texts reflect different periods in the history of Israel. I cannot here discuss each of them critically. This is done to some extent by HERMISSON, *Spruchweisheit*, 99; JAMIESON-DRAKE, *Scribes and Schools*, 150f.

2   *Wisdom*, 17.

3   METTINGER, *Officials*.—LIPIŃSKI, Scribes, 161–164, emphasizes the family as the setting of scribal education.

4   MCKANE, *Prophets*, 40–47. Differently WHYBRAY, *Intellectual Tradition*, 15–54; *idem*, Sage, 133f.

5   So e.g. HERMISSON, *Spruchweisheit*, 122–125, 188, 192; METTINGER, *Officials*, 145, including an account of other scholars; LANG, *Lehrrede, passim;* VON RAD, *Wisdom*, 11f; LANG, Schule, 186–201; *idem, Wisdom*, 7–12; SHUPAK, *RB* 94 (1987) 98–119.

6   LEMAIRE, *Écoles*, 7–33.—LEMAIRE, *ibid.*, 15, also discusses findings from Khirbet el-Qôm, but he does not use them as evidence for an actual school.

7   METTINGER, *Officials*, 143–157; SHUPAK, *RB* 94 (1987) 98–119.

8   *Écoles*.

9   *Intellectual Tradition*, 33–43. Cf. also *idem*, Prophecy, 181–199; *idem*, Social world, 233f.

10   *VT* 33 (1983) 257–270. Cf. also *idem, VT* 36 (1986) 13–36, trying to refute the assumption that many proverbial wisdom sayings originated at the royal court.

becomes all the more remarkable. A comparison with Egypt is relevant only when scholars take sufficient notice of the fact that this country was at a further stage of political sophistication than pre-exilic Israel. It is necessary to focus on a comparable stage in Egypt's development. And early Egyptian education was in the hands of the parents. The same educational system was therefore, according to Golka, the only one used during the initial stages of Israel's monarchy.

Lemaire responded by reinforcing his arguments concerning the biblical evidence and the inscriptions, and by presenting further historical and sociological comparison.[1] According to Lemaire, the cumulative force of different pieces of evidence from the OT, from the situation in Egypt during the time of the early Israelite monarchy and from archaeological and epigraphical findings points to the existence of schools in Israel even in pre-exilic times.

J.L. Crenshaw is more cautious.[2] The biblical evidence does point to the existence of literate persons, but it is not obvious where this literacy was acquired; the inscriptions brought out by Lemaire are less persuasive than sometimes maintained; the central position of the schools in Egytian and Mesopotamian life did have an influence on Israel, but the exact nature of those learned places remains unclear; the strong Egyptian influence evident in the lists of state officials cannot be denied, but the lists are striking in their silence about an official in charge of education. In assessing the evidence, Crenshaw adopts a sceptical position. He adds, however, that in reality Israelite education was far richer than the resulting account. The instruction of children by parents was certainly the primary means of education during the initial stage of the kingdom, but "it seems unwise to insist that all education occurred in the home, despite the paucity of evidence for royal schools."[3]

The debate has now moved into a stage of more detailed investigations. M. Haran and E. Puech have scrutinized the epigraphical findings.[4] While not at all denying that schools existed, they agree that the different inscriptions need to be treated with much caution. Not all abecedaries—not even the Gezer Calendar—can sustain the definition of school exercises composed in ancient Israel.

N. Shupak, a student of Haran, has studied the Egyptian parallels.[5] He acknowledges the limited value of the epigraphical data. However, the vocabulary of the biblical sages—especially in Proverbs—contains semantic equivalents with terms associated with Egyptian schools. Since contact with Egypt is evident during the Solomonic period, and since the administration created a need for officials, Shupak finds it reasonable to assume that "the first Hebrew schools were founded as early as the time of Solomon, and that the origins of these schools may be traced back to the educational tradition of Egypt."[6] In such schools, Proverbs served as a text book.

---

[1] *VT* 34 (1984) 270–281. Cf. also *idem, Sage,* 165–181; *idem, ABD* 2 (1992) 305–312.—LEMAIRE, *Écoles,* 72–83, relates the school hypothesis to the transmission of several biblical books and the formation of canon. For his view of 1, 2 Kings, see *idem, ZAW* 98 (1986) 221–236. However, as TALMON, Heiliges Schrifttum, 63f, points out, the connection between the formation of the canon and the schools is not evident.

[2] *JBL* 104 (1985) 601–615. Cf. also the review of Lemaire's book by CRENSHAW, *JBL* 103 (1984) 630–632.

[3] *JBL* 104 (1985) 614.

[4] HARAN, Literacy, 81–95; PUECH, Écoles, 189–203.

[5] *RB* 94 (1987) 98–119. The article builds on the author's dissertation *Selected Terms of Biblical Wisdom Literature Compared with Egyptian Wisdom Literature* (Hebrew). Hebrew University 1984. The dissertation was not available to me.

[6] *RB* 94 (1987) 118.

D.W. Jamieson-Drake develops in a monograph published in 1991 a new approach to the problem.[1] Since the data from texts, epigraphical remains and cross-cultural analogy are too allusive to be handled in a direct manner, Jamieson-Drake wants to place these data in the context of an archaeologically established and sociological framework. A study of the cultural level of the settlement, various public works and luxury items builds up the framework. The context achieved in this manner suggests that at the time of the Judahite state—which, according to Jamieson-Drake, cannot be before the eighth or seventh century—scribal training would have taken place in Jerusalem, but in quite a different manner than in Egypt and Mesopotamia.

All in all, although the biblical evidence is weak, it does not decisively speak against the assumption of the early existence of schools. The testimony about literate persons is not sufficient by itself, but the possibility that they were trained within a school cannot be rejected. The absence of a reference to an official in charge of education in the OT is noteworthy,[2] but it provides nothing more than an argument from silence. Concerning the lack of references to a school house in the OT,[3] we should remember that teaching could be given at private sites.[4] We also know from much later times, when the school system was further developed, that the open air could serve as a place of instruction.[5] The building does not define the school.[6]

The cumulative force of the observations made in epigraphical and extra-biblical areas of research sufficiently accounts, as it seems, for the hypothesis that elementary and scribal schools existed at an early time in ancient Israel. True, not all epigraphical findings testify to the existence of schools. Perhaps school education was provided only at some specific locations. But the epigraphical data are not entirely without value.[7] B. Lang points out that the virtual absence of scribal errors on about two hundred and fifty Hebrew ostraca indicates the educated skill of the scribes.[8] The education is too specified and accurate to be located only within the family. The references to education in surrounding cultures are likewise not to be pushed aside.[9] The data from

---

[1]   *Scribes and Schools.* For a review, see THIEL, *TLZ* 12 (1991) 898-900, who points out the possibility that scribal schools may have existed as early as during Solomon's reign (*ibid.,* 900).

[2]   Cf. 2 Sam 8:15–18 (1 Chr 18:14–17); 20:23–26; 1 Kgs 4:1–6. For discussion of the lists, see METTINGER, *Officials,* 7–11.

[3]   HERNER, *Erziehung,* 66; LEMAIRE, *ABD* 2 (1992) 310, regard 2 Kgs 6:1f as a reference to the school building. But this is an overinterpretation.—The house built on seven pillars in Prov 9:1 is probably not a school. Cf. e.g. AHLSTRÖM, *SEÅ* 44 (1979) 74–76.

[4]   Cf. 2 Kgs 4:38; 6:1, 32; Ezek 8:1; 14:1; 20:1; 33:31.—GEVARYAHU, *ASTI* 12 (1983) 5f, considers the tent of Moses (Exod 33:7–11; Num 11:24–26; Deut 31:14) as a place of teaching. But this is to stretch the evidence too far.

[5]   For the evidence from the rabbinic writings, see BÜCHLER, *JQR* 4 (1913–14) 485–491; KRAUSS, *JJS* 1 (1948–49) 82–84.

[6]   Cf. LEMAIRE, Sage, 167f.

[7]   GOLKA, *VT* 33 (1983) 263 n. 19, treats Lemaire's discussion about the epigraphical material in a footnote and concludes: "Wäre all diese Material an einem Ort, besonders in Jerusalem, gefunden worden, sähe die Beweislage schon ganz anders aus."

[8]   Schule, 191f. Cf. also PUECH, Écoles, 201.—CRENSHAW, *JBL* 104 (1985) 606f, explains this by the common reference to the simplicity of the Hebrew language. But such an argument neglects the standardized ortography and graphical uniformity of the ostraca.

[9]   For education in Mesopotamia, see CIVIL *ABD* 2 (1992) 301–305 (with lit.).

Egypt are especially important.[1] There seems to have been a deep knowledge of Egyptian culture during the Solomonic enlightenment.[2] If there was some influence from Egypt,[3] why would not the form of teaching be taken over to some degree together with the content? Since Israel could benefit from the long experience of a more developed nation, its educational structures might even have developed at a faster rate than Egypt's originally did.[4]

The crisis caused by the exile may have intensified educational measures.[5] Deuteronomy,[6] especially, reflects an eager interest in conveying religious teaching which promulgates Israel's monotheistic faith.[7] Perhaps Deut 6:4–9; 30:14 are indications that even the whole body of regulations (Deut 5–26) should be studied and learned by heart.[8] The many functions of the priests and the Levites after the restoration could hardly have been carried out without organized training. At this time, the temple school may have taken over much of the educational responsibilities earlier related to the court.[9] We may conclude that the cumulative force of the data makes it likely that *the ancient Israelite knew of teacher-pupil relationships manifested in more formal settings of education and professional training during the pre-exilic period and onwards.*

3.2. The School of Jesus ben Sira

Many scholars regard Sir 51:23, 29 as references to the school of Ben Sira. The Hebrew text from the Cairo Geniza (Cairo B) contains two especially important expressions:[10]

51:23	פנו אלי סכלים	Turn to me you foolish ones
	ולונו בבית מדרשי	and lodge *in my house of instruction.*
51:29	תשמח נפשי בישיבתי	My soul rejoices *in my yeshivah*
	ולא תבושו בשירתי	and you will not be ashamed at my song.

The two references are probably original. To be sure, Sir 50:27–29 seems to indicate the original conclusion of the book. And 11QPs^a 21:11–

---

[1] For literature on education in Egypt, see LEMAIRE, *Sage,* 169 n. 13. Cf. also the more recent treatment of early scribal education by the egyptologist SCHLOTT, *Schrift,* 201–206.

[2] METTINGER, *Officials,* 146–148.

[3] For a cautious assessment of the connections between Egypt and Israel, see KITCHEN, *Egypt and Israel,* 107–123.

[4] CRENSHAW, *JBL* 104 (1985) 609f.

[5] RIESNER, *Lehrer,* 159–198, summarizes the exilic and post-exilic situation.

[6] The late dating of Deuteronomy is not accepted by everybody. For a survey of the discussion, see KAISER, *Introduction,* 124–129, himself arguing for a late date.

[7] Cf. e.g. Deut 4:6, 10; 5:6f; 11:18–20; 17:19; 31:9–13. For the didacticism in Deuteronomy, see WEINFELD, *Deuteronomy,* 298–306. His observations are valid in spite of his different view on the dating of the book (*ibid.,* viii). For an emphasis on the monotheistic faith as a pedagogical object in Deuteronomy, see LANG, *Monotheism,* 42f. For an emphasis on the command to love (אהב) as Yahweh's specific (wisdom) teaching to his pupil Israel in Deut 6:5, see MCKAY, *VT* 22 (1972) 426–435.

[8] N. LOHFINK, *KatBl* 108 (1983) 91–96; *idem, BK* 39 (1984) 94.

[9] HERMISSON, *Spruchweisheit,* 131–133.

[10] For a list of the Hebrew MSS, see SKEHAN/DI LELLA, *Wisdom of Ben Sira,* 52f; B.G. WRIGHT, *No Small Difference,* 2–4.

17; 22:1, part of a collection of psalms from Qumran, contain Sir 51:13–
20b, 30b which, in turn, belong to the same alphabetic hymn as Sir 51:23,
29. According to J.A. Sanders, the editor of the Qumran scroll, the Qumranites ascribed the psalm to David, and the hymn can therefore not stem
from Ben Sira himself.[1] But H. Stadelmann has evaluated the subsequent
debate and pointed to the possibility that Ben Sira was in fact the actual
author.[2] The Qumranites' ascription of this psalm to David is not certain.
And significant parallels to the rest of Sirach appear within the hymn. As it
seems, the majority of scholars recognize today the hymn as an original
part of the book.[3] We may refer to further scholars than the ones Stadelmann has assessed. Alhough C. Deutsch does not take a stand in regard to
authorship, she finds several similarities between the presentation of the
sage in Sir 51:13–30 and in the rest of the book.[4] M.R. Lehmann's observations concerning the use of several texts from other parts of Sirach in the
Psalms scroll suggest that the Qumranites did not postulate a Davidic
authorship for the psalms in the scroll.[5] They rather regarded the scroll as
an apocryphal composition which freely included extra-canonical material
into the biblical psalms. A.A. di Lella pointed out that, just as the author of
Proverbs concluded his book with an alphabetic acrostic (Prov 31:10–31),
Ben Sira also closed his work with an alphabetic acrostic (51:13–30) of
twenty-three lines.[6] In this manner he created a counterpart to the poems of
twenty-two lines in 1:11–30; 6:18–37 and a frame to the book.[7] We have
sufficient reason for regarding Sir 51:23, 29 as part of the original composition from Ben Sira himself.

However, it is probable that Sir 51:23 originally contained a different
Hebrew expression for the school than the one given in Cairo B. P.W. Skehan argues for בית מוסר, "house of education."[8] Both the Greek (οἶκος παι-
δείας) and the Syriac (בית יולפנא) call for this original,[9] without suffix.[10]

---

1   *DJD* IV, 79–85, esp. 83. Cf. also J.A. SANDERS, *Dead Sea Psalms Scroll,* 112–
117, esp. 112f.
2   *Ben Sira,* 30–33. The articles by I. RABINOWITZ, *HUCA* 42 (1971) 173–184;
SKEHAN, *HTR* 64 (1971) 387–400, are of particular importance. Stadelmann did not take
notice of the study by MURAOKA, *JSJ* 10 (1979) 166–178. Although Muraoka is partially supportive of Sanders' (erotic) interpretation of the hymn, he proceeds from the assumption that "its common authorship with the rest of the book does not seem to be in
serious doubt" (*ibid.,* 166).
3   This is also the recent assessment of GILBERT, Book of Ben Sira, 83.
4   *ZAW* 94 (1982) 400–409.
5   *RevQ* 11 (1983) 239–251. An Hebrew version of this article was published in
Tarbiz 39 (1970) 232–247.
6   *CBQ* 48 (1986) 396. Cf. also SKEHAN/DI LELLA, *Wisdom of Ben Sira,* 576.
7   Sir 1:11–30; 6:18–37 are not alphabetic.
8   *HTR* 64 (1971) 397f. Cf. also SKEHAN/DI LELLA, *Wisdom of Ben Sira,* 578. A
similar proposal was made already by LÉVI, *L'Ecclésiastique* II, 229.
9   The Syriac version is essentially a translation from some form of the Hebrew text,
though influences from the Greek might also be present. See NELSON, *Syriac Version,*

Skehan can thus reconstruct a play on words (סורו [ἐγγίσατε] ... בית מוסר),[1] something to be observed also in 6:22. Since, as we have noticed, education (מוסר/παιδεία) is a central concern in Sirach, the proposal is not unlikely.[2] The expression in Cairo B is perhaps due to rabbinic revision of the text. We would expect also the reference to the joy of Ben Sira over his yeshivah in 51:29 to be due to the same revision,[3] but the translations do not propose an alternative reading here. "Yeshivah" may carry a non-technical sense. There are, as we have noticed, older texts that picture pupils as sitting in front (ישבים לפני) of their master (2 Kgs 4:38; 6:1; Ezek 8:1; 14:1; 20:1; 33:31).[4] Although the rabbinic literature reflecting tannaitic and amoraic times uses the term for a more institutional court,[5] it also maintains the non-technical sense of the term (m. ʾAbot 3:10).[6]

The statements in Sir 51:23, 29 are not metaphorical. The twofold reference to the location of instruction leads us to think of the actual house in which the sage met his pupils. It is perhaps significant that m. ʾAbot 1:4 attributes to Jose b. Joʿezer (c. 150 B.C.E.)—a contemporary of Ben Sira—a saying according to which the house should be a gathering place for sages.[7]

Sir 51:23, 29 thus indicate rather clearly that the account about a teacher-pupil relationship corresponded to the educational setting in a school. It is probable that this was the place where the pupils, Ben Sira's "sons," initially learned and transmitted the teaching of their authoritative teacher.

3.3. The School of the Righteous Teacher

Scholars have judged the possibility that the Qumranites performed a systematic study within a school setting variously. M. Delcor tried as early as in 1955 to collect data indicating the existence of a school—he speaks of בית המדרש—in which the Qumranites systematically learned to interpret the Torah.[8] The subsequent debate gave various answers.

Three contributions may be mentioned separately. After a detailed analysis of the scri-

---

6f, *passim.*—I write the Syriac with Hebrew letters because of convenience.

[10] GOODBLATT, *Rabbinic Instruction,* 93 n. 1, argues that the Greek and Syriac readings suggest בית מדרשי as original. But this way of arguing neglects the evident problems with the translations.

[1] The word סורו then replaces פנו at the beginning of 51:23 in Cario B.

[2] STADELMANN, *Ben Sira,* 306–308, points to the educational rather than purely scribal activity within the school.

[3] So RIESNER, *Lehrer,* 167.

[4] DEUTSCH, *ZAW* 94 (1982) 403, translates yeshivah with "instruction." This is misleading. Ben Sira usually employs other words when he speaks of instruction. And in view of 51:23, the location itself is probably referred to in 51:29.

[5] GOODBLATT, *Rabbinic Instruction,* 63–92, 263–265.

[6] Cf. also m. ʾAbot 2:7; b. Taʿan. 8a; b. Nid. 70b.

[7] Cf. ʾAbot R. Nat. A 6.

[8] *RB* 62 (1955) 66–75.

bal features in 1QIsa^a; 1QIsa^b; 1QS; 1QM; 1QH; 1QpHab, M. Martin arrived to the tentative conclusion that the MSS were transcribed or compiled in geographically separate and scribally different places. There would be no need to postulate "the operative presence of a sectarian scribal school at Qumrân."[1] R.A. Culpepper responded critically to Martin's caution. On the basis of additional data from archaeology and the scrolls, Culpepper concluded that "tentatively one may answer affirmatively" to the possibility that a school existed at Qumran.[2] Lemaire dealt with the issue in a separate article. On the basis of archaeology and literary data within and outside of the scrolls, he thinks that there was a school for adults at Qumran, "une sorte de *beit hammidrash essénienne.*"[3]

The lack of a clear consensus is due to the absence of clear data. In spite of Culpepper's attempt to use Martin's analysis as positive argument for a school at Qumran, the scribal features in some MSS do not yield sufficient information in any direction. They only show that educated scribes were active at Qumran, as does 4QTherapeia—probably a rather skilled writing exercise.[4] We do not know where the scribal abilities were acquired. Lemaire is correct to refrain from this line of argumentation. But other pieces of information are at hand.

One of the published ostraca might be an abecedaire.[5] But it is impossible to ascertain that someone at Qumran actually wrote it.[6] We cannot use it as evidence for an elementary school at Qumran. In addition, the small number of abecedaires found at Qumran is striking in view of the many such ostraca found at Murabba^cat.[7]

The accounts about Essenes in written sources originating outside of Qumran are not immediately useful here.[8] We must of course compare them with statements in the Dead Sea scrolls themselves.

Josephus provides three pieces of information. First, Vit. 10f mentions that Josephus received some education from the Essenes at the age of sixteen. Since Josephus was born 37–38 C.E. (Vit. 5),[9] it seems that it was possible to study the Essene doctrines in 53–54.

Vit. 10–12 is problematic in view of the chronology. Vit. 12 states that Josephus was only nineteen years old after receiving education from the Pharisees, the Sadducees and the Essenes and after living for three years with a certain Bannus. If Bannus was not an Essene,[10] we might assume that Josephus has idealized the picture. Perhaps he

---

[1]   *Scribal Character of the Dead Sea Scrolls* II, 696–715. Quotation from p. 714.
[2]   *School,* 156–158. Quotation from p. 166.
[3]   L'enseignement essénien, 191–203. Quotation from p. 203.
[4]   4QTherapeia is probably not a medical document. See correctly NAVEH, *IEJ* 36 (1986) 52–55. Cf. also GARCÍA MARTÍNEZ, *JSJ* 17 (1986) 242–244; GREENFIELD, *IEJ* 36 (1986) 118f.
[5]   DE VAUX, *RB* 61 (1954) 229, pl. 10a. Cf. also *DJD* III, 32.
[6]   LEMAIRE, L'enseignement essénien, 201.
[7]   *DJD* II, 91f, 175, 178f.
[8]   Cf. TALMON, *World of Qumran,* 17f; GARCÍA MARTÍNEZ/VAN DER WOUDE, *RevQ* 14 (1990) 527, 537f.
[9]   Cf. BILDE, *Flavius Josephus,* 29.
[10] LEMAIRE, L'enseignement essénien, 193.

spent only a very short time with the Essenes.[1]

Second, Bell. 2:120 speaks about the education of young children adopted by the Essenes. Although the reference to adoption is obscure,[2] the text expresses the view that the education should conform the children to the customs of the Essenes. This suggests that the Essenes provided training for the children. Third, Bell. 2:136 says that the Essenes are extraordinarily zealous in studying ancient writings that are useful for soul and body, such as those about the healing of diseases. Bell. 2:159 claims also that Essenes able to foretell the future are from their early years well trained in the study of the holy books. And Bell. 2:142 states that they should transmit their doctrines exactly as they received them and preserve the books of their group.[3] As it seems, the Essenes conducted, according to Josephus, a detailed and meticulous study of written texts in order to gain and transmit qualified knowledge and ability.

Philo gives an interesting remark. Omn. Prob. Lib. 80–82 says that the Essenes work on ethics with extreme care and instruct themselves constantly in ancestral laws, particularly setting aside the seventh day to hear the books read and expounded by an ancient method of inquiry. Although the information from Philo does not necessarily imply a school, it indicates that the Essenes were accustomed to a certain amount of scholastic study.

The data in the Dead Sea scrolls themselves are of course most important. The scrolls give no information about a school house. CD 20:10, 13 speak of בית התורה and 1QpHab 8:2; 10:3 of בית המשפט. But the latter expression reflects merely a conception about the future judgement. The former expression does not refer to any earthly institution. It cannot, as Lemaire assumes,[4] be equated with בית המדרש. Delcor's suggestion that מדרש in 1QS 8:26 is an abbreviation of בית המדרש is purely conjectural.[5]

There are however signs of a deliberate study within the community. 1QSa 1:6–9 provides the most important evidence. This messianic text, reflective of historical realities,[6] indicates the different stages and contents of education at Qumran.

1QSa 1:6f envisions that the whole community, even each person born in Israel, will receive instruction in the book of Hagi from youth onwards. Training in the book of Hagi—or Hagu—is essential for the community. It is a basic qualification for official positions of leadership (CD 10:6; 13:2

---

[1] Cf. BEALL, *Josephus' Description of the Essenes,* 34.

[2] There is no explicit report of such a custom in the Dead Sea scrolls. But cf. 1QH 9:34f.

[3] Cf. below p. 166.

[4] L'enseignement essénien, 197.

[5] *RB* 62 (1955) 73–75.

[6] Cf. SCHIFFMAN, *Eschatological Community,* 9.

[14:6–8]).[1]

This probably implies the basic reading of the Scriptures. Y. Yadin cautiously suggested that the book of Hagi was the Temple scroll composed by the Teacher. He identified this document also with several other books referred to in the scrolls.[2] But it is striking that while the scrolls frequently quote different parts of the OT, they never—as far as is possible know—quote from the Temple scroll.[3] This is indeed remarkable if it were to constitute an alternative or new torah to be read from youth on.[4] And it is difficult to establish that the Righteous Teacher wrote the Temple scroll. The document shows no concern to claim the authority of its real author.[5] It is God who delivers instruction,[6] probably to Moses.[7] It is also unlikely that the book of Hagi refers to a written and sectarian mishnah, as some think.[8] The mishnaic study usually belongs to a later stage of education, as the study of oral torah in the rabbinic schools. It is more likely that we should think of the reading of the Scriptures.[9] There are two indications in this direction. First, rabbinic texts claim that the young boys started their education by reading the Scriptures (m. ʾAbot 5:21).[10] And 1QSa 1:6 states that instruction in the book of Hagi is not restricted to the community only but re-

---

[1]   Cf. also 1QH 11:2, 21.

[2]   *Temple Scroll* I, 390–397. Cf. also the more popular version by *idem, Temple Scroll,* 222–229. Besides the book of Hagi, cf. the sealed book of the torah (CD 5:2–5); the torah sent to the wicked priest (4QpPsª 4:8f); the book of the second torah (4QCatenaª 1–4:14).

[3]   STEGEMANN, Origins of the Temple Scroll, 238f; *idem,* Temple Scroll, 129. For further literature, see below p. 151 n. 6.

[4]   The similarities between the Temple scroll on one hand, and the Damascus Document, the War Rule and the Commentary on Nahum on the other, do not prove that the Temple scroll is Qumranic, as claimed in SCHÜRER, *History* III, 412–414. Since the Temple scroll was read/heard at Qumran, it may of course have influenced the authors of other writings.

[5]   *Contra* WISE, *Temple Scroll,* 188f, 200.

[6]   Cf. CALLAWAY, *RevQ* 13 (1988) 246. Following with some modifications STEGEMANN, Origins of the Temple Scroll, 235–256, Callaway regards the Temple scroll as a scribal work to be dated between 450–200 B.C.E., at a time when the status of the biblical books would allow for "an improved law from Sinai" (*ibid.,* 250). Cf. also CALLAWAY, *RevQ* 14 (1990) 648; STEGEMANN, Temple Scroll, 126–136.

[7]   The Temple scroll never mentions Moses by name. 11QT 44:5 provides the clearest indication of Moses as the implied addressee. Aaron is here qualified as "your brother."

[8]   E.g. GINZBERG, *Eine unbekannte jüdische Sekte,* 71; J.M. BAUMGARTEN, *JSJ* 3 (1972) 10 n. 2; STEGEMANN, Origins of the Temple Scroll, 242.

[9]   So e.g. GOSHEN-GOTTSTEIN, *VT* 8 (1958) 286–288; I. RABINOWITZ, *JNES* 20 (1961) 112–114; SCHIFFMAN, *Halakhah at Qumran,* 44; GOIA, *Comunità,* 112 n. 83; SCHÜRER, *History* II 421 n. 41; LEMAIRE, L'enseignement essénien, 195; SCHIFFMAN, *Eschatological Community,* 15.

[10]   Also non-rabbinic texts indicate that young Jewish boys were well acquainted with the Scriptures. Cf. e.g. T. Levi 13:2; Philo, Ebr. 80f; Leg. All. 1:99; Leg. Gaj. 115, 210, 230; Praem. Poen. 162; Spec. Leg. 2:88, 228–230, 233, 236; 4:16, 150; Virt. 141; Ps.-Philo, Bib. Ant. 22:5f; Josephus, Ant. 4:211; Ap. 1:60; 2:178, 204.

quired for each Israelite. Second, the parallels between 1QS 6:6 and CD 13:2 might suggest that in the latter passage the book of Hagi refers to the Torah. It is most natural to relate "Hagi" or "Hagu" to meditation, הגה. The study focuses on the holy writings as a book of meditation.[1] Already the OT indicates such a view in a more limited way (Josh 1:8; Ps 1:2). It is therefore probable that the depiction of the future in 1QSa 1:6f reflects the conviction that the young boys should like all Israelites first of all, as a kind of elementary education,[2] learn to read the Scriptures.

1QSa 1:7f continues the account of the future by speaking of instruction "in the statutes of the covenant" (בחוקי הברית) and "in their precepts" (במשפטיהמה). The Qumranites probably believed that this advanced stage of education should involve a study of the teaching from the Righteous Teacher. It accords with references elsewhere in the scrolls. CD 20:29; 1QSa 1:5 speak also of the statutes of the covenant. CD 10:6 mentions besides the book of Hagi also the foundations of the covenant (יסודי הברית) as the object of study. They seem to denote particular precepts to be studied. The reference to the confession of failure to adhere to the statutes of the covenant in CD 20:29 is of particular interest. 20:30b, 33a take, with some variations, up the reference, and 20:28, 32 connect it with listening to the voice of the Teacher. 20:27f, 31f also connect adhering to the precepts (משפטים) with listening to the Teacher's voice.[3] When we read/hear this together with 1QSa 1:7f, listening to the Teacher and adhering to his teaching appear to be acts of study. This does not necessarily presuppose that the Teacher was alive. His voice may be heard in the traditions. But whether he was alive or not, persons regarding themselves as his pupils, read/heard,[4] perhaps even memorized,[5] the teaching they believed came from him.

1QSa 1:8 implies that the education lasted for ten years. It is not clear if this time of study also included the basic reading of the Scriptures or if the reading was completed before the ten years of education started. In any case, at the age of twenty,[6] the pupil, now mature for marriage,[7] completed his education and was enrolled to enter his duties.[8] After another five years, the person was ready to enter the important office of judge (CD 10:4–7; 1QSa 1:12f), and after five more years, the office of the guardian (CD

---

1 For the collective significance of ספר, see I. RABINOWITZ, *JNES* 20 (1961) 113.
2 Even GOIA, *Comunità,* 100, speaks of elementary instruction at Qumran, in spite of his emphasis (*ibid.,* 98) on the predominance of adult instruction.
3 Cf. below pp. 189f.
4 Cf. 1QSa 1:4f.
5 Cf. VINCENT, *SE* 3 (1964) 109.
6 Cf. Exod 30:14; 38:26.
7 Cf. BORGEN, *RevQ* 3 (1961) 267–277.
8 Cf. the enrollment referred to in CD 10:1; 15:5f. For discussion, see besides BORGEN, *RevQ* 3 (1961) 267–277; SCHIFFMAN, *Eschatological Community,* 16–20, also the early controversy between HOENIG, *JQR* 48 (1957–58) 371–375; *idem, JQR* 49 (1958–59) 209–214, and J.M. BAUMGARTEN, *JQR* 49 (1958–59) 157–160.

14:6–9; 1QSa 1:14–18).[1] The number of years is perhaps not exact. But 1QSa 1:6–9 indicates in any event that the qualifications for the important offices consisted in a profound knowledge attained through deliberate study of the Scriptures and the Teacher's ruling directives.

Also other data from the scrolls testify to the existence of a deliberate study connected with transmitting material from the Teacher. The advanced training in interpretation is related to the intense study (דרש) of the Torah. We saw above that some texts depict the Teacher as a scholar of the Torah (CD 6:7) and give other persons similar functions (1QS 6:6f; 8:11f), though without designating them as interpreters of the Torah. The interpretative rules of *the* interpreter of the Torah apparently served as important directives when Qumranites studied the Torah.

The existence of such a study is well attested. The root דרש is present numerous times in the scrolls. 1QS 8:14f pictures, in reference to Isa 40:3, the study of the Torah (מדרש התורה) even as preparing the way for God, and as commanded by God himself through Moses.[2] "To seek God" (דרש אל), a concept which appears already in the OT,[3] then related to a detailed scrutinizing of the Torah.[4] This study helped the Qumranite to discover the hidden things in the Torah (1QS 5:11).[5] The result of these efforts might have been (written) midrashim.[6] The term מדרש denotes primarily exegesis producing halakhah to which all members must conform (CD 20:6f; 1QS 8:25f),[7] though it is also used for haggadic exegesis of Ps 1:1 (4QFlor 1:14).[8] We gain the impression that some Qumranites performed a detailed and scholastic study on the basis of the Teacher's interpretative instructions and guidelines, aiming to seek out valid norms for the life of the community.

It is difficult to agree with L.H. Schiffman's contention that the occurrence of מדרש in 1QS 6:24 reflects a technical use of the term.[9] But J.T. Milik indicated long ago the possibility that the term is present as a title on different unpublished MSS from cave 4: on two MSS of the Community Rule, two of the Damascus Document and in a cryptic

---

[1]   For the various stages at Qumran, see SCHIFFMAN, *Eschatological Community*, 11–27.

[2]   Cf. DELCOR, *RB* 62 (1955) 66f.

[3]   Cf. Deut 4:29; Isa 9:12; 31:1; Hos 10:12; Amos 5:4, 6 and the discussion by ZOBEL, *Prophetie*, 90–100.

[4]   O. BETZ, *Offenbarung und Schriftforschung*, 16–18.

[5]   Cf. also 1QS 8:11f and the comments by BOCKMUEHL, *Revelation and Mystery*, 42–44.

[6]   Cf. SCHIFFMAN, *Halakhah at Qumran*, 58–60.

[7]   I cannot here discuss the relationship between different forms of interpretation at Qumran. BROOKE, *RevQ* 10 (1981) 483–503, proposes that the designation "Qumran midrashim" should be the main epithet under which the pesharim would be a sub-genre. But this may be too broad a use of the term. For literature on this subject, see SCHÜRER, *History* III, 420 n. 1.

[8]   Cf. BROOKE, *Exegesis at Qumran*, 149–156.

[9]   *Halakhah at Qumran*, 58f.

script A with square letters on the back of an unidentifiable MSS.[1] 4Q266 line 20, the end of the newly published last column of the Damascus Document, does contain (מ)דר(ש). The Genesis Apocryphon is also often called a midrash,[2] though it is sometimes regarded as pre-Qumranic.

The different data thus suggest that there existed certain scholastic settings at Qumran. There are signs of educational measures both on an elementary and an advanced level. On the advanced level, which is of most interest to us, Qumranites seem to have performed a deliberate study of the teaching from the Righteous Teacher. *The teaching believed to originate with the Teacher provided to some extent the more advanced education with an identity.* It was the object of study and guided the study of other objects as well. The accounts about a teacher-pupil relationship corresponded to a kind of educational setting. The school of the Righteous Teacher existed, in a sense.

3.4. The Schools of the Rabbis

The rabbinic literature contains numerous traces of a developed educational system, on the elementary as well as on the advanced level. It is true that the rabbis in principal maintained the biblical ideal (Deut 4:9f; 6:7, 20f; 11:18f; 32:7, 46) about the responsibility of the father to teach his son.[3] It was deeply rooted in antiquity.[4] But since many fathers were unable to fulfil this obligation either personally or by hiring private tutors, the boys usually went to a more organized form of education.[5]

The scripture school (בית סופר, בית ספר) provided the basic education in reading (מקרא) the Torah. According to an unattributed account in y. Ketub. 32c, Simeon b. Sheṭaḥ (c. 90 B.C.E.) was the first to decree that children should go to the scripture school. The more detailed account in b. B. Bat. 21a, attributed to Rab († c. 247 C.E), claims that after the ordinance of teachers for children (מלמדי תינוקות) in Jerusalem, Joshua b. Gamala (c. 60–70 C.E.) arranged that such teachers were appointed in each district and each town.[6] Whatever the origin of the basic educational institution, the rabbinic literature itself takes for granted that later scripture schools existed in practically every inhabited place of some size in Israel.[7]

---

[1]   *RB* 63 (1956) 61.

[2]   But cf. the discussion by EVANS, *RevQ* 13 (1988) 153–165.

[3]   Cf. e.g. m. Pesaḥ. 10:4; t. Ḥag. 1:2; t. Qidd. 1:11; b. Sukk. 42a; b. Nazir 29a; b. Qidd. 29b, 30a; b. B. Bat. 21a; Mek. on 13:13 (Lauterbach I, 164:91–165:96; 166:110–113); Sifre on Deut 11:19.

[4]   RIESNER, *Lehrer,* 102–110.

[5]   Cf. e.g. KRAUSS, *Talmudische Archäologie* III, 199f; MOORE, *Judaism* I, 316; GERHARDSSON, *Memory,* 57f; J. MAIER, *Geschichte der jüdischen Religion,* 112; SAFRAI, Education, 947; STRACK/STEMBERGER, *Talmud and Midrash,* 10.

[6]   For discussion of this account, see RIESNER, *Lehrer,* 200–206.

[7]   Cf. e.g. b. Giṭ. 58a; b. Sanh. 17b; y. Taʿan. 69a; y. Meg. 73d; y. Ḥag. 76c; y.

The teacher of the scripture school was of little independent importance. The texts usually call him סופר.[1] A real scholar was in tannaitic times no more a mere סופר, he was a חכם. The teacher of the scripture school did not have to produce a teaching giving him a highly respected position. It is also possible that the payment usually required and the increasing prominence of oral torah made him even less important.[2] The scripture school did not maintain its essential identity by reference to the individual teacher.

The elementary education, starting approximately at the age of five (m. ʾAbot 5:21), six (b. Ketub. 50a) or seven (b. B. Bat. 21a),[3] was followed by more advanced studies of interpretation (מדרש), and of certain other decrees (תקנות) and prescriptions (גזירות).[4] These studies took place in the wide-embracing institution of the college. During tannaitic and amoraic times, the college was in Palestine usually called בית המדרש, in Babylonia בי רב.[5] The advanced study might have started at the age of ten (m.ʾAbot 5:21) or somewhat later. The origin of the colleges is obscure,[6] but several texts attest their existence as early as in tannaitic times.[7]

The teacher during the first stages in a college could be a less distinguished mishnah teacher (משנה). Texts often refer to the colleges without further qualification or connect them merely with certain places. But there was also a more advanced study (תלמוד) at the feet of a recognized rabbi. And some texts identify the college by reference to a prominent teacher. The earliest archaeological evidence of a college mentions the leading rabbi. D. Urman has published an inscription on a decorated basalt lintel from Dabbura in Golan:[8]

אליעזר הקפר	Eliezer ha-Ḳappar
זה בית	this is his house

Ketub. 35c.

[1]   Cf. e.g. m. Soṭa 9:15; m. Qidd. 4:13; t. Meg. 4:38; y. Meg. 74a; y. Ḥag. 76c; y. Yebam. 13a. The teacher was sometimes also called מלמד תינוקות (Aram. מקרי דרדקי or מקרי ינוקי).

[2]   RIESNER, *Lehrer*, 185f.

[3]   Cf. e.g. SAFRAI, Elementary Education 151f; *idem,* Education, 952.

[4]   For definition of these terms, cf. CHAJES, *Student's Guide Through the Talmud,* 35–117; ELON, *EncJud* XV, 714; PATTE, *Jewish Hermeneutic,* 100–104.—A custom (מנהג), though important, was not part of oral torah. These customs were later collected in special books. Cf. ROTH, *EncJud* XII, 26–31.

[5]   The various other designations applied to the colleges are not entirely interchangeable. See GOODBLATT, *Rabbinic Instruction,* 63–154, 263–267.—ABERBACH, *HUCA* 37 (1966) 107–111, discusses the בית אולפנא as an even higher institute of learning.

[6]   There are references to an early college at the temple mount in Jerusalem (t. Sanh. 7:1) and probably in the Galilean village of Arab (y. Šabb. 15d). For other indications, see SAFRAI, Education, 962.

[7]   Cf. e.g. m. Ber. 4:2; m. Dem. 2:3; 7:5; m. Ter. 11:10; m. Šabb. 16:1; 18:1; m. Pesaḥ. 4:4; m. Beṣa 3:5; m. ʾAbot 5:14; m. Menaḥ. 10:9; m. Yad. 4:3, 4. In m. ʾAbot 1:4 a house of gathering (בית ועד) is referred to.—The common habit of mentioning Sir 51:23 as the earliest use of בית מדרש is probably erroneous, as we have seen.

[8]   *IEJ* 22 (1972) 21–23. Cf. *idem, EAEHL* II, 462, 464.

מדרשו   of instruction

שהלרבי   of the rabbi.

Although the building itself has disappeared completely, the inscription mentions clearly the school of R. Eliezer ha-Ḳappar, a scholar active towards the end of the second or the beginning of the third century C.E. Perhaps he is the scholar elsewhere called Bar-Ḳappara.[1] The lintel probably formed part of the main entrance to the school. As regards the Babylonian practice, D.M. Goodblatt observes that the basic designations for the place of instruction during the Sasanian period were forms of בי רב or of בי followed by the rabbi's name.[2] Similarly, person-oriented formulas intended to express situations of study and instruction are sometimes based on the semi-technical expression "in the presence of" (קמי), followed by the name of a certain rabbi.[3] They reflect further the centrality of the individual master. Sasanian Babylonia was, according to Goodblatt, not dominated by large academies. The place of education was instead identified by reference to the house of the teacher. Apart from the great college of the patriarch, the early colleges often depended upon the individual sage, as it appears.[4] The circle of disciples did not transcend its principal. Upon his departure or death, the group was normally disbanded and the pupils would gather around some other teacher or around one of the pupils who continued to instruct in accordance with the teacher.[5]

The rabbinic literature shows that the accounts about the teacher-pupil relationship corresponded to the actual existence of schools. *The colleges, in particular, were often schools in which the teacher himself provided the circle of disciples with its basic identity and coherence.*

4. Summary and Conclusions

Among various possible settings of transmission, this chapter concentrated on the one determined by the authority of a teacher. I intended to reconstruct a sociocultural situation in which the authority of a person considered in some way to be a teacher—whether alive or not—constituted the essential identity marker for the settings of transmission. To do this, it was necessary to focus on the related existence of two sociocultural phenomena:

---

[1] y. Šabb. 8a speaks of בית רבא דבר קפרא (Krotoshin ed. lines 41–42), perhaps a reference to the school of Bar-Ḳappara

[2] *Rabbinic Instruction,* 63–154, 263–267.

[3] GOODBLATT, *Rabbinic Instruction,* 199–220.

[4] Cf. GOODBLATT, *Rabbinic Instruction,* 267–272; SAFRAI, Education, 963; CO-HEN, *PAAJR* 48 (1981) 59; P.S. ALEXANDER, Orality in Pharisaic-rabbinic Judaism, 163f; STRACK/STEMBERGER, *Talmud and Midrash,* 12.

[5] Cf. e.g. the parallel accounts concerning R. Meir's disciples in b. Nazir 49b; b. Qidd. 52b; y. Qidd. 63a.

accounts about the teacher-pupil relationship and manifestations of the relationship in social settings.

There existed in ancient Israel and ancient Judaism several texts configuring significant teacher-pupil relationships. They appear in the Elijah/Elisha narratives, the writings of the later prophets, Sirach, the Dead Sea scrolls and the rabbinic literature. Various people, among whom there were the ancient transmitters, wrote and read/heard these texts as depictions of settings characterized by a specific didactic authority.

It is probable, generally speaking, that these brief accounts sometimes corresponded to social manifestations in the form of schools. Ben Sira, the Righteous Teacher and prominent rabbis provided individual groups of pupils with a basic identity externalized in educational settings. The ancient transmitters authoring and reading/hearing the accounts often thought of themselves as pupils in these schools. It is difficult to ascertain to what extent the accounts about a teacher-pupil relationship between a prophet and his follower(s) correlated with the existence of groups adhering to a particular prophet. But the redactional character of several prophetic books are explainable, at least, by reference to the activity of such groups. And the early existence of elementary and scribal schools shows that their existence would not be an entirely unique phenomenon in ancient Israel.

The field of cultural continuity in ancient Israel and ancient Judaism shows a *development* towards more organized schools. The accounts and the schools are usually easier to discern in later texts than in older ones. The development is probably due both to internal needs and external influences from the Greek-Hellenistic world. Nevertheless, *the cumulative force from a broad range of testimonies, ranging from pre-exilic times down to the amoraic period of rabbinic Judaism, shows that the phenomenon of settings determined by a didactic authority was deeply rooted in Matthew's socio-cultural situation.*

I have not discussed in this chapter if and how the settings correlated with the motives and the process of transmission. This is the task of the following two chapters. The settings provide the basic frame for the bodies of material to be used. It is now necessary to connect the impression given here with the person-oriented motives of transmission appearing within these settings. The next step is to inquire if and how the conceptions about the teacher motivated the transmission.

Chapter 2

Didactic Authority
and the Motives of Transmission

1. Introductory Remarks

The previous chapter pointed to the basic material of interest. The texts configuring accounts about the teacher-pupil relationship and testifying to the existence of certain schools also contain signs of basic motives of transmission. I will only broaden the scope of material somewhat further here. It is possible that indications are present also in texts not explicitly configuring a setting of transmission determined by didactic authority.

The issue of interest is how the transmitters' understanding of the teacher functioned to motivate the transmission, the person-oriented motives of transmission.[1] Within settings determined by the authority of a specific teacher, these motives may express themselves in at least three ways: as purely didactic motives, as didactic-biographical motives and as didactic-labelling motives.

2. The Didactic Motives

I understand "the didactic motives" as *prevailing interests in the teaching as an entity independent of the life and the status of the teacher*. It would be wrong to exclude these motives entirely from the ones oriented towards a person. The teacher was important and accorded authority. But the teacher was in these cases important only as a *carrier of tradition*, not as its originator. Although the sociologist J. Wach tended to idealize the distinction between master and disciple on one hand, and teacher and pupil on the other,[2] he clearly saw that within a purely didactic relationship the basic orienta-

---

[1] See the remarks in the introduction above p. 23.

[2] *JR* 42 (1962) 1–6. In the German original of the essay, Wach discusses references and literature more explicitly. See *idem, Meister und Jünger,* 47–75. The basic weakness of Wach's distinction is that it empties the master-disciple relationship of didactic implications and stresses too much the exclusive importance of the person of the master. Cf. also *idem, Sociology of Religion,* 133–137. A similar, though somewhat further elaborated, distinction is given by MENSCHING, *Soziologie der Religion,* 167–180.

tion is towards the teaching itself.[1] In principle, teacher and teaching are separated. Despite the importance of the teacher, the information in the teaching itself is the primary motive of transmission.

Didactic motives of transmission are of course present within all the didactic settings of transmission discussed above. A didactic setting often enhances the transmission to the level of a conscious and deliberate act. As concepts, "teacher" and "pupil" describe roles which enact transmission. The transmission is further stimulated if accounts about the teacher-pupil relationship correspond to social manifestations in the form of schools. A teacher normally exhibits authority motivating the transmission. However, there may be different emphases. A pupil may be interested in further aspects of a teacher than his teaching. I will discuss this in the following two sections of this chapter. In this section, *only those conceptions are of interest which maintain that the person at the centre of attention was essentially nothing but a teacher who handed on teaching to his pupils.*

2.1. Jesus ben Sira and the Wisdom Teaching

Although scholars have noticed that wisdom teachers did speak, write and act with certain authority,[2] some features in Sirach convey the unusual didactic rank of Ben Sira.[3] Three examples may suffice to illustrate this. First, in distinction to many other pieces of wisdom literature, Sirach does not conceal the identity of the teacher under the name of Solomon.[4] Solomon is not only the greatest among the wise in Sirach. He is also a person of questionable reputation (47:19f). People thought of him as the author of Sirach only much later.[5] Ben Sira's identity is instead clearly visible. His own colophon (50:27–29) forms an integral part of the book.[6] And this is not only due to the imitation of extra-Jewish devices of writing.[7] Such extra-Jewish influences are present also in wisdom literature concealing the identity of the author.[8] The lack of anonymity and pseudonymity is an indi-

---

[1]   Cf. e.g. WACH, *JR* 42 (1962) 1: "Let us speak of an ideal teacher-student relationship based solely on subject matter and not on the personalities of the teacher and student." Similarly MENSCHING, *Soziologie der Religion,* 169.

[2]   Cf. ZIMMERLI, *ZAW* 51 (1933) 181–192; E.L. DIETRICH, *ZRGG* 4 (1952) 293–296; CRENSHAW, Wisdom and Authority, 10–29 (with lit.).

[3]   Cf. GAMMIE, Sage, 370.

[4]   For Solomonic attribution in Jewish wisdom literature, see MEADE, *Pseudonymity,* 44–72.

[5]   Clement, Strom. II 5:24; VI 16:146; VII 16:105. But cf. Strom. I 4:27; I 10:47.

[6]   For the form of 50:27–29, cf. HASPECKER, *Gottesfurcht,* 89–93.

[7]   Cf. e.g. PAUTREL, *RSR* 51 (1963) 535; HASPECKER, *Gottesfurcht,* 91; MARBÖCK, *Weisheit im Wandel,* 168; HENGEL, *Jews, Greeks and Barbarians,* 121; SALDARINI, *Pharisees, Scribes and Sadducees,* 257; MACK, Sirach, 68; VON LIPS, *Weisheitliche Traditionen,* 102.

[8]   Cf. BLOMQVIST, Apokryfer, 187.

cation of Ben Sira's unusual importance.[1] Second, Ben Sira occasionally acts in an official context. He appears in front of the leaders and asks for their eager attention (33:16–19[G36:16a; 30:25–27]; 39:4).[2] Third, the central idea of Ben Sira's teaching implies a strong sense of authority. As the first known Jewish wisdom teacher, he explicitly identifies the object of his teaching—the Wisdom—with the Torah.[3] Even if other circles close to Ben Sira influenced this identification,[4] its consistent development and use in Sirach point to a teacher of an unusual rank.

2.1.1. The Prophetic Legitimation of Authority

A system of legitimation integrated within the teacher's own self-understanding gives the authoritative claims their validity in Sirach. The legitimation of Ben Sira's authority does not rest merely on the priestly office. Such a basis would not account sufficiently for the features exemplified above. It is necessary to turn to Ben Sira's view of his prophetic inspiration.

Ben Sira is strongly aware of his exceptional inspiration. This is most evident in the description of the ideal scribe in 39:6–11. In distinction to ordinary lay people (38:24–34), the normal scribe constantly tries to comprehend the Scriptures and the obscure meaning of the meshalim (39:1–3); he is taken into the service of the leaders (39:4) and spends all his time in a praying attitude (39:5). If the Lord is willing, the ordinary scribe will be filled with the spirit of understanding and produce the fruits of an *ideal* scribe (39:6–8)—a scribe to be praised for ever (39:9–11).[5] The connection between wisdom and spirit, and the related idea of wisdom as a divine gift (through the spirit), is a common theme in the OT and in later Jewish texts.[6]

---

[1] Cf. MACK, Sirach, 67; ENGBERG-PEDERSEN, Erfaring og åbenbaring, 93.

[2] G. MAIER, *Mensch und freier Wille*, 38f; HENGEL, *Judaism and Hellenism* I, 135, take this as an indication of Ben Sira's prophetic functions. STADELMANN, *Ben Sira*, 217, is correct to note the lack of prophetic allusions.

[3] Cf. 15:1; 19:20; 21:11; 24:23; 34(G31):8. For discussion, see MARBÖCK, *Weisheit im Wandel*, 81–96; *idem*, *BZ* 20 (1976) 1–21; SHEPPARD, Wisdom and Torah, 166–176; SCHNABEL, *Law and Wisdom*, 8–92; SCHIMANOWSKI, *Weisheit und Messias*, 38–61. Cf. also e.g. J.A. DAVIS, *Wisdom and Spirit*, 10–16; PREUSS, *Einführung*, 142–145; BOCKMUEHL, *Revelation and Mystery*, 63f, 68; VON LIPS, *Weisheitliche Traditionen*, 57–59, 149. For an attempt to refute the assumption that the Wisdom and the Torah were identified, cf. SANDELIN, *Wisdom as Nourisher*, 49–53.

[4] It is possible that the circle of scribes around Simeon II the Just (c. 210 B.C.E.) influenced the identification to some extent. Simeon's cosmic apprehension of the Torah is mentioned in m. ʾAbot 1:2.

[5] Cf. STONE, Ideal Figures, 577f.

[6] Cf. e.g. Gen 41:38f; Exod 28:3; 31:3; 35:31; Deut 34:9; 1 Kgs 3:28; Isa 11:2; Job 32:7f; Prov 1:23; Dan 2:20–23; 5:11f; Wis 1:5–7; 7:7, 21f, 27; 9:17; 2 Apoc. Bar. 44:14; 1 Enoch 5:8; 48:1; 49:3; Jub. 40:5; Pss. Sol. 17:37; 18:7; 1QH 12:11f; 13:18f; 14:13, 25; 11QPsª 27:3f, 11; Philo, Deus Imm. 2–3; Leg. All. 1:36–38; Plant. 23–24; Quest. in Ex. 2:7; Som. 2:252; Spec. Leg. 3:1–6. Cf. also the Jewish-Christian T. Sol. 22:1, 3; 26:6. For discussion, see VAN IMSCHOOT, *RB* 47 (1938) 23–49; RYLAARSDAM, *Reve-*

According to Sirach's creation theology,[1] which is more prominent than the creation theology of the wisdom literature in the OT,[2] all men are gifted with understanding to some extent (17:6f) and in possession of a spirit (30:15; 34[G31]:14; 48:12, 24). All men can strive for wisdom.[3] But in one passage, in 39:6, the spirit is an *exceptional* gift of the Lord. It is not merely creational here. It depends on the exceptional will of the Lord; it is a *donum superadditum.*[4] Ben Sira's testimony about his own activity in 50:27 uses identical terms as in 39:6 (הביע/ἀνομβρεῖν). Ben Sira considers himself to be an ideal scribe, exceptionally inspired by the Lord.

The belief in a unique possession of the spirit of understanding relates to a prophetic system of legitimation. To be sure, H. Stadelmann brings forward arguments to diminish the prophetic features in Sirach.[5] He fails however to convince entirely. It is true that Sirach never calls Ben Sira a prophet.[6] But this is no more but an argument from silence. Sirach never speaks explicitly of Ben Sira as a priest either, though the priestly category was, according to Stadelmann, essential for Ben Sira's understanding of himself. Stadelmann's vital argument for rejecting the prophetic features deals with Ben Sira's view of history.[7] In the lauditory review of the great men of Israel's history, the so-called *Laus Patrum* (44:1–50:24),[8] the prophets occur only within the period between the priestly triology in the desert (Moses, Aaron, Phinehas) and the post-exilic hierocracy. Accordingly, because of his view of history, Ben Sira cannot make prophetic claims. This scheme of the history is reminiscent of different texts which scholars often think reflect the view that prophecy was alive only for a limited time in Israel.[9] But the texts stem from different periods and situations. They hardly

---

lation, 99–118; DILLISTONE, *Int* 2 (1948) 275–287; HENGEL, Jesus als messianischer Lehrer, 166–177; STADELMANN, *Ben Sira,* 235–238; J.A. DAVIS, *Wisdom and Spirit,* 7–62; BOCKMUEHL, *Revelation and Mystery,* 57–68; VON LIPS, *Weisheitliche Traditionen,* 146f. For the NT, cf. 1 Cor 2:1–3:4 and the discussion of J.A. DAVIS, *ibid.,* 65–137.

    [1] Cf. MARBÖCK, *Weisheit im Wandel,* 134–151; LÖHR, *Bildung aus dem Glauben,* 69–95.

    [2] Cf. BOSTRÖM, *God of the Sages,* 85. A recent appreciation of the creation theology in Qoheleth is however given by M. SCHUBERT, *Schöpfungstheologie.*

    [3] Cf. 1:9f; 3:29; 6:23–37; 8:8f; 9:14, etc.

    [4] G. MAIER, *Mensch und freier Wille,* 37. Cf. also RICKENBACHER, *Weisheitsperikopen,* 195f; MARBÖCK, Schriftgelehrte Weise, 307f; STADELMANN, *Ben Sira,* 233f; BOCKMUEHL, *Revelation and Mystery,* 61; MENZIES, *Early Christian Pneumatology,* 69f, 76.

    [5] *Ben Sira,* 177–270.

    [6] Cf. STADELMANN, *Ben Sira,* 265.

    [7] *Ben Sira,* 188–216, 265–270.

    [8] For the delimitation of the hymn, see MACK, *Wisdom,* 195–198; LEE, *Form of Sirach 44–50,* 3–21.

    [9] The relevant texts are Ezek 13:9; Zech 13:2–6; Ps 74:9; Dan 3:38 (LXX); 9:24; 1 Macc 4:46; 9:27; 14:41; 2 Apoc. Bar. 85:3; Ap. 1:37–41; t. Soṭa 13:2; b. Yoma 9b; b. Soṭa 48b; b. Sanh. 11a; y. Soṭa 24b; Cant. Rab. on 8:9; S. ʿOlam Rab. 30.

represented a coherent dogma at the time.[1] Caution is therefore called for before we mould Ben Sira into this schematized model. Other considerations point in a different direction.

Sirach conveys numerous impressions of close relations between Ben Sira's teaching ministry and prophecy. First, in distinction to wisdom literature such as Job, Proverbs and Qoheleth, the Greek Sirach employs forms of προφητ- quite frequently, approximately twenty-one times.[2] Second, there are several texts showing that Ben Sira venerates the prophetic traditions and the prophetic office in Israel.[3] Third, although it is true that Sirach never presents Ben Sira's words as divine addresses,[4] W. Baumgartner showed long ago that a variety of prophetic forms are present in Sirach: the announcement of judgement (35:17–20[G32:22–26]), the invective and threat introduced by a woe (2:12–14; 41:8), the promise of salvation (47:22) and references to God's faithfulness in the past (2:10; 16:7–10).[5] Baumgartner concluded that Ben Sira himself intentionally imitated the prophets.[6] We may also notice the prophetic form of the prayer for the redemption of the people, shaped as a lament (36:1–17[G33:1–13a; 36:16b–22]).[7] Fourth, Sirach concludes the great hymn to the Wisdom—identified with the Torah—with a comparison between the teaching of Ben Sira and prophecy (24:33).[8] Fifth, scholars have suggested that Isa 11:2 was particularly influential for the view of the ideal scribe in Sir 39:6.[9] Although Stadelmann denies this,[10] it is at least evident that the Isaianic passage is intertextually present in other early Jewish writings.[11] Sixth, Sirach presents the report that Ben Sira provided education free of charge (51:25) as an allusion to Isa 55:1.[12] Seventh, the ideal scribe, Ben Sira and the Wisdom pour forth (הביע/ἀνομβρεῖν/ἐκφαίνειν) inspired teaching (16:25; 18:29; 39:6;

---

[1]   R. MEYER, *TDNT* VI, 812–819; SCHÄFER, *Vorstellung vom heiligen Geist,* 89–111, 143–146; LEIVESTAD, *NTS* 19 (1972–73) 288–299; AUNE, *Prophecy,* 103–106; GREENSPAHN, *JBL* 108 (1989) 37–49. Cf. also SANDNES, *Paul,* 43–47.

[2]   See, besides the LXX concordance, Rudolf SMEND, *Index,* 205; RICKENBACHER, *Weisheitsperikopen,* 169f.

[3]   Cf. 36:16(G36:21); 39:1; 46:1, 13, 15, 20; 47:1; 48:1–14, 22–25; 49:8–10.

[4]   Cf. VON RAD, *Wisdom,* 254; LANG, *Monotheism,* 151f.

[5]   *ZAW* 34 (1914) 186–189, 192–198.

[6]   LANG, *Monotheism,* 151f, rejects the idea that Ben Sira imitated the prophets, but without giving any arguments.

[7]   HENGEL, *Judaism and Hellenism* I, 134. The authenticity of this text is however debated. Cf. GILBERT, Wisdom Literature, 298 (with lit.).

[8]   The Hebrew is not available here. The Syriac reads "in prophecy" (בנביותא), thus indicating more than a comparison. The Greek (ὡς προφητείαν) reflects perhaps the original best. It creates a neat parallel to 24:32 (ὡς ὄρθρον).

[9]   G. MAIER, *Mensch und freier Wille,* 37; MARBÖCK, Schriftgelehrte Weise, 308.

[10]   *Ben Sira,* 238 n. 3.

[11]   Isa 42:1; 1 Enoch 49:3; Pss. Sol. 17:23, 29, 35, 37; 18:7. Cf. also T. Levi 18:7; T. Jud. 24:2f. For discussion, see HENGEL, Jesus als messianischer Lehrer, 168–175; RIESNER, *Lehrer,* 306–330.

[12]   This is admitted by STADELMANN, *Ben Sira,* 29, in a different context.

50:27).[1] The use of terms underlines the creative force of the teaching.[2] In addition, it is possible that 50:27c—a part of Ben Sira's colophon—originally contained ניבא,[3] not ניבע of Cairo B. This would have formed the parallel to הביע in 50:27d. If this is correct,[4] Ben Sira's inspired ministry is at least comparable to prophecy.

> The connections between prophetic and sapiential ideas are not new in Israel. We have seen that some of the prophets—Amos, Isaiah and Jeremiah—were perhaps associated with wisdom circles.[5] We may also detect the reverse. Job and Proverbs exhibit prophetic features.[6] And it is not necessary to assume a sharp distinction between different streams of ideas during the post-exilic period.[7] The temple school could use sapiential, prophetic and priestly notions without strict distinctions at this time.[8] In the (Egyptian) diaspora,[9] the Wisdom is even the source of prophecy (Wis 7:27; 11:1).

This is the picture of Ben Sira that emerges from Sirach itself. The ancient transmitters might have known about other aspects of the teacher. They were his pupils, his "sons." But they also knew him from reading/hearing his book. *Ben Sira, it seems, appeared to the ancient transmitters of Sirach as a person who delivered teaching and performed actions amounting to an authority valid by reference to prophetic legitimation.* The question is now if this didactic rank stimulated and guided the transmission of his teaching or if it was unrelated to the teaching itself and the transmission process.

2.1.2. The Authority and the Teaching

The teaching apparently carried an inherent value independently of Ben Sira. The pupils, who might have been the first transmitters, had practical occupations of their own (7:15), and once they had learned the teaching, the attachment to Ben Sira—the wearing-out of his door step (6:36)—was no longer essential. Accordingly, there are no episodal narratives about Ben

---

[1] The Hebrew of 18:29; 39:6 must be deduced from the Greek translation. Cf. also הביע/ἐξομβρεῖν in 1:19(G); 10:13 and the images employed in 24:30–33.

[2] MARBÖCK, Schriftgelehrte Weise, 308, 310.

[3] The arguments are listed by Rudolf SMEND, *Weisheit des Jesus Sirach erklärt,* 493f. Cf. similarly BOX/OESTERLY, *APOT* I, 512; BAUMGARTNER, *ZAW* 34 (1914) 186; HENGEL, *Judaism and Hellenism* II, 89 n. 199; ORTON, *Understanding Scribe,* 225 n. 15.

[4] Perhaps a similar confusion between נבנע/ὄμβρῳ and בנביא has arisen in 49:9. Cf. Rudolf SMEND, *Weisheit des Jesus Sirach erklärt,* 493f; BOX/OESTERLY, *APOT* I, 505.

[5] Cf. above pp. 39, 43, 57. See further VON LIPS, *Weisheitliche Traditionen,* 70–76. For a more sceptical assessment, cf. VAN LEEUWEN, Sage, 295–306.

[6] Cf. VON LIPS, *Weisheitliche Traditionen,* 77 (with lit.).

[7] Cf. the general discussion by STECK, *EvT* 28 (1968) 445–458.

[8] For the Hasidim, see HENGEL, *Judaism and Hellenism* I, 202–218, esp. 206.

[9] Most scholars locate the Wisdom of Solomon in Egypt. But cf. the arguments for Syria given by GEORGI, *JSHRZ* 3:4 (1980) 395–397.

Sira and there is no labelling process that validates Ben Sira as the only normative teacher from whom all teaching was to come. *The conceptions about the teacher did not directly motivate the transmission.* What purpose did Ben Sira's unusual claims for authority then serve? It remains to pay more attention to the polemic interaction with the Greek-Hellenistic environment.[1] Sirach reflects both Jewish and extra-Jewish influences. While T. Middendorp exaggerated the direct impact of Greek-Hellenistic thinking and neglected much of the international diffusion of ancient wisdom,[2] a number of echoes from extra-Jewish material—especially from the gnomic poetry of the famous Theognis of Megara (c. 500 B.C.E.)—appear.[3] But we should not, with Middendorp and others,[4] understand these echoes as the result of a *deliberate fusion* of Greek-Hellenistic and Jewish thoughts. As already Rudolf Smend pointed out,[5] and influential Sirach scholars such as V. Tcherikover, G. Maier, M. Hengel, J.T. Sanders, P.W. Skehan and A.A. di Lella have continued to argue,[6] Ben Sira's ministry was partly an attempt to counteract the heavy influence of alien thoughts upon the Jews in Jerusalem. It is not insignificant that Sirach was originally written in Hebrew.[7] The Greek language had already penetrated into Palestine, and at least one of the contemporaneous authors in Palestine—the so-called Pseudo-Eupolemus—wrote in Greek. The use of Hebrew is also striking in view of the possibility that Ben Sira had learned some of his literary skills in the Greek school.[8] Perhaps the repeated exhortation "say not" is as an indication of the polemical setting.[9] This setting is

---

1　Cf. already Rudolf SMEND, *Weisheit des Jesus Sirach erklärt*, xx: "Dies Selbstbewusstsein erklärt sich allein aus den ausserordentlichen Verhältnissen, unter denen Jesus Sirach wirkte."

2　*Stellung Jesu Ben Siras.* For criticism of Middendorp, see HENGEL, *JSJ* 5 (1974) 83–87; J.T. SANDERS, *Ben Sira and Demotic Wisdom*, 27–59. Cf. also KAISER, *VF* 27 (1982) 82f. The dissertation by H.-V. KIEWELER, *Ben Sira zwischen Judentum und Hellenismus.* Eine kritische Auseinandersetzung mit Th. Middendorp. University of Vienna 1987, was not available to me.

3　J.T. SANDERS, *Ben Sira and Demotic Wisdom*, 29–55, considers Theognis as the only author that Ben Sira read and used. Cf. also HENGEL, *Judaism and Hellenism* I, 149f, allowing for a somewhat broader, though indirect, influence.

4　Besides Middendorp, cf. e. g. PAUTREL, *RSR* 51 (1963) 535–549; MARBÖCK, *Weisheit im Wandel*, 160–173; GOLDSTEIN, Jewish Acceptance and Rejection, 72–75; NICKELSBURG, *Jewish Literature*, 64; VON LIPS, *Weisheitliche Traditionen*, 102.

5　*Weisheit des Jesus Sirach erklärt*, xx–xxviii.

6　TCHERIKOVER, *Hellenistic Civilization*, 144f; DI LELLA, *CBQ* 28 (1966) 139–146; G. MAIER, *Mensch und freier Wille*, 43–59; HENGEL, *Judaism and Hellensim* I, 138–153, 157–162; *idem, JSJ* 5 (1974) 83–87; *idem, Jews, Greeks and Barbarians*, 121–123; J.T. SANDERS, *Ben Sira and Demotic Wisdom*, 55–59; SKEHAN/DI LELLA, *Wisdom of Ben Sira*, 16, 46–50, *passim.* Cf. also e.g. KAISER, *VF* 27 (1982) 79–85; J.A. DAVIS, *Wisdom and Spirit*, 11, 157f n. 10; PREUSS, *Einführung*, 146f; M. SMITH, *Palestinian Parties*, 142; SANDNES, *Paul*, 142.

7　Cf. MACK, Sirach, 82.

8　See excursus 3 below.

9　5:1, 3f, 6; 7:9; 11:23f; 15:11f; 16:15(G16:17); 31(G34):12. Cf. PREUSS, *Einfüh-*

present in the background of several central concepts: wisdom comes from nowhere else but from the God of Israel;[1] the Wisdom found its permanent dwelling-place nowhere else but in Zion/Jerusalem (24:8–12); it is revealed nowhere else but in the Torah.[2] Accordingly, Sirach cautions about the futility of Greek-Hellenistic speculation and warns against false ways of seeking wisdom (3:21–24); it exhorts the wise man not to hate but to trust the Torah (33[G36]:2f); it pronounces woes over those who are prepared to compromise with Hellenism—to tread a double path (2:12)—and over those who completely forsake the Torah (41:8f).

In view of the polemical reflections in Sirach, it is conceivable that Ben Sira's elevated status was a means by which the teacher wanted to set himself over against the powerful didactic channels through which Greek-Hellenistic ideas were mediated to the Jews of Jerusalem. It is indeed probable that several *Jewish* wisdom schools existed in Jerusalem. The reference to different kinds of teachers in 37:19–26 may even indicate that these schools sometimes were in conflict with each other.[3] But the Jewish schools were probably not the primary reason for Ben Sira's emphasis on his own legitimate authority. In view of the antagonism against Greek-Hellenistic notions in Sirach, it is more likely that Ben Sira saw the *Greek* schools as the primary threat to the faith of Israel. In addition to the polemical thrust of several passages in Sirach, the cultural force of the Greek school system at this time makes it probable that Ben Sira's enhanced position was directed towards teachers propagating Greek-Hellenistic views. *Through the authoritative claims, Ben Sira wanted to attract students to himself, to the school (in the temple) that provided teaching in accordance with the faith of Israel. It was the teaching—not the teacher—that was the all important matter.*

Some indications in Sirach give further testimony of this. Just as the director of the Greek gymnasium had a particular responsibility for the young men in the third stage of education,[4] Ben Sira addressed men of young age, who started their quest for wisdom and were developing their sense of moral standards. And contrary to the practice in the Greek school,

---

rung, 146.

[1]   Cf. 1:1, 8–10, 26; 17:11; 24:3; 38:6; 43:33; 45:26; 50:23.

[2]   Cf. 15:1; 19:20; 21:11; 24:23; 34(G31):8. Further "polemical dogmas" in Sirach are discussed by DI LELLA, *CBQ* 28 (1966) 143–146; HENGEL, *Judaism and Hellenism* I, 138–150, 157–162.

[3]   HENGEL, *Judaism and Hellenism* I, 132.—The omission of Ezra from the *Laus Patrum* (44:1–50:24) is probably not due to a polemical attitude towards contemporary groups adhering to Ezra and his strict view on the purity of Israel's people. It depends perhaps on the fact that 49:11–13 intends to mention only persons involved in restoring Jerusalem and the temple So e.g. SNAITH, *Ecclesiasticus,* 247; STADELMANN, *Ben Sira,* 163 n. 1; SCHNABEL, *Law and Wisdom,* 27f; BEGG, *BN* 42 (1988) 17f. For a survey of various opinions, see SCHNABEL, *ibid.,* 26–28.

[4]   NILSSON, *Schule,* 54.

it was possible to receive Ben Sira's education free of charge (51:25).[1] The only payment was the labour put into the learning (51:28).[2] The polemical setting also makes it understandable why the pupils should seek eagerly for a wise teacher and attend his teaching constantly (6:35f). In view of the prevailing cultural atmosphere,[3] the early transmitters of Sirach probably detected these polemical indications in the book.

Excursus 3: *The Book of Sirach and the Greek Schools*

The Greek education was, generally speaking, well structured. Although significant variations may have existed due to different geographical and social factors, there were in principle three stages. After the primary education from the age of seven to twelve or fourteen, the ephebate followed. In addition to the literary training, this secondary level consisted of physical (and military) training in the gymnasium. In the third stage, the young men (οἱ νέοι) continued the education by studying subjects such as rhetoric and philosophy, until they reached the age of nineteen or twenty. An even higher learning was possible to attain in certain places.[4] The teachers usually received a salary, though the payment was sometimes low and irregular.[5]

Such well structured education exerted considerable cultural influence. The studies included literary education. Special teachers existed—at least theoretically—for each stage of the literary training, the grammatist (γραμματιστής) for the primary school, the grammarian (γραμματικός, κριτικός, φιλόλογος) for the secondary level and the rhetor (ῥήτωρ, σοφιστής) for the third stage.[6] Scholars have accordingly found libraries in close connection to the gymnasium.[7] There were also intimate relations between the schools and the cult.[8] Since the gymnasium was often an important establishment in the city,[9] the cultural impact of its education must have been considerable. The people often held the director (γυμνασίαρχος) of the school in high esteem, though they exchanged him each year. He occupied one of the most distinguished positions in

---

[1] This was the normal practice in Israel. Exceptions may be implied in Mic 3:11; Prov 17:16. But already Mic 3:11 indicates that the ideal practice was to give education without charge of money. The refusal to receive money for the advanced teaching of adults in rabbinic Judaism is well-known. Cf. e.g. m. 'Abot 1:13; m. Bek. 4:6; b. Ned. 37a, 62a. For discussion, cf. e.g. KRAUSS, *Talmudische Archäologie* III, 212f; Joachim JEREMIAS, *Jerusalem*, 112–116. For possible exceptions to this rule, cf. SCHÜRER, *History* II, 328.

[2] HARRINGTON, Wisdom of the Scribe, 186, interprets 51:28 as a reference to voluntary donation. In view of 51:25, it is better to understand it as a proverbial saying. So SNAITH, *Ecclesiasticus*, 261f.

[3] See further excursus 3 below.

[4] See NILSSON, *Schule*, 34–42; MARROU, *History of Education*, 102f. For the topics trained in the schools, see NILSSON, *ibid.*, 42–49; MARROU, *ibid.*, 150–216; CLARK, *Higher education*, 11–118.

[5] NILSSON, *Schule*, 52f; MARROU, *History of Education*, 145f.

[6] MARROU, *History of Education*, 160. Cf. also CLARK, *Higher education*, 11, 45; TORTZEN, Hvordan lærte oldtidens børn at læse og skrive?, 7.

[7] NILSSON, *Schule*, 51f; MARROU, *History of Education*, 187f; DELORME, *Gymnasion*, 331f.

[8] NILSSON, *Schule*, 61–75.

[9] DELORME, *Gymnasion*, 337–361. Cf. also I. NIELSEN, Undervisningens fysiske rammer, 77.

the city.[1] Also the building and the place itself was important. It was one of the primary locations for different forms of public life.[2] And the students maintained strong ties to the schools even after they had finished their education, often by means of associations.[3]

From one of the earliest accounts about the establishment of a gymnasium and ephebate in Syria and Palestine, we know that Greek schools existed in Jerusalem circa 175 B.C.E. (1 Macc 1:11–15; 2 Macc 4:9–15).[4] Although some scholars maintain that the establishment was not an intended act of hellenization,[5] the cultural force and impressiveness of this act should not be underestimated.[6] The accounts, though coloured by polemical interests, testify in this direction. They portray the establishment as the introduction of the customs of the Gentiles (1 Macc 1:13), as Jason's attempt to convert his fellow-countrymen to the Greek ways of life (2 Macc 4:10) and as a climax of the passion for Greek fashions (2 Macc 4:13). The report that Jason wanted to build the gymnasium under the citadel (2 Macc 4:12),[7] at the north-eastern corner of the temple area,[8] indicates perhaps the relation to the cult. The priests apparently showed an eager interest in the events taking place within the new establishment (2 Macc 4:14). Also large groups of the Jerusalemite population seem to have endorsed the school positively (1 Macc 1:11–15).

It is probable that Ben Sira himself knew about Greek schools and education already at the time of composing his book.[9] The establishment of a gymnasium in Jerusalem circa 175 B.C.E. presupposed the earlier existence of elementary schools and knowledge of Greek language and culture in at least some circles in Jerusalem. The enthusiasm of the Jerusalemites (1 Macc 1:11–15; 2 Macc 4:12–15) also points to a previous knowledge of Greek education. The Jews in the diaspora did not generally isolate themselves from Greek education,[10] and there is as early as in the third century B.C.E. some influence of Greek education in Palestine, even in Jerusalem.[11] Whatever the historical value,[12] it may be of some significance that Josephus (Ap. 1:176–182) much later wrote concerning Clearchus of Soloi, a pupil of Aristotle (c. 384–322 B.C.E.), that he believed his master to have met a Jew from Jerusalem who was

---

1   NILSSON, *Schule*, 53f, 87; MARROU, *History of Education*, 110.

2   NILSSON, *Schule*, 78–80, 85.

3   NILSSON, *Schule*, 75–78.

4   Cf. Ant. 12:241. For discussion, see BICKERMANN, *Gott der Makkabäer*, 59–65; NILSSON, *Schule*, 84; TCHERIKOVER, *Hellenistic Civilization*, 163–169; DELORME, *Gymnasion*, 198f; HENGEL, *Judaism and Hellenism* I, 70–78, 304f; GOLDSTEIN, *I Maccabees*, 117, 200; HENGEL, *Jews, Greeks and Barbarians*, 116; BRINGMANN, *Hellenistische Reform*, 66–68, 82–96, 145f; GOLDSTEIN, *II Maccabees*, 228–230; HENGEL/MARKSCHIES, *'Hellenization' of Judea*, 22; DORAN, Jason's Gymnasion, 99–109.

5   BRINGMANN, *Hellenistische Reform*, 67f, 82f, 145f. Cf. the review of Bringmann's work by APPLEBAUM, *Gnomon* 57 (1985) 191–193.

6   Cf. DORAN, Jason's Gymnasion, 99–109.

7   This is probably the meaning of "under the acropolis itself" (ὑπ' αὐτὴν τὴν ἀκρόπολιν).

8   HENGEL, *Judaism and Hellenism* II, 10 n. 81, 51 n. 131.

9   DI LELLA, *CBQ* 28 (1966) 140f, even suggests that Ben Sira knew Jason since Simeon II the Just—Jason's father—is praised as high priest in Sir 50:1–21.

10   HENGEL, *Judaism and Hellenism* I, 68f.

11   HENGEL, *Judaism and Hellenism* I, 59f, 63, 75f; *idem, Jews, Greeks and Barbarians*, 115; HENGEL/MARKSCHIES, *'Hellenization' of Judea*, 7, 22.

12   Cf. already LEWY, *HTR* 31 (1938) 205–235.

Greek not only in regard to the language but also in regard to the soul (Ap. 1:180). Through the excerpts of Alexander Polyhistor in Eusebius, Praep. Ev. IX 17:2–9, 18:2, we also know of an anonymous Jew (or Samaritan)—the so-called Pseudo-Eupolemus—who lived in Palestine at the time of Ben Sira and wrote his compositions in Greek.[1] Ben Sira may also have learned about the gymnasium during his journies (34[G31]:9–13).[2] A gymnasium existed already during the middle of the third century as close as in Antioch on the Orontes. And in Egypt there were gymnasia in Alexandria and at other places.[3] Perhaps he had even learned some of his literary skills at the feet of a rhetor. T.R. Lee has shown that the *Laus Patrum* (44:1–50:24) is reminiscent of the *encomium* (ἐγκώμιον), the rhetorical genre used by educated persons to praise men of reputation.[4] In any case, the sources suggest that *attractive schools propagating Greek-Hellenistic ideals existed close to the location of Ben Sira's ministry just after he had written his book. The early transmitters lived under conditions that promoted a polemical understanding of the elevated status which Sirach accords to Ben Sira.*

2.2. The Rabbis and Torah

As a matter of course, the advanced rabbinic teachers exhibited a dominating influence on their pupils. E. Bammel even suggests that the important rank of the teacher is the most characteristic feature of rabbinic Judaism.[5] This may be an overstatement. In any event, the rabbinic literature reflects in various ways how the pupils on their part acknowledged and validated the teachers.[6] But the teachers were not accorded an intrinsic authority. The issue of interest here is how the validation of the individual teachers ultimately related to the teaching itself—to torah in its various forms.

2.2.1. The Duty to Minister and Torah

The pupils performed a number of acts which implicitly validated the teacher. These acts were of uttermost importance. Several texts show that the

---

[1] For introductory discussion and literature, see ATTRIDGE, Historiography, 165f; SCHÜRER, *History* III:1, 528–531.

[2] Cf. 8:15f; 39:4; 51:3.—MIDDENDORP, *Stellung Jesu Ben Siras,* 170–173, tries to diminish the accuracy of this information. But J.T. SANDERS, *Ben Sira and Demotic Wisdom,* 41, correctly judges his explanation by reference to Odyssey 1:1–10 as "farfetched." And as MARBÖCK, *Weisheit im Wandel,* 162; LEE, *Form of Sirach 44–50,* 163, 244, remark, travels were of educational value in the Greek-Hellenistic world.

[3] DELORME, *Gymnasion,* 136–140.

[4] *Form of Sirach 44–50,* 81–245. Cf. also MACK, *Wisdom,* 128–137; SANDNES, *Paul,* 25.

[5] *Jesu Nachfolger,* 22: "Die Herausbildung des Lehrstands und der Rang, der ihm beigemessen wird, ist überhaupt das unterscheidende Phänomen der jüdischen Kulturgeschichte: das Judentum wird zum rabbinischen Judentum."

[6] For general discussion of the relationship between teacher and pupil in rabbinic Judaism, see KRAUSS, *Archäologie* III, 223–227; ABERBACH, Relations Between Master and Disciple, 1–24.

performance of such acts was an obligation which should take precedence over the duties to be carried out even to the father,[1] unless the father himself was a teacher.[2] In other instances, it is equated with fear of God (b. Pesaḥ. 22b; b. Qidd. 57a) or of heaven (m. ʾAbot 4:12).[3]

Most significant was the duty to minister (שימש) to the teacher.[4] Mek. on 12:1 (Lauterbach I, 14:151f) points out how Joshua ministered to Moses[5] and Elisha to Elijah.[6] It was accordingly of vital importance for a student to attend upon the needs of the rabbi.[7] Certain texts even claim that the rabbis considered those who did not fulfil this duty—no matter what knowledge had been acquired—like uneducated people, the עם הארץ (b. Ber. 47b; b. Soṭa 22a); they had no part in the world to come (ʾAbot R. Nat. A 36); they were liable to death (y. Nazir 56b; ʾAbot R. Nat. A 12; Der. Er. Zuṭ. 8).[8] The pupil was to do for the rabbi the same services as an ordinary slave,[9] though in order not to be mistaken for a non-Jewish slave he might at certain places be released from some menial tasks such as untying the sandals of the rabbi (b. Ketub. 96a).[10]

The duty to minister was not external to the actual studies.[11] On the contrary, it was an integral part of learning torah.[12] The action of the master, though occasionally idiosyncratic and exceptional, was normative teaching.[13] The pupil did not learn only by listening to the words.[14] He was also to observe and be a witness to his teacher's actions.[15] This is evident in many different texts. It occurs perhaps most clearly in the praise of the Torah added in m. ʾAbot 6. According to m. ʾAbot 6:6, the pupils learned the Torah through forty-eight qualifications, including the ministry to sages (שמוש חכמים).

---

1 Cf. e.g. m. B. Meṣ. 2:11; m. Ker. 6:9; t. B. Meṣ. 2:29; t. Hor. 2:5; b. Hor. 13a; y. B. Meṣ. 8d.—PESCE, *ANRW* II 25:1 (1982) 384 n. 109, stresses correctly that the obedience to the teacher did not exclude the respect for the father in rabbinic Judaism. It was a matter of setting the right priorities, not necessarily of choosing one or the other option.
2 Cf. e.g. m. B. Meṣ. 2:11; y. B. Meṣ. 8d.
3 Cf. also m. ʾAbot 1:3; b. Ketub. 96a.
4 Cf. ABERBACH, Relations Between Master and Disciple, 2f, 5–8.
5 Cf. Exod 24:13; 33:11; Num 11:28; Josh 1:1.
6 Cf. 1 Kgs 19:21; 2 Kgs 3:11.
7 Cf. e.g. b. Ber. 7b.
8 Further parallels are discussed by SPERBER, *Commentary,* 182f.
9 KRAUSS, *Archäologie* II, 101f; W.D. DAVIES, *Setting of the Sermon on the Mount,* 455.
10 DAUBE, *New Testament,* 266f, 277. For further references to the importance and significance of שמש, cf. STRACK/BILLERBECK, *Kommentar* I, 527–529.
11 Cf. ZUMSTEIN, *Relation du maître et du disciple,* 42f.
12 Cf. e.g. m. Dem. 2:3; m. B. Bat. 10:8; b. ʿErub. 13a; b. Ḥul. 54a; y. Šabb. 12c; y. Ḥag. 78d; y. Nazir 56b.
13 KIRSCHNER, *JSJ* 17 (1986) 70–79.
14 Cf. RENGSTORF, *TDNT* IV, 435.
15 GERHARDSSON, *Memory,* 181–187.

The integration of these acts into the torah study itself suggests that the basis of validation resided *outside* of the life and the status of the teacher. *Torah in its various forms, not the rabbi himself, was the focus of attention.* The teacher was of interest primarily as the embodiment of torah in words and deeds. This is consistent with the fact that knowledge of torah was by itself a sufficient quality for gaining certain respect and honour from others (m. ʾAbot 6:3; b. Pesaḥ. 113b). The fundamental basis for any kind of status was the knowledge of torah. *The implicit validation expressed in the act of ministering to the teacher was essentially not an acknowledgement of the life and the status of the teacher, but of the teacher's ability to transmit torah.*

2.2.2. The Ordination and Torah

The act of ordination (סמיכה),[1] which should probably not be distinguished too sharply from the act of appointment (מנוי) mentioned in the Palestinian Talmud,[2] was the most prominent manner to validate the rabbis. R. Ba (c. 270 C.E.)—also known as R. Abba b. Zabda—mentions R. Joḥanan b. Zakkai († c. 80 C.E.) as the first example in a row of rabbis practising the ordination (y. Sanh. 19a). But its actual origin is uncertain,[3] nor is it clear when it was discontinued.[4]

Although minor differences existed in the actual performance of the ordination, several general features testify to its institutional and official character. First, while the early teachers took the initiative to ordain a pupil themselves, later teachers needed the consent of the patriarch—either the patriarch alone or the patriarch together with the rabbinic sanhedrin (y. Sanh. 19a).[5] Perhaps there was even an official register of all the ordained persons.[6] The ordination was an official matter. Second, the ordination usually required the presence of at least three men. One of these men was himself ordained and the other two apparently served as witnesses (t. Sanh. 1:1; b. Sanh. 13b; y. Sanh. 19a).[7] The ordination was not merely a private affair. Third, the ordination was probably from the beginning performed through the laying on of both hands.[8] We should not doubt the originality of

---

1   The most important literature is listed in SCHÜRER, *History* II, 211f n. 42, and by D.P. WRIGHT, *JAOS* 106 (1986) 433f n. 2. Cf. also HRUBY, *MD* 102 (1970) 30–56.
2   LOHSE, *Ordination,* 28f.
3   Cf. the critical evaluation by WESTERHOLM, *Jesus and Scribal Authority,* 33–37.
4   Cf. NEWMAN, *Semikhah,* 144–154; HRUBY, *MD* 102 (1970) 55f; ROTHKOFF, *EncJud* XIV, 1142.
5   For discussion of the historical development implied in this text, see NEWMAN, *Semikhah,* 13–23; LOHSE, *Ordination,* 36–39; ALON, *Jews,* 401–410.
6   NEWMAN, *Semikhah,* 123–128.
7   STRACK/BILLERBECK, *Kommentar* II, 653; LOHSE, *Ordination,* 45; VON LIPS, *Glaube – Gemeinde – Amt,* 226. Cf. also m. Sanh. 1:1.
8   For discussion, see NEWMAN, *Semikhah,* 102–114.

this practice, as some do.[1] The fact that the act is called סמיכה, from סמך, "to lean,"[2] shows the close association between the ordination and the laying on of hands. The midrashim (Sifre on Num 27:18, 23; Sifre on Deut 34:9; Sifre Zuṭ. on 27:18) also testify that the biblical precedent to the act was the account about Joshua's authorization by Moses, which mentions the laying on of hands (Num 27:18, 23; Deut 34:9). In any case, we see the significance of this manner of ordaining through a comparison with other texts implying that some rabbis expressed doubts about the literal laying on of hands or that persons occasionally might have been ordained in their absence,[3] in spite of the sharp warnings against such a practice in b. Sanh. 14a. The "instrumental" aspect of the laying on of hands was not always very prominent, it seems. To be sure, the rabbis believed that the ordination conveyed the abilities of the ordainer to the one ordained.[4] But they hardly believed that these abilities were handed over *only* "through the hands." We would in that case expect the laying on of hands to be an unconditional means for the ordination on all occasions. The laying on of both hands in front of two witnesses functioned more as an act of demonstration. We might find this function already in the OT when Moses puts both his hands[5] on Joshua in front of the priest and the congregation (Num 27:18–23),[6] This function of the ordination is a further indication of its official character in rabbinic Judaism.

The institutional and official manner of validating the teachers resided in a high conception of torah. Of course, the ordination gave a certain status to the individual teacher. He could now become a member of the rabbinic court (m. Sanh. 4:4); he could be an elder (זקן) or rabbi (b. B. Meṣ. 85a; b. Sanh. 13b; Sifre on Num 11:16).[7] But the ordination also accorded a formal authority (רשות) to transmit torah. It gave the legitimate right to perform a *function*. The rabbis normally believed that Moses first ordained Joshua and that the chain back to Moses was secure through a continual succession

---

[1]　EHRHARDT, *JEH* 5 (1954) 125–130; FERGUSON, *HTR* 56 (1963) 13–16; A.T. HANSON, *TRE* 14 (1985) 417.

[2]　For discussion and literature on background of the term and the practice in the OT, see D.P. WRIGHT, *JAOS* 106 (1986) 433–439; WRIGHT/MILGROM/FABRY, *TWAT* V, 880–889.

[3]　Cf. b. Sanh. 13b; y. Bik. 65d.

[4]　This function is prominent according to e.g. NEWMAN, *Semikhah,* 2f; LOHSE, *Ordination,* 53–55; DAUBE, *New Testament,* 231, 245; ROTHKOFF, *EncJud* XIV, 1140f. Cf. also ZUMSTEIN, *Relation du maître et du disciple,* 24; SCHEDL, *Christologie,* 244–246; HANSSEN, *Handspåleggelsens funksjon,* 25f.

[5]　The laying on of the hand (sing.) in Num 27:18 may be interpreted as dual. Cf. PÉTER, *VT* 27 (1977) 50f; D.P. WRIGHT, *JAOS* 106 (1986) 435.

[6]　So D.P. WRIGHT, *JAOS* 106 (1986) 436; WRIGHT/MILGROM/FABRY, *TWAT* V, 884f. Cf. also Deut 34:9.

[7]　Cf. LOHSE, *Ordination,* 50–52; EHRHARDT, *JEH* 5 (1954) 129–131; FERGUSON, *HTR* 56 (1963) 16–19.

of ordained scholars.[1] The right procedure of succession—the ordination—was the guarantee and authorization for the faithful transmission of torah. Torah, not the individual rabbi, was the all important matter.

We see this focus on torah perhaps most clearly in the qualities demanded from the person to be ordained. It is difficult to know why certain gifted scholars did not receive the ordination (b. B. Meṣ. 85b–86a; b. Sanh. 14a; y. Taʿan. 68a).[2] But it is evident that those who were chosen to be ordained were the best pupils who had learned torah thoroughly. The rabbis ordained the pupils who were sitting in the first of the three rows of students in the rabbinic sanhedrin (m. Sanh. 4:4). It was a matter too important to be sold out to persons without proper qualifications (b. Sanh. 7b; y. Bik. 65d). The strong demands generally laid upon the one to be ordained even caused some attempts to evade the ordination.[3]

Some texts claim even that the ordination was an unconditional prerequisite for transmitting torah. Most striking is an account about R. Judah b. Baba († c. 135 C.E.) in b. Sanh. 13b–14a. In spite of the prohibition that Hadrian issued against the ordination, Judah ordained several of R. Akiba's pupils according to this account. The Romans slew Judah for this offence, but the all important matter was that traditional authority in matters of torah was secured.[4] And no one could nullify the ordination once it had been performed (b. Sanh. 30b).[5]

The ordination reveals in a way the minor independent importance attached to the life and status of the individual teacher. The institutional and official act of ordination served to validate the teacher, not some personal labels acknowledging some kind of intrinsic authority. This system of validation is consistent with the fact that *it was not the teacher himself who was at the centre of attention but the concept of torah. The ordination functioned as an official demonstration and acknowledgement of the teacher's capacity to transmit torah.*

2.2.3. The Titular Attribution "Rabbi" and Torah

Another way of validating the teacher, in addition to performing certain acts, was to ascribe him titles. As we saw in the previous chapter,[6] various forms of "Rabbi" (רבי) became the most prominent didactic title in rabbinic Judaism.[7]

---

1 Cf. STEMBERGER, *Judentum*, 86f.
2 Cf. NEWMAN, *Semikhah*, 95–97; LOHSE, *Ordination*, 37f.
3 Cf. e.g. b. Sanh. 14a; y. Bik. 65c–d. Discussion and further references are given by NEWMAN, *Semikhah*, 93f.
4 Cf. DAUBE, *New Testament*, 208.
5 NEWMAN, *Semikhah*, 97f. Cf. also LOHSE, *Ordination*, 35.
6 See above pp. 52f.
7 The most important literature on this topic is listed by SCHNEIDER, *EWNT* III,

The history of the titular use of רבי has been the object of some controversy between H. Shanks and S. Zeitlin, the former arguing for the existence of a pre-70 use and the latter claiming the absence of any real evidence for the early use of רבי as a title.[1] I do not need to enter into this debate here.[2] The term goes back on רבב, "to be many."[3] The adjective רב expresses the corresponding plentiness in quantity.[4] But it can also have a qualitative connotation, best translated with "great." Several texts apply it in this sense on persons occupying respected positions.[5] We find it already in the OT, especially in connection with the officials of the Assyrian-Babylonian army.[6] From the time before 70 C.E., we have one ossuary inscription (*CII* II, 1218) using it as a title, in this case for a certain Rab Ḥana (רב חנא).[7] Forms of רב were apparently used in a rather titular manner also in other languages throughout the ancient Near East.[8]

The rabbinic literature often expresses a qualitative understanding of רב. Several texts use it, for instance, to denote the lord in distinction to the servant or the slave.[9] There are likewise instances where the suffixes attached to רב carry a real pronominal meaning: the king is רבינו to the people (t. Sanh. 4:4); and not only Elijah (b. Ber. 3a) and the Messiah (b. Sanh. 98a) are called רבי,[10] but also the robber captain by his own accomplices (b. B. Meṣ. 84a). The term signifies the subordination under the legitimate authority of various figures.

The rabbinic writings use the term in the same qualitative sense also for

493. Cf. also MOORE, *Judaism* III, 15–17; I.L. RABINOWITZ, *EncJud* XIII, 1445; ZEITLIN, *JQR* 53 (1962–63) 345–349; VERMES, *Jesus the Jew,* 115–122; ELLISON, *NIDNTT* III, 115f; SCHÜRER, *History* II, 325f; RIESNER, *Lehrer,* 266–276; ZIMMERMANN, *Die urchristlichen Lehrer,* 72–75, 86–91; VIVIANO, *RB* 97 (1990) 207–218; RIESNER, Jesus as Preacher and Teacher, 186; LAPIN, *ABD* 5 (1992) 600–602.

1   SHANKS, *JQR* 53 (1962–63) 337–345; ZEITLIN, *JQR* 53 (1962–63) 345–349; SHANKS, *JQR* 59 (1968–69) 152–157; ZEITLIN, *JQR* 59 (1968–69) 158–160.

2   Cf. further below pp. 286f.

3   HARTMANN, *THAT* II, 715.

4   HARTMANN, *THAT* II, 719; BERLIN, *JBL* 100 (1981) 90–93.

5   Cf. STRACK/BILLERBECK, *Kommentar* I, 916; DALMAN, *Worte Jesu,* 274f; A. SCHULZ, *Nachfolgen,* 24f; LOHSE, *TDNT* VI, 961f; SHANKS, *JQR* 59 (1968–69) 152–155; HARTMANN, *THAT* II, 720f; HENGEL, *Charismatic Leader,* 43 n. 20; RIESNER, *Lehrer,* 268f; ZIMMERMANN, *Die urchristlichen Lehrer,* 86f.

6   Cf. e.g. רב מג (Jer 39:3, 13); רב טבחים (2 Kgs 25:8–11; Jer 39:9–13; 52:12–30); רב סריס (2 Kgs 18:17; Jer 39:3, 13; Dan 1:3); רב שקה (2 Kgs 18:17–37; 19:4, 8; Isa 36:2, 4, 11–13, 22; 37:4, 8). For further references, cf. SHANKS, *JQR* 59 (1968–69) 154.

7   Most of the relevant inscriptions up to the 7th cent. C.E. have been collected by COHEN, *JQR* 72 (1981) 1–17.

8   SHANKS, *JQR* 59 (1968–69) 153f. This is acknowledged also by ZEITLIN, *JQR* 59 (1968–69) 158.

9   Cf. e.g. m. Pesaḥ. 8:2; m. Sukk. 2:9; m. Giṭ. 4:4, 5; m. ʿEd. 1:13; m. ʾAbot 1:3; t. B. Qam. 11:2; b. Ber. 10a; b. Taʿan. 25b; b. Giṭ. 23b; Mek. on 12:1 (Lauterbach I, 8:82–84); Cant. Rab. on 1:1.

10   The Samaritans adressed God as רבי. Cf. DALMAN, *Worte Jesu,* 275.

the teachers. Its employment for the teachers becomes prominent in rabbinic writings.[1] Most significant is perhaps a saying—possibly very old[2]—attributed to Joshua b. Perahia (c. 104–78 B.C.E.) in m. ʾAbot 1:6. A person should provide himself with a רב.[3] It is therefore not surprising to find that the suffix in רבי can point specifically to "my" teacher[4] and that the term itself sometimes occurs independently of any following name.[5] It expresses a specific relationship between the teacher and his pupils.[6]

At some stage during the development, the titular connotations invaded the qualitative and relational appellation. The adjective became a proper title to be put in front of the name. A letter written by R. Sherira (c. 906–1006 C.E.)—the Gaon of the Pumbedithan academy—to the North African community of Kairouan circa 987 C.E. describes the history of the title.[7] It is indeed too late to serve as primary evidence for the tannaitic and amoraic periods. And it neglects—perhaps because of its official status—the unofficial use of the appellation. But it reflects accurately how different forms of רב became related to the institutional and official authorities.

The letter dates the earliest occurrence of the title "Rabbi" to the time of R. Johanan b. Zakkai († c. 80 C.E.) and connects it with the ordination. This is roughly consistent with the information in earlier sources. The title is there usually not prefixed to the names of the *old* sages. The use of the term as a title in front of the name comes to the surface during the first generation of tannas, such as R. Zadok, R. Eliezer b. Jacob and R. Hanina b. Dosa. We have seen that R. Johanan b. Zakkai is mentioned as the first teacher practising the ordination. And b. B. Meṣ. 85a takes it for granted that the gold-trimmed cloak put on the one ordained at the ceremony of the ordination was a token closely related to the bestowal of the title "Rabbi."[8] Here רבי no longer expresses the qualitative validation of a close relationship. It is a title. The pronominal meaning attached to the suffix carries no

---

1 HENGEL, *Charismatic Leader*, 43.

2 So RIESNER, *Lehrer*, 269; ZIMMERMANN, *Die urchristlichen Lehrer*, 87.

3 The text is given above p. 53. An identical statement in m. ʾAbot 1:16 is attributed to R. Gamaliel.

4 Cf. e.g. the expression רבי ותלמידי (m. Roš Haš. 2:9) and רבי מרי (b. Ketub. 103b; b. Mak. 24a) or merely, in greeting the teacher, רבי ומרי (b. B. Qam. 73b).

5 Cf. e.g. m. Pesaḥ. 6:2; m. Ned. 9:5; m. B. Qam. 8:6; b. Taʿan. 21a; ʾAbot R. Nat. A 14; Lev. Rab. 34:3, 14.

6 For other similar uses of רב—with or without suffix but always in a non-titular manner—in relation to different teachers, cf. e.g. m. Ber. 2:5–7; m. B. Meṣ. 2:11; m. ʿEd. 1:3; 8:7; m. ʾAbot 4:12; m. Ker. 6:9; m. Yad. 4:3; b. Ber. 63b.

7 An English translation of the relevant text portion is given by SHANKS, *JQR* 53 (1962–63) 338. Cf. also the German translation given by DALMAN, *Worte Jesu*, 272f. The Spanish and French recensions were not available to me. For general information about the letter, see STRACK/STEMBERGER, *Talmud and Midrash*, 7.

8 Cf. also b. Sanh. 13b. For comments, see NEWMAN, *Semikhah*, 117f; LOHSE, *Ordination*, 52; HRUBY, *MD* 102 (1970) 36f.

relational significance.[1]

In Babylonia, where the ordination was normally not practised indepen-dently of Palestine (b. Sanh. 14a),[2] the teachers were granted only the title "Rab" (רב).[3] The letter also says that certain eminent scholars were given the title "Rabban" (רבן) and describes this form of the title as superior to "Rabbi."[4] While רבן may originally have been equivalent with רב,[5] its re-striction to four outstanding scholars indicates the intensified connotation.[6] Only Gamaliel I Ha-Zaken, Johanan b. Zakkai, Gamaliel II and Simeon b. Gamaliel carry it.[7] Since the title for the patriarch—הנשׂיא—elsewhere re-places this title,[8] we may assume that it was the official designation for the head of the rabbinic sanhedrin.[9]

As a proper title, the various forms of רב carried their validating func-tion through the support from the official institutions, not through the inhe-rent qualities of the teacher. Although rabbinic Judaism reveals an aware-ness of the qualitative and relational aspects of רב, it also shows that the titu-lar attribution dominated. *The validation of the rabbinic teacher by means of titles did not primarily concern his own person. It concerned his function as a transmitter of torah.*

2.2.4. Discipleship and Torah

The rabbinic corpora do not concentrate traditions to one supreme rabbi only. Although some rabbis seem more important than others, they are not exclusive in any sense. The Mishnah mentions over one hundred and fifty rabbis.[10] And it has been estimated that the Babylonian Talmud increases

---

   [1]   The actual disappearance of the function of the suffix is clearly seen in the expres-sion "one Rabbi" (חד רבי) in y. Sota 24b (Krotoshin ed. line 59).

   [2]   Cf. NEWMAN, *Semikhah,* 129–143.

   [3]   L.I. RABINOWITZ, *EncJud* XIII, 1445. The title "Rab" is found also in Palestine (*CII* II, 857, 900, 1218). Cf. COHEN, *JQR* 72 (1981) 3, 6.

   [4]   Outside of the targumim, the Aramaic form רבון is reserved almost exclusively for God. For the Mishnah, cf. m. Taʿan. 3:8.

   [5]   HENGEL, *Charismatic Leader,* 42f n. 19.

   [6]   A possible interpretation of a passage at the very end of t. ʿEd. 3:4 would actually mean that a teacher was called "Rabbi" only as long as he was remembered as having disciples, while those whose disciples were forgotten (שׁכח) were called "Rabban." But t. ʿEd. 3:4 probably blurs the historical realities in this regard. The disciples of the teachers titled "Rabban" were not always forgotten. ZEITLIN, *JQR* 59 (1968–69) 159f, regards the statement as an explanatory interpolation. But cf. SHANKS, *JQR* 59 (1968–69) 155 n. 15.—NEUSNER, *Tosefta* IV, 309, translates with "praised" instead of "forgotten," per-haps (mis)reading נשתבחו for נשתכחו.

   [7]   For other possible carriers of this title, cf. SCHÜRER, *History* II, 326 n.13.

   [8]   DALMAN, *Worte Jesu,* 273; ZEITLIN, *JQR* 59 (1968–69) 158–160.

   [9]   For other possible meanings of the term, see GOODBLATT, *Rabbinic Instruction,* 286–288, claiming that it sometimes even denotes the disciples.

   [10] ALBECK, *Einführung,* 391–414.

the number to one thousand six hundred and ninety-one.[1] Some of them appear only occasionally. But the Talmud attributes specific significance to no less than seventy-eight rabbis. A focalization on one particular rabbi was apparently not a determinative force in the compilation of the rabbinic writings. Rabbinic literature is essentially collective.[2]

This redactional feature is in harmony with texts claiming that alternating teachers should be followed. A sage is the one who learns from everybody (m. ʾAbot 4:1).[3] A disciple of the house of Shammai, for instance, can follow the teaching of the house of Hillel (t. Sukk. 2:3). ʾAbot R. Nat. A 3 gives the explicit recommendation, attributed to R. Meir (c. 150 C.E.), that several teachers are to be consulted.[4] We should not diminish the importance of this recommendation because of the warning that R. Meir elsewhere issues against adhering to several teachers (ʾAbot R. Nat. A 8).[5] The plurality of teachers could of course have a confusing effect. In reponse to a statement by R. Ḥisda († c. 309 C.E.), claiming that whoever learns torah from (only) one master will never achieve success, it is said in b. ʿAbod. Zar. 19a–b that the adherence to one teacher is relevant for the learning of the specific and already formulated comment (גמרא) acquired orally.[6] This procedure would maintain unified modes of expression. The adherence to one teacher is apparently recommended in order to avoid fragmentation on the basic level of education.[7] Pedagogical concerns cause R. Meir's warning. As it seems, once the basic studies were completed and a more specialized training started, it was proper to consult several teachers.

Discipleship centred consequently on torah, not on a specific teacher. It meant not only to follow the *teacher* himself. Walking behind the teacher (הלך אחרי) was sometimes no more but an expression of reverence.[8] It may of course also express discipleship, but learning was ultimately learning

---

1 GOLDBLATT, Rabbis of the Babylonian Talmud, 81–89.
2 NEUSNER, *Rabbinic Traditions* III, 3. Cf. also E.P. SANDERS, *Paul and Palestinian Judaism*, 70f. This insight is well summarized by W.S. GREEN, What's in a Name?, 90: "No individual emerges as a 'whole person' in whom all wisdom and piety are centered and who might threaten or serve as a focus of resistance against the rabbinic collective itself."
3 Cf. also Sifre on Deut 11:22.
4 Cf. also b. Ber. 63b.
5 Cf. also b. ʿErub. 53a.
6 GERHARDSSON, *Memory*, 132. Cf. also GOODBLATT, *Rabbinic Instruction*, 270.
7 BACHER, *Agada der Tannaiten* II, 3f, 20f; KRAUSS, *Talmudische Archäologie* III, 220. Cf. more recently e.g. GOLDIN, Sidelights of a Torah Education, 186f.
8 Cf. e.g. t. Para 10:3; b. Ber. 23a–b, 24b; b. Šabb. 12b, 108b, 112a; b. ʿErub. 30a, 64b; b. Yoma 85a; b. Roš Haš. 34b; b. Ketub. 66b, 72b; b. B. Meṣ. 24b; b. Ḥull. 48a–b; y. Ḥag. 77a; y. B. Meṣ. 8c; y. ʿAbod. Zar. 40a; ʾAbot R. Nat. A 4; Mek. on 31:12 (Lauterbach III, 197:7–10); Sifre on Deut 31:14; Lev. Rab. 37:3. For discussion, see A. SCHULZ, *Nachfolgen*, 19–21; G. KITTEL, *TDNT* I, 213; ABERBACH, Relations Between Master and Disciple, 6f, 14f; HENGEL, *Charismatic Leader*, 51–53.

torah (תורה למד).[1] The all important duty of discipleship was not to follow a specific teacher, but to study and learn torah.[2]

The fact that rabbinic teachers did not themselves call students to follow them is in line with this. They could, at the most, invite persons to leave their own teaching and follow the teaching that they themselves delivered.[3] But this was not to enhance the individual rabbi himself. The general attitude was that the pupils were free to choose the teacher.[4] The pupils were in essence _disciples of torah_, not of a specific _teacher_. _Discipleship was primarily the learning of torah. And it was always essentially torah itself in its various forms that motivated the transmission._

Excursus 4: _The Rabbis and the Prophetic Spirit_

The view that the prophecy in the holy spirit ceased in Israel when the last of the OT prophets—Haggai, Zechariah and Malachi—died was common in rabbinic Judaism. There are some uncertainties about the cause and history of this conception.[5] But several texts reveal its prominence in the main stream of rabbinic Judaism.[6] The medium of direct revelation from heaven was no longer the inspired prophet or the rabbi. It was a heavenly echo (קול בת), though some would warn against attributing too much significance also to this (b. Ber. 51b–52a; b. ʿErub. 7a).[7]

While certain rabbis were considered worthy of the holy spirit, they did not receive it (t. Soṭa 13:3f; b. Sukk. 28a; b. B. Bat. 134a; ʾAbot R. Nat. A 14).[8] Claims of inspired leadership were suppressed and "rabbinized" in rabbinic Judaism.[9] The statement by R. Eliezer b. Hyrcanus (c. 90 C.E.) in b. ʿErub. 63a is characteristic. In response to the question if he was a prophet, he answers negatively by reference to Amos 7:14 and advises the questioner to keep to the tradition.[10] _The teacher was not an inspired mediator of new revelations; he was a transmitter of torah._

---

1 H.D. BETZ, _Nachfolge_, 13f; RENGSTORF, _TDNT_ IV, 402f; ZUMSTEIN, _Relation du maître et du disciple_, 16, 44; HENGEL, _Charismatic Leader_, 32, 51.

2 Cf. e.g. m. ʾAbot 1:13; 2:12, 14, 16; 4:5, 20; b. Yoma 35b; b. Sanh. 68a; ʾAbot R. Nat. A 3, 6.

3 Cf. b. B. Qam. 36b.

4 Cf. e.g. m. ʾAbot 1:6, 16.

5 For general discussion, see R. MEYER, _TDNT_ VI, 812–819; LEIVESTAD, _NTS_ 19 (1972–73) 288–299; AUNE, _Prophecy_, 103–106; SANDNES, _Paul_, 43–47. For rabbinic Judaism in particular, see MOORE, _Judaism_ I, 421f, _idem, Judaism_ III, 127; PARZEN, _JQR_ 20 (1929–30) 54–56; BONSIRVEN, _Judaïsme Palestinien_ I, 256f; SJÖBERG, _TDNT_ VI, 385f; SCHÄFER, _Vorstellung vom heiligen Geist_, 89–111, 143–146; URBACH, _Sages_, 564–567, 577–59; GREENSPAHN, _JBL_ 108 (1989) 37–49; BOCKMUEHL, _Revelation and Mystery_, 105–109; MENZIES, _Early Christian Pneumatology_, 92–96.

6 Cf. t. Soṭa 13:2; b. Yoma 9b; b. Soṭa 48b; b. Sanh. 11a; y. Soṭa 24b; Cant. Rab. on 8:9; S. ʿOlam Rab. 30.

7 For an extensive discussion of קול בת in rabbinic Judaism, see P. KUHN, _Offenbarungsstimmen_, 254–331.

8 Cf. also b. Sanh. 65b.

9 For this development in the traditions about Ḥoni the Circle Maker, see W.S. GREEN, _ANRW_ II 19:2 (1979) 619–647.

10 Cf. also y. Šeb. 36c; y. Giṭ. 43c; Sifra on 10:1; Lev. Rab. 20:6; Pesiq. Rab Kah. 26:7 (Mandelbaum's 2nd ed. 393).

There are indeed exceptions.[1] It is said that R. Gamaliel I Ha-Zaḳen (t. Pesaḥ. 1:27), R. Akiba (Lev. Rab. 21:8), R. Meir (y. Soṭa 16d) and R. Simeon b. Yoḥai (y. Šeb. 38d) did act under the influence of the holy spirit. There is also indication of the view that the gift of prophecy was passed on to—or not taken away from—the wise after the destruction of the first temple (b. B. Bat. 12a–b; S. ʿOlam Rab. 30)[2] or even that the word of the elders was of more worth than the word of the prophets (y. ʿAbod. Zar. 41c).[3] Some viewed the activity of the rabbis in close relation to the holy spirit and/or prophecy. Similar qualities are occasionally ascribed also to other persons. The statement attributed to Hillel in t. Pesaḥ. 4:14, claiming that all Israelites possessed the holy spirit, may be a late addition.[4] But the Israelites are at least said to be sons of the prophets.[5] There are also several texts suggesting that certain individuals were able to earn the holy spirit already now, as a present possession.[6] Certain variations within the belief that the holy spirit had ceased existed apparently. But the fact that four rabbis are attributed inspirational features does not significantly diminish the general non-inspirational system of validation. On no occasion do these passages indicate a major view.[7]

3. The Didactic-Biographical Motives

"The didactic-biographical motives" describe in this study *prevailing interests in the teaching as integrated within the life of a specific teacher.* They appear as longer or briefer episodal narratives in the third person. To be sure, purely didactic motives may also express themselves as narrations about episodes in the life of a teacher. But in these cases, the episodes do not relate to the life of a *specific* teacher. They serve instead as *typical* illustrations with only didactic intentions.[8] A didactic-biographical motive of transmission is at hand when the episodes show a higher degree of focus on a particular person.[9]

---

[1] Cf. STRACK/BILLERBECK, *Kommentar* II, 128f; SJÖBERG, *TDNT* VI, 386; SCHÄFER, *Vorstellung vom heiligen Geist,* 121–124, 147–149; HILL, *New Testament Prophecy,* 34f; AUNE, *Prophecy,* 104; GREENSPAHN, *JBL* 108 (1989) 47f; BOCK-MUEHL, *Revelation and Mystery,* 105f, 108f; BORING, *Continuing Voice,* 53.

[2] Cf. also m. ʾAbot 1:1.

[3] Cf. also b. B. Bat. 12a and the comments by KOOK, *Judaism* 21 (1972) 311f.

[4] Cf. SCHÄFER, *Vorstellung vom heiligen Geist,* 124f.

[5] Cf. b. Pesaḥ. 66a; y. Šabb. 17a; y. Pesaḥ. 33a.

[6] For references and discussion, see SCHÄFER, *Vorstellung vom heiligen Geist,* 118–121, 127–133, 148f.

[7] SCHÄFER, *Vorstellung vom heiligen Geist,* 123f, 148f.

[8] For the episodal narratives in the rabbinic literature, see excursus 5 below.

[9] I will deal primarily with a biographical *motivation* in transmitting material from the teacher—not with a literary genre, in which the typical function of the main character may be more emphasized.

3.1. The Elijah/Elisha Narratives

The interaction between Elijah and Elisha and between Elisha and the sons
of the prophets depicted in the texts contain factors that go beyond the didactic character of the situation. This is most evident in the Elisha narratives. There appears an interest in relating specific eschatological sayings to
Elisha.[1] These utterances are not purely didactic. They are authoritative
proclamations introduced with the messenger formula "thus says Yahweh"
(כה אמר יהוה).[2] And the followers use "man of God" (איש האלהים) and "my
lord" (אדני) to address Elisha (2 Kgs 4:40; 6:5). These utterances and addresses occur within episodal narratives depicting also the acts of the prophets. They reveal a concern that goes beyond the conception of Elisha as a
teacher with no more but a verbal form of instruction. *The integration of
words and deeds in the present texts suggests an interest to transmit the
words as intimately connected with the life of a prophet.*

I cannot here discuss the tradition and redaction history of the Eli-
jah/Elisha narratives at length. The Deuteronomist was probably responsible for incorporating the different stories about Elijah and Elisha into the
present composition.[3] But the Elijah/Elisha narratives reveal apparently
only a small amount of Deuteronomistic editing.[4] This may imply certain
post-Deuteronomistic additions.[5] Many scholars would however agree that
the Deuteronomistic historian had traditions of different kinds at his disposal. Although the narratives truly must have gone through a complex development, R.R. Wilson claims that they reflect—in spite of the diversity—
the same characteristic view of prophecy and that they were probably
created or shaped by groups which held common opinions about the behaviour and social roles of prophets.[6] I here proceed on these assumptions.

---

[1]   Cf. W. REISER, *TZ* 9 (1953) 321–338, and below p. 140.

[2]   2 Kgs 2:21; 3:16, 17; 4:43; 7:1.

[3]   I use the expression "Deuteronomist" (Dtr) as a comprehensive epithet for the final
redactor(s) of Deuteronomy, Joshua, Judges, First and Second Samuel and First and Second Kings. Regardless of the redactional history of the Deuteronomistic history, the *terminus a quo* for the final form of its major parts is probably given in 2 Kgs 25:27–30—
the release of king Jehoiachin c. 561 B.C.E.—and the *terminus ad quem* is fixed by the
lack of any indication of the rebuilding of the temple c. 520 B.C.E. For a survey of research, see WEIPPERT, *TRu* 50 (1985) 213–249; PREUSS, *TRu* 58 (1993) 229–264.

[4]   WILSON, *Prophecy,* 192. For the Elijah narratives, cf. the recent conclusion by
THIEL, Deuteronomistische Redaktionsarbeit, 171: "Die dtr. Bearbeitung der Elia-Über-
lieferungen erfolgte in erster Linie durch die Anordnung der Materialien ... und durch
ihre Umrahmung mit den Königsbeurteilungen ... In die Texte selbst hat die dtr. Redaktion nur an Einzelstellen eingegriffen."

[5]   Cf. STIPP, *Elischa,* 463–480; S.L. MCKENZIE, *Trouble with Kings,* 81–98, 148,
152. For critique of Stipp on this point, see BEGG, *CBQ* 51 (1989) 352f.

[6]   *Prophecy,* 194.

3.1.1. The Proposals of K. Baltzer and A. Rofé

K. Baltzer points to biographical features in the office and function of various prophets in ancient Israel.[1] Of most importance is the narration about the appointment, the "Einsetzungsbericht." The presence of these features reflect, according to Baltzer, an ancient biographical genre—an "Ideal-biographie"—known from early inscriptions in Egypt.[2] The Elijah/Elisha narratives show in spite of their legendary and secondary character traces of such a biography.[3] Especially prominent are the topoi of Elijah's total obedience to Yahweh and his legitimation as a prophet as well as the succession of the prophetical office from Elijah to Elisha.

Baltzer's proposal is problematic on two accounts. First, the topoi do not occur in the OT in a coherent narration. We find them at different places. The final redactors, at least, were not appreciative of the biographical genre.[4] Second, Baltzer does not discuss which persons that had the capacity and motive to create an ideal biography of Elijah and Elisha, and he does not consider it necessary to distinguish between items presented in the first person singular and those narrated in the third person. It seems more adequate to relate the biographical topoi to *motives* of transmission, instead of to a literary genre.

More recently, A. Rofé tried—unfortunately without relating his view to Baltzer's proposal—to give a classification of the narratives about the prophets.[5] Basing the classification on the content of the narratives, Rofé proposes twelve genres ranging from the short *legenda* to more elaborated forms.[6] He gives several examples from the Elijah/Elisha narratives, especially from the Elisha narratives. According to Rofé, the entire account about Elisha, from 2 Kgs 2—even from 1 Kgs 19:19–21—to 2 Kgs 13:19, represents an attempt to construct a *vita* out of the short *legenda* contained in six episodes about Elisha's miraculous acts (2 Kgs 2:19–22, 23f; 4:1–7, 38–41, 42–44; 6:1–7).[7] Initially the sons of the prophets handed down the brief episodes orally. Through an inherent "biographical drive,"[8] the brief episodes were subsequently expanded and arranged in an associative order

---

1 *Biographie*, 13–181.
2 *Biographie*, 20–23, 193.
3 *Biographie*, 95–105.
4 AUNE, *Literary Environment*, 43. For a similar critique of Baltzer in connection with the servant songs, see METTINGER, *Servant Songs*, 16f.
5 *Prophetical Stories*.
6 ROFÉ, *Prophetical Stories*, 8, claims to have worked with 12 distinct genres. He probably means the short *legenda*, the *reliquiae*, the literary elaboration or epigonic devolution of the *legenda*, the *vita*, the political *legenda*, prophetic historiography, prophetic biography, the ethical *legenda*, the *exemplum*, the parable, the epic and the martyrology.
7 *Prophetical Stories*, 13–51. Cf. earlier *idem*, *JBL* 89 (1970) 427–440.
8 Cf. ROFÉ, *JBL* 89 (1970) 436.

to form a written *vita* of the holy man Elisha.[1]

Rofé's suggestion concerning the formal classification of prophetic narratives has the advantage of not being based on a preconceived literary genre. He focuses on the content before determining the genre. It is difficult to imagine that literary forms developed independently of individuals intending to express certain ideas and convictions.[2] Although it must still remain questionable if we can here speak about actual genres,[3] Rofé makes it probable that *an underlying interest in the total impact of both the utterances and the actions held the transmission of Elisha's words and deeds together*.

3.1.2. The Sons of the Prophets and the Elisha Narratives

It is not evident when the sons of the prophets were first organized to form a proper fellowship. J.G. Williams thinks that Elijah was instrumental in this process,[4] but the evidence for Elijah's relation to them is restricted mainly to 2 Kgs 2:1–18. In any event, the expression "sons of (the) prophets" (בני [ה]נביאים) is used only for groups in the northern kingdom.[5] These groups are often present at ancient cult centres, such as Bethel (2 Kgs 2:3), Gilgal (2 Kgs 4:38) and Jericho (2 Kgs 2:5, 15).[6] They appear between the reign of Ahab (c. 869–850 B.C.E.) and the time of Amos—if the singular form of the expression in Amos 7:14 is accepted as referring to this kind of fellowship. This confines their existence to approximately 870–750 B.C.E.

There is certain indication that the groups exhibited some basic coherence. The term בן, "son," is often used to describe membership in certain social and professional groups.[7] The expression "sons of (the) prophets" probably implies that the individual person belonged to a group which was counted to the category of prophets.[8] True, it seems that some members possessed a house of their own and wife and children (2 Kgs 4:1–7). Perhaps Elisha himself had a house in Samaria (2 Kgs 5:3, 9). But there are also

---

[1]   According to ROFÉ, *Prophetical Stories,* 42f, an actual biography aspires to historical accuracy while a *vita* consists of embellished histories with accounts of miraculous acts and signs of faith.

[2]   Cf. already MUILENBURG, *JBL* 88 (1969) 5: "Exclusive attention to the *Gattung* may actually obscure the thought and intention of the writer or speaker."

[3]   Cf. VON RAD, *Theology* II, 36.

[4]   *JBL* 85 (1966) 345, 348.

[5]   For references, see above p. 38.

[6]   I cannot here dwell further on their relation to the cult. Cf. H.-C. SCHMITT, *Elisa,* 170–172.

[7]   HAAG, *TWAT* I, 675. Haag classifies the sons of the prophets as a professional group.

[8]   LINDBLOM, *Prophecy,* 70 n. 40. Cf. similarly WILLIAMS, *JBL* 85 (1966) 348, who also accounts for the expression in the singular in Amos 7:14.

texts suggesting that the groups ate and lived together (2 Kgs 4:38–44; 6:2). Possibly, as G. von Rad remarks,[1] the low economic status of the members was a contributing factor for the formation of the fellowship. The fact that Elisha is able to send out messengers from such a group testifies further to the coherence (2 Kgs 2:16–18; 9:1–10).[2] In addition, perhaps Amos 7:14 reflects a refusal to be associated with a specific group of prophets.[3] L. Rost even proposed that entrance into the fellowship must have been connected with a special ceremony and included the actual transference to new conditions,[4] though this is difficult to prove.[5]

Rofé thinks that the sons of the prophets initially began to tell brief stories about Elisha's miracles.[6] The close connection between Elisha and the sons of the prophets is not necessarily secondary.[7] But these "sons" were probably more than bands of admirers, as Rofé thinks.[8] It seems reasonable to assume that the sons of the prophets constituted rather coherent and definable groups capable of transmitting traditions about Elisha.[9]

Although Williams probably overstates the importance of Elijah, his picture of the social location of the sons of the prophets is conceivable.[10] The groups consisted, according to Williams, of those who separated themselves from society and devoted themselves to the service of the true God—Yahweh—under a leader who was *the* prophet and spiritual father.[11] The outer impulse for this concentration to one prophetic leader was the increasing conflict between the prophetic leadership on one hand, and the monarchic secularization of the military and the ancient Yahwist traditions on the other,

---

1   *Theology* II, 26.
2   Cf. also 2 Kgs 4:29–31.
3   Amos claims that he is—or was—not an ordinary prophet (לא נביא אנכי). His emphasis on not being a prophet's son (בן נביא) might then separate him from a prophetic group, not only from some lay supporters. However, the verse is much discussed. Some would regard it as an editorial addition. For a survey of interpretations, see BLENKINSOPP, *Prophecy*, 127 n. 23. For further literature, see VAN DER WAL, *Amos*, 230–234. Cf. also STOEBE, *VT* 39 (1989) 341–354; PFEIFER, *VT* 39 (1989) 497–503.
4   *TLZ* 80 (1955) 4.
5   If the sons of the prophets were recognized by a tattoo, a uniform and a tonsure, we have a further indicatation of the groups' coherence. But the texts usually adduced to support this assumption (1 Kgs 20:35, 38, 41; 2 Kgs 1:8; 2:23) do not allow any certain conclusion.
6   *Prophetical Stories,* 21f.
7   This is admitted by H.-C. SCHMITT, *Elisa,* 189f. To this question, cf. also RENDTORFF, *ZTK* 59 (1962) 154–158; H.-C. SCHMITT, *ZTK* 74 (1977) 261f, 269f; PORTER, Origins, 27f.
8   *Prophetical Stories,* 22. Cf. also H.-C. SCHMITT, *Elisa,* 189; HOBBS, *2 Kings,* 25, 27.
9   2 Kgs 8:4f says that Elisha's own young servant (נער) Gehazi—probably a leading person among the sons of the prophets—tells about (ספר) all the great deeds of Elisha. But WÜRTHWEIN, *Könige* II, 217, regards 8:4f as an interpolation.
10   *JBL* 85 (1966) 344–348.
11   As I indicated above, the plural expression בני [ה]נביאים does not necessarily indicate that the groups adhered to a long tradition of prophetic fathers. WILLIAMS, *JBL* 85 (1966) 348, explains it as "the awareness of many prophets under one prophet."

perhaps during the Omride dynasty.[1]

3.1.3. The Sons of the Prophets and the Elijah Narratives

The matter is even more complicated as regards the rather different Elijah narratives. Scholars are divided concerning the historicity of the relationship pictured between Elijah and Elisha in 1 Kgs 19:19–21 and 2 Kgs 2:1–18.[2] It is impossible here to bring an independent judgement on the issue. However, O.H. Steck proposes Elisha and the sons of the prophets as the initial carriers of the Elijah traditions.[3] Two factors speak, according to Steck, in this direction. First, the content and stylistic features in the material itself testifies to a level of sophistication that cannot appear within loosely structured groups. They require a more closed fellowship. Second, the fact that the Elijah narratives signal a focus on a prophetic figure and take into account the persecution of other prophets indicates the prophetic character of the group. Since Elijah himself was not directly associated with such a group, it is, according to Steck, most likely that the initial formation and elaboration of the Elijah narratives was connected with Elisha and the prophetic disciples around him. Steck realizes that it is difficult to think of the same group as responsible for the rather different material about both Elijah and Elisha. He suggests that a specific group of teachers were responsible for the transmission. The whole group became involved when the teachers delivered their lectures to other members of the fellowship.

Although Steck goes beyond what the texts actually show, his reflections are based on detailed work with the material itself. If he is correct, it was Elisha and his disciples that first formulated and carried the episodes about Elijah. In that case, *it is possible that the interaction between Elijah and Elisha and between Elisha and the sons of the prophets visible in the present*

---

[1]　The historicity of the Omrides in the Elijah/Elisha narratives is problematic. For Elijah, cf. the critical points given by H.-C. SCHMITT, *Elisa,* 183–187, and for Elisha, cf. J.M. MILLER, *JBL* 85 (1966) 441–454. The more general statement concerning the social location of the group by WILSON, *Prophecy,* 202, is sufficient for my purposes: "... members of this group were presumably peripheral individuals who had resisted the political and religious policies of the Ephraimite kings and who had therefore been forced out of the political and religious establishments."

[2]　H.-C. SCHMITT, *Elisa,* 109–119, 183–187, 189, represents some critical scholars arguing against any historical relationship between the two prophets. Elijah and Elisha are not representatives of the same religio-historical phenomenon and Elijah was not, like Elisha, involved in hostile actions against the Omrides. Cf. similarly ROFÉ, *Prophetical Stories,* 74.—HENTSCHEL, *Elijaerzählungen,* 325, 332, concludes that the connections between the Elijah and Elisha traditions were created only at a secondary, though pre-Dtr, stage.—Rudolf SMEND, Elia, 182, claims that although it is not unconceivable that a close relationship existed between Elijah and Elisha, the definite answer lies outside of what is possible to know.—FOHRER, *Elia,* 68; STECK, *Überlieferung,* 97, accept a basic historicity.

[3]　*Überlieferung,* 144–147.

accounts actually contained the embryo of biographical motives of trans-mission.

3.2. Episodal Narratives in the Later Prophets

The books of the later prophets contain three basic sorts of material.[1] First, there are sayings that the prophet proclaimed as a mouthpiece of Yahweh, either by speaking with the voice of Yahweh in the first person singular or by referring to Yahweh in the third person. Second, there are autobiographical accounts about the call and activity of the prophet. Third, there are series of episodal narratives concerning the prophet. Although the third group certainly takes a very minor place, it is of most interest here.[2]

Some books contain no such material at all. Most striking is perhaps Ezekiel. Not only are the numerous sign actions heavily overlaid with symbolic—dramatic[3]—interpretations.[4] With some minor exceptions (1:3; 24:24), the material also occurs as first person accounts. The composition does not explicitly reflect the interest of a third person.[5] No doubt, *the didactic and proclamative potentials that the authoritative words and illustrative deeds of the prophets contained constituted a major motive of trans-mission.* But this is not my prime concern here.

3.2.1. The Book of Amos

In the context of first-person accounts about Amos' visions, an episodal narrative occurs in 7:(9)10–17.[6] There is no general consensus about the extent and history of the different units in Amos.[7] But most scholars agree that a person closely associated with Amos shaped 7:(9)10–17.[8] The author

---

[1]   Cf. EISSFELDT, *Old Testament*, 147.
[2]   Scholars commonly refer to the episodal narratives as "Fremdberichte." But since—as we will see—these accounts often go back on texts formulated by close adherents of the prophets, this designation is inadequate.
[3]   Cf. STACEY, *Prophetic Drama*, 171–208.
[4]   Cf. e.g. 3:22–5:17; 12:1–11, 17–20; 21:11f, 23–29; 24:1–27; 33:21f; 37:15–28.
[5]   Of course, some material may be pseudonymous works by persons related to Ezekiel.—Joachim BECKER, Erwägungen zur ezechielischen Frage, 139f; *idem, Ez 8–11*, 136, uses the I-style of the book as an argument for its fictional and *entirely* pseudonymous character. But this way of arguing is problematic.
[6]   It is uncertain if 7:9 is part of this text-unit. Cf. e.g. BJØRNDALEN, Erwägungen, 237f n. 3.
[7]   For surveys of the discussion concerning the literary issues in Amos, see CHILDS, *Introduction*, 398f; AULD, *Amos*, 50–59.—VAN DER WOUDE, Prophets, 42f, calls for caution against too confident a use of redaction-historical methods in Amos.
[8]   So e.g. BOTTERWECK, *BZ* 2 (1958) 188; MAYS, *Amos*, 13, 134; RUDOLPH, *Joel – Amos – Obadja – Jona*, 252; WILLI-PLEIN, *Vorformen*, 59; KOCH et al., *Amos* I, 206; WOLFF, *Joel and Amos*, 108f, 308f; ZIMMERLI, *TLZ* 104 (1979) 485; STUART, *Hosea – Jonah*, 370; SATO, *Q und Prophetie*, 319, 401.—PFEIFER, *ZAW* 96 (1984) 116 n. 21, lists other scholars. PFEIFER, *ibid.*, 116–118, himself argues that the thought patterns in the text are characteristic of Amos and that it therefore stems from the prophet. But it

seems well informed and tells of a threat against Jeroboam II (c. 786–746 B.C.E.) which apparently never came true (7:11).[1] Although the verses contain language not present elsewhere in Amos,[2] they reveal an intimate knowledge about the language, style and themes of Amos himself.[3] A person well acquainted with the Amos tradition probably created 7:(9)10–17 at a rather early time.[4]

This is the only biographical piece in Amos.[5] It retells the words and depicts the deeds of Amos. Important words of a significant person occur within a narrative framework with biographical items. While the kerygmatic impressiveness and potentials of Amos' words could create a motive of transmission in some circles,[6] the biographical piece of material indicates—regardless of its function in the present context—that *a group of early transmitters cherished a certain biographical interest in Amos.*

3.2.2. The Book of Hosea

Hos 1:2b–6, 8f present an episodal narrative in the third person. 3:1–4 gives a parallel account in the first person.[7] The three first chapters of Hosea are more coherent than the rest of the book.[8] Although later additions are probably present (1:1; 1:7; 3:5),[9] most of the material consists of older biographical (Hos 1), oracular (Hos 2) and autobiographical (Hos 3) sections. The common subject matter—the matrimonial history of Hosea—unites the sections. I. Willi-Plein thinks that a person within a circle of close pupils of

---

seems strange that Amos should compose stories about himself in the third person. The thought patterns could as well express the studied thinking of a pupil of Amos, faithful to his master's teaching in form and content. Cf. below p. 177.

1   Cf. 2 Kgs 14:29. The threat against the house of Jeroboam in Amos 7:9 is in harmony with the violent death of Zechariah, the son of Jeroboam II (2 Kgs 15:8–10). Perhaps the redactors are responsible for this "extension" of the scene. So WOLFF, *Joel and Amos,* 108. But cf. the remark by GESE, Komposition, 82f.

2   Cf. ACKROYD, Judgment Narrative, 74–77.

3   See below p. 177.

4   WOLFF, *Joel and Amos,* 308, regards Amaziah as the subject of the scene. But as BJØRNDALEN, Erwägungen, 239 n. 5, remarks, it is then difficult to see why it was included in Amos at all.

5   Some believe that this text is part of a larger biography of Amos, including Amos 1:1. Some also see connections of different kinds to 1 Kgs 13:1–34; 2 Chr 25:14–16. Cf. ACKROYD, Judgment Narrative, 77–81. However, we are here left to mere speculations.

6   Cf. TUCKER, *Int* 27 (1973) 431: "One need not assume a formal body of disciples but only persons who heard and accepted as valid the word of Amos."

7   It is not necessary to discuss the exact relationship between the two accounts.

8   Cf. E.M. GOOD *SEÅ* 31 (1966) 29f, speaking of a careful (chiastic) compilation process.

9   For 1:1, cf. the superscriptions in Jer 1:1; Ezek 1:3; Joel 1:1; Jonah 1:1; Mic 1:1; Zeph 1:1; Hag 1:1; Zech 1:1; Mal 1:1. For discussion, see YEE, *Composition,* 56f (with lit.). For 1:7; 3:5, cf. the different views of WILLI-PLEIN, *Vorformen,* 117, 129; EMMERSON, *Hosea,* 88–95, 101–105; YEE, *ibid.,* 66.

Hosea created the basic unit of all the three chapters.[1] It does seem that one of Hosea's associates composed parts of the episodal narrative.[2] The author knows the name of Hosea's wife (1:3) and the time when the third child was born (1:8). The small biographical notice in 1:2b–6, 8f shows that the life of Hosea was of interest to his followers. In addition, even if a later editor composed the superscription in 1:1, he must have had some biographical data at his disposal—data which he perhaps attained through oral tradition or written catalogues.[3] Nowhere else is the father of Hosea referred to. It is indeed true that Hosea has no prominent place in the book. We find him mentioned by name only in 1:1f, where the third occurrence in 1:2b might come from his close followers. The inherent kerygmatic importance and potential of the words might indeed have created a motive of transmission. But it is one-sided to classify the narrative in chapter one as only kerygmatic, and not biographical.[4] Since the event and the kerygmatic word go together in these chapters, such a classification presents a false dichotomy.[5] It is the brief episode from Hosea's life that serves the message. By anchoring the sayings within his life, the author actually validated the prophetic master.[6] *Hardly anyone else but those who preserved an active interest in both the words and the life of Hosea would create an episodal narrative of this kind.*

3.2.3. The Book of Isaiah

An episodal narrative occurs in 7:1–17. It is part of the so-called memoirs of Isaiah (6:1–9:6).[7] Certain tensions are indeed visible in the present text.[8] And perhaps a later redactor added the historical setting in 7:1, though it functions well in the present context.[9] However, since we find no indication that the nucleus of the material ever occurred as a first-person report,[10] and since we can assume that the account reflects a real event,[11] we must take se-

---

1   *Vorformen*, 129, 244, 252. Differently Jörg JEREMIAS, *Hosea,* 19.
2   The phrase "Yahweh began to speak through Hosea" (תחלת דבר יהיה בהושע) in 1:2a is perhaps a later superscription for the transmission unit 1:2b–6, 8f. The repetition of "Yahweh" and "Hosea" in 1:2 might indicate this.
3   Cf. GEVARYAHU, Biblical Colophons, 46–51.
4   *Contra* MAYS, *Hosea,* 23.
5   VAN DER WOUDE, Prophets, 45.
6   YEE, *Composition,* 113–115.
7   See above pp. 39f.
8   HÖFFKEN, *TZ* 36 (1980) 321–337.
9   Cf. 2 Kgs 16:5 and the discussion by IRVINE, *Isaiah,* 135–138.
10   H. BARTH, *Jesaja-Worte,* 9 n. 18, makes literary operations in order to classify the unit as an "Eigenbericht." But cf. e.g. WILDBERGER, *Jesaja* I, 269f; HÖFFKEN, *TZ* 36 (1980) 332f; KAISER, *Isaiah 1–12,* 114f, 140f; WERNER, *BZ* 29 (1985) 2; RE-VENTLOW, *BN* 38/39 (1987) 63; HØGENHAVEN, *Gott und Volk,* 81; IRVINE, *ZAW* 104 (1992) 222f (with lit.); WERLITZ, *Studien,* 112–115.
11   WILDBERGER, *Jesaja* I, 273.

riously the possibility that some early followers of Isaiah formed the initial material during the Syro-Ephraimite war.[1] Although the life of the prophet is of minor importance in relation to the words of Yahweh,[2] the words do appear within a certain episodal context.[3]

The episodal narrative in 20:1–6 is well situated within the events of Ashdod's revolt against Assyria (c. 714–712 B.C.E.).[4] The composition shows a certain distance to Isaiah himself.[5] But H. Wildberger gives sufficient arguments for the assumption that the basic material comes from a well-informed author,[6] by other scholars called a disciple.[7] There is an intimate aquaintance with Isaiah's own diction.[8] The specific action of Isaiah has a symbolic, even dramatic,[9] purpose which might have increased the motive of composition and preservation.[10]

Isa 36–39 narrates about Isaiah's intervention when king Hezekiah (c. 715–686 B.C.E.) was facing the Assyrian threat. The present text is a self-contained unit with connections to other parts of Isaiah.[11] Legendary amplifications have probably been added. The unit was perhaps inserted at a rather late time.[12] However, while the exact relation to 2 Kgs 18:13–20:19 is still a matter of debate,[13] most scholars recognize that the texts are composite and build on earlier material.[14] Wildberger envisions an early narra-

---

[1]　Cf. WILDBERGER, *Jesaja* I, 270.

[2]　WOLFF, *Frieden,* 16; W. DIETRICH, *Jesaja,* 67, 69 n. 31.

[3]　K. BALTZER, *Biographie,* 112f.

[4]　Cf. BRIGHT, *History,* 281f.

[5]　Yahweh never addresses Isaiah directly. Cf. W. DIETRICH, *Jesaja,* 130–133; WILDBERGER, *Jesaja* II, 753f; HØGENHAVEN, *Gott und Volk,* 135f.

[6]　*Jesaja* II, 754. While Wildberger warns against regarding Isaiah's disciples as a closed fellowship (*Jesaja* I, 346), he allows the label of a school to be of some importance in the earliest redactional work (*Jesaja* III, 1545) and even agrees that Isaiah "einen S c h ü l e r k r e i s um sich hatte, den er mit der Verwaltung seiner Botschaft betraute" (*Jesaja* III, 1548).

[7]　E.g. MOWINCKEL, *AcOr* 11 (1933) 281; VERMEYLEN, *Isaïe* I, 325, *idem, Isaïe* II, 674.

[8]　See below p. 179.

[9]　Cf. STACEY, *Prophetic Drama,* 122–126.

[10]　GRAY, *Isaiah* I, 344, believes that this chapter constitutes a fragment of an early biography of Isaiah. This is of course impossible to prove.

[11]　Cf. ACKROYD, Isaiah 36–39, 3–21.

[12]　SEITZ, *Zion's Final Destiny,* however, argues that Isa 36–37, 38 originated in Isaiah—not in Kings—during the pre-exilic period. These chapters reveal a transitional character on matters of Zion and assist the movement into Isa 40–55 and the following. But for some critiqe of Seitz' dating, see CARR, What Can We Say?, 593–596.

[13]　Most scholars tend to believe that a redactor of Isaiah used—with some minor alterations and the exception of Isa 38:9–20—material from the Dtr. For discussion, see WILDBERGER, *Jesaja* III, 1370–1374, presenting arguments for the view that both texts utilize common sources; CAMP, *Hiskija,* 53–61; RUPRECHT, *ZTK* 87 (1990) 33–66; SEITZ, *Zion's Final Destiny,* 47–118, 149–191; SMELIK, *Converting the Past,* 93–128.

[14]　Cf. e.g. WILDBERGER, *Jesaja* III, 1374–1377; RUPRECHT, *ZTK* 87 (1990) 33–66. For Isa 36–37, cf. also CHILDS, *Assyrian Crisis,* 73–103; CLEMENTS, *Deliverance,* 53f.

tive.[1] The basic nucleus behind 36:1–37:9a, 37f is anchored within the events of Sennacherib's campaign (c. 701 B.C.E.). The composition was formed—on the basis of even earlier material—soon after the death of Sennacherib (c. 681 B.C.E.). Wildberger continues to argue that it exhibits a detailed knowledge of other Isaianic traditions and that a group thoroughly acquainted with the Isaiah tradition formed it.[2] Although two persons— Hezekiah and Isaiah—are at the centre of attention, the words of Isaiah (37:6f) occur again within a specific narrative context.

P.R. Ackroyd correctly notices that "the original status of the prophet is a necessary element in the continuing reinterpretation of his words."[3] It is of course true that Isaiah and his life do not constitute the *theological* focus of the book.[4] But the traditions behind the episodal narratives testify that some early followers were interested in both the words of and the episodes about Isaiah. Since it was the life of Isaiah—not of another person—that continuously served the message, the kerygmatic function of the episodal narratives in their present context excludes in no way an earlier biographical interest. An important question raised by Ackroyd concerns why Isaiah and not another prophet, such as Micah,[5] was enhanced to the extent that people created episodal narratives and attributed a whole collection of material to him.[6] A natural answer for the initial stages of this process appears when we recognize the early existence of disciples attached to Isaiah. *The transmission of the early Isaiah tradition was performed in awareness of the integrated importance of Isaiah's words and life.*

Of the so-called servant songs (Isa 42:1–4[–9]; 49:1–6[–12]; 50:4–9[–11]; 52:13– 53:12), the fourth one is a third person episode in which someone else than Yahweh speaks (53:1–6[–11a]). K. Elliger argued that since the servant is Second Isaiah, and since the song describes Second Isaiah's death, another person than Second Isaiah himself must have composed the unit. The similarities in terminology, style, and content with different parts of Isa 56–66—similarities not present in the other songs— suggested to Elliger that Third Isaiah was the individual author of the fourth song. He used the composition to close an extensive redactional activity within Isa 40–53.[7]

However, it is impossible to ascertain the biographical intention of the fourth song.

---

1   *Jesaja* III, 1391–1393. Cf. also *idem, TZ* 35 (1979) 35–47.
2   WILDBERGER, *Jesaja* III, 1391 states: "In solchen Kreisen muß die Erzählung entstanden sein." Cf. also ZIMMERLI, *Grundriß*, 174f: "Die in der Schule Jesajas entstandene Jesajalegende (Kap.36f.) ..." CLEMENTS, *Deliverance*, 54–71, believes that the original narrative was composed already during Josiah's reign (c. 640–609 B.C.E.). While he notices the interest in the prophecies of Isaiah revealed in the narrative, he is still reluctant to term the authors "Isaiah's disciples" (*ibid.*, 69f).
3   Isaiah I–XII, 27.
4   SEITZ, Isaiah 1–66, 116–122, spends considerable effort to refute such a theory.
5   Cf. Jer 26:17–19.
6   ACKROYD, Isaiah I–XII, 22–29.
7   *Deuterojesaja in seinem Verhältnis*, 6–27. Cf. also *idem, ZAW* 49 (1931) 138f. For Elliger's arguments regarding Third Isaiah as an individual disciple, see *idem, Einheit des Tritojesaia; idem, ZAW* 49 (1931) 112–141.

Even if we look away from the issue of authorship, the studies by T.N.D. Mettinger and others point to the difficulty of isolating the songs in form, structure and content from the rest of Isa 40–55,[1] where the servant is "Israel" (41:8f; 44:1f, 21).[2] If the fourth song deals rather with "Israel" than the life of Second Isaiah, it does not reflect a biographical interest.

3.2.4. The Book of Jeremiah

Like no other prophetic book, Jeremiah is permeated with episodal narratives about the prophet. They appear mainly in Jer 19–36 and 37–45.

The authorship of the episodal narratives is difficult to determine with certainty. The skilful literary features and the historical specificity of the material make it plausible that they originated within scribal circles around Jeremiah. Many scholars regard Baruch as to some extent the initial author of the so-called source B.[3]

The question concerning the tradition and redaction history behind Jeremiah is still a debated matter.[4] B. Duhm and S. Mowinckel gave the basic stimulus for this research—and for the habit of relating the biographical material to a source B. The application of source criticism on Jeremiah led Duhm to conclude that the book consists of three major sources:[5] (1) the poetic speeches of Jeremiah consisting of about two hundred and eighty verses and recorded within Jer 1–25, (2) the book of Baruch consisting of Jeremiah's biography of about two hundred and twenty verses and recorded within Jer 26–45 and (3) extensive supplements of approximately eight hundred and fifty verses, consisting of synagogue homilies and narrative material written under the influence of Deuteronomy, Ezekiel, Isa 40–55 and Isa 56–66 in order to explain the exile, and spread out in different parts of Jeremiah.

In his early work on Jeremiah, Mowinckel built on Duhm and used source analysis with even greater literary precision.[6] He distinguished four sources: (1) source A containing metrical oracles from Jeremiah, shaped by a careful editor and placed within Jer 1–25, (2) source B containing prose narratives concerning the prophet, written by an anonymous author and located mainly in Jer 19–20 and 26–44, (3) source C containing freely composed sermons in prose with strong Deuteronomistic language and style, located throughout Jer 1–45 and (4) source D containing the

---

1 METTINGER, *Servant Songs*. For an account of other recent scholars with similar interpretations, see HAAG, *Gottesknecht*, 138–141. Cf. also SAWYER, *JSOT* 44 (1989) 89–107; MATHEUS, *Lied*, 104–132. For critique of Mettinger, cf. HERMISSON, *TRu* 49 (1984) 209–222. MATHEUS, *ibid.*, 105–112, discusses both Mettinger's and Hermisson's view and is more positive to the former.

2 Cf. also 45:4; 48:20 and "Israel"—probably original—in the second song (49:3).

3 E.g. BIRKELAND, *Traditionswesen*, 49; MOWINCKEL, *Tradition*, 61; BRIGHT, *Jeremiah*, lxvii; EISSFELDT, *Old Testament*, 354f; RUDOLPH, *Jeremia*, xvf; J.A. THOMPSON, *Jeremiah*, 43; HOLLADAY, "Source B" and "Source C," 220; idem, *Jeremiah* II, 24, 286f. Cf. also DUHM, *Jeremia*, xiv–xvi; NICHOLSON, *Preaching to the Exiles*, 111–113; K. BALTZER, *Biographie*, 128; ROFÉ, *Prophetical Stories*, 114f.

4 For surveys of research, see HERRMANN, *TRE* 16 (1987) 574–580 (with further surveys listed on p. 583); HOLLADAY, *Jeremiah* II, 11–14.

5 *Jeremia*, xi–xx.

6 *Zur Komposition des Buches Jeremiah.*

oracles about the future now found in Jer 30–31. Some thirty years later, Mowinckel modified his position in two important matters:[1] he now believed that Baruch was the author of source B; and he now regarded the material as traditions from various traditionary circles, not as strictly literary sources.

G. Wanke's study of the material shows the difficulties in assuming a unified origin of all the narratives.[2] The episodal material occurring in different parts of Jer 19–36 has a complicated history.[3] It is not presented as a unified narrative. However, Wanke thinks also that the diction, structure and point of view in 26:1–28:17; 36:1–32 imply a single author behind the original narrative of these chapters.[4] While no real evidence can be adduced,[5] Wanke proposes Baruch as the author.[6] Baruch did have the motive, information and capability.[7]

As we saw in the previous chapter,[8] the texts claim that a supportive attitude to the person and message of Jeremiah existed also within broader scribal circles. This could account for the composition of biographical episodes by other persons than Baruch.[9] Such is probably the case with the rather unified narrative about the fall of Jerusalem in 37:1–43:7. On one hand, the text is suprisingly silent about Jeremiah's experiences in Egypt—experiences that Baruch as Jeremiah's companion in Egypt must have known about. On the other hand, the narrative is permeated with a specificity suggesting that the author was close to the events recorded.[10] There is, for instance, rather detailed information about Gedaliah's administration at Mizpah (40:7–41:18). Wanke's suggestion to locate the origin of the material within Gedaliah's administration[11] finds further support from the indication that Gedaliah was himself the grand-son of Shaphan, the scribe, and the son of Ahikam (40:5), the person who rescued Jeremiah (26:24). Gedaliah was apparently related to a family that was both supportive of Jeremiah and capable of the skilful features visible in the narrative. It is well conceivable that Gedaliah initiated the process of composition, and that there were persons around him to continue the work after his own death.

Wanke treats also the episodal narratives in 45:1–5; 51:59–64 as a unified cycle.[12]

---

1   *Tradition,* 61–63, 105 nn. 56, 61.
2   *Baruchschrift.*
3   The "biographical" material within this section has been variously identified. G. WANKE, *Baruchschrift,* 6–91, isolates 19:1–20:6; 26:1–24; 27:1–28:17; 29:1–32; 36:1–32.
4   *Baruchschrift,* 145.
5   Cf. MAY, *JBL* 61 (1942) 139f.
6   *Baruchschrift,* 147.
7   Cf. K. BALTZER, *Biographie,* 128.
8   See above pp. 43f.
9   DEARMAN, *JBL* 109 (1990) 419f.
10   Cf. SEITZ, *Theology in Conflict,* 232f.
11   *Baruchschrift,* 146.
12   *Baruchschrift,* 140–143

This is possible, though their unified character is not as evident.[1] The prophet is not in the centre of attention here. In line with the scribal custom of adding a colophon to a writing, J.R. Lundbom classifies these texts as extended colophons, most likely composed by Baruch and Seraiah and somewhat relocated in the MT.[2]

R.P. Carroll asks the important question what status the presentation of Jeremiah had in the book associated with his name.[3] Carroll's emphasis on the validating function of the growth of the Jeremiah tradition itself does not exclude a retrospective apprehension of the prophet.[4] It is true that Jeremiah is not always at the centre of attention.[5] But generally speaking, these episodal narratives do reflect an active interest in Jeremiah's life. Certain scholars think that this feature is strengthened by the occurrence of Jeremiah's own confessions (11:18–12:6; 15:10–21; 17:14–18; 18:19–23; 20:7–18),[6] some elements of which might reflect pre-Deuteronomistic elaborations by persons depending on the earlier Jeremiah tradition.[7] In any case, the biographical interest should not be put against the kerygmatic and theological function of the episodes. When the latter is in view, it is certainly reasonable to discuss whether they function, for instance, to portray the passion of Jeremiah and his friends[8] or to point to the reality of Jeremiah's prophetic existence (37:1–43:7) and demonstrate the truth of his proclamation (19:1–20:6; 26:1–24; 27:1–28:17; 29:1–32; 36:1–32).[9] For my purposes, the underlying biographical interest is of importance. While the diverse character of the different episodes causes scepticism in regard to a unified biographical genre,[10] the extensive intermingling of the prophet's words and the episodal narratives shows that *the early transmitters cherished Jeremiah's proclamation in connection with an active interest in his life, not just by adherence to his words.*[11]

3.2.5. The Book of Haggai

Among the remaining books of the later prophets only Haggai is of interest

---

1   Cf. HOLLADAY, "Source B" and "Source C," 219.

2   *JSOT* 36 (1986) 99–104. Lundbom's similar treatment of Jer 36:1–8 (*ibid.,* 104–106) is less convincing. The text is rather firmly anchored within the narrative. For a more general discussion of biblical colophons, cf. GEVERYAHU, Biblical Colophons, 42–59, though perhaps he draws too bold conclusions on the basis of merely comparative material.

3   *Jeremiah,* 33. Cf. also *idem, Chaos to Covenant,* 25–29.

4   Cf. CLEMENTS, Prophet, 214.

5   Cf. SEITZ, *Theology in Conflict,* 284f.

6   Cf. K. BALTZER, *Biographie,* 125; CHILDS, *Introduction,* 348.

7   ITTMANN, *Konfessionen,* 53–55.

8   So KREMERS, *EvT* 13 (1953) 122–140.

9   So G. WANKE, *Baruchschrift,* 155f.

10 *Contra* K. BALTZER, *Biographie,* 122–128; ROFÉ, *Prophetical Stories,* 109–111.

11 Cf. CHILDS, *Introduction,* 349.

as an extended narrative in the third person.[1] There are no accounts in the first person singular.

It is unlikely that Haggai himself was the author.[2] The other prophetical books make distinctions between accounts composed in the third person and in the first person singular. We may instead assume that other persons than the prophet himself composed the episodal narratives in the book.

While scholars have claimed that the editorial work in Haggai—and also in Zech 1–8—reflects a Chronistic milieu of composition,[3] with perhaps further Deuteronomistic and priestly traditions present in the framework,[4] H.W. Wolff observes that the narrative frames are distinct from Haggai's words and in themselves not uniform.[5] The episodal comments are built on special material available to the editor(s). Developing a suggestion by W.A.M. Beuken concerning a pre-Chronistic collection of Haggai's words,[6] Wolff proposes the early existence of five separate sketches ("Auftrittsskizzen") with an integrated presentation of the situation and the subject of the sayings.[7] In the form of a loosely organized collection ("Loseblattsammlung"), they served as the literary basis for the subsequent editorial activity.

If Wolff is correct, the words of Haggai were early integrated into episodal narratives depicting his historical situation. *Haggai's adherents combined their interest in the prophet's words with an interest in the prophet's life.*

Excursus 5: *Rabbinic Transmission and Episodal Narratives*

Rabbinic literature records only a minimum of episodal narratives about the rabbis.[8] The sayings usually appear without a narrative frame.[9] Personal details have been preserved only about a few rabbis.[10] Accordingly, there are no actual biographies.[11] The material giving information about a single rabbi is nowhere collected and presented as a comprehensive account. It is scattered throughout the rabbinic literature.[12] *The ex-*

---

[1] Jonah is of a different, legendary kind. The remaining prophetical books either contain merely the words of the prophets or are presented in the first person singular.

[2] *Contra* EISSFELD, *Old Testament*, 428f.

[3] BEUKEN, *Haggai – Sacharja 1–8*, 27–83, 331–334. Haggai and Zechariah are mentioned in Ezra 5:1; 6:14.

[4] MASON, *VT* 27 (1977) 413–421.

[5] *Studien*, 129–142. Cf. also *idem, TRE* 14 (1985) 356–358; *idem, Haggai*, 3–6.

[6] *Haggai – Sacharja 1–8*, 204f, 235. Beuken himself builds on the observations that Wolff made in his study of Hosea.

[7] The first sketch is found in 1:(2)4–11, 12b–13, the second in 2:15f, 18a, 19, the third in 2:3–9, the fourth in 2:11–14 and the fifth in 2:21b–23.

[8] So already G. KITTEL, *Probleme des palästinischen Spätjudentums*, 69.

[9] Cf. STRACK/STEMBERGER, *Talmud and Midrash*, 66f.

[10] SAFRAI, *ScrHier* 22 (1971) 209.

[11] Cf. LIGHTSTONE, *JJS* 31 (1980) 38; P.S. ALEXANDER, Rabbinic Biography, 40.

[12] Cf. W.S. GREEN, What's in a Name?, 79; NEUSNER, Rabbinic Biography, 88f; *idem, Talmudic Biography*, 1f.

istent rabbinic material does not reveal any biographical interest leading to the composition of episodal narratives.

Likewise, it is not possible to detect a biographical motive behind the personal anecdotes which do occasionally occur in various forms.[1] Although some anecdotes may contain a historical core,[2] and although the pupils sometimes formulated episodes to glorify the teacher,[3] the present trend of research—devised by J. Neusner and his students—has with sufficient detail and coherency pointed to the difficulty of attributing a general reliability to the biographical information.[4] The episodes about a certain rabbi are usually later than the halakhic material attributed to him.[5] The anecdotes have not been shaped, reshaped and communicated in order to convey exact historical information about a rabbi, but, for instance, for the purpose of supporting certain institutions, such as the school at Jamnia,[6] or defending an unfavourable event[7] or for other purely didactic purposes.[8] *The motive of rabbinic transmission was essentially non-biographical.*

4. The Didactic-Labelling Motives

"The didactic-labelling motives" are in this study *prevailing interests in the teaching as integrated within a process that enhanced the teacher to an exclusive status of authority by means of validating labels.* While the didactic and the biographical motives of transmission also contain validating processes, we do not find the extensive use of labels that extend the understanding of a person as teacher. Didactic-labelling motives are at hand when certain labels amplify the didactic conceptions significantly.

4.1. The Righteous Teacher and the Attribution of Labels

Although the Qumranites centred themselves around the conception of a scribal and priestly Teacher, they did not regard the Teacher as one among

---

[1] For different forms of anecdotes, see P.S. ALEXANDER, Rabbinic Biography, 20–24.

[2] Cf. GERHARDSSON, *Memory,* 181–189; SAFRAI, *ScrHier* 22 (1971) 210.

[3] P.S. ALEXANDER, Rabbinic Biography, 37.

[4] For a survey of this trend, see NEUSNER, Rabbinic Biography, 85–89. Other surveys are given by SALDARINI, Rabbinic Judaism, 451–454; SCHÄFER, *JJS* 37 (1986) 142f. Cf. also P.S. ALEXANDER, Rabbinic Biography, 39f.

[5] STRACK/STEMBERGER, *Talmud and Midrash,* 67.

[6] So, in reference to the function of the story about the escape of R. Joḥanan b. Zakkai from Jerusalem (b. Giṭ. 56a–b; ʾAbot R. Nat. A 4; ʾAbot R. Nat. B 6; Lam. Rab. on 1:5), SALDARINI, *JSJ* 6 (1975) 189–204, esp. 194f, 203. Cf. also SCHÄFER, *ANRW* II 19:2 (1979) 43–101.

[7] So, in reference to the function of the reshaping of the stories about the temporary replacement of R. Gamaliel II as president at Jamnia (b. Ber. 27b–28a; b. Bek. 36a; y. Ber. 7c–d; y. Taʿan. 67d), GOLDENBERG, *JJS* 23 (1972) 167–190, esp. 188f.

[8] Cf. W.S. GREEN, What's in a Name?, 85; STEMBERGER, *Talmud,* 171f; STRACK/STEMBERGER, *Talmud and Midrash,* 67f.

many. H. Stegemann emphasizes that the authority of the Teacher was rooted and inherent in his office as high priest.[1] But Stegemann does not recognize sufficiently that the Qumranites continuously validated the Teacher by means of various labels. Authority is, generally speaking, an expression of social relationships, and it needs to be approached from an interactionist perspective concerning acceptance and attribution of legitimacy by a group of followers.[2] In accordance with this, *I will focus on the authority of the Teacher as it emerges out of a process attributing and accepting legitimate domination through the use of validating labels.*

4.1.1. The Singularity of the Teacher

It is necessary first of all to ascertain that the labelling process actually concerned one specific person. Certain scholars assume that the adherence to the Righteous Teacher meant that the Qumranites were attached to *different* teachers assuming the role and office of "the Righteous Teacher."[3] The alternating manner in which the didactic figure is pictured in Damascus Document as compared with the pesharim suggests to these scholars that different persons entered the role and office.

The suggestion is partly supported by reference to the indefinite form מורה צדק in later Jewish sources. Besides the Karaites' use of this form for the coming Elijah,[4] six further instances from later Jewish writings have been brought into the discussion.[5] Most striking is the midrashic comment on Ps 102:18 in Midr. Pss. (Buber's ed. 216a). It speaks of the lack of a priest, a righteous teacher (לא כהן מורה צדק) in words strongly reminiscent of 4QpPsᵃ 3:15.

However, there are at least three objections. First, the texts are all late in comparison with the Dead Sea scrolls. Second, the use may reflect a creation which goes beyond or even is independent of the scrolls. Some of the references seem to be Jewish instances reflecting the Karaite use of the expression in reference to Elijah.[6] Only Midr. Pss. on 102:18 presents a pos-

---

1 'Teacher of Righteousness', 299–203, 207.
2 Cf. WEBER, *Wirtschaft und Gesellschaft*, 140, 655, who stresses that while charismatic authority is in itself independent, it creates among the followers a sense of duty ("Pflicht") to show their acceptance ("Anerkennung").
3 Cf. I. RABINOWITZ, *VT* 8 (1958) 398–404; BUCHANAN, *RevQ* 6 (1969) 553–558; *idem, RevQ* 9 (1977) 241–243; STARCKY, Maîtres de Justice, 249–256.
4 For references, cf. GINZBERG, *Eine unbekannte jüdische Sekte,* 306–309.
5 VON KÖLICHEN, *ZAW* 74 (1962) 324–327, found it in the 15th cent. MS Codex de Rossi 541 to S. ʿOlam Zuṭ. 226b. BUCHANAN, *RevQ* 6 (1969) 553–558, found it in Midr. Pss. on 102:18 and later, as he reports in *RevQ* 9 (1977) 241–243, in a 12th cent. document from the Cairo Geniza. SIEGEL, *RevQ* 9 (1978) 437–440, found it twice in Hebrew prayers concluding variant Pentateuchal readings. BREGMAN, *RevQ* 10 (1979) 97–100, found it in the MS of the Jewish Theological Seminary misc. 5029/acc. 0613, f. 64a–b.
6 SIEGEL, *RevQ* 9 (1978) 439f. Cf. also VON KÖLICHEN, *ZAW* 74 (1962) 326.

sible link to Qumran. But even in this case doubts remain. The expression
מורה צדק is probably a late addition to the text. M. Bregman observes that it
is missing in several MSS and ancient quotations of this passage.[1] And even
if it would be genuine, it seems to have been coined on the basis of 2 Chr
15:3 mentioning the lack of a priestly teacher (לא כהן מורה). It is therefore
not certain that it has anything to do with the scrolls at all. Third, in all the
instances outside of the Dead Sea scrolls, the definite article is missing in
front of צדק. It is missing only twice in the scrolls themselves (CD 1:11;
20:32). The vast majority of instances give the expression in the definite
form, indicating a certain specificity in the application of the term.

A study of the scrolls themselves causes further scepticism. Not only is
the frequent use of the definite article significant. The designation also varies somewhat in the scrolls. This would be unlikely if it was meant to serve
as an official title, but is understandable if a person conceptualized also by
other labels is the referent. Furthermore, the extensive use of charismatic
labels of validation overshadows the institutional connotations of the expression. This points to a person, not to an office.[2]

These considerations make it likely that *the expression* מורה הצדק *points
to one specific person*. The difference in the picture of the Teacher given in
Damascus Document as compared with the pesharim is not necessarily an
indication of different persons. It may instead be explained as alternating
ways of apprehending one and the same Teacher at different stages in the
history of the community.

4.1.2. The Expression מורה היחיד

The Teacher is twice qualified as היחיד. Once the combination מורה היחיד
occurs (CD 20:1) and once יורה היחיד (CD 20:14).

As a derivative of יחד, which etymologically may be related to אחד,
"one,"[3] this adjectival qualification is occasionally taken as a reference to
the unique status of the Teacher—the *only* Teacher.[4] M. Philonenko even
assumed that the term served in this sense as a messianic designation of Bar
Cochba.[5]

Although the numerical understanding of היחיד is possible from an etymological point of view, it becomes improbable when we look at the Dead

---

[1] *RevQ* 10 (1979) 97 n. 1.

[2] Cf. LAPERROUSAZ, *RevQ* 15 (1991) 267.

[3] Cf. DE MOOR, *VT* 7 (1957) 350–355; LOHFINK/BERGMAN, *TWAT* I, 211;
SAUER, *THAT* I, 104f; FABRY, *TWAT* III, 595–597.

[4] So e.g. SCHECHTER (ed.), *Documents of Jewish Sectaries* I, xliii, xliv; CHAR-
LES, *APOT* II, 800f, 820f; WALLENDORFF, *Rättfärdighetens lärare,* 67f; RIESNER, *Leh-
rer,* 264; STEGEMANN, 'Teacher of Righteousness', 209. Cf. also MURPHY–O'CON-
NOR, *RB* 79 (1972) 546 n. 6.

[5] *TZ* 17 (1961) 434f.

Sea scrolls themselves. The scrolls—especially the Community Rule—use various forms of (ה)יחד as a designation for the community.[1] The word is probably the Hebrew equivalent of (τὸ) κοινόν used for Greek associations,[2] though the Hebrew term does not carry strictly sectarian connotations.[3] A reference to אנשי היחיד, "men of היחיד," in CD 20:32 appears in close relation to the passages where the Teacher is qualified as היחיד. This expression has a parallel in 1QS 9:10, where the text reads אנשי היחד, "men of the community." Since היחיד and היחד sometimes were interchangeable,[4] it is likely, as most modern translators think,[5] that CD 20:1, 14 qualify the Teacher as the Teacher *of the community*. The context does not contradict such an understanding.[6]

The Qumranites labelled the Teacher *their own Teacher*. They were strongly aware of his importance for the community. It seems that they continuously thought of and remembered him as the Teacher standing at the centre of their common identity.[7]

4.1.3. The Designation מורה הצדק

The Qumranites were concerned to find a biblical basis for מורה הצדק. Scholars recognize either a phrase in Hos 10:12 (עד יבוא וירה צדק לכם)[8] or in Joel 2:23 (כי נתן לכם את המורה לצדקה),[9] or a combination of both,[10] as

---

[1] For discussion, see KOFFMAHN, *Bib* 42 (1961) 433–442; *idem, Bib* 44 (1963) 46–61; DOMBROWSKI, *HTR* 59 (1966) 293–307; WERNBERG-MØLLER, *ALUOS* 6 (1969) 56–81; J. MAIER, Zum Begriff יחד, 225–248; TALMON, *World of Qumran*, 53–60. For further literature, cf. FABRY, *TWAT* III, 595.

[2] DOMBROWSKI, *HTR* 59 (1966) 293–307. Cf. also HENGEL, Qumrān und der Hellenismus, 348f; WEINFELD, *Organizational Pattern*, 13f.

[3] Cf. WERNBERG-MØLLER, *ALUOS* 6 (1969) 56–81.—DOMBROWSKI, *HTR* 59 (1966) 293–307, stresses too much the community as a "Mystery Group" serving mainly "private ends" (*ibid.*, 296).

[4] SEGAL, *JBL* 70 (1951) 132, claims that היחיד is a medieval scribal correction. WERNBERG-MØLLER, *VT* 3 (1953) 311, 311f n. 1, regards it as a Samaritan pronunciation of היחד.

[5] Cf. CARMIGNAC/COTHENET/LIGNÉE, *Textes de Qumân*, 178, 180; LOHSE (ed.), *Texte aus Qumran*, 105; KNIBB, *Qumran Community*, 70 (but cf. also *ibid.*, 72); VERMES, *Dead Sea Scrolls in English*, 90.

[6] MURPHY-O'CONNOR, *RB* 79 (1972) 546 n. 6, refers to the polemical context and thinks that מורה and יורה are awkward explanatory additions to the original היחיד. However, the proposal of later additions is pure conjecture and the polemical context may also suggest an emphasis on the fact that it was the Teacher of this particular community that was "gathered in."

[7] If KOFFMAHN, *Bib* 42 (1961) 433–442 (cf. *idem, Bib* 44 [1963] 46–61) is correct to interpret the term יחד as a juridical designation for the community, we may add—though this is not done by Koffmahn herself—that היחיד carries a juridical overtone in regard to the Teacher's position over against the community. But this point is uncertain. Cf. the critique of Koffmahn by HENGEL, Qumrān und der Hellenismus, 348f n. 60.

[8] E.g. I. RABINOWITZ, *VT* 8 (1958) 397; J.M. BAUMGARTEN, *ANRW* II 19:1 (1979) 230; DIMANT, Qumran Sectarian Literature, 505.

[9] E.g. A. MICHEL, *Maître de Justice*, 266; SELLERS, *IEJ* 5 (1955) 93–95; MILIK,

the biblical background of the expression.[1]

As a verb ירה may exhibit three basic meanings: "to throw" or "to shoot," "to sprinkle" or "to rain" and—in hiphil—"to point out" or "to teach."[2] The MT, which is probably original,[3] conveys in both cases a meaning related to rain. This is most evident in the use of the noun in Joel 2:23. The immediate context reflects agricultural language and the second time מורה occurs in the same verse it is connected with heavy rain (גשם). Hos 10:12 uses the verb. The reference to rain is clearly present in Hos 6:3. The rabbis see in these instances a connection between rain and teaching.[4] Tg. Neb. Joel 2:23 makes a reference to an authoritative teacher of the end-time. It is common in different strata of Judaism to compare torah or wisdom teaching with images of water.[5]

There is unfortunately no clear testimony about how the Qumranites read/heard these passages.[6] 4QpHos[b] (4Q167) 5–6:2 might provide a small piece of information. As it seems, יורה of Hos 6:3 is in a comment on 6:4 rendered מוריהם. But there is no way to determine the significance of this. 1QH 8:16 gives some further information. There rain is used metaphorically (כיורה נשם) for what God has put on the lips of the speaker. It is parallelled by "living water" (מים חיים), which elsewhere is a description of the Torah (CD 19:34).[7] Accordingly, "water of lie" or "lying water" (מימי כזב) is an epithet for false teaching (CD 1:14f). These passages indicate that the Qumranites could understand the agricultural images in Hos 10:12 and Joel 2:23 as references to a teaching activity.

The whole expression מורה הצדק has a biblical basis. *It was a biblical label.* This attempt to ground the major designation for the Teacher within the OT reveals a manner of validation which relates the authority to what was held as sacred.

Ten Years of Discovery, 71 n. 2; O. BETZ, *Offenbarung und Schriftforschung,* 56, 115 n. 3; VERMES, *Scripture and Tradition,* 54.

[10] E.g. G. JEREMIAS, *Lehrer der Gerechtigkeit,* 312f; ROTH, *VT* 13 (1963) 91; CULPEPPER, *School,* 153; RIESNER, *Lehrer,* 306.

[1] A minority of scholars think that the community coined and used the term with no biblical background. So e.g. R. MEYER, Melchisedek, 230 n. 3; WOLFF, *Joel and Amos,* 63f; S. WAGNER, *TWAT* III, 919. In view of the prominence of biblical interpretation at Qumran, this would be surprising.

[2] S. WAGNER, *TWAT* III, 909–930.

[3] This is denied by WOLFF, *Hosea,* 180; *idem, Joel and Amos,* 55, 63f. For Joel 2:23, cf. already SELLERS, *IEJ* 5 (1955) 93–95; I. RABINOWITZ, *VT* 8 (1958) 397 n. 1. For a defence of the MT, see RIESNER, *Lehrer,* 304–306, though I do not agree that מורה/יורה should be translated "teacher/teaching" here (*ibid.,* 305).

[4] For references, cf. DALMAN, *Arbeit und Sitte* I, 122.

[5] Cf. e.g. Prov 13:14; 18:4; Sir 15:3; 24:21, 25–31; 1 Enoch 48:1; 49:1; m. ʾAbot 1:4, 11; b. Ḥag. 3a; b. B. Meṣ. 84b; b. Hor. 14a; Sifre on Deut 11:22.

[6] The passages are extant neither in the Hebrew scroll to the Minor Prophets from Murabbaʿat (Mur XII) nor in the Greek scroll from the cave of horror (8HevXII gr). The pesharim do not comment on the passages, although fragments of a commentary on Hosea (4QpHos [4Q166–167]) have been found.

[7] Cf. also CD 3:16; 6:4.

While the biblical basis of the label points to a certain manner of validating the Teacher, it does not reveal the actual connotations which the expression carried in the community. The expression מורה (ה)צדק(ה) is a construction with מורה in the construct state. The question is how to understand the *nomen rectum* (ה)צדק(ה). Does it denote the *object* of the Teacher's activity or does it exercise the *qualifying* affect of an adjective?

Considering the rather weak evidence for understanding the construction as an objective genitive,[1] we should give due attention to the arguments for reading/hearing the *nomen rectum* as an adjectival attribute. These arguments must of course build on the evidence from the scrolls themselves.[2] First, the adjectival understanding is possible from a philological point of view. There are uses of צדק as a *nomen rectum* elsewhere in the scrolls.[3] Of particular interest for our purposes are the adjectival attributes in CD 20:29–33. This text connects the precepts of God's covenant first with "his holy precepts" (חקי קדשו), "his righteous statutes" (משפטי צדקו) and "his true testimonies" (עדוות אמתו), and then with "righteous precepts" (חקי הצדק) of the מורה צדק.[4] Second, while the actual expression מורה הצדק is related to מטיף הכזב,[5] the Teacher is himself also put over against a priest who is qualified as "wicked," הכוהן הרשע.[6] An adequate counterpart would be someone who is "righteous." 1QpHab 9:9f; 11:4f use מורה הצדק in close relation to "the wicked priest," הכוהן הרשע.[7] Third, in connection with a further reference to הכוהן הרשע, 4QpPs^a 4:8 calls the Teacher "the righteous one," הצדיק, on the basis of Ps 37:32f.[8] 1QpHab 1:12f; 5:8f use perhaps an identical designation on the basis of Hab 1:4, 13.[9]

We should, it seems, interpret the genitive construction מורה (ה)צדק(ה) in an adjectival and qualitative sense. It is of course possible, and likely, that the Teacher did teach righteousness to the community. But this is not how the Qumranites understood the title as they confronted it in the scrolls. The primary function of the title was apparently not to denote the object of an

---

1   See excursus 6 below.
2   Two out of three arguments brought out by Jürgen BECKER, *Heil Gottes,* 174–176, to support his adjectival understanding of the term concern items outside of the Dead Sea scrolls.
3   Cf. CD 3:15; 20:11, 30f, 33; 20:33; 1QH 1:23, 26; 6:4, 19; 9:33; 1QS 1:13; 2:24; 3:1; 4:4, 9; 9:5; 1QSb 2:26. Even a most critical reading must accept that at least CD 20:33; 1QH 1:23; 9:33; 1QS 1:13 represent an adjectival use of צדק as *nomen rectum.*
4   Cf. CD 20:11.
5   See below p. 121f.
6   1QpHab 8:8; 9:9; 11:4; 12:2, 8; 4QpPs^a 4:8. Cf. also 1QpHab 8:16; 11:12.
7   I. RABINOWITZ, *VT* 8 (1958) 393 n. 3, claims that the Teacher's title must be in definite form in order to be comparable with הכוהן הרשע. But there is still a certain correlation between the two in the texts themselves.
8   The occurrence of לצדיק within the quotation in 4QpPs^a 4:7 makes it likely that the interpretation of the quotation in 4QpPs^a 4:8 uses הצדיק.
9   Cf. also the fact that the Qumranites are called בני (ה)צדק (1QS 3:20, 22; 4QS^e 9:14 [MILIK, *RB* 67 [1960] 414]) in distinction to בני עול (1QS 3:21).

action. It functioned to qualify the Teacher as righteous. He was the Righteous Teacher of the community.

What did this qualification imply to the Qumranites more precisely? The term צדק(ה) is frequent by itself.[1] The verb is used both in qal and hiphil.

Scholars understand this term variously. J.C. Reeves proposes that we should banish all theological connotations of the term and study it on the basis of the etymological meaning, "that which is legitimate, proper, true."[2] But this procedure is inappropriate if, as Reeves claims himself,[3] a *conceptual* study is intended. A concept involves more than the etymological meaning. Reeves neglects the context of the scrolls themselves. J. Weingreen gives the term a forensic flavor.[4] But only 1QH 12:19, where צדיק is used, provides such a significance, and only with an explicit forensic qualifier—"justified before you" (צדיק עמכה). The collective significance proposed by I. Rabinowitz, who translates the Teacher's designation with "the leader of the righteous," is even less likely, both in regard to etymology and the use of צדק(ה) in the scrolls themselves.[5]

The term צדק(ה) is theologically loaded in the scrolls. It is intimately related to God and his salvific action towards the community of the covenant.[6] 1QM 18:8 makes evident that God is himself צדק within the context of the covenant and acts in accordance with צדק. The action manifests itself as God creates and sustains salvation (1QS 10:11; 11:2–5, 12–14). J.A. Ziesler concludes rightly that "all cases of man's righteousness are in some sort of relation to God."[7]

This implies that the attribution of the term to the Teacher included theological connotations. *When the Qumranites labelled him "the Righteous Teacher," they acknowledged his relation to their sacred traditions and validated him as instrumental in God's salvific action towards themselves.*

Excursus 6: *G. Jeremias on the* מורה הצדק *Construction*

Although various scholars remarked on the significance of the מורה הצדק construction quite early,[8] G. Jeremias initiated the further discussion by presenting arguments for

---

1   For discussion and literature, see Jürgen BECKER, *Heil Gottes,* 37–189; STUHL-MACHER, *Gerechtigkeit Gottes,* 148–166; ZIESLER, *Meaning of Righteousness,* 85–94; O. BETZ, Rechtfertigung in Qumran, 17–36; KOCH, *THAT* II, 530; SEIFRID, *Justification,* 78–108.

2   *RevQ* 13 (1988) 292.

3   *RevQ* 13 (1988) 288.

4   *Bible,* 104–108.

5   *VT* 8 (1958) 393–398, quotation from p. 397.

6   For the salvific aspect, see Jürgen BECKER, *Heil Gottes,* 37–189. For the covenantal aspect, see ZIESLER, *Meaning of Righteousness,* 87–94; SEIFRID, *Justification,* 81–89.—STUHLMACHER, *Gerechtigkeit Gottes,* 148–166, relates the term to God's own character and tries, in addition, to prove that צדק(ה) אל is a technical expression in 1QS 10:25f; 11:12; 1QM 4:6. The last point is uncertain. Cf. the recent critique by SEIFRID, *ibid.,* 99–106.

7   *Meaning of Righteousness,* 94.

8   E.g. HONEYMAN, *JJS* 4 (1953) 131; VAN DER WOUDE, *Die messianischen Vor-*

the two main options.[1] He understood the expression as an objective genitive, though not excluding totally a qualitative aspect.[2] But the arguments he used for his option are not always convincing.[3]

Jeremias first refers to CD 6:10f, where יורה הצדק implies that צדק is the object of teaching.[4] However, in another context Jeremias notices the close parallel between this passage and the possible expectation of a *faithful* prophet in 1 Macc 14:41 (ἕως τοῦ ἀναστῆναι προφήτην πίστον).[5] This connection should at least cause some consideration about whether הצדק does not carry an adjectival sense also in CD 6:10f. Furthermore, although CD 6:10f refers to the priestly Messiah, it may be of some significance that 4QGenFlor (4Q252) 5:2–4—previously known as 4QPBless 2–4—speaks of a period of time until משיח הצדק, the branch of David, comes. Since the Davidic Messiah is nowhere in the scrolls said to be teaching righteousness, it is probable that the community, through allusion to Jer 23:5f; 33:15, used the text as a reference to the *legitimate* Messiah—the one from the branch of David.[6]

Second, Jeremias refers to Hos 10:12; Joel 2:23 as support.[7] Here צדק(ה) is (part of) the object of an action, though the constructions are slightly different from what we find in the scrolls.[8] However, while a connection to these texts is likely, it is impossible to know if the designation was coined on the basis of these two instances or if they were later adduced as exegetical support for an existing title. And moreover, the different forms of exegesis at Qumran reveal that the Qumranites often subsumed the original meaning and context of an OT passage under other considerations.

Third, Jeremias accurately points out that the designation was probably used as the opposing counterpart of מטיף הכזב.[9] In particular, Jeremias refers to CD 1:14f, stating that a scoffer arose "who shed over Israel waters of lies" (אשר הטיף לישראל מימי כזב), and to CD 6:1, claiming that his followers "prophesied lies" (ינבאו שקר). They indicate that מטיף הכזב and consequently מורה הצדק are objective genitives. However, כזב is not the object of action but an adjectival qualification of the water in CD 1:14f. Of the remaining instances of כזב in the scrolls,[10] only 1QS 10:22 uses the term clearly as an object, but then in a completely different context. Nor is CD 6:1 of much help. Here שקר occurs, not כזב. The remaining occurrences of שקר as verb (1QS 6:24) or noun[11] in the scrolls do not give any further aid. The expression מורה שקר appears in Isa 9:14;

---

stellungen, 171; I. RABINOWITZ, *VT* 8 (1958) 393; MILIK, *Ten Years of Discovery,* 76; CROSS, *Ancient Library,* 113 n. 3. Cf. also WEINGREEN, *Bible,* 102 (article originally published in 1961).

1 *Lehrer der Gerechtigkeit,* 308–317.

2 *Lehrer der Gerechtigkeit,* 315.

3 Cf. Jürgen BECKER, *Heil Gottes,* 174f.

4 *Lehrer der Gerechtigkeit,* 312.

5 *Lehrer der Gerechtigkeit,* 286. Cf. also 1 Macc 4:46.

6 The manner in which the Messiah frequently was called "righteous" in early Christianity, apocalyptic circles and the synagogue does not contradict my understanding of 4QGenFlor (4Q252) 5:2–4. For discussion and references, see DECHENT, *TSK* 100 (1927–28) 439–443; SCHRENK, *TDNT* II, 186f.

7 *Lehrer der Gerechtigkeit,* 312f

8 Hos 10:12 is close to CD 6:11, but צדק is indefinite in the former passage. Joel 2:23 has ל in front of צדקה.

9 *Lehrer der Gerechigkeit,* 313.

10 CD 8:13; 19:26; 20:15; 1QH 2:31; 4:10, 16; 1QpHab 2:2; 5:11; 10:9; 11:1; 1QpMic 8:10–4; 1QS 10:22. The verb is used in 1QH 8:16; 1QSb 1:4(?).

11 1QH 5:27; 7:12; 1QpHab 10:10, 12; 1QS 4:9, 21; 5:15; 4QpNah 2:2, 8.

Hab 2:18. But the context does not, as Jeremias claims,[1] concern so much the content of teaching as the quality of people. Rabbinic writings say that the prophets will be judged on the basis of Yahweh's directions in Deut 18:19f. This judgement, however, implies that even a prophet who withholds his prophecy (m. Sanh. 11:5) or teaches the right halakhah but bases it on an idol (m. Sanh. 11:6) is שׁקר. It is hardly the object of teaching itself that makes the prophet false.[2] Elsewhere נביא אמת, "a true prophet," is put against someone termed נביא שׁקר (b. Sanh. 90a). The Dead Sea scrolls contain numerous examples of אמת as the equivalent of צדק.[3] It is not at all clear, therefore, that מטיף הכזב is an objective genitive. There are reasons at least as strong for translating this designation with "the false prophet."[4]

Fourth, using an argument of A. Jaubert, Jeremias refers to 2 Pet 2:5; 1 Clem. 5:7 as support.[5] In the former passage Noah is as a messenger of righteousness guarded by God from the river, and in the latter passage Paul is said to be teaching righteousness. Needless to say, a Hebrew construction cannot be explained on the basis of Greek references which, in addition, do not have any evident connection with the scrolls.

4.1.4. The Prophetic Label

Although Josephus' account about the Essenes is not immediately applicable to the Qumranites, his account about their involvement in prophetic activities may be of some significance. Not only does he attest the close relationship between biblical study and accurate prophecy among the Essenes (Bell. 2:159). Besides mentioning John, the military commander (Bell. 2:567; 3:11, 19), he speaks also of three other Essenes being in possession of extraordinary prophetical gifts: a certain Simon interpreted a dream of Archelaus, the ethnarch of Judaea, to mean the imminent banishment of the ruler (Ant. 17:345–348; Bell. 2:111–113); a certain Menahem made predictions concerning Herod I the Great (Ant. 15:373–379); Judah the Essene predicted that Antigonus the Hasmonean would be killed at Strato's tower (Ant. 13:311–313; Bell. 1:78–80).

Josephus' account about the Essenes harmonizes in this case with the scrolls themselves. CD 2:12 portrays the OT prophets as God's anointed one(s) (משׁיחו), through whom he made known his holy spirit to Israel.[6] Their books constitute authorities which demand obedience (CD 7:15–18). And the Qumranites were convinced that God's spirit was present in their

---

[1]   *Lehrer der Gerechtigkeit,* 313.

[2]   Cf. also m. Sanh. 1:5; 11:1; b. Sanh. 89a–b.

[3]   Cf. e.g. CD 3:15; 20:29f, 31; 1QH 4:40; 1QM 13:10; 1QS 1:26; 2:24; 4:2, 24; 9:17; 1QSb 3:24; 1Q36 15:2.

[4]   For the prophetic connotations, see below p. 123.

[5]   *Lehrer der Gerechtigkeit,* 313f. Cf. JAUBERT, *RB* 65 (1958) 238f. JAUBERT, *ibid.,* 238, also refers to 1 Enoch 12:4; 15:1, where Enoch is called "scribe of righteousness." (The Greek version of 1 Enoch 15:1 has no reference to righteousness.)

[6]   LOHSE (ed.), *Texte aus Qumran,* 68f, renders the text to indicate that God taught Israel through "anointed ones of his holy spirit" (משׁיחי רוח קדשׁו). Cf. also CD 6:1; 1QM 11:7f.

midst.[1]

Although the scrolls never state it explicitly, the Qumranites probably attributed prophetic labels also to the Teacher. Perhaps they even attached a prophetic connotation to the term מורה itself. This connotation does not, however, emerge from its use in the OT. The prophetic writings attribute the term only to false prophets and oracles (Isa 9:14; Hab 2:18).[2] But there is perhaps an indirect prophetic connotation in the scrolls. The false prophet (CD 8:13; 19:25f; 1QpHab 10:9; 1QpMic 8–10:4),[3] known as the opponent of the Teacher,[4] probably carries his designation מטיף הכזב as a counterpart to מורה הצדק.[5] The term מטיף—a hiphil participle of נטף—has a prophetic connotation in Ezek 21:2, 7; Amos 7:16; Mic 2:6, 11. And much later, y. Ber. 3b uses Mic 2:6, 11 to prove that the words of the elders are more important than the words of the prophets. CD 4:19f indicates that especially Mic 2:6 provides the background for applying the designation on the Teacher's opponent in the scrolls. 1QH 4:16 consequently calls the followers of the מטיף הכזב "false prophets" (נביאי כזב).[6] It is therefore probable that the Qumranites attached a prophetic connotation also to מורה.

There are more circumstantial factors pointing in the same direction. Among the primary sources reflecting the Qumranites' conceptions about the Teacher,[7] the commentary on Habakkuk testifies most clearly to a prophetic labelling.[8] It attributes a prophetic inspiration to the Teacher—often in connection with picturing him as a wisdom sage:[9] in an almost apocalyptic fashion, all the secrets of the prophetic books were made known to him (1QpHab 7:4f); the knowledge was given directly from the mouth of God (1QpHab 2:2f), so that he, as a priestly Teacher, could interpret all the words of the prophets (1QpHab 2:7f), and even go beyond that which was revealed to the prophets themselves (1QpHab 7:1–8);[10] refusal to listen to

---

1   See H.-W. KUHN, *Enderwartung und gegenwärtiges Heil,* 120–139. Cf. also H. BRAUN, *Qumran und das Neue Testament* II, 252f; BRUCE, *ALUOS* 6 (1969) 54f. For the whole problem of רוח and its referent at Qumran, see SEKKI, *Meaning of Ruah.*
2   R. MEYER, Melchisedek, 234, mentions also Gen 12:6; Judg 7:14, but these instances are even more remote.
3   Cf. also CD 1:14f; 20:15; 1QH 2:31; 4:9f, 16; 1QpHab 2:1f; 5:11; 11:1(?).
4   Cf. G. JEREMIAS, *Lehrer der Gerechtigkeit,* 79–126.
5   G. JEREMIAS, *Lehrer der Gerechtigkeit,* 313.
6   Cf. also CD 6:1 (ונבאו שקר).
7   The "I" of the Hodayoth claims the possession of God's holy spirit in order to attain knowledge and insight (e.g. 7:6f; 12:11f; 13:18f; 14:13, 25; 17:26), particularly in order to understand certain secrets (2:13; 4:27f). Cf. P. SCHULZ, *Autoritätsanspruch des Lehrers der Gerechtigkeit,* 29–110, esp. 88–90.
8   Cf. G. JEREMIAS, *Lehrer der Gerechtigkeit,* 141.
9   The sapiential characteristics of the Teacher mentioned above pp. 49f relate closely to the prophetic inspiration. Cf. e.g. the comments about the Teacher by KÜCHLER, *Frühjüdische Weisheitstraditionen,* 93: "... seiner prophetisch-weisheitlichen Funktion und Botschaft ..."; SCHNABEL, *Law and Wisdom,* 204: "... a unique prophetic-apocalyptic wisdom." For Ben Sira, see above p. 46.
10   The statement that the Teacher has the capacity to go beyond the prophets indicates

the words of the Teacher parallels unfaithfulness to the covenant and profanation of God's name (1QpHab 2:4); faith in his teaching even determines the delivering from judgement at the end of times (1QpHab 8:1–3).

Scholars have often proposed that the Teacher fulfilled the function of the Moses of the end-time or a coming prophet like Moses,[1] though some remain sceptical.[2] The scrolls picture him first of all as the law-giver.[3] But three pieces of information make it probable that the community at an early stage of its history also waited for a coming prophet like Moses.[4] First, the scrolls mention Moses in connection with the OT prophets (CD 5:21–6:1; 1QS 1:3; 8:15f). The community would evidently not have objected to calling Moses a prophet. We know from extra-Qumranic texts also outside of Deuteronomy that Moses was sometimes regarded as a prophet (Hos 12:14; Sir 46:1; Wis 11:1). Second, the scrolls testify to the earliest use of Deut 18:18f as applied on the end-time. 4QTestim 5–8 quotes the text together with four other messianic proof-texts.[5] Num 24:15–17; Deut 33:8–11 refer apparently to the Messiah: the royal Messiah (4QTestim 9–13) and—implicitly—the priestly Messiah (4QTestim 14–20). Proof-texts are given for a triad of the end-time. One of the three is the awaited Mosaic prophet. Third, 1QS 9:11 mentions the eschatological triad together. The old statutes are to be valid "until the coming of a prophet and Messiahs of Aaron and Israel" (עד בוא נביא ומשיחי אהרון וישראל). In view of the proof-text in 4QTestim 5–8, this is probably an allusion to the coming of a prophet like Moses, not like Elijah.

As is well known, Deut 18:15, 18 are the basic texts for various expectations about Moses as a prophet. According to Deut 34:10–12, the promise of a future prophet like Moses was never fulfilled, in spite of the appearance of Joshua as the successor of

---

that the community did not put interpretative activity against prophetic inspiration. *Contra* e.g. SUTCLIFFE, *Monks of Qumran*, 60f; HILL, *New Testament Prophecy*, 41.

[1] E.g. WIEDER, *JJS* 4 (1953) 158–175; TEEPLE, *Mosaic Eschatological Prophet*, 51–56; VAN DER WOUDE, *Die messianischen Vorstellungen*, 84f; DUPONT-SOMMER, *Écrits esséniens*, 374f; SCHNACKENBURG, *SE* 1 (1959) 633f; O. BETZ, *Offenbarung und Schriftforschung*, 62–64; Joachim JEREMIAS, *TDNT* IV, 861; MEEKS, *Prophet-King*, 16–171; HAHN, *Christologische Hoheitstitel*, 367; K. SCHUBERT, Messiaslehre, 343–346; AUNE, *Prophecy*, 126; WISE, *Temple Scroll*, 185–187. For further references to older scholars, cf. G. JEREMIAS, *Lehrer der Gerechtigkeit*, 296f.

[2] The lack of clear evidence is stressed by G. JEREMIAS, *Lehrer der Gerechtigkeit*, 295–298. Cf. also CROSS, *Ancient Library*, 224f; WALLENDORFF, *Rättfärdighetens lärare*, 97–99; HILL, *New Testament Prophecy*, 42.

[3] E.g. CD 5:8, 21; 8:14; 15:2, 9, 12; 16:2, 5; 19:26f; 1QDM 1:1, 11; 2:5, 11; 4:3; 1QH 17:12; 1QM 10:6; 1QS 1:3; 5:8; 8:15, 22; 4QDibHamᵃ 5:14; 4QFlor 2:2f; 4Q266 line 6; 6Q15 3:4. Surprisingly, the Temple scroll does not mention Moses by name. But cf. 11QT 44:5.

[4] 11QMelch 18 does not contain any allusion to a prophet like Moses. See excursus 7 below.

[5] The texts are quoted in the order Deut 5:28f; 18:18f; Num 24:15–17; Deut 33:8–11; Josh 6:26.

Moses (Num 27:12–23; Deut 1:38; 31:7f, 23; 34:9).[1] It is probable that the ideal of a Mosaic prophet finds expression already in the OT.[2] In the later writings of early and rabbinic Judaism and the Samaritans several notions are attached to Moses, from conceptions of new Mosaic times and Moses as an ideal to the expectation of a future prophet like Moses or even—in spite of the account about Moses' death and burial (Deut 34:5–8)—the return of Moses himself, Moses *redivivus*.[3]

The pertinent question is if there are indications that the community identified the Teacher with the prophet referred to in 1QS 9:11. In addition to the prophetic labelling of the Teacher, there are two general considerations which make such an identification conceivable. First, CD 6:7 uses המחוקק, "the sceptre," for the Teacher.[4] This term carries not only didactic and scribal connotations. Sifre on Deut 33:21; Tg. Onq. Deut 33:21; Frg. Tg. Deut 33:21; Tg. Neof. Deut 33:21; Tg. Ps.-J. Deut 33:21 all apply it on Moses.[5] Second, there is a typological connection between the community and the Exodus generation. Moses and the Teacher are both leaders of an emigration.[6] *Since the Qumranites validated the Teacher with prophetic labels and related him to Moses in a general manner, it is conceivable that they also identified him with the coming prophet of 1QS 9:11.*[7]

It is unlikely that the Qumranites regarded the Teacher as the suffering servant of Isa 40–55. True, the suffering of the righteous one is a theme present in the scrolls.[8] It is possible that even more passages than the critical account by G. Jeremias allows for actually allude to the servant songs.[9] In addition, according to J. Starcky,[10] a scroll abbreviated 4QAhA pictures what seems to be the Aaronitic Messiah as suffering like the servant of the Isaianic servant songs.[11] However, the vast majority of texts ad-

---

1   Cf. also Josh 1:5; Sir 46:1. See further excursus 1 above.
2   For introductory discussion and literature, see WILSON, *Prophecy*, 157–166; CA-ZELLES, *TWAT* V, 32, 38–42. For an application of this motif on the book of Jeremiah, see SEITZ, *BZ* 34 (1990) 234–245.
3   Cf. e.g. TEEPLE, *Mosaic Eschatological Prophet*, 29–73; Joachim JEREMIAS, *TDNT* IV, 849–864; MEEKS, *Prophet-King*, 100–257; TIEDE, *Charismatic Figure*, 101–240.
4   See below pp. 126f.
5   The text quoted in CD 6:3f is Num 21:18. In the targumim to this passage, the chiefs who dug the well are the leaders of the people, the scribes. In later haggadic midrashim, the מחוקק of Num 21:18 is Moses. For references, cf. ROSMARIN, *Moses*, 20 n. 47; G. JEREMIAS, *Lehrer der Gerechtigkeit*, 272f.
6   Cf. e.g. CD 4:3; 6:5. G. JEREMIAS, *Lehrer der Gerechtigkeit*, 270f, gives further examples of this typological connection.
7   The frustrations caused by the death of the awaited prophet/Teacher will be dealt with below pp. 192f.
8   See RUPPERT, *Der leidende Gerechte*, 114–133, 185f; CARMIGNAC, Theologie des Leidens, 312–340; KLEINKNECHT, *Der leidende Gerechtfertigte*, 140–153.
9   G. JEREMIAS, *Lehrer der Gerechtigkeit*, 303, thinks that only 1QH 7:10; 8:35f allude to the servant songs.
10   *RB* 70 (1963) 492.
11   4Q285 frg. 7 lines 4–5 does not seem to refer to a suffering Davidic Messiah. See esp. VERMES, *JJS* 43 (1992) 85–90. Cf. also BOCKMUEHL, *TynBul* 43:1 (1992) 155–169; BETZ/RIESNER, *Jesus, Qumran und der Vatikan*, 103–110. This is now acknow-

duced in support are usually taken from the Hodayoth. The term "servant" (עבד) never occurs in explicit connection with the Teacher. The praying person in the Hodayoth and 1QS 11:16 uses it most often. The application of the term on the prophets is second in frequency (1QpHab 2:9; 7:5; 1QS 1:3; 4QDibHam[a] 3:12f; 4QpHos[a] [4Q166] 2:5). It is also used in the normal sense for a slave (CD 11:12; 12:10; 1QS 9:22) and for the slavery of the Israelites in Egypt (11QT 54:17). As applied to individuals, it is used for Moses (4QDibHam[a] 5:14) and David (1QM 11:2) only.[1] On the basis of the present evidence, it seems that the Qumranites did not regard the Teacher as the suffering servant.

4.1.5. The Messianic Label

The scrolls certainly attribute the function of studying and expounding the Torah, of making some kind of midrash,[2] to various individuals in the community. 1QS 6:6f tells about a man—a priest (1QS 6:3f)—who studies in the Torah (איש דורש בתורה) day and night within a group of ten men. 1QS 8:11f probably refers to the same person (איש הדורש).[3]

However, such an individual is never called דורש התורה, "interpreter of the Torah."[4] In spite of recent objections,[5] this expression seems to be a specific title for the Righteous Teacher in the scrolls. CD 6:7 suggests that the Teacher is *the* interpreter of the Torah.[6] A comparison with CD 1:11 points in this direction. The Righteous Teacher has been raised by God in order to guide the incipient community so that they will no longer be like blind men groping for the way. He is their guide. The chronological references in CD 1:1–11 and CD 6:2–11 are not clear enough to propose a distinction in time between the coming of the Teacher and the interpreter of the Torah.[7] There is actually a parallel connection. The community's attempt to seek God (דרשוהו)—in both cases the identical expression occurs—precedes in both contexts the appearance of the Teacher/interpreter of the Torah (CD 1:10; 6:6). Moreover, CD 6:7 explicitly identifies the interpre-

---

ledged in brackets also by EISENMAN/WISE, *Dead Sea Scrolls,* 29. But for a different view, cf. TABOR, *BARev* 18:6 (1992) 58f.

1   The occurrences of עבד in 1QSb 1:27; 1Q25 5:4; 1Q36 17:2 are too fragmentary in order to be of significance.

2   Cf. SCHIFFMAN, *Halakhah at Qumran,* 54–60.

3   Cf. O. BETZ, *Offenbarung und Schriftforschung,* 19–23; SCHIFFMAN, *Halakhah at Qumran,* 57.

4   G. JEREMIAS, *Lehrer der Gerechtigkeit,* 294, calls it an "Ehrentitel."

5   Cf. P.R. DAVIES, *Damascus Covenant,* 123f; *idem, Behind the Essenes,* 35, 47f; CALLAWAY, *History of the Qumran Community,* 107–113; MURPHY-O'CONNOR, Damascus Document Revisited, 380; P.R. DAVIES, *RevQ* 13 (1988) 314f; *idem,* Temple Scroll, 204–206; CALLAWAY, *RevQ* 14 (1990) 642f.

6   Cf. O. BETZ, *Offenbarung und Schriftforschung,* 23–36.

7   *Contra* P.R. DAVIES, *Damascus Covenant,* 124; CALLAWAY, *History of the Qumran Community,* 108f; P.R. DAVIES, *RevQ* 13 (1988) 314f; *idem,* Temple Scroll, 202; CALLAWAY, *RevQ* 14 (1990) 642f. Cf. correctly KNIBB, Teacher of Righteousness, 59f.

ter of the Torah with "the sceptre" (המחוקק). The "nobles of the people" (נדיבי העם)—the community—continued to study the Torah by the aid of the ordinances prescribed by the sceptre (CD 6:3f, 8–10). With G. Jeremias we must assume that this points only to one figure, the Righteous Teacher.[1] No other person exhibiting this authority is visible in the scrolls. The Teacher is the authoritative interpreter of the Torah and his teaching is to guide the continuous study and practice of the community.[2]

My understanding of CD 6:2–11 goes against the thesis of P.R. Davies.[3] He identifies the interpreter of the Torah in CD 6:7 with an unknown person in the initial history of the community and the future teacher in CD 6:11 with the Righteous Teacher.[4] He is of course not approaching the texts from the perspective of their *use* by the Qumranites, but from an entirely genetic and author-oriented perspective. The thesis builds on Davies' earlier study of the Damascus Document, arguing that the so-called Admonitions (CD 1–8, 19–20) are in essence pre-Qumranic.[5] The reference to the Teacher in CD 1:11 is due to later Qumranic redaction,[6] as are the references in CD 20:1, 14, 32.[7]

However, at least three questions remain. First, if the Qumranites inserted the reference to the Teacher in 1:11 and regarded the Teacher as identical with the future teacher of 6:11, why were the connotations of the end-time not expressed more clearly in 1:11? Because the Teacher was dead at this time? But then the second obstacle appears. If the death of the Teacher was a strong redactional force, why did the community maintain the clear allusions to the end-time in 6:11? A certain redactional modification is as plausible as the alleged insertion of 1:11. Third, if the reference to the Teacher in 1:11 was inserted on the basis of 6:11 and intended to speak about the same person, why were not identical designations used? Although יורה and מורה may of course be interchangeable,[8] the identification of the two would have been more natural if the definite article appeared in front of צדק also in 1:11. It seems more plausible that 1:11 was an integral part of the composition and that 6:7, 11 refer to two distinct teachers, one historical and one messianic.

The designation was probably connected with eschatological beliefs. The expression דורש התורה occurs also in CD 7:18; 4QFlor 1:11.[9] It is here attributed to the priestly Messiah. 4QFlor 1:11 speaks about the future. It applies 2 Sam 7:11–14 on the Davidic Messiah, who will appear together

---

[1]   *Lehrer der Gerechtigkeit,* 272: "Es ist deutlich zu erkennen, daß der Mechokkek nur den einen Lehrer darstellen kann, der in den Q.-Texten eine so überaus große Rolle spielt, der Lehrer der Gerechtigkeit."

[2]   Cf. STEGEMANN, 'Teacher of Righteousness', 203.

[3]   *RevQ* 13 (1988) 313–317. Cf. also *idem, Damscus Covenant,* 123f.

[4]   P.R. DAVIES, Temple Scroll, 205, now tends to regard the interpreter of the Torah as "an halakhic fiction."

[5]   *Damascus Covenant.*

[6]   *Damascus Covenant,* 199f.

[7]   *Damscus Covenant,* 173–197.

[8]   Cf. CD 20:1, 14.

[9]   4QFlor frg. 23 (*DJD* V, pl. 20) contains דורש. Perhaps this is an additional use of the designation.

with the interpreter of the Torah.[1] The quotation from and commentary on Deut 33:8–11—the passage that 4QTestim 14–20 gives as the biblical basis for the priestly Messiah—in fragments six and seven of the Florilegium provide a link for understanding the interpreter of the Torah as the priestly Messiah. Fragment five, line two, also contains a reference to the priestly Messiah—perhaps even to both messianic figures (ישראל ואהרון[י).[2]

Although part of the context of CD 7:18–20 concerns past events,[3] it is probable that also CD 7:18 refers to the same future figure. The messianic use of Num 24:15–17 is present.[4] The text identifies the interpreter of the Torah with the star of Jacob who, according to Num 24:17, will appear together with a sceptre (שבט) of Israel. The future reference is present not only in Num 24:17. Just as "coming" (הבא) is used to describe the appearance of the star (CD 7:19), so this verb occurs also elsewhere both as a participial (1QpHab 2:7, 10; 7:1)[5]—as in CD 7:19—and as an infinitive (1QS 9:11; 4QGenFlor [4Q252] 5:3) in connection with decisive future events.[6] Furthermore, it is well known that the present Testaments of the Twelve Patriarchs contain similar expectations about two Messiahs.[7] T. Levi 18:2f connects the star with the appearance of a new priest.[8] Aramaic fragments from the Testament of Levi (4Q213–214) and a Hebrew fragment from the Testament of Naphtali (4Q215) have been found at Qumran.[9] There are probably fragments from other Testaments as well.[10] It is likely, therefore, that the conceptions expressed in the Testaments influenced the messianic expectations of the community at some stage during its history.[11]

---

1 Cf. FLUSSER, *IEJ* 19 (1959) 104–109, though his identification of the interpreter of the Torah in CD 6:7; 7:18 with a successor of the community's founder is problematic. For further discussion, see BROOKE, *Exegesis at Qumran,* 197–205. For a summary, see VAN DER WOUDE, *TDNT* IX, 517–520.

2 Cf. BROOKE, *Exegesis at Qumran,* 204f, though he refers to frg. 4 instead of 5.

3 Cf. CALLAWAY, *History of the Qumran Community,* 109f.

4 For this use, cf. also 1QM 11:6f.

5 Cf. also CD 8:11; 4QpPs[a] 2:18.

6 Cf. G. JEREMIAS, *Lehrer der Gerechtigkeit,* 291f.

7 Cf. e.g. T. Reub. 6:8; T. Sim. 7:2; T. Levi 2:11; 8:11f; 18:1–14; T. Jud. 21:2–5; 24:1–6; T. Dan 5:10; T. Gad 8:1. Some of these instances may, however, be later interpolations. See below n. 11.

8 Cf. also T. Jud. 24:1. DE JONGE, *TDNT* IX, 513, regards it possible that T. Jud. 24:1–4 originally referred to Levi or an eschatological figure of his tribe. So also K. SCHUBERT, *WZKM* 53 (1957) 231f; VAN DER WOUDE, *Die messianischen Vorstellungen,* 215f.

9 See now EISENMAN/WISE, *Dead Sea Scrolls,* 136–141, 156–160.

10 Cf. SCHÜRER, *History* III, 775.

11 Cf. HULTGÅRD, *L'eschatologie des Testaments* I, 304–310. Some even conclude that the Testaments are of Essene origin. Cf. VAN DER WOUDE, *Die messianischen Vorstellungen,* 215; DUPONT-SOMMER, *Écrits esséniens,* 313–318; PHILONENKO, *Interpolations chrétiennes,* 3, 60, *passim.* The interpolations (e.g. in T. Reub. 6:8; T. Sim. 6:5, 7; 7:2; T. Levi 4:4; 10:2; 14:2; 18:7; T. Zeb. 9:8; T. Naph. 8:3; T. Ash. 7:3; T. Jos.

The Qumranites, it seems, used a designation for the priestly Messiah that was identical with one used for the Righteous Teacher. In a manner reminiscent of the description of the Teacher, CD 6:11 calls also the priestly Messiah יורה הצדק. CD 6:2–11 relates him to the historical Teacher, the interpreter of the Torah. The precepts of the Teacher are to be decisive until there appears someone called יורה הצדק at the end of days. There are two indications pointing to a messianic interpretation of יורה הצדק. First, a comparison with the use of the expression "until appears" (עד עמוד) in CD 12:23–13:1; 20:1 suggests a future messianic connotation.[1] Both passages depict the appearance of the two Messiahs. Second, the scrolls regularly use the expression "end of days" (אחרית הימים) in a future sense.[2] 4QFlor 1:11f is significant. As we have noticed, it gives a reference to the future coming of the Davidic and the priestly Messiah. It speaks of the seed of David, "which will appear" (העומד) together with the interpreter of the Torah on Zion "at the end of days" (בא]חרית הימים). If we acknowledge that CD 6:10f and 4QFlor 1:11f are parallel in some sense, we must identify יורה הצדק in the former passage with the coming interpreter of the Torah, the priestly Messiah.[3]

The understanding of the Teacher and of the future were inseparable in the conceptual world of the Qumranites. There are also other features showing that a merging of conceptions has taken place—especially in regard to the Teacher and the priestly Messiah: both the Teacher and the priestly Messiah come to "Damascus" (CD 6:5–7; 7:18f);[4] the priestly and the future significance the Righteous Teacher in 4QpPs[b] 1:4f are reminiscent of the priestly Messiah as the end-time teacher in CD 6:11. The Qumranites' conceptions about the two figures were apparently connected.

Although the labels discussed here carry no extensive validating function by themselves, the manner in which they influenced the ideas about the messianic future is significant. This does not mean that the Qumranites be-

---

19:11; T. Benj. 3:8; 9:3–5; 10:7; 11:2) hardly imply a Christian origin of the Testaments at large, as argued by DE JONGE in e.g. *NTS* 26 (1980) 508–524.

[1] For the future significance of עמד, cf. also CD 7:20; 4QFlor 1:11, 13; 4QpIsa[a] 8–10:17. For discussion, see G. JEREMIAS, *Lehrer der Gerechtigkeit,* 282.

[2] G. JEREMIAS, *Lehrer der Gerechtigkeit,* 282.

[3] I do not need to define the notion about the priestly Messiah as teacher more closely here. Some argue that the expectation about the coming of Elijah, based on Mal 3:23f, was decisive. See VAN DER WOUDE, *Die messianischen Vorstellungen, passim,* esp. 55, 74, 228f. The conception of a teaching Elijah is developed in the rabbinic literature. For basic references, cf. GINZBERG, *Eine unbekannte jüdische Sekte,* 304 n. 1; STRACK/BILLERBECK, *Kommentar* IV, 794–796; VOLZ, *Eschatologie der jüdischen Gemeinde,* 195–197; Joachim JEREMIAS, *TDNT* II, 928–934.

[4] I do not need to determine the exact significance of "Damascus" (CD 6:5, 19; 7:15, 19; 19:34; 20:12) here. My interpretation of CD 6:5–7; 7:18f only prevents me from identifying it with the Babylonian exile. Whatever its reference, it is apparently based upon an exegesis of Amos 5:26f (CD 7:15). For recent discussion, see CALLAWAY, *History of the Qumran Community,* 121–127; P.R. DAVIES, *RevQ* 14 (1990) 509–519.

lieved that the deceased Teacher would return in the appearance of a priestly Messiah at the end of times.[1] With my interpretation of CD 6:10f, there
are no texts supporting such a view. It would indeed be a unique notion in
the history of the Israelite people.[2] But the merging of the labels attached to
the Teacher and the priestly Messiah shows that the authoritative status of
the Teacher influenced the conceptions about the messianic age.[3] Terrest-
rial-historical experiences coalesced with celestial-spiritual utopia.[4] The labelling of the Teacher meant not only that he was connected with the sacred
traditions of the past, but also that the present conceptions about the Teacher influenced the expectations about the future. *The community transferred labels from the deceased Teacher to an awaited messianic teacher.*
This "transference of labels" reveals a contributing factor in the emerging
messianic conceptions. And it also points to the enduring status of the Teacher.

Excursus 7: *The Righteous Teacher and Melchizedek*

Ever since A.S. van der Woude published the Melchizedek Midrash (11QMelch),[5]
scholars have in different ways claimed that this document refers to the Teacher. R.
Meyer argues that the community understood the Teacher as the earthly prefiguration
of Melchizedek.[6] He gives four arguments: first, the LXX of Job 36:22b translates
מורה with δυνάστης; second, the Aramaic מרא or מרה is pronounced in an identical
manner as מורה; third, the connotations attached to מורה when it was pronounced aloud
at Qumran bring this term close to מלך; fourth, מלכי צדק and מורה צדק are parallel
constructions both in regard to the way they were written and in the way they were
heard.

This thesis is untenable. First, Meyer proceeds from the assumption that texts were
always understood only when they were heard. It should not be forgotten, however,
that the person reading the text either had it memorized or saw the actual words. Qumran was a literate community. The reader realized the difference in spelling. Second,
Meyer also assumes that identical phonology always carries with it identical meaning.
As is evident from many languages, this is not obvious. Third, Meyer does not take
account of how the scrolls actually use מר(י)א, or מרה as it is sometimes spelled. He
notices only the Greek translation of Job 36:22b. By itself, the term is used for God
(1QapGen 20:13, 15; 4QEn^b 1 IV:5; 11QtgJob 24:5[?], 7; 26:8[?]).[7] As may be ex-

---

[1] For a refutation of these theories, see G. JEREMIAS, *Lehrer der Gerechtigkeit*,
268–295.

[2] Although different individuals could be expected to reappear, they are not regarded
as coming Messiahs. The Christian view is not comparable. The belief in the reappea-
rance of Jesus was based upon a *past* experience of his resurrection. Cf. e.g. 1 Cor
15:12–18.

[3] Cf. M. BLACK, *SEÅ* 18–19 (1953–54) 86f; G. JEREMIAS, *Lehrer der Gerechtigkeit*, 295.

[4] So, in a different context, TALMON, *World of Qumran*, 300; idem, Concepts of
Māšîaḥ, 112.

[5] *OTS* 14 (1965) 354–373.

[6] Melchisedek, 228–239.

[7] Cf. FITZMYER, *Wandering Aramean*, 124f. I do not here need to discuss the pos-

emplified with the use in the Genesis Apocryphon, the same is also the case with the construct form.[1] There is not sufficient evidence to maintain that the Teacher was associated with Melchizedek himself.

Two different lines of reasoning claim that the herald (מבשר) of Isa 52:7, whom 11QMelch 18 describes as one anointed with the spirit ([מ]שׁיח הרו[ח]),[2] is the Teacher. M. de Jonge and van der Woude propose that "this משׁיח הרוח is the same figure as the נביא mentioned in 1QS ix 11."[3] The basic argument is that since the expression "anointed ones" is elsewhere used in different constructions (in the plural) for prophets (CD 2:12; 6:1; 1QM 11:7), the one anointed with the spirit in 11QMelch 18 should also be identified with the prophet of 1QS 9:11, who in view of Deut 18:18f in 4QTestim 5–8 is the Mosaic prophet. Although de Jonge and van der Woude do not draw the conclusion explicitly, the identification with the Teacher becomes natural from the indications that he was actually regarded as the awaited Mosaic prophet.

There is, however, one decisive argument against this proposal: nowhere is there an allusion to Deut 18:18f in the Melchizedek Midrash. There are instead two other significant passages. It is probable that the *lacuna* following 11QMelch 18 contained a reference to the anointed prince (משׁיח נגיד) of Dan 9:25.[4] This is likely since daleth, and perhaps also nun,[5] are visible in the MSS and since other possible references to Dan 9:24–27 appear (11QMelch 6/Dan 9:24 [לכפר עון]; 11QMelch 7/Dan 9:24–27). There is perhaps also an allusion to Isa 61:1, where someone anointed with the spirit of Yahweh is "to announce" (לבשׂר).[6] In 11QMelch 6 an unknown messenger proclaims freedom for them (קרא להמה דדר).[7] It seems probable that the herald is a messianic figure related to Dan 9:25 and Isa 61:1, but not to the awaited Mosaic prophet of Deut 18:18f.

Recognizing the messianic allusion, J.T. Milik proposes that the anointed herald is the Teacher.[8] This view presupposes, as Milik indicated elsewhere,[9] that the community attributed messianic labels to the Teacher. Milik presents three basic argu-

---

sible pre-Qumranic origin of some scrolls.

[1] The construct always refers to God (1QapGen 2:4; 7:7; 12:17; 21:2; 22:16, 21; 1Q20 2:5). There are also examples of the term with genitive suffix in the first person singular (מרי), both in reference to God (1QapGen 20:12, 14, 15; 22:32) and to human beings (1QapGen 2:9, 13, 24; 22:18). For מרא, cf. also 2QJN ar 3:3; 6Q23 2:2; 11QtgJob 5:1; 7:2; 11:2. For מרי, cf. also 1QTLevi ar 52:1; 4Q°Amram[b] 2:3 (מראי); 4QTLevi ar[a] 1:10, 18; 2:6. The reading is sometimes conjectural.

[2] For this reading, see YADIN, *IEJ* 15 (1965) 152f.—VAN DER WOUDE, *OTS* 14 (1965) 358, 366, first conjectured the article in front of שׁיח(מ), but he later adopted Yadin's proposal. Cf. DE JONGE/VAN DER WOUDE, *NTS* 12 (1965–66) 302, 306. This reading is now generally accepted.

[3] *NTS* 12 (1965–66) 307. They are followed by KOBELSKI, *Melchizedek and Melchireša‘*, 61f.

[4] The text would read: המבשׂר הו(אה) מ(שׁיח הרו(ח) אשׁר אמר דנ(יאל). Cf. FITZMYER, *Essays*, 250, 253, 265f. The continuation of the phrase is corrupt in the MSS. Perhaps a quotation (of Dan 9:25) followed.

[5] The nun is uncertain. It is not given by VAN DER WOUDE, *OTS* 14 (1965) 358; DE JONGE/VAN DER WOUDE, *NTS* 12 (1965–66) 302. It is accepted by e.g. FLUSSER, *CNI* 17 (1966) 24; CARMIGNAC, *RevQ* 7 (1970) 351, 357; MILIK, *JJS* 23 (1972) 98; FITZMYER, *Essays*, 248, 265; KOBELSKI, *Melchizedek and Melchireša‘*, 6, 21.

[6] Cf. M.P. MILLER, *JBL* 88 (1969) 468f.

[7] Cf. also Lev 25:10; Jer 34:8.

[8] *JJS* 23 (1972) 126.

[9] *Ten Years of Discovery*, 126.

ments: first, he mentions the reference to the last priest in 4QpHos[b] (4Q167) 2:3; second, he points to the didactic task of the herald in 11QMelch 20; third, he notices that 11QMelch 22, 24 present the herald as the founder of a congregation.

None of Milik's arguments is convincing. The reference to the last priest is certainly reminiscent of 4QpPs[b] 1:4f, where the Teacher seems to be a priest of the end-time. But 4QpHos[b] (4Q167) 2:3 is too fragmentary to secure an actual reference to the Teacher. Compared with 4QpPs[a] 2:17–19, the picture is quite contradictory. There Ephraim and Manasseh attempt to lay hands on the priest—probably the Teacher. In 4QpHos[b] (4Q167) 2:3 the last priest stretches out his hand to strike Ephraim. As to Milik's second argument, it is true that the herald is in 11QMelch 20 "to instruct them" (לה[ה]שכילמה).[1] But this teaching activity could also be performed by other figures than the Teacher, such as the priestly Messiah.[2] The third argument is without value since it builds on Milik's own conjectural reconstruction of the text in lines 22 and 24.[3] Line 22 is hopelessly corrupt, and even if it is possible that line 24 refers to the establishment of the congregation, it is far from clear in what relation the herald stands to this. In addition, the very claim that the Teacher actually founded the community is somewhat problematic.

Although the issue is difficult to determine, the most plausible identification of the herald is, as J.A. Fitzmyer cautiously proposes,[4] Melchizedek himself. In view of the exalted status attributed to him elsewhere in the Melchizedek Midrash,[5] it would be of no surprise if he was also given the function of the anointed herald of Isa 52:7.[6] The most probable actor in the proclamation of liberty in 11QMelch 6—the allusion to Isa 61:1—is indeed Melchizedek, perhaps mentioned at the end of the previous line. Although he was not of Aaronite lineage, we cannot exclude the possibility that the Qumranites somehow related his function at the end-time to the priestly Messiah.[7] Melchizedek was known as priest of the most high God, of אל עליון (Gen 14:18; Ps 110:4). Tg. Neof. Gen 14:18 pictures him even as a high priest.[8] In any case, the Melchizedek Midrash offers no insight into how the community labelled the Righteous Teacher.

---

[1] The imperfect (לה[י]שכילמה) is preferred by VAN DER WOUDE, *OTS* 14 (1965) 358, 366; DE JONGE/VAN DER WOUDE, *NTS* 12 (1965–66) 302; FITZMYER, *Essays*, 248.

[2] Cf. CD 6:11.

[3] In the text given by VAN DER WOUDE, *OTS* 14 (1965) 358, 366; DE JONGE/VAN DER WOUDE, *NTS* 12 (1965–66) 302; CARMIGNAC, *RevQ* 7 (1970) 351; FITZMYER, *Essays*, 248; KOBELSKI, *Melchizedek and Melchireša‛*, 6, Milik's lines 22 and 24 correspond to lines 23 and 25.

[4] *Essays*, 253f, 266. Fitzmyer is here not followed by his own student KOBELSKI, *Melchizedek and Melchireša‛*, 61f.—It may be symptomatic of the difficulties that STUHLMACHER, *Evangelium*, 144f, 148f, first endorsed the proposal given by de Jonge and van der Woude, but some years later in *idem*, Evangelium, 171 n. 32, abandoned it and accepted Fitzmyer's proposal.

[5] CARMIGNAC, *RevQ* 7 (1970) 363–369, argues that Melchizedek is only a terrestrial being in the Midrash. But for criticism, see DELCOR, *JSJ* 2 (1971) 133f.

[6] The merging of different exalted functions and the question of the possible identification of Melchizedek with the archangel Michael—including the correspondence between the names מלכי צדק and מלכי רשע, the latter being the name of Belial/Satan in 4Q‛Amram[b]; 4QBerakot A; 4QTeharot D—cannot be discussed here. For a full treatment, see KOBELSKI, *Melchizedek and Melchireša‛*, 49–98.

[7] Cf. FLUSSER, *CNI* 17 (1966) 23.

[8] For the veneration of Melchizedek (as high priest) in Nag Hammadi, cf. HELDERMAN, Melchisedeks Wirkung, 335–362; MÉNARD, *RevScRel* 64 (1990) 235–243, esp.

5. Summary and Conclusions

Among various possible motives of transmission, this chapter concentrated on the transmitter's understanding of the teacher, the person-oriented motives of transmission. Three basic categories have emerged.

1. Didactic motives are here prevailing interests in the teaching as an entity *independent* of the life and the status of the teacher. Sirach and the rabbinic literature reflect such motives. Sirach indicates that the unusual claims of Ben Sira belonged within a polemical struggle against views which the Greek schools in Jerusalem mediated to the fellow-Jews. Ben Sira was not concerned to attract students to his own person, only to the right kind of teaching. The conceptions about the teacher that Sirach conveyed to the transmitters did not function as motives in the process of preserving and elaborating the teaching. The teaching essentially remained independent of the teacher. Despite the authority of the teacher, the basic motive of transmisson focused on the inherent value of the teaching itself.

Rabbinic Judaism was more interested in the teachers as types than as individuals.[1] The integration of ministering acts into the actual study of torah implies that an authoritative status was accorded to the rabbis because they knew torah in its various forms. In addition, the validation through the ordination and the attribution of the title "Rabbi" yielded institutional and official support. The pupils were essentially disciples of torah, not of individual teachers. And the teacher was merely a carrier of torah, not its originator. All were in principle equal in regard to torah (Sifre on Deut 11:22).[2] The motives of transmission were external to the individual rabbi who gave the teaching. Just as torah was the basis of validation, so torah itself was also the basic motive of transmission.

2. Didactic-biographical motives are in this study prevailing interests in the teaching as *integrated within the life* of a specific teacher. The Elijah/Elisha narratives and episodal narratives in the later prophets reflect such motives. It is possible that the sons of the prophets initially formulated some of the narratives about Elisha. The interaction between Elisha and the sons of the prophets maintained in the present accounts contained in that case the beginning of didactic-biographical motives of transmission furthering the subsequent elaboration of the Elisha narratives now present in the Deuteronomistic history. The words and the specific deeds of Elisha might have been related to each other already at an early stage of transmission. In addition, if Steck is correct, the relationship between Elijah and Elisha and between Elisha and the sons of the prophets included didactic-biographical motives of transmission stimulating the emergence of narratives about the

---

235f.
[1] Cf. E.L. DIETRICH, *ZRGG* 4 (1952) 297.
[2] Cf. FRAADE, Early Rabbinic Sage, 430–432.

words and the deeds of both the prophets.

The later prophets contain episodal narratives. Going back on early formulations by close adherents to the prophets, they have either been inserted—with some expansion—into contexts of other text genres or elaborated with further narration. They portray significant sayings or deeds placed within the framework of episodes from the life of the prophet.

The episodal narratives show that didactic motives of transmission were sometimes related to biographical interests. There might be further indication of this, such as the beginning of virtual genealogies of the prophets.[1] It is also possible that the authority of the prophet was maintained through the creation of other sorts of texts containing, for instance, appeals to the prophet's transcendent commission or general tales in various forms about the prophet and his deeds.[2] The episodal narratives, however, often seem to go back on some early adherents of the individual prophet. They indicate that the accounts about the teacher-pupil relationship occasionally constituted the setting for an interest in the prophet's teaching as part of his specific life context.

3. Didactic-labelling motives are here defined as prevailing interests in the teaching as *integrated within a process that enhanced the teacher to an exclusive status of authority by means of validating labels*. The Dead Sea scrolls reflect such motives. The Righteous Teacher appears as a single individual functioning as the primary Teacher of the Qumran community. A group separating itself from institutional authorities needed to support the status of their leader with labels going beyond the ones taken from purely didactic and priestly officies and institutions. By applying מורה הצדק to the Teacher, the Qumranites accorded their leader with a status based on the sacred traditions and on God's righteous quality and salvific actions. The concept of the Mosaic prophet further associated the Teacher with the sacred traditions. The manner in which the community connected the interpreter of the Torah with the messianic future also implies that the Teacher was seen in relation to what was held sacred. In the context of a religious community, the reference to the sacred serves to define and support what is charismatic.[3] There was an extensive use of charismatic labels of validation in the Qumran community.

The motives of transmission are here manifest as an extensive broadening of the didactic relationship to include charismatic labels. The Teacher

---

1   Cf. e.g. Zeph 1:1.

2   LONG, Prophetic Authority, 6–16, 19. For the Jeremiah tradition, cf. BERGQUIST, *VT* 39 (1989) 130–133, 139.

3   Cf. the definition of "charismatic" by KEYES, Charisma, 1f: "I here take this term in its narrower and more original sense to connote a quality that others interpret as being itself sacred or as being a gift of the sacred, however sacred be understood in a particular cultural tradition, rather than in its broader sense as a label for any socially recognized extraordinary quality."

was to the Qumranites much more than merely one teacher among many others. The validated status made the Teacher and his teaching inseparable. The Qumranites did not subordinate the Teacher to the teaching. All teaching was to come from him. Although we find no evident interest in episodes from his life,[1] the conceptions about the Teacher's status were indispensible motives of transmission.

The reconstruction of Matthew's sociocultural situation of transmission points to three classes of person-oriented motives for transmitting traditions from a teacher. Although there is no development towards one specific category of transmission motives, there is *a phenomenological variety in the intensity of focus on the individual teacher.* This variety is divided on distinctive material reflecting the conceptions of different groups. But in principle, the motives were not always exclusive of each other. It should be possible to find them interacting within one social setting.

I have discussed how the settings fostered certain motives of transmission among the transmitters. This discussion was vital. Tradition and transmission concerns aspects broader than technical matters only. My approach includes the situation and interests of the transmitting person or group.[2] A basic notion in the present study is even that the process of transmission cannot be fully understood without some consideration of these factors. From the perspective of the settings and the motives of transmission outlined above, we can therefore now proceed to the actual process of transmission.

---

[1] For the restricted usefulness of the Hodayoth, see below pp. 150f.
[2] See the remarks in the introduction above pp. 20f.

Chapter 3

Didactic Authority
and the Process of Transmission

1. Introductory Remarks

The discussion in the previous chapter provided a threefold classification of the relevant material. I will structure the present chapter according to this classification. In some cases, however, the material does not yield much information concerning the actual transmission process. I will therefore not discuss Sirach here. It is indeed probable that Ben Sira's teaching was transmitted by the pupils in his school. There is also indication that the original text of Sirach was expanded. The Cairo A, the Long Greek, the Latin and the Syriac versions suggest this. The expansions might sometimes even go back on additions of Hebrew origin.[1] But there is no visible evidence of a continuous *elaboration* process. Sirach is to a large extent "Autorenliteratur," not "Überlieferungsliteratur."[2] In other cases, some additional material will provide valuable data. There is among the later prophets interesting information in texts that do not provide *explicit* references to settings determined by the authority of a teacher and to didactic-biographical motives of transmission. These texts are also of interest.

The purpose of this chapter is to study if and how the settings and the motives of transmission correlated with the discernable objects and acts of transmission.[3] This personal specificity within the transmission process may express itself in—at least—three different ways: in the process of identifying the traditions, in the means by which the traditions are carried and conveyed and in the preservation and elaboration of the traditions.

2. The Identification of Traditions

When I speak about "the identification of traditions," I am thinking of *procedures by which the transmitters marked and recognized the teaching as*

---

1   For a brief survey, see GILBERT, Book of Ben Sira, 88f.
2   For this distinction in a different connection, cf. LEVIN, *Verheißung des neuen Bundes,* 67.
3   See the remarks in the introduction above pp. 23f.

traditions from a specific teacher. There were indeed several other identification markers. The transmitters sometimes identified the units through various mnemonic aids: they grouped the material on the basis of factual and key-word associations, alphabetic order or midrashically—in the rabbinic literature according to the text of the OT; they provided a sign (סימן, σημεῖον) consisting of a brief (scriptural) text or a key-word of some kind.[1] These identity markers are not of primary significance for my study. They normally served as formal categories without the personal specificity of interest here.

2.1. The Rabbis and the Named Attributions

As we noticed in the introductory chapter, G. Kittel urged his readers to pay due attention to the fact that rabbinic Judaism, in distinction to early Christianity, incorporated traditions from a large number of teachers.[2] *The texts identify various statements often lacking an episodal frame through references to the names of the teachers.* We find "named attributions."

2.1.1. The Importance of the Attributions

The rabbinic literature abounds in named attributions. The frequency of this feature is consistent with the importance given to it.[3]

Rabbinic teachers often reveal their desire to be quoted on different occasions. Some texts even claim that the deceased teachers continue to exhibit their influence—"to make their lips move in the grave" (b. Yebam. 97a)—only when other teachers mention them by name as the ones who originally uttered a certain teaching.[4] A late statement in m. ʾAbot 6:6 represents a broad consensus:

כל-האומר דבר	Whosoever says a word
בשם אומרו	in the name of the one who said it
מביא גאלה לעולם	brings deliverance to the world.[5]

This is not an isolated occurrence. It is in harmony with what we often find in the Talmud and elsewhere.[6]

---

[1] GERHARDSSON, *Memory*, 141–156.
[2] See above pp. 14f.
[3] Cf. already PERLS, *MGWJ* 58 (1914) 311–322.
[4] Cf. also e.g. y. Ber. 4b; y. Šeqal. 47a; y. Moʿed Qaṭ. 83c; Tanḥ. B במדבר 27.
[5] The biblical basis mentioned is that Esther spoke to the king "in the name of" (בשם) Mordecai (Esth 2:22).
[6] Cf. e.g. b. Meg. 15a; b. Ḥull. 104b; b. Nid. 19b; Tanḥ B. במדבר 27.

2.1.2. The Function of the Attributions

The pertinent question is of course what function the attributions had within the transmission process. We gain information through the present rabbinic texts. J. Neusner has pointed to the paradox which the existence of the attributions constitutes in the rabbinic literature.[1] It is not insignificant, according to Neusner, that a literature which speaks collectively for all contains numerous passages assigned to the minority of one.

We must consider—at least—three features evident in the existing material.[2] First, we should notice the exceptions to the rule of attribution. Not all statements are attached to a name.[3] Some, though they are not numerous,[4] remain entirely anonymous. In other instances, "the wise" (החכמים) and other collective designations[5] occur as labels for the carriers of the traditions.[6] The inclusion of teaching not present in the Mishnah in the two Talmudim and other rabbinic texts is illustrative.[7] A statement of this kind—a baraita (ברייתא [מתניתא])—is often, though not always, anonymous. Whatever the exact age of these anonymous statements,[8] their presence within the rabbinic corpora shows that certain teaching spoke for itself, independently of any special teacher. Second, the attributions are not always consistent. There are several indications of this. Not only do the MSS often differ in the reading of the names.[9] It also happens in cases where the MSS are stable that one and the same saying occurs on the lips of different persons.[10] And a statement attributed to an amoraic rabbi in one text can elsewhere be classified as tannaitic teaching.[11] Sometimes the names might have been confused because they were similar.[12] But on other occasions, it seems that the rabbis were aware of the confusion. By including an alternative

---

1   *Talmudic Biography,* 1f.
2   Cf. W.S. GREEN, What's in a Name?, 80, 88; STRACK/STEMBERGER, *Talmud and Midrash,* 63–66.—Already BACHER, *Tradition und Tradenten, passim,* commented on the first two features. He also gave numerous references to relevant text.
3   For this problem, see already GUTTMANN, *HUCA* 16 (1941) 137–155.
4   Cf. NEUSNER, *Mishnah to Scripture,* 119.
5   See below p. 175.
6   Cf. e.g., with אמרו חכמים, m. Giṭ. 6:6; m. Ḥul. 3:6; m. Bek. 6:11; t. Yebam. 6:7(8); t. B. Meṣ. 3:14; Sifra on 4:35; 25:40. For references to other examples, cf. BACHER, *Tradition und Tradenten,* 156–170.
7   For discussion and references, see BACHER, *Tradition und Tradenten,* 235–242; DE VRIES, *EncJud* IV, 189–193; STRACK/STEMBERGER, *Talmud and Midrash,* 195f.
8   NEUSNER, *Mishnah to Scripture,* 117–123, concludes that they were not a separate body of traditions serving as a bridge from the Mishnah back to Scripture.
9   SALDARINI, *JBL* 96 (1977) 264 n. 22; STRACK/STEMBERGER, *Talmud and Midrash,* 64f.
10   BACHER, *Tradition und Tradenten,* 120–124.
11   BACHER, *Tradition und Tradenten,* 267–273.
12   BACHER, *Tradition und Tradenten,* 524–533.

name, some texts show explicitly that the names may have been confused.[1] Other texts mention that the teaching attributed to amoraic rabbis actually originated with a tanna.[2] The Babylonian Talmud sometimes leaves the exact attribution of certain teaching open. It introduces the statement with "if you want, say" (איבעית),[3] followed by an alternative name.[4] This inconsistency suggests that the transmitters of the rabbinic traditions did not consider it vital to relate the teaching to a specific teacher on all occasions. Third, the names have not determined—to any larger extent—how the transmitters finally ordered and presented the traditions in the present rabbinic corpora.[5] Although it happens that several sayings of one and the same teacher occur in close connection to each other,[6] the writings usually exhibit a structure based on thematic, formal or scriptural considerations. We often find various rabbis addressing a particular issue at stake.

These three features point to the non-biographical character of the rabbinic transmission process.[7] Neither the motive nor the actual process of transmission reveals a particular interest in relating traditions to the life of a particular rabbi. Although we may, with critical care, use the named attributions to envision the general history of rabbinic Judaism, they do not carry any primary biographical value.[8]

Why do the texts then include the named attributions? Perhaps because they were part of the tradition. It was surely sometimes important to show that a teaching was related to an especially prominent rabbi.[9] But it is also probable that the attributions served another function. The traditions became of course "personal" in this way. They emerged, after all, as teaching given by real persons. But as we saw in the previous chapter, it was essentially torah, not the individual rabbi, that was important. Central to the rabbinic understanding of torah transmission was the conviction that all teaching received its normativity through its relation to the past and the legitimate succession of tradition carriers.[10] An old statement often had a special dignity.[11] The names functioned as labels through which the teaching presented in the existing texts gained its "pastness" and "traditio-

---

1 BACHER, *Tradition und Tradenten*, 278f.
2 BACHER, *Tradition und Tradenten*, 279f.
3 For this translation, see BACHER, *REJ* 54 (1907) 273–275. Bacher here corrects his earlier proposal made in *idem, Die exegetische Terminologie* II, 4.
4 Cf. e.g. b. Ber. 5b; b. Ned. 78a. For further references, cf. BACHER, *Tradition und Tradenten*, 534–540.
5 Cf. NEUSNER, Rabbinic Biography, 88f.
6 BACHER, *Tradition und Tradenten*, 125–128.
7 See excursus 5 above.
8 Cf. KRAEMER, *HUCA* 60 (1989) 175–190.
9 Cf. the account of the Eliezer tradition below pp. 171–173.
10 See above pp. 92f.
11 Cf. PATTE, *Jewish Hermeneutic*, 15.

nality," its decisive basis in the past.[1] The labels may of course be historically correct. But the fact that the rabbis knew about the occasional confusion of the attributions shows that the intention was not only to give historical information. Rather, *the presence of the named attributions in the rabbinic literature gave the collective voice of the texts a legitimate basis in the
past.*

2.2. The Prophets and the Secondary Attributions

The prophetic teaching is usually attached to specific persons known from
the transmitted material itself. There are of course exceptions, such as in
Obadiah and Malachi.[2] But the Elijah/Elisha narratives and the books of the
later prophets usually identify the teaching by some kind of reference to the
individual prophet. There is, generally speaking, a substantial connection
between the teaching and the prophet.

Already the Elisha narratives show traces of a process that attributed
statements from the sons of the prophets to Elisha. W. Reiser claimed that
certain utterances introduced with the messenger formula actually originated with the sons of the prophets.[3] To some extent, the members of these
groups appear as independent prophets. 1 Kgs 20:35 tells that one of them
acted on a direct command of Yahweh. 20:41 calls him "one of the prophets."[4] It is remarkable—if Reiser is correct—that in spite of their independent activity and their use of the messenger formula (1 Kgs 20:42; 2 Kgs
9:6, 12), these sayings occur now—with one exception (1 Kgs 17:14)—on
Elisha's own lips (2 Kgs 2:21; 3:16, 17; 4:43; 7:1).[5]

This process of attribution is more evident in the writings of the later
prophets. It has here resulted in the attribution of complete literary corpora
to specific prophetic teachers. Other prophets than the main proponent are
mentioned only occasionally within the individual books. When it does happen, the other prophets serve a subordinated function: Hosea indeed regards
earlier prophets as instruments of Yahweh (6:5; 12:11), but the book does
not mention them by name; Jeremiah judges earlier prophets positively
(7:25; 25:4), but the book gives references to Micah of Moresheth, with an
allusion to one of his sayings (26:17–19),[6] and a certain Uriah, son of Shemaiah from Kiriath-jearim (26:20–23), only to defend Jeremiah. And rare-

---

[1]   W.S. GREEN, What's in a Name?, 87–90.
[2]   For Obadiah, cf. 1 Kgs 18:3–16; for Malachi, cf. Mal 3:1.—For Mal 1:1, cf. also
Zech 9:1; 12:1.
[3]   *TZ* 9 (1953) 336.
[4]   Cf. JOÜON, *RSR* 16 (1926) 309f.
[5]   To the question why this attribution took place, W. REISER, *TZ* 9 (1953) 337, responds: "Unseres Erachtens kann dafür nur jene massive Anschauung der Propheten-
jünger vom Prophetenmeister in Betracht kommen."
[6]   Cf. Mic 3:12.

ly—such as the mention of Isaiah in 2 Kgs 18:13–20:19—do the non-prophetic writings speak of the utterances and acts of the later prophets.[1] There is, for instance, a striking, and perhaps deliberate,[2] silence about Jeremiah and Ezekiel in the Deuteronomistic history. Most of the material has been concentrated to concern one specific prophet within one literary corpus.

These general observations point to a process in which the transmitters attributed prophetic teaching to a prophetic master at a secondary stage. We may speak of a process of "secondary attribution."[3] This expression denotes here the process that took place when *the transmitters elaborated new material by both building substantially on the earlier tradition and at the same time identifying their elaborations through reference to a person of dominating importance within the earlier tradition.* I distinguish between secondary attribution and "pseudonymous attribution," which identify the new material through reference to a person whose teaching had not functioned as a basis for the creation of the new material.[4] Pseudonymous material does not presuppose the use of an already identified tradition.[5]

Secondary attribution occurred in the elaboration of several prophetic traditions.[6] It is most evident in cases where the new material consisted of larger blocks, such as we find in Isaiah.

2.2.1. Second Isaiah and the Isaiah Tradition

Early Jewish authors regarded Isa 40–55 as an integrated part of the message from Isaiah of Jerusalem. They never attributed an independent status to it.[7] These people understood "(the) former things" (ראשׁנות[ה]), so often mentioned (41:22; 42:9; 43:9, 18; 46:9; 48:3),[8] as references to the prophecies of First Isaiah.[9] Although this understanding is difficult to ascertain

---

[1] For Jonah, cf. 2 Kgs 14:25.

[2] So BEGG, *IBS* 7 (1985) 139–164; *idem*, Non-Mention of Ezekiel, 340f.

[3] I have tried to find a better expression than the rather vague "secondary attribution." In a sense, pseudonymous attribution is also secondary. The Germans speak of "Deuteronymität," but the expression "deuteronymous attribution" is odd and may be confused with "Deuteronomic" and "Deuteronomistic."

[4] FISHBANE, *Biblical Interpretation*, 530–533, does not use this distinction. He speaks merely of pseudonymous or pseudepigraphic exegesis. The distinction may be implied when he differentiates between tendentious manipulation of authoritative names, rubrics and teaching on one hand, and non-manipulative amendment and elaboration of traditions on the other (*ibid.*, 536–539).

[5] For further discussion, see GNILKA, *Kolosserbrief*, 23–26. Cf. also P. MÜLLER, *Paulusschule,* 318.

[6] See below pp 176–183.

[7] Sir 48:22–25. Cf. SCHILDENBERGER, Sir 48:24f., 188–204.

[8] SEITZ, *Zion's Final Destiny,* 199, lists similar expressions.

[9] NORTH, "Former Things," 124; CHILDS, *Introduction,* 329; CLEMENTS, *Int* 36 (1982) 125.

as correct,[1] the unquestioned view of a coherent book indicates a reading/hearing that conceived a substantial relationship between the different sections.

Teaching of different kinds and origins certainly influenced Second Isaiah himself.[2] Some scholars have suggested an influence from teaching recorded in Hosea and Jeremiah.[3] The common exilic situation also allows for a possible influence from Ezekiel.[4] However, all these influences are now part of the Isaiah tradition. The texts give no explicit indication of the dependence on other prophetic authorities. Isaiah of Jerusalem was the only prophet to whom Second Isaiah attributed teaching exhibiting influence from other prophets.

Already this fact indicates that it would be wrong to claim that Second Isaiah was under no particular influence from the earlier Isaiah tradition.[5] On the contrary, it is likely that he was responsible for this attribution. As it seems, he understood and legitimized his whole ministry by reference to the old Isaianic tradition. Although Isa 40–55 does not amplify the picture of Isaiah of Jerusalem any further,[6] it is obvious that the traditions associated with him were of much importance. The modern interest in the redactional unity of Isaiah as a whole points in a way to a specific relationship between the anonymous individual behind large parts of Isa 40–55 and First Isaiah.[7] R.E. Clements, W. Brueggemann, R. Rendtorff, M. Fishbane, R. Albertz and R.J. Clifford, to mention a few, illustrate the terminological and thematic similarities between different parts of Isaiah.[8] Although some of these features might be due to late redaction(s) with unifying purposes,[9] certain resemblances are firmly anchored within the material and indicate

---

1   D. JONES, *ZAW* 67 (1955) 245f, proposes the testimony of the Isaianic school (8:16) as the former things. NORTH, "Former Things" 111–126, points in his influential essay to Second Isaiah's emphasis on the argument from prophecy and suggests the predicted coming of Cyrus (41:1–5, 21–29) as the original referent. According to North, later generations regarded certain prophecies of First Isaiah (13:17ff; 21:2ff) as the former things mentioned in 41:22; 42:9; 48:3.

2   WESTERMANN, *Isaiah 40–66*, 21–27.

3   WESTERMANN, *Isaiah 40–66*, 226–228; PAUL, Echoes of Jeremiah, 102–120; UNTERMAN, *Repentance*, 171–175; HOLLADAY, *Jeremiah* II, 86–88.

4   D. BALTZER, *Ezechiel und Deuterojesaja*, 179.

5   *Contra* FOHRER, *Introduction*, 375; KOCH, *Prophets* II, 119.

6   Cf. SEITZ, Isaiah 1–66, 116–122.

7   For surveys of research, see SWEENEY, *Isaiah 1–4*, 1–25; VERMEYLEN, L'unité du livre d'Isaïe, 11–27; SEITZ, *Zion's Final Destiny*, 26–32. In addition to the literature mentioned there, cf. STECK, *Abschluß der Prophetie*, 26–30, 80–87. This interest is not new. Cf. already e.g. HERZBERG, Nachgeschichte, 120; EISSFELDT, *Old Testament*, 345f; MELUGIN, *Formation*, 176–178.

8   CLEMENTS, *Int* 36 (1982) 117–129; BRUEGGEMANN, *JSOT* 29 (1984) 89–107; RENDTORFF, *VT* 34 (1984) 295–320; CLEMENTS, *JSOT* 31 (1985) 95–113; FISHBANE, *Biblical Interpretation*, 495–499; RENDTORFF, *Old Testament*, 198–200; idem, Jesaja 6, 73–82; ALBERTZ, Deuterojesaja-Buch, 241–256; CLIFFORD, *CBQ* 55 (1993) 1–17.

9   Cf. SWEENEY, *Isaiah 1–4*, 6f.

that Second Isaiah depended on the traditions he believed originated with Isaiah of Jerusalem.

A large number of important concepts and terms in Isa 1–39 recur in Isa 40–55.[1] Three examples may suffice. First, the vision of Yahweh as the holy one of Israel is at the centre of the Isaianic theology.[2] Since this notion appears only rarely elsewhere in the OT (2 Kgs 19:22 [=Isa 37:23]; Jer 50:29; 51:5; Pss 71:22; 78:41; 89:19), it constitutes a characteristic illustration of Second Isaiah's solidarity with vital elements in the Isaianic tradition known to him.[3] The notion is frequent in Isa 1–39. It occurs both in accusations (1:4; 5:19, 24; 30:11f, 15; 31:1) and eschatological words of salvation (10:20; 12:6; 17:7; 29:19, 23; 37:23).[4] Isa 40–55 adopts the eschatological and salvific use (41:14, 16, 20; 43:3, 14; 45:11; 47:4; 48:17; 49:7; 54:5; 55:5).[5] The firm basis of several instances in Isa 1–39 makes a later origin of the notion improbable.[6] Second, the Zion/Jerusalem terminology is present throughout Isaiah.[7] It is a key-concept in Isa 40–55 (40:2, 9; 41:27; 44:26, 28; 46:13; 49:14; 51:3, 11, 16f; 52:1f, 7–9).[8] It appears frequently also in Isa 1–39 (1:8, 27; 3:16f; 8:18; 10:12, 24, 32; 14:32, etc.). As it seems, Second Isaiah received this concept from the earlier Isaiah tradition and used it for his own purposes.[9] Third, the theme of Israel's blindness and deafness is central in Isa 40–55 (42:16, 18–25; 43:8f; 44:18; 48:8a).[10] The subject matter and the terms echo especially the important account about the prophetic commission in 6:9f.[11] Second Isaiah probably leaned on this vital text when he interpreted his own activity in the exilic situation. The condition of blindness and deafness still prevails, according to Isa 40–55, but it does not prevent the coming of the salvation.

---

[1] Cf. e.g. the following important concepts and terms: the "glory" (כבוד) of Yahweh in 3:8; 6:3 (35:2) and 40:5; 42:8, 12; 43:7; 48:11; "to comfort" (נחם) in 12:1; 22:4 and 40:1; 49:13; 51:3, 12, 19; 52:9; "witness" (עד) in 8:2; 19:20 and 43:9f, 12; 44:8f (55:4); "guilt" or "crime" (עון) in 1:4; 5:18; 6:7; 13:11; 14:21; 22:14 (26:21; 27:9); 30:13; 33:24 and 40:2; 43:24; 50:1 (53:5, 6, 11); "righteousness" ([ה]צדק) in 1:21, 26f; 5:7, 16, 23; 9:6; 10:22; 11:4f; 16:5 (26:9f); 28:17; 32:1, 16f; 33:5, 15 and 41:2, 10; 42:6, 21; 45:8, 13, 19, 21, 23f; 46:12f; 48:1, 18; 51:1, 5–8 (54:14, 17). It is possible that the occurrences put in brackets are later than Second Isaiah. But it is probable that most of the references reflect Second Isaiah's own adoption of the Isaiah tradition.
[2] J.J.M. ROBERTS, *Int* 36 (1982) 131.
[3] Cf. EATON, *VT* 9 (1959) 153.
[4] Cf. also 5:16; 6:3; 8:13; 10:17.
[5] Cf. also 40:25; 43:15.
[6] Cf. WILDBERGER, *Jesaja* I, 23f.
[7] Cf. VON RAD, *Theolgy* II, 155–169, 239f.
[8] Cf. D. BALTZER, *Ezechiel und Deuterojesaja*, 41–48; SEITZ, *Zion's Final Destiny*, 202–205.
[9] Cf. SCHREINER, Buch jesajanischer Schule, 153–155.
[10] Also Isa 35:5 points to the importance of this theme. STECK, *Heimkehr*, argues that Isa 35 was composed as an intentional bridge between Isa 1–11, 13–22 (23, 24–27), 28–34, 36–39 and Isa 40–55, 56–62.
[11] Cf. also 29:18; 32:3.

The early Isaiah tradition was not only used as a point of departure for an actualizing elaboration. It also constituted a valid basis through which Second Isaiah legitimized his own activity. But the dependence on the tradition is related to his anonymity.[1] Prophetic disciples were often anonymous, relying on the authority of the master visible in the transmitted material. We find this feature from pre-exilic times and onwards. It is especially clear in Isa 40–55 and might here be due to the increasing concern about prophetic authority which the exilic experiences caused.[2] The connections to the early Isaianic tradition suggest that the anonymity even was intentional. It is questionable if Second Isaiah ever understood himself as a poet "who outstripped his master."[3] Some scholars do continue to regard Isa 40–55 as an independent unit.[4] But perhaps it was never meant or circulated as such.[5] There is no superscription or formula marking a new beginning, and there are no texts giving secure information concerning Second Isaiah. References to historical settings are rare and vague.[6]

The most reasonable explanation of these data is, it seems, in terms of discipleship. Since prophetic disciples could themselves be creative prophets, the actualizing manner in which Isa 40–55 applies the tradition does not speak against such an explanation. Second Isaiah based the actualizing elaboration mainly on the tradition of one particular prophet. And he legitimized his own ministry by reference to one particular master.

It is of course necessary to remember the distance in time between First Isaiah and Second Isaiah. The discipleship did not include an immediate attachment to the master. It was "mediated" by tradition. We cannot know exactly how Second Isaiah came into contact with the Isaianic tradition. It is indeed difficult to explain why he chose Isa 1–39, generally speaking, as the basis of his preaching,[7] had he not been associated with some kind of group responsible for the Isaiah tradition. But for the moment, the question concerning the existence of a coherent Isaianic school transmitting the tradition through several centuries must be left open.[8]

It should suffice to conclude that Second Isaiah did internalize and use

---

1   Cf. MEADE, *Pseudonymity*, 34f.

2   WILSON, *Prophecy*, 291f.

3   D. JONES, *ZAW* 67 (1955) 237.

4   Cf. e.g. recently KRATZ, *Kyros*, 218.

5   Cf. MELUGIN, *Formation*, 176; CHILDS, *Introduction*, 329; CLEMENTS, *JSOT* 31 (1985) 101; ALBERTZ, Deuterojesaja-Buch, 242–248; SEITZ, *Zion's Final Destiny*, 29f, 147.

6   MELUGIN, *Formation*, 177, believes that someone deliberately eliminated all traces of the historical setting. But why were then the references to Cyrus not removed (44:28; 45:1)? And why was sufficient indication provided to give the prophecies an exilic date? Cf. ACKROYD, Isaiah 36–39, 4.

7   Cf. the discussion by ACKROYD, Isaiah I–XII, 21–29; ALBERTZ, Deuterojesaja-Buch, 254f, though they propose different explanations.

8   So also VERMEYLEN, L'unité du livre d'Isaïe, 17; STECK, *Tritojesaja*, 7.

central terminological and thematic features of the tradition attributed to Isaiah of Jerusalem. He regarded his ministry as an actualizing elaboration of the old Isaianic tradition, now applicable to the frustrated people of the exile. The authority of Second Isaiah's master was available through tradition.[1] Second Isaiah concealed his own identity and intentionally, it seems, located the validity of his oracles within the tradition from Isaiah of Jerusalem. *He both built substantially on the earlier tradition and identified his own elaborations through a person of dominating importance within the earlier tradition.*

2.2.2. Third Isaiah and the Isaiah Tradition

I will deal only with Isa 60–62 here.[2] Many scholars agree that these three chapters reflect the earliest nucleus of Isa 56–66.[3]

There are in particular two texts suggesting that Third Isaiah apprehended the commission and task in dependence on Second Isaiah. The two first person narratives in 61:1–3; 62:1–12 offer glimpses into the self-consciousness of Third Isaiah.[4] These texts present the commission and task as a catena of themes from Isa 40–55. The language of 61:1–3 might indicate some dependence on the nucleus of the servant songs (42:1–4[–9]; 49:1–6[–12]; 50:4–9[–11]; 52:13–53:12). This is the view of W. Zimmerli.[5] The text builds also on passages outside of the servant songs. It pictures the very commission of Third Isaiah in terms strongly reminiscent of various passages within Isa 40–55.[6] 62:1–12 exhibits the same dependence. 62:10f strongly reflects passages such as 40:3, 10; 49:22; 52:11.[7] The image of the watchmen (שמרים) in 62:6 reminds us of the group around Second Isaiah.[8] It expresses the task of Third Isaiah. Just as the walls of Zion are continually before Yahweh according to 49:16, the watchmen are to stand on the walls of Jerusalem day and night according to 62:6, never to be silent but con-

---

1 Cf. STECK, *Heimkehr*, 87–91. He uses the expression "überlieferungsbezogene Autorität" (*ibid.*, 90).
2 Isa 60–62 probably reflects a time when the temple was not yet rebuilt. Cf. esp. 60:13.
3 SEKINE, *Tritojesajanische Sammlung*, 25, 68–104. He regards only 60:14aβ as an interpolation (*ibid.*, 70–72).—STECK, *Tritojesaja*, 14–27, 119–139, regards Isa 60–62 as containing the oldest material within a fivefold literary pattern of growth. Its growth was closely related to the creation of Isa 40–55, according to Steck.
4 For the "I" in 61:1–3; 62:1, 6 as reflective of Third Isaiah (as an individual), see WESTERMAN, *Isaiah 40–66*, 299, ad loci.
5 *Gottes Offenbarung*, 227. Cf. also PAURITSCH, *Gemeinde*, 104.
6 For the (permanent) gift of the spirit, cf. 42:1 (Mic 3:8); for the bringing of "good news" (בשר), cf. 40:9; 41:27; 52:7; for certain acts of mercy in 61:1b, cf. 42:7; for the mission "to comfort" (נחם), cf. 40:1; 49:13; 51:3, 12, 19; 52:9; for the "year of favour" (שנת רצון), cf. 49:8; for the "faint spirit" (רוח כהה), cf. 42:3f.
7 Cf. also 62:11f with 54:1–6.
8 Cf. 52:8 and the comments above p. 42.

stantly functioning as a reminder to Yahweh. 61:1–3; 62:1–12 indicate therefore the desire to legitimize the commission and task by reference to the tradition and to apply Second Isaiah's promises of salvation to a later time.

The manner in which Third Isaiah unfolded the message confirms this. Restricting our observations to Isa 60–62, we find several quotations from Isa 40–55.[1] Some allusions indicate that the tradition recorded in Isa 40–55 penetrated and governed Third Isaiah's message in a profound way.[2] Scholars have judged the quotations and allusions differently. But since one and the same person hardly would plagiarize himself in this manner, it is difficult to assume they reflect a common author.[3] Zimmerli's influential study points to the stagnating significance of the original words.[4] Third Isaiah used them as conventional utterances. D. Michel suggests also that Third Isaiah regarded the tradition as quite fixed.[5] The tradition was for Third Isaiah a sacred text used as a basis for a kind of midrashic exegesis. Although Michel's argument is not entirely convincing,[6] it accords with the impression gained from the quotations and allusions. The manner in which Third Isaiah unfolded his message reflects the dependence on Second Isaiah and implies perhaps a rather exegetical interpretation of the tradition.[7]

Nevertheless, the new material of Third Isaiah appears ultimately as tradition from Isaiah of Jerusalem. Third Isaiah recognized the anonymity of Second Isaiah. We find no clear signs of a biographical interest in Second Isaiah himself.[8] Isa 60–62 consequently develops some of the elements from Isa 40–55 that go back on the early Isaiah tradition.[9] Although the important vision of Yahweh as the holy one of Israel falls somewhat into the background,[10] Isa 60–62 maintains its eschatological and salvific use (60:9,

---

1 Cf. Isa 60:4a and 49:18a; Isa 60:9bβ and 55:5bβ; Isa 60:13aβ and 41:19bβ; Isa 60:16b and 49:26b; Isa 62:11b and 40:10b.

2 Cf. Isa 60:4b and 43:6b; 49:12, 22; Isa 60:9a and 51:5b; Isa 60:10b and 54:7f; Isa 61:7 and 40:2b; Isa 61:8bβ and 55:3bα; Isa 61:10b and 49:18b, etc.

3 P.-E. BONNARD, *Second Isaïe,* 215. But cf. MAASS, "Tritojesaja?," 153–163.

4 *Gottes Offenbarung,* 217–233.

5 *TViat* 10 (1965–66) 213–230. Cf. also *idem, TRE* 8 (1981) 510.

6 D. MICHEL, *TViat* 10 (1965–66) 213–230, discusses Isa 62:1–5, 6f, 8f. However, it is uncertain if 62:1, 6 is, as Michel claims, a word of Yahweh. And nothing is proved by referring to unknown texts of Second Isaiah as the basis of the tradition (*ibid.,* 217). Michel's illustrations from 56:1–7; 58:1–12 are more convincing and make it credible that the same phenomenon could be found also in Isa 60–62.

7 FISHBANE, *Biblical Interpretation,* 289, rejects an exegetical intention in Third Isaiah and explains the quotations and allusions as due to "shared phraseology," which was later reapplied "in accordance with new tastes and cicumstances." This implies a narrower and more static view of exegesis than the one I assume here.

8 For the non-biographical character of the fourth servant song (52:13–53:12), see above pp. 109f.

9 See above p. 143.

10 PAURITSCH, *Gemeinde,* 230.

14).[1] And the frequency of the Zion/Jerusalem terminology indicates its continuing importance (60:14; 61:3; 62:1, 6f, 11).[2] Other key-concepts and terms from the early Isaiah tradition also occur in Isa 60–62.[3] The glory of Yahweh forms an essential part of the salvific proclamation (60:1f; 62:2).[4] And just as the task of prophets and of Yahweh was to comfort within the Isaianic traditions, so this motif is central in the commission of Third Isaiah (61:2).[5] We also find the concept of righteousness in the central texts about Third Isaiah's commission and task (61:3; 62:1f) and elsewhere (60:17; 61:10f).[6] As it seems, the watchmen of 62:6 regard their mission not only as a continuation of the task assigned to such persons in 52:8, but also in line with the commission given to a watchman already in 21:6–10.[7]

Second Isaiah's glorious message of salvation hardly answered to the realities within the post-exilic community.[8] In spite of the dissonant frustrations, Third Isaiah legitimized his commission and task by reference to the tradition attached to Second Isaiah. There was apparently a desire to protect Second Isaiah's message from being falsified by the historical realities and to reduce the cognitive tensions created by its promises. But Second Isaiah remained anonymous in the tradition. By adhering to Second Isaiah, Third Isaiah became involved in the tradition connected with Isaiah of Jerusalem. The tradition associated with the ancient prophet was the valid basis through which Third Isaiah ultimately legitimized his activity. There appears again a process of secondary attribution. *Third Isaiah built substantially on the earlier tradition and identified his own elaborations through the only person of dominating importance within the earlier tradition.*

Scholars sometimes divide also the book of Zechariah into distinguishable parts (Zech 1–8, 9–11, 12–14). However, while similarities between Zech 1–8 and the rest of the book exist, there is not sufficient evidence for assuming a common circle of transmitters using the earlier traditions in its own creative activity.[9] The lack of original interconnections makes such an assumption improbable.[10] Statistical analysis implies that at least Zech 12–14 originated independently of the previous chapters.[11] The identical opening (משא דבר יהוה) of the superscriptions in Zech 9:1; 12:1; Mal 1:1 is perhaps an indication that the final redactor of the book of the Twelve appended three anonymous

---

1   Cf. also 57:15.
2   Cf. also 59:20; 64:10; 66:7f, 10, 13, 20.
3   See above p. 143 n. 1.
4   Cf. also 58:8; 59:19; 66:18f.
5   Cf. also 66:13.
6   Cf. also 56:1; 57:12; 58:2, 8; 59:4, 9, 14, 16f; 63:1; 64:4f.
7   Cf. MEADE, *Pseudonymity,* 40.
8   CARROLL, *Prophecy,* 150–156.
9   *Contra* MASON, *ZAW* 88 (1976) 227–239.
10   So e.g. WILLI-PLEIN, *Prophetie am Ende,* 1; CHILDS, *Introduction,* 479–483; REDDITT, *CBQ* 51 (1989) 632. Cf. also recently BUTTERWORTH, *Structure,* 272–275, 291–297, though he elsewhere (*ibid.,* 304) seems to think of a basis for the continuing tradition.
11   RADDAY/WICKMANN, *ZAW* 87 (1975) 30–55.

collections—Zech 9–11; 12–14; Mal 1–3—to the last book (Zech 1–8) of a named prophet.[1]

2.3. The Righteous Teacher and the Anonymous Teaching

We should expect that the validation of the Righteous Teacher provided strong motives for a transmission with a high degree of personal specificity. Tradition and transmission concerned a venerated person, not merely impersonal items. It is all the more striking that both the Teacher himself and his teaching remain anonymous in the present texts. *The scrolls do not reveal the identity of the Teacher, nor do they identify his teaching.* The question arises how the Qumranites knew that they transmitted traditions from the Righteous Teacher.

2.3.1. The Anonymity of the Righteous Teacher

Various scholars challenge today the dominating view concerning the history of the community and present other proposals in regard to the historical identity of the Teacher.[2] These proposals are always very hypothetical.[3] And this is not without reason.[4] The extra-Qumranic sources are silent about the Righteous Teacher. At least, they do not refer to a person called the Righteous Teacher among the Essenes. And the scrolls themsleves—together with the archaeological data—do not allow a clear reconstruction of the community's history,[5] even less of the Teacher's own identity.

The Teacher's anonymity was perhaps intentional. Josephus, Bell. 2:145, 152, speaks about a certain lawgiver (νομοθέτης) whose name the Essenes—in addition to God's name—were forbidden to blaspheme. Neither Josephus nor the scrolls reveal such a veneration for Moses' name. The possibility

---

1   EISSFELDT, *Old Testament,* 440. Mal 1:1 probably takes the name from 3:1.

2   For a list of different proposals concerning the Teacher's historical identity, cf. SCHÜRER, *History* III, 436 n. 7, and excursus 8 below. For a survey of different reconstructions of the community's general history, see CALLAWAY, *History of the Qumran Community,* 12–15. A balanced alternative to the standard view is the so-called Groningen hypothesis. A recent summary of this hypothesis is given by VAN DER WOUDE, *SEÅ* 57 (1992) 95–101.

3   BURGMANN, *RevQ* 10 (1980) 317, correctly claimed that some of the recent suggestions betray "ein neues und höchst bedauerliches intellektuelles Verwirrspiel auf dem Felde von Qumrân." The critique concerns one of Thiering's books on Qumran. Cf. also the "absence of enthusiasm" expressed by VERMES, *JJS* 32 (1981) 29, and the recent criticism by BETZ/RIESNER, *Jesus, Qumran und der Vatikan,* 88–102, 121–138.

4   For some of the complicated methodological problems involved in working with the early history of the community, see P.R. DAVIES, Qumran Beginnings, 361–368.

5   CALLAWAY, *History of the Qumran Community,* 199–210, concludes his analysis of the different sources and hypotheses by allowing a only fragmentary and minimalistic reconstruction. Cf. also *idem, RevQ* 14 (1990) 639.

exists that Josephus thought of the name of the Righteous Teacher.[1] The evidence is admittedly slight. Josephus usually refers to Moses when he employs the term νομοθέτης.[2] And the scrolls never announce a prohibition against mentioning the Teacher's name.[3] But there is some further information suggesting that the anonymity perhaps was intentional after all. The Pythagoreans, with whom Josephus elsewhere compares the Essenes (Ant. 15:371),[4] avoided referring to their teacher by name.[5] And the Talmud occasionally implies that a sage honoured his father or teacher by not mentioning their names to the interpreter (b. Qidd. 31b).[6] These points are somewhat remote. But in view of the striking silence about the Teacher's identity in the scrolls themselves, the assumption that the Qumranites intentionally were silent about his name—at least in their written activity—is not entirely implausible.

2.3.2. The Anonymity of the Written Traditions

The Qumranites did not present the teaching as written traditions explicitly connected with the Righteous Teacher.[7] They did not order and/or identify the written material through references to the Righteous Teacher. While they may intentionally have concealed his actual name, it is surprising that they do not even attach any of his designations to a specific text portion.

Scholars have often regarded (parts of) various Dead Sea scrolls as compositions by the Righteous Teacher. Some suggested that the Teacher composed portions of the Damascus Document,[8] the War Rule,[9] the Community Rule[10] or the Rule of the

---

1 So DUPONT-SOMMER, *Dead Sea Scrolls*, 91; *idem, Écrits esséniens*, 42 n. 2, 103 n. 2, 369; REEVES, *RevQ* 13 (1988) 297f.

2 BEALL, *Josephus' Description of the Essenes*, 92–94. Cf. also DELCOR, *RB* 61 (1954) 550–553; SCHIFFMAN, *Sectarian Law*, 137.

3 DUPONT-SOMMER, *Écrits esséniens*, 103 n. 2, thinks that 1QS 6:27–7:2 refers to blasphemy of the Teacher's name. But this is far from evident.

4 Cf. also Hippolytus (c. 170–236 C.E.), *Ref.* IX 27:3. Direct influence from the Pythagoreans is unlikely. Cf. HENGEL, *Judaism and Hellenism* I, 243–247; CULPEPPER, *School*, 58–60 (with lit.); BEALL, *Josephus' Description of the Essenes*, 132.

5 DUPONT-SOMMER, *Dead Sea Scrolls*, 91; *idem, Écrits esséniens*, 42 n. 2. Cf. also CULPEPPER, *School*, 153 n. 45.

6 Cf. also b. Sanh. 100a.

7 Cf. ALLISON, *RevQ* 10 (1980) 268; P.R. DAVIES, *RevQ* 13 (1988) 317.

8 So e.g. TALMON, Oral Tradition and Written Transmission, 157.

9 So e.g. CARMIGNAC/GUILBERT, *Textes de Qumrân*, 85f. Cf. also CARMIGNAC/COTHENET/LIGNÉE, *Textes de Qumrân*, 11, 32.

10 So e.g. DUPONT-SOMMER, *Écrits esséniens*, 86f; MILIK, *Ten Years of Discovery*, 37; O. BETZ, *Offenbarung und Schriftforschung*, 35, 63; CARMIGNAC/GUILBERT, *Textes de Qumrân*, 14f, 85f; CARMIGNAC/COTHENET/LIGNÉE, *Textes de Qumrân*, 11, 32; PEUCH, *RevQ* 10 (1979) 111; CHARLESWORTH, Qumran Scrolls, xxxiv. Sometimes 1QS 8:1–16a; 9:3–10a is regarded as the earliest part of the Rule, perhaps composed by the Teacher. So MURPHY-O'CONNOR, *RB* 76 (1969) 531; *idem, RB* 81 (1974) 237. Cf. also NICKELSBURGH, *Jewish Literature*, 132; DOHMEN, *RevQ* 11 (1982) 92–94; P.R. DAVIES, *RevQ* 13 (1988) 317; KNIBB, Teacher of Righteousness, 54f.—ALLISON,

Congregation.[1] Some argued that 4QMMT, believed to be one of the most important writings from Qumran, is a halakhic letter perhaps written by the Teacher.[2] There are in particular two documents which scholars often understand as writings (partly) from the Teacher. It has been quite common to use the Hodayoth on the assumption that the Teacher authored some of the hymns.[3] This assumption builds on some form-critical considerations applied on the material. After initial studies in this direction by S. Holm-Nielsen and G. Morawe,[4] a number of theses under the supervision of K.G. Kuhn related the form-critical discussion to the identity of the "I" in the hymns. The studies by G. Jeremias, Jürgen Becker and H.-W. Kuhn were the most important ones. They agreed—with some variations—on a form-critical basis that some of the hymns came from the Teacher.[5] The more recent discussion has been diverse. Some studies make use of Jeremias', Becker's or Kuhn's conclusions in defining the personality of the Teacher;[6] other studies show a sceptical attitude.[7]

Certain scholars think that the Teacher composed the Temple scroll, or the Qumran torah.[8] Already Y. Yadin, the editor, did this implicitly.[9] As we have already noticed,[10] he cautiously identified the document with important books mentioned elsewhere in the scrolls and probed the possibility that Zadok, said to have found the sealed torah (CD 5:5), actually was the Teacher. B.Z. Wacholder, though critical of Yadin in some respects, claims more explicitly that a certain Zadok—a disciple of An-

---

RevQ 10 (1980) 257–268, tries to show that the Teacher authored 1QS 3:13–4:14.

1   So e.g. CARMIGNAC/COTHENET/LIGNÉE, *Textes de Qumrân,* 11, 32. Cf. also CARMIGNAC/GUILBERT, *Textes de Qumrân,* 85f.

2   So QIMRON/STRUGNELL, Unpublished Halakhic Letter, 400–407. Cf. also STRUGNELL, Qumran Scrolls, 99f, 103f, and the discussion below pp. 168f.

3   For a list of early scholars holding this view, cf. G. JEREMIAS, *Lehrer der Gerechtigkeit,* 168f n. 6.

4   HOLM-NIELSEN, *Hodayot;* MORAWE, *Aufbau und Abgrenzung der Loblieder.* The form-critical terminology of HOLM-NIELSEN, *ibid.,* 316–331, varies as he discusses the question of a plurality of authors and of literary genres. Cf. also *idem,* "Ich" in den Hodajoth, 220f. The basic form-critical distinction proposed by MORAWE, *ibid.,* 107–162, is between "individuelle Danklieder" and "hymnische Bekenntnislieder." Cf. also *idem, RevQ* 4 (1963) 323–356.

5   G. JEREMIAS, *Lehrer der Gerechtigkeit,* 171, thinks that the Teacher was the author of 2:1–19; 2:31–39; 3:1–18; 4:5–5:4; 5:5–19; 5:20–7:5; 7:6–25; 8:4–40. Jürgen BECKER, *Heil Gottes,* 51–55, proposes 2:1–19; 2:31–39; 4:5–5:4 (except 4:29–5:4); 5:5–19; 5:20–39; 6:1–36; 7:6–25; 8:4–40, and probably also 2:20–30; 3:1–18; 3:37–4:4; 7:1–5, as coming from the Teacher. H.-W. KUHN, *Enderwartung und gegenwärtiges Heil,* 22–24, classifies 2:1–19; 4:5–5:4 (except 4:29b–5:4); 5:5–19; 5:20–6:36; 7:6–25; 8:4–40 as "berichtende Loblieder des Offenbarungsmittlers" (*ibid.,* 23).

6   So most extensively P. SCHULZ, *Autoritätsanspruch des Lehrers der Gerechtigkeit.*—P.R. DAVIES, *Behind the Essenes,* 87–105, claims that whoever wrote the Hodayoth, the community understood the hymns—especially the autobiographical ones—as hagiographic compositions of and about the Teacher, and made use of them in the pesharim.

7   So in more recent years e.g. DOMBKOWSKI HOPKINS, *RevQ* 10 (1981) 331–336; B.P. KITTEL, *Hymns of Qumran,* 9f; DIMANT, Qumran Sectarian Literature, 523; SCHÜRER, *History* III, 453–455; CALLAWAY, *History of the Qumran Community,* 185–197; KNIBB, Teacher of Righteousness, 54; DAVIDSON, *Angels at Qumran,* 187f.

8   The former designation goes back to YADIN (ed.), *Temple Scroll* I, *passim,* and the latter to WACHOLDER, *Dawn of Qumran,* 21.

9   *Temple Scroll* I, 390–397. Cf. also *idem, Temple Scroll,* 222–229.

10   See above pp. 50, 72.

tigonus of Soko (c. 180 B.C.E.)—was the author of the document,[1] and perhaps also of Jubilees.[2] This Zadok composed the document a few years before 196 B.C.E., when he took office as the leader of a new group. M.O. Wise has recently argued that the Teacher gave the document its final content and shape.[3] The Teacher was an eschatological figure—the promised Mosaic prophet, a new Moses—who redacted four basic sources and, in addition, wrote his own portions of the document. The work on the Temple scroll is far from finished.[4] Some studies continue to connect it with the Teacher;[5] other studies exhibit a sceptical view in this regard.[6]

The primary argument for ascribing a certain text or document to the Teacher is the authority that the implied author of the scroll exhibits. Nowhere do we find the name or the title of the real author. S. Holm-Nielsen recognized that the "pertinent question" as regards the Hodayoth is not the one of authorship—the real identity of the "I"—but "what the purpose was in composing such psalms."[7] The Qumranites used them—whether privately or together—and the "I" became to them projections of the community's experiences.[8] They apparently used the Temple scroll as some kind of important torah. It is possible that the extraordinary claims emerging when they used these documents coloured their apprehension of the Teacher. But in that case this happened indirectly, not because of an explicit statement about the Teacher as the author.

However, the high degree of person-oriented motives of transmission makes it likely that there were channels besides the written records by which the Qumranites could recognize the traditions from the Teacher. They did not think of the Teacher as merely a wisdom teacher uttering anonymous sayings. Their interpretative activity and their salvation depended

---

[1]   *Dawn of Qumran,* 99–169, 202–212. Cf. excursus 8 below.
[2]   WACHOLDER, Ancient Judaeo-Aramaic Literature, 273f.
[3]   *Temple Scroll,* 179–189.
[4]   For surveys of research, see KAPERA, Review, 275–286; VAN DER WOUDE, *TRu* 54 (1989) 227–249; WISE, *Temple Scroll,* 2–33. Cf. also BROOKE, Introduction, 13–19.
[5]   Cf. e.g. REEVES, *RevQ* 13 (1988) 295f; WISE, *RevQ* 14 (1990) 606; SCHWEITZER, Teacher of Righteousness, 55–57.—LIGNÉE, *RevQ* 13 (1988) 340–344, believes that the Teacher was the author of Jubilees and the Temple scroll, but he identifies the Teacher with Judah the Essene, known from Ant. 13:311–313; Bell. 1:78–80.
[6]   See the discussion above p. 72. Cf. also the cautious remarks given in SCHÜRER, *History* III, 417, and by J. MAIER, *Temple Scroll,* 6f; VAN DER WOUDE, *TRu* 54 (1989) 244f, 248f. For criticism of Wacholder's identification of the sealed torah in CD 5:2–5, see VANDERKAM, *RevQ* 11 (1984) 561–570. Cf. also the response by WACHOLDER, *RevQ* 12 (1986) 351–368, and the further critical discussion by J. MAIER, *RevQ* 15 (1991) 231–241. For criticism of the dating of the scroll, with a preference for an early pre-Qumranic date, see STEGEMANN, Origins of the Temple Scroll, 235–256; *idem,* Temple Scroll, 126–136. Cf. also the review of various scholarly opinions by BROOKE, Introduction, 14f. For criticism of the presupposed unity of authorship, see CALLAWAY, *RevQ* 12 (1986) 213–222.
[7]   *Hodayot,* 316–348, quotation from p. 316. Cf. also *idem,* "Ich" in den Hodajoth, 217–220; DOMBKOWSKI HOPKINS, *RevQ* 10 (1981) 336–338.
[8]   Cf. THYEN, *Sündenvergebung,* 81–85.

on hearing his voice. There is no conclusive evidence that certain knowledge about the Teacher's life story was necessary for a correct understanding of his teaching. But the Qumranites regarded it as essential that the normative directives originated with the Teacher. There were presumably oral means of communicating the traditions' attachment to the Teacher. Written tradition does not always speak for itself.[1] In that case, the study of the written traditions within the school of the Righteous Teacher was only a part of the learning process. It was supplemented with oral instructions.

There is no evidence that the oral information was to be kept as a secret. The community was probably not a strictly separatist movement consisting of persons entirely isolated from their environment and in possession of secret knowledge.[2] At least three considerations speak against such an understanding of the community. First, there are foreign influences. M.Hengel has shown that the community was not untouched by the Greek-Hellenistic culture.[3] Second, while the Qumranites did possess an elite-consciousness, they also viewed themselves as part of the Israelite nation into which they were born.[4] We find not only a confessional community into which membership was attained by voluntary association. The Qumranites were in some sense open to define their identity in terms going beyond the borders of their own community. Third, it is not possible to maintain that the Qumranites cherished an esoteric form of knowledge available only to the full members of the community. They were indeed to seek out in the Scriptures the hidden things unknown to the people of Israel (1QS 5:11; 8:11f), but it is not evident that the knowledge thereby attained always was to remain limited to a smaller circle of people only;[5] they were indeed to communicate a certain kind of knowledge to (specific) persons within the community only,[6] but it is not evident that this was due to the esoteric character of the knowledge itself. It depended rather on the fact that men are more or less defiled and unable to attain knowledge. Outside of the community, there was defilement of spirit (CD 5:11) and only limited knowledge (1QS 3:2f); within the community, a spirit of holiness provided opportunity for increased knowledge (1QS 3:6–8; 9:3, 15f).[7] Even a member of the community who turned aside from what was commanded was excluded from the

---

1   Cf. ANDERSEN, Oral Tradition, 51.
2   Cf. the caution expressed by STEGEMANN, Die "Mitte der Schrift," 153–157.
3   Qumrān und der Hellenismus, 333–372.
4   Cf. TALMON, Jewish Sectarianism, 605–610.
5   Cf. the distinction between esoteric and public law adopted by P.R. DAVIES, The Temple Scroll, 206.
6   W.D. DAVIES, *HTR* 46 (1953) 121f, quotes 1QS 9:17, 22; 8:18 in order to prove the existence of secret knowledge. He adds 1QS 1:5, 11; 2:26; 5:3, 10 in order to show that a special truth was known to the members. 1QS 5:11f; 10:25 are interpreted similarly. Cf. also CD 15:10f; 1QS 4:6; 5:15f; Bell. 2:141.
7   J.A. DAVIS, *Wisdom and Spirit*, 43.

knowledge of the counsel until he had been purified from falsehood and walked in perfection of ways (1QS 8:16–19).[1] It is not possible to expound the issue further here. P. Wernberg-Møller has himself corrected his sectarian view of the community and shown to a number of further passages implying that the Qumranites did not regard their mysteries (רזים) as closely guarded secrets but communicated them also to other persons, irrespective of whether they were full members or not.[2] Although the Qumranites may have concealed the actual name of the Teacher, it is unlikely that the absence of personal identification markers in the written material depended on an intentional secrecy surrounding the traditions from the Teacher.

The motives of transmission, exhibiting a high degree of concentration on the Teacher, did not effect a strong personal specificity in the process of identifying the traditions in written material. When the Qumranites transmitted the traditions from the Righteous Teacher in writing, they did not identify them through a kind of personal attribution. They ordered and conveyed them as anonymous teaching and, as it appears within certain documents, occasionally even as integrated with teaching of a different origin.

Excursus 8: *The Historical Identity of the Righteous Teacher*

The cumulative force from the studies by scholars such as G. Vermes, G. Jeremias, H. Stegemann and J. Murphy-O'Connor,[3] though they disagree in individual issues, has provided the most influential view concerning the historical identity of the Righteous Teacher. They identify the Qumran movement in some sense with the Essenes mentioned in the classical sources.[4] This does of course not exclude the possibility that there were Essenes also elsewhere in Palestine.[5] Ant. 13:171 places the Essenes during the rule of the Maccabean high priest Jonathan reigning at the pontifical office from 152 until 142 B.C.E. This provides an independent indication that the "plant root" (CD 1:7) of the Essenes was born during the Hellenistic crisis in the early years of the second century B.C.E.[6] "Twenty years" later the Teacher appeared in order to organize the disillusioned community (CD 1:9–11). He came into conflict with the

---

[1]   For discussion of the association between the reception of the spirit and the entrance into the community in the Hodayoth, see MENZIES, *Early Christian Pneumatology,* 84–87.

[2]   *ALUOS* 6 (1969) 59–65.

[3]   Studies by these scholars have been listed in my bibliography. They all build on the archaeological work by de Vaux. See DE VAUX, *Archaeology and the Dead Sea Scrolls,* who here presents what he published in several earlier articles. For a survey of the research about the origin and development of the Qumran community, see VAN DER WOUDE, *TRu* 57 (1992) 225–253.

[4]   The texts are, with some exceptions (Ant. 13:298, 311f; 17:346; 18:11), easily available in VERMES/GOODMAN, *Essenes,* 19–99.—BEALL, *Josephus' Description of the Essenes,* evaluates the historical information of Josephus' account positively.

[5]   Although Omn. Prob. Lib. 76 says that the Essenes avoid cities, Philo himself (Hypothetica in Eusebius, Praep. Ev. VIII 11:1) and Josephus (Bell. 2:124) claim that they live in towns. Cf. also Ant. 13:311f; 15:373–378; 17:346; Bell. 2:567; 3:11; 5:145.

[6]   MURPY-O'CONNOR, *RB* 81 (1974) 215–244, thinks that "Damascus" in the Damascus Document points to the Babylonian pre-history of the community.

wicked priest, whom the pesharim often mention as the opponent of the community. Accepting that the wicked priest was a specific historical individual,[1] the most influential view deduces his identity from the indications that he first had some support among the pious Jews (1QpHab 8:8f) and later was killed by Gentiles (4QpPs^a 4:9f).[2] This twofold characteristic fits only Jonathan. It is probable that the Qumranites regarded him positively until he assumed the high-priestly office in 152 B.C.E., and thus became the wicked priest. 1 Macc 12:39–13:24; Ant. 13:187–209; Bell. 1:49 suggest that he was killed by Gentiles. It is therefore possible to detect the shadow of the Righteous Teacher, according to the standard view. Some propose that he was in the high-priestly office during the alleged *intersacerdotium* mentioned in Ant. 13:46; 20:237 as occurring between the death of Alkimos (c. 159 B.C.E.) and the nomination of Jonathan. The day of Atonement could hardly have been celebrated without participation of a high priest.[3] He may therefore have been the immediate predecessor of Jonathan in the high-priestly office—a high priest perhaps alluded to in 1 Macc 10:38.[4]

Since the early days of Qumran studies, other alternatives have appeared: D. Flusser argued that the description of Isaiah in the Martyrdom of Isaiah reflects the Teacher's destiny;[5] S. Mowinckel thought that the Assumption of Moses originated within the same circles as the Damascus Document and that the mysterious Taxo(n) in 9:1 was the Greek equivalent of מחוקק in Gen 49:10 and perhaps the Teacher at Qumran;[6] M. Philonenko identified the Teacher with the righteous man mentioned in Wis 2:12–20; 5:1–7;[7] J. Carmignac attempted in more recent years to substantiate his idea that the Teacher was Judah the Essene (Ant. 13:311–313; Bell. 1:78–80);[8] J.C. Trever has repeatedly suggested that the Teacher was the author/compiler of Daniel.[9] Others relate the Teacher to the NT and identify him with various persons, such as Jesus,[10] John the Baptist[11] and James the Just.[12]

The attempts to define the identity and name of the Teacher from indications within the scrolls are equally hypothetical. Wacholder refers to the Zadok mentioned in CD

---

[1] But cf. BROWNLEE, *JQR* 73 (1982) 3–9; VAN DER WOUDE, *JJS* 33 (1982) 349–359. For a refutation of van der Woude's thesis, see LIM, *JBL* 112 (1993) 415–425.— P.R. DAVIES, Qumran Beginnings, 366, denies the wicked priest all historical reality.

[2] Cf. also 1QpHab 8:16–9:2.

[3] STEGEMANN, *Entstehung der Qumrangemeinde,* 213–219.—This assumption is not accepted by VERMES, *JJS* 32 (1981) 28. For a critical assessment of Stegemann's use of the so-called *intersacerdotium,* see BURGMANN, *JSJ* 11 (1980) 135–176, claiming that there was an actual vacancy in the high-priestly office during 159–152 B.C.E. Cf. similarly SIEVERS, *Hasmoneans,* 75–77.—WISE, *RevQ* 14 (1990) 587–613, argues on a different basis than Stegemann that the Teacher served as the high priest during the *intersacerdotium.*

[4] So MURPHY-O'CONNOR, *RB* 83 (1976) 400–420. Cf. also WISE, *RevQ* 14 (1990) 606–613.

[5] *BIES* 17 (1952) 28–47.

[6] Hebrew Equivalent of Taxo, 92–96. Cf. also *idem, He That Cometh,* 300f.

[7] *TZ* 14 (1958) 81–88.

[8] *RevQ* 10 (1980) 235–246; *idem, RevQ* 10 (1981) 585f.

[9] *BA* 48 (1985) 89–102. Trever has developed his view in later articles.

[10] TEICHER, *JJS* 2 (1951) 97f; *idem, JJS* 3 (1952) 53–55.

[11] THIERING, *Redating the Teacher of Righteousness,* 212. Thiering has developed her view in later publications.

[12] EISENMAN, *James the Just in the Habakkuk Pesher.* Eisenman has developed his view in later publications.

5:5; 3Q15 11:3, 6, identifies him as a prominent disciple of Antigonus of Soko—Antigonus himself being a disciple of the high priest Simon II the Just (c. 200 B.C.E.)—and sees references to this Zadok in the rabbinic and the Karaite writings.[1] However, we have seen that CD 5:5, which is the most explicit reference to Zadok, was probably coined on the basis of the OT.[2] Wacholder's use of the rabbinic and the Karaite material is also problematic.[3]

W.H. Brownlee suggested tentatively that the Teacher was called Judah and as such referred to in 1QpHab 12:4f; 1QpMic 1:5.[4] The repeated "I thank thee, o Lord, because" (אודכה אדוני כי) in the Hodayoth is, according to Brownlee, also an allusion to Judah, since Leah gave her son the name Judah after saying "this time I thank Yahweh" (הפעם אודה את יהוה) according to Gen 29:35.[5] However, not only does Brownlee read far-fetched allusions into the texts. He also proceeds on the assumption that the Teacher was Judah the Essene (Ant. 311–313; Bell. 1:78–80)—an assumption which, as we saw, was especially endorsed by Carmignac.[6] While some have followed Carmignac in this regard,[7] the awkward chronology presupposed has led to severe criticism and rejection of his hypothesis.[8] *For whatever reason, the Qumranites did not reveal the identity of their great Teacher in their writings.*

3. The Means of Transmission

"The means of transmission" refers to *the media by which the verbal traditions were carried and conveyed.* I will not discuss the carriers of the traditions separately. We noticed in chapter one that some texts indicate the existence of (teachers and) pupils as possible carriers of traditions, and in

---

[1] *Dawn of Qumran,* 99–169. The primary rabbinic passages used are m. ʾAbot 1:3; ʾAbot R. Nat. A 5; ʾAbot R. Nat. B 10. The primary Karaite passages used are translated portions of the Arabic *Kitāb al-Anwār wal-Marāqib* (the Book of Lights and Watchtowers) by Abu Jusuf Jaʿqub al-Qirqisāni (10th cent. C.E.).
[2] See above pp. 50f.
[3] BASSER, *RevQ* 11 (1984) 549–560.—The possible relationship between the Dead Sea scrolls and the Karaites has been noticed ever since S. Schechter in 1896 found a number of Karaite writings together with the Damascus Document in the Cairo Genizah. An ancient letter from c. 800 C.E., discussed and partly quoted in German by EISSFELDT, *TLZ* 74 (1949) 597–600, also speaks of some books found 10 years ago in a rock-dwelling near Jericho. The relationship was discussed already by GINZBERG, *Eine unbekannte jüdische Sekte,* 206–220. Further literature is listed by BARDTKE, *TRu* 33 (1968) 204f; J. MAIER, *Geschichte der jüdischen Religion,* 231 n. 1. See also the recent discussion about the Karaites by SZYSZMAN, *Karaïsme,* including an account of the Essene heritage (*ibid.,* 34–48). For a review of Szyszman's book, see BURCHARD, *RevQ* 11 (1983) 279–285.
[4] In my system of referring to the commentary on Micah, Judah is mentioned in 1QpMic 8–10:5 (*DJD* I, 78).
[5] *JQR* 73 (1982) 27f.
[6] *RevQ* 10 (1980) 235–246; *idem, RevQ* 10 (1981) 585f.
[7] Cf. e.g. LIGNÉE, *RevQ* 13 (1988) 345.
[8] BURGMANN, *RevQ* 10 (1981) 553–578; MURPHY-O'CONNOR, *RevQ* 10 (1981) 579–585. For some criticism of both Carmignac and Brownlee, cf. TREVER, Qumran Teacher, 120 n. 68.

chapter two I substantiated this possibility by pointing to the person-oriented motives of transmission among the pupils of certain teachers. The
means of transmission concerns only the actual verbal traditions here.

Orality always influenced the means of transmission to some extent. We
are studying a sociocultural situation in which writing often related immediately to oral procedures. But there are also additional factors depending
on more specific circumstances. It is of particular interest to see how settings determined by the authority of a teacher and person-oriented motives
of transmission correlated with oral and written means of carrying and
conveying the traditions.

3.1. The Rabbis and Oral Transmission

The origin, history and significance of the notion about two torahs in rabbinic Judaism is a matter of scholarly discussion.[1] This section is most interested in oral torah. Although learning to read the written Torah from a
Hebrew text without vocalization certainly required the help of a teacher,[2]
oral means of transmission increased the importance of the teacher and the
need to memorize his teaching even further.

3.1.1. Written and Oral Torah

The rabbinic literature points in different ways to the conviction that torah
was given both in written form (תורה שבכתב) and orally (תורה שבעל פה).
The present texts associate discussions about the two torahs with early masters such as Hillel and Shammai (b. Šabb. 31a; ʾAbot R. Nat. A 15; ʾAbot R.
Nat. B 29), R. Gamaliel (Sifre on Deut 33:10)—whether Gamaliel I Ha-
Zaken (c. 30–40 C.E.) or Gamaliel II (c. 90 C.E.)—and R. Joḥanan b. Zakkai (Midr. Tann. 215 on Deut 33:10).[3]

Whatever the origin of this conviction, it implied two means of transmission in rabbinic Judaism, in writing and orally. The written Torah and
the act of written transmission was called מקרא. Oral, or memorized,[4] torah
and oral transmission was called משנה.[5] The former was a study in which

---

[1] For discussion, see SCHÄFER, *Studien*, 153–197 (with lit.). In addition to the literature mentioned there, see SAFRAI, Oral Tora, 35–119; E.P. SANDERS, *Jewish Law*,
97–130; STRACK/STEMBERGER, *Talmud and Midrash*, 35–49; P.S. ALEXANDER, Orality in Pharisaic-rabbinic Judaism, 159–184.—Neusner has repeatedly addressed these
problems in his numerous publications. Cf. e.g. NEUSNER, *Oral Tradition*. His
(alternating) view is discussed by E.P. SANDERS, *ibid.*, 110–115.
[2] SAFRAI, Education, 950f.
[3] Outside the rabbinic literature, Ant. 13:297 is most relevant. Cf. also Abr. 16; Leg
Gaj. 115; Spec. Leg. 4:150; Virt. 194; Hypothetica in Eusebius, Praep. Ev. VIII 6:9;
Ant. 10:51; 13:408.
[4] NEUSNER, *Memorized Torah*, 1; *idem*, *Oral Tradition*, ix.
[5] For the distinction between מקרא and משנה, cf. e.g. m. Qidd. 1:10; m. ʾAbot 5:21.

learning involved reading (קרא). The latter was a study in which learning involved repeating (שנה).[1]

The rabbinic literature gives in this manner a clear theoretical expression to the distinction between the two torahs and the two means of transmission. *In some ways, written and oral texts must have been used in interaction and interdependence.*[2] A pupil needed oral instruction in order to read the written Torah; oral torah often depended on the written Torah; and after all, oral torah finally did appear in writing. *But the clear statements about two torahs and two means of transmission imply that there was not an unconscious and entirely fluid interchangeability between the two, but a deliberate use of two means of transmission.* It is therefore legitimate to concentrate only on the oral transmission here.

3.1.2. The Rabbis and Oral Torah

The clear statements about oral torah and oral transmission give a significant characterization of the whole setting in which the traditions were carried and conveyed. It was essentially oral.[3] This must have increased the importance of the living teacher.[4] The baraita in b. ʿErub. 54b—the *locus classicus* for the oral transmission—gives the impression that from Moses and onwards the pupils must learn to repeat the statements of their teachers orally and word by word.[5] Just as Aaron learned from Moses, who himself had learned from the Omnipotent, each pupil must learn from the mouth of the teacher. This baraita probably reflects the procedure in the rabbinic colleges.[6]

An account about Hillel in b. Šabb. 31a illustrates the conviction that the pupils depended upon the teacher in regard to oral torah. Hillel teaches a proselyte the first four Hebrew letters on the first day. On the second day, he reverses the order of the letters. To the objection of the proselyte Hillel merely responds that the student has to rely on him in respect to the oral (torah) too.

An important teacher always exhibits a strong influence on young pupils. Although there was a general tendency to consult many teachers,[7] we consequently find also accounts implying that a close relationship between one

---

1   GERHARDSSON, *Memory,* 28f.
2   GERHARDSSON, *Memory,* 67–70. Cf. also *idem,* Gospel Tradition, 519–527.
3   Cf. e.g. BONSIRVEN, *Judaïsme Palestinien* I, 291; SAFRAI, Elementary Education, 154; GOLDIN, Sidelights of a Torah Education, 186; SAFRAI, Education, 966.
4   Cf. LENHARDT, *RSR* 66 (1978) 492–494; P.S. ALEXANDER, Orality in Pharisaic-rabbinic Judaism, 162–168.
5   NEUSNER, *JSJ* 5 (1974) 177; SCHÄFER, *Studien,* 187, stress the implication of this passage to repeat *verbatim.*
6   GERHARDSSON, *Memory,* 120f.
7   See above p. 97.

particular master and a pupil could develop. Of course, it was only as a carrier of oral torah that the teacher was important. But it happened that a pupil continued to stay in contact with his teacher as long as the old master was alive and to cherish him as his own teacher.[1] ᵓAbot R. Nat. A 14, for instance, tells about when R. Eleazar b. Arak (c. 90 C.E.) visits R. Joḥanan b. Zakkai on the death of Joḥanan's son. R. Eleazar, a distinguished teacher himself, addresses Joḥanan as "my teacher." Many texts also imply that it was a dramatic experience to realize the death of one's own teacher.[2] On certain occasions, it seems, a deceased scholar even appeared to be irreplaceable (y. Ber. 5c). The teachers were indispensible as carriers of oral torah.

When the pupil advanced from the elementary education in the scripture school and entered the advanced studies in the college, he therefore depended on the close contact with a teacher in order to acquire learning in oral torah. *The oral means of transmitting torah necessitated an interaction between teacher and pupil.*

3.1.3. The Rabbis and Memorization

The close contact with the teacher continued to direct the activity of the former pupil when he was himself to teach and transmit oral torah to others. The rabbinic literature discusses the circumstances under which qualified pupils were allowed to give their own halakhic judgements while their master was still alive: the person who taught his own halakhah in front of his own teacher was normally liable to death;[3] or he could give the halakhah, but only within proper distance from the teacher's residence.[4]

In any case, different passages suggest that when a (former) pupil gave his own teaching, he should keep to the instruction given by his master. A well known saying in m. ʿEd. 1:3 states it quite explicitly:

אדם חייב לומר	It is a man's duty to speak
בלשון רבו	with the tongue of his teacher.

It is possible that someone added this rule as an explanatory gloss to Hillel's use of a rather odd measurement.[5] But b. Šabb. 15a repeats it with the same commentary and other instances also apply it. At least one of them is au-

---

1 Cf. ABERBACH, Relations Between Master and Disciple, 11f, 18–21.
2 Cf. e.g. b. Ber. 42b–43a; b. Moʿed Qaṭ. 24a, 25b–26a; b. Ketub. 103b–104a; b. Sanh. 68a; y. Ber. 6a; y. Moʿed Qaṭ. 83a–d; y. B. Meṣ. 8d; y. Sanh. 20a; y. Hor. 47d; ᵓAbot R. Nat. A 25; Qoh. Rab. on 9:10.
3 Cf. e.g. b. Ber. 31b; b. ʿErub. 63a; b. Yoma 53a; y. Šeb. 36c; y. Giṭ. 43c; Sifra on 10:1; Sifre on Num 27:18; Lev. Rab. 20:6; Pesiq. Rab Kah. 26:7 (Mandelbaum's 2nd ed. 393).
4 Cf. e.g. b. Sanh. 5b; y. Šeb. 36c; y. Giṭ. 43c; Pesiq. Rab Kah. 26:7 (Mandelbaum's 2nd ed. 393f).
5 So e.g. STRACK/STEMBERGER, *Talmud and Midrash*, 44.

thentic (b. Bek. 5a).[1] The practice of maintaining the words of the tea-cher—to speak with his tongue—seems to have been in function already during tannaitic times.[2] There are also texts implying that a statement could be dismissed if it was not supported by the master's authority.[3]

The importance of oral torah and the need to maintain what the teacher said required that the traditions were remembered accurately. Numerous texts show that oral torah was carried by means of memorization. As is well known, the rabbis were utterly concerned to remember correctly the writ-ten Torah and oral torah.[4] Since oral torah was available only through li-ving teachers, it had to be memorized. Various measures were taken to counteract forgetfulness. For instance, y. Šeqal. 47a advises scholars to draw a mental picture of the author of a teaching. The author, so to say, stands besides the scholar uttering the teaching. Oral torah was easier to remember when it was related to the image of a real person. Memory of a concrete item is much better than of an entirely abstract item.[5]

R. Eliezer b. Hyrcanus (c. 90 C.E.) is perhaps the best example—probab-ly somewhat exceptional and idealized—of how someone carried oral torah by attachment to the traditions of his teacher. The rabbinic writings picture Eliezer's attachment to the early traditions and his teacher R. Joḥanan b. Zakkai.[6] Many texts maintain his reputation—as well as the reputation of his teacher—of not laying down any halkhic rule that he had not heard from his teacher.[7] According to m. Yad. 4:3, for instance, Eliezer confirms the out-come of a vote by reference to a tradition that he had heard from Joḥa-nan, who, in turn, had heard it from his teacher, all the way back to Moses on Sinai; and according to m. Neg. 9:3, he tries to limit the use of new halakhot by reference to what he has heard or not heard from the tradition.[8] This presupposes of course an exceptional ability to memorize. In m. ʾAbot 2:8 Joḥanan accordingly praises Eliezer for his excellent memory and compares him with a plastered cistern which loses not a drop.[9] According to b. ʿErub. 54b, Eliezer's own rule for helping the pupils to remember was the teacher's habit to repeat a teaching four times.

An absolutely strict adherence to the traditions from one's own teacher would of course have made any originality and growth within the oral

---

1 Cf. also b. Ber. 47a.
2 For examples, see GERHARDSSON, *Memory,* 132f.
3 Cf. e.g. b. ʿErub. 92a; b. Yebam. 43a; b. Nid. 62b.
4 GERHARDSSON, *Memory,* 122–170.
5 VANSINA, *Oral Tradition,* 171.
6 BACHER, *Agada der Tannaiten* I, 101f; GILAT, *EncJud* VI, 621; NEUSNER, *Elie-zer ben Hyrcanus* II, 219–223, 343–346; GILAT, *R. Eliezer ben Hyrcanus,* 474–479.
7 Cf. e.g. t. Yebam. 3:4; b. Yoma 66b; b. Sukk. 27b–28a; y. Yoma 43c.
8 For comments on the text, see NEUSNER, *Eliezer ben Hyrcanus* I, 301; GOLDIN, Sidelights of a Torah Education, 188f.
9 Cf. also ʾAbot R. Nat. A 14. For comments on the text, see NEUSNER, *Develop-ment,* 55; *idem, Eliezer ben Hyrcanus* I, 396f.

tradition impossible.[1] There must have been elaborations and some scholars must have introduced innovations.[2] The standardized language and the literary forms in the Mishnah and other rabbinic writings also show that the rule of stating a tradition in the words of the teacher was not decisive as a principle of literary compilation.[3] *It was essentially not the attachment to a particular rabbi that caused certain means of transmission.* This correlates with the purely didactic motives of transmission discussed in the previous chapter. Torah was at the centre, not the individual rabbi. *It was the conviction that torah is oral—not only written—and should be transmitted by oral means that caused the attachment to the teacher.*

3.2. The Prophets and the Interactive Means of Transmission

Despite the absence of clear statements about two means of transmission in the prophetic literature, the role played by written and oral tradition and transmission has been the object of much scholarly discussion.[4] The lack of clear evidence makes it necessary to deduce information from the material indirectly.

3.2.1. Written and Oral Traditions

The book of Isaiah provides perhaps the clearest indication of a written body of traditions. 8:16 parallels a torah to be sealed with a testimony (תעודה) to be bound (צור).[5] This adds a legal aspect to Isaiah's action. Nowhere in the rest of the OT do we find this object related to the same

---

1   Cf. GOLDENBERG, Originality in Talmudic Thought, 19–27.

2   Cf. SIGAL, *Halakah of Jesus,* 47–51.

3   Cf. W.S. GREEN, What's in a Name?, 80–83; NEUSNER, Rabbinic Biography, 88; *idem, Memorized Torah,* 112f, 115–117, 122, *passim;* STRACK/STEMBERGER, *Talmud and Midrash,* 44; P.S. ALEXANDER, Orality in Pharisaic-rabbinic Judaism, 176. For the same phenomenon in the Palestinian Talmud, see NEUSNER, Talmud's Authorship, 56–64.

4   For surveys, see NORTH, *ExpTim* 61 (1949–50) 292–296; KAISER, *Introduction,* 297–305; FOHRER, *Introduction,* 36–41; KOCH, *Formgeschichte,* 97–112. The written tradition and transmission were defended against the (Scandinavian) emphasis on oral tradition and transmission by GUNNEWEG, *Tradition.* For critique, see GERHARDSSON, *SEÅ* 25 (1960) 175–181. The Scandinavian contributions are summarized and evaluated by D.A. KNIGHT, *Rediscovering,* 217–399. Cf. also the discussion of tradition history by different Scandinavian scholars in JEPPESEN/OTZEN (eds.), *Productions of Time.* The prophets are treated by KAPELRUD, Traditio-historical Study, 53–66. Of importance is also the discussion on folklore and orality. For surveys, see FOLEY, *Theory of Oral Composition,* 84–86; CULLEY, Oral Tradition, 189–225, including also NT research. In addition to the literature mentioned there, cf. the contributions in NIDITCH (ed.), *Text and Tradition,* and E.F. DAVIS, *Swallowing the Scroll.* The whole problem of oral tradition and orality in different areas of the Israelite, Jewish and Greek antiquity has been discussed by various scholars in WANSBROUGH (ed.), *Jesus and the Oral Gospel Tradition.* The OT is treated by RÜGER, Oral Tradition, 107–120. See further below pp. 319–349.

5   Cf. above pp. 40f.

verb.[1] Nor is it elsewhere ever connected with the term תורה.[2] The term תעודה, used here and in 8:20,[3] occurs elsewhere only in Ruth 4:7. The context gives it there a legal connotation. The passage in Ruth concerns the reciprocal act of transferring sandals as a ratification of legal transactions.[4] Isaiah's action has a legal connotation.[5]

Although it is uncertain if תעודה actually denotes a literary genre of the prophetic words in 8:16,[6] there is reason to believe that the bound testimony and the sealed torah to some extent consisted of a literary deposit entrusted to the disciples.[7] The OT says elsewhere that literary documents were sealed (1 Kgs 21:8; Jer 32:10–14, 44).[8] Isa 29:11 compares the prophet's vision with the words of the sealed scroll (הספר החתום).[9] In 8:1f; 30:8 Yahweh tells the prophet to write down his message.[10] 30:8 is particularly instructive. The prophet faces rejection when the people refuses the torah of Yahweh (30:9–11). In this situation Yahweh commands Isaiah to "write it (כתבה) on a tablet (לוח) with (before) them (אתם) and inscribe it (חקה) upon a scroll (ספר), that it may be for a future day, to a witness (לעד) for ever." As we noticed earlier, the verse contains perhaps an allusion to Isaiah's disciples in 8:16.[11] There are also other similarities. The term תורה is again connected with Isaiah's action, and the action is again to function as a witness in time of rejection. It is difficult to avoid the impression that 30:8 presents a phenomenon similar to the one depicted in 8:16 as a literary procedure.

We could add other prophetic texts. Scholars have often understood Jer 36:2–32 as a report about the origin of a written tradition, with numerous attempts to identify the substance of the scrolls.[12] Although these attempts seem futile,[13] the passage clearly maintains that Jeremiah composed written

---

[1] The term צור mostly denotes the tying up of a purse (Deut 14:25; 2 Kgs 5:23; 12:11. Cf. also Ezek 5:3).

[2] The related term עדה is used together with תורה. The Mosaic torah then functions as a testimony. See D. JONES, *ZAW* 67 (1955) 234f; VAN LEEUWEN, *THAT* II, 218; OSWALT, *Isaiah*, 235.

[3] The occurrence in 8:20 probably depends on 8:16.

[4] VIBERG, *Symbols of Law*, 155.

[5] The hiphil of עוד might suggest that תעודה means "warning." This does not exclude a legal connotation. Cf. WILDBERGER, *Jesaja* I, 345; WATTS, *Isaiah* I, 122.

[6] *Contra* GEVERYAHU, *JBQ* 18 (1989–90) 65f.

[7] Scholars thinking of a literary deposit often identify it with the memoirs of Isaiah (6:1–9:6), or parts of it. Different proposals are listed by BOOGAART, *Restoration*, 92.

[8] Cf. also the enigmatic expression בספר התורה החתום in CD 5:2.

[9] This verse is often regarded as a later gloss. If this is the case, it illustrates that some of Isaiah's visions were associated with literary deposits quite early.

[10] Cf. ZIMMERLI, *TLZ* 104 (1979) 483f.

[11] See above p. 41.

[12] Cf. e.g. RIETZSCHEL, *Urrolle;* BAUMANN, *ZAW* 80 (1968) 350–373; KESSLER, *ZAW* 81 (1969) 381–383; HOLLADAY, *VT* 30 (1980) 452–467; DEARMAN, *JBL* 109 (1990) 403–421.

[13] HERRMANN, *TRE* 16 (1987) 574, calls it "ein aussichtsloses Unterfangen."

scrolls through Baruch. Other texts also claim that Jeremiah wrote down his message (29:1–32; 30:2; 51:60–64) or dictated to Baruch words to be written down in a book (45:1). There are similar accounts about Ezekiel. Some scholars think that Ezekiel was accompanied by a scribe;[1] others understand the rather technical manner in which the Ezekiel tradition apparently was elaborated as a sign of its literary character.[2] While these assumptions are difficult to prove, the texts claim that Ezekiel was acquainted with written media (2:9–3:3; 24:2; 37:16, 20; 43:11). Taken together,[3] these scattered pieces of information imply that written texts were used to transmit prophetic traditions.[4] The existence of scribal schools in ancient Israel,[5] suggesting that certain circles employed written media to transmit various verbal traditions, further substantiates the impression.

There is, however, no evidence that written transmission was separated from oral currencies in prophetic circles.[6] Some would even have faced practical difficulties with the act of writing and with finding writing material.[7] The prophets delivered their messages mainly orally. Isaiah's literary activity was probably not extensive: 8:1 tells only of four words put into writing; 30:8 speaks perhaps of no more than three, the cryptic end of 30:7.[8] It is likely that he supplemented the written deposit handed over to the disciples with some oral instruction.[9] The binding of a testimony and the sealing of a torah "among my disciples" (בלמדי) imply perhaps that the group of disciples was a social embodiment of the tradition.[10] It was present in their midst both in writing and orally. The rather extensive references to writing in Jeremiah are constantly related to oral procedures. The written texts reflect oral speech: the writing of Jeremiah is the recording of words spoken by Yahweh (30:2); the writing of Baruch is the recording of oral utterances from Jeremiah (36:4; 45:1)—words which Jeremiah even repeats from memory a second time (36:32). And the written texts are constantly actualized through oral and audible reading (36:3, 6, 8, 10–16, 21,

---

[1] WEVERS, *Ezekiel*, 12; BROWNLEE, *Ezekiel 1–19*, xxxvi.

[2] CLEMENTS, Chronology of Redaction, 287–294.—E.F. DAVIS, *Swallowing the Scroll*, argues the thesis that Ezekiel developed an archival speech form intentionally oriented toward subsequent reformulation of the tradition.

[3] Cf. also Hab 2:2.

[4] Cf. WIDENGREN, *Literary and Psychological Aspects*, 68–78; GUNNEWEG, *Tradition*, 32–41; LINDBLOM, *Prophecy*, 163f; ZIMMERLI, *TLZ* 104 (1979) 483–489.

[5] Cf. excursus 2 above.

[6] Cf. RÜGER, Oral Tradition, 113–119.

[7] Cf. PFEIFER, *VT* 41 (1991) 123–127, though he does not discuss oral tradition and transmission.

[8] ENGNELL, *SBU* I, 1144.

[9] Cf. EATON, *VT* 9 (1959) 149.

[10] Cf. the function of Isaiah and his children as signs and portents in 8:18. Perhaps the physical children of Isaiah were among the disciples. Cf. above p. 40.

23f; 51:61, 63).[1] There is an oral element both in composing and actualizing the written texts. The elaboration of the Ezekiel tradition not only shows to a process of literary character, but it may also reveal that certain material was internalized.[2] Some texts indicate the close connection between literacy and orality: written scrolls are coupled with images suggesting the internalization of texts (2:9–3:3);[3] writing needs oral explanation (37:16–28; 43:10f) or is followed by the command to speak in the form of a mashal (24:2f). The distinction between written and oral transmission is not to be drawn too sharply.[4]

Within the present OT scholarship, the old (German) literary criticism "has lost its general acceptance."[5] The assumption that the growth of the prophetic traditions reflects literary work with written sources is open to question,[6] as some scholars recognized long ago.[7] The distinction between oral and written media was fluid in ancient Israel—even within the whole ancient Oriental culture.[8] It is therefore difficult to regard the work of the prophetic disciples as an exclusively literary process.[9] To be sure, I have not been able to trace the historicity of each text here; nor was it possible to perform a detailed tradition-historical investigation of units in the prophetic writings.[10] But if I may still generalize somewhat, *the constant lack of a clear differentiation between written and oral media suggests that there was an interaction between literacy and orality.* This implies that the living settings in which the media *functioned as they were conveyed* also must be taken into account.

---

[1] Cf. also 29:29.

[2] WEVERS, *Ezekiel,* 26–28, stresses the oral means of transmitting the Ezekiel tradition.

[3] Cf. STACEY, *Prophetic Drama,* 174f.

[4] *Contra* CLEMENTS, Chronology of Redaction, 287. Clements relies entirely on studies by W.J. Ong. For an account of the interaction between literacy and orality from a phenomenological point of view, see ANDERSEN, Oral Tradition, 17–58.

[5] RENDTORFF, Historical Criticism, 302. Cf. also KNIERIM, Criticism, 128–136.

[6] This assumption becomes especially evident in the study of WILLI-PLEIN, *Vorformen.*

[7] NYBERG, *ZAW* 52 (1934) 241–254; *idem, Studien,* was one of the first scholars to see this in the OT. The changed view is reflected in Mowinckel's publications. In his study of Jeremiah, MOWINCKEL, *Zur Komposition des Buches Jeremiah, passim,* first worked on the assumption that there existed literary sources. Later, in *idem, Tradition,* 62, 105 n. 61, he believed that there were oral traditions within circles of transmitters. Some years later, RINGGREN, *ST* 3 (1949) 34, considered it to be established that oral and written transmission are complementary despite the lack of consensus on several other issues relating to the problem.

[8] For religio-historical accounts of the ancient Orient, see the different views of BIRKELAND, *Traditionswesen,* 7–13; WIDENGREN, *Literary and Psychological Aspects,* 11–56; E. NIELSEN, *Oral Tradition,* 18–38. Cf. also the cautious remarks by ENGNELL, *Call of Isaiah,* 57; *idem, Essays,* 8f, 165f; KOCH, *Formgeschichte,* 99f.

[9] Cf. ENGNELL, *Call of Isaiah,* 59f; *idem, Essays,* 168f.—RINGGREN, *TLZ* 91 (1966) 641–650, points out the need to combine several methods in OT exegesis.

[10] Already RINGGREN, *ST* 3 (1949) 34, 59, called for more detailed investigations.

3.2.2. The Prophet and the Oral Interaction of Traditions

The use of written and oral means of transmission may exhibit various emphasis depending on the transmitters.[1] It is probable that different circles of tradents transmitted in different ways because of alternating education.[2] This may, for instance, allow for the prominent existence of written documents within certain (scribal) circles.[3] However, *the traditions usually functioned as orally communicated material.* The transmitters were involved in an oral act of communicating a written or oral text. Some further—allegedly very general—considerations point to the functional interaction between the two media.

The actualization and handing over of a written or oral text was an oral event. Ancient texts were often committed to memory.[4] They were oral texts and their actualization and communication was bound to be oral. Transmission was oral.[5] The references in the prophetic writings imply that even written texts were communicated as oral texts. Silent reading was practised only rarely in antiquity.[6] People usually read aloud. The manner of speaking in Josh 1:8 illustrates the ancient practice:[7] meditating (הגה) on the book of the law day and night is equated with never allowing it to be separated from *the mouth.*

The reception of a text was consequently also connected with orality. *Orality related to aurality.* The texts should be heard. S. Talmon gives several examples from the OT.[8] The fundamental exhortation to Israel was that the people should hear the words of Yahweh by having them constantly present as oral and written words (Deut 6:4–9).[9] The texts were not only orally articulated and handed over. The delivery was also auricularly internalized by the recipient.

---

1   Cf. KIRKPATRICK, *Folklore Study,* 66f.

2   AHLSTRÖM, *HTR* 59 (1966) 69f. Cf. also ROFÉ, *Prophetical Stories,* 120f.

3   Cf. FISHBANE, *Biblical Interpretation,* 23–88.

4   For discussion and literature, see RIESNER, *Lehrer,* 119–123.

5   WIDENGREN, *Literary and Psychological Aspects,* 90f, admits that written texts often were "learnt by heart, read aloud and dictated." He still thinks that transmission was mainly a literary phenomenon separated from oral procedures. In my view, transmission also involved the oral act of communication.

6   BALOGH, *Philologus* 82 (1927) 84–109, 202–240.—BALOGH, *ibid.,* 220, concludes his broad survey of the texts: "Der Mensch des Altertums las und schrieb in der Regel laut; das Gegenteil war zwar nicht unerhört, doch immer eine Ausnahme." For recent discussion and further literature, see GITAY, *JBL* 99 (1980) 190–194; BARTHOLOMEW, *Semeia* 39 (1987) 69–96; BOOMERSHINE, *Semeia* 39 (1987) 47–68; GRAHAM, *Beyond the Written Word,* 31–33; ACHTEMEIER, *JBL* 109 (1990) 16f; GERHARDSSON, Gospel Tradition, 519f; TALMON, Oral Tradition and Written Transmission, 150; SLUSSER, *JBL* 111 (1992) 499.

7   Cf. L. KÖHLER, *ZAW* 32 (1912) 240.

8   Oral Tradition and Written Transmission, 148–156.

9   Cf. also Deut 9:1.

It is possible that oral traditions had a higher status than written traditions in ancient Israel,[1] as was later the case in early Christian, rabbinic and Greco-Roman environments.[2] Whatever the exact status of the means of transmission, there is some evidence that *written and oral media for carrying the tradition interacted with each other as communicative and oral speeches already in ancient Israel.*

How did this interactive means of transmission correlate with the settings and the motives of transmission reflected in the prophetic writings? It did not depend on a theoretical doctrine about the written and oral character of the tradition. The prophetic master was not important merely as a carrier of traditions that were to be oral by definition. In addition to the general dominance of orality, it probably depended on factors *inherent* in the traditions themselves. The traditions contained divine teaching given through certain prophets mentioned by name. The divine teaching was of vital importance to the transmitters, but it was, as we saw in the previous chapter, often important *as part of the life of specific prophets.* This importance of the traditions influenced the settings and the motives of transmission, which, in turn, furthered the interactive means of transmission. Written traditions of such importance could never be completely removed from the situation of the transmitters. They interacted with oral traditions. *The means of transmission depended to a certain extent on the attachment to the divine teaching given through specific prophets.*

3.3. The Righteous Teacher and the Written Transmission

In a rather recent lecture on oral tradition and written transmission at Qumran, Talmon closed with some comments on the transmission of the teaching from the Righteous Teacher.[3] Transmission took place, according to Talmon, as an audible reception of written texts reflecting the oral proclamation of the Teacher without major hermeneutical shifts. In view of the singular standing of the Teacher and his teaching, it is probable that the Qumranites collected and wrote down the Teacher's pronouncements quite early, and that these written texts "became part of the *Torah* which the Covenanters studied periodically, audibly proclaiming his message, both from memory and manuscript."[4]

It is significant that Talmon ends his discussion by relating the general problem of oral tradition and written transmission to the authoritative position of the Teacher and his teaching. Scholars usually pass over this question with silence. The oral pre-history of the written texts may, however,

---

1 RUPRECHT, *ZTK* 87 (1990) 55.
2 ACHTEMEIER, *JBL* 109 (1990) 3–27; L. ALEXANDER, Living Voice, 221–247.
3 Oral Tradition and Written Transmission, 157f.
4 Oral Tradition and Written Transmission, 158. Talmon refers here to 1QS 6:7f.

best be left open. There are no references to writing as a result of previous oral performances—such as we find in the prophetic literature. It is certainly legitimate to assume that the Teacher conveyed teaching by speaking. But the oral proclamation of the Teacher can only be defined if the written material that reflects his teaching is properly identified and isolated, and if oral techniques of composition are visible within this material. Both these steps involve a large amount of hypothetical presuppositions. In addition, there is some indication that the Teacher was a scribe.[1] But Talmon points out two other essential features: the dominance of written material at Qumran and the audibility of the texts. Since a theoretical distinction between oral and written tradition and transmission is missing in the scrolls, we must also here use the indirect testimony of the present texts as primary evidence and pay attention to the *function* of the traditions within the community.

3.3.1. The Written Teaching

Josephus tells about the prominence of written transmission among the Essenes. The person desiring to enter the group (αἵρεσις) does not obtain immediate admittance (Bell. 2:137). Among the various vows he has to make, "in addition, he swears to hand over (μεταδοῦναι) the doctrines to no one differently than as he received (μετέλαβεν) them ... and to preserve (συντηρήσειν) in like manner both the books of their group and the names of the angels" (Bell. 2:142).[2] Although Josephus might think that the doctrines are transmitted orally, he clearly states his view about the careful preservation of the books of the community. The evidence from Qumran itself does not contradict this depiction of the Essenes.[3]

The numerous fragments from the caves near Khirbet Qumran reveal the prominent use of written media within the community.[4] We cannot always be sure that the scrolls originated at Qumran. But it is probable that the Qumranites used them.[5] As we saw in chapter one, educated scribes seem to have been active at Qumran.[6] There was a thorough acquaintance with written texts.

The data from archaeology confirm this impression. The excavations have revealed the existence of a building where scribal activity was per-

---

[1]   See above pp. 49f.
[2]   Cf. also Bell. 2:136, 159.
[3]   BEALL, *Josephus' Description of the Essenes,* 85, 87–89.
[4]   I am not convinced by the new theories arguing that Khirbet Qumran contains the remnants of a villa or fortress unrelated to the scrolls. For a refutation of these views, see BETZ/RIESNER, *Jesus, Qumran und der Vatikan,* 67–76; SHANKS, *BARev* 19:2 (1993) 65–68; *idem, BARev* 19:3 (1993) 62–65.
[5]   Cf. TALMON, Oral Tradition and Written Transmission, 128 n. 3.
[6]   See above pp. 49f, 69f.

formed, the so-called scriptorium. Since this room belongs to period two in R. de Vaux's fivefold archaeological stratification,[1] it is reasonable to assume that a scriptorium existed at Qumran some time between 4 B.C.E. and 68 C.E.

As is well known by now, the archaeological work led by de Vaux brought forth indication of a location used for copying MSS.[2] In 1953, in a room, the ceiling of which had collapsed, the excavators discovered remnants from another room on the first floor. The findings consisted of different pieces of mudbrick. As they were put together, a long table emerged. It became evident that the fragments belonged to more than one such table. The room also contained a low bench and a platform with two cavities on its surface. Subsequently excavators found two inkwells—one made of earthenware and one of bronze—containing dried ink.[3] Although questions about the precise function of the furniture remain,[4] other hypotheses concerning this room remain unlikely.[5]

3.3.2. The Teacher and the Written Teaching

When Philo compares the Essenes with the Therapeutae, he points out that the latter had writings (συγγράμματα) from their founders (Vit. Cont. 29). A group comparable to the Essenes used, according to Philo, written media from the founders.

The wide diffusion of written texts and the scribal activity at Qumran make it likely that the Qumranites used written media to preserve the teaching of the Righteous Teacher as well. But it is difficult to substantiate this claim further. The traditions from the Teacher are anonymous in the written texts. Perhaps the Teacher's priestly task to make juridical decision and pronounce normative halakhah gives some confirmation.[6] This task is implicit in the use of various forms of ירה, and therefore in the didactic designation מורה.[7] Deut 17:10–12 equates the priest's teaching with judgement

---

[1] Cf. DE VAUX, *Archaeology and the Dead Sea Scrolls*, 1–45.

[2] DE VAUX, *RB* 61 (1954) 212. Cf. also *idem, Archaeology and the Dead Sea Scrolls*, 29–33.

[3] For pictures of the different items, see DE VAUX, *RB* 61 (1954) 206–236 pls. 9, 10b. The third inkwell on pl. 10b was not found in the same room (*ibid.*, 212 n. 1). Cf. also *idem, Archaeology and the Dead Sea Scrolls*, pl. 21.

[4] METZGER, *RevQ* 1 (1959) 509–515; PEDLEY, *RevQ* 2 (1959) 26–37. Cf. also P.R. DAVIES, *Qumran*, 44f.

[5] WINTON THOMAS, *ALUOS* 6 (1969) 10f, conjectures that the room was some kind of office. DRIVER, *ALUOS* 6 (1969) 23–27, proposes that the tables were merely refectory tables, but he does not offer any explanation for the two inkwells. Similar criticism may be labelled against the new proposal by Pauline and Robert Donceel-Voute, suggesting that the scriptorium was a Roman-style dining room. See SHANKS, *BARev* 19:2 (1993) 67.

[6] WEINGREEN, *Bible*, 108–112, puts teaching and the giving of halakhic pronouncements against each other. This is of course not necessary.

[7] See above p. 50.

(משפט) and claims that disobedience to the teaching should be punished by death. Other OT passages using forms of ירה for priestly teaching are not as evident in this regard, but it is possible to interpret them in a similar manner.[1] The LXX gives additional support. It frequently translates the hiphil of ירה with forms of νομοθετεῖν,[2] once with ἀποκρίνεσθαι (Mic 3:11). And Bell. 2:145, 152 say that the name of a certain lawgiver (νομοθέτης) is held in high esteem among the Essenes,[3] though it is, as we saw, uncertain if this refers to the Teacher. The rabbinic evidence is also of interest. Although מורה never became prominent as a title for teachers in the first centuries C.E.,[4] a number of instances with the hiphil of ירה testify to a use implying an enforcement of halakhah. The exegesis of Deut 17:8–13 in m. Sanh. 11:2; Sifre on Deut 17:12 gives the clearest evidence. There are further instances using the participial form—in the singular or the plural—in the same sense.[5] The stipulations of the priestly leaders were binding to the Qumranites.[6] CD 6:7–10; 20:27–34 show that also precepts of the Teacher were of uttermost significance.[7] It is consequently probable that the Qumranites thought that the Teacher, whom they regarded as a priest, had issued normative halakhah.

The Qumranites performed mishnaic studies on the basis of the written halakhah.[8] Scholars have, as we noticed, given various proposals concerning the presence of the teaching from the Teacher in the documents. The Temple scroll is a conceivable example of a written halakhah from the Teacher,[9] though we have already seen the difficulties in ascertaining who its author was. The strongest candidate is perhaps the document prescribing "some of the works (or words) of the Torah" (החורה [דברי or] מקצת מעשי) —usually referred to as 4QMMT.[10] E. Qimron and J. Strugnell, who were the prospective editors, claimed that it constitutes an important halakhic letter which the Teacher himself perhaps wrote and sent to the priests in Jerusalem.[11] R. Eisenman and M. Wise have presented an eclectic text divided

---

1 Cf. Lev 10:11; 14:57; Deut 24:8; 33:10; Ezek 44:23; 2 Chr 15:3. The use of 2 Chr 15:3 by WEINGREEN, *Bible,* 110; REEVES, *RevQ* 13 (1988) 293f, to prove the halakhic significance of מורה is somewhat circular. Weingreen's similar interpretation of Isa 9:14 (*ibid.,* 110f) is unconvincing.
2 Cf. Exod 24:12; Deut 17:10; Pss 24:8, 12; 26:11; 83:7; 118:33, 102, 104.
3 Cf. also Hypothetica in Eusebius, Praep. Ev. VIII 11:1 (ὁ ἡμέτερος νομοθέτης).
4 See above p. 52f.
5 Cf. e.g. m. ʾAbot 5:8; b. ʿErub. 63a; b. Pesah. 3b; b. Ketub. 79a.
6 Cf. e.g. 1QS 5:7–10; 9:7.
7 Cf. also 1QpHab 2:2; 8:1–3; 1QpMic 8–10:6f.
8 J.M. BAUMGARTEN, *JSJ* 3 (1972) 9.
9 WACHOLDER, *Dawn of Qumran,* 1–140.
10 KAPERA, Bibliography, 75–80, lists the studies and comments made on 4QMMT until 1991.
11 Unpublished Halakhic Letter, 400–407. Cf. also STRUGNELL, Qumran Scrolls, 99f, 103f.

on two letters and preceded by the calendrical exposition.[1] Two indications suggest a connection between 4QMMT and the Teacher.[2] First, 4QpPs[a] 4:8f relates the persecution of the Righteous (Teacher) by the wicked (priest) closely to "the torah which he sent to him" (התורה אשר שלח אליו). This could suggest that the Teacher sent a written document of special importance to the priestly authorities, though the text is not entirely clear at this point. Second, the implied author of 4QMMT exhibits unusual authority. He issues extra-biblical rules as halakhic interpretations of biblical proof-texts, using the first person plural. There is no discussion about the validity of the rules. The Dead Sea scrolls accord such an authority to no other person than the Righteous Teacher. In addition, although 4QMMT probably was sent from the community to another place,[3] fragments of no less than six separate MSS have been found in cave four (4Q394–399). It had apparently attained a public status of decisive value to the Qumranites.[4] They preserved it as normative tradition. Perhaps we have here an example of what was preserved, copied and studied as written tradition from the Righteous Teacher.

3.3.3. The Teacher and the Audibility of the Teaching

The biblical proof-text from Deut 18:18f, quoted in 4QTestim 5–8, states the importance of listening to the Mosaic prophet. As God's voice was once heard through his servant Moses,[5] so God will in the future put his words on the lips of the Mosaic prophet. The person who does not listen (שמע) to these words will be called to account before God.

The Qumranites probably regarded the Righteous Teacher as a prophet like Moses.[6] This conception implied an oral communication from the prophet to the community. While the proof-text stresses obedience first of all, it also describes the means of transmission in oral terms. Not only did the Qumranites think that the biblical Israel was urged to listen to Yahweh (1QM 10:3; 11QT 61:15),[7] but they were themselves also to listen to the Righteous Teacher speaking the words of God.[8]

---

[1] *Dead Sea Scrolls,* 190–192, 198f.

[2] Cf. e.g. STEGEMANN, Die "Mitte der Schrift," 160, 163; REEVES, *RevQ* 13 (1988) 296f; STEGEMANN, 'Teacher of Righteousness', 197, 209; TALMON, Oral Tradition and Written Transmission, 147f; BETZ/RIESNER, *Jesus, Qumran und der Vatikan,* 54.—SCHIFFMAN, *RevQ* 14 (1990) 435, speaks of the "leaders of the sect" as authors.

[3] Cf. CALLAWAY, *RevQ* 14 (1990) 649.

[4] TALMON, Oral Tradition and Written Transmission, 148.

[5] Cf. 4QDibHam[a] 5:13f.

[6] See above pp. 124f.

[7] Cf. also 1QDM 2:1; 11QT 56:11; 61:11; 64:6.— In 11QT 54:12–14 the testing of Israel concerns the question of loving (אהב) Yahweh "with all your heart and with all your soul" (בכול לבבכם ובכול נפשכמה), which implies walking after (הלך אחרי) him, serving (עבד) him and listening (שמע) to his voice.

[8] Cf. WISE, *Temple Scroll,* 187.

The scrolls accordingly describe the reception of the Teacher's instructions as an audible event. CD 20:28, 32 picture, in a parallel manner,[1] the recognition of certain statutes and precepts as listening to (שמע) and giving ear to (האזין) the voice (קול) of the (Righteous) Teacher. CD 20:33 implies that the Qumranites did not reject the righteous statutes which they heard (שמע). I have already illustrated the connection between CD 20:27–33 and 1QSa 1:6–9.[2] Hearing the voice of the Teacher was an act of study. 1QSa 1:1–5 envisions the assembling of all the members of the messianic community and tells about priests who "read into their ears" (קראו בא[וני]המה]) all the statutes of the covenant and all the precepts (1QSa 1:4f). This pictures the reading of not only the Scriptures, but also of the specific principles and teaching of the community.[3] CD 20:27, 29, 31 mentions statutes of the covenant and precepts in relation to hearing the voice of the Teacher. Transformed from a messianic vision into historical realities, this suggests that the written traditions of the community were read *and* heard. The written traditions from the Righteous Teacher were not devoid of oral and aural functions within the transmission process.[4] *The written means used for carrying the traditions related to aural means used for conveying them.*

The Qumranites understood the Righteous Teacher as *the* person with whom interpretative rules and halakhic regulations of normative value had originated. He was not merely one among many teachers carrying and interpreting traditions which by definition should be oral. The means of transmission depended on factors *inherent* in the traditions themselves. They contained vital rules and regulations. But the scribal character of the Qumran community makes it unlikely that there was, as in the prophetic transmission, an interaction between traditions preserved with written and oral media. The Qumranites preserved the teaching of the Righteous Teacher mainly by written media, it seems. And they probably copied and studied the written texts within the school.[5] In addition to the inherent value of the traditions, the notion that the rules and the regulations should come from the Teacher affected the means of transmission. There was a specific emphasis on *hearing* the voice of the Teacher. The written traditions should be audibly conveyed. *The means of transmission depended to a certain ex-*

---

1   Cf. below pp. 189f.
2   See above p. 73.
3   SCHIFFMAN, *Eschatological Community,* 13.
4   Cf. also CD 6:3; 1QH 4:24; 1QpHab 2:2(?).—TALMON, Oral Tradition and Written Transmission, 157f, believes that the phrases "and now listen" (ועתה שמעו) or "and now listen to me" (ועתה שמעו אלי) in CD 1:1; 2:2, 14 are prefaces to sermons delivered by the Teacher. This is possible. In 4Q525 1:1 the speaker starts perhaps (cf. the similar closure of the speech in 4Q525 1:12) with "and now listen to me" (ועתה שמעו לי). In 4Q298 1:1f the Maskil starts by calling "give ear to me" (האזי[נו לי) and with the command "listen" (ש[מע]ו).
5   This does not necessarily mean that the traditions were entirely fixed. Scribes could occasionally interpret—"improve"—the texts.

tent on attachment to the rules and regulations given by the Righteous Teacher.

4. The Preservation and Elaboration of Traditions

"The preservation and elaboration of traditions" concern *acts for maintaining and extending the object of transmission.* I leave the initial articulation of the transmitted texts out of consideration here. The material exhibits many different emphases. I am asking only about features that correlated with the settings and the motives described in chapters one and two.

4.1. The Rabbis and the Preservation of Torah

The theoretical emphasis on preserving oral torah suggests that the rabbis claimed to maintain torah in strict continuity with the received tradition. Although they did perform elaborative work, torah was to the rabbis *in principle preserved* torah. It is reasonable to ask how this picture of preservative transmission corresponded to the influence of specific masters.

4.1.1. The Definition and Collection of Legal Torah

The legal agenda of particular rabbis may *on certain occasions* give some information about the importance accorded to an individual teacher in the process of preserving torah. J. Neusner and his students have stressed that the teaching of a rabbi is best studied by focusing on the legal material.[1] Neusner considers it possible that one way—among others—to define and collect the legal material at a premishnaic stage would have been along the lines of a single authority's name.[2]

The legal teaching connected with R. Eliezer b. Hyrcanus (c. 90 C.E.) is particularly suitable for the present purpose. Neusner has himself devoted a separate study to it,[3] and his investigation has become the methodological paradigm for the work of other scholars. The material also represents the teaching of a person who is presented as prominent and influential. It consists of over three hundred items. Two hundred and twenty eight of them

---

[1] For a general comment, see NEUSNER, Rabbinic Biography, 86f, who also lists studies by himself and his students using this method (*ibid.,* 86 n. 3). Cf. also *idem, Talmudic Biography,* 7, and the remarks by W.S. GREEN, Introduction, 1–3; SALDARINI, Rabbinic Judaism, 452.

[2] Rabbinic Biography, 88.

[3] *Eliezer ben Hyrcanus* I–II. The detailed arguments are presented in more accessible form in *idem, Talmudic Biography.*—GILAT, *R. Eliezer ben Hyrcanus,* is not relevant here. He is not primarily interested in the development of the traditions (*ibid.,* 14).

are of legal character.[1] The material is large enough to allow some conclusions.[2]

Neusner makes three important observations. First, in spite of the opposition that Eliezer himself probably met, the traditions do not attribute conflicting and extraneous teaching to him until in later tannaitic and early amoraic times.[3] The views attributed to Eliezer in the best traditions are coherent. The teaching expressing the opinion of Eliezer in legal matters was defined quite early—perhaps before the Bar Cochba war (132–135 C.E.).[4] Second, there is not much indication that one diminished the importance of Eliezer's teaching by suppressing material originally attributed to him.[5] While this apparently did happen, its infrequency shows that his teaching was rather firmly defined and linked with his name. Third, there are reminiscences of collections containing Eliezer's teaching in the rabbinic writings.[6] Compilations of this kind usually serve as illustrations of a single principle of law. They reflect a thematic interest. But the Eliezer material contains indication also of collections which were not of the thematic type. R. Ila'i (c. 110), a disciple of Eliezer, refers with a threefold "I heard" (שמעתי) to three separate views of Eliezer in m. ʿErub. 2:6. R. Ila'i, it is said, looked for other disciples of Eliezer holding these views, but he found none. As it seems, he quoted from a collection the organizing principle of which was nothing else than Eliezer's name and authority.[7] The teaching was transmitted in clusters held together by the influence of Eliezer.

There are no signs that the Eliezer traditions were isolated in regard to literary form.[8] Most of them appear in six variations of the simple dispute form. The simple dispute is the characteristic form of the material connected with the houses of Shammai and Hillel.[9] The forms did not originate with Eliezer or with his disciples, nor with persons transmitting material from other teachers of the same generation. It is possible that the traditions related to certain rabbis of minor importance appeared in forms pertaining only to an individual teacher. J.N. Lightstone claims that the peripheral interest in R. Jose the Galilean (c. 110 C.E.) among the authorities producing the Mishnah and the Tosefta prevented the traditions attributed to him from being entirely standardized.[10] Some of the teaching assumed the fixed form

---

1 NEUSNER, *Eliezer ben Hyrcanus* II, 1–15.
2 NEUSNER, *JJS* 24 (1973) 65; idem, *Talmudic Biography,* 11f, admits the disadvantage of working with too small a body of material when he earlier studied the teaching connected with R. Joḥanan b. Zakkai. Cf. also SALDARINI, *JBL* 96 (1977) 266.
3 NEUSNER, *Eliezer ben Hyrcanus* II, 16, 63–91.
4 NEUSNER, *Eliezer ben Hyrcanus* II, 88.
5 NEUSNER, *Eliezer ben Hyrcanus* II, 205–224.
6 NEUSNER, *Eliezer ben Hyrcanus* II, 53–60.
7 Cf. also m. Šeb. 8:9f.
8 NEUSNER, *Eliezer ben Hyrcanus* II, 31f, 60.
9 Cf. NEUSNER, *Rabbinic Traditions* III, 5–14.
10 *Yosé the Galilean,* 166–169,186–188; idem, *JJS* 31 (1980) 37–45.

of independent sayings at a premishnaic stage. A group that was interested only in the single master transmitted the sayings. The transmitters did not intersect with others to any significant degree. But such evidence is not present within the Eliezer traditions. The formalized pattern of the rabbinic literature suggests that the general rule was the lack of forms which were specific to one teacher only.

One influence that a specific master could exhibit on the intention to perform preservative transmission was thus *the early definition and collection of legal teaching in accordance with his name and authority*. But it is impossible to draw any far-reaching conclusions about this phenomenon in rabbinic Judaism. The Eliezer tradition is rather special. And there is decisive and more general influence from another master, greater than Eliezer.

4.1.2. The Mosaic Origin of Torah

The rabbis cherished the view that all torah in principle originated with Moses at mount Sinai. Moses was the rabbi *par excellence*. It would surely be incorrect to call rabbinic Judaism "a conscious Mosaism."[1] The rabbis did not normally think that Moses was divine.[2] But they regarded him as the most authoritative teacher.[3] He was the supreme teacher of all Israel.[4] On several occasions, though not in the Mishnah,[5] the rabbinic literature refers to him plainly as "our teacher" (רבינו).[6]

As we see especially in b. ʿErub. 54b, it was vital for the rabbis that their teaching gave the impression of going back to Moses.[7] The ordination established the link down to the torah given by God to Moses at Sinai.[8] Reflecting the wide-spread custom of giving the teaching a spiritual genealogy, m. ʾAbot 1:1 places Moses at the head of the chain of tradition carriers.[9] Interpretations which *in reality* were new, were *in principle* preserved as traditions originating with Moses.[10] From him were both the written Torah and oral torah to come. Whatever was new, the rabbis believed, was

---

[1] *Contra* RENGSTORF, *TDNT* IV, 437. For criticism of this Mosaic notion, see ROTHKOFF, *EncJud* XII, 393.
[2] But for some minority circles, see MEEKS, Moses as God and King, 354–371. Cf. also *idem, Prophet-King,* 192–195.
[3] For numerous references to Moses as teacher in rabbinic literature, cf. ROSMARIN, *Moses,* 19 n.18 and n. 29, 26 n. 104, 27 n. 105 and n. 106.
[4] Cf. e.g. b. Roš Haš. 25b; Ruth Rab. 4:5; Tanḥ. B. ויקרא 4.
[5] ROTHKOFF, *EncJud* XII, 394.
[6] For references, cf. ROSMARIN, *Moses,* 27 n. 105.
[7] Cf. GERHARDSSON, *Memory,* 82, 120f; LENHARDT, *RSR* 66 (1978) 494–496.
[8] See above pp. 92f.
[9] Cf. BIKERMAN, *RB* 59 (1952) 44–54. In regard to the list in m. ʾAbot 1, he states (*ibid.,* 51): "A leur tour, les Pharisiens, après la mort de Hillel et de Shammai ... établirent la généalogie spirituelle de leur enseignement."
[10] Cf. BAMBERGER, *HUCA* 16 (1941) 97–113.

already inherent in the torah which God gave to Moses at Sinai.

Episodes and episodal statements make this need to claim a Mosaic origin more explicit. The most striking episode occurs perhaps in b. Menaḥ. 29b. Moses had been transported in time to attend the school of R. Akiba († c. 135 C.E). He felt disturbed at his inability to comprehend Akiba's teaching. It was then declared that Akiba had as a matter of fact received this teaching as a tradition from Moses at Sinai. And Moses was comforted. The episode shows that although the rabbis knew that certain teaching did not come from Moses, they still, in principle, held on to the Mosaic origin of their doctrines.[1] A statement in y. Peʾa 17a accordingly declares that whatever new teaching someone brings forth, it was already given to Moses.[2] It also happens that certain texts connect the persons giving the new teaching with Moses himself. According to Sifre on Deut 34:7, for instance, important masters like Hillel, R. Joḥanan b. Zakkai and R. Akiba lived for one hundred and twenty years, just as Moses did. In b. Beṣa 38b the name "Moses" functions even as an honorary title for distinguished teachers. These scattered episodes and episodal statements suggest that the relation to Moses validated the new teaching—and occasionally also the teachers themselves.

The aim to transmit all teaching as if it originated with Moses is evident also in more formal expressions attached to the material. The rabbis sometimes transmitted a new teaching explicitly as a tradition given to Moses at Sinai.[3] Many texts designate individual halakhic teaching as "halakhah (given) to Moses from Sinai" (הלכה למשה מסיני).[4] There are numerous examples in the Tosefta, the two Talmuds and the Sifra. The Mishnah uses the expression on three significant occasions (m. Peʾa 2:6; m. ʿEd. 8:7; m. Yad. 4:3). It always ends a chain of tradition carriers. The occurrence in m. Peʾa 2:6 is related to the school of R. Gamaliel I Ha-Zaḳen (c. 30–40 C.E.) and uttered by Nahum ha-Lablar. The chain of tradition carriers preceding the formula is here the longest of the three occasions,[5] reminiscent of the authorities listed in m. ʾAbot 1. The other two occurrences are related to the school at Jamnia and uttered by two disciples of R. Joḥanan b. Zakkai († c. 80): R. Joshua b. Ḥanania (m. ʿEd. 8:7) and R. Eliezer b. Hyrcanus (m. Yad. 4:3).[6] They link their own statements with the halakhah given to Moses at Sinai—regardless of the fact that the statements cannot be traced to

---

1 Cf. URBACH, Talmudic Sage, 137.
2 Cf. also b. Meg. 19b; y. Meg. 74d; Lev. Rab. 22:1; Qoh. Rab. on 1:10.
3 Cf. e.g. t. Peʾa 2:2; 3:2; t. Sukk. 3:1; b. Meg. 19b; y. Meg. 74d; Qoh. Rab. on 1:10.
4 For discussion, see BACHER, *Tradition und Tradenten,* 25–46; MOORE, *Judaism* I, 30, 256–258; *idem, Judaism* III, 76–79; JACOBS, *EncJud* VII, 1167; SCHÄFER, *Studien,* 161f, 184–186; SAFRAI, Halakha, 180–185; E.P. SANDERS, *Jewish Law,* 122f.
5 Cf. the somewhat shorter version in Tanḥ B. במדבר 27.
6 Cf. also t. Yad. 2:16.

any teacher between Joḥanan and Moses.[1] The formula functioned, at least among the rabbis themselves,[2] to validate halakhic statements which were not recorded in the Scripture or derived by hermeneutical rules.[3]

We cannot assume that all early definitions and collections of the traditions related to a certain rabbi always followed procedures similar to the ones in the Eliezer traditions. The validation of the rabbis and the adherence to the teachers were not ends in themselves. The tie between the teacher and his pupils was not exclusive, it was relative.[4] The tradition carriers could change. The necessary "pastness" of rabbinic traditions sometimes caused the attraction of certain teaching to early and famous authorities: collective groups could attract torah, such as the men of the great synagogue (האנשי כנסת הגדולה),[5] the scribes (הסופרים),[6] the wise (החכמים),[7] the elders (הזקנים) or the fathers (האבות);[8] also individual rabbis could attract sayings, such as Simeon b. Sheṭaḥ (c. 90 B.C.E.) and Hillel (c. 20 B.C.E.)[9] or the famous Abba Arika († c. 247 C.E.),[10] called Rab. This tendency has to do with the need to validate the teaching by anchoring it in the past.[11] The ultimate motive of transmission was not the teacher himself. It was torah— in all its manifestations—originally given to Moses at Sinai.[12] Through its association with the different carriers of torah, the teaching became part of what was given to Moses at Sinai. *The notion that all torah in principle originated with Moses, the most prominent rabbi of all, exhibited a decisive influence on the preservative intention in the transmission.* No matter how strong the impact of the various tradition carriers was, the teaching was always directly or indirectly related to Moses, "our teacher."

---

[1] Cf. GUTTMANN, *HUCA* 16 (1941) 141f; NEUSNER, *Development,* 53.

[2] E.P. SANDERS, *Jewish Law,* 124, argues that the general attribution to Moses was "a game played only among Rabbis, not used by Pharisees against Sadducees." I do not need to enter into this debate.

[3] SCHÄFER, *Studien,* 161f n. 25; E.P. SANDERS, *Jewish Law,* 122, point out that it was not the whole torah but only individual halakhot that were traced back to Moses in this manner. But in principle, the written Torah and oral torah in its entirety were held to be from Moses.

[4] Cf. LENHARDT, *RSR* 66 (1978) 499: "Chaque relation de maître à disciple est partielle, intérieure et inférieure à la richesse totale qui provient de l'unique source mosaïque."

[5] MOORE, *Judaism* I, 31–36; SCHÜRER, *History* II, 358f; SIGAL, *Halakah of Jesus,* 47.

[6] SCHÜRER, *History* II, 341f, E.P. SANDERS, *Jewish Law,* 115–117.

[7] GUTTMANN, *HUCA* 16 (1941) 144–154.

[8] PATTE, *Jewish Hermeneutic,* 15.

[9] NEUSNER, *Rabbinic Traditions* I, 242.

[10] RIESNER, *Lehrer,* 201.

[11] Cf. LENHARDT, *RSR* 66 (1978) 489–516. For the same tendency in early Pharisaic paradosis, see A.I. BAUMGARTEN, *HTR* 80 (1987) 73–77.

[12] Cf. URBACH, Talmudic Sage, 133.

4.2. The Prophets and the Elaboration of Traditions

The prophetic literature—as well as the OT at large[1]—presents preservation and elaboration as in constant interchange. This does not necessarily
mean that the two were indistinguishable. But there is no explicit and theoretical interest in the preservation as isolated from the elaboration. It is
therefore necessary to focus more on *the growth and expansion* of the
prophetic traditions.

The prophetic books contain several levels of additions. D.L. Petersen
proposes a fivefold stratigraphy for the pre-exilic prophetic books.[2] The
original oracles and narratives were supplemented with pre-exilic additions, deuteronomistic redaction, deutero-prophetic additions and expan-
sionistic textual traditions. My interest is directed towards the transmission
that correlated with a close adherence to the individual prophet and his teaching. In a certain sense, it is natural that any addition to a text is anchored
in existing material. I. Willi-Plein thinks that this phenomenon occurs in all
work with written texts.[3] I assume a personal specificity in the transmission
process when there is a more *substantial connection* between the basic
tradition on one hand, and the growth and expansion on the other. It may
also be present if the creative activity appeared *before the emergence of a
plurality of prophetic traditions and books,* to which more or less uniform
additions were made.[4] The pre-exilic and deutero-prophetic additions, according to Petersen's classification, are therefore of most interest. Some
post-exilic additions to the books of exilic prophets are also relevant.

4.2.1. The Interpretation of Traditions

In an attempt to trace the antecedents of early Jewish exegesis within the
Hebrew Bible, M. Fishbane argues for the existence of a genetic and inner-
biblical exegesis.[5] He categorizes the exegesis as scribal, legal, aggadic and
mantological. There are indeed extreme difficulties involved in any effort
to ascertain the temporal distance and the authorial differentiation between
the exegetical comment and the basic text.[6] But once we acknowledge the
question about genetic relations between texts, Fishbane's study appears as a
convincing illustration of how ancient traditions grew in dependence on
material formulated earlier. We may detect a similar, though more dyna-

---

[1] Cf. e.g. FOHRER, *ZAW* 73 (1961) 1–30.
[2] *Prophecy,* 14.
[3] *Vorformen,* 264.
[4] For instance, the superscriptions may have been added at a later time, sometimes
by the same (Dtr) editor of several books. Cf. GEVARYAHU, Biblical Colophons, 42–59;
G.M. GORDIS, Superscriptions, 69.
[5] *Biblical Interpretation.*
[6] ESLINGER, *VT* 42 (1992) 47–58.

mic, phenomenon within the prophetic traditions themselves. There was, with W. Zimmerli,[1] an *inner-prophetic process of transmission*, from the utterances of the prophet to the prophetic book. We have already noticed the dependence of Second and Third Isaiah on the Isaiah tradition. I will here rely on the detailed studies of some major scholars and illustrate how *the interpretation of the prophetic traditions* occurs at several scattered instances in the prophetic books.[2]

H.W. Wolff and, to some extent, Willi-Plein indicate how the early transmitters depended on the traditions from Amos when they added new formulations and when they created biographical notices.[3] A follower of Amos probably created the episodal narrative in 7:(9)10–17 on the basis of existing material attached to his master:[4] the threat of deportation against Israel in 7:11, 17[5] is rooted in Amos' own words (5:5b, 27; 6:7);[6] the proclamation formula "hear the word of Yahweh" (שמע דבר יהוה) in 7:16 might have been shaped on the basis of the prophet's own use of "hear" (שמע) to call for attention (3:1, 13; 4:1; 5:1);[7] the quotation in 7:16 is introduced with the participle "you are saying" (אתה אמר) as was the practice of Amos himself (4:1; 6:13);[8] the common messenger formula "thus says Yahweh" (כה אמר יהוה) in 7:17 was repeatedly used by Amos (1:3, 6, 13; 2:1, 6; 3:11, 12; 5:3, 4, 16).[9] We could mention also other texts pointing to the faithful labor of the early transmitters. Wolff thinks they were at work at a number of instances, either by redacting existing collections or by adding their own glosses and compositions (1:1b; 5:5a, 14f; 6:2, 6b; 7:9; 8:3–14; 9:7–10).[10] The language, style and themes are often reminiscent of Amos' own preaching.[11] A group of skilled followers apparently adhered to the traditions from their master in their own creative work.[12]

---

1   Prophetic Proclamation, 94 n. 48.
2   Interpretation is here conceived of as a broader activity than the mere exegesis of written texts. A more restricted view dominates the work by FISHBANE, *Biblical Interpretation*.
3   WILLI-PLEIN, *Vorformen*, 263f; WOLFF, *Joel and Amos*, 108f.—SATO, *Q und Prophetie*, 324–326, uses Wolff's observations and speaks of "Jüngerprophetie" (subdivided into "Fortprophetie" and "Kommentar-Prophetie") in dependence on the "Meistersprache."
4   See above pp. 105f.
5   The threat is both times given with identical words (וישראל גלה יגלה מעל אדמתו).
6   In regard to the authenticity of passages reflecting Amos' own diction, I follow WOLFF, *Joel and Amos, ad loci*.
7   Cf. also 8:4. WOLFF, *Joel and Amos*, 108, 325, attributes 8:4 to the school of Amos.
8   Cf. also 9:10. WOLFF, *Joel and Amos*, 109, 346, attributes 9:7–10 to the school of Amos.
9   Cf. also 1:9, 11; 2:4, which most scholar do not attribute to Amos himself.
10   *Joel and Amos*, 108–110.
11   SATO, *Q und Prophetie*, 324–326, uses 5:14f; 6:2; 9:8–10 to illustrate this phenomenon in the book of Amos.
12   LINDBLOM, *Prophecy*, 241, thinks that there were scribes among Amos' disciples.

Willi-Plein traces Hos 13:1–3 back to Hosea's disciples.[1] The reference to
the death of Ephraim (13:1) suggests a date around 721 B.C.E. There are
some peculiarities in these verses: "Ephraim" (13:1) often refers to the
whole of Israel in Hosea,[2] but here it denotes only part of Israel; "Baal"
(13:1) also occurs elsewhere, but sometimes in the plural.[3] There are also
similarities with the rest of the book: "their silver" (כספם) and "idols"
(עצבים) mentioned in 13:2 are reminiscent of 8:4; "craftsmen" (חרשים) as
the makers of idols in 13:2 are mentioned in the singular in 8:6; the statement that the people are "like morning mist, and like dew vanishing early"
(כענן בקר וכטל משכים הלך) in 13:3 has a parallel in 6:4. It is difficult, however, to ascertain that 13:1–3 depends upon the terminology used in the
earliest strata of the Hosea tradition. The actual terms "Ephraim"[4] and
"Baal" may go back to Hosea himself, but the similarities with 6:4; 8:4, 6
are open to several explanations. The complicated history behind the collections of sayings in Hos 4–14 makes it difficult to determine to what extent the early transmitters imitated the prophet in their own creative work.[5]
Nevertheless, it is at least possible that the peculiarities and the similarities
together imply that an early group of followers shaped the text somewhat
independently, but still on the basis of earlier material.

> Willi-Plein discovers a terminological dependence on several occasions in Hosea.[6]
> However, since she regards this "Prinzip der Verankerung" as valid for all textual
> work, she does not find it important to trace the additions back to a group of Hosea's
> followers or to locate the basic verses on which the additions depend within the ear-
> liest strata of the tradition. In many cases she even considers it impossible. Although
> she thinks that 4:1–9:9 was put together on mnemo-technical principles,[7] the process
> of compilation is "zeitlich kaum fixierbar."[8]

H. Wildberger estimated that circa 40% of the material in Isa 1–39 originated with the prophet himself.[9] Other scholars have attempted to locate
important additions.[10] Already S. Mowinckel searched for the origin of the
tradition behind certain texts within a pre-exilic activity during the Assy-

---

1   *Vorformen,* 221.—SATO, *Q und Prophetie,* 326f, uses these verses in order to demonstrate how the disciples in their "Fortprophetie" imitated the "Meistersprache."
2   It is used altogether 37 times in the book.
3   2:15, 19; 11:2. The singular occurs in 2:10, 18 (9:10).
4   WILLI-PLEIN, *Vorformen,* 236–241; YEE, *Composition,* 306.
5   Jörg JEREMIAS, *Hosea,* 19, states: "Die Schüler haben offensichtlich die Worte
des Meisters nicht primär für Außenstehende zusammengestellt, sondern für sich selber
bzw. für Leser, die mit der Botschaft Hoseas schon vertraut waren." Cf. also ANDER-
SEN/FREEDMAN, *Hosea,* 59.
6   *Vorformen,* 264.
7   *Vorformen,* 129–178. Cf. already NYBERG, *Studien,* 18.
8   *Vorformen,* 244.
9   *Jesaja* III, 1510.
10   For surveys of research, see VERMEYLEN, *Isaïe* I, 5–30; WILDBERGER, *Jesaja*
III, 1529–1547; LAATO, *Immanuel,* 6–31.

rian period.[1] H. Barth developed Mowinckel's observations and suggested a creative activity directed against the Assyrian power during the time of Josiah (c. 640–609 B.C.E.).[2] J. Vermeylen aimed in a part of his study to demonstrate how a pre-exilic group of Isaianic disciples transmitted and expanded a nucleus of Isaianic words.[3]

Other scholars try to show that the early disciples imitated the language, style and themes of Isaiah in their own creative work. R.E. Clements, while sceptical of labels such as "disciple" and "school of Isaiah," discusses 10:16–19, 33f; 14:24–27; 17:12–14; 29:5–8; 31:5, 8f from this perspective.[4] He builds on Barth's study and dates the passages to the reign of Josiah. They were created on the basis of Isaianic language visible in the earlier material. The authors elaborated Isaianic themes in a midrashic fashion, according to Clements. Also M. Sato, an NT scholar, makes use of Barth's observations.[5] He points to 9:1–6; 10:16–19; 30:27–33 as products from Isaiah's disciples active between the end of the prophet's activity (c. 701 B.C.E.) and the fall of the Assyrian empire (c. 612 B.C.E.). The texts are salvific utterances building on and developing Isaiah's own preaching.

Two additional texts in Isa 1–39 may exemplify the phenomenon further. The nucleus of the episodal narrative in 20:1–6 must have been formulated circa 712 B.C.E.[6] Some independence might be detected, as is natural even for the most faithful disciple.[7] But the combination of words and the existence of certain idioms also reflect dependence on Isaiah's own diction:[8] "sign and portent" (אות ומופת) in 20:3 are terms used together in the plural by Isaiah himself (8:18); "and they will be dismayed" (וחתו) in 20:5 represents Isaiah's own terminology (30:31; 31:4);[9] "and they will be ashamed of" (ובשו מן) in 20:5 is Isaianic (1:29); the reference to "hope" (מבט) in 20:5 may reflect dependence on Isaiah's frequent use of the verb in hiphil (5:12; 8:22; 18:4; 22:8, 11).

---

[1] The following texts were attributed to this activity: 9:1–6; 10:5–27a, 27b–34; 11:1–9; 14:24–27; 17:12–14; 29:5–8, 17–24; 30:27–33; 31:5–9; 32:1–8, 15–20; 37:22–37. See MOWINCKEL, *Jesaja*, 119–123; *idem, Jesaja-disiplene,* 46–56, 115, 138f; *idem, AcOr* 11 (1933) 280–284, 289; *idem, Tradition,* 74–76.

[2] *Jesaja-Worte,* 1–275.

[3] *Isaïe* II, 655–692.

[4] *Deliverance,* 44–51.

[5] *Q und Prophetie,* 327–330.

[6] See above p. 108.

[7] *Contra* T. COLLINS, *Mantle of Elijah,* 28, rejecting the general idea of faithful disciples as transmitters by reference to the fact that the words of the prophets were not left intact.

[8] WILDBERGER, *Jesaja* II, 753f. In regard to the authenticity of passages reflecting Isaiah's own diction, I follow, with some additional comments, WILDBERGER, *Jesaja* I–III, *ad loci.*

[9] Cf. also 7:8b.—It is possible that part of Isa 30:27–33 originated in the 7th cent. So MOWINCKEL, *Jesaja-Disiplene,* 51f, 139; H. BARTH, *Jesaja-Worte,* 92–103; CLEMENTS, *Isaiah 1–39,* 252–254; SATO, *Q und Prophetie,* 329.

Scholars have indeed judged the authorship and date of 11:1–5(–9)[1] differently, from its attribution to Isaiah himself[2] to options for its exilic or post-exilic origin.[3] Vermeylen presents a middle position.[4] He sees some indication for a date during the seventh century. The historical occasion might have been the enthronement of Josiah circa 640 B.C.E.[5] The text reflects the quest for authority which occurred when the eight years old boy was to succeed his assassinated father Amon,[6] "the stump of Jesse." If this is correct, the text may have originated quite early. Although the language shows peculiarities,[7] the Isaianic style is also present:[8] the pair "wisdom" (חכמה) and "understanding" (בין) in 11:2 is used elsewhere by Isaiah (5:21; 10:13; 29:14); the "poor" (דלים) and "afflicted" (עניים) in 11:4 are mentioned together by Isaiah (10:2); "to smite with the rod" (הכה בשבט) in 11:4 is an idiom perhaps employed by Isaiah (30:31);[9] "the waistcloth of his hips" (אזור חלציו) in 11:5 is characteristically used by Isaiah (5:27); the word "root" (שרש) used in 11:1 occurs also in authentic passages (5:24; 14:29f); "counsel" (עצה) in 11:2 is found in derivative forms on Isaiah's lips (5:19; 14:24–27; 28:29);[10] "strength" (נבורה) in 11:2 is utilized elsewhere (28:6; 30:15); "knowledge" (דעת) in the same verse is employed in different forms by Isaiah (1:3; 5:13; 6:9);[11] "to kill" (המית) in 11:4 is related to its use by Isaiah (14:30); "faith(fulness)" (אמונה) in 11:5 is also reported (by a disciple) to be required by Isaiah (7:9). As it appears, the pre-exilic disciples adhered to the prophet and his traditions.

Ending the account about the composition of scrolls containing Jeremiah's words, Jer 36:32 states that many words similar to Jeremiah's own were added. Without any attempt to identify a particular scroll, we may find the addition of words similar to Jeremiah's own within different prose sections of the so-called source C.[12]

---

1   The unity of 11:1–9 is disputed. Some regard 11:6–8(–9) as a later addition. Cf. e.g. H. BARTH, *Jesaja-Worte*, 60–63. I will therefore concentrate on 11:1–5.

2   For a list of scholars, cf. VERMEYLEN, *Isaïe* I, 269 n. 2. Cf. also LAATO, *Immanuel*, 203–205.

3   For a list of scholars, cf. VERMEYLEN, *Isaïe* I, 270 n. 1. Cf. also WERNER, *Eschatologische Texte,* 70–75.

4   *Isaïe* I, 269–275.

5   Cf. CROOK, *JBL* 68 (1949) 213–224, though she relates 9:2–7; 11:1–9 to the coronation and enthronement of Joash (2 Kgs 11) c. 837 B.C.E.

6   Cf. 2 Kgs 21:23f; 22:1f.

7   VERMEYLEN, *Isaïe* I, 273.

8   WILDBERGER, *Jesaja* I, 443.

9   But cf. above p. 179 n. 9.

10   Cf. also 10:12 and the comments by WILDBERGER, *Jesaja* I, 392f, 402.—It is possible that part of 14:24–27 represents redactional work done in the 7th cent. So MOWINCKEL, *Jesaja-Disiplene,* 49, 138; H. BARTH, *Jesaja-Worte,* 103–119; CLEMENTS, *Jesaja 1–39,* 145–147.

11   Cf. also 32:4 and the comments by WILDBERGER, *Jesaja* III, 1252–1254.

12   For the source terminology, see above pp. 110f. I adopt this terminology for the

W. McKane has brought the debate surrounding this material a step further.[1] Instead of the common comparisons between the prose in Jeremiah and the prose in other corpora, he stresses the need to concentrate on internal relations between the material within Jeremiah itself. McKane's studies suggest that the corpus grew through exegesis and commentaries on individual texts. This activity did not necessarily aim towards a coherency of the scroll as a whole. Jeremiah is, in McKane's view, an untidy accumulation of material to which many people contributed. W.L. Holladay has an entirely different approach to Jeremiah as a whole. Nevertheless, he also presupposes some kind of exegesis on already existing texts. In particular, he argued that the prose was generated by the poetry.[2] This fits indeed well with the fact that source C is now mingled with the poetic and biographical sections in Jeremiah.[3]

Although several scholars think that most of the poetry goes back to Jeremiah, there is more disagreement about the prose: H. Weippert attributes much of it to Jeremiah himself;[4] McKane is content neither with this view nor with the Deuteronomistic origin proposed by W. Thiel;[5] J. Bright concludes that the origin "must be sought among Jeremiah's intimates";[6] Holladay assumes that the prose was "Baruch's adoptation of Jeremiah's poetic message."[7] McKane's view of an exegetical growth suggests some kind of scribal activity. While Deuteronomistic redaction of several prophetic books is probable, the Deuteronomistic body of material exhibits no focus on a particular prophet. It is (deliberately) silent about Jeremiah,[8] and reveals no motive that would explain the detailed work with the Jeremiah tradition.[9] This motive was of course at hand among Jeremiah's own followers.[10]

McKane provides several examples of how poetic units, attributable to

---

sake of convenience, without adhering to a particular source-critical view.

[1] *Poetry and Prose,* 269–284; *idem, Jeremiah* I, xli–xcii. For an assessment of tradition- and redaction-historical work on Jeremiah, see LEVIN, *Verheißung des neuen Bundes,* 62–67.

[2] *JBL* 79 (1960) 351–367.

[3] Cf. WEIPPERT, *Prosareden,* 19f.

[4] *Prosareden,* 228f.

[5] *Poetry and Prose,* 269–275; *Jeremiah* I, xli–xlix. The thesis of the Dtr origin of the prose is especially connected with HERRMANN, *Heilserwartungen,* 159–241 (cf. *idem,* Jeremia – der Prophet, 197–214); NICHOLSON, *Preaching to the Exiles,* locating the Dtr activity to the exilic period in Babylon (*ibid.,* 116–135); THIEL, *Jeremia 1–25; idem, Jeremia 26–45;* HYATT, Jeremiah and Deuteronomy, 113–127; *idem,* Deuteronomic Edition, 247–267.

[6] *Prose Sermons,* 205. Cf. also *idem, Jeremiah,* lxx–lxxiii.

[7] "Source B" and "Source C," 220.

[8] Cf. BEGG, *IBS* 7 (1985) 139–164.

[9] WEIPPERT, *Prosareden,* 19f; STURDY, The "prose sermons," 149f.

[10] Cf. ENGNELL, *SBU* I, 1105f; DEARMAN, *JBL* 109 (1990) 419.

Jeremiah, generated exegesis in prose:[1] Jer 3:6–11 is based on 3:1–5, 12f;
Jer 5:18f on 5:15–17; Jer 7:29b–34 on 7:29a; Jer 9:11–15 on 9:9f; Jer 11:17
on 11:15f, etc. Holladay shows also—though with entirely different emphases—how expressions in poetry were repeated, elaborated and combined in
the prose material of source B and C.[2] Most striking are the poetic proto-
types with no parallels elsewhere in the pre-Jeremianic literature: the expression "gates of Jerusalem" (שערי ירושלם), occurring in prose four times
(1:15; 17:19, 21, 27), has its oldest prototype in Jeremiah's own poetry
(22:19); the different forms of the expression "the prophets who prophesy
lies in my name" (14:14, 15[f]; 23:[16] 25f [32]; 27:10, 14–16; 29:9, 21)
have a common poetic prototype (5:31); the expression "turn each one from
his evil (way)," found in similar phrasing six times in prose (18:11; 25:5;
26:3; 35:15; 36:3, 7), is utilized twice in poetic sections (23:14, 22). As it
seems, the early elaboration of the Jeremiah tradition consisted partly in the
interpretation of poetic material from the prophet himself.

Zimmerli's suggestion concerning a process of successive exegesis on a
kernel element implies the interpretative growth of the Ezekiel tradition.[3]
Such an activity is conceivable primarily within a group of prophetic
followers. S. Herrmann's and his student R. Liwak's hypothesis of a strong
Deuteronomistic influence on the Ezekiel tradition must again face the lack
of a clear motive as to why the Deuteronomist would show such an interest
in the prophet and his tradition.[4] The Deuteronomistic history is silent also
about Ezekiel, perhaps because of ideological differences.[5] And Clements is
hardly justified in diminishing the importance of Ezekiel's followers because of the creative interests evident in the elaboration.[6] A disciple may
indeed use his master's teaching with a certain amount of creativity.

We may use the connections between Ezek 16:1–43 and 16:44–63 as an
example. 16:1–43, reflecting a situation before the fall of Jerusalem in 587
B.C.E., has apparently served as the basis for the elaboration in 16:44–63,
reflecting a situation after the fall.[7] There are notable differences between
the sections. Not only is the figure of lovers in the original story abandoned. The restoration mentioned in 16:53–63 is in view of 16:40 also surprising. Yet 16:44–63 possesses only quasi-independent character: 16:44f
depends on 16:3; the references to the "covenant" (ברית) in 16:59–63 hark

---

1   *Jeremiah* I, lxii–lxix.
2   *JBL* 79 (1960) 354–368.
3   For the view of Zimmerli, see above pp. 60f.
4   HERRMANN, *Heilserwartungen,* 241–291; LIWAK, *Überlieferungsgeschichtliche
Probleme,* 205–219.
5   So BEGG, Non-Mention of Ezekiel, 340f.
6   Chronology of Redaction, 286.
7   ZIMMERLI, *Ezekiel* I, 69, *ad loc; idem,* Phänomen der "Fortschreibung," 176f.
Many modern scholars agree that 16:44–63 is later than 16:1–43. But cf. SWANEPOEL,
Ezekiel 16, 100f.

back to 16:8; the "remembering" (זכר) in 16:60, 61, 63 presents an intentional contrast to Jerusalem's lack of remembrance in 16:22, 43. The persons responsible for the elaboration show a profound understanding and appreciation of their teacher's thought.[1] A large number of additional instances could be adduced to illustrate the same phenomenon.[2] They all suggest that the Ezekiel tradition grew through an interpretative elaboration of material attributed to Ezekiel.

As it appears, *the elaboration of tradition consisted in a dynamic interpretation which adhered to the language, style and themes visible in the written and oral material from the prophet himself.* This implies, of course, that material was preserved. The body of traditions grew through close interaction between old and new material. The new material was not added as independent and foreign elements. The interaction presupposes even a certain internalization of the old material. The transmitted material was vitally important.[3] It was, in a sense, part of a routinization process.[4] An emerging group of adherents adopted it into their own work in their own situation. The disciples were stamped by their adherence to the teacher. In this way, *the settings and the motives of transmission correlated with the preservation and the elaboration of traditions.*

4.2.2. The Integration of Traditions

The inner-prophetic process of transmission also included interactions between *different* prophetic traditions. As Zimmerli points out,[5] traditions from earlier prophets influenced later prophets. This influence may have affected the transmitters as well. The inner dynamic of the preservation and interpretative growth of the tradition does not mean that the transmitters were isolated from all influences *external* to the transmitted material itself. It is probable that the early transmitters of a specific prophetic tradition came into contact also with traditions from other prophets.

An alien religious tradition can, generally speaking, either be assimilated by adaptation or refuted. This is well illustrated by E. Shils.[6] In the former

---

1 EICHRODT, *Ezekiel,* 41.
2 Cf. e.g. Ezek 23:28–30, 32–34, 36–49 based on 23:1–27; Ezek 26:7–14, 15–18, 19–21 based on 26:2–6; Ezek 29:6b–9a, 9b–16 based on 29:1–6a. Further examples and discussion are given by HOSSFELDT, *Komposition und Theologie,* 518–529.
3 Cf. ACKROYD, *ASTI* 1 (1962) 7–23.
4 WEBER, *Wirtschaft und Gesellschaft,* 275f, discusses the religious community and explains its emergence as due to routinization ("Veralltäglichung"): "Die 'Gemeinde' in diesem religiösen Sinn ... entsteht ... erst als ein Produkt der Veralltäglichung, indem entweder der Prophet selbst oder seine Schüler den Fortbestand der Verkündigung und Gnadenspendung dauernd sichern." Cf. also *ibid.,* 142–148, 661f. For the application of this theory on the prophetic material (Jeremiah), cf. CLEMENTS, *Prophet,* 214–220.
5 *Prophetic Proclamation,* 76.
6 *Tradition,* 97–99.

case, the assertation often follows that "the alien tradition was always contained within the challenged tradition."[1] This may even more be the case when the transmitters are especially attached to the tradition of one specific person. It may be essential to assert that all important teaching—no matter its actual origin—comes from the venerated master. I will here illustrate how the early transmitters integrated *influences from other prophets* into the tradition of the prophet they themselves adhered to.

Perhaps Hos 6:5; 12:11 include Amos among the earlier prophets acclaimed as instruments of Yahweh.[2] Several passages in Hosea are similar to passages in Amos.[3] It is possible that the young Hosea was himself in contact with Amos.[4] It is also possible that the early followers came into contact with Amos' traditions and placed the material on the lips of their own master.[5]

Let me exemplify. Some of Hosea's followers are probably responsible for certain Judaic elements in the book of Hosea. Willi-Plein and Jörg Jeremias think that carriers of the Hosea tradition fled to the southern kingdom circa 721 B.C.E. and continued the work of transmission there.[6] Willi-Plein, G.I. Emmerson and G.A. Yee point to signs of Judaic redaction in 4:15.[7] This verse is reminiscent especially of Amos 5:5.[8] As it appears in this particular case, Hosea's followers placed Amos' words, which initially were addressed to the northern kingdom, on the lips of Hosea and directed them to Judah, presumably before the fall of the southern kingdom.

Other instances are probably the result of *independent* work on *several* prophetic books. 8:14 and 11:10 may serve as examples. Some scholars trace the verdict formula in 8:14 back to Hosea himself.[9] But there are signs suggesting a later date for the verse:[10] the imperfect consecutive verbs differ from the style of the entire scene; the reference to Judah has not appeared since 6:11 and is unique in this chapter; Hosea never calls Yahweh "his creator" (עשׂהו), while comparable formulations occur in Isa 44:2; 51:13. However, the threat finds its closest parallel in Amos 2:4f, which most

---

1　SHILS, *Tradition*, 98.
2　So WOLFF, *TLZ* 81 (1956) 85; *idem, Hosea*, 120, 156f, 215.
3　Cf. Hos 4:15/Amos 4:4; 5:5; 8:13f; Hos 7:10b/Amos 4:6–11; Hos 8:14b/Amos 1:4, 7, 10, 12, 14; 2:2, 5; Hos 10:4b/Amos 5:7; 6:12; Hos 11:10a/Amos 1:2a; 3:4, 8; Hos 13:7f/Amos 5:18f.
4　Cf. WOLFF, *Hosea*, 89, 136.
5　It is not possible to decide *how* Hosea's disciples became acquainted with the Amos traditions. SATO, *Q und Prophetie*, 335f, speaks of contacts between different groups of disciples. This might be true in some cases, but it is difficult to prove.
6　WILLI-PLEIN, *Vorformen*, 251f; Jörg JEREMIAS, *Hosea*, 18.
7　WILLI-PLEIN, *Vorformen*, 135f, 244f; EMMERSON, *Hosea*, 77–83; YEE, *Composition*, 269–272, also listing a number of scholars of the same opinion (*ibid.*, 367f n. 25).
8　Cf. NISSINEN, *Prophetie*, 117, 219f.
9　So e.g. MAYS, *Hosea*, 124; EMMERSON, *Hosea*, 75; ANDERSEN/FREEDMAN, *Hosea*, 511f; STUART, *Hosea – Jonah*, 137. For its authenticity, cf. also RUDOLPH, *Hosea*, 169f.
10　Cf. WILLI-PLEIN, *Vorformen*, 170f, 244; YEE, *Composition*, 195f.

scholars regard as a Judaic addition.[1] Hos 11:10 is probably also an addition:[2] only this verse of the chapter contains statements about Yahweh in the third person; the terms "lion" (אֲרִיה) and "to roar" (שׁאג) never appear elsewhere in Hosea. They do appear in Amos 1:2; 3:4, 8. But since similar expressions are present on other occasions in the prophetic corpus (Jer 25:30; Joel 4:16), 11:10 may also stem from late work on several writings.

Interactions with other prophetic traditions are probably present in Isaiah. R. Fey argued that Isaiah himself knew the speeches of Amos.[3] The similarities might sometimes be due to the common cultural and religious situation.[4] But the connections between Isa 5:11–13 and Amos 6:1–7 are noteworthy. The striking similarities in context, form, and style pointed out by Fey are difficult to account for only by reference to common (wisdom) tradition.[5] D. Baltzer argued also that the Ezekiel tradition influenced Second Isaiah.[6] Holladay noticed that Isa 56–66 integrates part of the Jeremiah tradition.[7]

The transmitters of the Isaiah tradition did integrate material from other prophets. We see this most clearly in Isa 40–55. K. Elliger believed that Third Isaiah was responsible for much of the material in these chapters.[8] The coherent pattern of the final arrangement in Isa 40–55 warns us against assuming that there are extensive additions.[9] But Isa 60–62 uses Isa 40–55.[10] This makes it possible that Third Isaiah was to some extent involved in the shaping of Isa 40–55.

H.-C. Schmitt, a student of Elliger, finds a school theology employing Ezekiel traditions in Isa 40–55.[11] The most obvious example is perhaps 48:1–11. Many scholars agree that this unit contains additions.[12] There are several features pointing in this direction.[13] We may focus on 48:8b–10,

---

[1] But cf. R. GORDIS, *HTR* 33 (1940) 241–243; BOTTERWECK, *BZ* 2 (1958) 181.—W.H. SCHMIDT, *ZAW* 77 (1965) 174–178, thinks it is an addition by the Dtr.

[2] Cf. e.g. NISSINEN, *Prophetie*, 262.

[3] *Amos und Jesaja.*

[4] So e.g. WOLFF, *Amos' geistige Heimat*, 55–58; CLEMENTS, *Isaiah 1–39*, 15; E.W. DAVIES, *Prophecy and Ethics*, 36–38.

[5] *Amos und Jesaja*, 9–17.

[6] *Ezekiel und Deuterojesaja.*

[7] *Jeremiah* II, 88.

[8] *Deuterojesaja in seinem Verhältnis*, 103–219.

[9] WESTERMANN, *Isaiah 40–66*, 28; MELUGIN, *Formation*, 175.

[10] See above pp. 145f.

[11] *ZAW* 91 (1979) 43–61. Schmitt detects also influence from the Dtr.

[12] So e.g. DUHM, *Jesaia*, 332–336; MOWINCKEL, *ZAW* 49 (1931) 102f n. 4 (with some caution); ELLIGER, *Deuterojesaja in seinem Verhältnis*, 185–198; WESTERMANN, *Isaiah 40–66*, 194–199; SCHOORS, *God Your Saviour*, 283–292; WHYBRAY, *Isaiah 40–66*, 126–131; H.-C. SCHMITT, *ZAW* 91 (1979) 48–56; MERENDINO, *Der Erste und der Letzte*, 497–516.

[13] Also 48:4 contains redactional features. Cf. MERENDINO, *Der Erste und der Letzte*, 502. In particular, the four *hapax legomena*—"hard" (קשׁה), "sinew" (גיד), "neck" (ערף), "forehead" (מצח)—are striking because they represent terminology found in Ezek

which exhibits similarities with elements firmly anchored in the Ezekiel tradition.[1] The justification that 48:8a receives in 48:8b–10 is unusual within Isa 40–55.[2] This indicates perhaps that 48:8b–10 is an addition. Since this small unit also contains language found in Isa 56–66,[3] it is possible that Third Isaiah formed it. Most striking is the use of קרא in the pual (48:8b). We find this elsewhere only in Isa 58:12; 61:3; 62:2 and Ezek 10:13,[4] not in the earlier Isaiah tradition. A number of themes in 48:8b–10 are characteristic of Ezekiel: the notion that Israel was rebellious from the beginning in Isa 48:8b is central to Ezekiel's view of history in 16:1–43; 23:1–27(– 49); the saving of Israel "for my name's sake" (למען שמי) in Isa 48:9 never occurs elsewhere in Isa 40–55, but we find it in Isa 66:5 and, in a similar manner, in Ezek 20:9, 14, 22, 44;[5] the image of the furnace in Isa 48:10 appears in Ezek 22:17–22.[6] The Trito-Isaianic language and the similarities with concepts in the Ezekiel tradition—not in the Isaiah tradition—suggest that Third Isaiah integrated traditions from other prophetic authorities into the Isaiah tradition.

There are perhaps other examples of the same phenomenon, but they rest on even more hypothetical views about the origin of the passages. For instance, if we with Elliger think that the fourth servant song (52:13–53:12) was composed by Third Isaiah,[7] we may notice that the concept "to bear someone's guilt" (53:4, 11f) is central also in Ezek 4:4–6; 14:10; 18:19f; 23:49; 44:10, 12.[8] Similarly, if we with Elliger regard Isa 54–55 as Trito-Isaianic,[9] we may notice the resemblances between 55:7 and Ezek 3:18f and between 55:8f and Ezek 18:25–29.[10]

Several passages in Jeremiah acknowledge other prophets: 7:25; 25:4 re-

---

2:4; 3:7–9. However, this terminology is also found in the Dtr (Deut 9:6, 13; 10:16; 31:27; 2 Kgs 17:14. Cf. also Exod 32:9; 33:3, 5; 34:9; Judg 2:19; Jer 7:26; 17:23; 19:15) and it is therefore not certain that this verse stems from Isaianic disciples influenced by the Ezekiel tradition.

1 In regard to the authenticity of passages in Ezekiel, I follow ZIMMERLI, *Ezekiel* I–II, *ad loci*.

2 SCHOORS, *God Your Saviour*, 288, states that normally, according to Second Isaiah, "Israel has heard nothing about the coming things, because they are completely new." Here they hear nothing because they themselves were treacherous.

3 ELLIGER, *Deuterojesaja in seinem Verhältnis*, 194f.

4 It is impossible to determine at what editorial stage Ezek 10:13 was added. But there is no reason to regard it as an entirely foreign element in the Ezekiel tradition. Cf. ZIMMERLI, *Ezekiel* I, 255, though he wrongly refers to Ezek 9:13.

5 Cf. also Isa 48:11aβ LXX (τὸ ἐμὸν ὄνομα), by most scholars not regarded as original.

6 Ezek 22:17–22 might have employed Isa 1:22, 25 as a basis. Cf. ZIMMERLI, *Ezekiel* I, 462. However, the "furnace" (כור) mentioned in Isa 48:10; Ezek 22:18, 20, 22, does not figure there.

7 *Deuterojesaja in seinem Verhältnis*, 6–27. Cf. also *idem, ZAW* 49 (1931) 138f. For some critical comments, see above pp. 109f and the literature mentioned there.

8 Cf. ZIMMERLI, *Gottes Offenbarung*, 157–161.

9 *Deuterojesaja in seinem Verhältnis*, 135–167.

10 Cf. H.-C. SCHMITT, *ZAW* 91 (1979) 59 n. 79.

fer positively to them; 26:17–19 tells about Jeremiah's supporters defending the prophet through reference to Micah of Moresheth; 26:20–23 speaks about the fate of someone called Uriah, son of Shemaiah from Kiriath-jearim.

Jeremiah was himself influenced by older prophetic traditions.[1] But just as these acknowledgements serve only the characterization of Jeremiah,[2] the transmitters also integrated other prophetic traditions into the Jeremiah tradition. Allusions to the Micah tradition are normally not identified by reference to Micah himself in Jeremiah.[3] There are other examples of the integration. For instance, the similarities with Amos in certain prose sections testify to the creative labour of Jeremiah's followers: the expression "for evil and not for good" (לרעה ולא לטובה) in 21:10; 39:16; 44:27 appears in Amos 9:4, but not elsewhere in Jeremiah;[4] the phrase "(not) hear my words," occurring in various forms in 11:10; 13:10; 19:15; 25:8, has its only parallel in Amos 8:11.[5] We could refer to further influences from other prophets, such as from Hosea.[6]

Ezekiel was himself acquainted with older prophetic traditions.[7] But we find influences from various prophets also within the elaborative work of the transmitters. For instance, someone "familiar with the prophetic message"[8] added a quotation from Zeph 1:18 in Ezek 7:19 and presented it as part of Yahweh's speech to Ezekiel.

Scholars have noticed the relationship between Jeremiah and Ezekiel.[9] Ezek 7:26b, for instance, contains a rather close quotation of Jer 18:18. Ezek 16:44–63, added as an interpretation of 16:1–43,[10] may also here serve as an example. The persons responsible for introducing the image of the sisters did not come into contact with Ezek 23:1–27 only, even if this account would have existed in an early form depicting only one woman.[11] We find similarities also with Jer 3:6–11. There is even a common use of צדק in

---

[1] For Hosea and Jeremiah, see GROSS, *Verwandtschaft;* UNTERMAN, *Repentance,* 165f. For Amos and Jeremiah, see BERRIDGE, *TZ* 35 (1979) 321–341. But cf. also BEYERLIN, *Reflexe,* 103f, *passim,* arguing against Berridge that the reflections of Amos in Jeremiah are due to later redactions. For Jeremiah's general dependence on the prophets of the 8th and 7th cent., see HOLLADAY, *Jeremiah* II, 44–53.

[2] See above p. 140.

[3] For discussion of these allusions, see HARDMEIER, Propheten, 181–184.

[4] But cf. 29:11; 38:4.

[5] HOLLADAY, *JBL* 79 (1960) 364f.

[6] DEISSLER, "Echo" der Hosea-Verkündigung, 61–75.

[7] HOSSFELDT, *Komposition und Theologie,* 510–512; ZIMMERLI, *Ezekiel* I, 42–46.

[8] ZIMMERLI, *Ezekiel* I, 211.

[9] J.W. MILLER, *Verhältnis Jeremias und Hesekiels;* RAITT, *Theology of Exile.* Cf. also LUST, "Gathering and Return," 119–142; RENAUD, L'alliance éternelle, 335–339; VIEWEGER, *BZ* 32 (1988) 15–34; MENDECKI, *BZ* 35 (1991) 242–247.

[10] Cf. above pp. 182f.

[11] Cf. POHLMANN, *Ezekielstudien,* 215f.

Ezek 16:51f and Jer 3:11. Other passages in Jeremiah are also reflected: there is the combination of "to be ashamed" (בוש), "to be disgraced" (כלם) or "disgrace" (כלמה) and "to carry" (נשא) in Ezek 16:52 and Jer 31:19;[1] there is a combination of "to be ashamed" (בוש) or "shame" (בושה) and "disgrace" (כלמה) in Ezek 16:63 and Jer 3:25; "eternal covenant" (ברית עולם) is an expression present both in Ezek 16:60 and Jer 32:40; Ezek 16:60a is, as it seems, related also to Jer 2:2. The followers of Ezekiel integrated traditions from other prophets into the Ezekiel tradition.

These examples from several prophetic books must suffice here. Some of them may be open to discussion. It is always difficult to be certain about the different layers in a tradition- and redaction-historical reconstruction. But cumulatively there emerges a strong impression that early transmitters integrated influences from various prophets into the tradition of one specific prophet. There was not merely a principle, like the rabbinic view that all torah essentially came from Moses. The adherence to one prophet and his teaching did affect the actual transmission. This integration of traditions shows that *transmission was both open and closed.* On one hand, the traditions were not esoterically restricted to one specific group. They were known to persons outside of the group of transmitters. On the other hand, the early followers integrated teaching from other authorities into the tradition of their own prophetic master. They did not protect the tradition from alien influences. The master was attributed teaching of a different origin. The transmitters put the teaching on his lips and treated it as if it was already inherent in the old tradition. *The settings and the motives of transmission correlated with an elaboration that sometimes integrated external influences and made them into utterances internal to the tradition from one specific prophet.*

4.3. The Righteous Teacher and the Attraction of Teaching

There is no direct information about the preservation and elaboration of the teaching from the Righteous Teacher. The written traditions recorded in the Dead Sea scrolls are, as we have seen, anonymous. And there are neither theoretical emphases on the preservation of the teaching nor visible signs of an interchange between a basic tradition and its elaboration. Only indirectly, through a comparison of different documents, is it possible to discern somewhat vaguely how the setting and the motives of transmission correlated with an *attraction of other teaching* to the Righteous Teacher.

---

[1] Cf. also נשא, כלמה and כלם in Ezek 16:54.

4.3.1. The Problem of the Former Precepts

There is an apparent tension between 1QS 9:10f and CD 20:30–33. According to the former passage, the Qumranites will be judged "on the basis of the former precepts" (במשפטים הרשונים), in which the men of the community first were disciplined. The former precepts are valid until the coming of a prophet and two Messiahs. As I argued previously, the community probably thought that the Teacher was the eschatological—Mosaic—prophet mentioned here.[1] According to the latter passage, the Qumranites instructed themselves "in the former precepts" (במשפטים הראשונים), on the basis of which the men of the community were judged. This is strongly reminiscent of 1QS 9:10. But here the former precepts are connected with the Teacher's voice. While 1QS 9:10f relates the former precepts to directives given to the community *before* the appearance of the Teacher, CD 20:30–33 connects them with the Teacher's *own* instruction.

J. Murphy-O'Connor believes that the former precepts refer to statutes valid before the appearance of the Teacher in *both* 1QS 9:10 and CD 20:31.[2] CD 20:30–33 envisages, according to Murphy-O'Connor, four different criteria of judgement. The former precepts are part of the second criterion and the Teacher's voice of the third. The two criteria correspond to the first and the last in CD 20:8f.

There are several factors causing scepticism towards this interpretation of CD 20:30–33. One depends on a different understanding of CD 6:2–11. Murphy-O'Connor believes that the interpreter of the Torah in 6:7 was a person in the Babylonian pre-history of the community.[3] I have followed the view that it is the Righteous Teacher who in 6:2–11 issues precepts which will serve as rules until the coming of the priestly Messiah.[4] This suggests that CD 20:30–33 parallels the statements and makes judgement according to the former precepts an expression synonymous to listening to the voice of the Teacher.

There are also features in the context of CD 20:30–33. CD 20:27f defines the holding on "to these precepts" (במשפטים האלה) as listening to the Teacher's voice.[5] Indeed, the expression "they listened to the Teacher's voice" (ישמעו לקול מורה) in 20:28 gives the impression of being entirely synony-

---

[1]   See above p. 125.

[2]   *RB* 76 (1969) 530f; *idem, RB* 79 (1972) 547f; *idem, RB* 81 (1974) 238. Murphy-O'Connor is followed by e.g. POUILLY, *RB* 82 (1975) 525, though in *idem, Règle de la Communauté*, 28, he leaves the issue open; DOHMEN, *RevQ* 11 (1982) 91; P.R. DAVIES, *Damascus Covenant*, 183; *idem, RevQ* 15 (1991) 277, 281f. Cf. also *idem,* Halakhah, 47f.

[3]   Cf. Damascus Document Revisited, 380.

[4]   See above pp. 126f, 129f.

[5]   I understand מורה in 20:28 as a reference to the Righteous Teacher. See above p. 49.

mous with the phrase "they gave ear to the voice of (the) Righteous Teacher" (האזינו לקול מורה צדק) in 20:32.[1] The precepts of 20:27 are then closely connected with the Teacher mentioned in 20:28, just as the former precepts of 20:31 can be understood as connected with the Teacher mentioned
in 20:32.[2] The statements are closer to each other than Murphy-O'Connor
admits.

The use of identical terms in the four criteria separated by Murphy-
O'Connor indicates further the parallel significance of the statements: משפט
in 20:27 appears again in the first (20:30b) and the second criterion
(20:31b); חק in the initial confession of 20:29 recurs in the first (20:30b)
and the fourth (20:33a) criterion; צדק in 20:29 appears again in the first
(20:31a), the third (20:32b) and the fourth (20:33a) criterion. Identical
terms do not necessarily suggest identical meaning and significance. But the
lack of any explicit remark indicating a difference makes it most natural to
assume that the four statements describe parallel conceptions about the criterion of judgement.

As it seems, someone structured 20:30b–33a quite consciously as parallel
statements:

a.	ולא ירימו יד על חקי קדשו ומשפטי צדקו ועדוות אמתו
b.	והתיסרו במשפטים הראשונים אשר נשפטו בם אנשי היחד
b.	והאזינו לקול מורה צדק
a.	ולא ישיבו את חקי הצדק בשמעם אתם

a. And they did not raise hand against his holy statutes
   and his righteous precepts and his true testimonies.
b. But they instructed themselves *in the former precepts,*
   on the basis of which the men of the community were judged,
b. and they gave ear *to the voice of (the) Righteous Teacher.*
a. And they did not turn away the righteous statutes when they heard them.

After the summarizing introduction (20:27b–28a) and the following confession (20:28b–30a), the author created a parallel chiastic pattern: a negative statement followed by a positive and a positive followed by a negative.
The positive statements relate the former precepts and the voice of the
Righteous Teacher closely to each other.

All in all, the Teacher appears in the Damascus Document as the initiator
of the former precepts. Perhaps the reference to the last (precepts) in conjunction with the first in 20:8f indicates that the Teacher had issued ordinances at two decisive stages.[3] But the tension between 1QS 9:10f and CD
20:30–33 remains.

1	Cf. BOYCE, *RevQ* 14 (1990) 626f.
2	Cf. G. JEREMIAS, *Lehrer der Gerechtigkeit,* 164.
3	Cf. also T. Jud. 24:3.—LAPERROUSAZ, Les "ordonnances premières," 405–419;
idem, RevQ 13 (1988) 455–464, thinks that the Teacher actually issued decisive ordinances on two occasions.

4.3.2. The Attraction of Teaching

The tension may be explained if we approach the texts genetically, asking in what order they originated. It is probable that 1QS 9:10f reflects an early time in the history of the community. Scholars acknowledge today that the present Community Rule is a composite work with a pre-history.[1] 1QS 9:10f belongs to the oldest part. Murphy-O'Connor and J. Pouilly have convinced most scholars that we find the earliest unit in 1QS 8:1–16a; 9:3–10:8a—the so-called Manifesto representing a pre-Qumranic stratum.[2] The fact that 1QS 9:10f is missing in a copy of the Rule from cave four (4QSe) is not necessarily an indication that someone interpolated it later.[3] We would then expect the prophet to be mentioned also elsewhere in connection with the two Messiahs.[4] Scholars also often consider the Damascus Document as younger than the Community Rule,[5] though parts of the Damascus Document have been assigned a pre-Qumranic date.[6] It does seem that the Damascus Document occasionally makes use of the Rule.[7] Several passages express more clearly what is pre-supposed from the Rule.[8] A study of the community functionaries also shows that the stage of development reflected in the Rule is earlier than the one indicated in the Damascus Document.[9]

These brief considerations imply how the tension appearing at the reading/hearing of 1QS 9:10f and CD 20:30–33 may be genetically explained. It is not necessary to postulate the existence of separate, though related, groups with their own complex history and views.[10] It is quite possible that the two documents reflect various experiences in the collective history of

---

[1] For a survey of the most important contributions, see SCHÜRER, *History* III, 382–384.

[2] MURPHY-O'CONNOR, *RB* 76 (1969) 529–532; POUILLY, *Règle de la Communauté*, 15–34.—POUILLY, *ibid.*, 18, differs from Murphy-O'Connor in regarding 8:10b–12a as a later insertion. Cf. also POUILLY, *RB* 82 (1975) 524–526.—In SCHÜRER, *History* III, 383, it is stated that the unity of 1QS 8:1–16; 9:3–11 is "generally recognized as reflecting the most primitive concept of the Community."

[3] *Contra* CHARLESWORTH, Jewish Messianology, 232.

[4] For further arguments, see SCHIFFMAN, Messianic Figures, 120.

[5] Cf. SCHÜRER, *History* III, 395f: "Most ... authors ... generally consider CD to be somewhat younger than the Community Rule."

[6] P.R. DAVIES, *Damascus Covenant,* 201.—Murphy-O'Connor has in numerous articles dated different parts of the Damascus Document to a pre-Qumranic time. The earliest unit is the so-called Missionary document, delineated by MURPHY-O'CONNOR, *RB* 77 (1970) 201–229, to CD 2:14–6:1, later in *idem*, Damascus Document Revisited, 375, also including CD 6:2–11. STEGEMANN, *RevQ* 14 (1990) 409–434, regards CD 9–16 as the oldest part, older also than the Community Rule.

[7] WERNBERG-MØLLER, *JSS* 1 (1956) 110–128.

[8] DELCOR, *DBSup* IX, 847f.

[9] KRUSE, *RevQ* 10 (1981) 543–551.—The arguments of DIMANT, Qumran Sectarian Literature, 502f, suggesting that the Damascus Document is earlier than the Community Rule, are not at all compelling.

[10] *Contra* P.R. DAVIES, *RevQ* 15 (1991) 286. Cf. also *idem,* Halakhah, 38f.

the community and point to alterations in its conceptual world.[1]

I can only offer some general comments here. The community experienced the death of the Teacher at some stage during its history. Even if B.Z. Wacholder would be right to question the wide-spread assumption that the "gathering in" (האסף) in CD 19:35; 20:14 actually refers to the Teacher's death,[2] there is sufficient evidence that the Qumranites coped with his mortality (4QpPs[a] 4:8). At some stage he died. We do not know if his death was violent, involving crucifixion.[3] But it must have meant a shocking experience for the community.

1QS 9:10 expresses an expectation in which the coming of a prophet would be closely linked with the ultimate end and the coming of two Messiahs. A prophet—the Teacher—appeared and died, but the end was still not at hand. This experience did evidently not result in a change concerning the understanding of the Teacher's actual identity. While the two Messiahs continue to remain objects of expectation in the scrolls,[4] the prophet disappears.[5] The Qumranites did not mention him further as part of their expectation about the future. He had already come. At the time reflected in the major parts of the Damascus Document, a figure who fulfilled the role of a prophet like Moses had already appeared. It was the Teacher.

It is quite possible that some eschatological conceptions altered in view of the cognitive dissonance created through the death of the Righteous Teacher.[6] 1QpHab 7:1–8 suggests that the Qumranites struggled with the delay of the final end and reduced the dissonance between the reality and the ideal expectations by seeking biblical support for the view that the final age will be prolonged. The three figures of the end-time could therefore be sepa-

---

[1]   When the issue concerning the relationship between 1QS 9:10f and CD 20:30–33 is not related to a consideration of the identity ascribed to the prophet, a purely literary-historical solution may be proposed. The problem is recognized, though not discussed, by P.R. DAVIES, *RevQ* 15 (1991) 284. But cf. e.g. STEGEMANN, *RevQ* 14 (1990) 422f.

[2]   *RevQ* 13 (1988) 323–330. Wacholder thinks of the Teacher as the "gatherer" of the assembly, a function comparable to Moses'.

[3]   Alexander Janneus (c. 103–76 B.C.E.) was evidently the first Jewish ruler to employ crucifixion (Ant. 13:380; Bell 1:97. Cf. Ant. 13:410f; Bell. 1:113). This may be indicated in 4QpNah 1:4–8. But ROWLEY, *JBL* 75 (1956) 190, correctly points out—though he does not understand the commentary on Nahum in relation to Alexander Janneus—that the Teacher is nowhere mentioned here. For further discussion and literature, see HALPERIN, *JJS* 32 (1981) 32–46; ZIAS/CHARLESWORTH, Crucifixion, 273–289.

[4]   Cf. e.g. CD 12:23–13:1; 14:19; 19:10f; 20:1 (1QSa 2:12). In view of the plural expression in 1QS 9:11 (משיחי אהרון וישראל) it is probable that the singular expression ([משוח] משיח [מ]אהרון ו[מ]ישראל) in the instances mentioned here is to be rendered "Messiah of Aaron and (the Messiah) of Israel." For further discussion, see K.G. KUHN, Two Messiahs, 54–60; SCHIFFMAN, Messianic Figures, 116–129.

[5]   Cf. WIEDER, *JJS* 4 (1953) 171; VAN DER WOUDE, *Die messianischen Vorstellungen,* 84.

[6]   For an introduction to the theory of cognitive dissonance, see FESTINGER, *Cognitive Dissonance,* 1–31. From a different angle than the one adopted here, this theory was brought into the discussion concerning the apprehension of the Teacher by P.R. DAVIES, *RevQ* 13 (1988) 317. Cf. already earlier *idem, JBL* 104 (1985) 42.

rated in time. A prophet had come, and two Messiahs would appear at a later stage in the final age. If we follow the common interpretation of CD 19:35; 20:14 as referring to the death of the Teacher, we now see why the community was concerned to count the time from the gathering in of the Teacher until the appearance of the Messiah out of Aaron and the Messiah out of Israel (CD 19:35–20:1).[1]

It is conceivable, if I may hypothesize somewhat further, that these conceptions about the Teacher and the future effected the attraction of precepts to the Teacher. Although frustrated by the reality of the Teacher's death, the community did not give up the ideal of the Teacher fulfilling the role of the Mosaic prophet. In order to reduce the tension between the real and the ideal world, they enhanced the real Teacher to an ideal Teacher from whom all important teaching was to come. As the end-time was prolonged, *they ascribed elements of the past to him retrospectively.* The former precepts were originally issued before the Teacher appeared as a Mosaic prophet. But in an attempt to bring the real world closer to the ideal, the Qumranites ascribed the former preceps to the Teacher. He was the only normative Teacher of the community and of the school studying his teaching. *The setting and motives of transmission effected an attraction of the former precepts to the Teacher.*

5. Summary and Conclusions

From a broad range of various factors influencing the process of transmission, this chapter focused on the correlation between the settings and the motives of transmission described in the previous chapters on one hand, and the process of transmission on the other. The material as classified according to the pattern that emerged in chapter two reveals in different ways and with different emphases that a correlation existed in three major areas.

1. The identification of traditions has to do with the procedures by which the transmitters marked and recognized the teaching as traditions from a specific teacher. The material points to different and rather distinctive practices.

The named attributions appear as identification markers *substantially unconnected* with the content of the tradition. To judge from the present rabbinic corpora, the name of a rabbi functioned primarily to anchor torah in the past.

---

[1]   Cf. also CD 20:13–16; 4QpPs^a 2:6f. This explanation of the tension between 1QS 9:11 and CD 19:35–20:1 is not recognized by O. BETZ, *Offenbarung und Schriftforschung*, 63. But cf. SCHNACKENBURG, *SE* 1 (1959) 634; DOHMEN, *RevQ* 11 (1982) 93, though Dohmen claims that 1QS 9:11 originally came from the Teacher and was thought to refer to him only later; SCHWEITZER, Teacher of Righteousness, 79, 86f.

The secondary attributions suggest a more *substantial connection* with the transmitted material. The texts commonly believed to have originated with Second and Third Isaiah point to a process in which the elaboration both emerged in dependence on the previous material and assumed the identity of the person of dominating importance within the earlier tradition.

The existence of anonymous teaching shows that in spite of the vital importance of a teacher, the traditions may in themselves be *void* of personal identity markers. The high degree of concentration on the Righteous Teacher in the Dead Sea scrolls did not correlate with a strong personal specificity in the process of identifying the traditions in the written material. It was essential that the teaching originated with the Teacher. But his identity was not intimately linked with the substance of the recorded teaching. The community was probably sufficiently coherent to provide information concerning the identity of the traditions orally.

2. The means of transmission refers to the media by which the verbal traditions were carried and conveyed. The means often required or implied a significant relationship between teacher and pupil. Although the expressions of this feature are not distinctively different, they show different emphases.

The theoretical distinction between written and oral tradition and transmission, and the prominence of oral procedures for carrying and conveying the material, increased the importance of the teacher, but only as *a carrier of traditions.* The rabbinic literature implies that since the advanced learning of torah was to be attained in an oral setting, it was essential to establish close contacts with a teacher carrying torah and to develop practices for the accurate remembering of the material. The conviction that torah is oral and should be transmitted by oral means effected attachment to the teacher.

The teacher comes to the fore in cases where written and oral traditions interacted as they were *conveyed.* The teacher is here important as a person inherent in the tradition itself. There were probably both written and oral media for carrying the prophetic message. But the prophetic literature contains indications that the actualization, handing over and reception of the texts were oral events. Written and oral traditions interacted as texts which were read and heard. The interaction depended partly on the vital importance of traditions containing the divine teaching given *through specific prophets.* Written and oral traditions of such importance constantly *interacted* in an oral currency of transmission.

There are also cases with no theoretical distinction and no visible interaction between written and oral tradition. Even within a highly literate group of transmitters, the influence of the teacher emerged as the written traditions were *conveyed.* The Qumranites favoured written media to carry the traditions. But the actualization, handing over and reception of texts constituted also in this case oral events. *Literacy did not abolish orality.*

Although there was no interaction between written and oral media to carry the tradition, there was an audible reading of the written material. The audibility of the written texts depended partly on the attachment to the rules and regulations *of the Righteous Teacher*. The voice of the Teacher had to be heard. Written traditions of such importance constantly *returned* to an oral currency of transmission.

3. The preservation and elaboration of traditions concern acts for maintaining and extending the object of transmission. Sometimes these acts correlated with the settings and the motives of transmission. With due regard to the hypothetical steps involved in individual cases, there emerges cumulatively a conceivable pattern of emphases.

The adherence to a specific master resulted occasionally in the early definition and collection of traditions. The transmitters preserved the teaching in accordance with the name and authority of their master. But since the master was essentially only a carrier of torah, there was also the more general principle of attributing all teaching to one originator. According to the rabbinic writings, the two influences were not contradictory: the former constituted a *sporadic* influence on the collection and ordering of the preserved material; the latter was a *basic need* to validate everyting—also the elaborations—as in principle preserved from Moses.

The growth and expansion of the prophetic material exhibit influences from the settings and the motives of transmission. The preserved tradition functioned as a fundamental basis and catalyst for elaboration. Various texts in the prophetic literature imply an early, inner-prophetic process of transmission. It expresses itself in two ways: as a dynamic interpretation of traditions already linked to the prophet and as an integration of influences from other prophets into the tradition of one specific authority. The settings and the motives of transmission effected an *interpretative development* and an *integrative concentration* of the tradition.

The adherence to a specific teacher also effected the subsequent attraction of teaching to him. The Dead Sea scrolls contain neither any principles about the preservation nor visible traces of the interpretative or the integrative elaboration. But they do indicate that the frustrations caused by the historical realities did not at all diminish the ideal conceptions about the Righteous Teacher. In order to reduce the frustrations, the Qumranites altered the conceptions about the future and made use of the Teacher's undisputed status among them. His authority, manifested in the setting and the motives of transmission, effected a *retrospective attraction* of former teaching to him.

The reconstruction of Matthew's sociocultural situation reveals various patterns of how settings determined by didactic authority and person-oriented motives of transmission correlated with the objects and acts of transmission. I have not been able to trace a development implying that one pat-

tern is closer to Matthew than others.

The first part of my investigation is thus complete. In a general and synthetic fashion, I have tried to reconstruct the primary sociocultural situation of transmission in the Matthean community and focused especially on the three issues mentioned in the introduction. We have seen that the settings, the motives and the process of transmission contain several patterns of interest for the purpose of this investigation. The reconstruction sets the stage for a study of the transmission of the Jesus tradition in the Matthean community. The patterns emerging in each chapter were inherent in Matthew's own sociocultural situation and provide therefore the basic model for examining the transmission in the Matthean community.

Part Two

**Jesus as Teacher and Transmission
in the Matthean Community**

Chapter 4

Jesus as Teacher
and the Setting of Transmission

1. Introductory Remarks

We saw in chapter one that Matthew was part of a sociocultural situation developing—among other things—settings of transmission determined by the authority of a specific teacher. There were accounts about the teacher-pupil relationship and there were manifestations of the relationship in the form of social settings—schools.

Did the Matthean community have a similar setting of transmission? The evidence comes from material somewhat different than the one investigated previously. Matthew provides only an account of the teacher-pupil relationship. There is no explicit discussion of schools. And the account does not consist merely of small pieces of information but is an important part in *the story of a narrative*. Literary theorists define "setting" as the geographical, temporal and social features which give the characters and the events their narrative context.[1] The setting describes the general locale, the historical time and the social circumstances in which characters appear and events take place. This is not the kind of setting relevant for the present study. The teacher-pupil relationship does not only provide a narrative context to the characters and the events. The characters *are* to some extent teacher and pupils and the events *are* to some extent teaching and understanding.[2] The teacher-pupil relationship is part of the story itself. I am first of all interested in a "didactic story line" narrated as a relationship between a specific teacher and a group of pupils. *The aim of this chapter is to examine the basic didactic story line that Matthew depicts as a teacher-pupil relationship. This depiction is thought of as a general index to Matthew's own setting of transmission in the community.*[3]

The didactic story line thus consists of two factors. There is a teacher and there are pupils serving as recipients of his teaching. These two elements

---

[1] ABRAMS, *Glossary of Literary Terms*, 172. Cf. also CHATMAN, *Story and Discourse*, 138–145; POWELL, *What Is Narrative Criticism?*, 69–75. For an application on Matthew, see KINGSBURY, *Matthew as Story*, 28–30.

[2] POWELL, *What is Narrative Criticism?*, 69, says that "settings are never presented as espousing a particular point of view." This is done by characters in the story.

[3] See the remarks in the introduction above pp. 29f.

are embodied in certain characters of the story. The didactic story line can not be studied separated from the characterization of persons. *It is necessary to ask about the basic didactic traits that Matthew attributes to Jesus and the disciples.*

2. Jesus as διδάσκαλος

Scholars estimate the importance of the notion about Jesus as teacher in Matthew variously.[1] While some regard the didactic designation as the "most appropriate title,"[2] others remain sceptical and even negative about the general importance of any didactic traits given to Jesus in Matthew.[3] The latter group of scholars often rely—sometimes implicitly—on a synoptic comparison according to the two-source hypothesis. They have observed that Matthew maintains[4] or adds[5] such terms as διδάσκαλος and ῥαββί only when persons who are not positively related to Jesus use them.[6] When a didactic designation occurs on the lips of characters revealing a confessing attitude towards Jesus in the alleged source(s), Matthew either replaces it with κύριε[7] or omits it altogether.[8]

This view is too simple. Besides relying on a rather static fashion of making the synoptic comparison, it also gives undue attention to the didactic

---

[1]   For studies devoted primarily to this aspect in Matthew, see GASTON, *Int* 29 (1975) 24–40; BEARE, *SE* 7 (1982) 31–39; BRÄNDLE, *RevistEspir* 43 (1984) 187–209; PILCH, *BibTod* 25 (1987) 23–28; ZELLER, *Jesus als vollmächtiger Lehrer*, 299–317; LINCOLN, *Matthew—A Story for Teachers?*, 103–125. Studies devoted to teachers and teaching in the NT generally also refer to the didactic perspective in Matthew. Cf. e.g. NORMANN, *Christos Didaskalos*, 23–44; J. DONALDSON, *JQR* 63 (1972–73) 288; BLANK, *TQ* 158 (1978) 163; FRANCE, Mark and the Teaching of Jesus, 106–109; H.-F. WEISS, *EWNT* I, 767; GRASSI, *Teaching the Way*, 86–95; DOWNING, *NTS* 33 (1987) 447; RIESNER, *Lehrer*, 249–251, 367; ZIMMERMANN, *Die urchristlichen Lehrer*, 144–193; PERKINS, *Jesus as Teacher*, 72–84; VIVIANO, *RB* 97 (1990) 209f; KARRER, *ZNW* 83 (1992) 3f, 16–18.

[2]   GASTON, *Int* 29 (1975) 38.

[3]   Cf. e.g. KILPATRICK, *Origins*, 80; MEYE, *Jesus and the Twelve*, 39–42; D.R. BAUER, *Structure*, 35.—FRANCE, Mark and the Teaching of Jesus, 109, describes the teacher language in Matthew as "almost derogatory." But cf. *idem, Matthew: Evangelist and Teacher*, 257.

[4]   Matt 19:16/Mark 10:17/Luke 18:18; Matt 22:16/Mark 12:14/Luke 20:21; Matt 22:24/Mark 12:19/Luke 20:28; Matt 22:36/Luke 10:25; Matt 26:49/Mark 14:45.

[5]   Matt 8:19/Luke 9:57; Matt 9:11/Mark 2:16/Luke 5:30; Matt 12:38/Mark 8:11/Luke 11:16. For Matthew's special material, cf. 17:24; 26:25.

[6]   Already by BORNKAMM, End-Expectation, 41, made this observation. It has often been repeated by other scholars.

[7]   Matt 8:25/Mark 4:38/Luke 8:24 (ἐπιστάτα); Matt 17:4/Mark 9:5/Luke 9:33 (ἐπιστάτα); Matt 17:15/Mark 9:17/Luke 9:38; Matt 20:33 (9:28)/Mark 10:51. Cf. also Matt 8:19 with Matt 8:21 and Matt 26:22 with Matt 26:25.

[8]   Matt 20:20/Mark 10:35; Matt 21:20/Mark 11:21; Matt 24:1/Mark 13:1. Cf. also Matt 19:20/Mark 10:28.

designations only. As a first step towards some clarification, it is necessary to consider more carefully the use of both the basic designation depicting Jesus as teacher and the terms portraying his didactic deeds. An adequate appreciation of the didactic trait attributed to Jesus cannot neglect one of the two. *Matthew characterizes Jesus not only by means of designations and titles, but also by informing the readers/hearers about what Jesus does.*

The primary terms describing the basic trait of Jesus as teacher are different forms of διδάσκαλος and of the related verb διδάσκειν and noun διδαχή.[1] The depiction of Jesus as teacher is of course not restricted to uses of these terms only. As we will see in the following chapters, there are other relevant terms and concepts as well. But the didactic connotation of other terms and concepts depends to a higher degree on factors that are specific within the context of the story. *These three terms—διδάσκαλος, διδάσκειν and διδαχή—carry for the Greek readers/hearers an inherent didactic meaning and are the most important means for characterizing Jesus as teacher.*[2] I therefore start the inquiry by focusing on them separately.

W. Schenk has in his study *Die Sprache des Matthäus* developed a methodological basis for word-statistical inquiries in the gospel narratives. His redaction-semantical method goes beyond the normal use of word statistics. It takes seriously the fact that words attain their primary meaning intertextually—only as parts of various kinds of texts—and that the work of an author should be analysed in relation to the reception of texts.[3] Although I will not pursue all the steps proposed by Schenk, the basic aim of this section is, as far as I can see, in harmony with his method. I will discuss some aspects of the didactic terminology used by the author of a narrative.[4] Since it is today evident that the creation and reading/hearing of all texts relate implicitly or explicitly to other textual worlds,[5] I will compare the text passages in which the didactic terms appear with material both external and internal to Matthew's narrative itself.

---

[1] The terms ῥαββί (23:7, 8, 26:25, 49) and καθηγητής (23:10) carry in Matthew connotations which are either negative or go beyond the purely didactic ones. I will discuss them in the next chapter.

[2] For some important uses of διδάσκαλος in the Greco-Roman world, see excursus 9 below.

[3] SCHENK, *Sprache des Matthäus*, 2, states: "Die *Textverarbeitung* eines Autors wird durch *Rezeptionsanalyse* der jeweiligen *Intertextualität* bestimmt." Cf. also the source-oriented elaboration of the word-statistical method proposed by J. FRIEDRICH, *Gott im Bruder?*, 9–13; GUNDRY, *Matthew*, 2–5; J.H. FRIEDRICH, *ZNW* 76 (1985) 29–42.

[4] For the importance of the author in narrative criticism, see above pp. 30f.

[5] For a comparison between author-oriented redaction history and reader-oriented intertextuality, cf. VORSTER, Intertextuality and Redaktionsgeschichte, 15–26. Since the authors of the synoptic gospel narratives also were readers/hearers and interpreters of other texts, the difference between the two methods is perhaps not to be stressed to the extent that an author-oriented intertextuality becomes totally inconceivable.

2.1. The Basic Material

Since the didactic terms are the primary means of characterizing Jesus as teacher, I will present their distribution separately. I will read the material "intersynoptically," trying to take the other synoptics into account without making false conclusions on the assumption of static genetic relationships.[1] There is no reason to isolate the *creation* of Matthew's narrative from traditions reflected in Mark and Luke.

Matthew employs διδάσκαλος twelve times altogether.[2] All instances refer explicitly or implicitly to Jesus.[3] Within an intersynoptic perspective,[4] the material occurs in the triple tradition, the double tradition and Matthew's special material.[5] The use of διδασκάλος harmonizes with Mark and/or Luke in seven cases.[6] From a total of twelve, this is somewhat more than half. On certain occasions, Matthew is alone among the synoptics in using διδάσκαλος in reference to Jesus. This is the case in the remaining five instances: three are specific to Matthew in spite of the presence of the traditions in one or both of the other synoptics;[7] the term appears twice in the special material.[8]

On other occasions, διδάσκαλος is absent in Matthew while present in one or both of the other two synoptics: corresponding terms are three times missing altogether in Matthew when Mark records them;[9] κύριε appears

---

1　I will state my view of the relationship between the synoptic gospel narratives in chapter 6, esp. pp. 331f.

2　8:19; 9:11; 10:24, 25; 12:38; 17:24; 19:16; 22:16, 24, 36; 23:8; 26:18.

3　The reference to Jesus is implicit in 10:24, 25 and probable in 23:8.

4　For Jesus as teacher in Mark, see MEYE, Messianic Secret and Messianic Didache, 57–68; NORMANN, *Christos Didaskalos*, 1–23; MEYE, *Jesus and the Twelve*, 30–87; R.H. STEIN, *ZNW* 61 (1970) 91–94; J. DONALDSON, *JQR* 63 (1972–73) 287f; FRANCE, Mark and the Teaching of Jesus, 101–136; H.-F. WEISS, *EWNT* I, 766f; RIESNER, *Lehrer*, 251–252; VIVIANO, *RB* 97 (1990) 207–218; ROBBINS, *Jesus the Teacher*, 75–196; SCHOLTISSEK, *Vollmacht*, 119–125, 213f. For Jesus as teacher in Luke, see SAGGIN, *VD* 30 (1952) 208f; GLOMBITZA, *ZNW* 49 (1958) 275–278; OEPKE, *TDNT* II, 622f; NORMANN, *ibid.*, 45–54; J. DONALDSON, *ibid.*, 288f; BACHMANN, *Jerusalem und der Tempel*, 261–289; H.-F. WEISS, *ibid.*, 767f; GRIMM, *EWNT* II, 93f; RIESNER, *ibid.*, 247–249.

5　There are no substantial reasons for accepting alternative readings in the passages containing didactic terminology related to Jesus in Mark and Luke. I will discuss textcritical problems in Matthew as we proceed.

6　Matt 10:24, 25/Luke 6:40; Matt 19:16/Mark 10:17/Luke 18:18; Matt 22:16/Mark 12:14/Luke 20:21; Matt 22:24/Mark 12:19/Luke 20:28; Matt 22:36/Luke 10:25; Matt 26:18/Mark 14:14/Luke 22:11. The presence of the term constitutes in Matt 22:36/Luke 10:25 a minor agreement against Mark 12:28.

7　Matt 8:19/Luke 9:57; Matt 9:11/Mark 2:16/Luke 5:30; Matt 12:38/Mark 8:11/Luke 11:16 (but cf. Matt 16:1).—I am not certain that HAHN, *Christologische Hoheitstitel*, 84, is correct when he claims that Matthew never adds διδάσκαλος to his sources.

8　17:24; 23:8.

9　Matt 19:20/Mark 10:28; Matt 20:20/Mark 10:35; Matt 24:1/Mark 13:1.—Mark 5:35/Luke 8:49; Mark 9:38/Luke 9:49 (ἐπιστάτα); Mark 12:32; Luke 5:5 (ἐπιστάτα); 7:40; 8:45 (ἐπιστάτα); 11:45; 12:13; 17:13 (ἐπιστάτα) are missing altogether in Matt-

twice in Matthew when both the other synoptics have διδάσκαλε—or ἐπιστάτα as Luke sometimes prefers.[1] Of these five cases, the absence is peculiar to Matthew in three.[2] It is twice in agreement with Luke.[3]

Various forms of διδάσκειν occur in Matthew altogether fourteen times: nine times the verb refers to Jesus' own action;[4] three times it concerns a future action of other persons with positive traits;[5] once, in an OT quotation, it describes negatively the action of Pharisees and scribes (15:9); once it refers to the instruction that the chief priests and the elders give to the soldiers (28:15). The nine occurrences of the verb as a description of Jesus' actions as well as the three occurrences of the verb as a description of the actions of other persons with positive traits are of most interest here.

The presence of the verb harmonizes with Mark and/or Luke six times.[6] From a total of twelve, this constitutes half of the instances. In the remaining six instances, the verb appears in Matthew alone: twice Matthew is the only one to give it within traditions that are recorded in some form also in one or both of the other synoptics;[7] four times it belongs to Matthew's special material.[8]

There are also four passages in which the verb is missing in Matthew while present in Mark[9] or Luke.[10] In none of these instances the absence is peculiar to Matthew alone. It is always in agreement with one of the other synoptics.[11]

On five additional occasions, Matthew has another verb than one of the other synoptics. Instead of διδάσκειν in Mark, Matthew has forms of δεικνύειν,[12] λαλεῖν[13] or even, it seems, θεραπεύειν.[14] In three of these cases, Luke also gives a different term.[15] The other two are part of texts which

hew. Within the double tradition (Matt 10:24f/Luke 6:40; Matt 8:19/Luke 9:57), there is no instance of an absence of the term in Matthew.
1 Matt 8:25/Mark 4:38/Luke 8:24 (ἐπιστάτα); Matt 17:15/Mark 9:17/Luke 9:38.
2 8:25; 17:15; 20:20. There is no Lukan parallel to 20:20.
3 Matt 19:20/Luke 18:21; Matt 24:1/Luke 21:5 (but cf. Luke 21:7).
4 4:23; 5:2; 7:29; 9:35; 11:1; 13:54; 21:23; 22:16; 26:55.
5 5:19 (*bis*); 28:20.
6 Matt 7:29/Mark 1:22; Matt 9:35/Mark 6:6b; Matt 13:54/Mark 6:2; Matt 21:23/Luke 20:1; Matt 22:16/Mark 12:14/Luke 20:21 (*bis*); Matt 26:55/Mark 14:49 (cf. Luke 19:47; 21:37). The use of the term in Matt 21:23/Luke 20:1 constitutes a minor agreement against Mark 11:27.
7 Matt 4:23/Mark 1:39/Luke 4:44; Matt 5:2/Luke 6:20 (cf. Mark 3:13a).
8 Matt 5:19 (*bis*); 11:1; 28:20.
9 Matt 21:13/Mark 11:17; Matt 22:42/Mark 12:35.
10 Matt 4:17/Luke 4:15; Matt 12:9/Luke 6:6.
11 Matt 21:13; 22:42 are in this regard in agreement with Luke 19:46; 20:41. Matt 4:17; 12:9 belong to the triple tradition and are in this regard in agreement with Mark 1:14; 3:1.
12 Matt 16:21/Mark 8:31.
13 Matt 13:3/Mark 4:2; Matt 17:22/Mark 9:31.
14 Matt 14:14/Mark 6:34; Matt 19:2/Mark 10:1.
15 Matt 14:14/Luke 9:11 (λαλεῖν, ἰάεσθαι); Matt 16:21/Luke 9:22 (λαλεῖν); Matt

Luke does not record at all.[1] Luke 12:12 uses διδάσκειν for the activity of the spirit, while Matt 10:19 gives διδόναι. Matthew is here in agreement with Mark 13:11. Matthew never uses another term when both Mark and Luke have διδάσκειν.[2]

Matthew also utilizes the terms διδαχή (7:28; 16:12; 22:33) and διδασκαλία (15:9). Twice the former describes Jesus' teaching (7:28; 22:33). Once it refers to the teaching of Jesus' opponents (16:12). The term διδασκαλία is this time taken from Isa 29:13 (LXX). Of interest are here only the two occurrences of διδαχή in 7:28; 22:33.

Matthew shares one of the relevant occurrences of διδαχή with both the other synoptics (Matt 7:28/Mark 1:22/Luke 4:32). The other is present in a verse not found in Mark or Luke (22:33).[3] The term appears in Mark at four additional instances. The whole text (Mark 1:27; 11:18)[4] or the term itself (Matt 13:3/Mark 4:2; Matt 23:1f/Mark 12:38) is missing in Matthew. Luke does not use διδαχή in any of these cases.[5]

From a more general perspective, we may thus conclude that the material exhibits both traditional and redactional features. The large number of instances that Matthew shares with the rest of the synoptics makes it probable that the evangelist received a number of the occurrences from traditions already present as oral or written texts. The material was tradition material, present as intertextual references which influenced the creation of the story. Matthew was a reader/hearer of the traditions. But *the evangelist did not take over the didactic terms in the tradition mechanically.* While it is possible that some didactic terms were missing already on a pre-Matthean stage,[6] the synoptic comparison implies that the author noticed certain didactic elements in the tradition specifically. The material appearing only in Matthew indicates further that it was not a matter primarily of minimizing the didactic terms, but of using them in accordance with special purposes. In order to discover these purposes, I will first study the use of the didactic terms within the narrative structure of Matthew's story and then ask for the connotations attached to them within the world of the story itself.

17:22/Luke 9:43 (λαλεῖν).

1   But for Matt 13:3, cf. Luke 5:3 (διδάσκειν).

2   The remaining instances in which Mark and/or Luke have διδάσκειν are part of passages not present in Matthew. Cf. Mark 1:21/Luke 4:31 (but cf. Matt 4:13); Mark 2:13; 6:30 (cf. Luke 9:10a); Luke 5:17 (cf. Mark 2:1); 11:1; 13:10, 22, 26 (but cf. Matt 7:22); 19:47 (cf. Mark 11:18); 21:37; 23:5.

3   But cf. Mark 11:18 (Luke 20:39).

4   For Mark 11:18, cf. Matt 22:33.

5   Cf. Luke 4:36; 8:4; 19:48; 20:45.

6   DUPONT, Le point de vue, 251, notices that the absence of διδάσκειν and διδαχή in Matthew is parallelled in Luke.

2.2. Jesus as Teacher within the Narrative Structure

The importance of the didactic traits ascribed to Jesus in Matthew becomes evident when we take notice of how the relevant terms appear within the narrative structure of the story. Literary theorists have often commented upon the obvious insight that the initial information focalized by the narrator provides the point of view from which to apprehend the following story until further information supplements or corrects the initial impression.[1] The introduction, amplification and closure of the didactic terms within the narrative structure of Matthew's story are consequently primary means to convey the essential importance of the didactic traits ascribed to Jesus.

2.2.1. The Narrative Introduction of the Didactic Terms

The beginning of the narrative presents the manner according to which Jesus, as the main character of the story, is to be perceived.[2] Matthew subsequently moves on to the arrest of John the Baptist and Jesus' withdrawal to Galilee (4:12–16).[3] Nowhere does Matthew's narrator refer to Jesus as a teacher in the beginning of the narrative. The story does not concern merely one teacher among many others. Jesus carries as teacher a specific authority based on his extraordinary origin and identity. This has to be clear to the readers/hearers before any didactic characterization of Jesus can be introduced.[4]

The narrator significantly introduces the didactic traits as Jesus is to start his major proclamative activity. We find two structural strategies making this clear. To begin with, in the very first summary of Jesus' active ministry in 4:23, the narrator mentions the teaching activity specifically. He does this in spite of the non-didactic focalization of Jesus in the beginning of the whole narrative. He will, with some minor variations, repeat the formula appearing here in 9:35, and partly in 11:1b. It will function as the narrator's explicit reminder of the basic characteristics of Jesus' ministry. The teaching is the first element in the triad consisting of teaching, preaching

---

[1] STERNBERG, *Expositional Modes,* 93f, *passim;* GENETTE, *Narrative Discourse,* 189–198; ECO, *Role of the Reader,* 7; FUNK, *Poetics,* 212–226. Cf. also the discussion about sequence and causality by CHATMAN, *Story and Discourse,* 46f, and about the frame of an artistic text by USPENSKY, *Poetics,* 137–151. For an overview of this debate among literary theorists, see PARSONS, *Departure of Jesus,* 151–155; *idem, Semeia* 52 (1990) 11–31.

[2] Cf. HOWELL, *Inclusive Story,* 115–128; SCOTT, *Semeia* 52 (1990) 83–102.

[3] For a separate discussion about the narrative function of withdrawal in Matthew, see D. GOOD, *NovT* 32 (1990) 1–12, though the hypothesis about the relation of this motif to wisdom christology remains uncertain.

[4] The next chapter will explore further the labelling of Jesus as an extraordinary teacher. See below pp. 276–306.

and healing (4:23; 9:35) or in the pair teaching and preaching (11:1b).[1] This is all the more striking in view of the important beginning of the narrative depicting Jesus—just like John the Baptist (3:1f)—as preaching (κηρύσσειν) without any reference to teaching (4:17). The structural prominence of the didactic trait in these programmatic summaries shows that the didactic story line is of prime importance in the depiction of Jesus' total ministry on earth.

Further, the non-didactic focalization of Jesus in the beginning of the narrative stands in sharp contrast to the presentation of Jesus' first extended speech in 5:1–7:29. Until this moment, the readers/hearers have confronted mainly an episodal narration about Jesus. There are some significant utterances by Jesus himself. They appear as responsive (3:15; 4:4, 7, 10) or non-responsive (4:17, 19) sayings. Although these utterances are important, they are also brief and thoroughly embedded in the narration. But in 5:1–7:29 the narration gives way to a longer speech, and the only narration given (5:1f; 7:28f) conveys the impression of a teaching situation. The actual speech confirms this impression (5:19). When for the first time Jesus speaks extensively in Matthew, he speaks as a teacher.

Through these two structural strategies, the narrator introduces additional information in regard to Jesus' earthly ministry. It implies that *although Jesus is essentially much more than the didactic terms can express, his active ministry is from the out-set partly a comprehensive didactic event.*

2.2.2. The Narrative Amplification of the Didactic Terms

Jesus' ministry contains a number of individual events. A narrative usually contains several actions and happenings arranged in a particular temporal and causal sequence. They constitute the "events."[2] The events appear in a certain order, each event has a certain duration in the sense that some events are told more quickly than others and the events occur with a certain frequency. These components constitute the "narrative time" in which the events take place.[3] The amplification of the didactic terms in the narrative structure points to a number of individual teaching events which gradually build up the comprehensive didactic event.

The didactic terms become more frequent and amplified after their important introduction in 4:23; 5:2, 19; 7:28f. The narrator reminds the rea-

---

1   Cf. e.g. RENGSTORF, *TDNT* II, 139; FLENDER, *EvT* 25 (1965) 704; DAVIES/ALLISON, *Matthew* I, 413.

2   CHATMAN, *Story and Discourse*, 43–95. Cf. also POWELL, *What Is Narrative Criticism?*, 35–42. For an application on Matthew, see KINGSBURY, *Matthew as Story*, 3–9.

3   GENETTE, *Narrative Discourse*, 33–160. For an application of narrative time to gospel research, see CULPEPPER, *Anatomy*, 51–75.—CHATMAN, *Story and Discourse*, 62f, calls this "discourse time."

ders/hearers about Jesus' teaching activity (9:35; 11:1; 13:54). And before the narrative moves towards the suffering, death and resurrection of Jesus (16:21), it presents Jesus as διδάσκαλος on five occasions.[1] The next phase intensifies the impression further. The most frequent use of the didactic terms appears after the narrative has depicted Peter's important declaration about Jesus at Caesarea Philippi (16:13–20) and "from that time on" (ἀπὸ τότε) goes on more explicitly to the suffering, death and resurrection of Jesus in Jerusalem (16:21).[2]

Matthew's narrative here reveals the importance of the terms gradually as it multiplies their frequency during its last phase. This strategy becomes especially apparent in 23:8 and 26:18, both using the term διδάσκαλος in reference to Jesus. The narrative has prepared Jesus' own use of διδάσκαλος in 23:8. The term occurs in 17:24; 19:16. Jesus now approaches the kernel events in Jerusalem—the city that the narrative programmatically indicates already in 16:21, moves further towards in 17:24; 19:1; 20:17f and which is within immediate reach in 21:1.[3] The remaining instances of the didactic terms appear once Jesus has entered Jerusalem, the centre of opposition and rejection.[4] The narrative frequently depicts Jesus as a teacher, presumably active close to the temple (21:23; 26:55).[5] The readers/hearers again perceive διδάσκαλε as the opponents' way of addressing Jesus in 22:16, 24, 36. Between 22:24 and 22:36, the narrator also speaks about the crowds' amazement over Jesus' teaching (22:33). The didactic events are frequent. The speech given by Jesus in Matt 23, not ending until the formula in 26:1 occurs,[6] then informs the readers/hearers about the didactic designations in a decisive manner. The repeated use of the didactic terms in the previous narrative has prepared Jesus' utterance in 23:8–10. This passage comes in at a crucial point in the didactic story line of the narrative. Jesus *is* a διδάσκαλος, but not one among the many Jewish teachers. He is *the* teacher—the only teacher of the disciples.[7]

The MSS have treated 23:8 somewhat variously.[8] The replacements of μὴ κληθῆτε with μηδένα καλέσητε and the following ῥαββί with διδάσκαλον ἐπὶ τῆς γῆς in

---

1   8:19; 9:11; 10:24, 25; 12:38.
2   17:24; 19:16; 21:23; 22:16, 24, 33, 36; 23:8; 26:18, 55; 28:20.
3   Cf. MATERA, *CBQ* 49 (1987) 250f; HOWELL, *Inclusive Story*, 145–149.
4   Cf. 2:3, 15:1, 16:21; 20:18. In 23:37 Jesus speaks of Jerusalem explicitly in negative terms.
5   The phrase ἐν τῷ ἱερῷ ἐκαθεζόμην διδάσκων in 26:55 has been the object of textual rearrangement in the MSS. Some minuscules (*f*¹) omit διδάσκων. The reason for this procedure is difficult to estimate, but external witnesses (ℵ, B, L, Θ) support the reading given in the 26th edition of Nestle-Aland.
6   The concluding function of this formula, with the much discussed πάντα, probably relates to the composite speech in Matt 23 and 24–25 only, not to all the speeches in Matthew. See HELLHOLM, *SEÅ* 51–52 (1986–87) 87f.
7   For further discussion of 23:8–10, see below pp. 284–290, 299–302.
8   Cf. HOET, *"Omnes autem vos fratres estis,"* 8f.

23:8a are weakly attested and clearly secondary. The same is the case with the addition of ὁ χριστός (ὁ ἐν τοῖς οὐρανοῖς) in 23:8b and the replacement of ἀδελφοί with μαθηταί in 23:8c. The support for the replacement of διδάσκαλος with καθηγητής in 23:8b is stronger, especially through Sinaiticus *prima manus* and second corrector.[1] But διδάσκαλος, which the first correctors of Sinaiticus and Vaticanus give, is probably original. It is the more difficult reading. The double occurrence of forms of καθηγητής in 23:10 might have caused the change.

After this decisive moment in the narrative structure, the readers/hearers are capable of correctly understanding the final instance of διδάσκαλος in 26:18. Jesus here tells his disciples to refer to him merely as ὁ διδάσκαλος.[2] This is the first and only time that the definite form occurs without any further qualifier such as αὐτοῦ or ὑμῶν. Jesus should be referred to merely as "the teacher." *The readers/hearers know at this point in the narrative structure how to fill ὁ διδάσκαλος with the right connotations,*[3] and no further explanation is therefore required. These implications are of course not evident to the anonymous man to whom Jesus tells the disciples to go. But for the readers/hearers of Matthew, ὁ διδάσκαλος is at this point a clear reference to the only teacher of the disciples. They now realize fully the significance of the term διδάσκαλος, and consequently no more instances of this designation appear.

2.2.3. The Narrative Closure of the Didactic Terms

Just as the beginning of a narrative is of importance, so is of course the end.[4] The necessary implications of the choices previously made between different possibilities in the narrative usually become evident at the closure.[5] The "process of declining or narrowing possibility," as S. Chatman puts it,[6] comes to its inevitable end.

Ever since the important Marburg lecture delivered by O. Michel in 1950,[7] scholars have often noticed that 28:16–20 forms the climax of the whole Matthean narrative.[8] Although it opens up some possibilities not

---

[1]   ZEITLIN, *JQR* 53 (1962–63) 346; MICHAELS, Christian Prophecy and Matthew 23:8–12, 306, 309, prefer this reading.

[2]   The omission of ὁ διδάσκαλος λέγει in some MSS (A, Φ) is, judging from the external support, secondary.

[3]   The discussion whether Matt 26:18/Mark 14:14/Luke 22:11 reflects a christological use of διδάσκαλος, as claimed by HAHN, *Christologische Hoheitstitel,* 79f, or not, as RIESNER, *Lehrer,* 253f, argues, can be addressed anew from this perspective, taking the narrative structure of each gospel story seriously.

[4]   For different proposals about the function of narrative endings, see PARSONS, *Departure of Jesus,* 66–71.

[5]   GOODMAN, *Structure of Literature,* 13f.

[6]   *Story and Discourse,* 46.

[7]   I am using the English translation: Conclusion of Matthew's Gospel, 30–41.

[8]   The literature on this pericope is enormous. See G. WAGNER (ed.), *Bibliography,* 386–394. Cf. also more recently the structural importance attached to 28:16–20 by e.g.

clearly resolved earlier in Matthew,[1] it also gives the final interpretation of various elements which were introduced previously. In a more recent study devoted to the literary design of Matthew, D.R. Bauer mentions the notions of Jesus' authority and the universalism as coming to a climax and refers to the inclusio which the narrative creates through the correspondence between 1:23 and 28:20 in the conception of "God (or Jesus) with us".[2]

The teaching is also an element recurring at the closure of the narrative.[3] Just as Jesus teaches the disciples at the first extended presentation of his own words (5:1f; 7:28f),[4] so he now commands them—as part of their commission to make (other) disciples (μαθητεύειν)—to teach (διδάσκειν) the nations (τὰ ἔθνη) to observe everything (τηρεῖν πάντα) that he has commanded (ἐντέλλεσθαι) them (28:19f). This didactic part of the commission harks back to 5:19 in particular.[5] Jesus there exhorts the disciples not to set aside (λύειν) "one of the least of these commandments" (μίαν τῶν ἐντολῶν τούτων ἐλαχίστων) when they themselves teach (διδάσκειν) them to the others (οἱ ἄνθρωποι). As I will argue later,[6] "these commandments" probably refer to Jesus' own teaching—especially in the Sermon on the Mount.[7] In that case, Matthew contains another climatic inclusio which concerns the story line about Jesus as teacher. *The process of narrowing potential possibilities throughout Matthew's narrative ends partly in the command that Jesus' teaching activity is to continue in the future mission of the disciples.*

2.3. Jesus as Teacher within the Story

The location of the didactic terms within the narrative structure does not reveal the connotations assigned them apart from the sequential arrange-

---

T.L. DONALDSON, *Jesus on the Mountain,* 170–190; LEVINE, *Social and Ethnic Dimensions,* 165–192.

[1] Cf. POWELL, *NTS* 38 (1992) 190f.

[2] *Structure,* 115–127.

[3] HUBBARD, *Matthean Redaction,* 90f. For the structural importance of teaching in Matthew, cf. e.g. MEIER, *Vision of Matthew,* 45–48; O.S. BROOKS, *JSNT* 10 (1981) 2–18; LINCOLN, Matthew—A Story for Teachers?, 103–125.

[4] For the disciples as the primary addressees of the Sermon on the Mount, see below pp. 224–226.

[5] Cf. BANKS, *JBL* 93 (1974) 239 n. 46; *idem, Jesus and the Law,* 222 n. 2; O.S. BROOKS, *JSNT* 10 (1981) 7; BAASLAND, *TTK* 1 (1983) 8; RIESNER, *Lehrer,* 459; ORTON, *Understanding Scribe,* 159; SCHNACKENBURG, "Jeder Schriftgelehrte," 62; LINCOLN, Matthew—A Story for Teachers?, 115.

[6] See below pp. 291–294.

[7] The MSS vary in 5:19. The omission of the second half of the verse (ὃς δ' ἂν ποιήσῃ καὶ διδάξῃ οὗτος μέγας κληθήσεται ἐν τῇ βασιλείᾳ τῶν οὐρανῶν) in some uncials (ℵ*, D, W) is most significant. However, the external support for this reading is not strong enough. The omission can be explained as an *homoioteleuton,* the copyist passing from the first occurrence of κληθήσεται ἐν τῇ βασιλείᾳ τῶν οὐρανῶν in 5:19a to the second in 5:19b.

ment of the narrative.[1] Although the narrative structure reflects the existence of a text composer not enslaved under specific literary forms and genres, it is evident that the narrative itself is not devoid of literary patterns.
These patterns constitute part of the components whereby Matthew built his
narrative in order to present the story. Without implying any form- and
tradition-historical conclusions,[2] I will ask about the connotations of the
didactic terms by focusing on their location within certain grammatical and
form-critical patterns.[3]

Matthew's narrative also depicts certain persons. Through various means
of telling or showing the readers/hearers about different traits attached to
the persons, it characterizes them in a certain paradigmatic manner.[4] They
may be "round" characters exhibiting a number of traits and behaving in an
unpredictable manner; they may be "flat" characters showing only a few
traits and being rather predictable in their behaviour;[5] they may be "stock"
characters possessing only one trait throughout the story.[6] The connotations
attached to the didactic terms depend also on the characterization of the persons using them.

2.3.1. The Foundational Connotation of the Didactic Terms

The structural importance of the terms characterizing Jesus as teacher implies that they are foundational in the story. They do not give only a random
characterization of Jesus. Grammatical and form-critical features confirm

---

[1]   I refrain from speaking about the "plot" of the story. As is evident from discussions by e.g. MATERA, *CBQ* 49 (1987) 233–253; HOWELL, *Inclusive Story,* 110–114;
CARTER, *CBQ* 54 (1992) 463–481; KINGSBURY, *Int* 46 (1992) 347–356; POWELL,
NTS 38 (1992) 187–204, the term "plot" needs a clear definition accepted by a large
number of scholars before it can serve as a helpful instrument in the interpretation. For a
discussion related to gospel research, with the most important literature, see CULPEPPER,
Anatomy, 77–98.

[2]   In principle, I make a distinction between "form criticism," i.e. the *textinternal* isolation of a formal unit, and "form history," i.e. the *textexternal* definition of the history of
the forms at a pre-synoptic stage. The isolation of a formal unit within an existing text—
the "Sitz im Text"—does not automatically imply that it was also a pre-synoptic unit within a particular life setting of the community—the "Sitz im Leben." For a broader discussion of this problem in relation to Matthew, see FRANKEMÖLLE, *Bib* 60 (1979) 153–
190.

[3]   I do not think that the presence of Greek rhetorical forms in a gospel narrative excludes the presence of Hebrew forms, such as the mashal. In the modern form-critical
discussion, the two often represent different scholarly approaches to forms. The former
focuses primarily on the communicative function of a form, the latter primarily on the
(variating) content.

[4]   CHATMAN, *Story and Discourse,* 107–138. Cf. also CULPEPPER, *Anatomy,* 101–
148; POWELL, *What Is Narrative Criticism?,* 51–55. For an application on Matthew, see
KINGSBURY, *Matthew as Story,* 9–28.

[5]   FORSTER, *Aspects of the Novel,* 93–106; ABRAMS, *Glossary of Literary Terms,*
23. Cf. also CHATMAN, *Story and Discourse,* 131f.

[6]   ABRAMS, *Glossary of Literary Terms,* 179.

this observation.

The tenses in the twelve instances of διδάσκειν are significant. They express certain aspects of the action from the viewpoint of the speaker.[1] The present tense of the term itself appears in eight cases.[2] It mostly serves as a modifyer in the form of a present participle. We find the periphrastic imperfect in 7:29. 11:1 uses it as an infinitive; 22:16 as indicative. Further, the imperfect indicative occurs twice (5:2; 13:54) and the aorist subjunctive, describing the activity of other persons, twice (5:19 [*bis*]). The verb thus depicts Jesus' teaching activity from an internal perspective and as in constant process, whether it occurs in the present tense as without beginning or end or in the past tense as iterative.[3]

From the nine cases in which the *narrator* uses διδάσκειν or διδαχή, eight appear in basic formulaic texts expressing a summarizing comment.[4] As we have already noticed, διδάσκειν occurs twice as the primary element of three in the programmatic summaries (4:23; 9:35). While the position of the summaries gives them the function of an inclusio to Matt 5–9, the triadic formula itself points to the whole programme for Jesus' active ministry in Matthew's story.[5] The terms are also present four times in summarizing statements related to the formula occurring after Jesus' major speeches:[6] two of the instances belong to summarizing statements in 7:28, 29 and refer to a previous speech; the two others belong to statements in 11:1; 13:54 and refer to the subsequent narrative, though without defining the actual teaching more closely. The verb appears also in 5:2 as part of a summary description of the following speech. And the noun διδαχή is in 22:33, as in 7:28, present as a comment referring to the previous teaching, but in this case without connection to an actual formula.

The narrator uses διδάσκειν with a more restricted view only in 21:23. He employs it merely in the frame of the pericope about Jesus' authority. The use of the participle (διδάσκοντι) shows however that the teaching is also here a continuous act not restricted to an indvidual incident only.

F. Van Segbroeck thinks that διδάσκοντι is secondary in 21:23 and due to harmonization with Luke 20:1.[7] But this is unlikely. The omission of the verb in the majority

---

[1] FANNING, *Verbal Aspect,* 84: "Verbal aspect in NT Greek is that category in the grammar of the verb which reflects the focus or viewpoint of the speaker in regard to the action or condition which the verb describes." Cf. also BOMQVIST/JASTRUP, *Grammatik,* § 252.

[2] 4:23; 7:29; 9:35; 11:1; 21:23; 22:16; 26:55; 28:20.

[3] For these aspectual functions of the tenses, see FANNING, *Verbal Aspect,* 101–103, 244–249.

[4] BERGER, *Formgeschichte,* 331–333, prefers to call such a text a "Basis-Bericht" instead of a "Summar." But since some of these texts do function as condensed descriptions of Jesus' active ministry, I will here continue to use the term "summary."

[5] Cf. GERHARDSSON, *Mighty Acts,* 23; GUELICH, *Sermon on the Mount,* 42.

[6] Cf. the formula in 7:28; 11:1; 13:53; 19:1; 26:1.

[7] *Bib* 49 (1968) 175 n. 4.

of the old Latin witnesses and some Syrian translations as well as in part of the transmission of Origen's writings is not sufficient external support. The omission is probably secondary and perhaps due to harmonization with Mark 11:27.

Thus the predominant grammatical and form-critical features of διδάσκειν and διδαχή show that *the didactic terms carry a foundational connotation as a positive description of extended parts of Jesus' active ministry.* Nowhere do they depict Jesus' didactic actions from an external perspective implying that the actions were merely instantaneous or isolated events.[1] The narrative never speaks about Jesus' didactic actions from this perspective, in spite of the dominance of the aorist as the narrative tense in Matthew.[2] It narrates about Jesus' actions from an internal perspective as a foundational and ongoing aspect of his whole ministry on earth. The fact that διδάσκειν and διδαχή mostly occur within summarizing comments by the narrator and that Jesus himself singles out the teaching specifically when he looks back on his activity (26:55) is in line with this foundational aspect.

2.3.2. The Normative Connotation of the Didactic Terms

The foundational connotation correlates with a normative connotation attached to the terms. Matthew presents the foundational connotation from a normative point of view. The normative connotation supplements the foundational. This becomes evident from Jesus' own use of the didactic terms and the form-critical location of διδάσκαλος.

Jesus is the main character in the Matthean story. Although there always emerges a positive picture of him, the great number of traits by which he is characterized make him into a round character. He is not a standardized but a real person in the story.[3] What Jesus says and does constitute the normative point of view in accordance with which the readers/hearers evaluate various elements in the story.[4]

From a total of twelve occurrences of διδάσκαλος, Jesus uses the term four times referring to himself (10:24, 25; 23:8; 26:18). In addition, four of the twelve relevant instances of διδάσκειν appear on the lips of Jesus (5:19 [*bis*]; 26:55; 28:20). The opponents' use of the verb is reduced to a minimum.[5] Nowhere is there an indication that Jesus would reject the

---

1 For the aspectual meaning of the aorist, see FANNING, *Verbal Aspect,* 86–98.

2 FANNING, *Verbal Aspect,* 253f

3 KINGSBURY, *Matthew as Story,* 10, 12.

4 For Jesus' ideological (evaluative) point of view as concurring with the one of the implied author, see KINGSBURY, *JSNT* 21 (1984) 4–7; *idem, JSNT* 25 (1985) 63–65; *idem, Matthew as Story,* 33–37; HOWELL, *Inclusive Story,* 179–203. Kingsbury's thesis is that Jesus represents God's evaluative point of view as the normative one. Kingsbury is in this regard followed by POWELL, *What Is Narrative Criticism?,* 24, 48, 54; *idem, NTS* 38 (1992) 199. But for critique of Kingsbury on this point, see HILL, *JSNT* 21 (1984) 38–42; HOWELL, *ibid.,* 186f.

5 Cf. 22:16.

terms. On the contrary, *Jesus—the main character whose point of view is normative in the story—acknowledges the terms providing the didactic characterization.* The occurrences of διδάσκαλος in 10:24, 25; 23:8 belong to individual units which are form-critically distinguished. They appear in two speeches of Jesus (10:5–11:1; 23:1–26:1).[1] The two instances in 10:24f belong to a unit (10:24f) reminiscent of independently circulating maxims (γνῶμαι, *sententiae*),[2] or aphoristic meshalim.[3] Luke 6:40 uses a mashal similar to the one in Matt 10:24f within a different context. The employment of the didactic terminology within an aphoristic mashal shows that the Matthean Jesus can use common didactic metaphors, which by themselves may vary in application,[4] to describe his relationship with the disciples positively.[5] 23:8 occurs within an epideictic speech of blame in the grand style.[6] This verse is part of an indvidual unit (23:8–12) having the appearance of a rule[7] given as a deliberative exhortation to the disciples.[8] A correct understanding of the didactic characterization is apparently an essential communicative purpose of the story.[9] *On the occasions when Jesus uses* διδάσκαλος *in a speech, the location of the term in the particular forms of the individual units supports the normative connotation.*

---

[1] For the "speech" as a form-critical designation, cf. BERGER, *Formgeschichte,* 67–80.

[2] For further definition of γνώμη and *sententia,* see LAUSBERG, *Handbuch,* 431–434, 540. For the form-critical aspects of the terms, cf. BERGER, *Formgeschichte,* 62–67.

[3] Cf. GERHARDSSON, *NTS* 34 (1988) 339–342; *idem,* Narrative Meshalim, 289f; *idem, NTS* 37 (1991) 323.—BULTMANN, *Geschichte der synoptischen Tradition,* 107, classifies Matt 10:24 among the secular meshalim. He regards 10:25 as added to 10:24 during the pre-Matthean transmission process (*ibid.,* 90).

[4] See above pp. 158f. Cf. also e.g. b. Ber. 58b; Sifra on 25:23; Exod. Rab. 42:5; Midr. Pss. on 27:4 (Buber's ed. 113b); Tanḥ. B. לך לך 23.

[5] BORNKAMM, End-Expectation, 41, uses this text to claim that Jesus "ceases to be a διδάσκαλος in the Jewish sense." While this is true for the Matthean story as a whole, Matt 10:24f cannot be used as evidence.

[6] GRAMS, Temple Conflict Scene, 51, 60–64. Cf. similarly KENNEDY, *New Testament Interpretation,* 74.

[7] BULTMANN, *Geschichte der synoptischen Tradition,* 154, calls it a "Gemeinderegel." But this term introduces textexternal considerations into the form too soon. It is also probable that 23:9 concerns not merely internal matters, but the relationship between the disciples (community) and persons outside of the Christian group.

[8] In spite of the broader audience presented in 23:1, it is probable that Jesus turns to the disciples in 23:8. See below p. 227.

[9] For the three rhetorical "species" (γένη, *genera*), see Aristotle, Rhet. I 3:3, and the discussion by LAUSBERG, *Elemente der literarischen Rhetorik,* 18f; *idem, Handbuch,* 52–61. For further references and literature, cf. WATSON, *Invention,* 9f nn. 63–79.—BERGER, *Formgeschichte,* 18f, uses the Greek expressions (συμβουλευτικὸν γένος, ἐπιδεικτικὸν γένος, δικανικὸν γένος) to classify the three rhetorical situations. In Berger's terminology, 23:8–12 is one of several examples of "symbuleutische Argumentationen" (*ibid.,* 100). I use the expressions "deliberative," "epideictic" and "judicial" rhetoric.

2.3.3. The Interactive Connotation of the Didactic Terms

In the Greek literature, the term διδάσκαλος carries in itself normally neither a negative implication nor validating significance. The basic meaning is merely "teacher," and the context of each Greek text sometimes gives it various further connotations, sometimes negative and sometimes positive.[1]

In the Matthean story, the foundational and normative connotations of the didactic terms find their concretization in texts showing that Jesus interacts as διδάσκαλος with various characters. The use of διδάσκαλος in certain rhetorical forms and by certain characters shows that it carries a basic interactive connotation.

The occurrence of διδάσκαλος in specific forms of communicative speech gives a first indication. Although some text-units are difficult to isolate and give an exact classification, nine of the twelve instances of διδάσκαλος appear in units at least reminiscent of the chreia.[2] According to the rhetorician Aelius Theon of Alexandria (1st cent. C.E.), "a chreia is a concise statement or action which is well aimed, attributed to a specified character or something analogous to a character" (Progymnasmata 5).[3] If we do classify the nine units as chreiai, we should also notice that all nine are, to be more precise, responsive chreiai. The individual unit consists of a significant verbal response to a previous utterance from a character interacting with Jesus. In eight cases the didactic term occurs in one of the sayings to which Jesus responds directly or indirectly. In 26:18 it is part of Jesus' response. It is possible to divide these chreiai further into three groups according to the intention of Jesus' response. Either it conveys certain information (9:10–13; 17:24–27; 22:15–22, 34–40; 26:17–19)[4] or it corrects

---

1 See excursus 9 below.
2 8:18–22; 9:10–13; 12:38f; 17:24–27; 19:16f; 22:15–22, 23–33, 34–40; 26:17–19. With the exception of 26:17–19 and some different isolation of the units, BERGER, *Formgeschichte,* 81, also classifies all these texts as chreiai. For 8:18–22, see MACK/ROBBINS, *Patterns of Persuasion,* 70–74.
3 According to SPENGEL (ed.), *Rhetores Graeci* II, 96 lines 19–21, the Greek text reads as follows: χρεία ἐστὶ σύντομος ἀπόφασις ἢ πρᾶξις μετ' εὐστοχίας ἀναφερομένη εἴς τι ὡρισμένον πρόσωπον ἢ ἀναλογοῦν προσώπῳ. (The recent critical edition of Theon's Progymnasmata by J.R. BUTTS, *The Progymnasmata of Theon. A New Text with Translation and Commentary.* Claremont Graduate School 1987, was not available to me. But cf. HOCK/O'NEIL [eds.], *Chreia,* 82.) I understand μετ' εὐστοχίας as modifying the preceding, not the succeeding. So also ROBBINS, Chreia, 2 n. 5. For further comments on the chreia, cf. e.g. DIBELIUS, *Formgeschichte,* 150–164; FISCHEL, Studies in Cynicism, 372–374; BERGER, *Formgeschichte,* 82–93; HOCK/O'NEIL (eds.), *ibid.,* 3–60; ROBBINS, *ibid.,* 1–23; MACK/ROBBINS, *Patterns of Persuasion,* 11–18, *passim;* ROBBINS (ed.), *Ancient Quotes,* xif; SANDERS/DAVIES, *Studying the Synoptic Gospels,* 146–162; LAUSBERG, *Handbuch,* 536-540. Further literature is listed by HOCK/O'NEIL (eds.), *ibid.,* 49 n. 1.—MACK, *Rhetoric,* 43–47, treats the chreia only in passing. For critique of Mack on this point, see WATSON, *Bib* 72 (1991) 118.
4 As BERGER, *Formgeschichte,* 92, notices, the chreia form does not in itself make a distinction between information given to the disciples and to the opponents. For a recent

(8:18–22; 19:16f) or refutes (12:38f; 22:23–33) something in the previous statement. The responsive character of these chreiai shows that διδάσκαλος is not a confessional label. We do not find it in exclamations validating Jesus' prominence and christological status. There are no non-responsive chreiai containing διδάσκαλος and there are no instances of the term in the narrator's comments on the different episodes. It is present primarily within responsive chreiai expressing a dialogue between Jesus and different characters. *The primary location of διδάσκαλος within responsive chreiai implies that it connotes a dialogical interaction.*

Jesus often interacts with persons outside of the group of disciples. In three out of twelve cases of διδάσκαλος, the person using the term, though not antagonistic to Jesus, reveals no attitude of confessional belief (8:19; 17:24; 19:16). The texts depict the characters as "one scribe" (εἷς γραμματεύς) addressing Jesus directly, as "the tax-collectors" (οἱ τὰ δίδραχμα λαμβάνοντες) referring to Jesus as "your teacher" (ὁ διδάσκαλος ὑμῶν) in an address to Peter and as "someone" (εἷς)—later (19:20, 22) identifed as "the young man" (ὁ νεανίσκος) with many possessions—addressing Jesus directly. The latter two characters occur only here in the Matthean story and function as stock characters. The utterance of one scribe in 8:19 points to a desire to follow Jesus, but not to actual faith. This is evident also from the answer which Jesus gives in 8:20.[1] In none of these three instances does the text reveal an attitude of confessional belief on the part of the characters using διδάσκαλος for Jesus. The term expresses merely that they *interact* with Jesus as teacher.

Characters with evident negative traits use διδάσκαλος in five further cases.[2] They represent the religious leaders of the Jewish people. Although Matthew often depicts the Jewish leaders as a united front against Jesus, there are certain distinctions which make it appropriate not to treat them as a single character.

With one exception (23:26), Matthew always speaks of the Pharisees as a collective group.[3] No individual Pharisee occurs. They form a flat character exhibiting only a few traits. The traits carry negative implications. Evilness is the root trait of the Pharisees.[4] Throughout the Matthean story,

---

overview of various designations proposed for units expressing a conflicting or scholastic dialogue, see W. WEISS, *"Eine neue Lehre,"* 3–18, who himself prefers the conventional German terms "Streitgespräche" and "Schulgespräche." For his discussion of the chreia, cf. *ibid.,* 317–329.

1   See below pp. 303f, 311f.
2   9:11; 12:38; 22:15f, 23f, 34–36.
3   They are mentioned 29 times in Matthew.
4   KINGSBURY, *CBQ* 49 (1987) 57–73, proposes evilness as the root trait of all religious leaders in Matthew Cf. also *idem, Matthew as Story,* 17–24.

they reject Jesus' person and ministry and appear as his main opponents.[1] They use διδάσκαλος on four occasions, either directly (9:11; 12:38)[2] or indirectly through others (22:15f, 34–36).[3] When they speak *about* Jesus as διδάσκαλος, they are alone (9:11); when they *address* Jesus, they appear together with other characters. Their use of the term indicates *an interaction of conflict.*

The participle in 22:16 alternates in the uncials between λέγοντες (C, D, W, Θ) and λέγοντας (ℵ, B, L), presenting either the Pharisees themselves or the disciples of the Pharisees—together with the Herodians—as the grammatical speaker. The criteria for deciding the original reading give no unanimous guidance.[4] However, Sinaiticus and Vaticanus do provide strong external support for the accusative. Judging from the internal criteria, it is possible that a desire to harmonize with the parallels (Mark 12:14; Luke 22:21) or with the normal practice reflected elsewhere in Matthew explains the alternation from λέγοντας to λέγοντες.[5]

Matthew does not subordinate all the scribes under the general category of the religious leaders.[6] D.E. Orton points out that if we take into account both Matthew's work with the tradition and his independent use of the term γραμματεύς, it becomes evident that he has a clear notion of who the scribes are and what they should ideally be.[7] Matthew indeed refers to them frequently,[8] but not only as a collective group. There are two references in the singular (8:19; 13:52).[9] And 13:51f; 23:34—to some extent also 8:19[10]— show a certain positive estimation of the scribe(s).[11] They constitute a round character. The scribes possess a variety of traits and give the impression of being real people which are not absolutely predictable in their

---

[1] Cf. e.g. KILPATRICK, *Origins,* 121; HUMMEL, *Auseinandersetzung,* 12–14; LÉGASSE, L'"antijudaïsme," 418.

[2] Some MSS omit ὁ διδάσκαλος ὑμῶν in 9:11. The external testimony shows that this is secondary. It is probably due to harmonization with Mark 2:16/Luke 5:30.

[3] In view of the rather strong external support for νομικός in 22:35, I accept it as the original reading, perhaps taken over from the tradition (cf. Luke 10:25). But it is impossible to be entirely certain. Cf. METZGER, *Textual Commentary,* 59.

[4] The 26th edition of the Greek NT has altered the reading of the previous edition from λέγοντας to λέγοντες.

[5] While Matthew elsewhere uses λέγοντας only in 21:15, he uses λέγοντες approximately 46 times.

[6] *Contra* e.g. HUMMEL, *Auseinandersetzung,* 12–22; WALKER, *Heilsgeschichte,* 11–33; VAN TILBORG, *Jewish Leaders,* 1–6; COOK, *Jewish Leaders,* 21–25; GARLAND, *Matthew 23,* 43–46; KINGSBURY, *CBQ* 49 (1987) 57–73; idem, *Matthew as Story,* 17–24; FRANCE, *Matthew: Evangelist and Teacher,* 218–223.

[7] *Understanding Scribe,* 23–38.

[8] They are referred to 23 times, if we count also 22:35.

[9] Cf. also 22:35.

[10] See below pp. 239f, 303f, 311f.

[11] ORTON, *Understanding Scribe,* 35, 137–163. Cf. already HUMMEL, *Auseinandersetzung,* 17f, 27f.—WALKER, *Heilsgeschichte,* 17–29; SCHENK, *Sprache des Matthäus,* 66f, argue that there is no positive estimation of the scribes in Matthew at all. However, their interpretation of 8:19; 13:52; 23:8–10, 34 is not convincing.

behaviour. They once appear as representatives of the religious leaders addressing Jesus with διδάσκαλε (12:38).[1] They are here present together with the Pharisees and reveal the intention to oppose Jesus.[2] One trait applied rather explicitly to the scribes in Matthew is that they constitute the teachers of the people and of Jesus' opponents.[3] This characterization makes it probable that they signal an interaction between two didactic characters when they approach Jesus with διδάσκαλε. The opponents do not adhere to the one and only teacher. They send forward their own teachers to confront Jesus. This gives an additional didactic connotation to διδάσκαλος. It is not only a conflict term. It sometimes implies a more specific *conflict between different teachers.*

The Sadducees are always a collective group in Matthew.[4] With the exception of 22:23, 34, they constantly occur as the second part in the formula "the Pharisees and Sadducees" (οἱ φαρισαῖοι καὶ σαδδουκαῖοι). The lack of the article in front of σαδδουκαῖοι shows that Matthew thinks of them in close relation with the Pharisees. 22:34 also mentions the Pharisees and the Sadducees together, though without use of the formula. Instead of indicating a distinction between the two parties,[5] 22:34 depicts them as united against Jesus.[6] There is no remark that the two groups carry separate traits. The collective treatment of the Sadducees and their constant subordination to the Pharisees show that the Sadducces function as a stock character. They are an impersonal group and their behaviour within the story is highly predictable.

However, their presence in the story is not accidental. The close connections between the Pharisees and the Sadducees are peculiar to Matthew and reflect some work on the tradition.[7] In dependence on G.D. Kilpatrick, R. Hummel proposes that the Sadducees represent heretics in Matthew.[8] It is

---

[1]   If νομικός is the original reading of 22:35, an additional instance of a scribal character addressing Jesus with διδάσκαλε is found in 22:36.
[2]   The same is the case with the νομικός in 22:34–36.
[3]   2:4; 7:29; 17:10; 23:2, 7, 13, 16. Cf. also 15:9. For the didactic trait of the scribes, Pharisees and Sadducees, cf. WALKER, *Heilsgeschichte,* 18–23; SCHENK, *Sprache des Matthäus,* 67f.
[4]   3:7; 16:1, 6, 11, 12; 22:23, 34.
[5]   *Contra* ZAHN, *Matthäus,* 643; MCNEILE, *Matthew,* 324; LOHMEYER, *Matthäus,* 328; WALKER, *Heilsgeschichte,* 15f; SCHWEIZER, *Matthäus,* 277; G. MAIER, *Matthäus-Evangelium* II, 227; FRANCE, *Matthew: Evangelist and Teacher,* 222.
[6]   HUMMEL, *Auseinandersetzung,* 19; GUNDRY, *Matthew,* 447; PATTE, *Matthew,* 313; SCHENK, *Sprache des Matthäus,* 71; GNILKA, *Matthäusevangelium* II, 259; KVALBEIN, *Matteusevangeliet* II, 170.
[7]   The other synoptics refer to the Sadducees only within the discussion about the resurrection (Mark 12:18/Luke 20:27). Cf. HUMMEL, *Auseinandersetzung,* 18f; WALKER, *Heilsgeschichte,* 11; VAN TILBORG, *Jewish Leaders,* 2f.
[8]   KILPATRICK, *Origins,* 120f; HUMMEL, *Auseinandersetzung,* 19f.—HUMMEL, *ibid.,* 20, proposes a historicizing interest behind the mention of the Sadducees, but he does not consider their function within the Matthean story.

perhaps no coincidence that four out of five references to the Pharisees and Sadducees in Matthew occur within a context dealing with false teaching (16:5–12).[1] If this observation is valid,[2] the Sadducees add a further characteristic to the opponents. Their presence indicates that the opponents' teaching is false. On one occasion, the Sadducees address Jesus with διδάσκαλε (22:23f). This is the only instance in Matthew where they appear alone as actors.[3] Their opinion about the resurrection expressed in 22:23–28 can apparently not be connected with the view of the Pharisees.[4] The Sadducees' use of διδάσκαλε in addressing Jesus gives the term an additional connotation. Jesus' ministry takes place in *an interaction of conflict between his own true teaching and the opponents' false teaching.*[5]

Out of twelve occurrences of διδάσκαλος, eight occur on the lips of characters expressing a lack of faith or a thoroughly negative estimate of Jesus' person and teaching. But this does not give the term a derogatory connotation.[6] The foundational and normative connotations that the Matthean story attaches to the didactic terms obstruct such a negative understanding. Its use by these characters shows merely that the designation is of minor importance as a confessional and validating label for Jesus. Rather, there emerge two variations of the basic interactive connotation of διδάσκαλος. First, *as a teacher Jesus dialogues* with various characters. It is natural that a teacher discusses his teaching with others and responds to their reactions. Second, *as a teacher Jesus enters into open conflict.* The conflict consists occasionally of an open opposition from false teachers. The didactic trait is a polemical device pointing to Jesus as the only normative teacher.

Excursus 9: *The Greek Use of* διδάσκαλος

For an ancient Greek-speaking person, διδάσκαλος was of course the most natural

---

1   16:1, 6, 11, 12.

2   STRACK/BILLERBECK, *Kommentar* IV, 344, mention that the term "Sadducee" (צדוקי) often replaced the original term "heretic" (מין) in rabbinic texts. Cf. also more recently e.g. SALDARINI, *Pharisees, Scribes and Sadducees,* 226; STEMBERGER, *Pharisäer, Sadduzäer, Essener,* 41f, 48. This would imply that people associated the Sadducees with heretics also much later.

3   The same was apparently the case in the tradition. Cf. Mark 12:18/Luke 20:27.

4   KILPATRICK, *Origins,* 120; HUMMEL, *Auseinandersetzung,* 19, claim that Matthew did not, in distinction to Mark and Luke, think of the Sadducees as a group always rejecting the resurrection. But this claim cannot be supported by 22:23.

5   I do not need to discuss the Herodians who appear together with the disciples of the Pharisees addressing Jesus with διδάσκαλε (22:16). Their presence is probably due to tradition (Mark 12:13). Matthew never refers to them elsewhere, perhaps even omitting such references deliberately (cf. Matt12:14/Mark 3:6 [Matt 16:6/Mark 8:15]). For the most important proposals and literature concerning their historical identity, see HILLYER, *NIDNTT* III, 441–443. Hillyer does not discuss the suggestion that the Herodians were Essenes. For a survey and critique of this proposal, see W. BRAUN, *RevQ* 14 (1989) 75–88. Cf. also the recent and positive evaluation of the hypothesis by O. BETZ, *Jesus and the Temple Scroll,* 76–78.

6   *Contra* FRANCE, Mark and the Teaching of Jesus, 108f.

term to use as a designation for a teacher. We find it already in the Homeric hymns, of which the major ones perhaps derive from the seventh or sixth century B.C.E.[1] The fourth hymn to Hermes uses it (Hymn. Merc. 556).[2] The term occurs also in the writings of the pre-Socratic philosopher Heraclitus of Ephesus (c. 535–475 B.C.E.)[3] and of Aeschylus of Eleusis (c. 525–456 B.C.E.), the first of the Attic dramatists.[4] It appears abundantly in later Greek literature, inscriptions, papyri and the writings of Philo and Josephus.[5] The LXX uses it only twice (Esth 6:1; 2 Macc 1:10). In general, διδάσκαλος *denoted a person or a personified item conveying information or skills to others by superior knowledge and ability.*[6]

A.F. Zimmermann has supplemented and corrected R.H. Rengstorf's earlier evaluation of the Greek use of διδάσκαλος.[7] Zimmermann distinguishes four important fields of application: to an adviser in both a positive and negative sense, to teachers in the elementary schools, to teachers of a specific art or ability (τέχνη) and to religious or philosophical teachers. In distinction to Rengstorf, Zimmermann also points out that the employment varies and not always expresses an intellectual systematization.[8]

Two observations are of special interest. First, διδάσκαλος *was in itself neutral in regard to the positive or negative estimation of a person.* It did not, on one hand, carry negative implications. This is most evident in its use for Greek gods of different kinds. Such a utilisation of the term occurs already in early texts.[9] Justin Martyr († c. 165 C.E.) is also revealing. He does not only think of Jesus as teacher,[10] but calls Hermes the interpreter of logos and "teacher of all" (πάντων διδάσκαλος) and appeals in this way to the familiarity with the sons of Zeus (Apol. I 21:2).[11] There are, in addition, examples from the first century C.E. showing that the Greek-speaking people called also the god of the Jews διδάσκαλος.[12] But it is also evident, on the other

---

1   LESKY, *PWSup* XI, 824–831.
2   In the introduction to the LCL edition, EVELYN-WHITE dates the 4th hymn to the early 6th cent. See Hesiod, *Homeric Hymns,* xxxviii.
3   Cf. e.g. frgs. 57, 104 (DIELS/KRANTZ [eds.], *Fragmente* I, 163, 174).
4   Cf. e.g. Eum. 279; Prom. 109, 324, 375; Sept. c. Theb. 573.
5   For references, cf. REISCH, *PW* V, 401–406; PREISGKE, *Papyrusurkunden* I, 371; LSJ, 421; RENGSTORF, *TDNT* II, 148–151; KIESSLING (ed.), *Papyrusurkunden* IV, 567f; *idem* (ed.), *Papyrusurkunden* suppl. I, 73; RENGSTORF (ed.), *Concordance to Flavius Josephus* I, 487; MAYER, *Index Philoneus,* 77; W. BAUER, *Wörterbuch,* 385f; ZIMMERMANN, *Die urchristlichen Lehrer,* 76–86 (with lit.). The further material in the *Thesaurus Linguae Graecae* computer database does not significantly alter the general impression.
6   ZIMMERMANN, *Die urchristlichen Lehrer,* 76.
7   RENGSTORF, *TDNT* II, 148–151; ZIMMERMANN, *Die urchristlichen Lehrer,* 76–86.
8   ZIMMERMANN, *Die urchristlichen Lehrer,* 89–91. For a similar criticism of Rengstorf's discussion about μαθητής, see WILKINS, *Concept of Disciple,* 14.
9   Cf. e.g. Plato, Menex. 238b (διδασκάλους αὐτῶν θεοὺς ἐπηγάγετο).
10   Cf. e.g. Apol. I 4:7; I 15:5; I 19:6; I 21:1; I 46:1; Dial. 108:2. For further references and discussion, see NORMANN, *Christos Didaskalos,* 107–125. The emphasis on Jesus as teacher is partly due to Justin's own activity as teacher. To this subject, see NEYMEYR, *Die christlichen Lehrer,* 16–35 (with lit.).
11   Cf. RENGSTORF, *TDNT* II, 136, 157; NORMANN, *Christos Didaskalos,* 114 n. 49.
12   Cf. e.g. Philo, Congr. 114; Mut. Nom. 270; Rer. Div. Her. 19; Sacr. AC. 65; Vit. Mos. 1:80. Cf. also Rer. Div. Her. 102. For the concept of being a disciple of God in Philo, see WILKINS, *Concept of Disciple,* 101f.

hand, that διδάσκαλος did not serve in itself as an honorary appellation or title. It carried no inherent validating function. The foremost evidence of this is the use with a negative referent. Examples do not only appear in older literature,[1] such as in (Socrates' and) Plato's (c. 428–348 B.C.E.) well known denouncing of the term as related to the Sophists' conception of a teacher (Ap. 33a).[2] Examples occur also in later Jewish writings, e.g. in the works of Philo and Josephus.[3]

Second, *in the first century C.E., διδάσκαλος had acquired a connotation relating to religious and philosophical teachers.* The Syrian rhetorican and satirist Lucian of Samosata (c. 120–180 C.E.) speaks somewhat later of all philosophers as διδάσκαλοι (Hermot. 68). It is more difficult to find evidence from the first century philosophers. Epictetus (c. 50–130 C.E.) does speak of himself as διδάσκαλος (Diss. I 9:12),[4] but mostly he prefers παιδευτής.[5] But this use is frequent among the Greek-speaking Jews of the first century C.E. Philo's application of the term to a religious teacher is best exemplified with Moses, whom Philo regards as the greatest and most perfect of men in every respect (Vit. Mos. 1:1). He exceeded all the Greek teachers (Vit. Mos. 1:21). Spec. Leg. 1:59 consequently speaks of Moses as a teacher of truth (ἀληθείας ... διδάσκαλος). And Gig. 54 calls Moses "a teacher of divine rites" (ὀργίων ... διδάσκαλος θείων). Josephus' alternating use of the term also included an application to religious teachers (Ant. 18:16; 20:41, 46)—even false ones (Ap. 2:145; Vit. 274)—and to philosophers (Ap. 1:176). Here it is not primarily Moses who is the teacher, though Josephus calls him the teacher of Joshua (Ant. 3:49). Among the three groups of Jewish teachers mentioned by Josephus,[6] especially the Pharisees are called διδάσκαλοι.[7] On the basis of Josephus, Zimmermann interprets even the pre-70 ossuary inscriptions CII II, 1266b (ΔΙΔΑΣΚΑΛΟΥ)—and probably also 1268 (ΔΕΣ..ΚΑΛΟΥ) and 1269 (ΘΕΜΝΤΟΣΔΕ-ΕΣΚΑΛΟΥ)[8]—as referring to Pharisaic teachers.[9] Scholars have, however, not always accepted Zimmermann's interpretation.[10]

---

[1]   Cf. e.g. Heraclitus, frgs. 57, 104 (DIELS/KRANTZ [eds.], *Fragmente* I, 163, 174); Aeschylus, Sept. c. Theb. 573; Euripides (c. 480–406 B.C.E.), Andr. 946; Lysias (c. 445–380 B.C.E.) 12:47, 78; 14:30.

[2]   For discussion of the teacher-disciple relationship in Plato, see RENGSTORF, *TDNT* II, 150; *idem, TDNT* IV, 396f, 417–421; WILKINS, *Concept of Disciple,* 15–22.

[3]   Cf. e.g. Spec. Leg. 3:11; Ant. 1:61; 17:334.

[4]   Cf. also Diss. II 21:10. For discussion of Epictetus as teacher and of his school, see CULPEPPER, *School,* 135–141; NEYMEYR, *Die christlichen Lehrer,* 220–224.

[5]   Cf. Diss. I 9:12, 18, 19; II 19:29. He prefers the term ἀνδράποδον for his followers. Cf. CLARK, *Higher education,* 90; WILKINS, *Concept of Disciple,* 39f.

[6]   For a general account of the Pharisees, Sadducees and Essenes as teachers according to Josephus, see G. MAIER, Die jüdischen Lehrer, 260–270.

[7]   ZIMMERMANN, *Die urchristlichen Lehrer,* 84f.

[8]   CII II, 1269 is divided in two lines between ΘΕΜΝΤΟΣΔΕ and ΕΣΚΑΛΟΥ.

[9]   *Die urchristlichen Lehrer,* 69–75, 85f. Cf. also RIESNER, *Lehrer,* 273.—The ossuary inscriptions functioned to identify the bones which some time after the burial were put into a small chest, an ossuary. Cf. e.g. KANE, *JSS* 23 (1978) 268–270; SIL-BERMAN, *BARev* 17:3 (1991) 73f.

[10]   Cf. e.g. KARRER, *ZNW* 83 (1992) 12 n. 54.

3. The Disciples as Pupils of Jesus

Discipleship is a central concern in Matthew. Several recent studies make this evident.[1] Although it is possible for a teacher to exhibit his functions in interaction with various discussion partners only, the Matthean Jesus appears together with a defined group of disciples.

Being a disciple is not necessarily the same as being a pupil. A disciple may follow a person or a cause without receiving any particular information from a teaching master. Discipleship is not always a didactic category. *We must ask specifically about the didactic traits attributed to the Matthean disciples. The characterization of the disciples as persons receiving and understanding Jesus' teaching constitute one such trait.* It corresponds directly to the depiction of Jesus as teacher.[2]

3.1. The Disciples as Recipients of Jesus' Teaching

Working partly on the assumption that Matthew deliberately changed Mark and Q in a certain fashion, M.J. Wilkins points out that a major device in the inclusion of the term μαθητής was to create units where Jesus delivers some kind of teaching to the disciples.[3] The teaching is of varying kind and it is not always described by a didactic term—with forms of διδάσκειν or διδαχή. But it usually consists of certain information or instruction that Jesus conveys to the disciples, often in response to something they say or ask for.[4] To substantiate this view further, I will study the characterization of the disciples as recipients of Jesus' teaching in the story itself.

3.1.1. The Didactic Connotation of the Basic Terms

The occurrence of the term μαθητής[5]—and sometimes also μικρός and ἀδελφός[6]—and of verbs such as ἀκολουθεῖν, μαθητεύειν, μαθητεύεσθαι and

---

1 See WILKINS, *Concept of Disciple,* 126–224, and the literature referred to there. Cf. also PATTE, Prolegomena, 1–54; LINCOLN, Matthew—A Story for Teachers?, 103–125; R.A. EDWARDS, Characterization, 1305–1323.

2 For the disciples as (future) teachers themselves, see below pp. 238–261.

3 *Concept of Disciple,* 165f.

4 WILKINS, *Concept of Disciple,* 165 n. 181, claims that μαθητής is a signal word for discipleship instruction in the following cases: 8:21, 23; 9:27; 10:42; 12:49; 13:10; 15:23; 16:5; 17:6, 10; 18:1; 19:10; 21:20; 24:3; 26:8, 40, 45. (The reference to 9:27 should probably be 9:37.) It is however not always evident that the disciples are here given instruction in the proper sense. Textcritical uncertainties exist in 20:17; 26:20.

5 It occurs approximately 73 times. Textcritical uncertainties exist in 20:17; 26:20.

6 For μικρός, cf. 10:42 (11:11); 18:6, 10, 14. For ἀδελφός, cf. especially 12:48–50; 23:8; 28:10. The attempt by ZIMMERMANN, *Die urchristlichen Lehrer,* 160–163, to diminish the importance of ἀδελφός in relation to the disciples builds on too sharp a distinction between tradition and redaction.

μανθάνειν[1] indicates the prominence of discipleship in Matthew. But they exhibit a broad semantic spectrum, implying that various connotations are attached to the interaction between Jesus and his followers.

The general connection between Jesus as teacher and discipleship is implicit in such pericopes as 8:18–22 and 19:16–22. Someone approaches Jesus as teacher specifically (8:19; 19:16), and Jesus responds by speaking about what it means to follow him (8:20; 19:21). Although the terms for discipleship do not carry a uniform didactic meaning in themselves, there are certain didactic connotations attached to them in Matthew.

The term μαθητής is often associated with the appearance of Jesus as teacher. There are three especially relevant pieces of information. First, the initial impression provided by the narrative structure implies a certain connection between the conception of the disciples and of Jesus as teacher. The first time the narrator uses μαθητής for the whole group of disciples, he relates it closely to an activity of Jesus described with διδάσκειν (5:1f). The primacy effect, which is not contradicted by the subsequent narrative,[2] is that the disciples are pupils taught by Jesus. Second, all four times when Jesus uses διδάσκαλος in reference to himself, he speaks to the disciples (10:24, 25; 23:8; 26:17f).[3] An indirect extension of the addressee to an anonymous person exists only in 26:18. Jesus never speaks of himself directly as teacher to anyone but to the disciples. Third, the outsiders identify Jesus twice as the teacher of the disciples (ὁ διδάσκαλος ὑμῶν), who are held responsible for Jesus' actions (9:10f; 17:24).[4] They acknowledge Jesus as the teacher of his own followers.

Jesus is thus constantly characterized as the teacher of his disciples. This is the view expressed by the narrator, Jesus himself and the outsiders. It is true that only other persons than the disciples address Jesus with διδάσκαλε. And Jesus indeed gives teaching to various characters. But Jesus is essentially not the teacher of the Jewish people as a whole in Matthew. As we saw, the crowds and the opponents have their own scribal teachers appearing in sharp contrast to Jesus. He is first of all the teacher of his own group of followers. Through the association between μαθητής and διδάσκαλος/διδάσκειν, the disciples appear as followers of Jesus the teacher.

There is also a certain didactic connotation attached to the basic verbs used for the learning process. From an intersynoptic perspective, these terms appear to be important in Matthew: the two instances of μαθητεύεσθαι occur either in the special material (13:52) or as a likely change of the tra-

---

[1]   For ἀκολουθεῖν, cf. 4:20, 22; 8:19, 22(f); 9:9; 10:38; 16:24; 19:21, 27f. For μαθητεύειν, cf. 28:19. For μαθητεύεσθαι, cf. 13:52; 27:57. For μανθάνειν, cf. (9:13) 11:29; 24:32.

[2]   The second, third, fourth and fifth time μαθητής appears (8:21, 23; 9:10, 11), it is clustered around an explicit address or reference to Jesus as teacher (8:19; 9:11).

[3]   For the disciples as addressees of 10:24, 25; 23:8, see below pp. 226f.

[4]   Cf. DAUBE, *NTS* 19 (1972–73) 11–15.

dition (27:57);[1] one of the three instances of μανθάνειν belongs to the special material (11:29), and one is part of a probable addition to the tradition (9:13).[2] Matthew inherited the term from Mark only once (24:32).[3] The terms in 13:52 (μαθητεύεσθαι) and 24:32 (μανθάνειν) are connected with the disciples' reception of Jesus' teaching. It is true that these terms are much less frequent than μαθητής. But this statistical fact should not lead to the conclusion that discipleship is totally void of a learning process and concerned with a commitment to Jesus' person only.[4] The use of μαθητεύεσθαι and μανθάνειν testifies in a different direction, and there is no reason to separate the verbs from the noun μαθητής itself.[5] Discipleship is not a general activity without clear concepts in Matthew. It is connected with a didactic story line in which the disciples are pupils receiving teaching from their master.

The didactic connotation is clearest in the use of μανθάνειν.[6] Jesus uses the verb as part of an explicit command to the disciples in 24:32: "learn the mashal" (μάθετε τὴν παραβολήν). The earlier instances of the verb show that it connotes the learning of some specific teaching. 9:13 uses it in the expression "go and learn" (πορευθέντες δὲ μάθετε). This is strikingly reminiscent of the rabbinic command "go (and) learn" (צא [ו]למד) the Scriptures.[7] The Pharisees have previously referred to Jesus as διδάσκαλος (9:11), and he now urges them to go and learn a specific lesson from the Scriptures. In 11:29 Jesus calls people to learn from himself. The allusions to wisdom motifs in 11:28–30 are well known and give the command to learn a specific connotation related to Jesus' role as teacher.[8] It is perhaps also significant that all three instances of μανθάνειν use the aorist, implying an active and specific decision to learn.[9]

It is not certain that μαθητεύεσθαι in 13:52 should be rendered as a transitive passive,

---

[1] Cf. Mark 15:43/Luke 23:51. The rest of the NT uses only μαθητεύειν (Matt 28:19; Acts 14:21), not μαθητεύεσθαι.

[2] Cf. Mark 2:17/Luke 5:32.

[3] Cf. Mark 13:28.

[4] RENGSTORF, *TDNT* IV, 406, suggests this for all the synoptics, to some extent. But see already FASCHER, *TLZ* 79 (1954) 332f, and recently for Matthew more specifically WILKINS, *Concept of Disciple,* 159.

[5] ALBRIGHT/MANN, *Matthew,* lxxvii; STRECKER, *Weg der Gerechtigkeit,* 192f, make a distinction between the μαθητής of history and μαθητεύεσθαι as used in relation to others than the twelve. But see U. LUZ, Disciples, 109; PRZYBYLSKI, *Righteousness,* 108–110; WILKINS, *Concept of Disciple,* 161; FRANCE, *Matthew: Evangelist and Teacher,* 261.

[6] Cf. also μαθητεύσατε used with the explicative διδάσκοντες in 28:19f.

[7] Cf. e.g. Num. Rab. 8:4. For comments on the formula, see BACHER, *Terminologie* I, 75; STRACK/BILLERBECK, *Kommentar* I, 499. Cf. also e.g. DAUBE, *New Testament,* 433; STENDAHL, *School of Matthew,* 129.

[8] For a full treatment of 11:25–30 within its historical and literary context, see DEUTSCH, *Hidden Wisdom.* For further discussion, see below p. 303.

[9] Cf. WILKINS, *Concept of Disciple,* 160.

"being made a disciple" or even "being instructed."[1] Although this would in some sense strengthen the didactic connotations even further, it is more plausible that the expression is an intransitive medium, "being or becoming a disciple," with the following dative indicating in respect to what or to whom the person is or becomes a disciple. This seems to have been the primary Greek use of μαθητεύεσθαι,[2] and there is no reason here to interpret Matthew from some alleged Semitic constructions.[3] This use possibly appears also in the letters of Ignatius on two out of three occasions.[4] In addition, it may be of significance that some copyist of Matt 27:57 rendered the original ἐμαθητεύθη with intransitive active ἐμαθήτευσεν.[5] However, the substantial difference between the two grammatical possibilities is not to be unduly stressed.[6] In Matthew being a disciple means being an instructed pupil.

Thus, the disciples are recipients of Jesus' teaching. They do not adhere to his person only. *The contextual location of the terms for discipleship gives them certain connotations which imply that the disciples receive teaching as the pupils of Jesus.* They are expected to learn the information he provides.

3.1.2. The Disciples and the Major Speeches of Jesus

As is well known, Jesus' teaching appears in Matthew to a large extent in the speeches. They stand out as vital collections in which Jesus speaks about matters of special importance. The fictional addressees of these speeches are consequently the recipients of major aspects in Jesus' teaching in a special way.

5:3–7:27, the Sermon on the Mount, is especially important. The introduction of the Sermon presents for the first time the disciples as a group of pupils (5:1). And it is the only extended presentation of Jesus' activity that is formally framed by διδάσκειν (5:2; 7:29) and called διδαχή (7:28).[7]

The crowds and the disciples are present at the speech (5:1; 7:28). Within

---

[1] This is the rendering of most scholars. Cf. e.g. TRILLING, *Israel,* 145f; WILKENS, *TZ* 20 (1964) 323; KINGSBURY, *Parables of Jesus,* 126f; COPE, *Matthew,* 25; WILKINS, *Concept of Disciple,* 160; ORTON, *Understanding Scribe,* 231 n. 9.

[2] Cf. BDF, § 148:3, who regard the term as an intransitive deponent. But the transitive use occurs in Matt 28:19.

[3] ORTON, *Understanding Scribe,* 231 n. 9, uses an observation of DALMAN, *Worte Jesu,* 87, suggesting that the middle form would have no exact Semitic equivalent. But Orton should also note how DALMAN, *ibid.,* 87, continues: "Aber wahrscheinlich gehört der Ausdruck dem griechisch schreibenden Schriftsteller an."

[4] Eph. 3:1; Rom. 5:1 use the verb without dative. In Eph. 10:1 the verb is connected with a dative (ὑμῖν) and may be interpreted as a passive. So apparently W. BAUER, *Wörterbuch,* 985, though he interprets the similar constructions in Matt 13:52; 27:57 as deponents.

[5] The normal meaning of μαθητεύειν τινι is "to be a disciple of someone." Cf. LSJ, 1072.

[6] Cf. GUNDRY, *Matthew,* 281; SCHNACKENBURG, "Jeder Schriftgelehrte," 61f.

[7] Cf. also 22:33 with the previous (22:16, 24) and the subsequent (22:36) use of didactic terms.

5:11–7:23 Jesus often changes between giving the address in the second person plural and in the second person singular.[1] Since the alterations do not follow the substance of the argument, they probably reflect a purely stylistic technique. We will see that there are indeed other stylistic features concerning the addressees which are of more significance. But the constant change between the plural and the singular does not seems to indicate that Jesus is turning to different audiences.[2]

Yet scholars often discuss to what extent the Sermon addresses various audiences.[3] The reference to the crowds in 5:1 and 7:28 forms an inclusio implying their constant presence as the audience of the Sermon.[4] However, they are not addressed by the Sermon in the same sense as the disciples are. They are only "potential disciples," who have not accepted the life of discipleship—and who will apparently not accept it.[5] Jesus merely presents to them the conditions that pertain to this kind of life.[6] The radical demands of the Sermon are the conditions for the life as Jesus' disciple.

The disciples mentioned in 5:1 as those who actually approach (προσέρχεσθαι) Jesus are the primary addressees.[7] Besides the substance of the Sermon, there are at least three formal indications suggesting that Jesus speaks primarily to his disciples. First, although Jesus uses the second person plural already in 5:11, the emphatic ὑμεῖς in 5:13, 14 shows that he now turns to his disciples specifically. A similar technique occurs as a more explicit reference to the disciples in the other speeches of Jesus. Matt 13 mentions first the crowds as addressees (13:2f) and says subsequently that the

---

1   The changes between the plural and the singular occur in 5:11, 23, 27, 29, 32, 39b, 43, 6:2a, 2b, 3, 5, 6, 7, 17, 19, 21, 24; 7:3, 6. The initial and concluding text-units (5:3–10; 7:24–27) are generalized statements in the third person, without the joining of an explicit address.

2   *Contra* MINEAR, *Matthew,* 46.

3   G. LOHFINK, *Bergpredigt,* discusses the subject at length.

4   Cf. 22:33 expressing the crowds' amazement over Jesus' διδαχή.

5   Cf. 26:47, 55; 27:15, 20, 24.—This speaks against the view of MINEAR, *ATRSup* 3 (1974) 28–44; *idem, Matthew,* 57, suggesting that the crowds represent lay Christians. 26:55; 27:15, 24 are not merely taken over passively from the tradition. Cf. Matt 26:55/Mark 14:48/Luke 22:52; Matt 27:15/Mark 15:6. Matt 27:24 is peculiar to Matthew and shows together with 27:25 that ὄχλος and λαός are to some extent interchangeable in Matthew. For a recent attempt to account for the ambiguous role of the crowds in Matthew, see CARTER, *CBQ* 55 (1993) 54–67.

6   MINEAR, *ATRSup* 3 (1974) 33; *idem, Matthew,* 46, 61; WEDER, *"Rede der Reden,"* 35–37; STRECKER, *Sermon on the Mount,* 25f; WILKINS, *Concept of Disciple,* 149f; WOUTERS, *"... wer den Willen meines Vaters tut,"* 274–280, regard the crowds as a secondary object for the teaching in the Sermon. GUELICH, *Sermon on the Mount,* 59; LAPIDE, *Bergpredigt,* 17, underestimate their presence when they consider them merely as a neutral chorus and illustrative background with little or no theological significance.

7   FASCHER, *TLZ* 79 (1954) 334, asks if Matthew's use of προσέρχεσθαι in 5:1; 13:36; 15:12, 23; 17:19; 18:1; 24:1, 3; 26:17 reflects the rabbinic use of בוא to describe the pupils' approach to the teacher. This is possible, but difficult to prove. It is, after all, a rather common term used also elsewhere in Matthew. For another suggestion, see below p. 303 n. 9.

disciples approach (προσέρχεσθαι) Jesus (13:10). 13:18 then introduces the emphatic ὑμεῖς in reference to the disciples as a distinct group.[1] Similarly, 23:1 speaks of both the crowds and the disciples as addressees of Jesus' speech. 23:8 again marks the shift of attention to the specific group of disciples by means of the emphatic ὑμεῖς.[2] Second, Jesus qualifies the addressees of the Sermon specifically in 6:30. He calls them "you of little faith" (ὀλιγόπιστοι). This is a Matthean description of the disciples.[3] Third, although Jesus does not use the term ἀδελφός in direct address, its frequency in the Sermon is noteworthy.[4] Matthew uses it for the disciples elsewhere. This is especially evident in 12:48–50; 23:8; 28:10 .[5]

The disciples are therefore the primary recipients of Jesus' teaching in the Sermon on the Mount. Jesus does inform the crowds about the demands of discipleship. But in the Sermon itself, he primarily addresses those who have already accepted the call to follow him.[6]

In 10:5b–42, the missionary speech,[7] Jesus speaks to the disciples only (10:1–5a). He instructs (παραγγέλειν, διατάσσειν) his twelve disciples (10:5a; 11:1).

There is a stronger concentration on the actual instructions in Matthew than in the tradition.[8] While the narrator introduces the missionary speech by stating that Jesus sent out the twelve (10:5a), he subsequently reports neither that they actually went out nor that they came back: 11:1 closes the speech by referring to that Jesus instructed (διατάσσειν) the disciples, but without mentioning that they went out after being instructed; 12:1 speaks again of the disciples, but without indicating that they had come back from a mission. In comparison with Mark and Luke, this is peculiar to Matthew.[9] The speech is instead framed by statements about Jesus' own activity. They precede (9:35) and close (11:1) the speech. This suggests, to some extent, a specific relationship between the task of Jesus and the task of the disciples.[10]

---

1   Cf. also 13:11 (ὑμῖν δέδοται γνῶναι).
2   Other emphatic uses of ὑμεῖς in reference to the disciples may be present in 16:15; 19:28; 24:33, 44.
3   See below pp. 231f.
4   5:22 (*bis*), 23, 24, 47; 7:3, 4, 5. Cf. OVERMAN, *Matthew's Gospel,* 135.
5   Cf. also 18:15 (*bis*), 21, 35; 25:40
6   G. LOHFINK, *Bergpredigt,* 33–35, claims that since the crowds are constantly present, the Sermon is not teaching about discipleship. But this is to overestimate the importance of the crowds and to neglect some indication to the contrary in and around the Sermon.
7   I will use the expression "missionary speech" because of convenience. For the inadequacy of this expression, or "missionary discourse," when it comes to describing the actual content of the section, cf. S. BROWN, *ZNW* 69 (1978) 73 n. 1, preferring "central section"; U. LUZ, *Matthäus* II, 79, preferring "Jüngerrede."
8   Cf. BEARE, *JBL* 89 (1970) 2f.
9   Cf. Mark 6:12/Luke 9:6; Mark 6:30/Luke 9:10a.
10   S. BROWN, *ZNW* 69 (1978) 77–79, 85; FRANKEMÖLLE, Mission, 126. Cf. also WEAVER, *Missionary Discourse,* 125f, though she neglects the fact that Jesus does not

The disciple is ultimately to be like his teacher.[1] He is the teacher's emissary. The focus on the instruction itself implies that the actual mission is yet to be carried out. In spite of Jesus' recommended restriction of mission to the Jews of Israel only (10:5f), the missionary speech is open to the future.[2] The future tenses in 10:17–22—and also the aorist subjunctives (10:19)—strengthen this impression and imply that Jesus envisions a future persecution of his disciples.

As it therefore appears, the missionary speech does not depict an actual mission activity. Jesus gives specific instructions to the disciples. He is himself the active person and the disciples are expected to learn from him in preparation for their own future mission activity.

The remaining speeches also give the impression of being addressed—at least to a large extent—to the disciples. As we noted, in 13:10 the disciples approach Jesus specifically, who immediately turns to them with an emphatic ὑμῖν δέδοται γνῶναι. He gives them special explanation in 13:18–23, 36–43 and poses in 13:51 finally the question about their understanding. In 18:1–35 the disciples only are in view. As in 5:1; 13:10, 36, they—or Peter as their representative—approach (προσέρχεσθαι) Jesus in order to receive his teaching (18:1, 21).[3] 23:2–25:46 mentions indeed several addressees: a reference to the crowds and the disciples precedes the speech (23:1);[4] in 23:13–36 Jesus speaks to the scribes and the Pharisees; in 23:37–39 the children of Jerusalem are in view.[5] It is possible that the alternating addressees represent a stylistic feature, as in the Sermon on the Mount. In that case, Jesus speaks merely *about* the scribes, the Pharisees and the children of Jerusalem in the form of a direct address to them.[6] It is significant that the disciples are again singled out. In 23:8–12 Jesus addresses the disciples as a specific group. This is indicated by the emphatic ὑμεῖς δέ (23:8a), by the occurrence of ἀδελφοί (23:8c) and by 23:11f, the two parts of which are used elsewhere in exhortations to the Matthean disciples (18:4; 20:26). The group of disciples clearly become the exclusive addressee in 24:1–3. As in 13:10, 36, they approach (προσέρχεσθαι) Jesus in the middle of a speech and

---

give the twelve the specific task to teach here. For this important restriction, see below pp. 258f.

[1] Cf. 10:24f.

[2] S. BROWN, *ZNW* 69 (1978) 75; LEVINE, *Social and Ethnic Dimensions*, 46, 196f. Cf. WEAVER, *Missionary Discourse*, 150f, 152f, who claims that the universal commission in 28:18–20 is for the implied reader the ongoing fulfilment of 10:5b–42.

[3] Cf. W. PESCH, *Matthäus der Seelsorger*, 18f, 45f; W.G. THOMPSON, *Matthew's Advice*, 71, 204f.

[4] For discussion of the audience, see GARLAND, *Matthew 23*, 34–41.

[5] There is a change in 23:37b–39 from an address in the second person singular, directed to Jerusalem, to an address in the second person plural.

[6] MINEAR, *ATRSup* 3 (1974) 36; *idem, Matthew*, 116, considers the woes against the scribes and the Pharisees and the lament over Jerusalem as primarily addressed to the disciples.

ask for special information about a specific issue (24:3).

In short, *Jesus' major speeches are directed mainly to Jesus' own disciples*. Jewish crowds are also often present. But the speeches are not preaching aimed for an audience of outsiders first of all. They are mostly information to the disciples. The disciples are the primary recipients of Jesus' teaching. They are his pupils.[1]

3.2. The Understanding of Jesus' Teaching

As a matter of course, a pupil normally tries to understand the teaching of his teacher. Although this understanding is not always a necessary prerequisite for the transmission of the teaching, the Matthean disciples are pupils of a teacher whose words concern their present and future situation immediately. What Jesus teaches is vitally important to them. The understanding of Jesus' teaching is therefore an essential part of Matthew's characterization of the disciples as pupils.

3.2.1. The Terminological Concentration

The central term describing the understanding is συνιέναι (συνίειν).[2] We do not find the same importance attached to this term in Mark and Luke as in Matthew.[3] There is in most cases no evidence that the term comes from the tradition. From a total of nine occurrences of the term, only 13:13; 15:10 reveal some influence from the tradition in the use of συνιέναι.[4] The remaining occurrences in the other synoptics usually point to the disciples' lack of understanding.[5] These instances are in Matthew either absent altogether or present as positive depictions of the understanding which the disciples do achieve.[6]

The term συνιέναι appears as the terminological focus of all discussions about the understanding in Matthew. 13:14f implies that it was generated by Isa 6:9f. G. Barth points out that there are also other expressions depicting

---

[1] It may also be of significance that the non-therapeutic miracles are in distinction to the therapeutic miracles constantly worked for the disciples only. They reveal something and lend authority to the disciples. See further GERHARDSSON, *Mighty Acts,* 53f, 60–62, 66.

[2] 13:13, 14, 15, 19, 23, 51; 15:10; 16:12; 17:13. Textcritical problems occur in 13:13, but they do not rule out the probability that συνιέναι is original.—For the different conjugations used in the NT, cf. CONZELMANN, *TDNT* VII, 892f.

[3] CONZELMANN, *TDNT* VII, 893, claims even that συνιέναι is theologically significant only in Matthew.

[4] Cf. Matt 13:13/Mark 4:12/Luke 8:10; Matt 15:10/Mark 7:14.

[5] Mark 6:52; 8:17, 21. (Mark 4:9 did not originally contain συνιέναι.) Cf. also the same conception expressed with other terms in Mark 4:13; Mark 9:6/Luke 9:33; Mark 9:10; Mark 9:32/Luke 9:45, etc. Luke 18:34 uses συνιέναι to reference the disciples' lack of understanding. But cf. also Luke 24:45.

[6] Cf. Matt 16:9, 12 with Mark 8:17, 21.

the understanding or the lack of understanding in Matthew.[1] But in each case listed by Barth, συνιέναι is present in the context and governs the other expressions: γινώσκειν (13:11) is followed by συνιέναι (13:13);[2] the word-pair βλέπειν/ἀκούειν (13:13–17) and παχύνειν (13:15) are also related to συνιέναι (13:13, 14, 15); ἀσύνετος (15:16) and νοεῖν (15:17) are part of a pericope headed by a command containing συνιέναι (15:10); both νοεῖν (16:9, 11) and ἐπιγινώσκειν (17:12) are followed by conclusions governed by συνιέναι (16:12; 17:13). *The concept of understanding is terminologically concentrated to συνιέναι.* It appears as the main term describing the ultimate acquisition of Jesus' teaching in Matthew.[3]

3.2.2. The Pedagogical Concern of the Understanding

Both times when the disciples are explicitly assumed to learn in some sense (μανθάνειν, μαθητεύεσθαι), the teaching is given in the form of brief parables, narrative meshalim.[4] In 24:32 it is evident that the object of learning is the mashal about the fig tree. 13:51f conveys the impression that every scribe is or becomes a disciple for the kingdom of heaven on the basis of (διὰ τοῦτο) understanding the previous meshalim.[5] Although it is possible that the expression "these things" (ταῦτα πάντα) carries an apocalyptic connotation in 13:51,[6] its prime reference is to the narrative meshalim which Jesus has just given and explained.[7] 13:34 uses the same expression in direct reference to what Jesus says in the form of meshalim.

The terminological concentration of the concept of understanding further strengthens the impression that there is a certain connection between

---

1 Law, 109.
2 Cf. SCHENK, *Sprache des Matthäus*, 138.
3 Cf. ORTON, *Understanding Scribe*, 145.
4 SCOTT, *Hear Then the Parable*, 35, defines a parable as "a *mashal* that employs a **short narrative fiction** to reference a symbol." STERN, *Parables in Midrash, passim*, focuses on the "midrashic mashal"—with its application, the "nimshal"—and stresses its narrative function in midrash. It is then a short step to call the NT parables "narrative meshalim." So GERHARDSSON, *NTS* 34 (1988) 341f. Cf. also *idem*, Narrative Meshalim, 290; *idem*, *NTS* 37 (1991) 323.
5 For the force of διὰ τοῦτο in 13:52, see ORTON, *Understanding Scribe*, 141–144. Cf. also e.g. DUPONT, Nova et vetera 60; KÜNZEL, *Gemeindeverständnis*, 177; GUNDRY, *Matthew*, 281; SCHNACKENBURG, "Jeder Schriftgelehrte," 60; LAMBRECHT, *Treasure*, 173.
6 So ORTON, *Understanding Scribe*, 146f.—Orton's counting is however incorrect, it seems. From 12 instances of the expression (including the reverse order of the words) in Matthew, 5 occur in apocalyptic contexts (23:36; 24:2, 8, 33, 34). The remaining appear in 4:9; 6:32, 33; 13:34, 51, 56; 19:20. Orton does not mention 23:33 and finds two occurrences of the expression in 6:33.
7 GUNDRY, *Matthew*, 281, seems to think that 13:56 also refers to the meshalim. But 13:53 has introduced a new scene. The expression is in 13:56 linked to Jesus' wisdom and mighty acts mentioned in 13:54. Both verses use πόθεν in the beginning of the question.

the disciples' learning and the use of meshalim. The references to the understanding are generally linked with a mashal requiring explanation. The term συνιέναι occurs either within the explanation of the mashal itself (13:19, 23) or in the larger framework of the meshalim (13:13–15, 51; 15:10). In 16:12; 17:13 the understanding focuses on an image—the yeast of the bread and the coming of Elijah—which is in itself known to the disciples but in need of further comment in regard to its application. 15:15f calls the disciples ἀσύνετοί because they ask for some explanation of a mashal. Jesus' meshalim are the prime object of the understanding.

However, it is difficult to accept the assumption that the object of the understanding is ultimately restricted merely to the fictional narratives and images. The disciples appear as pupils of Jesus in major parts of the Matthean story. 13:19 defines the ultimate object of the understanding as the word of the kingdom, and 13:23 as the word. Elsewhere the object concerns Jesus' opinion about the traditions of the elders (15:1–20), about the teaching of the opponents (16:5–12) or about John the Baptist (17:9–13). The actual object of the understanding goes beyond the meshalim and consists at the end of all that Jesus teaches and preaches in Matthew.[1] The narrative meshalim serve essentially as didactic aids—tools—for illuminating the mysteries of the kingdom.[2]

This suggests that *it is Jesus' fictional manner of speaking that causes the Matthean emphasis on the understanding.* The narrative meshalim are to help the disciples understand Jesus' teaching and preaching. Understanding them means understanding the word of the kingdom. But they are not in themselves always immediately open to full understanding. They need to be explained. *The understanding is consequently a pedagogical concern* in the characterization of disciples as pupils.

3.2.3. The Pedagogical Means of the Understanding

G. Strecker proposes that Matthew's emphasis on the full understanding reflects the intention to idealize the disciples as representatives of an unrepeatable holy past.[3] To be sure, the Matthean concept of history indeed involves many complicated issues.[4] But Strecker's suggestion seems unsatisfactory under closer scrutiny. It is necessary to discuss Matthew's insistence on the full understanding of the disciples *together* with his less ideal depiction of their faith and his presentation of the means for achieving the un-

---

[1]   Cf. G. BARTH, Law, 109f, though he underestimates the fictional manner of conveying the ultimate object of the understanding.

[2]   GERHARDSSON, Illuminating the Kingdom, 282f, 295f, 299.

[3]   *Weg der Gerechtigkeit,* 193f; *idem,* Concept of History, 73.

[4]   For a survey of the most important contributions, see FRANCE, *Matthew: Evangelist and Teacher,* 198–201. Cf. also the recent study by LEVINE, *Social and Ethnic Dimensions.*

derstanding.

It is true that nobody but the disciples will achieve the full understanding (13:51; 16:12; 17:13). Jesus states explicitly that the crowds do not understand (13:13–15).[1] And the opponents are blind leaders (15:14; 23:16, 24).[2] 15:10 implies that the crowd should try to understand,[3] but there is no subsequent report that it did understand. The focus is instead on the fact that Jesus explains the mashal to the "ignorant" (ἀσύνετοι) disciples (15:15–20). Discipleship is indeed the basic means of understanding fully Jesus' teaching.

However, the faith of the disciples is not the inevitable means of reaching understanding. They are men of little faith (ὀλιγόπιστοι).[4] Just as rabbinic writings occasionally speak of those of little faith (קטני אמנה, מחוסרי אמנה) as doubting within the larger framework of adherence to God,[5] the concept of little faith describes in Matthew the scepticism which Jesus' closest followers sometimes may express. They act cowardly (8:26); they doubt that Jesus would rescue or accept them (14:31; 28:17);[6] they are frightened (14:30; 17:6), indignant (20:24; 26:8), terrified (14:26), etc. Jesus gives the harshest possible response to Peter's rebuke of him (16:22f). Matthew includes even Judas, the betrayer, among those called disciples (10:4; 26:14, 47). There are also other negative traits present in large parts of the story.[7] Faith is not the primary means for achieving understanding. And it is not possible, with Barth,[8] to claim that the understanding is the presupposition of faith in Matthew. The doubts remain to the end of the narrative. The understanding of the disciples illustrated in Matthew has evidently not abolished all the doubts.[9] Jesus leads the disciples to the full understanding of his teaching, but their faith is and remains subject to weakness.[10] The faith

---

1 Several scholars consider 13:14f as a later gloss. So e.g. GNILKA, *Die Verstockung Israels,* 103f; *idem,* Das Verstockungsproblem, 119, 127; STENDAHL, *School of Matthew,* 131; ROTHFUCHS, *Erfüllungszitate,* 23f; STRECKER, *Weg der Gerechtigkeit,* 70 n. 4. But there is no textcritical justification for this. For arguments in favour of its original presence in Matthew, see GUNDRY, *Use of the Old Testament,* 116–118.
2 21:45 pictures the understanding of the opponents merely with γινώσκειν, not συνιέναι.
3 This is one of the few instances that Matthew probably took over from the tradition. Cf. Mark 7:14.
4 6:30; 8:26; 14:31; 16:8; 17:20.
5 Cf. e.g. b. Soṭa 48b; Mek. on 16:4, 19f, 27 (Lauterbach II, 103:27; 116:12; 120:84). Further references are given by STRACK/BILLERBECK, *Kommentar* I, 439.
6 GRAYSTON, *JSNT* 21 (1984) 105–109. Cf. also OBERLINNER, "... sie zweifelten aber," 375–400.
7 Cf. 15:23; 19:13; 26:40, 45, 56.
8 Law, 113, 116. Cf. also SHERIDAN, *BTB* 3 (1973) 247.
9 R.A. EDWARDS, Uncertain Faith, 59.
10 H. KLEIN, Glaubensverständnis, 37, states: "Obwohl Matthäus nie vom Wachsen des Glaubens redet, dürfte er doch gemeint haben, daß man Glauben fördern, Kleinglauben langsam überwinden kann." But the flow of the Matthean narrative itself does not express this view.

expected of the disciples is that kind of trust which is required by persons who themselves are to perform miracles. In this sense the disciples fail to believe. Persons who are not counted among Jesus' close followers express another kind of faith which does not fail.[1] This is an expression of trust in the powers of Jesus to work therapeutic miracles.[2] But such faith never relates directly to understanding. It is expressed by other persons than the ones achieving understanding. With the possible exception of 16:8f,[3] the understanding is not immediately connected with faith.[4] As things are presented in Matthew,[5] it is neither promoted by faith nor does it promote faith.

To be sure, we should indeed not think that the understanding is merely the result of an intellectual effort.[6] Three considerations make this especially clear. First, in spite of referring in 13:13 to the inherent obduracy of the crowds as the reason (ὅτι) for speaking with meshalim,[7] Jesus states in 13:11 that the ability of knowing the mysteries of the kingdom of heaven has been given (δέδοται) to the disciples. The statement is followed by an aphoristic mashal implying the consequences of the gift (13:12).[8] The disciples do not have an inherent ability—as opposed to the inherent obduracy of the crowds—to understand. It is essentially not something which they can achieve by their own efforts. Knowledge of the mysteries—the understanding—is the result of revelation. Second, the understanding involves the very centre of man's inner life—his heart:[9] the heart has grown dull when people do not understand (13:15a); the heart is the instrument of understanding (13:15b); the heart is the place where the word of the kingdom is

---

1   Cf. 8:10; 9:2, 22, 28f; 15:28; 17:15.

2   For the connection between faith and mighty acts, see GERHARDSSON, *Mighty Acts,* 47–51, 62–65; HELD, Miracle Stories, 275–296. Cf. also ZUMSTEIN, *Condition du croyant,* 234–238.—SHERIDAN, *BTB* 3 (1976) 247–249; G. BARTH, Law, 112–116; U. LUZ, Disciples, 103f, 107; GIESEN, Krankenheilungen, 92–97, do not give due attention to the distinction between the different aspects of faith.

3   In comparison with Mark 8:17, it is noteworthy, however, that συνιέναι is not used in the negative statement in Matt 16:9, only in the positive depiction in 16:12, which is not present in Mark at all.

4   Cf. U. LUZ, Disciples, 103f. More recently U. LUZ, *Matthäus* II, 447f, does not seem to regard 16:8f as an exception to the separation of the understanding from faith.

5   VERSEPUT, *JSNT* 46 (1992) 3–24, argues that the depiction of the disciples' little faith as contrasted to their understanding in the narrative is intended to impart a cognitive element to the faith of the reader. For my purposes, it is not necessary bring the text pragmatic questions into the analysis at this point.

6   Cf. G. BARTH, Law, 110.

7   This is a Matthean emphasis. Both parallels (Mark 4:12/Luke 8:10) use ἵνα. Cf. WILKENS, *TZ* 20 (1964) 311f. For an extensive discussion of the problems involved, see GNILKA, *Die Verstockung Israels,* 89–115; *idem,* Das Verstockungsproblem, 119–128.

8   For the general and proverbial character of the mashal, cf. e.g. Prov 1:5; 9:9; 11:24; Dan 2:21; 4 Ezra 7:25; b. Ber. 55a; Qoh. Rab. on 1:7.

9   BEHM, *TDNT* III, 611–613, gives numerous NT examples of the heart as the centre of man's inner life to which God turns.

first sown (13:19).[1] The understanding should be an undivided act of the heart.[2] It means the complete internalization of Jesus' words.[3] Third, the understanding has its spontaneous manifestation in active practice. It concerns not only the intellect. The one who understands is the one who indeed (ὅς δή) brings forth fruit (13:23). Understanding is doing (ποιεῖν).[4] Only the one who shows actions corresponding to the word of the kingdom has truly understood.[5]

But revelation also makes use of conventional means of teaching. It was a normal pedagogical habit to deliver specific teaching to the persons closest to the teacher. As we saw in the previous part of the study, already Isa 8:16 speaks of a torah which the prophet gives to his own disciples only.[6] Esoteric teaching was a pedagogical means in various ancient circles eager to achieve wisdom.[7] Although the Qumranites did not develop a sectarian teaching for its own sake, there is evidence that they avoided conveying certain doctrines to persons outside of the community.[8] Josephus' report about the Essenes in Bell. 2:141 confirms this. There are also other examples, both from Jewish practices in some apocalyptic and rabbinic circles and the diaspora as well as from practices in some philosophical schools and mystery religions.[9]

In spite of implying that the understanding is basically a divine gift, Matthew mostly pictures it as the result of special teaching which Jesus gives to the disciples only.[10] It is not correct to emphasize the revelatory character of the understanding without paying attention to the pedagogical means of achieving it.[11] Revelation also comes in unveiled words of interpretation.[12] In 13:36; 15:15 the disciples ask Jesus about the meaning of the meshalim. And the explanation of the meshalim that Jesus gives in 13:18–23, 37–43 is the basis for their affirmative answer to the question of under-

---

[1] Cf. also 15:8.

[2] Cf. GERHARDSSON, *NTS* 14 (1967–68) 176, who refers to the divine demand of the Shemaᶜ to love God with your whole heart (Deut 6:5), i.e. with both the good and the evil inclination of your heart (m. Ber. 9:5).

[3] Cf. P. BONNARD, Matthieu, 3.

[4] For the connection between bringing forth fruit and doing, cf. 3:8, 10; 7:17–19; 13:26; 21:43 and CHARETTE, *Recompense,* 121–140.

[5] Cf. U. LUZ, *Matthäus* II, 318: "Verstehen des Wortes vom Reich gibt es nur für den, der es mit dem Gehorsam, der Praxis verbindet."

[6] See above pp. 40f.

[7] See MCKANE, *Prophets,* 94–101.

[8] Cf. CD 15:10f; 1QS 4:6; 5:15f; 8:18; 9:16f and the discussion above pp. 152f.

[9] See RIESNER, *Lehrer,* 481f (with lit.). Cf. also already DAUBE, *ExpTim* 57 (1945–46) 175–177.

[10] Cf. 13:10–23, 36–52; 15:15–20; 16:9–12; 17:10–13.

[11] *Contra* G. BARTH, Law, 106–109, who builds too much on Matthew's treatment of Mark 4:34. Cf. similarly WILKENS, *TZ* 20 (1964) 311; SHERIDAN, *BTB* 3 (1973) 244.

[12] Cf. GERHARDSSON, *NTS* 14 (1967–68) 165, 188.

standing in 13:51. The connection between the special teaching and the understanding becomes even more explicit later in Matthew. Jesus' questioning of the disciples' understanding in 15:16; 16:9a precedes the teaching he gives in 15:17–20; 16:9b–11. And immediately after he has given the teaching in 16:9b–11; 17:11f, the narrator reports that the disciples now (τότε) did understand (16:12; 17:13). Also outside of the major passages dealing explicitly with the understanding, Jesus gives the disciples special information.[1] They receive special teaching more frequently in Matthew than in any other gospel narrative.[2]

The understanding of the disciples is therefore not merely part of something ideal and unrepeatable. *The understanding appears both as an important gift internalized in the lives of Jesus' disciples and as a normal result of conventional pedagogical means to teach.* The two need to be held together. The disciples understand fully because they have been given the gift of understanding and after they have been properly instructed by Jesus. The depiction of the means for achieving a full understanding contributes therefore to the characterization of the disciples as Jesus' attentive pupils.

4. Summary and Conclusions

This chapter tried to answer the question if the Matthean community had a setting of transmission similar to the ones described in the first chapter of the present investigation. It was necessary to discuss the basic didactic story line that Matthew depicts as a teacher-pupil relationship.

The essential factors contributing to the didactic story line were the existence of persons characterized as teacher and as pupils. The characterization of Jesus as teacher is significantly introduced, amplified and closed in the narrative structure of Matthew. The connotations of the didactic terms themselves show that the didactic trait is foundational and normative for Jesus' active ministry, pointing, more concretely, to a dialogical and polemical interaction with other characters than the disciples. But the disciples are the actual pupils of Jesus. They receive Jesus' teaching and aim ultimately to understand it. Conventional pedagogical procedures for understanding the teaching are not opposed to the revelatory gift of its total internalization. They are aids for understanding fully the mysteries of the kingdom.

Jesus is primarily the teacher of his own chosen disciples. To be sure, the didactic story line depicts him also as a teacher handing over teaching to other persons: he teaches openly; he enters into discussions and conflicts. But he addresses his teaching mainly to his own disciples. They are his pupils, expected in a special way to carry—first by receiving and understan-

---

[1] Cf. e.g. 16:13–28; 17:19f, 25–27; 19:23–20:19; 21:21f; 26:26–29.
[2] U. LUZ, Disciples, 102.

ding—his teaching. In this teacher-pupil relationship, *Jesus is as teacher the essential identity marker for a group of pupils.*

The question then arises to what extent the didactic story line provides an index to the author's setting of transmission in the community. Did the teacher-pupil relationship in the story correspond to a social manifestation in the form of a school? M. Smith stated bluntly that no one establishes a school in the NT.[1] This is true when we look for explicit statements only. As far as Matthew is concerned, there is, to be sure, no clear statement that the author belonged to a school. The fiction of the story itself gives no such remark, nor is there any direct information to this end from other sources.

But there is more circumstantial evidence. The school hypothesis is normally based on form-critical considerations claiming that specific forms of texts correspond to specific life settings. This way of arguing is similar to the one concerning the early existence of prophetic schools.[2] It is in a sense rather circular—as most reconstructions of historical phenomena to some extent have to be. According to K. Stendahl, whom Smith did give some credit,[3] the sophisticated use of the OT quotations is the primary evidence from Matthew's narrative itself for the existence of a school.[4] Although such a hypothesis is not historically implausible at all,[5] it remains essentially within the boundaries of an assumed correlation between the form and the life setting.

It is also possible to argue for the existence of a school by assuming a connection between the didactic story line and the author's understanding of his own situation. What is important, after all, is how the ancient persons themselves thought of their situation. The Matthean story is not totally closed to the extra-textual world of the real author. With the voice of the implied author, Matthew sometimes "opens" the boundries of the story. He refers to the reader (24:15) and to his own day (27:8; 28:15). One way of reaching to the situation of the author is to assume that Matthew intended the reading/hearing of the story to involve a certain amount of *identification with its characters.*

The story claims that Jesus the teacher had a specific group of pupils to whom he handed over his teaching. Jesus remains, of course, a unique and ideal figure. But the disciples exhibit—generally speaking—traits that some of the Christian readers/hearers in the Matthean community were likely to share. The disciples are not merely ideal figures of the past. The rea-

---

1 *JBL* 82 (1963) 174.
2 See above p. 63.
3 *JBL* 82 (1963) 173 n. 10.
4 *School of Matthew,* 42, 142, 203–206. Cf. also CULPEPPER, *School,* 217–219.
5 STENDAHL, *School of Matthew,* 30–35, 183–202, substantiates his hypothesis with some general considerations and a discussion of the pesher exegesis at Qumran. For criticism of Stendahl's school hypothesis, see GÄRTNER, *ST* 8 (1954) 22–24; GUNDRY, *Use of the Old Testament,* 155–159.

ders/hearers may have felt an "idealistic empathy" for Jesus and a "realistic empathy" for the disciples.[1] They saw themselves in the disciples; they could identify with them. If this empathy has some reference to the situation of the evangelist himself, it suggests that *the author, as a user of his own text, recognized the didactic story line and identified himself as one among Jesus' disciples and pupils.* He "included" himself in the story; he thought of himself as associated with a school established by Jesus, regardless of whether this understanding was—by the standards of the modern scholar—historically correct or not. It was not the school of Matthew. It was essentially the school of Jesus. It was to Jesus, the only teacher, that Matthew continuously adhered. He believed himself to be among the pupils who, in a special way, were expected to receive and understand Jesus' teaching, also in the face of opposing and conflicting views from outsiders. *Matthew therefore shared in the field of cultural continuity developing towards clearer accounts of the teacher-pupil relationship and more organized schools.*

The evidence presented in this chapter does not allow for a more concrete picture of the author's setting of transmission in the community. It does not generate clear conclusions about how the setting related to the general communal situation of the evangelist. I have only discussed the setting *in* the community, without defining it more clearly. Matthew understood this setting to be determined by Jesus' didactic authority. I do find it difficult to assume that all the members of the community identified with all the didactic traits of the disciples—especially with the task of understanding. Is it not likely that there were Christians relying on the fuller understanding of other fellow-Christians in the Matthean community? I do think that the didactic traits point to a special group of transmitters in a special setting. But in order to substantiate such an assumption further, I must investigate also other aspects of the transmission visible in Matthew. It is first necessary to study more closely the motives of transmission emerging within this setting.

---

[1]   I have borrowed this distinction from POWELL, *What Is Narrative Criticism?*, 56f, who speaks about the idealistic and the realistic empathy of the implied reader.

Chapter 5

Jesus as Teacher
and the Motives of Transmission

1. Introductory Remarks

The second chapter showed that Matthew lived in a sociocultural situation exhibiting three categories of person-oriented motives for transmitting traditions from someone considered to be a teacher: the didactic, the didactic-biographical and the didactic-labelling motives of transmission.[1] The three categories represent the impression from material reflecting the conceptions of different groups in ancient Israel and ancient Judaism. But in principle, they are not exclusive of each other.

Did Matthew cherish similar motives of transmission? Although Matthew certainly contains material originating at different times and with various people, its final form reflects the conceptions of a person related to a rather coherent group of transmitters—the school of Jesus in the Matthean community. *The aim of this chapter is to investigate to what extent an interest in Jesus' teaching itself, in Jesus' teaching as integrated within his life and in Jesus' teaching as integrated within a labelling process interacted as motives of transmission.*[2]

The motives related to Matthew's understanding of Jesus as teacher cannot easily be isolated from other factors. Jesus was not only a teacher to Matthew. Nevertheless, a conception of Jesus as teacher implies a more conscious transmission of his teaching. It enacts transmission, in a sense. Without denying the importance of other christological aspects in Matthew, *I will pay attention only to motives emerging from a study of traits, techniques and labels with evident didactic implications.*

2. The Didactic Motives

In an attempt to determine Matthew's motives of transmission, P.-G. Müller stresses the importance of the final commission in 28:19f.[3] The disciples should continuously teach in accordance with what Jesus as their only tea-

---

1 For the definition of the three categories, see above pp. 79f, 99, 114.
2 See the remarks in the introduction above p. 23.
3 *Traditionsprozeß,* 157–161.

cher had commanded. The activities in the Matthean community remained bound to Jesus' own teaching. Consequently, Jesus' teaching had to be transmitted.

Scholars have often hinted at the importance of the disciples' future teaching activity in Matthew.[1] A.T. Lincoln even suggests that we should read the whole Matthean narrative as a story for potential teachers.[2] The disciples are gradually prepared for their future teaching mission. Lincoln connects the story line about the education of the disciples with the one about Israel and the Gentiles and the one about Jesus. The disciples function as the character with whom the implied reader can identify most easily, without neglecting other major story lines.[3]

If we regard Matthew as a reader/hearer of his own narrative, Lincoln's study substantiates Müller's basic thesis. The latter stresses the enduring normativity of Jesus' teaching and the former the disciples as future teachers. It is possible to develop these aspects further. *The didactic motives become evident when we study how Matthew depicts both the preparation of the disciples for a future teaching mission and the remaining validity of the teaching once given by Jesus.*

2.1. The Disciples as Scribes

We saw in the previous chapter that the disciples appear as pupils expected to understand Jesus' teaching partly through normal pedagogical procedures. Jesus is the only person performing teaching in a positive sense. The disciples remain pupils.

The situation changes after Jesus' death and resurrection. Jesus now extends the task of teaching to his eleven disciples. Their commission to disciple all the nations includes teaching (28:19f). They do not cease to be disciples. But as Jesus' disciples they are also to be teachers.

This important closure of the narrative is not unexpected.[4] In addition to the repeated characterization of the disciples as pupils of Jesus, there are also passages pointing to their future activity as teachers. It is possible that Jesus' promise in 4:19 to make the disciples fishers of men imply their edu-

---

[1] Cf. P.F. ELLIS, *Matthew*, 137; MINEAR, *ATRSup* 3 (1974) 28–43; KÜNZEL, *Gemeindeverständnis*, 176; O.S. BROOKS, *JSNT* 10 (1981) 2–18; GRASSI, *Teaching the Way*, 86–95; U. LUZ, *Disciples*, 103; R.A. EDWARDS, Uncertain Faith, 47–61; DOYLE, *RB* 95 (1988) 34–54; PATTE, Prolegomena, 30–34; OVERMAN, *Matthew's Gospel*, 127–136, 152f.—WILKINS, *Concept of Disciple*, 162f only speaks of 28:19 as revealing a central purpose in the gospel. He does not pay much attention to the preparation of 28:19f earlier in the narrative, in spite of being positive on a linear analysis of Matthew (*ibid.*, 6f, 126f) and calling it "a manual on discipleship" (*ibid.*, 172).

[2] Matthew—A Story for Teachers?, 103–125.

[3] Lincoln overstates his case to some extent, in my opinion. Teaching is, after all, only one part of the comprehensive task of discipling. The story may also contain aspects that are not immediately related to the education of the disciples as teachers.

[4] Cf. above pp. 208f.

cation as teachers.[1] Also the aorist subjunctives addressed to the disciples in 5:19 may suggest that a teaching activity is something to be expected in the future. But the scribal characters mentioned in 8:19; 13:52; 23:34 provide more explicit information.[2]

2.1.1. The Anonymous Scribe

8:19 belongs to 8:18–22.[3] A scribe expresses the desire to follow Jesus as teacher wherever Jesus may go. The occurrence of ἀπέρχεσθαι also in 8:18 shows that the immediate implication of this desire is to follow Jesus to the other side of the sea. But the use of ἀκολουθεῖν in 8:19, 22 indicates that the scribe also wants to follow as a disciple.[4] The following pericope (8:23–27) confirms this. It concerns the issues about discipleship (8:23)[5] and lack of faith.[6] The dialogue between Jesus and the disciples is at the centre.[7] This structure has been worked out with uttermost care.[8] It shows that Jesus' exclamation about the little faith of the disciples is essential.[9] 8:18–22 therefore also illustrates an aspect of discipleship. In a conventional way,[10] the scribe expresses the desire to take on the obligations of sharing the teacher's life and ministering to his needs.

This does not imply that the scribe is an actual disciple. Until this moment in the narrative, Matthew has not given the scribes any positive traits.[11] True, in bringing out five arguments for regarding the scribe as a disciple, R.H. Gundry represents a rather large number of scholars.[12] But the argu-

---

[1]   Cf. also 13:47–50.—The expression "fishers of men" does of course not contain a didactic meaning in itself. And it is not possible, with WUELLNER, *"Fishers of Men,"* 214, to speak of "Matthew's theology of men-fishing."

[2]   Cf. ORTON, *Understanding Scribe,* 137–163, though he pays too little attention to 8:19, which he discusses elsewhere (*ibid.,* 35–37).

[3]   A somewhat different variant of the episode occurs in Luke 9:57–60, but without διδάσκαλε.

[4]   Cf. KINGSBURY, *JBL* 97 (1978) 59f, 62.

[5]   This emphasis is most evident in Matthew. Cf. Mark 4:36/Luke 8:22. See BORNKAMM, Stilling of the Storm, 54f. Cf. also THEISSEN, *Wundergeschichten,* 290; KINGSBURY, *JBL* 97 (1978) 62; GERHARDSSON, *Mighty Acts,* 55; HELD, Miracle Stories, 201f; U. LUZ, Wundergeschichten, 154.

[6]   BORNKAMM, Stilling of the Storm, 55f.

[7]   Mark 4:40/Luke 8:25 gives Jesus' question about faith after the calming of the storm.

[8]   If we read πλοῖον (8:23) without the article, 8:23–27 consists of 72 words—36 in 8:23–25 and 36 in 8:26f. The centre occurs exactly between the disciples' prayer and Jesus' reply. According to GERHARDSSON, *Mighty Acts,* 53, the same division appears when the syllables are counted, with 83 syllables in each part of the pericope. For a discussion of other (possible) numerical patterns in this pericope, cf. SCHEDL, *Christologie,* 160–163.

[9]   GERHARDSSON, *Mighty Acts,* 54f, mentions christology, faith and discipleship as of central importance in 8:23–27.

[10]   See above pp. 53, 77, 89f, 96–98. Cf. also A. SCHULZ, *Nachfolgen,* 106.

[11]   Cf. 2:4; 5:20; 7:29.

[12]   *Matthew,* 151f.

ments are not convincing.[1] There are factors suggesting that this scribe is not one of Jesus' disciples. In correlation to εἰς γραμματεύς, the narrator uses ἕτερος δὲ τῶν μαθητῶν in 8:21, not—as would be more consistent—ἕτερος δὲ μαθητής. The difference between the two expressions is perhaps not all that significant, but it could imply that only the second actor is one of the disciples.[2] The use of διδάσκαλε by the scribe and κύριε by the other person from the group of disciples is in harmony with this correlation. The disciples never address Jesus with διδάσκαλε elsewhere in Matthew.

At the same time, the scribe is not one of the opponents. The most decisive argument against such a view is that Matthew would hardly allow the opponents to express the desire to follow Jesus without additional comments concerning their negative objectives.[3] And when Matthew elsewhere pictures the scribes as Jesus' opponents, he usually speaks of them as a group.[4] In 8:19—and also 13:52—he refers to an individual scribe. Perhaps εἰς is more than an indefinite article, indicating that among the many scribes there is at least one expressing a real desire to follow Jesus.[5]

The scribe is neither one of the disciples nor one of the opponents. He is an anonymous scribal character.[6] He functions as a paradigm for all teachers—whatever their exact identity may be—who are eager to become pupils of Jesus.[7]

---

[1] The arguments are (1) the portrayal of the crowd, from which the scribe comes, as consisting of disciples, (2) Matthew's use of εἰς for emphasis, (3) the fact that Matthew is not calling the scribe one of "their" scribes, (4) the implication of the matching phrase in 8:21 and (5) the reference to scribes in 13:52; 23:34. Argument three and five have been sufficiently criticized by KINGSBURY, *NTS* 34 (1988) 47f. Concerning the first argument, we may note that there is neither anything in 8:18 suggesting that the crowd consists of disciples nor anything in 8:19 stating explicitly that the scribe came out of the crowd. As to the second and fourth arguments, the emphasis and the matching phrase can be interpreted either way.

[2] Cf. KILUNEN, *NTS* 37 (1991) 275.—In order to refute the assumption that this correlation points to the scribe as one of the disciples, KINGSBURY, *NTS* 34 (1988) 48, minimizes too much the reciprocal relationship between the two expressions.

[3] KINGSBURY, *NTS* 34 (1988) 52, claims that the scribe is an outsider because the expression "the son of man," which Jesus uses in 8:20, elsewhere occurs almost exclusively with a view to such persons. Cf. also *idem, JSNT* 21 (1984) 22–32; *idem, JSNT* 25 (1985) 68–74; *idem, Matthew*, 61–65; *idem, Matthew as Story*, 95–103; *idem, Matthew: Structure, Christology, Kingdom*, xxii–xxiv, 113–122. But Matthew uses in fact "the son of man" most frequently with the disciples as addressees. See GEIST, *Menschensohn*, 24–31. Cf. also MEIER, *Vision of Matthew*, 68 n. 41; HILL, *JSNT* 6 (1980) 2f; U. LUZ, *Matthäus* II, 497; *idem, Christologie*, 226 n. 15; *idem, JSNT* 48 (1992) 5, 12 n. 21, 19. For further discussion of Jesus' response in 8:20, see below pp. 303f, 311f.

[4] The only possible exception is 22:35. But the term γραμματεύς is not used here.

[5] Luke 9:57 indicates the acting character with τις only.

[6] ZUMSTEIN, *Relation du maître et du disciple*, 226; *idem, Condition du croyant*, 62, 156.

[7] KILUNEN, *NTS* 37 (1991) 276–279, partly recognizes this function of the scribe. But he prefers to regard him as the "'Stammvater' der 'christlichen Schriftgelehrten'" (*ibid.*, 278). Kilunen also points out that the distinction between Jewish and Christian scribes should not be pushed too far.—WALKER, *Heilsgeschichte*, 27, speaks of the scribe as a "Paradigma der Nachfolge," though he rejects any notion suggesting that the

2.1.2. The Understanding Scribe

The next time a single scribe appears is in 13:52. The mention of "every scribe" (πᾶς γραμματεύς) is a general reference to the disciples. Matthew now develops the scribal paradigm and applies it on a well-known character, namely the disciples.

While it is possible that the expression contains an implicit reference to Matthew himself,[1] there is no conclusive evidence that only a more limited or a different group than the disciples is in view. The context speaks against this assumption.[2] We have already seen that the disciples' understanding is central in the previous context and that their new understanding is the basis on which Jesus gives the mashal concerning becoming or being a scribe for the kingdom of heaven.[3] The disciples' understanding qualifies them to be scribes.[4] An ideal scribe was expected to understand (Sir 39:6, 9), especially the meshalim,[5] and in Matthew the disciples are the ones brought to understanding. 5:19 confirms this connection between the scribes and the disciples. Just as 13:52 speaks of every scribe becoming or being a disciple for the kingdom of heaven, so 5:19 includes persons with a future teaching function in the kingdom of heaven. The disciples are the scribes of the kingdom. Also 23:8–10 addresses the disciples as teachers.

2.1.3. Prophets, Wise Men and Scribes

23:34 further depicts scribes in a positive sense. Jesus speaks of sending prophets (προφήτας), wise men (σοφούς) and scribes (γραμματεῖς) to the Jewish people.[6]

It is difficult to separate the three into entirely distinctive groups.[7] The

___

paradigm is applied to Jesus' disciples (*ibid.*, 24–29).

[1] This is a common assumption. Cf. e.g. HOH, *BZ* 17 (1926) 266–269; LÉGASSE, *RB* 68 (1961) 490; DUPONT, Nova et vetera 62; GOULDER, *Midrash and Lection*, 13–27; BEARE, *Matthew*, 317; SCHNACKENBURG, "Jeder Schriftgelehrte," 67; ORTON, *Understanding Scribe*, 165–168.

[2] U. LUZ, *Matthäus* II, 362–366, thinks that the scribes represent a specific group and that the disciples are transparent for the whole community. He consequently points to the difficulties in relating 13:52 to its (previous) context. Already MCNEILE, *Matthew*, 205; E. KLOSTERMANN, *Matthäusevangelium*, 125, noticed contextual problems.

[3] See above pp. 229, 233f.

[4] So e.g. ZAHN, *Matthäus*, 502f; ALLEN, *Matthew*, 154f; SCHLATTER, *Matthäus*, 450; DUPONT, Nova et vetera, 60f; KINGSBURY, *Parables of Jesus*, 126; BEARE, *Matthew*, 317; SCHWEIZER, *Matthäus*, 205; GUNDRY, *Matthew*, 281; FRANCE, *Matthew*, 230f; ORTON, *Understanding Scribe*, 141–151, *passim*. Cf. also SCHNACKENBURG, "Jeder Schriftgelehrte," 60f.

[5] Cf. above pp. 47, 81.

[6] As becomes evident in 23:36f, the object of reproach now includes the Jewish people as a whole. See HARE, *Jewish Persecution*, 151f; *idem, Matthew*, 271.

[7] *Contra* e.g. KILPATRICK, *Origins*, 110f, 126; STRECKER, *Weg der Gerechtigkeit*, 37f; SAND, Propheten, 173–184; MANSON, *Sayings of Jesus*, 239.—HUMMEL, *Auseinandersetzung*, 27f, 32, distinguishes between prophets and scribes in 24:34. SCHWEI-

mention of wise men and scribes probably serves as one comprehensive reference to teachers.[1] The distinction between a scribe (סופר) and a wise man (חכם) in the rabbinic literature is hardly evident in Matthew. The rabbis differentiated between "scribe" as a designation for an early rabbi and "wise man" as a designation for a contemporary rabbi,[2] or between the scribe as an elementary teacher and the wise man as a teacher at the more advanced level.[3] Matthew does not mention the scribes before the wise men, as would be expected if the former distinction was present. And in view of the rather negative use of σοφοί in 11:25, it is difficult to assume that 23:34 employs it for a special class of advanced teachers. It is not impossible that the mention of wise men and scribes was taken over from the tradition,[4] though we cannot be sure.[5] In any case, the close connections between the concept of a wise man and a scribe are evident elsewhere, especially in early wisdom literature.[6] These connections have deep roots in the ancient educational system in Israel.[7] Even Enoch, the scribe (1 Enoch 12:4; 15:1; 92:1),[8] is depicted as a man who aquired wisdom (Jub. 4:17).[9] In the light of this background, it seems somewhat artificial to see distinctively separate groups of wise men and scribes in Matt 23:34.

It is even possible that the whole triad of prophets, wise men and scribes is a stylized expression. The OT, Sirach and the Dead Sea scrolls testify to certain connections between prophets and wisdom circles.[10] Prophets and teachers appear together also in Christian texts such as Acts 13:1; Did. 15:1f.[11] In addition, Jewish texts speaking about the persecution of the

---

ZER, *Matthäus*, 114–117, emphasizes that all three refer to the disciples, but he also claims that they reflect, together with the righteous ones, specific gifts and services in the community.

[1] So with various emphases e.g. HILL, *NTS* 11 (1964–65) 296f; STECK, *Israel*, 291 n. 3, 313 n. 2; VAN TILBORG, *Jewish Leaders*, 68, 140; KÜNZEL, *Gemeindeverständnis*, 170; GARLAND, *Matthew 23*, 175 n. 48; BURNETT, *Jesus-Sophia*, 173–176; ORTON, *Understanding Scribe*, 155.

[2] Cf. e.g. b. Qidd. 30a; y. Šeqal. 48c.

[3] See above p. 76.

[4] Luke 11:49 mentions merely prophets and apostles. It is easier to assume that Luke changed an original reference to wise men and scribes to apostles than that Matthew did the reverse.

[5] Cf. GARLAND, *Matthew 23*, 174f.

[6] This is evident on certain occasions also in the rabbinic literature. R. Meir is called חכם וסופר in b. Giṭ. 67a.

[7] Cf. above pp. 39, 43, 46, 49f, 64.

[8] Cf. also 4QEnGiants^a 2:4; 4QEnGiants^b 2:14 (2:21f); Tg. Ps.-J. Gen 5:24; 2 Enoch 36:3 (short rec. MS A according to *OTP* I, 161).

[9] Most scholars date Jubilees to the 2nd cent. B.C.E. Cf. e.g. SCHÜRER, *History* III, 311–313.—For discussion of Enoch as a scribe, see ORTON, *Understanding Scribe*, 77–99, who also includes a discussion of the later Enochic literature; J.J. COLLINS, *Sage*, 344–347.

[10] See above pp. 39, 43, 57, 82–84, 123f.

[11] Cf. also Did. 11:10f; 13:1f.—For the didactic aspects of the prophetic ministry in the early church, see HILL, *Christian Prophets*, 108–130. For discussion of the relations between the prophets and the (sedentary) teachers in the Didache, see NEYMEYR, *Die*

prophets sent to Israel mention prophets, wise men and scribes respectively.[1] The Testaments of the Twelve Patriarchs present prophets (T. Levi 16:2; T. Juda 18:5; T. Dan 2:3), wise men (T. Levi 13:7) and scribes (T. Levi 8:17) as preachers and teachers to Israel.[2] Since Matthew does not give any remark about separate meanings of the three terms, it is probable that they are conventional expressions. In that event, the evidence available suggests that they served as a comprehensive description of Jesus' emissaries, and the distinction between teachers and prophets appears to be fluid.[3]

The triad is in a sense parallel to the prophets and the righteous men (δίκαιοι) appearing in 23:29 as the object of Jewish veneration. The fact that 23:30 mentions only the prophets and 23:35 only Abel, the righteous one,[4] shows that there is no essential distinction between the prophets and righteous men. A traditional expression connected with the suffering of the prophets occurs also here. T. Levi 16:2; T. Dan 2:3 relate the prophet and the righteous man closely as the common object of neglect and persecution. Matthew elsewhere uses the two as one comprehensive expression for the emissaries of Jesus (10:41) and for the former messengers (13:17) [5] The emphatic ἐγώ of Jesus in 23:34 apparently involves an aspect of correlation to a previous sending. The triad he now sends out represents the continuation of the former mission by the prophets and righteous men.[6]

23:29–36 is in this way held together.[7] The Jewish leaders venerate the prophets and the righteous men and claim to have no part in the persecution of the prophets (23:29f). But nevertheless, their treatment of Jesus' emissaries shows that they actually continue the act of persecution against the prophets and the righteous men (23:31–34). Thus *all* the righteous blood will come upon them and their contemporaries (23:35f). This does not mean that the righteous ones are especially singled out,[8] but that the persons

---

christlichen Lehrer, 149–152; SCHÖLLGEN, *BN* 52 (1990) 19–26, the latter objecting to Neymeyr's view concerning the sedentary character of these teachers.

[1] STECK, *Israel,* 208, 291 n. 3.

[2] T. Levi 8:17 mentions a triad of priests, judges and scribes.

[3] Even BORING, *Continuing Voice,* 70, who stresses the importance of the prophets, acknowledges that the relations between prophets and teachers in the Matthean community remain unclear.

[4] The reference to Abel as the righteous one is similar to the targums. See LE DÉAUT, *Bib* 42 (1961) 31, 34; MCNAMARA, *Palestinian Targum,* 159. Besides the targumic texts to Gen 4:3–16, cf. e.g. Heb 11:4; Ant. 1:53.

[5] HILL, *NTS* 11 (1964–65) 296–302, regards δίκαιοι in Matthew as a quasi-technical term for teachers. So also SAND, Propheten, 177. But the traditional character of the expression "prophets and wise men" makes it difficult to assume that δίκαιος refers to a specific teacher in 10:41. And elsewhere, when Matthew uses δίκαιος by itself (1:19; 5:45; 9:13; 13:43, 49; 23:28, 35; 25:37, 46; 27:[4] 19 [24]), there appears a rather variating application of the term.

[6] ORTON, *Understanding Scribe,* 156, thinks that γραμματεῖς here carries also a polemical function against the sending by the Jewish leaders. But this is not evident.

[7] SAND, Propheten, 173, poses an unnecessary distinction between 23:29–32 and 23:34–36, with 23:33 functioning as a connecting link.

[8] *Contra* SAND, Propheten, 179, who neglects the significance of πᾶς in both 23:35

sent in former as well as present times are one group. With this interpretation, the following reference to the prophets and those who are sent (23:37) becomes natural and harks back to the envoys of previous and present generations. Prophets, wise men and scribes constitute together another traditional expression for all the persecuted envoys sent to the Jewish people.

Matthew indicates in several ways that Jesus' disciples are in view here. First, 5:11f connects their persecution with the treatment of earlier prophets. The disciples are related to the notion about the violent fate of the prophets. Second, 10:41 speaks of a prophet and a righteous person to illustrate the reception of the disciples. Third, 10:5, 16 use ἀποστέλλειν for the sending of the disciples.[1] This is the verb found also in 23:34. Fourth, 10:16f introduces an exhortation to the disciples with ἰδοὺ ἐγὼ ἀποστέλλω[2] and continues by mentioning the flogging in the synagogues. This probably constitutes an independent addition to the tradition.[3] It is similar to 23:34. Fifth, the way Jesus is treated is the way the emissaries will be treated.[4] As part of the persecution of the envoys, 23:34 mentions flogging and crucifixion.[5] It refers to the treatment of the present emissaries.[6] The disciples are also to carry a cross (10:38; 16:24). Both flogging and crucifixion are linked with the destiny of Jesus himself. The first and only time the two terms (μαστιγοῦν, σταυροῦν) occur together outside of 23:34, they describe the treatment of Jesus (20:19). The envoys of 23:34 will experience a persecution reminiscent of Jesus' own sufferings.[7] The remark in 23:35, that all the righteous blood shed (ἐκχύννειν) on earth will come upon the present generation, points in the same direction. The Jewish people is responsible for the blood of Jesus. While the blood is to Jesus' followers the blood of the covenant shed (ἐκχύννειν) for many for the forgiveness of sins (26:28), the people as a whole acclaim that they take the blood of Jesus upon themselves

---

and 23:36.

[1] 10:2 calls the disciples ἀπόστολοι. Since there are no signs of an independent interest in this term elsewhere in Matthew—it was perhaps taken over from the tradition (cf. Luke 6:13)—and since it is connected with the corresponding verb in 10:5, 16, it probably carries a non-titular sense here.

[2] Perhaps Jer 8:17 (LXX) exhibited some influence. Jer 8:8 connects wise men and scribes closely. Cf. above p. 43 and ORTON, *Understanding Scribe,* 154.

[3] Cf. Luke 10:3; 11:49. Matt 10:17 does not have an actual parallel in Mark and Luke.

[4] Cf. 10:24f.

[5] Since the Jews did not use the crucifixion as a legal form of capital punishment, HARE, *Jewish Persecution,* 91, considers σταυρώσετε to have been "clumsily added to the completed gospel by an early glossator." But the external support for this assumption is missing. Although παραδιδόναι normally implies that the Jews (20:19; 26:2) or Pilate (27:26) cause the crucifixion, the possibility that also σταυροῦν here—as in Acts 2:36; 4:10—is used in a causative sense has not been conclusively refuted by HARE *ibid.,* 89f. See GUNDRY, *Matthew,* 470.

[6] Cf. KÜMMEL, Die Weherufe, 139.

[7] VAN TILBORG, *Jewish Leaders,* 69.—GARLAND, *Matthew 23,* 177f, claims that the flogging and persecution imply the guilt of the Jews for the death of Jesus. But Jesus' own fate does not explicitly enter into the picture here.

and their children (27:24f).[1] They are responsible for the blood of Jesus and for that of all the emissaries. The prophets, wise men and scribes are in fact Jesus' disciples.

The sending of Jesus' envoys is not restricted to a specific time in the history of Israel.[2] It is open to the present and the future.[3] Jesus speaks in 23:34 of the sending in the present tense (ἀποστέλλω) and of the persecution in the future tense (ἀποκτενεῖτε, σταυρώσετε, μαστιγώσετε, διώξετε). He tells in 23:35 about the consequences in the aorist subjunctive (ἔλθῃ) and as a result of an activity presented with a present participle (ἐκχυννόμενον). The full implications of the disciples' mission as scribes is yet to become a reality.

23:34 is the last positive reference to scribes in Matthew. The application of the scribal paradigm on the disciples is combined with an openness to the present and future time. Together with 8:19; 13:52, it prepares the disciples' commission to teach in 28:19f and implies that *a scribal teaching activity is to be carried out by Jesus' disciples.*

2.2. Peter as Didactic Authority

How does the disciples' teaching relate to the teaching once given by Jesus? 16:13–20 provides a further aspect of the didactic motives of transmission. Although there is no explicit mention of teachers here, the pericope depicts an extension of a foundational didactic authority from Jesus to Peter.

2.2.1. The Extension of Authority

The handing over of the keys of the kingdom of heaven to Peter in 16:19 is a figurative expression for the formal bestowal of authority. The image of the key(s) often implied authority. Isa 22:22, which some scholars believe influenced Matt 16:19,[4] is an early and clear testimony of this use. We could also refer to texts from later times.[5] If the temple was in some sense the model of the early church,[6] the motif of the keys of the temple is of interest.[7] In a tradition recorded in various texts trying to explain the destruc-

---

1 Cf. also 27:4.

2 *Contra* e.g. STECK, *Israel,* 306, 313 n. 2, 314 n. 3; WALKER, *Heilsgeschichte,* 25f, who claim that the sending is only relevant as a historical event during the time of Israel.

3 Cf. HILL, *NTS* 11 (1964–65) 296; KÜNZEL, *Gemeindeverständnis,* 95, 169; GARLAND, *Matthew 23,* 176. (The present participle referred to by Garland occurs in 23:35, not 23:34.)

4 So e.g. EMERTON, *JTS* 13 (1962) 325–331; NICKELSBURG, *JBL* 100 (1981) 594; OVERMAN, *Matthew's Gospel,* 138.

5 See Joachim JEREMIAS, *TDNT* III, 750.

6 Cf. HOFFMANN, Petrus-Primat, 422f; B.P. ROBINSON, *JSNT* 21 (1984) 90–93, 96. Robinson's tradition-historical reconstruction is however difficult to follow.

7 See LACHS, *Rabbinic Commentary,* 256; OVERMAN, *Matthew's Gospel,* 138. Cf.

tion of the temple, the false stewards—the priests—are commanded to cast the keys of the sanctuary to the highest heaven and give them back to the Lord so that he himself may guard the temple (2 Apoc. Bar. 10:18).[1] The keys are here an image of the authority over a religious community.

Immediately after (ἀπὸ τότε) the bestowal of authority, Jesus starts explaining his impending suffering, death and resurrection (16:21). Perhaps even "the gates of Hades" in 16:18 refers to the following passion and death.[2] Jesus claims in that case that not even his own passion and death will hinder the future realization of the church.[3] In any event, the bestowal of authority and Jesus' passion and death apparently belong together in Matthew.[4] As M. Weber pointed out, an important factor in the routinization of charisma is the problem of the transferral of authority that must take place at the death of the leader. One way for the leader to deal with this problem is to appoint the person who will carry the authority further.[5] This would be part of the less purposive institutionalization inherent in most human interaction.[6] As Jesus now approaches his death, he extends authority to Peter.[7]

2.2.2. The Didactic Aspect of Peter's Authority

The second image used in 16:19 defines the nature of the authority more precisely. Although we would expect that a reference to opening and closing followed after the mention of the keys,[8] it is the image of binding (δεῖν) and loosing (λύειν) that further describes the authority.

The meaning and connotation of the imagery is difficult to determine. However, we find no evidence in Matthew that it carries connotations related to magical authority[9] or to a certain authority over Satan and satanic

---

also the Enoch-Levi tradition (1 Enoch 12–16; T. Levi 2–7), which NICKELSBURG, *JBL* 100 (1981) 575–600, discusses as a background of Matt 16:13–19.

[1] Cf. also Paral. Jerem. 4:3f; b. Taʿan. 29a; y. Šeqal. 50a; ʾAbot R. Nat. A 4; Lev. Rab. 19:6; Pesiq. R. 26 (Friedmann's ed. 131a).

[2] WILKINS, *Concept of Disciple*, 194 n. 95.

[3] The closest referent of αὐτῆς in 16:18 is ἐκκλησίαν, not πέτρᾳ.

[4] The suggestion of CULLMANN, *Petrus*, 199–206, that Luke 22:31–34 indicates the original setting of Matt 16:17–19 within the passion, is however too hypothetical. For criticism, see OBRIST, *Echtheitsfragen*, 61–63; GUNDRY, *NovT* 7 (1964) 1–9.

[5] Among 6 different ways to deal with this problem, WEBER, *Wirtschaft und Gesellschaft*, 143, speaks of "Nachfolgerdesignation seitens des bisherigen Charisma-Trägers und Anerkennung seitens der Gemeinde."

[6] Cf. HOLMBERG, *Paul and Power*, 175–178.

[7] Since Jesus is irreplaceable and as the risen Lord will continue to be with his disciples, the Weberian notion is not to be applied too strictly. WEBER, *Wirtschaft und Gesellschaft*, 664, shows awareness of this.

[8] As in Isa 22:22. To be noted, however, is that the LXX occasionally—though not on this occasion—translates the term that Isa 22:22 MT uses for opening, חתפ, with λύειν. Cf. Gen 42:27; Isa 5:27; 14:17; 58:6; Jer 47:4 (MT 40:4); Ps 101:21 (MT 102:21); Job 39:5.

[9] *Contra* CONYBEARE, *JQR* 9 (1896–97) 468–470; DELL, *ZNW* 15 (1914) 38–46.

beings.[1] There are essentially three options available.[2] It either carries its frequent and basic meaning of putting into chains and setting free[3]—often in connection with death—or its related but rare connotation of imposing and removing a religious ban (m. Mo'ed Qaṭ. 3:1f; b. Mo'ed Qaṭ. 16a)[4] or the frequent rabbinic connotation of declaring by halakhic teaching what is forbidden and permitted.[5]

The first option finds support in the use of δεῖν and λύειν elsewhere in Matthew. The terms conveys in 21:2—the only instance besides 16:19; 18:18 in which δεῖν and λύειν appear together—the basic meaning of putting into chains and setting free.[6] H.W. Basser argues that the image in 16:19—and also in 18:18 and, by extension, John 20:23—refers to having the bonds of death set in place or loosened.[7] But he builds perhaps too much only on philological considerations related to the use of אסר and פתח (התיר) in the OT.[8] If his interpretation implies that the forgiving of sins is the means by which a person is loosened, we should also note that this forgiveness was usually the prerogative of God himself.[9] No intermediary is needed in Matthew.[10] This objection also speaks against interpreting 16:19 on

---

Cf. also DULING, *Forum* 3:4 (1987) 7f, 11f, 21f. For criticism of this suggestion, see DALMAN, *Worte Jesu,* 177; BÜCHSEL, *TDNT* II, 60.

[1]   *Contra* HIERS, *JBL* 104 (1985) 233–250. Cf. also BOHREN, *Kirchenzucht,* 52–55; NICKELSBURG, *JBL* 100 (1981) 592. The only indication of this background in Matthew is the ambiguous reference to Hades in 16:18 (HIERS, *ibid.,* 242f). But this is hardly sufficient. The image of the key in Rev 1:18; 20:1 (HIERS, *ibid.,* 244)—Rev 9:1 could perhaps also be mentioned—is not relevant for understanding Matt 16:19. Peter is given the key of the kingdom of heaven, not of Hades. For some further criticism, see MARCUS, *CBQ* 50 (1988) 450; U. LUZ, *Matthäus* II, 465 n. 90.

[2]   Besides the magical and demonic background referred to, scholars often put forward other suggestions. DULING, *Forum* 3:4 (1987) 6–12; DAVIES/ALLISON, *Matthew* II, 635–639, list various proposals.

[3]   Cf., with either both or one of the terms, e.g. Isa 58:6; Pss 102:21 (LXX 101:21); 146:7 (LXX 145:7); Job 36:13; 39:5; CD 13:10; 1QH 11:32; 1QS 10:17; Bell. 2:28; b. Ber. 5b.

[4]   Cf. also Bell. 1:111, which parallels διώκειν τε καὶ κατάγειν with λύειν τε καὶ δεσμεῖν as actions of the Pharisees increasing in power during the reign of Alexandra.

[5]   Most relevant are the instances using the image of binding and loosing without an object. Cf. e.g. the binding by the school of Shammai and the loosing by the school of Hillel in m. Ter. 5:4; m. Pesaḥ. 4:5; t. Yebam. 1:11; y. Šabb. 4a. STRACK/BILLERBECK, *Kommentar* I, 740f, give other references, including instances with objects consisting of persons and things. DERRETT, *JBL* 102 (1983) 114, gives examples from the contemporary Arabic-speaking world.

[6]   For this sense of δεῖν in Matthew, cf. 12:29; 14:3; 22:13; 27:2.

[7]   *JBL* 104 (1985) 297–300.

[8]   In addition to philological considerations, BASSER, *JBL* 104 (1985) 299f, claims that this application of the image became prominent in the 3rd cent. Didascalia Apostolorum of the Syrian church. But as VON CAMPENHAUSEN, *Kirchliches Amt,* 141 n. 4, points out, its use there does not exclude a didactic implication of the image.—The criticism of Basser by MARCUS, *CBQ* 50 (1988) 450f, is misconceived. See BASSER, *CBQ* 52 (1990) 307f.

[9]   DERRETT, *JBL* 102 (1983) 115f.

[10]   But cf. John 20:23.

the background of Tg. Neof. Gen 4:7[1] or as an extension of vows to a "monopoly of salvation."[2]

Since it seems that the great ban (חרם) was not practised during the first century C.E., the second alternative would imply that Matthew uses the terms on the background of the little ban (נידוי)—a partial and temporary expulsion.[3] The little ban, however, finds only weak attestation outside of the NT, and its presence in Matt 18:18 is by no means certain.[4] The juxtaposition of earth and heaven in both 18:18 and 18:19 shows, at least, that binding and loosing relates to common prayer. No one has an inherent right to pronounce a ban. But even if 18:18 should imply this kind of right for a group of people, the verse does not rule out a use of the image suggesting an authority to teach.[5] The situation in 18:18 gives disciplinary connotations to the image. 16:19 has no such context.

This leaves us to consider the didactic interpretation of the image in 16:19. Besides the fact that the rabbinic literature uses binding (אסר) and loosing (התיר Aram. שרא) primarily for the teaching by which something is declared forbidden and permitted,[6] Matthew itself supports this interpretation. First, the pericope about the yeast of the Pharisees and the Sadducees occurs immediately before our passage only in Matthew (16:5–12). And the yeast is the teaching (διδαχή) from which the disciples should keep away. This does not determine the full meaning of 16:13–20, of course. But only rarely do scholars give this observation sufficient attention in discussing the image of binding and loosing.[7] This contextual location of 16:19 suggests that the authority given to Peter partly concerns an issue about who is to deliver the right kind of teaching.

Second, the relation to the image about the keys of the kingdom of heaven is significant. The connection is present only in 16:19—not in 18:18 and John 20:23. Although this image primarily concerns authority, the rabbinic literature occasionally relates it to teaching and learning. According to b. Šabb. 31a–b, Rabbah b. Huna († c. 322 C.E.) compares the key with know-

---

1 *Contra* DÍEZ MACHO, Palestinian Targum, 231. Cf. also VERMES, *Studies*, 123f.

2 *Contra* FALK, *JJS* 25 (1974) 99.

3 For discussion and classification of the texts, see FORKMAN, *Religious Community*, 92–98. I do not need to take a stand on Forkman's assumption that the ban concerned questions of purity before 70 C.E. (*ibid.*, 97f).

4 FORKMAN, *Religious Community*, 126f, 130f; G. BARTH, *ZNW* 69 (1978) 171.

5 Cf. STRACK/BILLERBECK, *Kommentar* I, 738; CULLMANN, *Petrus*, 230; SCHWEIZER, *Church Order*, 59; VON CAMPENHAUSEN, *Kirchliches Amt*, 138, 141; HUMMEL, *Auseinandersetzung*, 61f; CULLMANN, *TDNT* VI, 108; KRETZER, *Herrschaft der Himmel*, 28; BLANK, *Concilium* 9 (1973) 177; BORNKAMM, "Bind" and "Loose," 88, 93; CLAUDEL, *Confession*, 376f; U. LUZ, *Matthäus* II, 465. Among these scholars, Strack/Billerbeck and Cullmann do not think that the didactic connotations are dominant in 16:19.

6 Even BÜCHSEL, *TDNT* II, 60, admits this, in spite of his preference (*ibid.*, 61) for the second option mentioned above.

7 But cf. C. KÄHLER, *NTS* 23 (1976–77) 37; SCHENK, *BZ* 27 (1983) 74; MARCUS, *CBQ* 50 (1988) 451f.

ledge in torah. To have this knowledge but no fear of Heaven is like having the key to the inner rooms but not to the outer.[1] The rabbinic interpretation of Isa 22:22 is also of interest. It is possible that this text influenced Matt 16:19 at some stage.[2] On one occasion the rabbinic literature clearly relates it to teaching activity. Sifre on Deut 32:25 states that the locksmith (המסגר) in 2 Kgs 24:16 is the teacher whose authoritative decisions are comparable to the decisive opening and closing mentioned in Isa 22:22.[3] The Isaianic verse occasionally implied teaching, it seems. It is difficult to ascertain if some early form of the rabbinic interpretation is present in Matt 16:19.[4] Yet, not only does the mention of the opponents' teaching in the previous context suggest a didactic interpretation of the keys, but 23:13 points in the same direction. Jesus blames the scribes and the Pharisees for locking (κλείειν) people out of the kingdom of heaven. The dissonance between what they say and what they do shows that their teaching is false and an obstacle to those who try to learn by listening to their words and observing their deeds.[5] The image of locking the kingdom of heaven describes here a misuse of the teaching authority. This verse even makes the giving of the keys to Peter in 16:19 somewhat polemical.[6] Peter, not the Jewish leaders, is given the legitimate authority to teach. Both images in 16:19 imply therefore teaching activity and teaching authority. Matthew depicts an extension of Jesus' authority *to teach*.

2.2.3. The Foundational Aspect of Peter's Authority

The asyndetic opening of 16:19 does not indicate that this verse is merely an unconnected appendix to the previous statement.[7] Following M. Black,[8] scholars often understand the asyndeton in general as a semitism reflecting Aramaic diction. This is also a common explanation of the asyndeton in 16:19.[9] The asyndetic construction would then hardly imply that 16:19 is unconnected to the previous verse as regards the content. Although we may

---

1 Luke 11:52 speaks of the key of knowledge which the lawyers have taken away.
2 EMERTON, *JTS* 13 (1962) 325–331. Isa 22:22, however, uses סגר/פתח, not the rabbinic אסר/התיר.
3 BASSER, *JBL* 104 (1985) 298, discusses the parallels. The passages also explain the function of the craftsman (החרש). BASSER, *ibid.*, 298f, believes that a distinction was made between two types of scholarly enterprises in the talmudic period: חרש, which implies the theoretical interpretation of the Torah, and מסגר, which implies lectures promulgating decisive halakhah.
4 Cf. BASSER, *JBL* 104 (1985) 299.
5 Cf. 23:2–7.
6 So also Joachim JEREMIAS, *TDNT* III, 751, who goes on to define the authority in judicial terms.
7 *Contra* CARAGOUNIS, *Peter,* 86, 104. Cf. the criticism by SAND, *TRev* 88 (1992) 30.
8 *Aramaic Approach,* 55–61.
9 Cf. e.g. WILCOX, *NTS* 22 (1975–76) 80; B.P. ROBINSON, *JSNT* 21 (1984) 86.

not always think of an asyndeton as a semitism,[1] we should notice in this case that 16:18 and 16:19 are substantially connected. The future verb construction δώσω in 16:19 picks up οἰκοδομήσω in 16:18 and the image of the keys relates to the building of a house,[2] and in a contrasting sense also to the gates of Hades.[3]

The foundation of the church, "this rock," is connected with Peter himself. There is, to be sure, no compelling philological reason for assuming that the word-play between πέτρος and πέτρα means that the latter is entirely identical with the former, perhaps not even if we refer to the Aramaic.[4] But nor is it evident that πέτρα refers only to the christological confession in 16:16.[5] Philology does not exclude the possibility that the rock is associated with Peter—in some qualified sense.[6] Matthew itself provides information which cannot easily be set aside.[7] Jesus directs his pronouncement both before and after the word-play to Peter personally. We find no explicit remark suggesting a change of reference. Furthermore, Peter is undoubtedly the nearest antecedent of ταύτῃ τῇ πέτρᾳ. Unless something in the context specifies another referent, the nearest antecedent is to be preferred to a more distant one. If 16:19 implies that Jesus extends his teaching authority to Peter, 16:18 points to the foundational function of Peter's teaching authority as Jesus will build his church.[8]

The foundational aspect of Peter's teaching authority relates to his position among the other disciples. There is a combination of a *personal* and a *representative* depiction of Peter in Matthew.

On one hand, the extension of teaching authority to Peter is congruent with the importance attributed to him elsewhere.[9] 10:2 is significant. Peter is in distinction to both

---

[1] See M. REISER, *Syntax und Stil,* 138–162, 165–167. Cf. also the cautious conclusion by BEYER, *Semitische Syntax* I, 237: "Über die Herkunft der ntl. Belege (...), ob semitisch oder griechisch, läßt sich also nichts sagen."

[2] Cf. e.g. CULLMANN, *Petrus,* 228f; HUMMEL, *Auseinandersetzung,* 61; U. LUZ, *Matthäus* II, 455.

[3] Cf. MARCUS, *CBQ* 50 (1988) 446.

[4] CARAGOUNIS, *Peter,* 9–57, 116f.

[5] This is the thesis of CARAGOUNIS, *Peter.* Unfortunately Caragounis did not discuss the lengthy study of Peter's confession by CLAUDEL, *Confession.*—For references to similar—though not identical—interpretations already in the early (mainly eastern) church, see LUDWIG, *Primatworte,* 54f, 57. Cf. also CULLMANN, *Petrus,* 180; GERHARDSSON, Nycklamakten, 57; BROWN/DONFRIED/REUMANN (eds.), *Peter,* 93 n. 216; U. LUZ, *Matthäus* II, 476f; *idem, NTS* 37 (1991) 419–421. For similar interpretations among more recent scholars, cf. e.g. ALLEN, *Matthew,* 176; MCNEILE, *Matthew,* 241; MUNDLE, *NIDNTT* III, 384f.

[6] CLAUDEL, *Bib* 71 (1990) 572; MEIER, *CBQ* 53 (1991) 492f, criticize the claim of CARAGOUNIS, *Peter,* 90, 116, that πέτρος and πέτρα must be strictly contradistinguished because of the philology.

[7] The observations have been repeated often. See e.g. WILKINS, *Concept of Disciple,* 192, though he does not pay attention to the ambiguity of the philological observation (*ibid.,* 189–192).

[8] For further discussion of ταύτῃ τῇ πέτρᾳ, see below pp. 278f.

[9] WILKINS, *Concept of Disciple,* 173–216, 232–240, discusses and tabulates the

parallels (Mark 3:16/Luke 6:14)—and also to Acts 1:13—referred to as "first" (πρῶτος). This is not merely a numerical information.[1] The narrator does not continue to number the other disciples. And 4:18–22 would in that case require that also Andrew was mentioned as "first." The narrator gives a *qualitative* remark about Peter's importance within the larger group of disciples. There are also other factors pointing to the prominence of Peter. From an intersynoptic perspective, the naming is distinguished in Matthew. Matthew mentions Peter's name explicitly in cases where one or both of the other synoptics refer to him only implicitly (Matt 26:35/Mark 14:31)[2] or where they have only a general reference to the disciples (Matt 15:15/Mark 7:17; Matt 18:21/Luke 17:4). The name appears on other occasions more clearly, either through an explicit specification that "Simon" is the one who is called "Peter" (Matt 4:18/Mark 1:16)[3] or through a full reference to "Simon Peter" instead of merely "Peter" (Matt 16:16/Mark 8:29/Luke 9:20) or through a preference for "Peter" instead of "Simon" (Matt 8:14/Mark 1:29/Luke 4:38). Sometimes we find the other synoptics mentioning several disciples by name while Matthew names only Peter (Matt 8:14/Mark 1:29; Matt 26:37/Mark 14:33). This suggests an occasional concentration upon Peter.[4] There is also special Matthean material associated with Peter (14:28–31; 16:18; 17:24–27). Matthew indeed depicts Peter both positively and negatively.[5] The last impression of Peter is even his progressive and public denial—the third time even cursing (26:74)— of Jesus (26:69–75).[6] Peter is a round character exhibiting a variety of conflicting traits. But whether presented positively or negatively, his individuality is accentuated. Peter does not fill a typical function which any of Jesus' followers in principle can assume.[7] Matthew is interested in Peter as an individual person.

On the other hand, he is also a representative of all the disciples. What Peter says, all the disciples say (26:35). In comparison with the other synoptics, there is sometimes even an absence of any mention of Peter in Matthew.[8] From an intersynoptic perspective, either the attention becomes focused on Jesus (Matt 9:22f/Mark 5:37f/Luke 8:51) or Peter becomes one in the group of all the disciples (Matt 21:20/Mark 11:21; Matt 24:3/Mark 13:3).[9] The latter feature is perhaps relevant also for the striking absence of any reference to Peter in Matt 28:7 as compared with Mark 16:7.[10] And as we know, almost everything otherwise said of Peter is also said of several or all of the disciples.

---

relevant material. I differ only slightly from his classification.

[1]   Contra STRECKER, *Weg der Gerechtigkeit*, 204 n. 1; HOFFMANN, Petrus-Primat, 428; SCHWEIZER, *Matthäus*, 153.

[2]   The inclusion of πέτρος in some variants of Mark 14:31 is probably secondary.

[3]   Cf. Luke 5:8, 10.

[4]   In regard to Matt 8:14/Mark 1:29, we should notice that also Luke 4:38 discloses a certain concentration on Peter.—In regard to Matt 26:37/Mark 14:33, we should observe that while in Matt 26:40 Jesus speaks to Peter as a representative of several disciples, in Mark 14:37 he speaks to Peter only. Thus the impression is somewhat reversed.

[5]   Cf. the illustrative graph by WILKINS, *Concept of Disciple*, 240. WILKINS, *ibid.,* 211, claims even that Matthew purposely accentuated this tension in the presentation of Peter.

[6]   GERHARDSSON, *JSNT* 13 (1981) 46–66.

[7]   Contra STRECKER, *Weg der Gerechtigkeit*, 205f; WALKER, *Heilsgeschichte*, 118.

[8]   WILKINS, *Concept of Disciple*, 206–208, discusses the texts.

[9]   In regard to Matt 24:3/Mark 13:3, we should notice that Luke 21:7 does not mention any specific disciple either.

[10]   Luke 24:6–9 does not mention Peter either. But cf. Luke 24:12, 34. For other possible explanations of this feature in Matthew, cf. Joachim JEREMIAS, *Neutestamentliche Theologie,* 291; WILKINS, *Concept of Disciple,* 207f. There is no external support for

16:13–20 exhibits a mixture of both perspectives. On one hand, Jesus speaks in 16:17–19 to Peter personally, in the singular. He does not—as in 15:15f; 26:40f—respond to Peter by giving the address in the second person plural. Furthermore, 16:16 constitutes the only occasion when the narrator refers to Peter as "Simon Peter." This is the proper presentation in view of Jesus' subsequent use of first "Simon" (16:17) and then "Peter" (16:18). It also harks back to the two occasions when the narrator explained that Simon is the one called Peter:[1] once when he introduced Peter for the first time (4:18) and once when he depicted him as first among the disciples (10:2).[2] There is perhaps also a correspondence between σὺ εἶ in 16:16 and 16:18.[3] The expression κἀγὼ δέ σοι λέγω in 16:18 points to an emphasis caused by σὺ εἶ which Peter used when he spoke to Jesus in 16:16. Peter first uses σὺ εἶ for Jesus personally and Jesus then uses it for Peter personally. Peter is not merely a type.[4] Jesus addresses him as an individual.

On the other hand, Jesus addresses Peter as part of the larger group of disciples. References to all the disciples frame the dialogue between Peter and Jesus (16:13–15, 20). Peter replies in 16:16 to a question which Jesus actually posed to all the disciples. And the dialogue itself resembles statements elsewhere related to all the disciples: the confession of Jesus as the Son of God in 16:16 is almost identical with what the disciples confess in 14:33; the blessing of Peter in 16:17 is reminiscent of the blessing of the disciples' eyes and ears in 13:16; the authority to bind and loose in 16:19 is, in a sense, further extended to all the disciples in 18:18.

The combination of these personal and representative features is perhaps partly due to the importance accorded to Peter in Matthew's environment.[5] But this explanation still leaves open the question of Peter's theological position in the Matthean story. And it is hardly sufficient to relegate Peter's personal importance to a temporal, salvation-historical primacy.[6] Besides the general difficulties of ascertaining a rigid salvation-historical perspective in Matthew,[7] the authorization of Peter in 16:18f points to the future,

---

deleting Peter in Mark 16:7.

[1] Cf. KINGSBURY, *JBL* 98 (1979) 74, though his conclusion concerning the salvation-historical primacy of Peter does not necessarily follow from this observation.

[2] It is therefore questionable if σὺ εἶ πέτρος in 16:18 depicts an actual giving of the name, as claimed by e.g. CULLMANN, *Petrus,* 15f, 197f; BROWN/DONFRIED/REUMANN (eds.), *Peter,* 90 n. 210; SCHWEIZER, *Matthäus,* 222.

[3] CARAGOUNIS, *Peter,* 86, 110f, recognizes the juxtaposition but denies its significance. But cf. VÖGTLE, *BZ* 2 (1958) 94; WILCOX, *NTS* 22 (1975–76) 75, 82, though his tradition-historical conclusions do not necessarily follow from this observation.

[4] *Contra* BLANK, *Concilium* 9 (1973) 176f.

[5] Cf. U. LUZ, *NTS* 37 (1991) 425.—It is difficult to ascertain if the elevation of Peter is an actual polemic against claims in Matthew's environment. See T.V. SMITH, *Petrine Controversies,* 156–160.

[6] *Contra* KINGSBURY, *JBL* 98 (1979) 76–83. Cf. also CLAUDEL, *Confession,* 382f, 387.

[7] Cf. the sceptical remarks by SENIOR, *Matthew,* 35f; U. LUZ, *TRE* 12 (1984) 597; FRANCE, *Matthew: Evangelist and Teacher,* 199f, and below pp. 259–261.

not the past. Future verb constructions (οἰκοδομήσω, δώσω) describe the building of the church and the giving of the keys. Neither is the authority to bind and loose yet a full reality.[1] The conditional construction with the two aorist subjunctives (δήσῃς, λύσῃς) shows that the extension of the teaching authority is something to be expected, but not a reality at the time of speaking. And we cannot deny the futuristic implication of the two periphrastic future perfects (ἔσται δεδεμένον, ἔσται λελυμένον), though perhaps the avoidance of the simple future passive indicates that the future teaching will be a result of what has already been decided in heaven.

The combination of the two features suggests instead that Peter represents Jesus' disciples precisely through his singularity as a historical person.[2] He is an individual character epitomizing the remaining group of disciples—except of course for Judas.[3] *16:17–19 portrays Peter—the foundation of the church—as the historical person through whom Jesus' teaching authority legitimately is to be extended to the rest of the disciples.* True, it is difficult to ascertain that 16:17–19 depicts Peter's unique investment as the guarantor and bearer of revelation.[4] The evidence for the existence of such a form elsewhere is meagre.[5] Nor can we claim that Peter is the supreme rabbi of the church.[6] Jesus' own teaching continues to be normative within a brotherhood of followers (5:19; 23:8–10; 28:20). And the task to bind and loose is at the end not the prerogative of Peter only (18:18). But Peter's authority to teach is more than "a historicized literary cliché."[7] It anchors the disciples' teaching in the teaching given in the past history of Jesus himself. It is foundational. *The disciples will through Peter remain bound to the foundational teaching that Jesus has given once and for all.* They will perform their teaching on a legitimate basis in the past history.

---

1   Cf. SCHNACKENBURG, Petrus, 123; MARCUS, *CBQ* 50 (1988) 453f.

2   HOFFMANN, Petrus-Primat, 429, 432; U. LUZ, *Matthäus* II, 468f. Cf. also R. PESCH, *Simon-Petrus*, 142–144; DAVIES/ALLISON, *Matthew* II, 651; ROLOFF, *Kirche*, 163f.

3   Cf. WILKINS, *Concept of Disciple*, 198, 210f, who points to the personal, representational and exemplary function of Peter.

4   *Contra* C. KÄHLER, *NTS* 23 (1976–77) 46–56. He is followed by R. PESCH, *Simon-Petrus*, 98f; SCHENK, *BZ* 27 (1983) 71f; SCHNACKENBURG, Petrus, 122.

5   For critical comments, see KINGSBURY, *JBL* 98 (1979) 75 n. 26; CLAUDEL, *Confession*, 344f.

6   Already STREETER, *The Four Gospels*, 515, called Peter "the supreme Rabbi" of the church in Antioch. DOBSCHÜTZ, Matthew, 25, called him a "Christian chief rabbi." Cf. also HUMMEL, *Auseinandersetzung*, 63; BORNKAMM, "Bind" and "Loose," 94; GNILKA, *Matthäusevangelium* II, 66.—It is difficult to claim on the basis of e.g 15:15; 16:19; 17:24–27; 18:21 that Matthew links Peter in a special way with halakhic questions. So e.g. KILPATRICK, *Origins*, 38, 95f; HUMMEL, *ibid.*, 59, 63; MUNDLE, *NIDNTT* III, 384; R. PESCH, *Simon-Petrus*, 142f; SCHENK, *BZ* 27 (1983) 70; SYREENI, *JSNT* 40 (1990) 5. For criticism, see KINGSBURY, *JBL* 98 (1979) 81 n. 45; U. LUZ, *Matthäus* II, 467; *idem, NTS* 37 (1991) 426.

7   SYREENI, *JSNT* 40 (1990) 5.

2.3. Jesus' Teaching as the Historical Basis of Mission

The close relationship between the teaching of the disciples and the teaching of Jesus becomes further evident through Matthew's depiction of the *object* of mission. The final extension of the didactic activity in 28:19f concerns also the recipients of the teaching, not only the performers. The participial construction διδάσκοντες αὐτούς refers back to μαθητεύσατε πάντα τὰ ἔθνη and explains it together with βαπτίζοντες αὐτούς. For the first time in the Matthean narrative, the teaching activity is to reach all the nations.[1]

The story line depicting the disciples as future teachers is connected with the story line extending the recipients of the teaching. The two coalesce in 28:19f. But we see this connection also through the rather ambiguous preparation earlier in the narrative. There are both a contrasting particularisation and an implicit extension in regard to the objects of Jesus' and the disciples' mission.

2.3.1. The Particularisation of Mission

The most evident contrast earlier in the narrative is the ethnic particularisation of Jesus' and the disciples' mission. Jesus not only applies the exclusive (οὐκ ... εἰ μή) principle of addressing no other ethnic group than the lost sheep of Israel to his own ministry in 15:24, but he also gives the principle, though in a somewhat milder form (μᾶλλον),[2] as a directive to the disciples in 10:6.[3] The command is coupled with a prohibition against going to the Gentiles (ἔθνη) and the Samaritans (10:5b). It is a strict principle. Jesus and his disciples were not to address any other than the Jewish people of Israel.

Also the teaching activity has a restricted group of recipients earlier in the narrative. 28:20 describes the teaching with διδάσκειν. We can distinguish two separate addressees of Jesus' teaching depicted with διδάσκειν.

---

[1]   I will speak of "extension" and "nations" without deciding if the extension to all the nations in 28:19f constitutes an actual *break* with the Jewish people or a *broadening continuation* including both Jews and Gentiles, as already LINDBLOM, *Jesu Missions-och dopbefallning*, 142–158; TRILLING, *Israel*, 26–28, proposed. My understanding of 10:23; 23:34 suggests a future mission among the Jewish people. But a full answer would have to consider also other texts. For interpretations of the term ἔθνος, ἔθνη, see the discussion between HARE/HARRINGTON, *CBQ* 37 (1975) 359–369, and MEIER, *CBQ* 39 (1977) 94–102.—LEVINE, *Social and Ethnic Dimensions*, 186–239; WONG, *Interkulturelle Theologie*, 96, 98–108, supplement this linguistic debate by considering the theology of the whole gospel narrative. Cf. also e.g. FRANKEMÖLLE, *Jahwebund*, 119–123; FRANCE, *Matthew: Evangelist and Teacher*, 235–237; HARRINGTON, *Matthew*, 414f.

[2]   TRILLING, *Israel*, 99–101; U. LUZ, *Matthäus* II, 88, 91, believe that 10:5b–6 is traditional and that the stricter variant in 15:24 is Matthew's own creation. But this is difficult to ascertain.

[3]   9:36 indicates that "the lost sheep of Israel" primarily refers to harassed crowds of the Jewish people. Cf. LEVINE, *Social and Ethnic Dimensions*, 56f.

The Jewish people are often present as a *general* addressee of the teaching. Matthew refers to them either explicitly, as οἱ ὄχλοι (5:1; 7:28f),[1] or implicitly, as the population of Galilean cities (11:1) and as those present in the synagogues of Galilee (4:23; 9:35; 13:54) and at the temple area in Jerusalem (21:23; 22:16; 26:55). The narrator once mentions explicitly the disciples as addressees (5:2). They are the *primary* addressees of the Sermon on the Mount.[2] Jesus' teaching activity described with διδάσκειν does not reach the nations here.

We gain the same impression from the geographical locations of the activity described with διδάσκειν.[3] Matthew mentions four places: the synagogue(s), the cities, the mountain and the temple. In these cases, Matthew always speaks of "their" synagogue(s): in 4:23 the pronoun does not have a proper grammatical antecedent but refers implicitly to the inhabitants of Galilee; in 9:35 it refers to the people in the cities and villages where Jesus went about, still in Galilee;[4] in 13:54—also here without an actual grammatical antecendent—it refers to the population of Jesus' home territory. 11:1 speaks of "their" cities. This probably harks back to the cities and villages that the narrator mentioned as locations of Jesus' teaching in 9:35. The mountain is the place of teaching in 5:1. This is also implicit in 7:29–8:1. Later in the narrative, when Jesus has entered Jerusalem (21:1–11), the temple area is the place of teaching. 21:23; 26:55 state it explicitly. In 22:16 it is implicit.

The teaching is restricted to various places within Israel. With the exception of the mountain,[5] they are typically Jewish. The synagogues and the temple are religious centres of the Jews, and even the cities are qualified as "their" cities. Jesus' teaching activity never goes beyond the borders of Israel. He performs it in places especially related to the Jewish people of Israel.

Excursus 10: *Teaching in Summaries and Individual Cases*

The geographical location of Jesus' teaching described with διδάσκειν exhibits a certain ambiguity in Matthew. While the programmatic summaries in 4:23; 9:35 and the summarizing statement in 13:54 locate the teaching within the synagouge(s), the actual performance of the teaching never takes place in the synagogues but on the mountain or in the temple.

An intersynoptic reading offers an explanation of this ambiguity to some extent. The parallels to 4:23 mention that the preaching (κηρύσσειν) of Jesus took place "in their

---

[1] The presence of people from Decapolis among the many crowds (4:25) gathering around Jesus in 5:1 does not fall outside of this pattern, as implied by WONG, *Interkulturelle Theologie,* 51. See correctly G. LOHFINK, *Bergpredigt,* 25–29.
[2] See above pp. 224–226.
[3] Cf. TRILLING, *Israel,* 131–137.
[4] Jesus does not leave Galilee until in 19:1.
[5] For critique of the alleged Sinaitic connotations of the mountain in 5:1, see excursus 12 below.

synagogues" (Mark 1:39) or "in the synagogues of Judea" (Luke 4:44). And 13:54 is in agreement with both parallels giving the reference to the synagogue in the singular (Mark 6:2/Luke 4:16).

Another part of the explanation concerns the *confessional language* used in passages summarizing the ministry of Jesus. Matthew does not merely take over summaries and summarizing statements from the tradition. The summarizing comments by the reliable narrator are important clues to Matthew's own conception of the story. It is then understandable that Matthew here goes beyond the situation depicted in individual cases.[1] The same impression emerges when we compare summarizing statements concerning Jesus' mighty acts with the depiction of his therapeutic activity in individual cases. In the summarizing passages expressing a confessional attitude towards Jesus, the language of praise takes over. They magnify and generalize Jesus' mighty acts.[2] The rhetorical situation of the summaries and the summarizing statements is strongly epideictic.[3] In regard to the teaching, they not only magnify and generalize, but also add information not present elsewhere in Matthew.

2.3.2. The Extension of Mission

There is also some indication that the total effect of Jesus' ministry ultimately will go beyond any ethnic particularism. Matthew prepares the final extension in 28:19f earlier in the narrative. The most *explicit* anticipation is the positive estimate of the Gentiles' faith in Jesus' miraculous power. 8:5–13 shows how the believing trust of a Gentile overcomes Jesus' principal restriction. The presence of the saying about many people from east and west (8:11f) before the report about the actual miracle (8:13) gives the episode an anticipatory character indicating that Jesus' total ministry will finally reach the Gentiles. 15:21–28 illustrates how Jesus relativizes the hard principle of 15:24 to an initial reluctance.[4] As in 8:5–13, the believing trust of a Gentile finally defeats Jesus' hesitation. And this pericope also concludes with the report that Jesus actually performed the therapeutic miracle (15:28).

There are also a number of *implicit* anticipations. Perhaps already the programmatic depiction of Jesus as son of Abraham in 1:1 is significant.[5] Abraham is not only the father of the Jews. Matthew mentions him in contexts reflecting a certain distance to the people of Israel (3:9; 8:11).[6] According to the OT, Abraham was to be the father of

---

1   Cf. BERGER, *Formgeschichte,* 332: "Gegenüber diesen grundlegenden Berichten sind die Einzelszenen mehr oder weniger stark verselbständigt."

2   GERHARDSSON, *Mighty Acts,* 24, 34.

3   BERGER, *Formgeschichte,* 331–333, treats the summary ("Basis-Bericht") as part of the epideictic genre.

4   Cf. FRANCE, *Matthew: Evangelist and Teacher,* 234.

5   It is grammatically possible to regard David—not Jesus—as the son of Abraham in 1:1. But whether indirectly or directly, Matthew does link Jesus with Abraham. Cf. 1:2, 17.

6   Cf. also 22:32.—WIESER, *Abrahamvorstellungen,* 94–98, does not acknowledge this motif and stresses that the texts are taken from the tradition and therefore reflect only vaguely the Matthean perspective. But certainly, traditions can be incorporated as meaningful inter-texts.

(Gen 17:4f) and a blessing for (Gen 18:18; 22:18) many nations (גוים, ἔθνη),[1] and these motifs were kept alive and embellished in later Jewish texts (1 Macc 12:21; Sir 44:19, 21; Ant. 12:226)[2] and the NT (Rom 4:12, 16–18; 9:7f; Gal 3:7–9, 14, 16, 29).[3] Rabbinic texts associate Abraham with the proselytes (גרים). They speak of him as a proselyte (Mek. on 22:20 [Lauterbach III, 140:31f, 36–41]), the first of proselytes (b. Sukk. 49b; b. Ḥag. 3a) or the father of proselytes (Tanḥ. B. לך לך 6).[4] Through the reference to Abraham, Matthew may imply that the ministry of the messianic king of the Jews—the son of David—ultimately concerns also other nations. The mention of the four women in the following genealogy—Tamar (1:3), Rahab (1:5), Ruth (1:5) and the wife of Uriah (1:6)—perhaps strengthens the initial impression,[5] though this is uncertain.[6] In any event, the following narrative contains several implicit anticipations: certain men from the east are the first to worship the king of the Jews (2:11); Jesus performs a miracle among Gentile swineherds and is ultimately asked to leave the region, presumably because the time has not yet come for a mission outside of Israel (8:28–9:1); the ethnic particularism in 10:5b–6 is put in tension with a temporal openness (10:16–22) including an indirect testimony to the nations (10:18);[7] the ministry of the Isaianic servant is positively connected with the nations (12:18d, 21);[8] in the form of narrative meshalim, Jesus alludes to the extension of the people to be included in the kingdom of God (21:28–22:14) and claims—in Matthew alone— that the kingdom will be given to a nation producing its fruits (21:43);[9] as a testimony to the nations, the gospel of the kingdom will be preached in the whole inhabited world (24:14), including also the gospel as the deeds done towards Jesus (26:13);[10] the centurion and—in Matthew only—the persons with him guarding Jesus perceive the supernatural portents at Jesus' death as an indication that Jesus was God's son (27:51–54), which in Matthew probably functions as the Gentiles' recognition of Jesus' divine sonship.[11]

There are also anticipations that are oriented more specifically towards the teaching activity mentioned 28:20. The location of Jesus' teaching in Galilee is not only an indication of its restriction to the Jewish people, but

---

[1] Cf. also Gen 12:3 (משפחות, φυλαί).

[2] Cf. also Ant. 14:255.

[3] The NT understanding of Gen 22:18 follows the LXX which implies not that the nations of the earth will bless themselves (התברכו) in Abraham's seed, but that they will be blessed (ἐνευλογηθήσονται) in the seed of Abraham. Cf. Acts 3:25; Gal 3:8.

[4] Cf. also t. Ber. 1:15; b. Šabb. 105a; y. Bik. 64a. For discussion of various (and separate) Jewish conceptions about Abraham, see WIESER, *Abrahamvorstellungen,* 153–179.

[5] So e.g. W.D. DAVIES, Jewish Sources, 503.

[6] DAVIES/ALLISON, *Matthew* I, 170–172; U. LUZ, *Matthäus* I, 93f, discuss briefly the major interpretations of these women. For recent discussion (by women), cf. LEVINE, *Social and Ethnic Dimensions,* 59–88; WAINWRIGHT, *Feminist Critical Reading,* 60–69, 160–170, 174f.

[7] Cf. S. BROWN, *ST* 31 (1977) 29; *idem,* ZNW 69 (1978) 79, 87–90.

[8] Cf. TRILLING, *Israel,* 126f; HAHN, *Mission,* 109f.

[9] The singular form of ἔθνος may have been caused by a contrasting allusion to Dan 2:44.

[10] Cf. also 13:38 and the comments by TRILLING, *Israel,* 124–126.

[11] Cf. e.g. VERSEPUT, *NTS* 33 (1987) 547f; KINGSBURY, *Matthew as Story,* 89f, each pointing to the importance of the pericope, though with different emphases.—The absence of the definite article cannot be taken as an argument against the importance of the soldiers' utterance. Cf. e.g. GUNDRY, *Matthew,* 578.

also a sign that the teaching will extend beyond the borders of the Israelite community. On the basis of the prophecy from Isa 8:23–9:1, Galilee appears as the territory of the nations in 4:15. This definition does not imply merely that Galilee had Gentile inhabitants[1] or that Jesus addressed other nations. It shows that the activity of Jesus will ultimately affect the nations.[2] In Galilee Jesus will meet his disciples after his death and resurrection (26:32; 28:7, 10); in Galilee the final extension of the teaching takes place (28:16, 19f).

There are also significant connections between 5:19 and 28:19f.[3] Only these two passages refer to the teaching activity of disciples with the term διδάσκειν. A certain extension of the recipients of the teaching is noticeable on both occasions. 28:19f mentions them as "the nations," 5:19 quite generally as "men" (ἄνθρωποι). Of course, the term ἄνθρωπος does not possess a fixed meaning to be applied to all occasions in Matthew. Its more restrictive and negative use in 10:17 is therefore not to be put over against 5:19. Here 5:13, 16 cause the term.[4] And the fact that 5:14 calls the disciples "the light of the world" suggests a rather broad connotation of ἄνθρωπος.[5] Although the mention of "men" in 5:19 does not automatically imply an extension to the nations, we should notice that Matthew uses a general term, giving no qualifying limitation.

2.3.3. The History About Jesus

It is necessary to interpret the story line extending the recipients of the teaching together with the story line depicting the disciples as future teachers. Both coincide in 28:19f. The disciples now become teachers and the teaching now reaches the nations. A comparison with the missionary speech in Matt 10 shows that this convergence is not accidental. After telling the disciples not to go beyond the ethnic borders of the Israelite people (10:5b–6), Jesus instructs them about their preaching and healing activity (10:7f), but not about their teaching activity. Matthew has no statement like Mark 6:30 indicating that the disciples were teaching already during Jesus' public ministry. The Matthean Jesus is the only active teacher before his death and resurrection. The assignment given to the disciples in Matt 10 points to a specific relationship between the task of Jesus and the task of the disciples.[6] Since some important comments about Jesus' own teaching frame the missionary speech (9:35; 11:1), the fact that the speech itself does not include the teaching in the assignment of the disciples is striking. As it seems, Matt-

---

[1]   *Contra* KRETZER, *Herrschaft der Himmel,* 79.

[2]   OGAWA, *L'histoire de Jésus,* 60f; DAVIES/ALLISON, *Matthew* I, 384f; U. LUZ, *Matthäus* I, 171.

[3]   Cf. above p. 209 and below pp. 291f.

[4]   Cf. also 4:19.

[5]   Cf. TRILLING, *Israel,* 126; FRANKEMÖLLE, Mission, 125.

[6]   See above pp. 226f.

hew reserves the task to teach for Jesus alone. The disciples will teach only when they have fully learnt Jesus' teaching and when the mission is to reach beyond the ethnic particularisation.[1]

S. Brown argues that the tension between the ethnic particularisation and the universalistic extension reflects two missions advocated by different parties in the Matthean community, and that Matthew himself, though recognizing the particularistic tendencies, wanted to encourage the universalistic group.[2] This proposal does not convince. Besides the hypothetical steps involved in attributing certain texts to certain social groups constructed on the basis of some tensions in the text itself,[3] it is difficult to prove that 10:5b–6 expresses an opinion that is merely respected as dominical tradition but not regarded as normative.[4] Nor does M.D. Goulder's assumption that the restriction to the Jewish people was applicable only to the twelve while the commission to go to all the nations was intended for the whole church resolve the tension.[5] This suggestion accepts on one occasion the fictional addressees of the text but replaces on another the disciples with the church.

The convergency of the two elements in 28:19f relates to *the historical dimension in the story*. The narrator, reflecting Matthew's own standpoint, tells the story from a perspective acknowledging the reality of the final extension. From this point of view, the Matthean story is history. The story claims to contain past history.[6] Matthew is a story about Jesus' history.

Two major alternatives propose different stages in the history as *salvation history*. G. Strecker, R. Walker and J.P. Meier—though they differ on individual points—are the major proponents of a threefold pattern.[7] It includes the time of preparation, the time of Jesus and the time of the church. J.D. Kingsbury is the main proponent of a two-stage history.[8] The history contains the time of Israel and the time of Jesus. Neither of the suggestions is entirely satisfactory when applied to my problem.[9] To be sure, a change does appear in the extension of the didactic mission in 28:19f. But this change has been prepared by anticipatory events. The time of Jesus contains in itself various stages and the time of the church is thoroughly embedded in the past history. An adequate model needs to take account of the pastness and unrepeatable aspects of Jesus' earthly ministry as well as the openness of the history to future occasions. The sug-

---

1 For the connection between the exousia of Jesus and the teaching activity of the disciples, see below pp. 283f.
2 *ST* 31 (1977) 21–32. Cf. also *idem, ZNW* 69 (1978) 89f; *idem, NovT* 22 (1980) 215–221. Brown now seems to go beyond the historical reconstruction and ask about the psychological reality behind the tension in the narrative. See *idem*, Universalism, 388–399.
3 For an emphasis on the methodological issues involved in studying the mission in Matthew, see FRANKEMÖLLE, Mission, 103–109, 115–120.
4 T.L. DONALDSON, *Jesus on the Mountain*, 212; WEAVER, *Missionary Discourse*, 162f n. 53, offer some further criticism of Brown.
5 *Midrash and Lection*, 343.
6 Cf. the remarks in the introduction above pp. 25f.
7 WALKER, *Heilsgeschichte*, 114–127; STRECKER, *Weg der Gerechtigkeit*, 41–242; MEIER, *CBQ* 37 (1975) 203–215; *idem, Law and History*, 25–40; *idem, Vision of Matthew*, 26–39; STRECKER, Concept of History, 67–84.
8 *Matthew: Structure, Christology, Kingdom*, 25–37.
9 The matter has become even more complicated since the introduction of narrative criticism in gospel studies. Cf. HOWELL, *Inclusive Story*, 55–92.

gestion by U. Luz makes it easier to integrate all the complexities of history.[1] In his conception, Matthew is an inclusive story which maintains the history in its pastness. The history in the story is indirectly transparent for the experiences of the present community. The history in indvidual pericopes may be directly transparent for the contemporary Christian individual.

There is a distance between the "now" of the author and the history about Jesus. The repeated use of αὐτῶν in reference to the Jewish places of Jesus' teaching indicates this.[2] In three out of four instances (4:23; 9:35; 11:1; 13:54), the term is peculiar to Matthew (9:35; 11:1; 13:54). Elsewhere, in contexts of opposition and persecution,[3] Matthew qualifies the synagogue(s) with αὐτῶν (10:17; 12:9) or, in a direct address by Jesus, with ὑμῶν (23:34).[4] The lack of a clear grammatical antecedent in 4:23; 9:35; 13:54 reveals the fixed nature of the expression. "Their" city in 22:7 refers to Jerusalem as the city of the Jewish people. There is not only a distance to the places of the Jewish leaders,[5] but to the Jewish people as a whole.[6] Jesus taught in locations different from Matthew's present place of existence.[7]

The contrasting preparation of 28:19f is also the basic principle during the active ministry of Jesus. The ethnic particularisation is not casual in the story. Even where the faith of Gentiles convinces Jesus to help them, there is an initial reluctance to go beyond the ethnic borders of the Israelite people. The particularism is the basic rule, to which Jesus made only occasional exceptions. And the basic summaries give no hint that Jesus would extend his ministry to the Gentiles. They report instead that he performed the teaching activity among the Jews of Israel (4:23; 7:28f; 9:35; 11:1; 13:54).[8]

Although there is a distance between the "now" of the author and the history about Jesus' mission among the Jews, the history is acknowledged. By placing the extension of the performers and the recipients of teaching in

---

[1] Cf. e.g. U. LUZ, Disciples, 98–128; *idem, TRE* 12 (1984) 597; *idem,* Wundergeschichten, 149–165; *idem, Matthäus* II, 64–68; *idem,* Christologie, 221f.

[2] See above p. 255.

[3] Cf. HARE, *Jewish Persecution,* 80–114.

[4] Cf. also the synagogues as the location of the Jews' deplorable activities in 6:2, 5; 23:6. For discussion, cf. already KILPATRICK, *Origins,* 110f, who interprets this feature by reference to the berakhah against the heretics (המינים ברכת), though this interpretation is today difficult to ascertain.—HUMMEL, *Auseinandersetzung,* 28–31, understands the synagogues merely as of the Pharisees, while WALKER, *Heilsgeschichte,* 33–35, understands them as of all Israel.

[5] *Contra* T.L. DONALDSON, *Jesus on the Mountain,* 206–208.

[6] FRANCE, *Matthew: Evangelist and Teacher,* 223–227.

[7] Cf. also 28:15.—TAGAWA, *NTS* 16 (1969–70) 149–162, proposes Matthew's community consciousness as the primary explanation for the seemingly contradictory picture of the relation between Jews and Gentiles. However, he moves too quickly from the textual world to the real world of the Matthean community and neglects the historical dimension in the story itself. This is also the basic weakness of the study by WONG, *Interkulturelle Theologie,* explaining the picture as an attempt to address a multicultural community by means of an intercultural theology.

[8] Cf. TRILLING, *Israel,* 137.

Jesus' final commission, Matthew presents the disciples' teaching to the nations as an on-going activity decisively prepared in the history about Jesus.[1] The preparation is a historical foundation for a present activity. But Matthew does not give the foundation through the chronological ordering of historical events eventually leading to the final extension. History does not consist of past stages in the successive unfolding of salvation-history; it is not abolished and swallowed up by the present. Matthew gives an actualized historical drama about Jesus. The mission among the Jewish people is part of the history about Jesus located in the past but actualized and transparent for the contemporary and future time. As such, Jesus' history remains the basis for the mission to all the nations.[2] And the teaching that Jesus once gave among the Jewish people remains the foundation for the didactic aspects of the universal mission.[3]

In this way, the story reflects Matthew's didactic motives of transmission. The didactic and scribal activity of the disciples, with Peter as the personal link back to Jesus' own teaching authority, receives a decisive historical basis. Jesus' teaching remains the norm of all teaching activity. But the teaching does not come directly from the risen Lord. The foundational aspect of the teaching authority that Jesus extends to Peter reflects a transmission process that focused on the teaching given by Jesus once and for all.[4] The teaching gained its normative function within a specific historical context in the past. It was a historical foundation. *The teaching that Jesus gave in the past was of decisive importance in the teaching activities of the Matthean community. This motivated the transmission of the Jesus tradition.*

3. The Didactic-Biographical Motives

Jesus is the central character in a story narrating about him in the third person. Matthew not only attributes teaching to Jesus, but his didactic characterization of Jesus appears within an episodal narration about Jesus.

I will not deal with the emergence and definition of the literary genre of

---

1 WEAVER, *Missionary Discourse,* 152f, points to the fusion of the world of the story and the world of the implied reader in 28:20. I would rather speak of history reaching into the "now" of the author as a user—reader/hearer—of his own text.

2 For the binding connection to Israel, see HAHN, *Mission,* 109–111; FRANKEMÖLLE, Mission, 112f.

3 Cf. GASTON, *Int* 29 (1975) 40: "Matthew wrote a Gospel which consciously presents a Jesus of the past who speaks to his church in the present, not a Christian but a Jewish Jesus."

4 I find it difficult to determine what exactly Peter's teaching authority depicted in the story corresponded to in the Matthean community. Are we to think of an office, of a tradition associated especially with Peter or of nothing at all? The risk of making a "referential fallacy" is evident here.

the gospel narratives.[1] L. Hartman points out that an adequate genre classification needs to account for several features in a literary piece of work: its
linguistic expressions, its general manner of presentation, the basic intention of its message and its reception and use.[2] I will concentrate on the
biographical items encoded within the story only. To be sure, C.H. Talbert
has revitalised the old view associating the gospel narratives with the biographical literature—the βίοι—in the Greco-Roman world.[3] P.L. Shuler
even suggests that the *bios* factor in Matthew is reminiscent of the "laudatory biography," which conforms to the rhetorical genre known as *encomium*.[4] However, even if we would accept Shuler's general deliniation of a
biographical genre called "laudatory biography,"[5] it is still difficult to
mould the intentions of Matthew's message into this pattern.[6] In particular,
Shuler's own emphasis on the sharp distinction between biography and history—whether accurate or not—is an obstacle to his thesis.[7] Shuler does not
consider the well-known discussions about the (salvation-)historical dimensions visible in Matthew as authorial intentions.[8] The Matthean story
does, as we just saw, reflect a fundamental desire to present an unrepeatable
history about Jesus.[9] A. Dihle—a most recognized expert in this field—
even considers the historical dimension in all the gospel narratives as a distinctive feature setting them apart from the Greek biographies.[10] Be that as
it may. *I will leave the question concerning the literary genre of Matthew
open.* Shuler has pointed—perhaps accurately—to several biographical
features in Matthew.[11] But instead of interpreting them from the external

---

[1] For surveys of genre criticism on the gospel narratives, see GUELICH, Gospel
Genre, 185–204; DORMEYER, *ANRW* II 25:2 (1984) 1545–1581; *idem, Evangelium,*
26–194; BLOMBERG, *Themelios* 15 (1990) 40–42; BURRIDGE, *What are the Gospels?,*
3–25, 82–106.

[2] *AARSU* 21 (1978) 11–22.

[3] *What Is a Gospel?*—In the most recent and complete discussion of the gospel narratives and the Greco-Roman biography, BURRIDGE, *What are the Gospels?,* argues that
while the gospel narratives diverge from Greco-Roman βίοι, they do not do so to any
greater extent than βίοι do from one another.

[4] *Genre.* Shuler is followed by e.g. BERGER, *Formgeschichte,* 347 (cf. also
BERGER, *ibid.,* 370f); PUSKAS, *Introduction,* 118–126.

[5] But cf. the criticism by DOWNING, Analogies, 51–54; BURRIDGE, *What are the
Gospels?,* 88f; STANTON, *Gospel,* 65; *idem,* Matthew: βίβλος, εὐαγγέλιον, or βίος?,
1198.

[6] For cautious assessments by specialists in classical philology, see DIHLE, Evangelien, 383–411; CANCIK, Bios und Logos, 115–130.

[7] *Genre,* 37–43, 108.

[8] SHULER, *Genre,* 32–34, admits the role of the author's intent in the construction
of a literary text.

[9] Cf. U. LUZ, *Matthäus* I, 27f: "Am wichtigsten ist, daß Mt nicht die *typische* Geschichte eines vorbildlichen Menschen, sondern die völlig *einmalige* Geschichte Gottes
mit dem Menschen Jesus erzählt." Cf. now also *idem, ZNW* 84 (1993) 171–174.

[10] Evangelien, 404–407.

[11] SHULER, Genre(s), 459–483, 495f, has extended his view to all the biblical gospel narratives. But for criticism, see STUHLMACHER, Genre(s), 484–494.

perspective of an over-all genre,[1] *I will only ask for a biographical interest inherent in the message of the story itself.*[2] The two most important summaries in Matthew—the programmatic ones in 4:23; 9:35—indicate how Matthew integrates the didactic portrayal of Jesus into other aspects of Jesus' active ministry. The initial reference to teaching (διδάσκειν) occurs together with preaching (κηρύσσειν) and healing (θεραπεύειν). The three terms serve as condensed descriptions of Jesus' major activities. I will therefore focus on them separately and ask how they relate to each other in the narrative as a whole.

3.1. The Teaching and the Narrated Law

In the previous chapter, we noticed the importance and connotations of some terms characterizing Jesus as teacher. The two programmatic summaries use διδάσκειν for part of his activity. The totality of Jesus' teaching in Matthew is of course not limited to instances of this term only. But as a first step to distinguish the didactic-biographical motives of transmission, I will define the units in which the didactic terms appear and ask about episodal features connected with the depiction of Jesus in them.

3.1.1. The Teaching as Law and Morality

Scholars have often pointed out that Jesus' teaching concerns law and morality.[3] The units presenting the teaching with διδάσκειν or διδαχή confirm this.[4] The narrator gives an explicit didactic classification only in regard to the Sermon on the Mount (5:2; 7:28f), large parts of which concern law and morality. But what Jesus elsewhere says in his identity as teacher (διδάσκαλος) is of course also teaching. In the pericope concerning the requirements for eternal life, the rich young man addresses Jesus as teacher in 19:16. Jesus' response in 19:17–21 is certainly proper teaching. 22:16 states in general terms that Jesus teaches the way of God. The term διδαχή refers in 22:33 back to the discussion about the paying of taxes and the resurrection (22:15–32). The occurrence of διδάσκαλε in 22:24 confirms the didac-

---

1   E.D. HIRSCH, *Validity*, 68–126, stresses the importance of genre definition and claims that "an interpreter's preliminary generic conception of a text is constitutive of everything he subsequently understands" (*ibid.*, 74). But as KINGSBURY, *Matthew*, 12f, points out, the assumption that the genre definition is a vital condition for comprehending the meaning and purpose of all literature should be balanced with an awareness of the small peculiarities in each piece of literature and the various purposes for which one and the same genre can be employed.

2   ALLISON, Matthew: Structure, 1203–1221, asks for what he calls Matthew's "biographical impulse" by focusing on revelation as belonging to Jesus' whole life and on ethics as in need of Jesus to be imitated.

3   So especially SIGAL, *Halakah of Jesus*.

4   Of course, as is seen most clearly in 28:15, the didactic terms do not refer only to teaching of law and morality.

tic classification of the discussion. The use of the same address in 22:36 indicates that also the discussion about the greatest commandment in the Torah (22:34–40) is proper teaching. These are the units explicitly classifying what Jesus says as teaching. And they concern law and morality.

To be more precise, Jesus' utterances concern in these cases either the interpretation of the Scriptures or doctrinal matters of conduct or both together. It is too narrow to claim that the teaching always has to do with the interpretation of the Scriptures—the discussion concerning the paying of taxes does not directly. Similarly, the teaching does not always concern doctrinal matters of conduct—the discussion about the resurrection does not. Jesus' teaching concerns both the interpretation of the Scriptures and doctrinal matters of conduct. *We can describe Jesus' teaching as "law and morality" only when we take these terms in a broad and general sense.*

3.1.2. The Episodal Frames and Narratives

The teaching as here defined is communicated with words. These words often stand out as the most significant element in a pericope. But Matthew does not depict Jesus as teacher merely by means of brief and casual introductions followed by an important midrashic exposition or halakhic statement. Matthew sometimes even mentions the teaching activity without actually presenting it.[1] The use of ποιεῖν in connection with teaching in 21:23, 24, 27 shows that it is a matter of what Jesus says *and* does. We find a close relationship between verbal teaching and episodal comments in Matthew.

Episodal comments are present both in the introductions and the conclusions to the teaching. In 5:1f the narrator prepares the readers/hearers for the following Sermon by means of a short remark about where the teaching is given and who listens to it. Since 7:28–8:1 harks back to the introduction, the episodal comments are essential to the presentation of the teaching itself. In 19:16; 22:17, 24–28, 36 a question posed by characters whose traits the narrator has commented upon introduces the teaching. These episodal features in the introductions are significant when we compare them with the rabbinic literature. The normal introduction to the legal teaching of a rabbi does not contain episodal elements.[2] It is a brief statement, mostly—but not always—mentioning merely the name of the teacher. And the presentation of the teaching does not depend on it. Matthew presents the teaching differently.

Episodal comments also conclude the teaching. They often concern the reactions of the people.[3] Such comments occur after the Sermon on the

---

1 Cf. 4:23; 9:35; 11:1; 13:54; 21:23; 26:55.
2 See above pp. 137–140. Cf. also excursus 2 above.
3 Generally speaking, the gospel narratives do not record specific reactions to Jesus' teaching. See DILLON, *LumVit* 36 (1981) 135–162.

Mount (7:28), the teaching about eternal life (19:22),[1] the question about the paying of taxes (22:22) and the resurrection (22:33). 22:33 is reminiscent of the reaction depicted in 7:28.[2] Only the teaching about the greatest commandment in the Torah (22:37–40) ends—in contrast to Mark 12:32f—without any reference to the reaction of the audience. But in the remaining cases, the teaching is not isolated from narrated conclusions about its effects.

If we broaden the perspective somewhat, it becomes evident that while Jesus' words mostly dominate the scene, there are exceptions. A long episodal narrative in 1:1–2:23, where Jesus does not speak at all, introduces the whole story. And towards the end, after the arrest in 26:47–56, Jesus says only a few words (26:64; 27:11, 46; 28:9f), until he finally commissions the disciples (28:18–20).

Matthew gives not only episodal narratives containing (almost) no logia.[3] We find also units with both episodal elements and Jesus-sayings. It is well known, to be sure, that Matthew—when compared with the other synoptics—often reduces episodal elements and focuses on the sayings.[4] But there are also certain passages in which the episodal material does not seem to be abbreviated.[5] The narration becomes more prominent as Jesus approaches his death. In some important passages, the episodal elements in units containing sayings of Jesus are largely in agreement with Mark.[6] In other instances, the episodal elements are in Matthew more extensive than in Mark and Luke.[7]

Episodal features have occasionally a value independent of the Jesus-sayings. For instance, the episode in 8:28–9:1 does not include any of the words that Jesus utters in Mark 5:1–20/Luke 8:26–39.[8] The brief ὑπάγετε, which is not present in the parallels, is not structurally significant. The narrated episode has a value of its own. Further, although Jesus' question in 20:32 occurs also in Mark 10:51/Luke 18:41, the episode in 20:29–34 does not include the other words of Jesus present in Mark 10:46–52/Luke 18:35–43.[9] The question of the Matthean Jesus is not structurally emphasized. The prayer of the blind men in 20:31b forms the centre.[10] And at the end, the

---

1 Cf. also the reaction of the disciples in 19:25.
2 Cf. also 13:54, though there is no account of what Jesus actually said here.
3 Cf. also 4:23–25; 9:32–34; 12:15–21; 15:29–31.
4 Cf. already HAWKINS, *Horae Synopticae,* 158–160. See further below pp. 374f.
5 E.P. SANDERS, *Tendencies,* 84–87, 150f, warns against the generalization that Matthew consistently abbreviated Mark.
6 Cf. e.g. Matt 26:26f/Mark 14:22f; Matt 26:30/Mark 14:26; Matt 26:47/Mark 14:43.
7 Cf. e.g. Matt 26:1–5/Mark 14:1f/Luke 22:1f; Matt 27:45–54/Mark 15:33–39/Luke 23:44–48.
8 Mark 5:8; Mark 5:9/Luke 8:30; Mark 5:19/Luke 8:39.
9 Mark 10:49; Mark 10:52/Luke 18:42. Cf. also Matt 9:27–31 containing three utterances of Jesus (9:28, 29, 30).
10 Without κύριε in 20:30, the phrase οἱ δὲ μεῖζον ἔκραξαν λέγοντες, ἐλέησον

pericope records an action of Jesus, not an utterance.

These observations should not cause us to neglect the obvious fact that what Jesus says is of most importance in Matthew. I will discuss this in the next chapter.[1] But they do show that Jesus' legal teaching is not void of episodal elements. It is essentially not only isolated words of instruction. It happens; it is an event; it is part of a unique life-story. Jesus himself is the ultimate centre of the entire tradition. The words that Jesus utters as teacher of law and morality interact therefore with the episodal features. Together with the occasional prominence of similar elements elsewhere in Matthew, *the episodal features in passages presenting Jesus as teacher reflect an interest to integrate his legal teaching within a total conception of his life.*

3.2. The Teaching and the Preaching Event

The two programmatic summaries in 4:23; 9:35 and the summary statement in 11:1 mention the act of teaching together with the act of preaching (κη-ρύσσειν). This is unique in the synoptic gospel narratives.[2] Although Mark and Luke refer to both teaching and preaching, they do not connect the two in this manner.[3] The parallels to 4:23 speak only of preaching in the synagogues (Mark 1:39/Luke 4:44).[4] Matthew regards the synagogues as the places of teaching and the gospel of the kingdom as the content of preaching,[5] indicating that the latter qualifies the former in regard to its content. The parallels to 9:35 speak either of teaching (Mark 6:6) or preaching (Luke 8:1), but not of both together. Matthew relates the two closely, in a way not evident in the other synoptics.[6] The question here is if he provided the content of Jesus' teaching with an additional aspect connected with a broader interest in the life of Jesus.

ἡμᾶς, κύριε, υἱὸς Δαυίδ forms the centre of 20:29–34. There are 34 words before the phrase and 34 after. The numerical pattern is 34+10+34=78.

[1] See below pp. 369–378.

[2] In the rest of the NT, διδάσκειν and κηρύσσειν are directly connected only in Acts 28:31; Rom 2:21.

[3] They seem to be entirely synonymous in Mark. Cf. Mark 1:21f with Mark 1:14, 38f and Mark 6:30 with Mark 3:14; 6:12. The arguments for a distinction brought out by MEYE, *Jesus and the Twelve,* 55f, 60, are not convincing.—Acts 28:31 represents only an occasional linking of the two, because Acts 8:12; 28:23 do not maintain the distinction between preaching the kingdom of God and teaching about Jesus. Luke seems to use also εὐαγγελίζεσθαι and διδάσκειν synonymously. Cf. Luke 20:1; Acts 5:42; 15:35 (17:18f; 20:20, 24) and the comments by e.g. B.F. MEYER, *Aims of Jesus,* 70; BARRETT, *School,* 102.

[4] Cf. also Acts 9:20.

[5] Cf. SCHWEIZER, *Matthäus,* 43; GUELICH, *Sermon on the Mount,* 44f. Schweizer's emphasis on the consistent distinction between teaching in the synagogues and preaching *in the streets* is not evident in Matthew.

[6] G. FRIEDRICH, *TDNT* III, 713; MCDONALD, *Kerygma and Didache,* 5f, do not give due consideration to this distinctive feature in Matthew.

3.2.1. The Teaching as Preaching

There are significant overlappings between teaching and preaching.[1] The content of the proclamation contains elements of teaching.[2] The preaching does not announce the acts of God only,[3] but it carries within itself an imperative call for repentance (3:2; 4:17; 12:41). Just as the teaching in the Sermon on the Mount ends with a call for commitment (7:24–27), so the proclamation is a call for active decision—"ein Entscheidungsruf."[4] The preaching moves the readers/hearers in the direction of a didactic apprehension of the kerygma. There is a didactic kerygma.[5]

By the same token, kerygmatic connotations are present in the teaching.[6] This is most evident in the Sermon on the Mount, which Matthew defines as teaching (5:2, 7:28f). Although the beatitudes (5:3–12) contain implicit imperatives and to some extent are ethical,[7] together they function first of all as initial blessings. 5:3, 10 even refers to the kingdom of heaven, the primary object of the preaching.[8] 11:5 seems to confirm the kerygmatic implication of the beatitudes by maintaining the tradition that the gospel was preached (εὐαγγελίζεσθαι) to the poor.[9] It might also be of significance that 5:19; 13:52 relate the disciples as future teachers to the kingdom of heaven. The content of Jesus teaching does more than presuppose the content of the preaching. It *is* to some extent preaching.

3.2.2. The Preaching as Narrated Gospel Event

The overlappings between teaching and preaching do not imply that the preaching ceases entirely to be an important entity of its own. C.H. Dodd proposed a strict distinction between the content and activity of teaching and of preaching in early Christianity.[10] This distinction has now given way

---

[1]   *Contra* BORNKAMM, End-Expectation, 38 n. 1, who argues that διδάσκειν and κηρύσσειν represent a strict distinction between the law and the kingdom of God.

[2]   STENDAHL, *TLZ* 77 (1952) 719, uses the expression "das unkerygmatische Kerygma."

[3]   *Contra* SCHLATTER, *Matthäus,* 121: "Der Lehrende spricht von dem, was der Mensch zu tun hat, der Ausrufende von dem, was Gott tun wird."

[4]   STRECKER, *Weg der Gerechtigkeit,* 127.

[5]   Cf. VINCENT, *SJT* 10 (1957) 262–273.

[6]   STENDAHL, *TLZ* 77 (1952) 719, would include this under "das kerygmatische Nicht-Kerygma."

[7]   Many regard the beatitudes as ethical requirements. But see GUELICH, *JBL* 95 (1976) 415–434; *idem, Sermon on the Mount,* 109–111; BROER, *Seligpreisungen,* 96–98; DAVIES/ALLISON, *Matthew* I, 439f. Cf. also KIEFFER, Weisheit und Segen, 36–43; HAGNER, Righteousness, 103.

[8]   Cf. 3:1f; 4:17, 23; 9:35; 10:7; 24:14.

[9]   Cf. Luke 7:22 and the discussion by KVALBEIN, *Jesus og de fattige,* 293–319. For the connections between Matt 11:5 and the beatitudes, see STUHLMACHER, *Evangelium,* 219, 222f. For the background of the close relationship between κηρύσσειν and εὐαγγελίζεσθαι, see STUHLMACHER, *ibid.,* 230f n. 5a.

[10]   *Apostolic Preaching,* 7f, 53, *passim.*

to a recognition of significant overlappings between the two.[1] But certain distinctions remain in Matthew.

There is a distinction in regard to the performers of the action. While no other person but Jesus himself gives teaching in a positive sense, Jesus is not the only one preaching. John the Baptist is the first person to preach in the narrative structure (3:1), and subsequently both Jesus (4:17, 23; 9:35; 11:1) and the disciples (10:7, 27) perform this action. Jesus (4:17) and the disciples (10:7) reiterate the preaching of John the Baptist (3:2). Rhetorically—perhaps by deliberate comparison (σύγκρισις)[2]—this points to the continuity of the preaching by the three characters.[3] 12:41 even mentions the proclamation of Jonah. Just as the preaching of John the Baptist and Jesus concerns the call for repentance, so did Jonah's.[4] This might reflect a distinction going beyond the formal manner of presentation merely.[5] Although the future teaching depends entirely on Jesus himself, the preaching goes back not only to Jesus and his disciples, but to John the Baptist,[6] and even further.[7]

There is a difference in regard to the addressees. The preaching addresses mostly the Jewish people, explicitly or implicitly.[8] In the two last instances mentioning preaching (24:14; 26:13), Matthew refers to the whole world as the addressee. The preaching is never for the disciples only. It addresses or will address those outside of Jesus' group of followers.[9]

Matthew contains much more teaching than preaching.[10] The preaching never occurs in definable blocks. Only small capsule-summaries indicate its content, either with a short description (4:23; 9:35; 24:14; 26:13) or with a pointed utterance (3:1f; 4:17; 10:7).

The narrative structure also exhibits a distinction. While Jesus' teaching activity continues also when the narrative moves towards rejection and suffering,[11] Matthew says nothing further about his preaching after 11:1. J.D.

---

[1] For recent discussion, see MCDONALD, *Kerygma and Didache*, 4–7 (with lit.).

[2] So STANTON, *Gospel*, 81f.

[3] Cf. MACK/ROBBINS, *Patterns of Persuasion*, 21f.

[4] Perhaps Jonah 3:2, 4 (LXX) caused the use of κήρυγμα.

[5] *Contra* FLENDER, *EvT* 25 (1965) 706; STRECKER, *Weg der Gerechtigkeit*, 175; U. LUZ, *Matthäus* I, 183.

[6] For the similarities between the ministry of John and Jesus, cf. also e.g. 3:7 with 23:33 and 3:10 with 7:19 and the comments by ERNST, *Johannes der Täufer*, 157, 183–185; WEBB, *John the Baptizer*, 56f, 60.

[7] For a salvation-historical account of the similarities and dissimilarities between John and Jesus, cf. MEIER, *JBL* 99 (1980) 383–405.

[8] Cf. 3:5; 4:23–25; 9:35; 10:6; 11:1

[9] Cf. HAHN, *Mission*, 104f.

[10] SAND, *Matthäus-Evangelium*, 108, claims that the whole gospel narrative could be called διδαχή. But this classification does no justice to the narrative features in Matthew. DODD, *Apostolic Preaching*, 53, described the matters more accurately: Matthew "combines *kerygma* with *didaché*, and if we regard the book as a whole, the element of *didaché* predominates." Cf. also BLANK, *TQ* 158 (1978) 163.

[11] Cf. 19:16–22; 21:23; 22:15–40; 26:55.

Kingsbury is not entirely correct to claim the same structural significance for both activities and assume that after 11:1 the teaching is merely an unimportant item rejected by the Jewish leaders:[1] 19:16–22 directs the teaching to a rich young man, who must be a Jew judging from his question, without any motif of hostility; 22:22 does not depict the opponents' reaction in an outright negative manner; 22:33 does not fill the crowds' reaction with connotations of conflict. As it seems, after 11:1 Jesus preaches no more in Matthew. The preaching is to be retained in the future mission to the world (24:14; 26:13). But the teaching continues throughout Jesus' active ministry.[2]

The gospel makes the preaching activity into something more than the mere proclamation of words. Four instances show that the preaching consists of the gospel: in 4:23; 9:35 it consists of "the gospel of the kingdom" (τὸ εὐαγγέλιον τῆς βασιλείας), in 24:14 of "this gospel of the kingdom" (τοῦτο τὸ εὐαγγέλιον τῆς βασιλείας) and in 26:13 of "this gospel" (τὸ εὐαγγέλιον τοῦτο). Although later writings close to Matthew understand "gospel" as referring to a written account (Did. 8:2; 11:3; 15:3f),[3] we should not identify "this gospel (of the kingdom)" occurring in Matt 24:14; 26:13 without grammatical correlation with the written gospel itself.[4] In both instances the gospel is an oral event (κηρύσσειν, λαλεῖν).[5] And the preaching always represents the oral proclamation of a decisive event involving the nearness of the kingdom (3:1f; 4:17; 10:7). The preaching is the explicit manifestation of "this gospel (of the kingdom)" in Matthew.[6] It becomes a dynamic gospel event not restricted to the boundaries of mere words and utterances.

This gospel centres on Jesus' whole ministry and life. The telling of "this gospel" in 26:13 involves a narration about the deeds done towards Jesus.

---

1 *Parables of Jesus*, 29f; idem, *Matthew: Structure, Christology, Kingdom*, 20f.

2 To some extent, KINGSBURY, *Matthew: Structure, Christology, Kingdom*, xi, xviii, recognizes this, but he does not consider it significant.

3 Cf. also Ign. Phld. 5:1f; 8:2; 9:2; Smyrn. 5:1; 7:2 and the comments by e.g. HENGEL, *Mark*, 54; DORMEYER, *Evangelium*, 17f.—2 Clem. 8:5 seems to relate gospel to a written account (λέγει γὰρ ὁ κύριος ἐν τῷ εὐαγγελίῳ). But cf. the scepticism regarding the identification with any of the canonical gospel narratives expressed (again) by KOESTER, *Christian Gospels*, 7f, 16–18.—Justin, Apol. I 66:3, is the first to use the plural εὐαγγέλια to refer to gospel books, the ἀπομνημονεύματα τῶν ἀποστόλων. The term is probably original here. See L. ABRAMOWSKI, Die "Erinnerungen der Apostel," 341. For Justin's use of the singular, cf. Dial. 10:2; 100:1.

4 *Contra* e.g. DIBELIUS, *Formgeschichte*, 264 n.1; SCHNIEWIND, *Matthäus*, 241; HAHN, *Mission*, 105; BAUMBACH, *TLZ* 92 (1967) 893; WALKER, *Heilsgeschichte*, 81 n. 24; STANTON, Matthew as a Creative Interpreter, 287; GRASSI, *BTB* 19 (1989) 23, 28f; KINGSBURY, *Matthew: Structure, Christology, Kingdom*, 130f; STANTON, Matthew: βίβλος, εὐαγγέλιον, or βίος?, 1194f.

5 STRECKER, *Weg der Gerechtigkeit*, 128f; GNILKA, *Matthäusevangelium* II, 388.

6 The absence of the reference to the kingdom in 26:13 is probably not as significant as STRECKER, *Weg der Gerechtigkeit*, 129, assumes. He thinks "this gospel" refers to the passion narrative. Cf. also SCHNIEWIND, *Matthäus*, 258; STUHLMACHER, *Evangelium*, 242.

The consistent qualification of the gospel also shows the christological focus. Unlike Mark,[1] Matthew never uses εὐαγγέλιον without further qualification. The impression—as may occur in Mark 1:1; 8:35; 10:29—that the gospel is an entity besides Jesus does not emerge.[2] The gospel is realized in the integrated impact of the words of Jesus and the narration about him.[3] A prophecy about one who *prepares* the way (3:1–3) follows John's preaching, but a passage pronouncing the *fulfilment* of prophecy (4:15–17) precedes Jesus' initial preaching. Jesus is not the proclaimer of the gospel only; he is also the one who is proclaimed through the telling of his ministry and life as the fulfilment of prophecy.

With these connotations attached to the preaching, the overlappings between teaching and preaching affects the former significantly. The content of Jesus' teaching contains within itself the preaching of the dynamic gospel event including Jesus' own ministry and life. *The presentation of the teaching as linked with the preaching reflects Matthew's interest to integrate Jesus' words of instruction within the narration about his whole life.* Teacher and teaching were inseparable. Without an account of the dynamic gospel event, Jesus' teaching was for Matthew incomplete. The words needed the episodal setting.

3.3. The Teaching and the Healing Activity

The two programmatic summaries in 4:23; 9:35 mention teaching also together with healing (θεραπεύειν). This is peculiar to Matthew.[4] Mark 1:39 speaks of healing briefly.[5] But healing is there connected with preaching, not teaching. There is no other immediate connection between the two.[6] The interesting question is how Matthew elsewhere relates Jesus' didactic and therapeutic activity.

3.3.1. The Teaching as Healing

There are several general features suggesting a connection between teaching and healing.[7] First, in 4:24f Jesus heals the sick people, and subsequently these people are present as the audience of the teaching in the Sermon on the Mount (5:1; 7:28–8:1).[8] Second, two didactic designations

---

1   Cf. Mark 8:35; 10:29; 13:10; 14:9; 16:15.
2   Cf. STUHLMACHER, *Evangelium*, 238–240.
3   Cf. STRECKER, *Weg der Gerechtigkeit*, 129; SCHWEIZER, *Matthäus*, 115; KINGS-BURY, *Matthew: Structure, Christology, Kingdom*, 130f, 133; U. LUZ, *Matthäus* I, 182.
4   Cf. COMBER, *JBL* 97 (1978) 431; GUELICH, *Sermon on the Mount*, 47.
5   In a sense, Jesus' teaching authority is connected with healing also in Mark. Cf. Mark 1:21–28 and the comments by SCHOLTISSEK, *Vollmacht*, 122–124.
6   Cf. Luke 4:44; Mark 6:6/Luke 8:1.
7   Cf. GERHARDSSON, *Mighty Acts*, 23, 40, 46, 51; BEARE, *SE* 7 (1982) 31–39.
8   Cf. G. LOHFINK, *Bergpredigt*, 23, 29–31.

(8:19; 9:11) occur within the collection of nine or ten miracle episodes in Matt 8–9. To be sure, these chapters include other material as well (8:18–22; 8:23–27; 9:9–13; 9:14–17), and the themes are indeed to be studied with regard to the narrative structure of the story.[1] But the inclusio created by 4:23; 9:35 gives a general indication that Matt 8–9 deals mainly with Jesus' therapeutic deeds. Third, although the people in Jesus' hometown react on his teaching, the result is that Jesus does not perform many mighty acts there (13:53–58). Fourth, one of Jesus' first actions in the temple—after cleansing it—is the performance of therapeutic miracles (21:14), and this is one of the factors arousing the anger of the temple authorities (21:15f). But afterwards, no further miracle is mentioned. Matthew says instead that Jesus was continuously teaching in the temple, and this is (also) the cause for the opponents' question about Jesus' authority (21:23).[2] Fifth, the miracle stories reveal an interest in the words of Jesus. Just as the words of teaching in the Sermon on the Mount are called λόγοι (7:24, 26, 28),[3] so are some of the miracles made effective by a λόγος from Jesus (8:8, 16).[4] And as is well known since the study of H.J. Held,[5] these episodes exhibit a concentration on the dialogues and the words of Jesus. When Jesus performs a miracle, he also teaches. This is true also for the non-therapeutic miracles.

A tradition-historical consideration may add to the picture. The primary label used to explain Jesus' therapeutic miracles—but not the non-therapeutic ones—is the servant of God.[6] 8:16f relates the activity to Isa 53:4 and 12:15–21 to Isa 42:1–4.[7] If we go beyond the christological titles,[8] we notice that the concept of Jesus as God's servant plays an important role in Matthew.[9] Some Jewish texts reveal that the servant of God (as Messiah) is also a didactic figure of wisdom.[10] Already B. Duhm saw a reference to the servant as torah teacher in Isa 42:1–4—especially in 42:1 (משפט) and 42:4

---

[1] U. LUZ, Wundergeschichten, 149–165.
[2] Cf. also 26:55.
[3] Cf. also 24:35.
[4] Cf. also 15:23.
[5] Miracle Stories, 168–211, 233–237. Cf. also e.g. GATZWEILER, Les récits de miracles, 212f; GERHARDSSON, *Mighty Acts,* 40f, 46f, 53.
[6] GERHARDSSON, *Mighty Acts,* 24–27, 88–91; HELD, Miracle Stories, 259–264.
[7] Cf. also 11:2–6.
[8] Cf. FRANCE, *Matthew: Evangelist and Teacher,* 298–302.
[9] GERHARDSSON, *ST* 27 (1973) 73–106; Sacrificial Service, 25–35; HILL, *JSNT* 6 (1980) 2–16; SCHNACKENBURG, "Knecht," 203–222. For Isa 42:1–4 and its importance in Matt 12, cf. COPE, *Matthew,* 32–52; NEYREY, *Bib* 63 (1982) 457–473; VERSEPUT, *Rejection,* 194–204.
[10] Isa 50:4 (LXX); Tg. Neb. Isa 11:1f, 42:7; 50:4; 53:5, 11. Cf. also the wisdom ascribed to an important figure in 1 Enoch 49:2–4; Pss. Sol. 17:23, 29, 35, 37, 42f; 18:4–9; T. Levi 18:7 (perhaps interpolation). For the Dead Sea scrolls (11QMelch 6, 18, 20; 4QAhA), cf. above pp. 125, 131f. Cf. also 4QMess ar 1:6–8.—The messianic interpretation is sometimes uncertain. Cf. SEIDELIN, *ZAW* 35 (1936) 204, 219 (on Tg. Neb. Isa 50:4f), 225 (on Pss. Sol.). For the connections between "messiah" and "servant" in Tg. Neb. Isa 43:10; 52:13, see CHILTON, *Glory of Israel,* 90–94, concluding that "the meturgeman attests a primitive exegesis common to Judaism and Christianity" (*ibid.,* 94).

(מ‎שׁפמ, ‎ולחותו).[1] Others have followed Duhm.[2] Although Matthew agrees to a large extent with the LXX in translating מ‎שׁפמ with κρίσιν and ‎ולחותו with καὶ τῷ ὀνόματι αὐτοῦ,[3] we should not exclude the possibility that the Isaianic text carries a didactic connotation in Matthew. Taking its cue from the reference to the spirit of wisdom in Isa 11:1–4, such a connotation seems to be behind allusions to Isa 42:1ff in 4QMess ar 1:6–10; 1 Enoch 49:2–4.[4] And in Matthew, the servant's ministry to the nations (12:18d, 21) finds part of its realization in the future teaching activity of the disciples (28:20).[5]

These general features are not accidental. Jesus explains his therapeutic actions and defends them *as teacher*. After all, the combination of teaching and healing in one person was not common in the ancient Jewish world,[6] nor outside of the Jewish world.[7] Although the Pharisees hold the disciples responsible for the action of their teacher,[8] Jesus himself gives the defence in 9:10–13. Of importance is the quotation, or translation,[9] of Hos 6:6. Despite its covenantal background of steadfast love in the OT[10] and its halakhic use in rabbinic literature,[11] Hos 6:6 is not the basis for halakhah here.[12] It concerns Jesus' entire vocation and ministry.[13] 9:13 links the quotation to an ἦλθον-saying by means of γάρ.[14] Just as in 12:7f, a self-referential statement from Jesus supports the quotation. The quotation is christological. It refers mainly to Jesus' exemplary activity. The quotation concerns mercy. Mercy is indeed one of the weightier matters in the Torah (23:23), but a special relationship also exists between Jesus' therapeutic miracles and the

---

1 *Jesaia*, 285–287.
2 W.D. DAVIES, *Setting of the Sermon on the Mount*, 133–137. Cf. also e.g. ELLI-GER, *Deuterojesaja*, 217–219; RIESNER, *Lehrer*, 307.
3 The text as a whole agrees neither with the MT nor with the LXX nor with the targum. For discussion, see GUNDRY, *Use of the Old Testament*, 110–116; STENDAHL, *School of Matthew*, 107–115, 198; ROTHFUCHS, *Erfüllungszitate*, 72–77, 123f.
4 HENGEL, *Jesus als messianischer Lehrer*, 173, 178f; RIESNER, *Lehrer*, 309f, 323f.
5 Cf. MCCONNELL, *Law and Prophecy*, 124; VERSEPUT, *Rejection*, 202; KINGS-BURY, *Matthew: Structure, Christology, Kingdom*, 95. Kingsbury, however, minimizes the importance of the (implicit) servant christology in Matthew.
6 KAMPLING, *BZ* 30 (1986) 237–248.
7 DOWNING, *NTS* 33 (1987) 446f.—Apollonius of Tyana, active in the 1st cent. C.E., could of course be mentioned. For discussion of the person and teaching of Apollonius, including a phenomenological comparison with the early Christian understanding of Jesus, see PETZKE, *Apollonius von Tyana*, 161–229. But according to the recent study by KOSKENNIEMI, *Apollonios von Tyana*, scholars have often overestimated the importance of Apollonius for the NT.
8 Cf. DAUBE, *NTS* 19 (1972–73) 11f.
9 Cf. HILL, *NTS* 24 (1978) 108f.
10 Cf. HILL, *NTS* 24 (1978) 109f, 118; FRANCE, *Matthew*, 168.
11 Cf. STRACK/BILLERBECK, *Kommentar* I, 499f.
12 *Contra* e.g. HUMMEL, *Auseinandersetzung*, 38f; HILL, *NTS* 24 (1978) 111; GNILKA, *Matthäusevangelium* I, 332.
13 LOHMEYER, *Matthäus*, 174; ARENS, *The ἦλθον-Sayings*, 56–59; GUNDRY, *Matthew*, 168; HELD, *Miracle Stories*, 258; VERSEPUT, *Rejection*, 169f; PATTE, *Matthew*, 128; U. LUZ, *Matthäus* II, 45.
14 Cf. MCNEILE, *Matthew*, 119f; LOHMEYER, *Matthäus*, 173.

request for mercy.[1] When Jesus therefore as teacher urges the Pharisees to go and learn what the Scriptures really say about mercy, he is actually defending his therapeutic deeds.

The request in 12:38 confirms this. The scribes and the Pharisees approach Jesus as teacher. The question about Jesus' legitimation concerns his therapeutic activity. The previous healing of the blind and mute demoniac (12:22) has triggered a demand for legitimation. The healing leads to the question if Jesus is the Son of David[2] and to the accusation that Jesus casts out the demons only by Beelzebul (12:23f). Just as rabbinic teachers sometimes are to validate an unusual halakha (b. B. Meṣ. 59b) or a prophecy (b. Sanh. 98a)[3] by giving a sign (אות, סימן), Jesus is as teacher[4]—not Messiah[5]—asked for a sign (σημεῖον) of some kind.[6] The sign usually served to ascertain the genuine legitimation of a person, action or event.[7] Considering the belief that persons appearing with prophetic claims should validate themselves with a sign from God,[8] it is understandable that the opponents now expect Jesus, who acted beyond the normal behaviour of a teacher, to confirm that he is a teacher who performs therapeutic miracles legitimately.

Excursus 11: *Prophets and Signs*

The wide-spread assumption that a prophet should validate himself by a sign from God is evident in various texts from different times. Moses was regarded as the prophet *par excellence* and as such believed to have brought incomparable signs and wonders (Deut 34:10–12). Consequently, other prophetic figures were to validate their utterances or actions by signs from God (1 Sam 2:34; 10:7, 9; 1 Kgs 13:3, 5; 2 Kgs 19:29; 20:8f; Isa 7:11). The same belief later comes to the surface in some rabbinic writings (y. Sanh. 30c; Exod. Rab. 9:1).

However, the signs were not automatically guarantees of truth. We see this already in Deut 13:1–3, and it is behind certain passages in the Dead Sea scrolls (11QT 54:8–

---

1 Cf. 9:27; 15:22; 17:15; 20:30f. Besides these instances where mercy is related to a therapeutic miracle, mercy is spoken of only in 5:7; 6:2–4; 18:33.

2 This should perhaps be read/heard against the background of Jewish notions about Solomon, son of David, as exorcist. The most important text is Ant. 8:45–49. For discussion and further references, see the positive evaluation by FISHER, Son of David?, 82–97; LÖVESTAM, SEÅ 37–38 (1972–73) 196–210; BERGER, NTS 20 (1973–74) 5–9, and the more cautious assessment by DULING, HTR 68 (1975) 235–252; idem, NTS 24 (1978) 408f; GERHARDSSON, *Mighty Acts*, 87; DULING, BTB 22 (1992) 109, 112. Cf. also SCHÜRER, *History* III, 375–379 (with lit.).

3 Cf. also Tanḥ. B. וישלח 8.

4 Cf. R.A. EDWARDS, *Sign of Jonah*, 103; FRANCE, *Matthew*, 212; PATTE, *Matthew*, 180.

5 *Contra* e.g. MCNEILE, *Matthew*, 181; E. KLOSTERMANN, *Matthäusevangelium*, 111; A. JONES, *Matthew*, 151; HUMMEL, *Auseinandersetzung*, 126; GNILKA, *Matthäusevangelium* I, 464.

6 The sign did not have to be a miracle. The term σημεῖον is never used for miracles in the synoptic tradition.

7 LINTON, ST 19 (1965) 116, 118–128.

8 See excursus 11.

16),[1] the NT (Mark 13:22/Matt 24:24; Rev 16:13f; 19:20), Josephus' writings (Ant. 20:97–99, 168–172, Bell. 2:259–263; 6:285f) and the rabbinic literature (Sifre on Deut 13:2). Probably Matthew did not expect his readers/hearers to believe that a sign automatically would have altered the opponents' negative understanding of Jesus' previous miracle.

3.3.2. The Healing as Visual Teaching

There are texts implying that Matthew prefers to mention therapeutic actions instead of giving the expected reference to teaching. In 15:29 Jesus goes up on the mountain and sits down. This is reminiscent of 5:1. But while in 5:2 the disciples approach Jesus and he teaches them, in 15:30 many crowds approach Jesus and he heals them. And in 4:25 the crowds that Jesus healed follow him and are present at the teaching delivered to the disciples (5:1; 7:28f). But in 8:1–4; 12:15; 14:13f; 19:2, their following leads to a therapeutic miracle.[2] An intersynoptic reading of certain passages gives the same impression. 14:14; 19:2 do not in distinction to Mark 6:34; 10:1 state that Jesus teaches the crowds. He heals them.[3]

Since the indications listed above and 9:10–13; 12:38 point towards a positive relationship between teaching and healing, this preference does not imply a strict distinction between the two aspects of Jesus' ministry. It is instead due to the various objects of Jesus' action. The recurring feature in all the passages depicting the therapeutic activity is that the action is aimed towards groups or individuals who are neither actual disciples of Jesus nor in total opposition to him. The disciples are nowhere the object of therapeutic miracles.[4] From sixteen instances of θεραπεύειν, the object of the action is stated thirteen times:[5] in nine cases, it is stated in general terms as consisting of all the sick persons of the people (λαός) or the crowd(s) (ὄχλος, ὄχλοι);[6] in four other instances, the object is an individual person—whether a son (παῖς)[7] of a Gentile (8:7) or an anonymous blind and mute person (12:22) or the son of someone from the crowd (17:16, 18). When such persons listen to Jesus' verbal teaching (διδάσκειν, διδαχή), it causes merely amazement (7:28; 22:33) and grieving rejection (19:16–22). But when Jesus "addresses" them with the therapeutic miracles, they are out of their minds (ἐξιστάναι), marvelling (θαυμάζειν) and giving glory (δοξάζειν) to the God

---

1   Cf. also 11QT 61:1–5.
2   Cf. also 20:29–34.
3   Luke 9:11 mentions that Jesus both spoke (λαλεῖν) to the crowds and healed them.
4   GERHARDSSON, *Mighty Acts,* 43, 49–51.
5   It is not stated in 9:35; 10:1; 12:10.
6   So with minor variations in 4:23, 24; 8:16; 10:8 (healing expected to be performed by the disciples); 12:15; 14:14; 15:30; 19:2; 21:14.
7   For παῖς as son here, see U. LUZ, *Matthäus* II, 14 n. 17.

of Israel (12:23; 15:31).[1] The references to the blind that see (12:22; 15:31) also illustrate the positive recognition of Jesus as a result of his therapeutic actions.[2] By contrast, there is no difference between the opponents' response to Jesus' verbal teaching and to his therapeutic miracles. Just as the former causes hostile reactions (13:54–57; 21:23),[3] so do the therapeutic miracles (12:10, 14, 24; 21:15f).[4] As it appears, the therapeutic activity is a kind of visual teaching which Jesus gives to outsiders who are not overtly hostile.

This kind of teaching also contains proclamative elements. It is related to the preaching of the kingdom of heaven, the gospel event.[5] Accordingly, the term (διὰ)σῴζειν appears in relation to the therapeutic activity (9:21, 22 [bis]; 14:36). This term links Jesus' activity as healer with the whole purpose of his name and ministry as indicated in 1:21.[6] But whereas the preaching with words is silenced when the narrative moves towards opposition, the therapeutic miracles continue to accompany the verbal teaching as its kerygmatic counterpart.

The therapeutic miracles contain visual teaching which Jesus addresses to those who cannot fully apprehend the significance of the verbal teaching related to a life in discipleship. They give Jesus' comprehensive teaching activity an additional proclamative aspect. The persons addressed experience parts of the salvific reality to be present in Jesus as a therapeutic teacher. To be sure, the verbal teaching dominates. Matthew states only rarely that Jesus' words effect healing for the people.[7] And while teaching, preaching and healing are mentioned together in 4:23; 9:35, healing is not part of the summary in 11:1. Similarly, while Jesus gives the task of healing to the disciples in 10:1, 8, he does not explicitly commission them to heal in 28:19f.[8] But nevertheless, the therapeutic miracles are observable actions with a message. They represent the preaching of the kingdom in deeds and provide the teaching with another kerygmatic element. *The Matthean story reflects an interest in Jesus which goes beyond the concentration on his didactic words only and incorporates the therapeutic deeds into the teaching itself.*

---

1   Cf. also 9:8, 33.
2   Cf. also 9:30; 11:5; 20:34. In 13:13–16 the giving of meshalim is related to healing (ἰᾶσθαι) of ears and eyes. For further discussion, see LOADER, *CBQ* 44 (1982) 570–585.
3   Cf. also 26:55.
4   Cf. also 9:34.
5   Cf. GIESEN, Krankenheilungen, 87f; G. LOHFINK, *Bergpredigt,* 29–31, though they present different views concerning the relationship between teaching, preaching and healing.
6   Cf. also 8:25; 10:22; 14:30; 16:25 (18:11); 19:25; 24:13, 22; 27:40, 42, 49 and the discussion by KJÆR-HANSEN, *Jesus,* 329–345.
7   Only in 13:15 is healing (ἰᾶσθαι) the direct result of verbal teaching. But the meshalim in Matt 13 are not explicitly classified as διδαχή, in distinction to what we find in Mark 4:1f. For different explanations of this, cf. KINGSBURY, *Parables of Jesus,* 28–31, 131; DUPONT, Le point de vue, 250–259; LAMBRECHT, *Treasure,* 155f, 158.
8   Cf. KJÆR-NIELSEN, *Heilung und Verkündigung,* 135f.

4. The Didactic-Labelling Motives

Several scholars have observed that the high conception of Jesus' person served as a prominent motive of transmission in early Christianity.[1] An even more precise motive is at hand when the high conception is directly connected with an understanding of Jesus as teacher. This is reflected in Matthew. Jesus is a teacher, but not merely one teacher among many. He appears within a significant framework of labels defining and validating his status as teacher.

The christological features in the Matthean story will here serve as testimonies of a labelling process. Although some scholars take the perspective from the narrative structure of the story into account as a means of conceiving the Matthean christology,[2] the common procedure is still to relate Jesus to God and to man. The book *Calling Jesus Names* by B.J. Malina and J.H. Neyrey now supplements this common procedure. The two authors analyze the titles of Jesus in terms of their social value. There is not only a christology "from above" or "from below," but also "from the side." The christology reflects a process of positive and negative labelling by groups marked by the relation of inside and outside, centre and periphery.[3] Although I will continue to give the internal features of the story due consideration, the focus of interest here involves a perspective similar to the one of Malina and Neyrey. *As a reflection of Matthew's didactic-labelling motives of transmission, I will ask how the positive and negative labelling visible in the story defines and validates Jesus' status as teacher.*

4.1. The Labellers

The labellers are the persons in the story who validate Jesus by means of labels. When we focus on the labelling connected with the didactic characterization only, there emerges a rather clear demarcation of those who recognize and validate Jesus' didactic status.

4.1.1. Disciples and Believers

The characterization of Jesus as teacher occurs occasionally in a significant conjunction with the use of κύριος. Both διδάσκαλος and ῥαββί/ῥαββουνί are treated similarly in this case. While 8:19 uses διδάσκαλε as an address to

---

[1] So, with various emphases, e.g. RIESENFELD, Gospel Tradition, 63–65; GERHARDSSON, *Memory*, 332; LARSSON, *Vorbild*, 32f; GERHARDSSON, *Tradition and Transmission*, 41; *idem, Origins of the Gospel Traditions*, 48f; HENGEL, Jesus als messianischer Lehrer, 170; RIESNER, Elementarbildung, 219; *idem, Lehrer*, 39f, 351f; *idem, Jesus as Teacher and Preacher*, 209; *idem,* Teacher, 808.

[2] Cf. KINGSBURY, *Matthew as Story*, 43–58, 95–103; U. LUZ, Christologie, 221–235; QUESNEL, *Jésus-Christ*, 165–199.

[3] MALINA/NEYREY, *Calling Jesus Names*, xf, 35–42.

Jesus, 8:21 uses κύριε; while 26:22 gives the expression μήτι ἐγώ εἰμι, κύριε, 26:25 employs μήτι ἐγώ εἰμι, ῥαββί. An intersynoptic reading supports the pattern. Matthew is twice alone against Mark[1] and twice in agreement with Luke against Mark[2] in giving no didactic address at all. And even more significantly, κύριε appears instead of a didactic address to Jesus three times in Matthew as compared with both Mark and Luke[3] and once in Matthew and Luke as compared with Mark.[4]

The use of κύριος is philologically reasonable.[5] In spite of the rather technical and titular connotation attached to the negatively loaded ῥαββί in Matthew,[6] κύριος might initially have suggested itself on the basis of the early Semitic use of רבי in the sense "my great" as related to מרי, "my lord." There are connections between forms of רב and מ ר in certain fragments from Qumran: 4QEn[b] 1 III:14 mentions Raphael and Michael speaking of God as "our great lord" (מרנא רבא); 4QEn[d] 1 XI:2—unfortunately somewhat corrupted at this point—twice blesses the "lord of greatness" (מרא רבותא); 1QapGen 2:4 tells about Lamech commanding his wife Bitenosh "by the great lord" (במרה רבותא). Rabbinic writings reveal an awareness of the fact that רבי essentially means "my great" and sometimes use the term for teachers almost as a synonym of מרי.[7] There is not sufficient evidence to suggest an entirely parallel development of the two terms as used for Jesus in the earliest strata of the gospel tradition.[8] But it is possible that Matthew's consistent way of relating the didactic designations to κύριος, and not to another label, initially depended on an understanding coloured by Semitic connotations.

The use of κύριος instead of διδάσκαλος and ῥαββί/ῥαββουνί is more than a stylistic variation. The term κύριος occurs also elsewhere and carries flexible and auxiliary connotations. Contrary to the opinion of several scholars,[9] Kingsbury has demonstrated that κύριος as used for Jesus does not function as a fixed christological title of majesty.[10] It normally appears in the vocative and serves as a relational term validating the superior status of Jesus in a general manner. The exact dignity and christological implication are not fixed. The use of this rather vague label is suitable in order not to nullify the didactic portrayal of Jesus.[11] *Jesus does not cease to be a tea-*

---

1 Matt 20:20/Mark 10:35; Matt 21:20/Mark 11:21.
2 Matt 19:20/Mark 10:20/Luke 18:21; Matt 24:1/Mark 13:1/Luke 21:5.
3 Matt 8:25/Mark 4:38 (διδάσκαλε)/Luke 8:24 (ἐπιστάτα); Matt 17:4/Mark 9:5 (ῥαββί)/Luke 9:33 (ἐπιστάτα); Matt 17:15/Mark 9:17 (διδάσκαλε)/Luke 9:38 (διδάσκαλε).
4 Matt 20:33 (cf. 9:28)/Mark 10:51 (ῥαββουνί)/Luke 18:41.
5 Cf. RIESNER, *Lehrer*, 250.
6 See below pp. 284–287.
7 Cf. e.g. b. Ketub. 103b; b. B. Qam. 73b; b. Mak. 24a.
8 See FITZMYER, *Wandering Aramean*, 117, with the decisive argument that there is no known instance of מרי in which the suffix has lost its significance, as רבי sometimes has.
9 E.g. TRILLING, *Israel*, 21–51, FRANKEMÖLLE, *Jahwebund, passim;* BORNKAMM, End-Expectation, 41–43.
10 *Matthew: Structure, Christology, Kingdom*, 103–113. Cf. also GERHARDSSON, *Mighty Acts*, 85f; SCHENK, *Sprache des Matthäus*, 307f.
11 Kingsbury does not draw this conclusion.

cher when he is called κύριος.[1] Rather, he is as teacher attributed an extraordinary status.[2]

The common denominator of the six passages using κύριε in connection with a didactic address elsewhere in Matthew or in the other synoptics is the occurrence of the label on the lips of the disciples (8:21, 25; 17:4; 26:22) or persons showing trust in Jesus' miraculous powers (17:15; 20:33 [cf. 9:28]). Such characters never address Jesus with διδάσκαλε in Matthew. Only those who are Jesus' own disciples—except Judas (26:25, 49)—or acknowledge his miraculous powers validate his unique status as teacher in Matthew.

4.1.2. Peter

As we have already noticed,[3] Peter is according to 16:17–19 the person through whom Jesus' teaching authority legitimately will remain normative in the disciples' future teaching. This appointment depends on Peter's recognition of Jesus' unique status. We see this in the same pericope. Although Peter is the foundation of the church, the word-play between πέτρος and πέτρα implies that it is not merely the question of a simple identification between the two. The term πέτρα occurs elsewhere in Matthew. Its use in 7:24f is interesting.[4] 7:24f is related to 16:18. It not only uses πέτρα twice, but the image centres in 7:24 as in 16:18 around both πέτρα and οἰκοδομεῖν. Building on a rock illustrates in 7:24f the practice—the full internalization—of Jesus' words. The suggestion of interpreting 16:18 together with 7:24f has the advantage of taking seriously the semantic field provided by the Matthean narrative itself.

The demonstrative pronoun ταύτῃ in front of τῇ πέτρᾳ in 16:18 indicates a specific reference connected with Peter as the rock. If there is an allusion back to 7:24f, it may be possible to regard the pronoun as an echo of μου τοὺς λόγους τούτους.[5] But it is more natural to assume that the pronoun has an immediate referent in the context. Since we think of Peter as the rock, the pronoun must imply a certain qualification connected with Peter himself.[6] In 7:24f the rock is part of an expression illustrating the full recognition of Jesus' words—internalized knowledge. In 16:13–20 the basic issue has to do with Jesus' identity revealed to Peter. The blessing of Peter in

---

[1]　*Contra* BORNKAMM, End-Expectation, 41.
[2]　Cf. STRECKER, *Weg der Gerechtigkeit,* 126, though his emphasis on the eschatological importance attributed to the teaching by means of calling the teacher κύριος limits the labelling process to an activity related to ideological factors only.
[3]　See above pp. 245–253.
[4]　Cf. KILPATRICK, *Origins,* 39; BLANK, *Concilium* 9 (1973) 175; GUNDRY, *Matthew,* 334; SCHENK, *BZ* 27 (1983) 73; CROSBY, *House of Disciples,* 50–53; MARCUS, *CBQ* 50 (1988) 444.
[5]　So GUNDRY, *Matthew,* 334.
[6]　Cf. WILKINS, *Concept of Disciple,* 193.

16:17 forms the structural centre of the whole pericope.[1] It is not a matter of Jesus' identity only,[2] but of knowledge revealed to Peter. 16:16 shows that Peter knows who Jesus is. It has been revealed to him,[3] and because of the revelation he is blessed and made the rock of the church. Peter's function as the rock is therefore intimately linked with the special insight given to him by the Father. The following pericope in 16:21–23 confirms this. When Peter does not think the thoughts of God but of men, he becomes a stumbling stone (16:23).[4] The phrase σκάνδαλον εἶ ἐμοῦ occurs in Matthew only,[5] and through this utterance Matthew creates an antithetical counterpart to μακάριος εἶ in 16:17. Peter does not utter revealed knowledge in 16:22. In such a case, he is not even ironically thought of as a rock.[6] He is the opposite. It is on the basis of the christological understanding revealed by the Father that Jesus makes Peter the rock of his church. Jesus ultimately remains the foundation of the church.[7] It is "this Peter," the one who has been given the correct understanding of Jesus' identity, that is the rock of the church.[8]

The labeller is here one of those who themselves will teach others. The individual who is to carry Jesus' teaching ministry further must have internalized the words and deeds of his teacher and been given knowledge about the teacher's true identity. As I concluded in the previous chapter, Matthew saw himself as one of Jesus' disciples and pupils. He was probably one of the future teachers depicted in the story. *The portrayal of the disciples as labellers reflects Matthew's own interest in integrating Jesus' teaching within a labelling process enhancing Jesus' status as teacher.*

4.2. The Didactic Exousia of Jesus

In what way did Matthew then enhance Jesus as teacher? The use of the term ἐξουσία is a first indication. Derived from ἔξεστιν, the Greek term essentially means "the ability and possibility to perform an action," and even further "the right, power and authority to do something."[9] Matthew uses it

---

1   In the text accepted in the 26th edition of Nestle-Aland, the phrase ὁ Ἰησοῦς εἶπεν αὐτῷ, μακάριος εἶ, Σίμων Βαριωνᾶ, ὅτι σὰρξ καὶ αἷμα οὐκ ἀπεκάλυψέν σοι ἀλλ᾽ ὁ πατήρ μου ὁ ἐν τοῖς οὐρανοῖς forms the centre of 16:13–20. Before and after this phrase there are 67 words. The numerical pattern of the pericope is 67+23+67=157.
2   CARAGOUNIS, *Peter,* 95f, emphasizes the importance of 16:20.
3   *Contra* SCHENK, *BZ* 27 (1983) 76, who claims that the lack of the accusative of the object to ἀπεκάλυψέν σοι shows that the revelation concerns all that has been said from 4:17 and onwards. The gospel is the gospel of Peter. Cf. also C. KÄHLER, *NTS* 23 (1976–77) 57. For some criticism of Schenk, cf. CARAGOUNIS, *Peter,* 76 n. 41, 104.
4   Cf. HOFFMANN, Petrus-Primat, 426.
5   Cf. Mark 8:33.
6   *Contra* STOCK, *BTB* 17 (1987) 64–69.
7   Cf. also 21:42(–44).
8   OBRIST, *Echtheitsfragen,* 126–130, considers this understanding as the common protestantic one, but adds that some catholics propose similar views.
9   Cf. LSJ, 599; FOERSTER, *TDNT* II, 562f; W. BAUER, *Wörterbuch,* 562–564.

eight times in reference to Jesus.[1] Once it also describes what Jesus gives to his disciples (10:1).[2] With the exception of 9:8 and the special material in 28:18, the instances have parallels in one or both of the other synoptics.[3] 7:29; 21:23–27 and, to some extent, 28:18 connect it most evidently with a teaching activity. These three instances point to significant aspects of Jesus' teaching authority.

4.2.1. The Didactic Exousia as Universal Dominion

Matthew leads the readers/hearers to a full understanding of Jesus' didactic exousia. When he first introduces Jesus' exousia in 7:29, he connects it closely with Jesus' teaching activity. Unlike in Mark 1:22,[4] the exousia here refers back to an extended presentation of Jesus' teaching. While Matthew subsequently expands this initial impression to include motifs concerning the forgiving of sins (9:6, 8) and healing (10:1), he first focalizes on the didactic exousia manifested in Jesus' teaching.

21:23–27 mentions Jesus' exousia four times (21:23 [*bis*], 24, 27). It is the essential topic of the pericope. Jesus' final words in 21:27 (ἐν ποίᾳ ἐξουσίᾳ ταῦτα ποιῶ) hark back to his first words in 21:24 and to the initial question of the chief priests and elders of the people in 21:23 (ἐν ποίᾳ ἐξουσίᾳ ταῦτα ποιεῖς). The whole pericope is framed by the question of Jesus' exousia. It concerns a specific didactic activity.[5] The setting in 21:23, presenting Jesus as teaching in the temple, is the immediate occasion for the question of the Jewish authorities.[6]

In distinction to 7:29, the didactic exousia now appears together with other aspects of Jesus' active ministry. The expression ταῦτα ποιεῖν is appended to the issue concerning the exousia. It is not merely a matter of what Jesus says as teacher, but also of what he does.[7] The expression probably relates to all that Jesus has done since he came to Jerusalem: the triumphal entry (21:1–11), the cleansing of the temple (21:12f), the healing (21:14), the cursing of the fig tree (21:18–22) and the teaching in the temple (21:23).[8] They all represent acts implying a special exousia. The initial mention of the exousia in 7:29 suggests that the didactic aspect remains essential. But as the narrative has developed, Jesus' didactic exousia has become associated with matters broader than the words of teaching only.

---

[1] 7:29; 9:6, 8; 21:23 (*bis*), 24, 27; 28:18.

[2] The term is used also in 8:9.

[3] Cf. Mark 1:22/Luke 4:32; Mark 2:10/Luke 5:24; Mark 6:7 (cf. 3:15)/Luke 9:1; Mark 11:28 (*bis*)/Luke 20:2 (*bis*); Mark 11:29; Mark 11:33/Luke 20:8.

[4] Cf. SCHOLTISSEK, *Vollmacht*, 120–122.

[5] Cf. e.g. DAUBE, *New Testament*, 221; SCHWEIZER, *Matthäus*, 267; GUNDRY, *Matthew*, 419; SAND, *Matthäus*, 427f; GNILKA, *Matthäusevangelium* II, 216.

[6] Cf. also 13:54, though the term ἐξουσία is not used in this case.

[7] Cf. HILL, *Matthew*, 296; SCHNACKENBURG, *Matthäusevangelium* II, 201.

[8] Cf. MEIER, *Matthew*, 238.

In 28:18, towards the very end of the narrative, Jesus himself closes the use of ἐξουσία by pointing to its all-embracing character. Without controversial and polemical implications, Jesus now states that he has been given all exousia. The continued references to *all* the nations (28:19), *all* that Jesus has commanded (28:20a) and *all* days (28:20b) strengthen the emphasis on *all* exousia. This emphasis is also congruent with the mention of both heaven and earth. Jesus has indeed been ascribed exousia also previously in the narrative. But it is always qualifed in a certain sense: he teaches "as" (ὡς) one having exousia (7:29); it is "on earth" (ἐπὶ τῆς γῆς) that he has the exousia to forgive sins (9:6, 8); the opponents' question concerning "this exousia" (τὴν ἐξουσίαν ταύτην) has to do with specific actions in Jerusalem (21:23). The narrative exhibits a development preparing the final mention of the exousia.[1] The didactic exousia ultimately includes aspects that concern not only the verbal teaching and other parts of Jesus' earthly ministry, but everything in heaven and on earth. It resides in the universal exousia finally attributed to the risen Jesus.

4.2.2. The Didactic Exousia as Personal Quality

The contrast between Jesus and the scribes in 7:29 does not concern a distinction between the unordained Jesus speaking as if he had the authority (רשות) of an ordained rabbi and the elementary teachers (סופרים) of the Jews.[2] There is no evidence in Matthew that the rabbinic use of סופר for the elementary teacher determines the connotation of γραμματεύς. And Jesus' teaching in the Sermon on the Mount goes beyond any teaching normally given by later rabbis. The contrast between the didactic exousia of Jesus and of the scribes is not based on formal systems of validation. Nor can we explain it by reference to a particular christological title to which Jesus would conform.[3] The titles do not define Jesus in the story. Jesus' person defines the titles.[4] The significance of the teaching in the Sermon depends on Jesus' own person.[5] The teaching contains claims that set it apart from all other teaching and point to a didactic exousia carried by Jesus' own person.

21:23–27 suggests further an exousia residing in Jesus' person. This is implied not only in the question of the Jewish authorities, but also in the re-

---

[1] I focus on Matthew's use of ἐξουσία only. The development in the use of this term is not opposed to the authority that Jesus exhibits in other ways throughout the narrative, e.g. in 11:25–30.

[2] *Contra* DAUBE, *New Testament,* 205–223, though his discussion is focused primarily on Mark as reflective of earlier traditions.

[3] MEIER, *Vision of Matthew,* 64, suggests that in view of its occurrence in the rest of the gospel narrative, the exousia is the one of the son of man. Similarly GEIST, *Menschensohn,* 342. But as U. LUZ, Christologie, 226, 228, points out, there are no references to the son of man in the Sermon on the Mount itself.

[4] Cf. KECK, *NTS* 32 (1986) 370f, stressing that the titles do not generally so much interpret the Jesus event as the Jesus event interprets the titles.

[5] STRECKER, *Sermon on the Mount,* 26.

sponse of Jesus in 21:28–32. While Jesus refers to John's baptism in 21:25, he speaks of believing John himself in 21:32. Together with 3:15 this probably means the acknowledgement of the way of righteousness which John brought through his preaching and conduct.[1] The concise expression πισ-τεύειν αὐτῷ used three times by Jesus in 21:32 shows that John's ministry was inseparable from John's person, just as Jesus' ministry points to an exousia carried by Jesus' own person.

28:18 makes evident that the exousia is a quality given to Jesus independent of his actions. There is no explicit connection to his previous words or deeds in the narrative. Jesus merely states that all exousia has been given to him. By referring to other texts, scholars frequently try to mould Jesus' exousia in 28:18 into specific christological patterns.[2] Cumulative evidence from Matthew itself must of course support the parallels adduced.[3] And the only explicit connection between the giving of exousia to Jesus and a closer definition of Jesus' identity in Matthew itself is the reference to the exousia of the son of man in 9:6.[4] But the discussion here appears in a polemical context. Moreover, the exousia is not like in Dan 7:13f connected with universal dominion, but with an exousia to forgive sins on earth, which the crowds, according to the narrator's comment in 9:8, think has been given to men.[5] 9:6, 8 do not confirm the common assumption that Jesus' exousia in 28:18 is the one of the Danielic son of man.[6] It is more likely that 28:18 is connected with 11:27.[7] In particular, ἐδόθη μοι πᾶσα ἐξουσία in 28:18 is reminiscent of πάντα μοι παρεδόθη ὑπὸ τοῦ πατρός μου in 11:27.[8] This

---

[1] Cf. PRZYBYLSKI, *Righteousness*, 94–96; GIESEN, *Christliches Handeln*, 41–77; HAGNER, Righteousness, 117f; WOUTERS, " ... *wer den Willen meines Vaters tut,*" 65f, 221, 225f.

[2] GEIST, *Menschensohn*, 104–120, discusses the most important proposals. In addition, T.L. DONALDSON, *Jesus on the Mountain*, 171–190, relates the exousia to a christologically reinterpreted vision of the Zion eschatology.

[3] HARTMAN, Scriptural Exegesis, 144, though suggesting that 28:18f implies a reference to Dan 7:14, insists that "the meaning must be found from the context and not from an interpretative tradition."

[4] It is not necessary for my purposes to decide if 9:6 as a whole or merely partly is a comment by the narrator. Cf. DAVIES/ALLISON, *Matthew* II, 51, 93f.—References to the son of man occur of course also elsewhere in Matthew. But the other instances do not explicitly mention the designation in relation to Jesus' exousia.

[5] Cf. PAMMENT, *NTS* 29 (1983) 120; HARE, *Son of Man*, 140f; *idem, Matthew,* 100.—I cannot see that CARAGOUNIS, *Son of Man*, 190 n. 293, has conclusively refuted this "inexcusably bad exegesis." It is not merely "the astonished and unenlightened crowd" that speaks in 9:8. It is the narrator commenting on the reaction of the crowds. And why, if 9:6 identifies Jesus with the heavenly being of Dan 7:14, has 9:8 at all, as it seems, been deliberately (re)formulated (cf. Mark 2:12/Luke 5:26) to refer to the exousia given to men?

[6] *Contra* GEIST, *Menschensohn*, 117f. For further arguments against a dependence on Dan 7:13f in Matt 28:18, see VÖGTLE, *SE* 2 (1964) 269–277.

[7] Cf. LANGE, *Das Erscheinen des Auferstandenen*, 152–167; GEIST, *Menschensohn*, 113–116.

[8] Cf. also the use of οὐρανός and γῆς in 28:18 and 11:25, and πατήρ/υἱός in 28:19 and 11:27.

verse does not by itself stress a particular Son (of Man) christology. The term υἱός is quite natural when God is referred to as "Father."[1] The point of the verse is that since Jesus has been given all the hidden knowledge of the Father, his words and deeds are authorized as revelation.[2] 11:27 legitimizes Jesus' teaching as revelation handed over (παραδιδόναι) directly from the Father, not from tradition. When we read/hear 28:18 in conjunction with 11:27, it includes an aspect of special transcendental authorization.[3]

Matthew consistently attributes exousia to Jesus' own person. The exousia is intrinsic. It is one with Jesus, depending on the authorization of none but God. The attribution is not based on external qualifications suggesting a formal basis on which the exousia is considered valid. Matthew acknowledges Jesus' exousia as a personal quality given directly from God.[4]

4.2.3. The Didactic Exousia as Identity Marker

The didactic exousia functions in two ways as an identity marker in Matthew. On one hand, it polemically defines who is outside of the group of Jesus' adherents. Jesus' exousia is a matter of amazement and dispute:[5] the crowds are amazed at Jesus' teaching in 7:28f, because it points to an exousia which their own scribes do not have;[6] Jesus discusses in 21:23–27 with the opponents and refuses to give them a direct answer. The polemical situation becomes even clearer when we consider the narrative meshalim in 21:28–32, 33–43(–44); 22:1–14 suggesting the exclusion of the Jewish people.[7] Especially the first of these meshalim, present only in Matthew, is directly connected with 21:23–27. In addition to placing the importance of doing at the centre (21:31) and thus harking back to 21:23, 24, 27, it picks up the reference to John the Baptist and points to the consistent failure of the Jewish people to believe him. Outsiders do not recognize Jesus' exousia.

On the other hand, Jesus' didactic exousia defines the identity and activity of the adherents themselves. The final and all-embracing exousia is the prerogative (οὖν) of the mission to the nations,[8] involving—in addition to baptizing[9]—the disciples' teaching ministry (28:19f). Not until Jesus has been

---

[1]   Cf. U. LUZ, *Matthäus* II, 209: "Es ist also 'der Vater', der das Gegenüber 'des Sohns' rhetorisch – und nicht religionsgeschichtlich – fordert."
[2]   Cf. DEUTSCH, *Hidden Wisdom*, 33f.
[3]   LINDBLOM, *Jesu missions- och dopbefallning*, 74–77; M. MÜLLER, *"Menschensohn,"* 121, deny that 11:27 relates to 28:18 since there is a difference in what is given to Jesus. But they do not discuss the formal similarities between the two verses.
[4]   BOCHEŃSKI, *Was ist Autorität?*, 17–21, stresses that authority has aspects of both quality ("Eigenschaft") and relationship ("Beziehung"). It is "Status in Beziehung" (*ibid.*, 17f).
[5]   Cf. KINGSBURY, *Matthew as Story*, 125.
[6]   Mark 1:22 did not originally contain αὐτῶν.
[7]   Cf. FRANCE, *Matthew: Evangelist and Teacher*, 139f.
[8]   HUBBARD, *Matthean Redaction*, 84.
[9]   Cf. HARTMAN, *Till Herrens Jesu namn*, 120–124.

given all exousia is it possible to extend the mission to all the nations. In 10:1 the disciples are given exousia to perform therapeutic actions. Of course, this does not mean that they are expected to perform miracles independent of Jesus. But there is a difference in comparison with the didactic exousia. Although Jesus extends his teaching authority to Peter and the other disciples, he never says explicitly that he gives them the exousia to teach. In regard to their teaching activity, the exousia remains exclusively bound to Jesus' person. Jesus is in 28:19f the risen one, always to be with the disciples. And the teaching of the disciples represents a direct manifestation of Jesus' own exousia.[1] Since the commission opens up the narrative to the situation of Matthew himself, it seems that Jesus' didactic exousia, now integrated within a cosmic perspective, continued to manifest itself in the teaching activities of the Christian community. *The attribution of a didactic exousia to Jesus' person defined the identity and activity of the transmitting teachers in the Matthean community. They were the ones continuing to manifest Jesus' didactic exousia in their own teaching activities.*

4.3. The Didactic Designations

Certain didactic designations accentuate further the didactic exousia attributed to Jesus. There are both negative and positive designations. The negative labelling establishes what Jesus as teacher is not and the positive labelling centres on Jesus' validated teaching authority.

4.3.1. The Negative Didactic Designation

The term ῥαββί occurs four times in Matthew: 23:7 concerns the scribes' and the Pharisees' desire to be called in this manner; 23:8 exhorts the disciples not to use the term for themselves; 26:25, 49 give it in Judas' address to Jesus. The other synoptics parallel the presence of the term only once (Matt 26:49/Mark 14:45).

> The term exhibits certain similarities with the other gospel narratives. There are especially two constant features. First, it is a term mostly *reserved for Jesus*. From a total of eleven occurrences of ῥαββί in the NT outside of Matthew,[2] it refers to Jesus ten times.[3] Only John 3:26 uses it for John the Baptist. The related, but probably intensified, form ῥαββουνί occurs twice, both times referring to Jesus (Mark 10:51, John 20:16). Second, the whole gospel tradition is unanimous in using ῥαββί/ῥαββουνί as an *address*. The terms never appear in third person accounts about Jesus. The evangelists never say "Rabbi Jesus." In view of the frequent use of such a manner of speaking in the rabbinic literature, this silence in the gospels is noteworthy. Jesus' identity goes beyond rabbinic categories. The terms do not function as confessional labels im-

---

[1] Cf. TRILLING, *Israel*, 25.
[2] It is not used outside of the gospel narratives.
[3] Mark 9:5; 11:21; 14:45; John 1:38, 49; 3:2; 4:31; 6:25; 9:2; 11:8.

plying christological views.[1] These two general aspects of ῥαββί/ῥαββουνί are not substantially different in Matthew.

The synoptic tradition on which Matthew builds to a large extent gives both ῥαββί/ῥαββουνί and διδάσκαλος a similar didactic connotation. They not only appear together without high christological significance[2] in John 1:38; 20:16,[3] but the didactic use of ῥαββί/ῥαββουνί is present also in Mark.[4] To be sure, although Mark often uses διδάσκαλος for Jesus,[5] none of the instances using ῥαββί/ῥαββουνί gives a direct Greek translation with διδάσκαλος. B.T. Viviano accordingly suggests that ῥαββί/ῥαββουνί carries no didactic connotation in Mark but is roughly equivalent to κύριος—a use found in Aramaic texts from Qumran and in the targumic translations of Genesis in Targum Onqelos and Targum Neofiti I.[6] Viviano takes this feature in Mark as an explanation why Matthew sometimes replaced the Markan ῥαββί/ῥαββουνί with κύριε.[7] However, although Viviano's suggestion is philologically possible, none of the four Markan instances using ῥαββί/ῥαββουνί exhibit any direct relation to κύριος. And where κύριε elsewhere occurs as an address to Jesus (7:28), the possessive pronoun μου is not present. It would be natural sometimes to find κύριε μου, had the term been closely related to the non-technical ῥαββί/ῥαββουνί in Mark. Nor is there a possessive pronoun on other occasions having additional forms of κύριος in reference to Jesus (5:19; 11:3).[8] In addition, with the possible exception of 10:51, the use of ῥαββί/ῥαββουνί does not reveal a confessional attitude of the speaker. In spite of the fact that ῥαββί/ῥαββουνί is never directly related to forms of διδάσκαλος, it is indeed probable that these terms serve primarily to characterize Jesus as teacher in Mark.[9]

Matthew breaks the semantic equating of ῥαββί/ῥαββουνί and διδάσκαλος. The readers/hearers encounter ῥαββί for the first time in 23:7.[10] It is the designation by which the scribes and the Pharisees love to be saluted. In 23:8 Jesus exhorts the disciples not to act like the scribes and the Pharisees and call themselves ῥαββί. Jesus uses ῥαββί in the negative statement and

---

[1]   Cf. FRÖVIG, *Das Selbstbewusstsein Jesu,* 16f, 43f; DODD, Teacher and Prophet, 53; LOHSE, *TDNT* VI, 965; RIESNER, *Lehrer,* 253f.

[2]   Cf. R.E. BROWN, *John,* 75, 77f, 1010.—BEASLEY-MURRAY, *John,* 375, states that in John 20:16 the didactic term expresses Mary's deep veneration of Jesus. This is true in a sense (cf. OLSSON, *Structure,* 220f). But when Mary subsequently tells the disciples about Jesus, she says instead that she has seen τὸν κύριον (20:18).

[3]   Cf. also John 3:2.

[4]   9:5; 10:51; 11:21; 14:45. Luke does not use ῥαββί/ῥαββουνί.

[5]   Mark 4:38; 5:35; 9:17, 38; 10:17, 20, 35; 12:14, 19, 32; 13:1; 14:14.

[6]   *RB* 97 (1990) 207–218. Cf. also LAPIN, *ABD* 5 (1992) 601.

[7]   Mark 9:5/Matt 17:4; Mark 10:51/Matt 20:33 (cf. 9:28).

[8]   Cf. also 2:28; 12:37. Forms of κύριος is also used metaphorically (12:9; 13:35) and in OT quotations (1:3; 11:9; 12:11, 29f; 12:36). Mark 13:20 alludes to God.

[9]   Cf. MEYE, *Jesus and the Twelve,* 36.

[10]   The use of μέγας in 5:19b is hardly a play on the literal meaning of רבי, as GUNDRY, *Matthew,* 82, suggests. Such a play would go against the exhortation in 23:8–10. And furthermore, to what would then ἐλάχιστος in 5:19a correspond?

διδάσκαλος in the positive. The reason for the change is not necessarily that ῥαββί means "my teacher."[1] As is evident from the parallel statement in 23:10, using the same didactic term both times, ῥαββί and διδάσκαλος correspond to each other, though with different connotations. Most likely, Jesus avoids ῥαββί in 23:8b because it is located in a self-referential phrase.[2] The Matthean Jesus does not think of himself as ῥαββί. Instead he prefers διδάσκαλος.[3]

26:25, 49 consequently use ῥαββί negatively. No other character than Judas uses the term to address Jesus in Matthew. This restriction is present in Matthew only. Judas is a flat character in the Matthean story. True, as is evident especially from 27:3–10,[4] Matthew has special interest in Judas' feeling of remorse and suicide. But his root trait is determined by the constant references to him as the betrayer.[5] Judas' question in 26:25 parallels the disciples' question in 26:22, with the significant difference that Judas uses ῥαββί and the disciples κύριε. And Jesus' extended answer to the disciples' question in 26:23f is in sharp contrast to his abrupt σὺ εἶπας in 26:25. Also 26:49 carries negative connotation in its use of ῥαββί. Judas greets Jesus with ῥαββί. He thus greets Jesus exactly as the ordinary Jewish teachers prefer to be saluted (23:7). He regards Jesus as one among many Jewish teachers. Jesus' response in 26:50 is consequently negative. It is as brief and abrupt as the one in 26:25, and the term ἑταῖρε, by which Jesus addresses Judas, has already acquired derogatory connotations in Matthew.[6] The readers/hearers have confronted it twice (20:13; 22:12), and each time the relationship between the speaker and the one addressed has been scorned by the latter.

Matthew's distinction between ῥαββί and διδάσκαλος probably depends on the emerging official and titular connotations attached to רבי in Judaism.[7] H. Shanks' and S. Zeitlin's controversy about the early pre-70 use

---

[1] *Contra* RIESNER, *Lehrer,* 271; ZIMMERMANN, *Die urchristlichen Lehrer,* 172f.

[2] Since Matthew uses διδάσκαλος, which elsewhere always refers to Jesus, it is unlikely that 23:8b refers to God as teacher, as claimed by e.g. LÉGASSE, *RB* 68 (1961) 335 n. 58; PATTE, *Matthew,* 322. For its possible reference to God on a pre-Matthean level, cf. SCHNIEWIND, *Matthäus,* 228; BARBOUR, *ExpTim* 82 (1970–71) 140; Joachim JEREMIAS, *Neutestamentliche Theologie,* 166 n. 6; BULTMANN, *Geschichte der synoptischen Tradition,* 154; DERRETT, *Bib* 62 (1981) 377; SCHWEIZER, *Matthäus,* 281.

[3] Cf. FRANKEMÖLLE, *Jahwebund,* 99f; LAPIN, *ABD* 5 (1992) 601.

[4] For literature, see GARLAND, *Study on the Passion Narratives,* 109f. Cf. also VOGLER, *Judas Iskarioth,* 65–70; MATERA, *Passion Narratives,* 105–107; KLAUCK, *Judas,* 92–101; FORNBERG, *Jewish-Christian Dialogue,* 21; LIMBECK, *Matthäus-Evangelium,* 287–293; VAN TILBORG, Matthew 27.3–10, 159–174; MACCOBY, *Judas Iscariot,* 44–49.

[5] 10:4; 26:25, 46, 48; 27:3.

[6] For different interpretations of ἐφ' ὃ πάρει, see the proposals listed by SENIOR, *Passion Narrative,* 125f, VOGLER, *Judas Iskarioth,* 64f; GNILKA, *Matthäusevangelium* II, 418.

[7] Cf. W.D. DAVIES, *Setting of the Sermon on the Mount,* 297f; OVERMAN, *Matthew's Gospel,* 44–48.

of רבי as a title has been taken up and developed in more recent years.[1] In dependence on G. Dalman's early observations,[2] R. Riesner and A.F. Zimmermann point to the distinction between a use of the term as a reverential appellation, where the pronominal meaning of the suffix carries its full significance, and as a proper title.[3] The former existed already before 70 and is the one reflected in the synoptic gospel narratives. The latter is a post-70 development. This distinction reflects accurately the evidence available from outside of the NT. There is no pre-70 testimony of רבי as a title, neither in writings nor in epigraphical material.[4] The rabbinic literature suggests that the title became prominent only during the first generation of tannas.[5] But it remains questionable if Matthew reflects the non-titular use. 23:7 suggests an employment of ῥαββί as a title. Jesus accuses the scribes and the Pharisees of loving to be called ῥαββί by the people. A nontechnical use implies a close relationship between master and pupil and cannot serve to describe a general custom performed by the people in general. Moreover, in 23:8 ῥαββί occurs in the singular, in spite of the fact that Jesus addresses several persons and uses the plural (καθηγηταί) in the corresponding phrase in 23:10a.[6]

As it seems, ῥαββί functions as a negative titular label in Matthew. It sets Jesus apart from other Jewish teachers claiming the official Jewish title. Matthew validates Jesus negatively, as not being a rabbi in any sense.[7]

4.3.2. The Positive Didactic Designation

Matthew uses καθηγητής as a positive designation directly connected with the portrayal of Jesus as teacher. It occurs twice in 23:10—once in the negative exhortation to the disciples and once in the reference to Christ's unique position as teacher.[8] In spite of the parallel structure of 23:8–10, 23:10 does not repeat the didactic terminology of 23:8. The term is not attested elsewhere in the NT. In addition, it occurs on the lips of Jesus, the normative character of the story, in a unit intended as a deliberative exhortation. It is

---

1 Cf. above p. 94.
2 *Worte Jesu,* 272–280.
3 RIESNER, *Lehrer,* 266–276; ZIMMERMANN, *Die urchristlichen Lehrer,* 72–75, 86–91.
4 Cf. COHEN, *JQR* 72 (1981) 1–17.
5 See above pp. 95.
6 Cf. HAENCHEN, Matthäus 23, 140.
7 *Contra* MARQUET, *Christus* 30 (1983), 94, who claims that Jesus appears in Matthew as "un rabbin d'un genre particulier."
8 There is no external evidence indicating that 23:10 is a later interpolation, as claimed by WELLHAUSEN, *Matthaei,* 117. Cf. also ZEITLIN, *JQR* 53 (1962–63) 346. In that case, we would also expect to find it quoted among early Christian authors. But neither MASSAUX, *Influence de l'Évangile de Saint Matthieu,* 673, nor W.-D. KÖHLER, *Rezeption des Matthäusevangeliums,* 562, list any such use of 23:10.—The alternative word order εἰς γάρ ἐστιν ὑμῶν ὁ καθηγητής is probably a secondary attempt to create an exact parallel to 23:8b, 9b.

therefore a decisive interpretative element in Matthew.

The term is present in extra-biblical Greek literature, inscriptions and papyri.[1] Generally speaking, it designates a guide or a leader of some kind.[2] C. Spicq has discussed most of the relevant material.[3] J. Gluckner and B.W. Winter supplement Spicq's investigations.[4] The term often refers to teachers during the first centuries C.E. The Epicurean philosopher Philodemus of Gadara (c. 110–28 B.C.E.) gives perhaps the clearest—though somewhat early—evidence. On several occasions he uses the term for persons active within some kind of didactic setting.[5] Papyri from the first and second centuries C.E. point in the same direction.[6] Gluckner and Winter suggest that the term often connotes a private tutor who teaches for a fee at various levels, but without close attachment to official or permanent establishments.[7] It carries also connotations of honour. In Alex. 5:4 Plutarch (c. 50–120 C.E.) says that while young Alexander was appointed many nurturers, disciplinarians and teachers (τροφεῖς καὶ παιδαγωγοὶ καὶ διδάσκαλοι), Leonidas was called τροφεὺς Ἀλεξάνδρου καὶ καθηγητής because of his dignity and prominent family relationship. It sometimes refers even to prominent philosophers acting as teachers of individuals. Already Dionysius of Halicarnassus (c. 30 B.C.E.) speaks in Th. 3 of Plato as the καθηγητής of Aristotle.[8] And in Quom. Adul. 70E Plutarch mentions Ammonius, a philosopher residing in Athens, as his own καθηγητής. In Alex. Fort. Virt. 327E he also speaks with great respect of Aristotle as the καθηγητής of Alexander.[9] Herode's inscription to Secundus recorded in *SEG* XXIII, 115 speaks of the rhetor as (τὸν ἑαυτο(ῦ φίλον) ... (κα)θηγητ(ήν). While dated to about 150 C.E., it implies similar connotations of honour.[10]

The available material gives us no reason to assume that the term is related to a Semitic equivalent in Matt 23:10. No known text uses καθηγητής on the basis of a corresponding Semitic term. It does not occur in any of the Greek-Jewish writings. 2 Macc

---

[1] For references, see PREISGKE, *Papyrusurkunden* I, 713; LSJ, 852; KIESSLING (ed.), *Papyrusurkunden* suppl. I, 132; W. BAUER, *Wörterbuch*, 789. The material in the *Thesaurus Linguae Graecae* computer database does not significantly alter the general impression.

[2] LSJ, 852; SPICQ, *Lexicographie* I, 389.

[3] *RB* 66 (1959) 390–393; *idem, Lexicographie* I, 389–391.

[4] GLUCKER, *Antiochus*, 127–134; WINTER, *TynBul* 42 (1991) 152–157.—Only Gluckner adds a few references not noted by Spicq. WINTER, *ibid*, 152 n. 4, claims that Spicq did not examine P. Oxy. 2190. This is wrong. See SPICQ, *Lexicographie* I, 390.

[5] Ir. 19:14; Περὶ παρρησίας 31:11; 45:5; 52:6f; 80:2f, etc.

[6] Cf. e.g. P. Oxy. 930:6, 20 (a letter to Ptolemaeus from his mother, dated to the 2nd or 3rd cent. C.E.); P. Oxy. 2190:7f, 15, 24, 26, 31 (a letter to Theon, dated to late 1st cent. C.E.).

[7] GLUCKER, *Antiochus*, 127–134; WINTER, *TynBul* 42 (1991) 152–157.

[8] Cf. also 1 Amm. 5, where Dionysius speaks of Aristotle as καθηγούμενος Ἀλεξάνδρου.

[9] Thes. 18:2 even speaks about the god at Delphi commanding Theseus to make Aphrodite his καθηγεμόνα.

[10] Cf. also *SEG* XXIII, 117 (τὸν ἑαυτ[οῦ κα]θηγη[τήν ...]). SPICQ, *Lexicograpie* I, 390f, mentions other funeral inscriptions made by pupils in honor of their καθηγητής.

10:28 uses καθηγεμών in a metaphorical sense, and Bell. 3:497 uses καθηγεῖσθαι to denote a leading military action. But even these texts have no Semitic basis.[1] It is therefore striking that scholars continue to postulate a Semitic term for an earlier stage of the tradition in Matt 23:10. The proposals abound,[2] מורה being the most common.[3] Certainly, מורה is frequent in the Dead Sea scrolls. But the scrolls do not reveal any Greek rendering of it. It did not even become a prominent didactic designation in the first centuries C.E.[4] The decisive argument against the proposal is that the LXX never translates מורה with καθηγητής.[5] If מורה were the original behind καθηγητής in Matt 23:10, we would expect such a correspondence to exist also in the LXX, especially since scholars often refer to OT texts containing מורה as influential for this background.[6] It is at least as probable, as already Dalman believed,[7] that καθηγητής carries no Semitic connotation in Matthew. The artificiality of Dalman's hypothesis is for some reason obvious to J.D.M. Derrett.[8] But the question is if it is not more artificial to postulate that "some semitic term has been rendered in this way"[9] without the possibility of any justification.

The use of καθηγητής implies that Matthew labels Jesus as a teacher of a higher dignity than the ordinary διδάσκαλος.[10] This honorary label qualifies in its context Jesus in two ways. First, it suggests that Jesus the teacher provides his disciples with more than mere information. He is also their guide and leader,[11] which even goes beyond his function as a moral example.[12] Teacher and teaching become inseparable. There are blind leaders (ὁδηγοὶ τυφλοί) in Matthew,[13] represented in the same chapter by the scribes and the Pharisees (23:16, 24).[14] In distinction to these blind leaders, Jesus as teacher the only legitimate leader. Second, the personal and pri-

---

[1] The attempt by SCHLATTER, *Matthäus*, 671, to relate καθηγεῖσθαι in Bell. 3:497 to מנהיג is purely conjectural.

[2] For different proposals, see SAGGIN, *VD* 30 (1952) 211f; SPICQ, *RB* 66 (1959) 392.

[3] So even SPICQ, *RB* 66 (1959) 392; *idem, Lexicographie* I, 391. Cf. more recently e.g. RIESNER, *Lehrer*, 263; ZIMMERMANN, *Die urchristlichen Lehrer*, 163; VIVIANO, *JSNT* 39 (1990) 13.

[4] DALMAN, *Worte Jesu*, 276; G. JEREMIAS, *Lehrer der Gerechtigkeit*, 316.

[5] Cf. GLUCKER, *Antiochus*, 425, though in his subsequent treatment of Matt 23:2–12 (*ibid.*, 426–448), he overestimates the positive significance of ῥαββί and neglects the unique features of Jesus as teacher in Matthew.

[6] SPICQ, *RB* 66 (1959) 392; *idem, Lexicographie* I, 391, mentions Isa 30:20; Joel 2:23; Hab 2:18; Prov 5:13; Job 36:22.

[7] *Worte Jesu*, 276, 279. Cf. more recently e.g. HOET, *"Omnes autem vos fratres estis,"* 15f, 19, 134; GNILKA, *Matthäusevangelium* II, 272 n. 10.

[8] *Bib* 62 (1981) 380f n. 44.

[9] DERRETT, *Bib* 62 (1981) 381 n. 44.

[10] Cf. GNILKA, *Matthäusevangelium* II, 277.—ZAHN, *Matthäus*, 650, mentions a similar connotation of καθηγητής, but he is more interested in finding the Semitic equivalent.

[11] G. MAIER, *Matthäus-Evangelium* II, 242f, overestimates this observation and sees an allusion to church leaders.

[12] Cf. SAGGIN, *VD* 30 (1952) 212.

[13] Cf. Jesus' description of the Pharisees in 15:14.

[14] Cf. W. MICHAELIS, *TDNT* V, 99.

vate aspects of καθηγητής are present in Matthew.[1] The group of disciples is according to 23:8f a brotherhood with one heavenly Father. Within this intimate setting, Jesus is not a teacher validated by means of official and institutional titles. While his didactic exousia is universal, he functions as the personal teacher of his disciples.

Thus, καθηγητής functions in Matthew as a positive label acknowledging Jesus the teacher as the personal guide and leader of the disciples. It reflects part of Matthew's own didactic validation of Jesus. He was for Matthew more than an ordinary teacher. *Jesus was as teacher also Matthew's personal guide and leader.* This validation defined further the identity and activity of the group of transmitters to which Matthew belonged. There was to them no other teacher with normative status. *Jesus was the only normative teacher in a quantitative sense.* Matthew was part of an intimate circle—a brotherhood—finding its identity in Jesus' exclusive teaching authority. The labelling process therefore set up certain limits to any authoritative pretensions from teachers inside and outside of the group. This must have meant that the teaching of other persons became subordinated to what the only normative teacher had said and done. *Jesus' exclusive status as teacher motivated a focus on what was believed to represent his words and his deeds only.*

4.4. The Didactic Christology

The expression "didactic christology" denotes here the positive assessment of Jesus' role and status in terms of existing Jewish categories for teachers and teaching. The didactic exousia and designations define and acknowledge Jesus' role and status as teacher. But they do not reveal exactly to what didactic category the role and status amount. It is necessary to ask about broader patterns into which Matthew integrates the didactic exousia and designations.

L.E. Keck points out that the scholarly preoccupation with the christological titles is inappropriate for understanding Jesus' interpreted identity and significance.[2] This is true also of Matthew.[3] Since Jesus identifies himself as messianic teacher in 23:10, it would indeed be tempting to interpret his didactic activity from the Jewish expectation—though not very prominent—that the Messiah would appear as a teacher at the end-time.[4] But the messianic appellation appears also elsewhere in Matthew—fifteen or sixteen times.[5] And the context does not, in these cases, provide a didactic conno-

---

1   Cf. WINTER, *TynBul* 42 (1991) 157.
2   *NTS* 32 (1986) 368–370.
3   For the limited importance of the appellations related to the mighty acts of Jesus in Matthew, see GERHARDSSON, *Mighty Acts,* 82, 91f.
4   For the Jewish expectation of Messiah as (wisdom) teacher, see RIESNER, *Lehrer,* 304–330.
5   Only some MSS of 16:21 include the term.

tation.[1] Kingsbury claims that Jesus accomplishes the teaching ministry as Son of God and with divine authority.[2] But in order to establish the priority of the Son of God designation, Kingsbury frequently minimizes the importance of other appellations by reference to indications in the narrative, such as the depiction of the audience. As it seems, christology pervades the whole story. The narrative itself provides the basic interpretative key to the christological appellations.[3]

4.4.1. The Teaching as Commandments

Matthew often uses the term ἐντολαί, "commandments," to denote the statutes given by God in the Torah.[4] When the Torah is viewed as a collective entity, νόμος is used.[5] The former term often occurs in didactic contexts. There is a consistent connection between ἐντολή and units depicting Jesus as teacher (19:17; 22:36, 38, 40) or the opponents' teaching activity (15:3–9). The commandments constitute the normative basis of teaching about legal matters.[6]

Matthew regards some of Jesus' teaching as commandments. The use of both ἐντέλλεσθαι and τηρεῖν in 28:20 makes it likely that Matthew not always uses the former in a general manner merely.[7] It points to Jesus' teaching as commandments.[8] These should be the basis of the disciples' teaching—an understanding that Ignatius apparently shared (Eph. 9:2; Rom. *inscr.*).[9]

It is therefore conceivable that the expression "one of the least of these commandments" (μίαν τῶν ἐντολῶν τούτων ἐλαχίστων), which the future teachers according to 5:19 are not to set aside, refers to some of Jesus' teaching. We have already noticed the similarities between 5:19 and 28:19f.[10] And E. Baasland has pointed out the weakness of certain arguments normally used for interpreting the expression as referring to the Mosaic commandments.[11] There are also features in the expression which speak posi-

---

1 KINGSBURY, *Matthew: Structure, Christology, Kingdom*, 96–99.
2 *Matthew: Structure, Christology, Kingdom*, 60f.
3 Cf. U. LUZ, Christologie, 223, 235.
4 15:3; 19:17; 22:36, 38, 40.
5 5:17f; 7:12; 11:13; 12:5; 22:36, 40; 23:23. Cf. also 15:6 (א*, b, C, etc.).
6 BAASLAND, *TTK* 1 (1983) 7, suggests that ἐντολή is a polemical concept and limited to the Decalogue (15:3f; 19:17–19a) and the love commandment (19:19b; 22:36–40). But this is hardly a consistent pattern. 19:17 is not evidently polemical and 19:7 introduces also the commandment from Deut 24:1—outside of the Decalogue—with Moses "commanded" (ἐνετείλατο), not, with Moses "says," as Baasland claims.
7 The verb is used in 4:6; 17:9; 19:7; 28:20. Cf. also 15:4 (א*, b, C, etc.).
8 Cf. also 19:17 (τήρησον τὰς ἐντολάς).
9 Cf. also Phld. 1:2.—Rom. 3:1 refers to the Christian activity of teaching (διδάσκειν) and making disciples (μαθητεύειν) in connection with giving commandments (ἐντέλλεσθαι).
10 See above pp. 209, 258.
11 *TTK* 1 (1983) 1–12. Baasland himself cautiously favours the interpretation which relates the commandments closely to Jesus' teaching.

tively in favour of understanding "these commandments" as referring to some of Jesus' teaching.[1]

It is of importance that Jesus qualifies the commandments as "the least."[2] The term ἐλάχιστος refers in two out of three cases elsewhere in Matthew to the disciples (25:40, 45),[3] just as μικρός often has a similar reference (10:42; 18:6, 10, 14).[4] In 5:19aα Jesus speaks of the commandments and not the disciples as "the least." But why does he add the qualification at all? 5:18 gives no justification. Jesus mentions there small items of the Torah merely. One iota or one stroke of a letter cannot constitute a commandment. And it would indeed be suprising to find the Matthean Jesus claiming with no further comments that the one who practises and teaches the Mosaic commandments will be called great in the kingdom of heaven. If Matthew's use of ἐλάχιστος elsewhere is of some importance for understanding 5:19, "the least of these commandments" must connote the commandments which the disciples are to practise when they teach others. And 28:19f states that they should teach the nations to keep what Jesus himself has commanded.

Since ἐλάχιστος carries a derogatory connotation in 5:19aβ,[5] it is probable that Jesus ironically refers to certain commandments disregarded by the opponents.[6] This is perhaps an independent application of the rabbinic discussion about certain commandments of greater (מצות חמורות) and lesser (מצות קלות) importance, reflected in 23:23.[7] 11:28–30 supplies the ironic connotation with further aspects. While the rabbinic view is that the yoke represents the kingdom of heaven and the commandments (m. Ber. 2:2),[8] in Matthew the yoke is the teaching of Jesus himself. When Jesus' teaching— the kingdom and the commandments in one event—is viewed from the standpoint of the opponents, it is of the least importance. It does not burden the people but is easy and light.[9] The ironical hint in 5:19 also makes the connection to 5:20 (γάρ) understandable.[10] The righteousness exceeding

---

[1]   H.D. BETZ, *Sermon on the Mount,* 46–51, also regards 5:19 as referring to Jesus' commandments, but in line with his form-critical view of the Sermon, he restricts the perspective to the Sermon itself only.

[2]   Cf. LOHMEYER, *Matthäus,* 111; BANKS, *JBL* 93 (1974) 238–240; *idem, Jesus and the Law,* 222f; RIESNER, *Lehrer,* 458f.

[3]   It occurs also in 2:6.—The criticism by SCHWEIZER, Matthew's Church, 138f, against interpreting 25:40, 45 as referring to the disciples is not convincing. See J. FRIEDRICH, *Gott im Bruder?,* 239–249.

[4]   Cf. also 11:11 and the discussion by G. BARTH, Law, 121–125. Cf. already O. MICHEL, *TSK* 108 (1937–38) 401–415, though his discussion is primarily aimed towards an understanding of Jesus himself.

[5]   BAASLAND, *TTK* 1 (1983) 6.

[6]   Cf. H.D. BETZ, *Sermon on the Mount,* 49f.

[7]   This influence is denied by BAASLAND, *TTK* 1 (1983) 5.

[8]   Cf. accepting the נזירות in Mek. on 20:3 (Lauterbach II, 238:8–10).

[9]   Cf. also 23:4.—The ὅτι in 11:29b marks the reason, not the object, of learning. The emphasis is on the source rather than the content of learning.

[10]   BAASLAND, *TTK* 1 (1983), 2–4, shows that the argument of 5:19 relates primarily to 5:16 and 5:20, not 5:17f.

that of the scribes and the Pharisees is the one that adheres to and practises also the disregarded exposition of the Torah contained in some of Jesus' teaching. If the disciples fail in this regard, they will be called neither least nor great in the kingdom of heaven, they will not enter it at all. 5:19 emphasizes ironically that this kind of teaching is not to be set aside. It is the norm for all practice and further teaching.[1]

There exists of course a certain kind of connection between the smallest items of the Torah in 5:18 and "the least of these commandments."[2] But the connection does not, as I just stated, imply that the latter is merely identical with the former. The demonstrative pronoun—"*these* commandments"—requires no such understanding.[3] The pronoun qualifies Jesus' words in a general manner also in 7:24, 26, without precise indication of the referent. A similar use is present elsewhere in Matthew (24:14; 26:13). 24:35 may indicate a different kind of identification. The verse is strongly reminiscent of 5:18. The main difference is that it is the words of Jesus, not one iota or one stroke of a letter, that remain. 7:24, 26 identify Jesus' teaching with his words. And the possibility of a parallel significance of Jesus' words and Jesus' commandments emerges from the parallel between God's word and God's commandment in 15:3, 6.[4] The implication would be that "these commandments" are actually the words of Jesus contained in the Sermon on the Mount, most likely in the Antitheses, to be more precise. The smallest items of the Torah will indeed not pass away as long as heaven and earth remain. Even the smallest little sign in the Torah prevails in Jesus' teaching, which will continue to manifest itself in the future mission of the disciples.[5]

Matthew thus portrays some of Jesus' teaching as commandments. Although the opponents regard them as of little importance, the disciples are to use them as the prevailing basis for practising and teaching the Torah. Just as the Johannine literature refers both to keeping (τηρεῖν) Jesus' commandments (John 14:15, 21; 15:10; 1 John 2:3f) and to keeping (τηρεῖν,

---

[1] m.ʾAbot 4:20 expresses the view that learning is not to be acquired from the small ones (הקטנים). Although the term refers to young persons and does not, like μικρός in Matt 10:42; 18:6, 10, 14, illustrate meekness, this view might give a further ironical connotation. As it seems, y. Moʿed Qaṭ. 82d indicates a similar view, and here the small ones (הקטנים, זעירייא) might represent certain unimportant teachers.

[2] This is denied by BAASLAND, *TTK* 1 (1983) 5f. But cf. e.g. LJUNGMAN, *Das Gesetz erfüllen*, 48f; GUELICH, *"Not to Annul the Law,"* 248–250; MEIER, *Law and History*, 91f, though they overestimate the importance of τούτων.

[3] G. BARTH, *Law*, 66 n. 2, thinks that the general reference of the demonstrative pronoun is a semitism. It is difficult to be sure.

[4] For λόγον as the original reading in 15:6, see METZGER, *Textual Commentary*, 39.

[5] R.F. COLLINS, *Matthew's ἐντολαί*, 1344–1347, understands "the least of these commandments" as those other commandments which are pale in insignificance beside the twofold great commandment in 22:34–40. While I regard the Antitheses themselves as commandments, Collins regards them as examples of Jesus' teaching on the commandments of the Torah. He does not, in my opinion, pay sufficient attention to the similarities between 5:19 and 28:20 and to Matthew's use of ἐλάχιστος.

ποιεῖν) God's commandments (1 John 3:22, 24; 5:2f), Matthew also gives Jesus' teaching the highest possible status. It equals the word of God.

4.4.2. The Authoritative ἐγώ

We already touched on the Antitheses.[1] The ἐγώ of Jesus in 5:21–48 is the ἐγώ of a teacher. The didactic setting emerges clearly in the frames of the Sermon (5:1f, 7:28f). If my understanding of 5:19 and its immediate context is correct, it is reasonable to ask if the ἐγώ of Jesus in the sixfold antithetical construction (5:21f, 27f; 31f, 33f, 38f, 43f) also corresponds to a status equalling divine authority.

Scholars have often claimed that the antithetical construction reflects certain patterns in the rabbinic literature. These assumptions go back on observations made by S. Schechter, M. Smith and D. Daube.[2] Only Smith draws (non-)christological conclusions. But if their proposals are correct, we may be inclined to understand the teacher of the Antitheses in terms of an authoritative rabbi merely.

Schechter proposed that the formula תלמוד לומר ... אני שומע in Mekilta explains the construction in Matthew. The rabbinic expression suggests, according to Schechter, that the words of Scripture at the first glance might be conceived of as having a particular meaning, but when the context or the wording of the sentences are considered a different meaning emerges. The Matthean Jesus warns the disciples that they might hear the literal sense of the OT too closely. There is a teaching saying (תלמוד לומר) that the words must not be taken in such a sense. Since the formula was a strictly rabbinic idiom, it was not accurately translated into Greek.

Smith paid attention to certain tannaitic parallels to the counterdemand.[3] The expression ἐγὼ δὲ λέγω is, according to Smith, parallel to ואני אומר which introduces a contradictory halakhic opinion in some rabbinic writings. It is not possible, Smith argues, to find evidence for the peculiarity of Jesus in the antithetical construction. Jesus is here merely one among many self-confident rabbis.

Daube developed Schechter's proposal. The thesis of the antithetical construction corresponds to the rabbinic שומע אני which introduces a false interpretation of Scripture. As for the counterdemand, Daube saw the nearest rabbinic equivalent in the use of אמרת. Rabbinic writings use it to refute a false interpretation by reference to another text from Scripture or by logical deduction. Since the formula was well established in the first half of the second century C.E., it must be considerably older and may in an earlier and slightly different variant have served as the source of Matthew's pattern.

The parallels from the rabbinic literature are, however, only remotely relevant for understanding Matthew.[4] The Matthean formula is different

---

[1] LAPIDE, *Bergpredigt,* 49, prefers to call the Antitheses "Superthesen." Because of convention, I will speak of "Antithesis/Antitheses" when a complete unit or 5:21–48 as a whole is meant, and of "thesis" and "counterdemand" when the different parts of the antithetical construction, which is part of each Antithesis, is under consideration.

[2] SCHECHTER, *JQR* 10 (1897–98) 11 n. 3; *idem, JQR* 12 (1899–1900) 427f; M. SMITH, *Tannaitic Parallels,* 27–30; DAUBE, *New Testament,* 55–62.

[3] Cf. already DALMAN, *Jesus-Jeschua,* 68.

[4] For discussion of the rabbinic parallels, see BACHER, *Die exegetische Termino-*

from all the rabbinic constructions referred to. Schechter and Daube tried to account for both parts of the Matthean formula. But nowhere do the parallels contain all the elements present in Matthew. In particular, the first person singular with the emphatic ἐγώ, so important in Matthew, does not appear in conjunction with אמר. Rather, it occurs together with שמע. Nor does ἐρρέθη have a counterpart in the alleged parallels. Smith deals with the counterdemand only. To be sure, ואני אומר is in itself formally close to ἐγὼ δὲ λέγω. But it does not suffice to isolate one part of the construction in the search for parallels.[1] Both elements must be viewed together. Smith does not give any example of ואני אומר together with שמע as its counterpart. In addition to formal differences, the declaratory character of Jesus' speech sets it apart from strictly scholarly discussions about the interpretation of Scripture.

Jesus' didactic ἐγώ cannot, therefore, be reduced to reflect the authority of a prominent rabbi merely. The rabbinic parallels might have interacted with the Matthean construction.[2] But the evident differences imply that the formula is at the end an independent creation which should be read/heard within the context of the Matthean narrative itself.

The christological significance of ἐγώ is thus an integrated part of the Matthean formula and as such related to its corresponding expression in the thesis. The structure shows that the focal point of the two parts occurs in the two verbs of saying:

ἠκούσατε ὅτι   ἐρρέθη   τοῖς ἀρχαίοις
              ἐγὼ δὲ λέγω   ὑμῖν.

The term ἐρρέθη is central in the thesis. It is the only element recurring in all the six Antitheses.[3] In addition, Matthew often uses it elsewhere in the participial form. Its importance is especially evident in the introduction to ten of the eleven formula quotations,[4] but also in 3:3; 22:31; 24:15 as com-

---

logie I, 190 n. 2; MCCONNEL, *Law and Prophecy*, 41f; LOHSE, "Ich aber sage euch," 191–196; SUGGS, *Wisdom*, 111f; HOWARD, *Ego*, 189–191; MEIER, *Law and History*, 133f n. 21; HÜBNER, *Gesetz*, 231–236.—SUGGS, Antitheses, 442, has withdrawn his complete rejection of the parallels.

1   GUELICH, *NTS* 22 (1975–76) 455; *idem, Sermon on the Mount*, 185.

2   Schechter, Smith and Daube did not discuss who created the Matthean formula. The dominant opinion when Smith and Daube published their studies was that of BULTMANN, *Geschichte der synoptischen Tradition*, 142–144, according to whom the pattern was inherited from the tradition and then elaborated. Today this is an open matter. Cf. the different views of BROER, *BZ* 19 (1975) 50–63; SUGGS, Antitheses, 433–444; GUELICH, *NTS* (1975–76) 444–457; STRECKER, *ZNW* 69 (1978) 36–72; KOSCH, *Tora*, 258–275. I will discuss this further below pp. 391–395.

3   From a formal point of view, it is difficult to regard the second and third Antitheses as one.

4   1:22, 2:15, 17, 23; 4:14; 8:17; 12:17; 13:35; 21:4; 27:9.—Even STRECKER, *Weg der Gerechtigkeit*, 50f, 84f, admits that the introductory formula of the formula quotations is not from the tradition, though he believes that the quotations themselves come from a special source. For further discussion of the introductory formula, see ROTHFUCHS, *Erfüllungszitate*, 27–56; SOARES PRABHU, *Formula Quotations*, 46–63.

pared with Mark 1:2/Luke 3:4; Mark 12:26/Luke 20:37; Mark 13:14/Luke 21:20. The term introduces the words of God in Scripture. Just as the rabbinic literature often uses the niphal of אמר in such introductions,[1] so ἐρρέθη functions as a divine passive in Matthew.

If ἐρρέθη constitutes the vital point determining ἐγὼ δὲ λέγω structurally, the construction portrays Jesus as a teacher more confident than any rabbi or other human teacher ever heard of.[2] Since ἐρρέθη and ἐγὼ δὲ λέγω are different both in the tense used and in the presupposed speaker, the antithetical construction conveys a double impression. The relation between the aorist (ἐρρέθη) and the present tense (λέγω) implies perhaps a temporal distinction. The location of τοῖς ἀρχαίοις as a counterpart to ὑμῖν confirms this impression.[3] Jesus addresses the eschatological moment of his audience. More evidently, Jesus' didactic ἐγώ amounts to divine categories.[4] It corresponds to a divine passive. It is not necessary to discuss the content of each Antithesis here. The repeated construction itself shows that Jesus' teaching carries an importance to be compared with what God himself has said.

Excursus 12: *Jesus and the Mountain of Teaching*

Jesus pronounces according to 5:1 his authoritative ἐγώ as he sits on a specific mountain (τὸ ὄρος). This location has given cause to at least two suggestions implying other christological conceptions.

It has often been argued that the location is reminiscent of mount Sinai, which would relate Jesus' teaching to the law issued there by Moses.[5] Although the scholars affirming this connection do not always interpret the ἐγώ of the Antitheses in Mosaic categories, it is a reasonable assumption that if the location contains Mosaic allusions, so

---

1   BACHER, *Die exegetische Terminologie* I, 6; *idem, Die exegetische Terminologie* II, 10.

2   4QMMT, perhaps composed by the Righteous Teacher (cf. above pp. 168f), relates "we reckon/say" (אנחנו חושבים/אומרים) to "you know" (אתם יודעים). But this hardly amounts to a literary pattern. Furthermore, the author of 4QMMT merely puts himself over against other torah teachers, not God.—As WEDER, "But I say to you ...," 215f, points out, the Matthean construction also goes beyond the prophetic messenger formula. Cf. also *idem, "Rede der Reden,"* 180–102. Jesus is not prominently pictured as a prophet in Matthew at all. See below p. 364.

3   Cf. GUELICH, *Sermon on the Mount,* 179f.

4   It is therefore difficult to agree with H.D. BETZ, Christology, 191–209, claiming that there is a lack of christology in the Sermon on the Mount and that the self-references "merely conform to Jesus' role as a teacher" (*ibid.,* 193). The christology of the antithetical construction is implicit in the very structure of the text, and not only "a matter of presupposition or consequence" (*ibid.,* 193 n. 6).

5   Cf. e.g. E. KLOSTERMANN, *Matthäusevangelium,* 33; KILPATRICK, *Origins,* 108; BLAIR, *Jesus,* 134; LOHMEYER, *Matthäus,* 75f; Joachim JEREMIAS, *TDNT* IV, 871; DAHL, *Matteusevangeliet* I, 64; FRANKEMÖLLE, *Jahwebund,* 97; SALAS, *CD* 188 (1975) 10–12; G. BARTH, *TRE* 5 (1980) 608; *idem,* Law, 157f; BORNKAMM, End-Expectation 35; GUNDRY, *Matthew,* 66, 138; LAPIDE, *Bergpredigt,* 16f; GNILKA, *Matthäusevangelium* I, 109; ALLISON, *ExpTim* 98 (1987) 203–205; PATTE, *Matthew,* 61; DAVIES/ALLISON, *Matthew* I, 423f; G. LOHFINK, *Bergpredigt,* 31; GRASSI, *BTB* 19 (1989) 25; FORNBERG, *Matteusevangeliet* I, 76; U. LUZ, *Matthäus* I, 197f, 416; M. DAVIES, *Matthew,* 48.

does the ἐγώ of the Antitheses.

The most precise argument refers to the expression ἀνέβη εἰς τὸ ὄρος in 5:1. From a total of twenty-five instances, the LXX uses forms of ἀναβαίνειν εἰς τὸ ὄρος nineteen times in the Pentateuch,[1] thirteen of these in reference to an action by Moses.[2] In most of these thirteen cases, Moses climbs mount Sinai.[3] To this we could add that καταβάντος δὲ αὐτοῦ ἀπὸ τοῦ ὄρους in 8:1 is reminiscent of when Moses descends mount Sinai.[4] However, the LXX does not use ἀναβαίνειν εἰς τὸ ὄρος as a fixed idiom always including allusions to mount Sinai and Moses. Even within the Pentateuch, we find the expression related to other persons climbing, or actually not climbing, a mountain.[5] And the mountain is not always mount Sinai.[6] Outside of the Pentateuch, the LXX links the expression neither with Moses nor with Sinai,[7] but primarily with various persons going up to mount Zion.[8] And Matthew does not restrict the expression only to situations where Jesus is to teach. It occurs also in other contexts (14:23; 15:29), and instead of ἀναβαίνειν other verbs sometimes appear with εἰς τὸ ὄρος (21:1; 26:30, 28:16). In regard to καταβάντος δὲ αὐτοῦ ἀπὸ τοῦ ὄρους in 8:1, it is sufficient to notice that the same motif occurs with a different implication in 17:9. It has a different wording than in 8:1 and includes also the action of three disciples. The expressions are fixed neither in wording nor in reference.

A further argument builds on the notice that Jesus sits down when he teaches. In opposition to this argument, some have claimed that the Jewish literature never depicts Moses as a sitting teacher.[9] But it is true that b. Meg. 21a discusses the verb יֹשֵׁב in Deut 9:9 and probes the possibility that Moses taught sitting.[10] However, besides the problem of dating the rabbinic tradition, this argument makes too much out of a single word. The sitting posture was after all the natural position for a teacher during the second half of the first century C.E. Although a baraita in b. Meg. 21a implies that scholarly discussions had been conduced in standing posture since early times, it also suggests that the sitting position was the normal one after the death of R. Gamaliel I Ha-Zaken (c. 30–40 C.E.).[11] Accordingly, Matt 26:55 says, in distinction to Mark 14:49/Luke 22:53, that Jesus is sitting also when he teaches in the temple. And Matthew presents Jesus as sitting down on several other occasions when he speaks to the crowds and the disciples.[12] The term καθίζειν carries no inherent allusion to mount Sinai and Moses in Matthew.

Thus, *just as the rabbinic connotations of the didactic ἐγώ are vague and remote, so are the Mosaic ones.* Although a certain Moses typology may be present in, for in-

---

[1] Exod 19:3, 12, 13 (with ἐπί); 24:12, 13, 15, 18; 34:1, 2 (with ἐπί), 4; Num 27:12; Deut 1:24, 41, 43; 5:5; 9:9; 10:1, 3; 32:49.

[2] Exod 19:3; 24:12, 13, 15, 18; 34:1, 2, 4; Num 27:12; Deut 9:9; 10:1, 3; 32:49.

[3] In Num 27:12; Deut 32:49 it is not mount Sinai.

[4] Cf. Exod 19:14; 32:1, 15; 34:29. These instances usually employ καταβαίνειν ἐκ τοῦ ὄρους. Only Exod 32:15 uses ἀπό.

[5] Exod 19:12, 13; Deut 1:24, 41, 43; 5:5.

[6] Deut 1:24, 41, 43 refer to the hill country.

[7] Isa 2:3; Mic 4:2; Hag 1:8 (with ἐπί); Ps 23:3; 1 Macc 5:54; 7:33.

[8] So in all cases except Hag 1:8.

[9] So e.g. LANGE, *Das Erscheinen des Auferstandenen*, 442.

[10] ALLISON, *ExpTim* 98 (1987) 203f; DAVIES/ALLISON, *Matthew* I, 424; W.D. DAVIES, Jewish Sources, 506.

[11] Cf. e.g. m. ʾAbot 1:4; 3:2, 6; ʾAbot R. Nat. A 6. In Luke 4:20 Jesus sits down and expounds the Scripture after reading it standing.—For discussion of the baraita in b. Meg. 21a, see ABERBACH, Change from a Standing to a Sitting Posture, 277–283.

[12] 13:1f; 24:3. Cf. also 15:29.

stance, Matt 1–2,[1] the arguments put forward in regard to 5:1 do not convince.[2]

T.L. Donaldson gives extensive support to a second proposal.[3] With the exception of 14:23, the scenes situating Jesus on a mountain are, according to Donaldson, based on a dominating Zion typology.[4] The Sermon on the Mount is the messianic interpretation of the Torah for the eschatological community. It represents the fulfilment of a christologically reinterpreted Zion eschatology.

In regard to 5:1, Donaldson's case depends on three arguments.[5] First, the depiction of the gathering of the Israelite people around Jesus in 4:23–5:1 builds on the expectation of a great gathering on mount Zion, where Israel will be constituted as the people of God. Second, Jesus issues a new torah, or gives the Torah a new role, on the mountain. This relates to the Zion motif. Third, 5:14b alludes to the new Jerusalem established as the centre of the restored people. The disciples and the crowds constitute the eschatological city of God.

The first two arguments, though not unlikely as observations in themselves, are too general in order to carry much weight. The third is the decisive one, as Donaldson himself recognizes. But this is also the most problematic one. It is difficult to ascertain that G. von Rad and K.M. Campbell were correct in identifying the city in 5:14b with the new Jerusalem.[6] Several commentaries on Matthew published after that Donaldson presented his dissertation imply that this proposal is not as generally accepted as Donaldson believes.[7] We would at least expect the definite articles in front of πόλις and ὄρους.[8] Neither von Rad nor Campbell comments on this absence.[9] But even if this interpretation is accepted, it is not "but a simple step"[10] to draw the connection between the mountain in 5:14b and 5:1. To begin with, the lack of the definite article in front of ὄρους in 5:14b is strange in view of its presence in 5:1. Furthermore, the emphasis of 5:14b is within the context of 5:13–16 not on a city or a mountain itself, but on the *visibility* of a city on a mountain. 5:14b merely illustrates 5:14a. Finally, it is difficult to maintain, without additional qualification, that 5:13–16 addresses the same audience as in 5:1, i.e. the disciples *and* the crowds as the eschatological people of God. No doubt, the Sermon as a whole is directed to both the disciples and the

---

[1]   Cf. e.g. SOARES PRABHU, *Formula Quotations,* 7f, 288–292; R.E. BROWN, *Birth of the Messiah,* 112–116; SAITO, *Mosevorstellungen,* 58–60.

[2]   FRANCE, *Matthew: Evangelist and Teacher,* 186–189, 313, acknowledges the importance of the Moses typology in Matt 2 but denies altogether the importance of the mountain motif in 4:8; 5:1; 15:29; 17:1; 24:3; 28:16. For further critique, cf. e.g. W.D. DAVIES, *Setting of the Sermon on the Mount,* 85f, 93, 99; GIBBS, *SE* 4 (1968) 45; LANGE, *Das Erscheinen des Auferstandenen,* 442–444; BANKS, *Jesus and the Law,* 231f; T.L. DONALDSON, *Jesus on the Mountain,* 111–114; STRECKER, *Sermon on the Mount,* 24f; KINGSBURY, *Matthew: Structure, Christology, Kingdom,* 91.

[3]   *Jesus on the Mountain.* Cf. already SCHMAUCH, *Orte der Offenbarung,* 76–80.

[4]   Cf. 4:8; 5:1; 15:29; 17:1; 24:3; 28:16.

[5]   *Jesus on the Mountain,* 116–118.

[6]   VON RAD, *EvT* 8 (1948–49) 447; CAMPBELL, *SJT* 31 (1978) 358–363.

[7]   Cf. e.g. FRANCE, *Matthew,* 112 n. 2; SCHNACKENBURG, *Matthäusevangelium* I, 50; SAND, *Matthäus,* 105; DAVIES/ALLISON, *Matthew* I, 475; NEPPER-CHRISTENSEN, *Matthæusevangeliet,* 67f; FORNBERG, *Matteusevangeliet* I, 71, 81; U. LUZ, *Matthäus* I, 223; HARE, *Matthew,* 45.

[8]   Cf. GUNDRY, *Matthew,* 77; SCHENK, *Sprache des Matthäus,* 375; DAVIES/ALLISON, *Matthew* I, 475; FORNBERG, *Matteusevangeliet* I, 71; U. LUZ, *Matthäus* I, 223.

[9]   The attempt by G. LOHFINK, *Bergpredigt,* 144f, to diminish this problem deals with the absence of the article in front of πόλις only, not ὄρους.

[10] T.L. DONALDSON, *Jesus on the Mountain,* 118.

crowds.[1] But within the Sermon itself, Jesus turns primarily to the disciples.[2] The possible allusion to mount Zion in 5:14b does not, therefore, concern all the people of Israel gathered as the new eschatological city around Jesus, but only the limited group of persons who have accepted the call to discipleship. If the argument based on 5:14b does not convince, *the assumption that the location of Jesus' teaching activity on the mountain relates him to a christologically reinterpreted Zion eschatology has to be treated with caution.*

4.4.3. The Only Teacher

23:8–10 is a vital point in the didactic story line.[3] Together with the aphoristic mashal in 23:11f,[4] it forms an exhortation concerning the disciples' relationship to teaching authorities.

A didactic christology is present implicitly in two ways. The first has to do with the father terminology. 23:9 uses a reference to the heavenly Father as a basis for not calling others "father." We do not know exactly who the persons being called "father" are. Their identity is indicated only by ὑμῶν,[5] which either qualifies πατέρα—"do not call (anyone) your father on earth"—or functions as a partitive genitive—"do not call (anyone) among you father on earth."[6] The former alternative emphasizes the disciples' relationship to persons outside of their own group, the latter the internal relationship. The former is probably to be preferred. Elsewhere Matthew often attaches πατήρ to genitive pronouns.[7] The separation of πατήρ from the pronoun in 23:9 is perhaps due to an attraction of πατέρα to ἀδελφοί in 23:8c. Moreover, the active voice of καλεῖν is remarkable when compared with middle voice in 23:8, 10. We would expect an exact parallel to the other two statements, were the internal relationship between the disciples in view also in 23:9.[8]

The term πατήρ probably refers to teachers—not just any person of authority[9] or any great men of previous generations[10] or Abraham, Isaac

---

1   Cf. 7:28f.

2   See above pp. 224–226.

3   See above pp. 207f.

4   23:8–12 consists, rhetorically speaking, of three enthymemes concluded by a maxim. Cf. GRAMS, Temple Conflict Scene, 52, 61; VINSON, Enthymemes, 125, 136.

5   The MSS supporting ὑμῶν are stronger than the ones supporting ὑμῖν. It is also unlikely that ὑμῶν is an aramaism for an original ὑμᾶς. See ZIMMERMANN, *Die urchristlichen Lehrer,* 165.

6   With e.g. Joachim JEREMIAS, *Abba,* 44, I understand μή as μηδένα.

7   Cf. e.g. 2:22; 4:21, 22; 5:16, 45, 48; 6:1, 4, 6, 8, 9, 14, 15, 18, 26, 32; 7:11, 21; 8:21, etc.

8   Cf. Joachim JEREMIAS, *Abba,* 45.

9   *Contra* HOET, *"Omnes autem vos fratres estis,"* 128–133. Cf. also COLUNGA, "A nadie llaméis padre," 333.

10   *Contra* Joachim JEREMIAS, *Abba,* 44f; *idem, Neutestamentliche Theologie,* 73, 166 n. 6; MICHAELS, Christian Prophecy and Matthew 23:8–12, 306.

and Jacob[1] or the physical father.[2] The context deals with teaching authorities. Although there is a tendency to avoid "father" as a designation for rabbinic teachers,[3] the habit of depicting the relationship between a teacher and his pupils as one between a father and his sons occurs already in the OT—especially in the wisdom literature, including Sirach.[4] In the rabbinic literature the designation appears in close connection to the name of teachers from earlier generations.[5] Their primary function was to carry the tradition. Gal 1:14; Ant. 13:297, 408 accordingly refer to certain teaching as the tradition of the fathers.[6] This background makes it likely that Jesus exhorts the disciples not to show undue respect for the teachers transmitting the opponents' teaching.

The father terminology takes its cue from God as the heavenly Father. The ultimate reason for the exhortation not to call anyone "father" is the unique position of the heavenly Father. But the references to Jesus as teacher in 23:8b, 10b parallel this explanatory clause. Matthew enhances Jesus' unique status as teacher with God himself, the heavenly Father, as the point of reference. Just as he depicted Jesus' didactic ἐγώ in relation to what was said by God, he now presents Jesus as a teacher whose status is comparable to the one of the Father.

The threefold εἷς is a second sign of an implicit didactic christology. Matthew uses it in presenting the cause of the exhortation—twice with εἷς γάρ ἐστιν (23:8b, 9b) and once with ὅτι ... ἐστιν εἷς (23:10b). H.-J. Becker brings attention to this threefold pattern in a study of 23:1–12 on the background of rabbinic texts.[7] It constitutes, according to Becker, an allusion to the first part of the Shemaᶜ in Deut 6:4 (אחד יהוה/κύριος εἷς ἐστιν). Becker bases his view on certain reminiscences of the Shemaᶜ in 23:3f, 5–7. The pattern of three in 23:8–10 could also anticipate the threefold formula in 28:19. If Becker has not overstated his case, the Shemaᶜ carries a christological dimension. The adherence to Jesus as teacher relates to the confession of the one and only God.[8]

The interpreted Shemaᶜ as a whole plays an important role in Matthew.[9]

---

[1] *Contra* TOWNSEND, *JTS* 12 (1961) 56–59. Cf. also SCHWEIZER, *Matthäus,* 282.

[2] Cf. LOHMEYER, *Matthäus* 340; ZIMMERMANN, *Die urchristlichen Lehrer,* 167f.

[3] See above p. 53.

[4] See above pp. 37 n. 9, 47f. For the Dead Sea scrolls, cf. above p. 52.

[5] See above p. 53. Cf. also SCHRENK, *TDNT* V, 977f.—VIVIANO, *JSNT* 39 (1990) 14, refers in this connection to the Greek synagogue inscription from Stobi (northern Macedonia)—probably dating to the 3rd cent. C.E.—speaking of the father of the synagogue at Stobi (ὁ πατὴρ τῆς ἐν Στόβοις συναγωγῆς). See further HENGEL, *ZNW* 57 (1966) 176–181, with numerous references to other (relatively late) inscriptions using similar designations (*ibid.,* 177 nn. 102, 103).

[6] The Mishnah tractate Pirqe ʾAbot, "sections of the fathers," should also be mentioned, unless the title means simply "fundamental principles" (of the Mishnah).

[7] *Auf der Kathedra des Mose,* 170 n. 2, 203f.

[8] Cf. also KARRER, *ZNW* 83 (1992) 17f.

[9] The basic texts are Num 15:37–41; Deut 6:4–9; 11:13–21. For the rabbinic interpretation of Deut 6:5, see especially m. Ber. 9:5; Sifre on Deut 6:5. STRACK/BILLER-

Numerous studies by B. Gerhardsson have made this evident.[1] Matthew understands large parts of Jesus' activity and destiny as true obedience to Israel's confession of faith, the Shema𝑐. Jewish readers/hearers would certainly perceive the threefold εἰς as connected with ἐστιν on the background of the Shema𝑐. Each pious, adult and male Jew internalized it as a confession recited every morning and evening (m. Ber. 1:1–4) in Hebrew or any other language (m. Soṭa 7:1; t. Soṭa 7:7)—perhaps also in Greek.[2] The detailed discussions about the Shema𝑐 in the Mishnah as well as the reports that the priests in the temple recited it (m. Tamid 4:3; 5:1) and that the houses of Shammai and Hillel discussed it (m. Ber. 1:3) point to its early use—in some form at least.[3]

The christological application of the Shema𝑐 is present already earlier in Matthew. The yoke of Jesus in 11:29 is certainly to be read/heard on the background of such Jewish wisdom traditions as the ones in Sir 6:23–31; 51:26.[4] But precisely Sir 6:26 shows that the yoke of Wisdom relates to the Shema𝑐. Ben Sira tells the pupil to draw near to the Wisdom "with your whole soul" (ἐν πάσῃ ψυχῇ σου) and to keep her ways "with your whole power" (ἐν ὅλῃ δυνάμει σου).[5] The connection between the yoke and the Shema𝑐 is explicit in the rabbinic literature. The recital of the Shema𝑐 means "to accept the yoke of the kingdom of heaven" (קיבל עול מלכות שמים).[6] First the yoke of the kingdom of heaven is accepted, and then the yoke of the commandments (m. Ber. 2:2; Mek. on 20:3 [Lauterbach II, 238:8–10]).[7] In Matt 11:29 the yoke is not the yoke of Wisdom or of the kingdom of heaven. It is the yoke of Jesus himself, from whom the invited ones are to learn.[8] The background suggests that Jesus invites persons to learn his teaching after they have confessed his unique and absolute status.[9]

A christological application of the Shema𝑐 is perhaps present also in 19:17. Matthew does not only omit Deut 6:4,[10] or allusions to it.[11] A possible allusion does occur in the εἰς ἐστιν ὁ ἀγαθός of 19:17.[12] There might

---

BECK, *Kommentar* I, 905–907, list other (parallel) texts. SCHÜRER, *History* II, 454 n. 143, gives literature on the subject.

[1] See The Shema𝑐, 275–293, and the literature mentioned there.

[2] Cf. y. Soṭa 21b mentioning the recital of the Shema𝑐 in Greek at Caesarea.

[3] Cf. also Ant. 4:212f, though it does not refer to the Shema𝑐 explicitly.

[4] Cf. DEUTSCH, *Hidden Wisdom,* 115f, 133–135.

[5] Sir 6:23–31 does not like 51:26 express the image of the yoke with ζυγός, but with words like πέδη (6:24, 29), κλοιός (6:24, 29) and δεσμός (6:25, 30).

[6] Cf. e.g. m. Ber. 2:2, 5; b. Ber. 61b. Further references are listed by STRACK/BILLERBECK, *Kommentar* I, 177f. For discussion, cf. e.g. H.-J. BECKER, *Auf der Kathedra des Mose,* 145f, 161–164.

[7] Cf. ABRAHAMS, *Studies* II, 9.

[8] Cf. GERHARDSSON, *SEÅ* 37–38 (1972–73) 136f.

[9] Cf. also 10:32f.

[10] Cf. Matt 22:37/Mark 12:29, 32. The absence is in agreement with Luke 10:26. For discussion, see DAUBE, *New Testament,* 247–250.

[11] Cf. Matt 9:3/Mark 2:7/Luke 5:21.

[12] 19:17 is besides 23:8–10 the only instance in Matthew where εἰς and ἐστιν are di-

be a deliberate oscillation between Jesus and God here. The absence of a reference to God prevents the misunderstanding that Jesus is not good—a conclusion that could be drawn from Mark10:18/Luke 18:19.[1] Jesus' answer in 19:17 implies that only the one who is good can teach about what is good. And Jesus himself gives the following teaching.[2] In addition, the teaching shows that the goodness required of the young man means keeping the commandments to the extent of giving up the possessions. This accords with the interpretation of the Shema` to love God with all your might.[3] And it is here a condition for being a disciple of Jesus (19:21). 19:17 seems to oscillate between relating the Shema` to God and to Jesus as teacher.

The reason why the disciples according to 23:8–10 should abstain from attributing the didactic labels to themselves or any other person is therefore that they have taken the obligations of God and Jesus upon themselves. They have no teaching authority apart from their dependence on Jesus. Jesus' disciples are to abstain from claiming or relying on the authority of human teachers, because adherence to Jesus as teacher equals adherence to the one and only God.

4.4.4. The Wisdom

F. Christ and M.J. Suggs have sharpened the debate about Jesus as the Wisdom of God in Matthew.[4] Some scholars have accepted and developed their proposal—especially as presented by Suggs—that Jesus is the Wisdom in Matthew;[5] others have remained more cautious,[6] even sceptical.[7] The issue relates to Matthew's didactic christology. C. Deutsch emphatically argues for a connection between the depiction of Jesus as teacher and the wisdom christology in Matthew and claims that as teacher of wisdom Jesus *is* the

---

rectly connected.

[1] Cf. BANKS, *Jesus and the Law,* 160f; BEARE, *Matthew,* 394; SCHWEIZER, *Matthäus,* 252; COULOT, *Jésus et le disciple,* 110f.

[2] There is no evidence in Matthew that the goodness of the Torah is in view, as COPE, *Matthew,* 111–119, claims on the basis of Prov 3:35; 4:2, 4; 28:10; m. ᾽Abot 6:3. Cope is followed by R.F. COLLINS, Matthew's ἐντολαί, 1327.

[3] Cf. GERHARDSSON, *SEÅ* 37–38 (1972–73) 140; *idem, Ethos,* 50.

[4] CHRIST, *Jesus Sophia;* SUGGS, *Wisdom.* The major difference between the two is that while Christ believes that Jesus was the Wisdom already in Q, Suggs argues that Matthew created this identification by altering Q, where Jesus was merely the envoy of Wisdom.

[5] E.g. HAMERTON-KELLY, *Pre-existence,* 67–83; J.M. ROBINSON, Jesus as Sophos and Sophia, 1–16; BURNETT, *Jesus-Sophia;* DEUTSCH, *Hidden Wisdom; idem, NovT* 32 (1990) 13–47; D. GOOD, *NovT* 32 (1990) 7–10, 12. Cf. also the review by STRECKER, *TLZ* 98 (1973) 519–522.—The dissertation by F.T. GENCH, *Wisdom in the Christology of Matthew.* Union Theological Seminary 1988, was not available to me.

[6] E.g. W.G. THOMPSON, *CBQ* 33 (1971) 145f; VON LIPS, *Weisheitliche Traditionen,* 280–290; PREGEANT, Wisdom Passages, 469–493.

[7] The most extensive critique of Suggs is given by JOHNSON, *CBQ* 36 (1974) 44–64. Cf. also the brief review by GOULDER, *JTS* 22 (1971) 568f.

Wisdom personified, the Wisdom incarnated.[1]

The most important text implying some kind of connection between the characterization of Jesus as teacher and wisdom speculations is 11:25–30. Deutsch demonstrates the dominating presence of motifs related to wisdom concepts in Jewish texts from the second temple and tannaitic periods.[2] Supplementary or alternative suggestions appearing after Deutsch's study do not alter the view significantly.[3] In addition to the tentative and utterly hypothetical reference to Paral. Jerem. 5:32 as a possible background of Matt 11:25–30, D.C. Allison proposes Exod 33:12f; Deut 34:10 as important texts behind Matt 11:27.[4] The similarities between what Jesus says and what is said about Moses in these texts are indeed noteworthy. But they apply primarily to Jesus' reciprocal and exclusive knowledge.[5] As Allison elsewhere admits,[6] they do not exclude the presence of wisdom motifs in 11:25–30. B. Charette's proposal of a prophetic background to 11:28–20 is less convincing.[7] The presence of μανθάνειν (11:29) clearly evokes didactic, not quasi-political, connotations of the yoke. And 12:1–14 illustrates immediately what the easy yoke means. Wisdom motifs are clearly present and related to the characterization of Jesus as teacher, especially in 11:28–30 appearing in Matthew only.[8] By inviting persons to himself and to his own yoke, Jesus assumes the functions of Wisdom herself.

8:19f also exhibits a possible connection between the characterization of Jesus as teacher and wisdom motifs. Jesus is for the first time in Matthew addressed διδάσκαλε. The desire of the scribe using the address points to an insufficient understanding of the conditions involved in following this specific teacher.[9] Jesus' response contains elements contrasting the statement of the scribe:[10] the scribe approaches Jesus as a teacher, but Jesus refers to himself as the son of man; the scribe wishes to follow Jesus to certain places, but Jesus says that he has no place to rest his head. Jesus' answer does not

---

[1]   *Hidden Wisdom,* 134f, 139, 142; *idem, NovT* 32 (1990) 37f, 46.

[2]   *Hidden Wisdom,* 55–143.

[3]   It is unfortunate that STANTON, *Gospel,* 354–377, does not enter into debate with the more recent studies but merely reproduces an earlier article in which he denies the presence of wisdom motifs in 11:28–30.

[4]   *JTS* 39 (1988) 477–485.

[5]   ALLISON, *JTS* 39 (1988) 481–483, mentions also the promise of rest in Exod 33:14 and Matt 11:28 and points out that just as Moses was meek according to Num 12:3 and later Jewish traditions, so is also Jesus according to Matt 11:29.

[6]   DAVIES/ALLISON, *Matthew* II, 272, 287, 295. Unfortunately Allison presents no real discussion with Deutsch.

[7]   *NTS* 38 (1992) 290–297.

[8]   DEUTSCH, *Hidden Wisdom,* 113–139.

[9]   On the basis of the Pentateuch (LXX) and Hebrews, J.R. EDWARDS, *JBL* 106 (1987) 65–74, thinks that προσέρχεσθαι, which is used in 8:19, denotes a cultic approach to objects or persons representing the presence of God in Matthew. However, texts such as Matt 17:7; 27:58; 28:18 require further explanation. Cf. also above p. 225 n. 7.

[10]   Cf. MACK/ROBBINS, *Patterns of Persuasion,* 71.

focus on the comparison with the animals.[1] Such a misunderstanding of Jesus' statement 8:20 has fostered various proposals concerning the background and significance of the expression "the son of man."[2] The focus is instead on Jesus' homelessness. 8:28–9:1 illustrates this further. After performing a miracle, Jesus is asked to leave the neighbourhood (8:34). In view of the fact that Jesus appears to be rather domiciled elsewhere in Matthew,[3] the reference to the homelessness points beyond itself. Homelessness was a well-known characteristic of the Wisdom.[4] Through the reference to the homelessness of the son of man, the readers/hearers realize that "this man,"[5] the teacher speaking, is in some sense like Wisdom herself.[6] Jesus tells the scribe about the special destiny that a life as his disciple would involve.[7] The scribe cannot expect merely to attend to a teacher who travels from various school houses, and subsequently to move on to consult other teachers of reputation. Following Jesus, the teacher, means to learn while sharing his homelessness and life-long destiny. The aphoristic mashal in 10:24f expounds this further. When for the first time the readers/hearers encounter Jesus as explicitly addressed διδάσκαλε, they discern a teacher who is like the didactic majesty of Wisdom herself.

Matthew nowhere specifies the relationship between Jesus and the Wisdom of God. The term σοφία occurs in 11:19; 12:42; 13:54. Only 11:19 speaks of the Wisdom personified. While Luke 7:35 states that the Wisdom is vindicated by her children, Matt 11:19b claims that she is vindicated by her deeds (ἀπὸ τῶν ἔργων αὐτῆς).[8] 11:19b may form an inclusio with 11:2 mentioning the deeds of the Messiah (τὰ ἔργα τοῦ χριστοῦ). But granted there is a real inclusio,[9] a clear identification of Jesus with the Wisdom does still not emerge. 11:19b has the appearance of a generally recognized mashal.[10] An aphoristic mashal often corresponds rhetorically to a maxim. While located at the end for rhetorical purposes, the mashal functions logi-

---

[1] Cf. CASEY, *JSNT* 23 (1985) 5.

[2] COLPE, *TDNT* VIII, 432; GNILKA, *Matthäusevangelium* I, 311, point to different proposals.

[3] Cf. 2:11, 23; 4:13; 9:1. Jesus is also located in a home in 9:10, 28; 13:1, 36; 17:25. Already LURIA, *ZNW* 25 (1926) 282–286, noticed this, though with the conclusion that 8:20 must stem from a contradictory (Aramaic) source.

[4] Cf. most explicitly 1 Enoch 42:1–3, though perhaps, as DEUTSCH, *NovT* 32 (1990) 28, believes, this is an interpolation. Cf. also Job 28:21; Prov 1:20–33; Bar 3:9–4:4; 4 Ezra 5:9–12; Sir 24:7; 1 Enoch 94:5.

[5] Cf. KINGSBURY, *JSNT* 25 (1985) 73.

[6] Cf. already ARVEDSON, *Mysterium Christi*, 210f n. 9.

[7] Cf. already FRÖVIG, *Das Selbstbewusstsein Jesu*, 53.

[8] The reading ἀπὸ τῶν τέκνων is probably a secondary harmonization with Luke.

[9] Cf. the critical remarks by VERSEPUT, *Rejection*, 116.

[10] For examples of similar conceptions in Jewish liteature, cf. JOHNSON, *CBQ* 36 (1974) 57f.—LEIVESTAD, *JBL* 71 (1952) 179–181, believes that Jesus is quoting a proverb referring ironically to the wisdom of the Jews. But Leivestad fails to bring out such Jewish proverbs.

cally as the rationale for Jesus' previous response to John the Baptist.[1] Because the Wisdom is vindicated by her own deeds, Jesus answers merely by recounting his ministry of healing and preaching (11:4–6) and by pointing to the Jewish rejection of both John and himself (11:7–19a).[2] The premise that Jesus, who is greater than John, actually *is* the Wisdom never occurs. The emphasis is on the ministry which is rejected. This suggests no more than a *function* making Jesus' mission Wisdom's own.[3]

The other two instances of σοφία agree with their synoptic parallels in using the term to qualify Jesus' active ministry. 12:42 ascribes wisdom to Solomon.[4] It implies that wisdom is present in Jesus' ministry to an even higher degree. Since there is nothing to suggest a personification of Jonah's proclamation, to which 12:41 compares Jesus, the statement that something greater than Solomon is here points to a function rather than an actual identification with the Wisdom.[5] 13:54 presents Jesus' teaching as the immediate cause for a question concerning the origin of his wisdom and mighty deeds.[6] The discussion about Jesus' wisdom appears on the lips of those who do not believe. And they regard it as a quality visible in his ministry.

It is possible, but less certain, that 23:34–36, 37–39—and according to F.W. Burnett also 24:1–31[7]—further associate Jesus, who here speaks as a transhistorical person, with the Wisdom.[8] The basic observation is that an emphatic ἐγώ occurs in 23:34 instead of ἡ σοφία τοῦ θεοῦ present in Luke 11:49. However, the only way to turn this observation into an argument for identifying Jesus with the Wisdom is to depend entirely on a theory according to which Matthew at this point changed the Q source visible in Luke's version. Although this is not implausible, there is in this case no sufficient substantiation from Matthew itself. The alleged changes in the sources actually make the only explicit reference to the Wisdom disappear.

The most prominent didactic label therefore validates Jesus. An implicit use of categories taken from Jewish conceptions about the Wisdom of God further defines the ministry of Jesus as teacher. The function suggests status.[9] Matthew's depiction of Jesus as teaching decisive commandments, as speaking with an authoritative ἐγώ, as referring to himself as the only normative teacher and as assuming the functions of the Wisdom establishes a didactic christology. As part of a "christology from the side," it reflects a labelling process which assessed and validated Jesus' role and status as tea-

---

1   For this function of a maxim in a different context, see MACK/ROBBINS, *Patterns of Persuasion,* 78–80.

2   This is reinforced in 11:20–24.

3   Cf. U. LUZ, *Matthäus* II, 189, 218; PREGEANT, Wisdom Passages, 490.

4   Cf. Luke 11:31.

5   Cf. the careful statement by KIEFFER, *SEÅ* 44 (1979) 142: "Mer än Salomo representerar Jesus visheten."

6   Cf. Mark 6:2.

7   *Jesus-Sophia,* 112–354

8   SUGGS, *Wisdom,* 13–29, 58–71.

9   Cf. DUNN, *Christology,* 205, and more generally AALEN, *SEÅ* 37–38 (1972–73) 35–46; *idem, Kristologien,* 26–28, 117–122.

cher by reference to divine categories. *Jesus was to Matthew qualitatively the only normative teacher. This must have constituted the strongest possible motive of transmission.*

5. Summary and Conclusions

This chapter addressed the question if Matthew cherished person-oriented motives of transmission similar to the ones described in chapter two. Since this part of my study deals with the conceptions of a person related to one rather coherent group of transmitters, the issue concerned to what extent the different motives evident in *various* groups in the sociocultural field of transmission interacted in *one* group represented by *one* person. It was necessary to investigate certain traits, techniques and labels in Matthew as reflections of the didactic, the didactic-biographical and the didactic-labelling motives of transmission.

1. There is an evident interest in Jesus' verbal teaching, reflecting didactic motives of transmission. The disciples are not merely pupils of Jesus; they are also future scribes. Peter is the foundational link back to Jesus' own teaching authority. The teaching that the disciples will give is not received only directly from the risen Lord. The future teaching activities will be based on the teaching that Jesus gave within a specific historical situation once and for all.

This suggests certain motives of transmission that *focused on the teaching itself.* There was for Matthew an inherent value in Jesus' teaching. What Jesus said was important as part of an event that occurred in history. It was not overshadowed entirely by the present. But the didactic motives related to certain activities. Matthew was also concerned to transmit Jesus' teaching for *the present purpose of teaching others.*

The practical interest in Jesus' verbal teaching does not necessarily mean that the transmission and the teaching activities were entirely fused. A fusion of the two would hardly have maintained the object of transmission at the historical distance as part of a past event. Matthew itself also suggests that there were scribes in the community. They seem to have constituted a special group to which Matthew belonged. And the previous chapter showed that there were persons with the task of understanding Jesus' teaching. These persons were probably scribes, as 13:51f indicates in particular.[1] It is true, we do not find traces of persons responsible for preserving the tradition only, without studying and trying to understand it. But Matthew's depiction of the scribes and the concept of understanding seems to reflect a situation where a group of specialists studied and tried to comprehend the past tradition *before* teaching it to others. It is—and was—after all quite

---

[1]   See further above pp. 229, 233f, 241 and below pp. 323f.

normal for a teacher to prepare his teaching lessons in this way. And it was probably in this separate setting—the school of Jesus in the Matthean community—that transmission in the sense of preservation and elaboration of the Jesus tradition took place.

2. The didactic-biographical motives of transmission are visible as episodal and narrative elements inherent in the presentation of Jesus' teaching as law and morality, as preaching and as healing. Jesus' teaching contains *within itself* biographical elements.

This suggests motives of transmission that *integrated the teaching within the life of a specific teacher*. Matthew must have cherished further interests than the transmission of Jesus' words only. The purely didactic motives cannot sufficiently explain the presence of these biographical features in the tradition. There was no interest in the verbal teaching independent of the teacher's life. The teaching and the biographical elements were inseparable. The desire to transmit Jesus' verbal teaching *necessarily* involved the desire to locate his words within the setting of his life. *Matthew's story indicates the concern and necessity to transmit Jesus' verbal teaching as integrated within the account about his ministry and life.*

3. The didactic-labelling motives appear in the story as the attribution labels validating Jesus' status as a teacher. The use of ἐξουσία in connection with the didactic characterization points to a teaching authority of universal dimension, accorded to Jesus' person by transcendental legitimation. Certain didactic designations identify Jesus' teaching authority further both negatively and positively. Jesus is not one of the ordinary Jewish teachers appropriating the title "Rabbi." He is the prominent didactic guide and leader of a brotherhood. The exousia and the designations point to a specific status. And there is accordingly a didactic christology assessing and validating Jesus' role and status in terms of divine categories.

This suggests motives of transmission that *integrated the teaching within a process that enhanced the teacher to an exclusive status of authority by means of validating labels*. There was no interest in the verbal teaching independent of the teacher's status. Matthew himself was one of the labellers and belonged to a group concerned to manifest Jesus' own exousia in its own teaching activities. He adhered to Jesus as the qualitatively and quantitatively one and only normative teacher. This must have motivated the transmission in at least two ways. *Since Jesus was a qualitatively unique teacher, it must have been generally essential to transmit his words and deeds. And since Jesus was also a quantitatively unique teacher, it must have been important to transmit his words and deeds as if they were isolated from the utterances and actions of other persons inside and outside of the community.* Teacher and teaching were inseparable in Matthew's didactic-labelling motives of transmission.

Matthew thus shared in the sociocultural situation exhibiting person-orien-

ted motives of transmission. But within the comparative perspective provided by the first part of this study, there are also specific and *contrasting* features. The cumulative presence of all three motives of transmission in one group represented by one person levelled the phenomenological variety in the intensity of focus on the individual teacher present in the sociocultural situation. None of the other groups adhering to a teacher in ancient Israel and ancient Judaism discloses such strong person-oriented motives of transmission. *The three motives of transmission worked together cumulatively in Matthew's transmission of the Jesus tradition.* The didactic motives did not stand alone. They always interacted with the didactic-biographical and the didactic-labelling motives of transmission.

It becomes increasingly clear that the transmission of the Jesus tradition cannot be adequately accounted for by focusing merely on technical matters in the present texts. A static comparison of different stages in the transmission gives only a partial picture, no matter what source theory we adopt. The transmission took place within a setting completely dominated by the authority of Jesus, the only teacher, and it was performed by persons actively interested in Jesus' teaching, life and status. The transmission had a *social setting* and was held together by a strong *motivating engagement.*[1] Transmission of items carrying such special significance is, generally speaking, different from the procedures appearing when items of no apparent interest to the transmitters are involved.[2] It is now adequate, therefore, to ask how the setting and motives of transmission correlated with Matthew's actual treatment of the Jesus tradition.

---

[1] Cf. the remarks above pp. 20f, 135.

[2] Cf. e.g. the account about rumor transmission by ABEL, *JR* 51 (1971) 280, though his article as a whole reflects a low estimation of the early Christian capacity to remember by memorization.

Chapter 6

Jesus as Teacher
and the Process of Transmission

1. Introductory Remarks

The reconstruction of Matthew's sociocultural situation in chapter three revealed various patterns of how settings determined by didactic authority and person-oriented motives of transmission correlated with the objects and acts of transmission. There were three major areas in which the correlation was especially evident: the identification of traditions, the means of transmission and the preservation and elaboration of traditions.[1] I referred to this correlation as the "personal specificity" in the transmission process. Because of the transmitters' variating settings and motives of transmission, the three areas exhibited different emphases.

Did Matthew's setting and motives of transmission cause a similar personal specificity in the transmission of the Jesus tradition? And in that case, are there within the patterns of similarity also significant differences depending on the cumulative presence of the person-oriented motives of transmission? *The aim of this chapter is to study the personal specificity in the process of identifying traditions, of carrying and conveying traditions by different means and of preserving and elaborating traditions.*[2]

Of course, numerous factors influenced the transmission. C.H. Lohr argued that several techniques evident in Matthew's written narrative reflect oral composition and transmission.[3] Lohr paid most attention to the formulaic language through which the sources were adapted to the stereotyped style of oral tradition. These techniques are not in themselves of interest here. If my observations in the previous chapters are correct, the transmission took place within a setting that the Matthean story identifies as the school of Jesus and was performed by persons aiming to convey Jesus' teaching as linked to his own life and status. *I will here concentrate only on features that correlated with the didactic setting and the person-oriented*

---

[1] For a clarification of what I mean by these three areas, see above pp. 136f, 155f, 171.

[2] See the remarks in the introduction above pp. 23f.

[3] *CBQ* 23 (1961) 403–435. Cf. already DOBSCHÜTZ, Matthew, 19–24, though he drew different conclusions.

motives of transmission.

The focus will be on the sayings of Jesus. We have seen that Jesus' teaching in its totality contains biographical elements within itself. But I will not treat the episodal frames and narratives independent from the Jesus-sayings. The biographical elements point to a desire to transmit Jesus' verbal teaching within the setting of his life. Since Jesus' life is an essential part of his teaching, the sayings cannot be separated from the episodal frames and narratives without being distorted as to their meaning and significance. *The episodal frames and narratives are then of interest as they relate intimately to what Jesus says.*

2. The Identification of Traditions

Jesus is the main speaker in Matthew. There is an evident and consistent identification of utterances as sayings of Jesus himself. The traditions are not anonymous, as is the case with the teaching of the Righteous Teacher in the Dead Sea scrolls. Just as the rabbinic literature usually attaches teaching to the name of a teacher, Matthew identifies sayings through *named attribution*. He attaches them to Jesus' name.

Further comparison with the rabbinic literature shows that the consistent attribution of sayings to only one teacher is not such an obvious procedure as modern readers of the NT might be accustomed to think. Truly, several important persons must have given valuable teaching in the early Christian communities. But their voices are not identified in the gospel narratives.[1] Jesus is the main speaker. To clarify this peculiar feature somewhat further, *I will study how Matthew, as a reflection of the transmission process, identifies Jesus-sayings and relates utterances of other persons to the all-important presentation of Jesus.*

2.1. The Named Attribution to Jesus

There are several variations in the way Matthew attributes sayings to Jesus. In a rough twofold classification, we may distinguish between instances in which the Matthean narrator either directly or indirectly, but in the same sentence, mentions Jesus' name, and instances in which he uses only a verb—sometimes with the definite article serving as a pronoun[2]—indicating that Jesus is going to speak.[3] The former procedure directs the attention

---

[1]   Cf. already EASTON, *Gospel,* 113f.

[2]   Only 21:27 uses αὐτός to introduce a Jesus-saying.

[3]   I have counted altogether 137 separate introductions to Jesus-sayings in Matthew. In cases where the saying is "interrupted" by utterances of another character (cf. e.g. 15:21–28;) or the narrator's comments (cf. e.g. 26:36–46), I have counted each separate

to the person speaking, while the latter focuses more directly on the actual saying—without of course neglecting the speaker's identity entirely. The narrator explicitly mentions Jesus by name in 56–57% of his introductions to the Jesus-sayings.[1] In 73–74% of these instances, he mentions the name directly together with the finite verb expressing that Jesus is going to speak. For my purposes, the *importance* and *function* of this named attribution in the transmission process is of interest.

2.1.1. The Importance of the Attribution

The mention of Jesus' name is often a deliberate means to identify a saying. It is not casual or due merely to certain needs of clarification. It often happens in one and the same pericope that the narrator first describes various circumstances or Jesus' actions without mentioning Jesus' name and later introduces the decisive Jesus-saying with a statement that contains Ἰησοῦς.[2] While he depicts the circumstances and the actions in more general terms, he specifically identifies the utterance as a saying from Jesus. We also find the narrator repeating Jesus' name in introductions to two sayings following closely upon each other. These repetitions are of course present especially in the dialogues. But they are not always necessary for the sake of clarifying who is speaking.[3] By contrast, brief utterances of Jesus that are not of the same essential significance are thoroughly embedded in the narration. They are often not directly identified by reference to Jesus' name.[4]

It even happens that the mention of the name implies an emphatic stress on the identification of Jesus as speaker. This is perhaps most evident in 8:22.[5] The verse forms the climax of 8:18–22,[6] the two scenes of which are held together by the catchwords ἀπέρχεσθαι (8:18, 19, 21) and ἀκολουθεῖν (8:19, 22).[7] The introduction ὁ δὲ Ἰησοῦς λέγει αὐτῷ in 8:22 corresponds chiastically to καὶ λέγει αὐτῷ ὁ Ἰησοῦς in 8:20. But it is perhaps more than a structural feature. Jesus responds in 8:20 merely by means of a common

---

introduction.

[1]   In 14:16, 27 Ἰησοῦς is textcritically uncertain. I have included them in my counting. Some MSS not followed in the 26th edition of Nestle-Aland also use Jesus' name to introduce a Jesus-saying. Cf. variant readings of 8:3, 7; 9:12; 12:25; 13:51; 15:16; 17:11, 20; 18:2; 22:20, 37, 43; 24:2. I consider all of them as secondary.

[2]   Cf. 4:12–17; 8:1–4, 5–13; 9:14–17; 11:2–6; 13:54–58; 17:14–17; 18:21f; 19:13–15; 20:20–22; 21:15–17, 18–22, 23–27; 22:23–33; 24:3–8.

[3]   Cf. 4:7 with 4:10; 8:10 with 8:13; 8:20 with 8:22; 15:32 with 15:34; 16:6 with 16:8; 17:7 with 17:9; 17:25 with 17:26; 19:18 with 19:21; 19:23 with 19:26, 28; 26:31 with 26:34; 28:9 with 28:10.

[4]   Cf. 8:7, 32; 12:13; 14:18, 29; 20:21.

[5]   Ἰησοῦς is probably original in 8:22. There is a strong external support (א, B, C, *f*¹, 33). The omission in some MSS might be due to influence from Luke 9:60.

[6]   MACK/ROBBINS, *Patterns of Persuasion,* 70–74, classify it as a double chreia. Cf. also BERGER, *Formgeschichte,* 81, 86f.

[7]   Cf. further COULOT, *Jésus et le disciple,* 18; KINGSBURY, *NTS* 34 (1988) 45f.

aphoristic mashal which he applies to himself. Plutarch's well-known use of the image concerning the safe refuge (φολεός) of the wild beasts roaming over Italy in distinction to the homelessness of men fighting and dying for Italy (Tib. Gracch. 9:4f) is certainly applied on a specific military situation. Yet, its use by Plutarch shows that this is a general saying which can be used in various contexts and with different speakers.[1] By contrast, only Jesus can give the decisive command "follow me" (ἀκολούθει μοι) in 8:22. Instead of placing Jesus' name after the finite verb, the narrator therefore puts it first. Together with the scribe's initial desire to follow Jesus expressed in 8:19, the implication appears that discipleship is not the object of free choice. It is the result of a call coming from no one else but Jesus.[2]

It is not impossible that the neat structure of 8:18–22, with the emphatic identification of the final Jesus-saying, is the result of Matthew's work on the tradition. Luke 9:57–60 would probably reflect to a larger extent the same structure and identification had these features been present in the tradition. In any case, it is striking that from all the Matthean units which introduce a Jesus-saying by name and which have a parallel saying in Mark and/or Luke,[3] 50–51% are within an intersynoptic perspective alone to portray a narrator who identifies the saying by directly or indirectly mentioning Jesus' name. This is to be compared with the fact that Matthew is alone *not* to include Jesus' name only in 15% of all the instances which introduce the saying *without* explicitly mentioning the name and which have a parallel saying in Mark and/or Luke.[4] Of all the sayings in Matthew which do not have a clear parallel in Mark and Luke,[5] the narrator introduces 57–58% by referring to Jesus by name, while he uses merely a verb—sometimes together with a pronoun—in 42–43% of the instances. Individual cases might be open to various tradition-historical explanations. And not all instances can be isolated as parts of separate units in the tradition. But the cumulative impression emerging from all these introductions is clearly that *Matthew's work on the tradition strengthened the named attribution of the Jesus-sayings.* The sayings are Jesus' own words.

---

[1]   Cf. HAHN, *Christologische Hoheitstitel,* 44; BULTMANN, *Geschichte der synoptischen Tradition,* 27, 102 n. 2. Cf. also *idem,* Ergänzungsheft, 37. The further texts from the OT and from Homer adduced by ZUMSTEIN, *Relation du maître et du disciple,* 224, are not to the point. But cf. Philo, Abr. 31.

[2]   KINGSBURY, *NTS* 34 (1988) 49, 56f, believes that the scribe is a negative character because he himself takes the initiative to follow Jesus—in contrast to such call episodes as 4:18–20, 21f; 9:9, in which Jesus is the one who first summons. But this conclusion is not necessary. Cf. above p. 240.

[3]   Of 76 instances introducing a saying by reference to Jesus' name in Matthew, 57 have a parallel utterance from Jesus in at least one of the other synoptics.

[4]   Of 61 instances introducing a saying only with a verb in Matthew, 47 have a parallel utterance from Jesus in at least one of the other synoptics.

[5]   Of totally 137 instances containing introductions to Jesus-sayings in Matthew, 33 are without a parallel in any of the other synoptics.

2.1.2. The Function of the Attribution

E.P. Sanders concludes his detailed survey of the proper names in the synoptic tradition by observing that "in most of the instances in which Matthew has a proper name where Mark or Luke has a noun or pronoun, the proper name is 'Jesus'."[1] But the addition of the name is not merely a general tendency. The most prominent use of Ἰησοῦς in Matthew is precisely to present Jesus as the speaking subject. It is a term employed primarily by the narrator. Characters within the story use it only rarely,[2] and never in the vocative.[3] F.W. Burnett estimates that from the undisputed instances having Jesus as the subject, 81,5% present him in the act of speaking, answering or having just spoken.[4]

The use of Ἰησοῦς points first of all to a historical person. The Matthean narrator never identifies the sayings by employing a christological title. Ἰησοῦς is the term he uses. By contrast, the Lukan narrator uses ὁ κύριος to introduce a Jesus-saying in a number of cases,[5] mostly—but not always (Luke 17:6)—in the special material.[6] In Matthew, however, only Ἰησοῦς appears. And this name has not been taken from a mythical context. Already long ago, A. Deissmann refuted any idea of a cultic use of the Greek transcriptions of ישׁוע, derived from the early and later recurrent יהושׁע,[7] in pre-Christian times.[8] Nor is there sufficient evidence for assuming that the "Joshua christology" later emerging in some early Christian writings[9] depended on the existence of a Joshua myth in ancient Judaism.[10] Ἰησοῦς is essentially a personal name.[11] *The sayings are rooted in a historical person carrying the name of a historical individual.* The named attribution to Jesus

---

1   *Tendencies*, 185.
2   21:11; 26:69, 71; 27:17, 22; 28:5. Cf. also 27:37.
3   KJÆR-HANSEN, *Jesus*, 304–306.
4   Characterization and Christology, 589.
5   Cf. Luke 7:13; 10:1f, 41; 11:39; 12:42; 13:15; 17:6; 18:6.
6   Cf. FOERSTER, *TDNT* III, 288.
7   Cf. KJÆR-HANSEN, *Jesus*, 81–100.
8   The Name 'Jesus', 3–11.
9   Justin Martyr († c. 165 C.E.) is an early representative. Cf. e.g. Justin's justification for the messianic interpretation of the blessing of Judah (Gen 49:10) in Dial. 120:3: "For all of us from all the Gentiles do not wait for Judah, but Ἰησοῦν, the one who also led your fathers out of Egypt" (καὶ γὰρ Ἰούδαν πάντες οἱ ἀπὸ τῶν ἐθνῶν πάντων οὐ προσδοκῶμεν, ἀλλὰ Ἰησοῦν, τὸν καὶ τοὺς πατέρας ὑμῶν ἐξ Αἰγύπτου ἐξαγαγόντα).

10   FOERSTER, *TDNT* III, 290–293.—In an unpublished paper R.A. Kraft cautiously adduces some Samaritan and Qumranic texts not considered by Foerster. But even if these questionable references are taken into account, the evidence does not amount to the existence of an actual "Joshua messianology" in the main stream of ancient Judaism.

11   DEISSMANN, The Name 'Jesus', 11, concludes: "Thus when in the New Testament a Galilean Jew bore the name *Jesus* it was only one instance among dozens of authenticated similar cases and among hundreds of others. At first his name had only the character of a plain personal name." For Matthew more specifically, see KINGSBURY, *Matthew: Structure, Christology, Kingdom*, 84f.

locates the sayings within a historical situation of the past.

To some extent, this corresponds to a similar phenomenon in the rabbinic literature. In that context the named attribution serves to give the teaching its "traditionality," its fundamental and authoritative basis in the past, as I concluded in chapter three.[1]

But there are also striking differences. To start with, the narrative form of the story gives the name an emphatic connotation. A fact seldom noticed is the consistent presence of the definite article in front of Ἰησοῦς. Of all the introductions to Jesus-sayings that contain Ἰησοῦς, only two give the name without the definite article (21:1; 28:9), and in both cases some MSS include it.[2] Although ancient Greek writers vary, the normal practice at the time is to use the article anaphorically.[3] It points back to a person already named or assumed to be known. It is therefore not the special significance of Jesus' name *itself* that causes the article. In Matthew it remains essentially a personal name of a historical individual. The narrator introduces also sayings of other characters with the definite article in front of the name.[4] And outside of the gospel narratives and Acts, in texts where narrative anaphora does not explicitly come into view, the nominative Ἰησοῦς is always anarthrous, also in cases where no appositional words are added.[5] The emphatic connotation emerges rather out of the presentation of the story in the form of a narrative.[6] Therefore, the presence of the definite article in the narrative strengthens the referential stability of the name.[7]

It is also probable that Ἰησοῦς carries an emphatic connotation unrelated to the anaphoric function of its definite article in the narrative. In 1:21 an angel gives the name Ἰησοῦς a decisive interpretation. 1:21–25 connects the soteriological implications of Ἰησοῦς with Ἐμμανουήλ. The parallel between καλέσεις τὸ ὄνομα αὐτοῦ Ἰησοῦν (1:21), καλέσουσιν τὸ ὄνομα αὐτοῦ Ἐμμανουήλ (1:23) and ἐκάλεσεν τὸ ὄνομα αὐτοῦ Ἰησοῦν (1:25), with the formula quotation in 1:23 exactly in the middle of the unit,[8] shows that Ἰησοῦς and Ἐμμανουήλ interpret each other.[9] The name Ἰησοῦς is given a

---

[1]   See above pp. 139f.

[2]   Some MSS omit the article also in 20:32; 23:1. This may reflect Semitic idiom. The nominative Ἰησοῦς is usually anarthrous in the LXX, also in cases where no appositional phrase is added (Exod 17:10, 13; 32:17; Josh 1:10, 12; 3:1, 5, 6, 9, etc.). Cf. M. BLACK, *Aramaic Approach,* 95; HOFFMANN/VON SIEBENTHAL, *Grammatik,* § 134b.

[3]   Cf. e.g. MOULTON, *Grammar,* 83; HOFFMANN/VON SIEBENTHAL, *Grammatik,* § 134a.

[4]   Cf. e.g. the introductions to sayings of John the Baptist (3:14; 11:2f; 14:4) and Peter (14:28; 15:15; 16:22; 17:4; 18:21; 19:27; 26:33, 35).

[5]   Cf. 1 Thess 4:14; Heb 6:20; 7:22; 13:12; 1 John 2:22; 4:15; 5:1, 5; Rev 22:16.

[6]   Cf. BDF, § 260.

[7]   Cf. BURNETT, Characterization and Christology, 589.

[8]   1:21f and 1:24f contain 33 words each. There are no serious textcritical problems.

[9]   Cf. KJÆR-HANSEN, *Jesus,* 292–297.

pronounced "semantic inscription."[1]
Although the name of Jesus indeed denotes a historical person, it is also emphatic. The narrative form of the story and the name itself imply this. There exists therefore a striking contrast between Jesus' name and the names attached to sayings of rabbis in the rabbinical literature. We do not find a large number of teachers whose different names are mentioned and whose various sayings are subordinated to the collective voice of the text in Matthew.[2] There is one name above all other names! This feature in Matthew must reflect the transmission process, to some degree. Jesus' name was the uncomparably most important means to identify the traditions. *The one carrying the name Ἰησοῦς was the only teacher and from him, the transmitters believed, all normative tradition ultimately emerged.*

2.2. The Sayings of Other Characters

There are several characters in Matthew. Jesus is not the only actor speaking, and his sayings are not, as in the rabbinic literature, presented in isolation from episodal narration about what other persons say and do. For the issue at hand, it is of interest to see how the identification of sayings given by other persons related to the dominating presentation of Jesus in the process of transmission.

2.2.1. The Material

There are, in fact, many characters speaking in Matthew besides Jesus. A broad classification points to thirty-four different speakers:

Table 1

Jewish leader(s)	2:5f; 9:3, 11; 9:34; 12:2, 10, 24, 38; 15:2; 19:3, 7; 21:16, 23, 25b–26, 27, 31, 41; 22:16f, 21, 24–28, 36, 42; 26:5, 62, 63, 65f, 68; 27:4b, 6, 42f, 63f; 28:13
disciple(s)	8:21, 25b; 13:10, 36, 51; 14:15, 17, 33; 15:12, 23, 33, 34; 16:14; 17:10, 19; 18:1; 19:10, 25; 21:20; 24:3; 26:8f, 17, 22
Peter alone	14:28, 30; 16:16, 22; 17:4, 25, 26; 18:21;

---

1   Cf. BURNETT, Characterization and Christology, 591–295.

2   DEISSMANN, The Name 'Jesus', 16–26, points even to the tendency in the history of the NT texts to obliterate or make unrecognisable Ἰησοῦς where it occurs as the name of another person. He refers esp. to variants in Matt 27:16f; Luke 3:29; Acts 7:45; 13:6; Col 4:11. In addition, he believes that the name was originally present in Mark 15:7, with reference to Barabbas, and in Phlm 23f, with reference to Jesus Justus mentioned in Col 4:11. Cf. also TAYLOR, *Names of Jesus,* 5f. I have not been able to verify Deissmann's view in all cases. For the general, though apparently limited, influence of christology upon textual transmission, see HEAD, *NovT* 35 (1993) 105–129.

	19:27; 26:33, 35, 70, 72, 74
the people, the crowds	8:27; 9:33; 12:23; 13:54–56;[1] 21:9, 10,[2] 11; 27:21b, 22b, 23b, 25
John the Baptist	3:2, 7–12, 14; 14:4
Pilate the governor	27:11, 13, 17, 21a, 22a, 23a, 24, 65
an (the) angel	1:20f; 2:13, 20; 28:5–7
two blind men	9:27, 28; 20:30, 31, 33
Judas Iscariot	26:15, 25, 48, 49; 27:4a
a (the) centurion (and those with him)	8:6, 8f; 27:54
people standing (passing) by	26:73; 27:40, 47, 49
the devil (tempter)	4:3, 6, 9
a Canaanite woman	15:22, 25, 27
the young man	19:16, 18, 20
a heavenly voice	3:17; 17:5
John's disciples	9:14; 11:3
a servant-girl	26:69, 71
a man of the crowd	17:15f
wise men	2:2
Herod the king	2:8
a leper	8:2
one scribe	8:19
demoniacs	8:29
the demons	8:31
a ruler	9:18
a bleeding woman	9:21
an anonymous person	12:47[3]
Herod the tetrarch	14:2
Herodias' daughter	14:8
the Zebedees' mother	20:21
the Zebedees	20:22
two false witnesses	26:61
the wife of Pilate	27:19
the soldiers	27:29.

The different speakers appearing besides Jesus are not equally frequent and significant. It is immediately evident that the Jewish leaders and the disciples—with Peter as the personal representative mentioned by name—often occur as characters attributed sayings of various kinds. John the Baptist gives the longest unbroken utterance (3:7–12).

2.2.2. The Function of the Sayings of Other Characters

The sayings of other characters reveal significant differences compared to the ones attributed to Jesus. They are usually brief. There are no examples

---

[1] I.e. those gathered in the synagogue of Jesus' home-town.
[2] I.e. the people of all Jerusalem.
[3] This verse is textcritically uncertain.

of various sayings collected to constitute one comprehensive speech. The most extended utterance is the one ascribed to John the Baptist in 3:7–12.[1] But in the vast majority of cases, the sayings are contained within one single verse.[2]

They are also often without a well-aimed significance in the argument of the context. Most of the thirty-two utterances of the Jewish leaders are as statements, questions, answers or requests regularly subordinated to an all-important Jesus-saying.[3] With the possible exception of 2:5f,[4] the remaining ones are thoroughly embedded within episodal comments developing the negative characterization of the Jewish leaders.[5]

The same subordinated status is evident also in the sayings uttered by positive characters apart from Jesus. Among the twenty-three utterances attributed to the disciples, only the confession in 14:33 appears as a statement not immediately followed by other words of Jesus himself. Similarly, with the exception of the confession in 16:16, the fourteen utterances ascribed to Peter are mostly simple questions (18:21; 19:27), answers (17:25, 26), requests (14:28, 30) or wrongly aimed statements.[6] From the remaining cases, the most pointed sayings are ascribed to John the Baptist in 3:2, 7–12, an (the) angel in 1:20f; 28:5–7, the centurion and those with him in 27:54 and a heavenly voice in 3:17; 17:5. Some other sayings, though of less independent importance, could also be mentioned.[7] But the majority of the utterances do not by themselves carry the pointed significance usually so characteristic of Jesus' own sayings.

Even the significant sayings that remain gain their importance by directly testifying about Jesus.[8] They never deal with other doctrinal or ethical matters, as Jesus may do in his own speeches and sayings. The focus on Jesus sometimes seems to have been a deliberate force in the reshaping of the tradition. The important saying of John the Baptist in 3:2 occurs already at the beginning of the pericope. With some changes, it was taken over from the utterance ascribed to Jesus in Mark 1:15. In Matthew it receives its force from being the preaching of Jesus himself (4:17), and further, from being the preaching that Jesus expects his disciples to give (10:7). The extended utterance of John in 3:7–12 was probably, with some freedom, put together

---

[1] It consists of approximately 120 words. Textcritical uncertainties occur esp. in 3:12.

[2] From a total of 145 separate utterances, 131 are contained within one verse.

[3] So the utterances in 9:3, 11; 12:2, 10, 24, 38; 15:2; 19:3, 7; 21:16, 23, 25b–26, 27, 31, 41; 22:16f, 21, 24–28, 36, 42; 26:63.

[4] Note however that the common introduction to the formula quotations (1:22, 2:15, 17, 23; 4:14; 8:17; 12:17; 13:35; 21:4; 27:9) is not used here.

[5] So the utterances in 9:34; 26:5, 62, 65f, 68; 27:4b, 6, 42f, 63f; 28:13.

[6] 16:22; 17:4; 26:33, 35, 70, 72, 74.

[7] Cf. 2:2; 9:33; 15:27; 20:33; 21:9, 11(?); 27:25

[8] Cf. 1:20f; 2:5f; 3:2, 7–12, 17; 14:33; 16:16; 17:5; 27:54; 28:5–7.

out of some separate units.[1] In the unit emerging in Matthew, the accusing words in 3:7–10 are immediately followed and interpreted by statements about the one who is more powerful than John (3:11f), not as in Luke 3:7–9, 10–14 by further discussions about what the crowds should do. In 3:17; 17:5 the heavenly voice speaks openly about Jesus in the third person (οὗτός ἐστιν) as being the Son of God. Mark and Luke give such a third person reference only at the transfiguration (Mark 9:7/Luke 9:35), while at the baptism (Mark 1:11/Luke 3:22) they restrict the address to Jesus only (σὺ εἶ). The almost identical confession of the disciples and of the centurion and those with him in 14:33 and 27:54 was probably incorporated from Mark 15:39. But by inverting υἱὸς θεοῦ into θεοῦ υἱός, which apart from Matt 27:43 is not attested elsewhere in the NT, Matthew created a certain emphasis on the divinity of Jesus' sonship.[2] The confession in 16:16 shows through its attribution to Simon Peter instead of Peter merely—as in Mark 8:29/Luke 9:20—a close association with the disciple himself. But in Matthew the confession depends on Jesus' ultimate affirmation. Peter gives in Matthew a longer and fuller christological utterance than in the other synoptics. And the confession is immediately attached to Jesus' own blessing in 16:17, which constitutes the structural centre of 16:13–20.[3] And finally, while the saying of the angel(s) in Matt 28:5–7/Mark 16:6f/Luke 24:5–7 always concerns Jesus' resurrection, Matthew exhibits in comparison with Mark a stronger focus on the resurrection.[4] Its mention in 28:5b–6, including the reference to what Jesus himself said (καθὼς εἶπεν), appears at the centre of 28:1–10.[5] It is also accentuated by the repetition of ἠγέρθη—together with the probably original addition of ἀπὸ τῶν νεκρῶν—in 28:7.[6]

In short, *the sayings attributed to other characters than Jesus are in Matthew usually very brief and insignificant or entirely focused on Jesus.* Other characters never give important teaching on doctrinal and ethical matters. Significant attributions to specific individuals do appear—especially to John the Baptist and, to some extent, Peter. But even these sayings gain their force by their constant association with Jesus. They function to build up the characterization of him.

The identification of the sayings indicates in two ways how the setting and motives of transmission correlated with the process of transmission.

---

[1] For Matt 3:7–10, cf. Luke 3:7–9; for Matt 3:11f, cf. Mark 1:7f/Luke 3:16f.

[2] Cf. MOWERY, *NovT* 32 (1990) 195–199.

[3] See above pp. 278f.

[4] It remains uncertain, however, if Mark 16:1–8 is the only text behind Matt 28:1–10.

[5] According to the text accepted in the 26th edition of Nestle-Aland, the statement Ἰησοῦν τὸν ἐσταυρωμένον ζητεῖτε· οὐκ ἔστιν ὧδε, ἠγέρθη γὰρ καθὼς εἶπεν· δεῦτε ἴδετε τὸν τόπον ὅπου ἔκειτο forms the centre of 28:1–10. Before and after this statement, there are 78 words in the pericope, which contains 173 words altogether. The numerical pattern is 78+17+78=173.

[6] Cf. NEIRYNCK, *NTS* 15 (1968–69) 175; GNILKA, *Matthäusevangelium* II, 491.

First, *the Jesus tradition was in its main elements transmitted isolated from the sayings of other characters.* G. Kittel stressed, as we saw in the introduction, that this was the case already from the beginning in early Christianity as a whole.[1] The fact that the Jesus tradition is normally not quoted explicitly outside of the gospel narratives may be an indication that it was in fact transmitted separated from other early Christian material.[2] It certainly provides no reason for rejecting the very existence of an authentic oral tradition.[3] However, as far as Matthew is concerned, the identification of traditions suggests in a general manner that *there was no entirely free incorporation and integration of traditions from other persons into the Jesus tradition.* We have noticed the striking historical fact that the voice of Jesus dominates completely in Matthew. The named attribution to Jesus is strongly accentuated. This is a general indication, but I will substantiate it further below when discussing Matthew's aim to preserve the Jesus tradition. Second, the manner of presenting the material suggests that *the sayings from other characters did not carry a status independent of Jesus' teaching during the transmission.* Not even important and pointed utterances from others could be separated from the Jesus tradition in its Matthean form. Matthew treated those sayings of other characters that did enter into the body of transmitted material as integrated within the tradition identified by reference to Jesus himself. They were essentially *Jesus* tradition.

3. The Means of Transmission

Matthew contains no explicit information about the means by which the Jesus tradition was carried and conveyed. A discussion comparable to the theoretical emphasis on oral teaching and oral transmission in rabbinic literature is absent. The case is more as in the prophetic literature and the Dead Sea scrolls, where the means of transmission is of no theoretical interest and the oral/aural actualization, handing over and reception of various kinds of texts convey the voice of the teacher. We may consequently find information about the means of transmission only indirectly.

This is not an easy way to go. More than twenty years ago, E. Güttgemanns objected to the levelling of the distinction between the oral character of pre-synoptic genres and the written gospel narratives.[4] In more recent years, W.H. Kelber has developed Güttgemanns' objection and brought the

---

[1] *Probleme des palästinischen Spätjudentums,* 69 n. 3.
[2] GERHARDSSON, Weg der Evangelientradition, 81, 83. A possible exception is Acts 20:35, though as PLÜMACHER, *ZNW* 83 (1992) 270–275, points out, this is perhaps merely a reminiscence influenced first of all by Thuc. II 97:3f.
[3] *Contra* TEEPLE, *JBL* 89 (1970) 63.
[4] *Offene Fragen,* 69–166, 252.

strict dichotomy between orality and literacy,[1] with Mark's alleged disruption of the oral currency on the pre-synoptic level, into the centre of debate.[2] B.W. Henaut, while critizising Kelber's dichotomy, goes as far as to claim that the oral phase is forever lost behind a series of gospel texts and pre-gospel sources.[3] Nevertheless, others take seriously that literate and oral societies and communities exist in a continuity, not in a dichotomy.[4] Scholars are also aware of the complicated relationship between literacy and orality as information technologies. R. Finnegan, one of the most respected experts in this field, stresses throughout her collection of studies that specific social and cultural factors play a more crucial role than literacy and orality—or modern telecommunications—in conditioning human actions. There can be no sharp division between literate and oral societies. She concludes that "on the topics of oral and written transmission there are no simple and generalizable answers or even clear-cut definitions."[5] Scrutiny of a number of texts from various corners in the ancient Israelite, Jewish-Hellenistic and Greco-Roman world shows that written compositions can be used to deliniate oral traditions only with much caution.[6] The issue needs to be considered anew from case to case.

I will approach the problem in a way which is in agreement with my view of Matthew's narrative as a reflection of the transmission process. P. Achtemeier, to mention one, focuses on the indications in written compositions which point to the way the author himself wanted his material to be performed.[7] Such a study reveals indirectly how the author conceptualized the means of transmission. I will combine this approach with the common "source-oriented" question concerning the media of transmission. As a first step, *I will study how Matthew encoded the means of transmission into his story. The authorial conceptions emerging out of the story will then lead to a consideration of how Matthew actually incorporated previous texts— written and oral—into his own structural arrangement and narrative.*

---

[1]   Kelber uses the term "textuality" instead of "literacy." But since the terms "text" and "texture" may refer to a "web" of meanings expressed also by oral media, I prefer the term "literacy."

[2]   *The Oral and the Written Gospel.*

[3]   *Oral Tradition.*

[4]   Cf. ROSENBERG, *Oral Tradition* 2:1 (1987) 74.

[5]   *Literacy,* 174.

[6]   This is one of the major conclusions that several independent scholars agreed upon after two conferences about oral tradition before, in and outside of the gospel narratives. See WANSBROUGH (ed.), *Jesus and the Oral Gospel Tradition,* 12. The variety of contributing scholars and studied texts gives this conclusion its force. Cf. my review in *STK* 69 (1993) 85–87.

[7]   *JBL* 109 (1990) 3–27. Cf. also already LOHR, *CBQ* 23 (1961) 403–435, and more recently DEWEY, *Int* 43 (1989) 32–44; HENDERSON, *JBL* 111 (1992) 283–306.

3.1. Verbal and Behavioural Transmission in the Story

Matthew speaks about two means of appropriating Jesus' teaching, through hearing (ἀκούειν) and doing (ποιεῖν). When teaching is carried on, it becomes a tradition which is transmitted. Hearing and doing therefore correspond to what B. Gerhardsson calls "verbal tradition" and "behavioural tradition."[1] The two aspects of the tradition imply two means of transmission: by words and by actions.

As we saw in the discussion of the didactic-biographical motives of transmission, Matthew exhibits an interest that goes beyond the mere concentration on words and incorporates the therapeutic deeds into the teaching itself. There is a kind of visual teaching. Matthew's emphasis on hearing and doing as means of appropriating the teaching is broader. It relates to the totality of Jesus' teaching by word and deed. It is of interest to look at this emphasis as an index to the author's understanding of the verbal and behavioural means to transmit the Jesus tradition.

3.1.1. Hearing the Teaching of Jesus

Forms of ἀκούειν occur approximately sixty-three times in Matthew.[2] In at least twenty-eight cases, the term refers in one way or the other to hearing the words of Jesus.[3] It is not a technical term for receiving teaching. The use is variated. But some instances are more significant than others.

Jesus speaks in 7:24, 26 of hearing his words. The words denote Jesus' teaching in the Sermon on the Mount. 7:15ff discloses indeed that Jesus subordinates hearing to doing.[4] I will explore this fact below. Yet the audible means of appropriating the teaching is not unimportant. Hearing receives its significance from two angles. First, the emphasis on hearing relates intertextually to the beginning of the Shemaᶜ.[5] Although Matthew never quotes the call to hear in Deut 6:4, he allows the interpreted Shemaᶜ to play an important role below the surface of the story.[6] He uses it to interpret Jesus'

---

1   Gospel Tradition, 501f.

2   STRECKER, *ZNW* 69 (1978) 45, counts 66 occurrences. But see GUNDRY, *Matthew,* 641; MORGENTHALER, *Statistik,* 70; SCHENK, *Sprache des Matthäus,* 383; U. LUZ, *Matthäus* I, 36. Additional instances are present in some MSS of 11:15; 13:9, 43; 15:31. Mark has 44 and Luke 65 occurrences. For the significance of hearing and teaching in Mark, see MEYE, *Jesus and the Twelve,* 49–51.

3   7:24, 26; 10:27; 11:4, 15; 13:9, 16, 17 (*ter*), 18, 19, 20, 22, 23, 43; 15:10, 12; 17:5; 19:22, 25; 20:24; 21:33, 45; 22:22, 33; 26:65; 27:47. Cf. also 11:5; 12:19, 42; 13:13–15. SCHENK, *Sprache des Matthäus,* 382–386, mentions other semantically related terms. For our purposes, only οὖς (10:27; 11:15; 13:9, 15 [*bis*], 16, 43) is of some interest, though this term is always connected with ἀκούειν in Matthew.

4   Cf. already 7:12.

5   Cf. excursus 13 below.

6   See above pp. 300–302 and below pp. 361–364.

obedience to God and the disciples' obedience to Jesus. The latter aspect is of interest here. 11:29; 19:17; 23:8–10 suggest that Jesus' followers should conform to the Shema^c in their obedience to Jesus.[1] It is therefore possible that Jesus' advice to hear his teaching gains its force through a confessional text implying a fundamental religious duty of obedience to Jesus. Second, 7:24, 26 speak of hearing in a context dealing partly with the appropriation of tradition.[2] The Antitheses contain repeated references to what the audience had previously heard (5:21, 27, 33, 38, 43). It is true that ἀκούειν is not central in all the antithetical constructions. It is not even present in 5:31. Nevertheless, we may perceive a certain relationship between what Jesus says and what the audience had heard was said (by God) to those of ancient times. The listeners had heard the Torah, we may assume, as it was read and expounded to them. They appropriated the tradition through hearing a text and its exposition, the torah tradition. Jesus places his own utterances in connection with this.[3] The relation between what was heard and what Jesus says suggests that hearing Jesus' words connotes in 7:24, 26 a means of appropriating the tradition.

The pertinent question is of course whether ἀκούειν carries a connotation of memorizing in Matthew. The Shema^c connects the call to hear with an emphatic demand that the people, by various measures, should remember the words of Yahweh and pass it on to following generations (Deut 6:6–9; 11:18–21).[4] It is probable that some kind of memorizing is involved in this call.[5] This use of שמע becomes prominent in tannaitic and amoraic texts. The term there often denotes the active hearing and learning of a biblical text together with its exposition or of a halakhic tradition.[6]

It is impossible to decide with certainty if hearing implies memorizing in Matthew. In many cases it obviously does not. It simply means listening passively. The opponents, for instance, hear various utterances of Jesus.[7] Of course, this does not mean that they memorize them. Even a foolish man hears Jesus' words (7:26). Nevertheless, listening to Jesus is an important act, even called for by God (17:5), when the disciples are concerned. Restricting the observations here to the use of ἀκούειν, we may find indication that a connotation of memorizing is, it seems, occasionally present.

Hearing is on several occasions in Matthew a preliminary act. It must involve or be followed by other steps in order to effect the full appropriation of Jesus' words. 7:24, 26 relate hearing to doing. Hearing is in 10:27 a pre-

---

1   See above pp. 300–302.
2   Cf. H.D. BETZ, *Sermon on the Mount*, 4.
3   For a fuller discussion of the antithetical construction, see below pp. 391–396.
4   Cf. also Num 15:37–40.
5   Cf. RIESNER, *Lehrer*, 122f.
6   BACHER, *Die exegetische Terminologie* I, 189–192; *idem, Die exegetische Terminologie* II, 189–192. Cf. also *idem, Tradition und Tradenten*, 9–15.
7   Cf. 15:12; 21:45; 22:22; 26:65.

requisite for preaching. The disciples "must become hearers of Jesus before they can be preachers."[1] A most important connection, which in most cases is Matthean,[2] is that hearing should aim towards understanding (συνιέναι). 13:13 states that one may hear but still neither hear nor understand.[3] This suggests that there exists a kind of hearing which is not passive listening, but which leads ultimately to understanding. The right kind of hearing must be done with attention.[4] It should be an active step towards understanding. God's command that the disciples should listen to Jesus (17:5) relates therefore to their subsequent understanding (17:13). The narrative meshalim, in particular, emphasize the close connection between hearing and understanding.[5] The active hearing is the first step towards the understanding which the disciples do achieve (13:51).[6] Perhaps the Matthean introduction in 13:24, 31, παραβολὴν παρέθηκεν αὐτοῖς, even contains technichal transmission terminology.[7]

When we view the story as an index to Matthew's own understanding of the transmission, we may here detect a distinction in the appropriation of the narrative meshalim, at least. Others have argued on the basis of different observations that the transmitters memorized the basic text first and reflected on its meaning subsequently.[8] It is true that folklore studies in the line of M. Parry and A.B. Lord have often made generalizing claims that memorizing in the sense of a word-for-word repetition is uncommon in oral cultures.[9] Such claims cause some biblical scholars to reject the notion that early Christian transmitters memorized a basic text.[10] But due attention should also be paid to Finnegan's pluralistic model of oral literature. She

---

1 HORST, *TDNT* V, 553. Cf. similarly GNILKA, *BibLeb* 2 (1961) 76.

2 13:14, 15 (OT quotation) do not have any clear parallels. 17:13 has no parallel. In Matt 13:19/Mark 4:15/Luke 8:12; Matt 13:23/Mark 4:20/Luke 8:15, Matthew alone has references to understanding. Only in Matt 13:13/Mark 4:12/Luke 8:10; Matt 15:10/Mark 7:14 are both terms present also in the parallels. For Matthew's view on the understanding of the disciples, see further above pp. 228–234.

3 In 15:10 Jesus exhorts the crowd to hear and understand, while the Pharisees apparently hear without understanding (15:12). In 21:45 the opponents' understanding of a narrative mashal, which is introduced with the command to hear (21:33), is of a different kind. The understanding is therefore described with γινώσκειν, not συνιέναι.

4 Cf. the repeated formula ὁ ἔχων ὦτα ἀκουέτω in 11:15; 13:9, 43.

5 Cf. 13:13–15, 19, 23, 51; 15:10.

6 Cf. also 16:12; 17:13. In spite of the command to hear and understand in 15:10, it is not stated in the following verses whether the crowd did eventually understand or not.

7 Cf. 1 Tim 1:18; 2 Tim 2:2.

8 Cf. VINCENT, *SE* 3 (1964) 114–116; GERHARDSSON, *NTS* 14 (1967–68) 188; *idem, NTS* 19 (1972–73) 19; RIESNER, *Lehrer*, 369f, 374–377; *idem*, Jesus as Teacher and Preacher, 205.

9 GOODY, *Domestication*, 118 states: "Reproduction is rarely if ever verbatim." This represents the view of several scholars influenced by the so-called "oral-formulaic school." For an overview of the most important contributions of this school, see FOLEY, *Theory of Oral Composition*.

10 Cf. e.g. KELBER, *The Oral and the Written Gospel*, 27; SELLIN, *EvT* 50 (1990) 317f.

not only asserts that variability rather than verbal identity of orally transmitted pieces is common,[1] but also stresses specifically that there are notable exceptions.[2] The performance of a text does sometimes depend on the
previous composition and exact memorization. Even Lord himself noticed,
somewhat to his regret, that once the art of writing entered into the
situation of the Balkan singers, people began to memorize a written or an
oral text word-for-word.[3] They no longer memorized only certain formulas and themes of a song. This procedure of *verbatim* memorization was
clearly present in those parts of antiquity where writing was known.[4] And
Matthew knew how to write. It is possible that the task of memorizing and
understanding certain texts was given to some trained specialists in the community. The disciples' affirmative response to the question of understanding is emphatically linked (διὰ τοῦτο) with the task of a scribe being or becoming a disciple for the kingdom of heaven (13:51f).[5] Just as the scribe
according to Sir 39:2f is to understand the meshalim,[6] so perhaps the scribal
functionaries of the community had a special responsibility to reveal the
significance of memorized narrative meshalim. Scribal features of literacy
then interacted with the oral culture and made memorization of rather fixed
texts possible. As it seems, Matthew pictures an early Christian community—with its specialists—actively hearing Jesus' teaching with the aim of
(later) understanding it.[7]

3.1.2. Doing the Teaching of Jesus

Forms of ποιεῖν occur approximately eighty-six times in Matthew.[8] Only
one aspect of doing is of importance here, namely when it functions as a
means of appropriating Jesus' teaching.[9]

---

[1]   *Oral Poetry,* 54–58.—KELBER, *The Oral and the Written Gospel,* 27, pays attention only to this point in Finnegan's study. ONG, *Orality and Literacy,* 62–64, rejects
Finnegan's findings but acknowledges other examples of *verbatim* memorization among
oral peoples.

[2]   Cf. e.g. *Oral Poetry,* 73–86, 142; *idem, Literacy,* 90, 158, 166f, 172f.—FINNE-
GAN, What is Oral Literature?, 243–282, presents a concise critique of the generalizations
within the oral-formulaic school. She bases it on her own field-work.

[3]   *Singer of Tales,* 109, 129f, 136f. Cf. also *idem,* Memory, 460. This practice was
for Lord incompatible with a sense of orality and traditionality.

[4]   See GERHARDSSON, *Memory,* 123–130; RIESNER, *Lehrer,* 441–443; HARRIS,
Literacy, 30–33.

[5]   Cf. ORTON, *Understanding Scribe,* 137–153.

[6]   Cf. also Sir 1:25; 3:29 (13:26[G]); 20:20; 38:33; 47:15, 17 and above pp. 47, 81.

[7]   Cf. the famous observation by MANSON, *NTS* 1 (1954–55) 58, that "the early
Church remembered better than it understood." I would add that they did also try to understand.

[8]   MORGENTHALER, *Statistik,* 133; *idem,* Beiheft, 10, 14; SCHENK, *Sprache des
Matthäus,* 246; U. LUZ, *Matthäus* I, 49.—GUNDRY, *Matthew,* 647, counts only 84. The
two occurrences in 7:18 are somewhat uncertain. Mark has 47 instances; Luke 88.

[9]   SCHENK, *Sprache des Matthäus,* 245–248, discusses other terms semantically re-

A general correlation between verbal and behavioural *acts of teaching* appears on several occasions in Matthew.[1] First, 5:19bα combines the teacher's task to do and to teach. Doing is here the positive counterpart of setting aside (λύειν) one of the least of these commandments in 5:19aα. This structural relation between λύειν and ποιεῖν suggests that also the former term primarily describes an act that accompanies the teaching. The close correspondence between doing and teaching becomes even clearer as 5:19aα first describes the false act of setting aside the commandments and subsequently adds "and teaches accordingly" (καὶ διδάξῃ οὕτως). The teacher normally teaches in accordance with his actions. Second, 5:16 testifies in the same direction. In 5:13 Jesus starts to emphasize the disciples' exemplary function in relation to other people. 5:16 then makes evident that the good deeds of the disciples should serve as a kind of moral proof to men. 5:19a relates to this and speaks of the disciples' actions and teaching in relation to men. We may add that the reference to salt in 5:13—possibly also the reference to light in 5:14–16[2]—perhaps indicates the didactic function of the disciples,[3] though we cannot be sure.[4] Salt was occasionally thought of as the wisdom of the scribe (m. Soṭa 9:15).[5] Third, 7:15–20 warns certain persons by stating that a tree can only be known by the fruit it produces (ποιεῖν). It is not impossible to regard this warning as aimed against prophetic persons whose actions miscredit their words.[6] The action and the teaching go hand in hand and give testimony to each other, whether positively or negatively. Fourth, while 21:23 presents Jesus as teaching in the temple, the following question and answer (21:24, 27) concern what Jesus is doing. The teaching is part of a larger framework dealing with Jesus' actions.[7] Fifth, the close connection between teaching and doing is evident also in 23:2f, 5.[8] Jesus reacts against the discrepancy between what the opponents say and do,[9] regardless of his seemingly positive attitude to their words here.[10] Their words must be accompanied by adequate acts.

The correlation between verbal and behavioural acts of teaching puts a

---

lated to ποιεῖν in Matthew.

1 Elsewhere in the NT, a similar connection is present only in Acts 1:1.

2 For light as wisdom (law), see AALEN, *Die Begriffe 'Licht' und 'Finsternis'*, 175–178, 183–192. Cf. also CONZELMANN, *TDNT* IX, 323–327.

3 So NAUCK, *ST* 6 (1952) 165–178, esp. 177.

4 Cf. the criticism of Nauck by LATHAM, *Symbolism of Salt*, 226f.

5 Cf. also b. Qidd. 29b speaking of someone's son as bright and "salty" (ממולח). For other references from the rabbinic literature and the early church, cf. NAUCK, *ST* 6 (1952) 166–170.

6 Cf. the discussion of 7:15–23 below p. 361.

7 Cf. above p. 280.

8 Cf. also 6:1.

9 Cf. also 23:23.

10 GARLAND, *Matthew 23*, 46–55, concludes that 23:2f serves merely as a rhetorical stratagem which sets the scene for the following impeachment.

similar emphasis on a correlation between hearing and doing as means of *appropriating* the teaching. There is, to be sure, not much explicit evidence of actual imitation in Matthew or elsewhere in the synoptic tradition. Matthew never states in plain words that Jesus is an ethical model to be imitated (μιμεῖσθαι).[1] But there is plenty of implicit evidence.

We find a general emphasis on doing in Matthew.[2] The Shemaᶜ, so important as an inter-text, puts the threefold command to act in love after the initial call to hear (Deut 6:5).[3] Doing is in Matthew a religious act expressing obedience to the will of God. The active practice of the Father's will is the essential identity marker of Jesus' true family (12:50). Jesus shows this attitude of obedience himself (26:39, 42) and teaches his disciples to exhibit a similar disposition in their prayer (6:10). It has implications for the future admisson to the kingdom of heaven (7:21).[4]

Obedience to God is inseparable from obedience to Jesus. 12:49 defines Jesus' true family more narrowly than Mark 3:34. It consists of the disciples only. The will of the Father is done within Jesus' true family. 25:31–46 suggests that actions done towards Jesus and his followers determine decisions concerning eternal life.

Obedience expresses itself first of all in doing—practising—the *words* of Jesus. Jesus points in 7:21 to the importance of doing the will of his heavenly Father and continues in 7:24–27 by stressing the importance of performing his own words. Jesus' words reveal the will of God. Practising the words of Jesus means to do the will of the heavenly Father. This is the all-important act,[5] even taking precedence over hearing. Already 7:12 points to the importance of doing. 7:15ff makes it the dominating theme. In 7:24–27 it is practising, not only hearing, the words of Jesus that makes the difference between the wise and the foolish man.

Doing is a means of appropriating the verbal teaching in the fullest sense. It is not merely the subsequent result of learning acquired previously by other means. Doing is part of the learning process itself in Matthew. In distinction to Luke 6:47–49, Matthew speaks in 7:24–27 of the wise man (ἀνὴρ φρόνιμος) and the foolish man (ἀνὴρ μωρός). The term φρόνιμος denotes in Matthew the wise and reflecting—even serpentine—person.[6] The wise man in 7:24 acquires learning by hearing *and* doing, by sense-perception, reflection *and* practice.[7] The one who hears without acting accordingly is

---

1 A. SCHULZ, *Nachfolgen*, 252–270, 332. Cf. also LARSSON, *Vorbild,* 39; H.D. BETZ, *Nachfolge,* 2f, 43; MOHRLANG, *Matthew and Paul,* 76.

2 For a basic classification of ποιεῖν in Matthew, see SCHENK, *Sprache des Matthäus,* 246–248.

3 Cf. also Num 15:39f; Deut 11:13.

4 Cf. also 18:14; 21:31.

5 Cf. excursus 13 below.

6 Cf. 10:16; 24:45; 25:2, 4, 8, 9.

7 Cf. H.D. BETZ, *Sermon on the Mount,* 6.

μωρός. Matthew employs this term elsewhere.[1] Most significant is its use as a negative counterpart to φρόνιμος in 25:1–13.[2] The contrast implied here shows that the wise persons are accepted, while the foolish ones are rejected altogether, in spite of calling Jesus κύριε (25:10–12). Persons calling Jesus κύριε are rejected also within the close context of 7:24–27. In 7:21–23 Jesus excludes them from the kingdom of heaven, because they do not act according to the Father's will. As it seems, the foolish ones know about Jesus; they had listened to his teaching and even prophecied and performed miracles in his name. But Jesus eventually rejects them, because they do not act according to his words revealing the will of the Father. Jesus' rejection shows that they had actually not learned anything at all. Doing is not simply the result of learning. It is the very means by which learning becomes effective in the total process of appropriating and internalizing Jesus' verbal teaching.[3] Without doing, learning is meaningless and ultimately no real learning at all![4]

Obedience expresses itself also as imitation of Jesus' *behaviour*. In 9:14; 12:1f Jesus is held responsible for the behaviour of the disciples and in 9:11; 17:24 the disciples are, in turn, approached with questions concerning the behaviour of their teacher.[5] The disciples are to imitate Jesus in their active ministry of preaching (10:7, 27) and of performing mighty acts (10:1, 8; 17:14–20; 21:21).

The imitation of Jesus has a moral significance. Just as God is an example motivating behaviour (5:48), there is an ethical dimension in Matthew's christology.[6] Jesus invites people to himself and to his teaching since he is gentle and humble in heart (11:28–30).[7] He is the perfect example.[8] His disciples are to imitate his service of God and of men (20:26–28; 23:11).[9] Servanthood is the essence of discipleship.[10] The disciples are even to carry a cross, in a sense (10:38; 16:24).[11]

---

[1]   5:22; 23:17 (19); 25:2, 3, 8. Cf. also μωραίνειν in 5:13.

[2]   25:2, 3f, 8f.

[3]   BERTRAM, *TDNT* IV, 842, states that in 7:24–27; 25:1–13 one learns to distinguish between what is wise and foolish by testing. But more accurately, one learns by doing.

[4]   Is there a further connection between the salt that looses its taste, "becomes foolish" (μωραίειν) in 5:13 and the foolish (μωρός) man in 7:26? The question deserves further investigation.

[5]   See DAUBE, *NTS* 19 (1972–73) 1–15.

[6]   GERHARDSSON, Sacrificial Service, 29; *idem, ET* 42 (1982) 124f.

[7]   MOHRLANG, *Matthew and Paul,* 76f. Cf. also LARSSON, *Vorbild,* 39; G. BARTH, Law, 104.

[8]   Cf. GERHARDSSON, *Ethos,* 54–60.

[9]   LARSSON, *Vorbild,* 39; GERHARDSSON, Sacrificial Service, 26, 29f; MOHRLANG, *Matthew and Paul,* 76. Cf. also A. SCHULZ, *Nachfolgen,* 252–265; H.D. BETZ, *Nachfolge,* 34.

[10]   Cf. KINGSBURY, *Matthew as Story,* 139–144.

[11]   Cf. also 23:34. See further LARSSON, *Vorbild,* 40–42; A. SCHULZ, *Nachfolgen,*

There are texts relating the imitation to didactic situations more specifically. 5:17 is of special importance. Scholars disagree about whether the two verbs (καταλύειν, πληροῦν) describe Jesus' verbal or behavioural teaching.[1] It is possible that this disagreement poses false alternatives.[2] A strict distinction between Jesus' words and Jesus' deeds is not present in Matthew.[3] The structure suggests that 5:17 concerns primarily what Jesus is doing,[4] though not in total separation from his verbal teaching.[5] The negative statements in 5:17, centring around καταλύειν, parallel the negative statements in 5:19a, centring around λύειν and διδάσκειν. This shows that the term καταλύειν relates to doing, without excluding the verbal teaching. The positive statement in 5:17 expressed with πληροῦν is consequently structurally connected with ποιεῖν and διδάσκειν in 5:19b. The term πληροῦν therefore also relates to doing, without excluding the verbal teaching.[6]

Jesus' behaviour functions in the argumentation of the context as a kind of proof supporting a case concerned with the action of the disciples. 5:13–16 stresses the good deeds of the disciples as visible testimony to other men. 5:17 then refers to the example from Jesus' own behaviour. 5:18 presents the theoretical basis. Jesus' ethos correlates with his logical reasoning.[7] 5:19 returns to the deeds—and the teaching—of the disciples. It applies (οὖν) the proofs to the future actions and teaching of the disciples. 5:20 relates (γάρ) the deeds of the disciples to moral righteousness,[8] which—in a manner

---

265–269; GERHARDSSON, *Sacrificial Service*, 32. Cf. also H.D. BETZ, *Nachfolge*, 34; G. BARTH, *Law*, 105.

[1] For various proposals, see LJUNGMAN, *Das Gesetz erfüllen*, 19–36; MCCON-NELL, *Law and Prophecy*, 14–17; U. LUZ, *ZTK* 75 (1978) 413f; BROER, *Freiheit vom Gesetz*, 26f; DAVIES/ALLISON, *Matthew* I, 485f; U. LUZ, *Matthäus* I, 232.

[2] Cf. LJUNGMAN, *Das Gesetz erfüllen*, 20, 34–36; U. LUZ, *ZTK* 75 (1978) 416; *idem, Matthäus* I, 236; WONG, *Interkulturelle Theologie*, 39–42.

[3] G. BARTH, *Law*, 69; DAVIES/ALLISON, *Matthew* I, 486 n. 11, do not pay sufficient attention to this and reject therefore unduly the interpretation which takes 5:17 as primarily referring to Jesus' obedience within the totality of his ministry.

[4] LJUNGMAN, *Das Gesetz erfüllen*, 19, 52f, 54, stresses also the use of γίνεσθαι in 5:18.

[5] For a similar view based primarily on the use of καταλύειν and πληροῦν in relation to νόμος in other Greek literature, see U. LUZ, *ZTK* 75 (1978) 415; *idem, Matthäus* I, 235.

[6] The influential proposal by DALMAN, *Jesus-Jeschua*, 53–58, claiming that καταλύειν and πληροῦν are equivalents of בטל and קים, is criticized by LJUNGMAN, *Das Gesetz erfüllen*, 29–32.

[7] For the use of ethos as a rhetorical proof, see Aristotle, Rhet. I 2:3f; I 8:6; II 1:7; Cicero, De Orat. II 43:182–184; Orator 37:128; Quintilian, Inst. Orat. VI 2:8–19. Cf. further the comments by LAUSBERG, *Elemente der literarischen Rhetorik*, 35; *idem, Handbuch*, 141f. For an application to the gospel narratives, see MACK/ROBBINS, *Patterns of Persuasion*, 69–84.

[8] So PRZYBYLSKI, *Righteousness*, 80–87; GIESEN, *Christliches Handeln*, 143–146; HAGNER, Righteousness, 111; WOUTERS, *"... wer den Willen meines Vaters tut,"* 228–248.—POPKES, *ZNW* 80 (1989) 1–23, tries to show that righteousness was part of the instruction given to the newly baptized within the school of the Matthean community.

exemplified in the following Antitheses (5:21–48)—is to go beyond the one of the opponents. The context thoroughly embeds 5:17 in a discussion about the deeds of the disciples.[1] The aorist subjunctive μὴ νομίσητε in 5:17, which is not evidently polemical,[2] might suggest that the Matthean Jesus addresses a thought that may occur in the future.[3] When the disciples themselves will act and teach, Jesus' own practice of fulfilling the Law and the prophets—the totality of the Scriptures—remains the example to be imitated.[4] 5:17 points to Jesus' own behaviour as the model.[5]

The emphasis on practising Jesus' teaching—both his verbal and behavioural teaching—suggests that Matthew and his circle of transmitters carried the Jesus tradition also through practical actions. The tradition and the transmission were not only verbal. *There existed behavioural tradition and transmission interacting with verbal tradition and transmission.* Hearing was the means of appropriating the words; doing was the means of appropriating both the words and the behaviour of Jesus.

This points to a dominating impact of orality and to a correlation with the person-oriented motives of transmission. W.J. Ong remarks that in oral cultures words are not part of a separate world but continuous with the rest of life.[6] The words and the actions form a unity. Matthew's world was not at all devoid of literacy. Yet, *the words of the Jesus tradition never lived a life entirely of their own.* The vital centre of Matthew's world concerned the teaching as well as the life and status of Jesus. The motives of transmission did not emerge out of an interest in the teaching as an impersonal object. They focused on the teaching of a venerated person exhibiting influence over the present situation. *The word of the tradition related to the existence and was enacted in the life of the transmitters themselves.* This integration of verbal and behavioural transmission does not, as might be assumed, contradict the notion of a group of specialists especially authorized with the task of transmission. It shows rather that the transmitters did not hear (and memorize) the words of the Jesus tradition in *total* isolation from the rest of life in the community. They also embodied and materialised the Jesus tradition in the various activities of the community. *Hearing and*

---

[1]   *Contra* BROER, *Freiheit vom Gesetz*, 27f, who restricts the contextual perspective to 5:18 and therefore interprets 5:17 as a reference to the teaching of Jesus. He detects in 5:19 "ein nicht unerheblicher Wechsel der Perspektive" (*ibid.*, 51).

[2]   *Contra* G. BARTH, *Law*, 67. See correctly U. LUZ, *ZTK* 75 (1978) 412; *idem*, *Matthäus* I, 232. Cf. also GUELICH, *"Not to Annul the Law,"* 217f, 228.

[3]   MEIER, *Law and History*, 65f, 81f.

[4]   MCCONNELL, *Law and Prophecy*, 10–14; G. BARTH, *Law*, 92f; GUELICH, *Sermon on the Mount*, 141–143. Cf. also SAND, *Gesetz*, 33, 183–187, though he wrongly claims that the Talmud knew only of a twofold division of the Scriptures (*ibid.*, 33 n. 5).

[5]   U. LUZ, *ZTK* 75 (1978) 416, states in connection to 5:17 "daß in der matthäischen Christologie der Lehrer und das Vorbild Jesus eng zusammengehören und daß auch beim Jünger Lehren und Tun zusammengehört."

[6]   *Semeia* 39 (1987) 14.

doing—the verbal and the behavioural means of transmission—constituted an integrated means to transmit the Jesus tradition.

Excursus 13: *Hearing and Doing as Didactic Duties*

The custom of hearing religious teaching was of course a wide-spread ancient phenomenon occurring in various settings. It was deeply rooted in Matthew's Jewish culture.[1] The basic expression of this attitude occurs in the Shemaᶜ (Num 15:37–41; Deut 6:4–9; 11:13–21). Deut 6:4 introduces the confession with the call to hear (שׁמע).[2]

It was especially important for a pupil to listen to his teacher. The call to hear is a frequent component in the directives concerning the attitude towards the teacher. It was part of the teacher's call for the attention of the pupils, the "Lehreröffnungsruf." R. Riesner points out that this call is present in old Egyptian school texts, pre-exilic wisdom writings, Deuteronomy, introductions to prophetic oracles, Sirach, the Testaments of the Twelve Patriarchs and the Talmud.[3] To be sure, we may question if all these texts actually reflect a teaching situation. But there is certainly sufficient evidence to claim that many of them relate to such settings. We could add the evidence from the Dead Sea scrolls: CD 1:1; 2:2, 14; 4Q525 1:1 use "and listen now" (ועתה שמעו) as some kind of preface; similarly, 4Q298 1:1 uses "give ear to me" (האזי]נו לי) and 4Q298 1:2 "listen" (שׁ[מע]ו).[4] *Listening to the teacher was the duty of the pupil.* It was the essential means of receiving teaching in broad spectra of didactic settings.[5]

Doing the teaching is also a didactic duty. It is the duty of the teacher to give practical examples and it is the duty of the pupil to do—to practise—the teaching.

The first aspect is evident in the wide-spread ancient conviction that teaching should be given both by theoretical words and by practical illustrations, by precept and example.[6] We find occasional evidence of this conviction already in the OT, but it is worked out most fully in the rabbinic literature.[7] The pupils should not acquire the teaching by only hearing the words of the teacher. They should also observe him, be witnesses. The broad diffusion of practical illustrations appears also in the Greek-Hellenistic world. The giving of examples (*exempla, παραδείγματα*) from history, custom and imaginative worlds was a well-known rhetorical device used to develop inductive logic. Both Aristotle (c. 384–322 B.C.E.), Cicero (c. 106–43 B.C.E.) and Quintilian (c. 35–95 C.E.) discuss it.[8] The Greek literature of the Jews accordingly praises Moses—the teacher *par excellence*—for combining the methods of precept and

---

[1]   Cf. G. KITTEL, *TDNT* I, 217–219; SCHULT, *THAT* II, 981f.

[2]   Cf. also Deut 11:13.

[3]   *Lehrer,* 120, 376. Cf. also SCHULT, *THAT* II, 977f.

[4]   For more explicit references to the importance of listening to the Righteous Teacher, cf. CD 20:28; 1QpHab 2:2(?); 4QPsᵃ1:19 and above p. 170.

[5]   RENGSTORF, *TDNT* IV, 434f, defines listening as the true function of the rabbinic pupil and regards the duty to minister (שׁמשׁ) as an expression merely of external submission. But this is misleading. Ministering was also a vital part of the learning process itself. See above pp. 90f.

[6]   Cf. DAUBE, *New Testament,* 67–89.

[7]   See above p. 90.

[8]   Aristotle, Rhet. II 20:1–9; Cicero, Inv. I 30:49; Quintilian, Inst. Orat. V 11:1–44. Cf. LAUSBERG, *Elemente der literarischen Rhetorik,* 134; idem, *Handbuch,* 227–235. For the relation between the speaker's ethos and his function as a model to be imitated (μιμεῖσθαι) in basic rhetorical theory, see MACK/ROBBINS, *Patterns of Persuasion,* 41–44.

example (Ep. Arist. 131; Ap. 2:171–173).[1]

The second aspect of teaching and doing concerns the fact that doing is an important means of appropriating and internalizing the teaching. Hearing is not sufficient. As we saw, the Shema⁣ᶜ combines the initial call to hear with the command to act in love. Several texts thus speak about doing the Torah.[2] The whole concept occurs in various ancient Jewish writings. Wis 6:18 identifies the love of Wisdom, which in a sense here represents the Torah,[3] with nothing less than the observance (τήρησις) of her laws. And the combination of hearing and practising the word of Jesus occurs in early Christian literature also outside of Matthew (Luke 6:47, 49; Jas 1:22–25).[4]

Doing is even the most important matter in the total appropriation of the Torah. Philo, Praem. Poen. 79, implies that doing, which is carried out by your own life, is more important than merely hearing the divine commandments and precepts. And Josephus, Ant. 20:44, suggests that doing the Torah is superior to reading (ἀναγινώσκειν) it. Sayings ascribed to tannaitic rabbis confirm this view. Practising the Torah is not only a necessary implication of study, but even the most essential matter in its total appropriation. The Mishnah ascribes this view to early rabbis such as Shammai (m. ᵓAbot 1:15), R. Simeon b. Gamaliel (m. ᵓAbot 1:17), R. Ḥanina b. Dosa (m. ᵓAbot 3:9) and R. Eleazar b. Azariah (m. ᵓAbot 3:17).[5] Only subsequently, perhaps under the pressures of time, did the study in itself become an increasingly important matter (b. Qidd. 40b).[6] But *when Matthew wrote his story, practising the teaching was the most important duty of the pupil.*[7]

3.2. Literacy and Orality in the Use of the Traditions

The verbal and behavioural means of transmission reflect Matthew's own understanding of the process. The conclusions concerning their integrated presence in the life of the community sets the stage for looking at how Matthew actually used the traditions at his disposal. We cannot observe Matthew's behavioural transmission today, of course. The tradition consists now entirely of words, and we can therefore study only the verbal tradition and transmission.

The relationship between the synoptic gospel narratives is a matter of intense scholarly

---

1 Cf. Philo, Op. Mund. 1–2, praising Moses because he disdains the one-sided extremes of other legislators and refrains both from stating abruptly what should be practised or avoided and from inventing myths himself or acquiescing in those composed by others. For Josephus' emphasis on the combination of both methods in the education of children, cf. Ap. 2:204, probably basing the practice on Deut 6:7; 11:19.

2 Cf. e.g. Deut 28:58; 29:28; 1 Macc 2:67; Sir 19:20; 1QpHab 7:11; 8:1; 12:4f; 4QpPsᵃ 2:14, 22. Cf. also Rom 2:13.

3 SCHNABEL, *Law and Wisdom*, 133.

4 Cf. also Joh 13:17.

5 See VIVIANO, *Study*, 27f, 29f, 75–77, 82–86, also discussing the parallels. For the equal importance of studying and practising, cf. e.g. m. ᵓAbot 5:14.

6 See VIVIANO, *Study*, 105–109, also discussing the parallels.

7 U. LUZ, *Matthäus* I, 412f, considers it significant that the rabbinic literature speaks of *studying* and doing while Matthew speaks of *hearing* and doing. But if hearing occasionally implies active remembrance in Matthew, this distinction is not all that sharp.

discussion.[1] I will proceed on the assumption that there is sufficient evidence for the view, still in some form held by the majority of scholars,[2] that Matthew knew a version of Mark's narrative and that the material which Matthew's narrative shares only with Luke's narrative reflects another (flexible) body of tradition—the Q material.[3] In addition, part of the unparallelled material seems to be traditional,[4] though it is often difficult to define the exact units. Some would argue that Matthew had other definable traditions at hand. For instance, G. Strecker believes that the formula quotations (1:22f, 2:5f, 15, 17f, 23; 4:14–16; 8:17; 12:17–21; 13:35; 21:4f; 27:9f) constituted "eine alttestamentliche Zitatensammlung";[5] D. Wenham concludes his analysis of Jesus' eschatological speech with the assumption that it existed (in Greek) as an elaborate pre-synoptic gospel which "was used independently by Matthew, Mark and Luke";[6] H.D. Betz argues that the Sermon on the Mount as found in Matthew was "a presynoptic source that has been preserved in its entirety."[7] But both Strecker's and Betz' theories have been subjected to much criticism.[8] And Wenham's suggestion, though calling for some caution in regarding Q as one expanding source,[9] does not necessarily imply a rejection of the entire two-source hypothesis, as Wenham himself recognizes.[10] It is indeed also possible that Matthew knew of the Markan tradition through various other (oral) channels than the written account.[11] But I cannot account for all possible influences. I only intend to study how Matthew incorporated the main streams of tradition—Mark, the Q material and the M material.

3.2.1. The Written Traditions

Matt 1–13 exhibits the largest amount of freedom in the use of Mark. These chapters are therefore particularly useful for studying how Matthew used the tradition. The *Markan tradition* appears in the following order:[12]

---

[1]   For a survey of the most important, recent contributions, see BYRSKOG, *Nya testamentet och forskningen,* 49–52.

[2]   For a recent defence, see R.H. STEIN, *Synoptic Problem,* 29–138.

[3]   Since I am not certain that we can speak of Q as an actual "source"—or as a "sayings gospel," as J.M. ROBINSON, Sayings Gospel, 361–388, esp. 371f, proposes—at any stage of its development, I prefer to speak merely of the "Q material."

[4]   S.H. BROOKS, *Matthew's Community,* 25–110.

[5]   *Weg der Gerechtigkeit,* 50.

[6]   *Jesus' Eschatological Discourse,* 365.

[7]   *Sermon on the Mount,* 90.

[8]   For surveys of other proposals than the one of Strecker, see SENIOR, *Matthew,* 37–46; STANTON, *ANRW* II 25:3 (1985) 1930–1934; FRANCE, *Matthew: Evangelist and Teacher,* 176–181. For the present purposes, it is also to be noted that these quotations never appear as part of Jesus' own teaching.—For criticism of Betz, see CARLSTON, *CBQ* 50 (1988) 47–57; STANTON, Origin and Purpose, 181–187; FORNBERG, *SEÅ* 53 (1988) 123f.

[9]   Cf. RIESNER, *TZ* 46 (1990) 82f.

[10]   *Jesus' Eschatological Discourse,* 1.

[11]   Cf. recently DUNN, Matthew's Awareness, 1349–1359, venturing the hypothesis that Matthew had access to variant oral versions of much of Mark's material, versions which lacked the details of Markan redaction.

[12]   The brackets around the Matthean and the Markan passages indicate that in spite of the Markan parallel, the Matthean version probably builds also or primarily on an alterna-

Table 2

Matthew	Mark
3:1–6	1:3–6
(3:11f	1:7f)
3:13–17	1:9–11
(4:1–11	1:12f)
4:12–17	1:14f
4:18–22	1:16–20
4:23	1:39
(5:13	9:50)
(5:15	4:21)
5:29 (cf. 18:9)	9:47
5:30 (cf. 18:8)	9:43
(5:32 [cf. 19:9]	10:11f)
6:14	11:25
(7:2	4:24)
7:28f	1:22
8:1–4	1:40–45
8:14f	1:29–31
8:16	1:32–34
8:18, 23–27	4:35–41
8:28–9:1	5:1–20
9:2–8	2:3–12
9:9–13	2:13–17
9:14–17	2:18–22
9:18–26	5:21–43
9:27–31 (cf. 20:29–34)	10:46–52[1]
(9:34 [cf. 12:24]	3:22)
9:35	6:6b
9:36 (cf. 14:14)	6:34
10:1	6:7
10:2–4	3:16–19
(10:9–14	6:8–11)
10:17f (cf. 24:9)	13:9
(10:19f	13:11)
10:21f (cf. 24:10, 13)	13:12f
(10:26	4:22)
(10:37 [cf. 19:29]	10:29)
(10:38f [cf. 16:24f]	8:34f)
10:42	9:41
(11:10	1:2)
12:1–8	2:23–28
12:9–14	3:1–6
12:15f	3:7–12

---

tive tradition (Q) recorded also in Luke. Possible doublets in Matthew are given in brackets after the Matthean passages.

[1] Cf. also Mark 8:22–26.

(12:22–30 [cf. 9:32–34]	3:22–27)
12:31	3:28
(12:32	3:29)
(12:38f [cf. 16:1–2a, 4]	8:11f)
12:46–50	3:31–35
13:1–9	4:1–9
13:10f	4:10f
13:12 (cf. 25:29)	4:25
13:13	4:12
13:18–23	4:13–20
(13:31f	4:30–32)
13:34	4:33f
13:53–58	6:1–6a.

In the basic framework of the narrative, Matthew depends on the Markan account. The table shows that basic blocks of Markan material are reproduced in almost the same order. With some omissions, Matthew follows Mark's account up to Mark 1:39. At this point, Matthew leaves the Markan context and inserts the Sermon on the Mount. After the Sermon, he returns to Mark 1:40ff. Matt 8–9 contains mainly a collection of nine or ten miracle stories. Matthew here uses Mark 1:40–45 and 2:3–12 to introduce the first episode of the two parts of this fourfold composition (8:1–17; 8:18–9:1; 9:2–17; 9:18–34).[1] He continues the Markan order in 9:9–13, 14–17 and includes Mark 2:13–17, 18–22, in spite of the fact that these pericopes do not describe Jesus' mighty acts. Another departure from the Markan context appears at 9:18ff. But Matthew returns to Mark 2:23ff in 12:1ff and, with some transpositions and omissions, follows the Markan tradition to the end of the parable chapter. And from 14:1ff to the end of the narrative, he reproduces almost all Markan pericopes in the order they occur in Mark.

The broad agreement in the structural framework shows that a version of Mark's narrative was available to Matthew in written form. The exact wording of the Marcan account which Matthew used is not always evident.[2] And we cannot exclude the possibility that some traditions now present in Mark were available to Matthew also through other (oral) channels. But

---

[1]   With some minor variations (the division between 8:34 and 9:1 instead of 9:1 and 9:2 and the inclusion of 9:35), this structure is followed by e.g. BURGER, *ZTK* 70 (1973) 284–287; KINGSBURY, *CBQ* 40 (1978) 562; U. LUZ, Wundergeschichten, 150. A somewhat different division (8:1[2]–17; 8:18–9:17; 9:18–31; 9:32–34) is given by W.G. THOMPSON, *CBQ* 33 (1971) 368; GERHARDSSON, *Mighty Acts,* 39; HELD, Miracle Stories, 248f. A structure based on the Sermon on the Mount, as proposed by MOISER, *ZNW* 76 (1985) 117f, is unlikely. The correspondences between Matt 5–7 and 8–9 are too vague.

[2]   The minor agreements between Matthew and Luke against Mark are of course open to different explanations, even if the essentials of the two-source hypothesis is accepted. Cf. R.H. STEIN, *Synoptic Problem,* 123–127; *idem, CBQ* 54 (1992) 483–485. One explanation would be that Matthew and Luke used a version of Mark different from the one available today. So e.g. J.P. BROWN, *JBL* 78 (1959) 215–227; GLASSON, *JBL* 85 (1966) 231–233.

there is no doubt that in the Matthean community the Markan version of the Jesus tradition was carried primarily by means of a written text.

The units perhaps belonging to the *Q material* can be divided into sixty-nine items.[1] The following table presents them in the Lukan order:[2]

Table 3

Item no.	Luke	Matthew
1.	3:7–9	3:7–10
2.	3:16b–17	3:11f (cf. Mark 1:7f)
3.	4:1–13	4:1–11 (cf. Mark 1:12f)
4.	6:20b–21	5:3, 6, 4
5.	6:22f	5:11f
6.	6:27f	5:44
7.	6:29f	5:39f, 42
8.	6:31	7:12
9.	6:32–36	5:46f, 45, 48
10.	6:37f	7:1f (cf. Mark 4:24)
11.	6:39	15:14
12.	6:40	10:24f
13.	6:41f	7:3–5
14.	6:43f	7:16f/12:33
15.	6:45	12:35
16.	6:46	7:21
17.	6:47–49	7:24–27
18.	7:1f, 6b–10	7:28a; 8:5–10, 13
19.	7:18–23	11:2–6
20.	7:24–28	11:7–11 (cf. Mark 1:2)
21.	7:31–35	11:16–19
22.	9:57–60	8:19–22
23.	10:2–12	9:37f; 10:16, 9–10a, 12f, 11b, 10b, 7f, 14f
24.	10:13–15	11:21–23
25.	10:16	10:40
26.	10:21f	11:25–27
27.	10:23f	13:16f
28.	11:2–4	6:9–13
29.	11:9–13	7:7–11
30.	11:14f	9:32–34/12:22–24 (cf. Mark 3:22)
31.	11:17–23	12:25–30 (cf. Mark 3:23–27)
32.	11:24–26	12:43–45
33.	11:29–32	12:39f, 42, 41
34.	11:33	5:15 (cf. Mark 4:21)
35.	11:34f	6:22f
36.	11:39–44	23:25f, 23, 6f, 27f (cf. Mark

---

[1] This division into items is provisional and made for analytical purposes only.

[2] The brackets around the Lukan and the Matthean units indicate that the assignment of the whole item to Q is less certain than in other cases. Possible overlappings with Mark are given in brackets after the Matthean units.

		12:37b–40)
37.	11:46–52	23:4, 29–32, 34–36, 13
38.	12:2–9	10:26–33
39.	12:10	12:32 (cf. Mark 3:29)
40.	12:11f	10:19f (cf. Mark 13:11)
41.	12:22–31	6:25–33
42.	12:33f	6:19–21
43.	12:39f	24:43f
44.	12:42–46	24:45–51
45.	12:51–53	10:34–36
46.	12:58f	5:25f
47.	13:18–21	13:31–33 (cf. Mark 4:30–32)
48.	13:24	7:13f
49.	13:25–27	7:22f
50.	13:28f	8:11f
51.	13:34f	23:37–39
52.	(14:16–24	22:1–10)
53.	14:26f	10:37f
54.	14:34f	5:13 (cf. Mark 9:50)
55.	(15:4–7	18:12–14)
56.	16:13	6:24
57.	16:16	11:12f
58.	16:17	5:18
59.	16:18	5:32
60.	(17:1	18:7 [cf. Mark 9:42])
61.	17:3f	18:21f
62.	17:6	17:20
63.	17:23f	24:26f
64.	17:26f	24:37–39a
65.	17:33	10:39
66.	17:34f	24:40f (cf. Mark 13:35)
67.	17:37b	24:28
68.	(19:12–27	25:14–30)
69.	22:28–30	19:28.

Any discussion of the Q material is beset with a number of uncertainties. It is difficult to determine if it was carried by written or oral media, or both. Most recent experts on Q tend to think of a (growing) written body of material.[1] But other informed scholars, such as R.H. Stein,[2] call for caution. They point out that the evidence is far from conclusive and prefer to maintain that Q—here mostly seen as a common designation for a variety of material—was mainly oral.[3]

---

[1]   SCHMITHALS, *Einleitung*, 218; SAND, *Matthäus-Evangelium*, 1, give the impression that modern scholarship thinks of Q as an oral product. I do not share this evaluation of recent research. Cf. e.g. POLAG, *Christologie*, 1; WEGNER, *Hauptmann*, 277–286; KLOPPENBORG, *Formation of Q*, 42–51, URO, *Sheep Among the Wolves*, 2; SATO, *Q und Prophetie*, 16f; KOSCH, *Tora*, 28f.

[2]   *Synoptic Problem*, 103–108.

[3]   In his recent commentary on Matthew's special material, WREGE, *Sondergut*, 10–

There is significant indication that Matthew did know of some Q material in written form. Table three shows that Matthew and Luke share a common order of certain items.[1] We can see this in certain *blocks* of items. The common order is most evident in the blocks consisting of items no. 1–5, 13–14, 16–18, 19–21, 43–44, 63–64. We also find a common order within *separate* items containing groups of sayings or longer sayings. Such is the case especially in items no. 22, 29, 31, 38, 47. To this we may add V. Taylor's observation that there is a large measure of agreement in order when each of the major speeches in Matt 5–7, 13, 18, 23–25 and the remainder of Matthew are compared individually with the Lukan parallels.[2] Although even such a comparison does not yield an exact and entirely continuous agreement in order throughout each speech, as Taylor recognizes,[3] there is a significant degree of correspondence in groups and series of passages.

What the table does not show is that sometimes there also exists a significant word-for-word correspondence.[4] As examples, we may mention Luke 11:9f/Matt 7:7f and Luke 16:13/Matt 6:24. In the former case, all words are identical; in the latter, there is a difference only in one word. Other instances with a high degree of verbal agreement also exist.[5]

The two aspects of agreement—the order and the word-for-word correspondence—are most easily accounted for if we assume that some of the Q material was available to Matthew in written form. To be sure, the agreement could also occur within a process of oral transmission including exact memorization. J.S. Kloppenborg begs the question, it seems, when he rejects such a notion entirely by stating, without discussing the sources and the literature, that there is no evidence of oral techniques of transmission in primitive Christianity or contemporary Judaism.[6] The decisive argument is

---

12, maintains the position, probably shaped under the influence of his teacher Joachim JEREMIAS, *ZNW* 29 (1930) 147–149, that Q is more like a field of various traditions ("Traditionsbereich") than a literary document. Cf. also his earlier discussion in *idem, Überlieferungsgeschichte,* 2f.

1 For a survey of the earlier discussion about the order in Q, see KLOPPENBORG, *Formation of Q,* 64–72.

2 *Essays,* 90–118.

3 *Essays,* 97.

4 For a survey of earlier discussion about the verbal agreements, see KLOPPEN-BORG, *Formation of Q,* 42–44.

5 Cf. Luke 3:7b–9/Matt 3:7b–10; Luke 6:41f/Matt 7:3–5; Luke 7:22f/Matt 11:4–6; Luke 7:24b–28/Matt 11:7b–11; Luke 10:13–15/Matt 11:21–23a; Luke 10:21b–22/Matt 11:25b–27; Luke 11:24–26/Matt 12:43–45; Luke 12:42b–46/Matt 24:45–51a; Luke 13:34f/Matt 23:37–39.

6 *Formation of Q,* 44.—KLOPPENBORG, *ibid.,* 45, continues his sweeping arguments by claiming that "early Christian literature betrays no trace of the institutions and professional classes of memorizers which an accurate transmission of oral tradition would require and which later rabbinic Judaism presupposed." He supports his statement with a reference to the old and polemical article by M. SMITH, *JBL* 82 (1963) 169–176. Kloppenberg must at least—to mention only this issue—account also for more recent investigations pointing in a different direction. Cf. e.g. ZIMMERMANN, *Die urchristlichen*

instead, it seems, that if these features of agreement are the result of oral tradition and transmission, there must have been a significant "feedback" of literacy upon orality,[1] to the extent that literacy superimposes itself upon the signs of orality.[2] When that is the case, we must consider it as more likely that part of the material was actually carried by means of written media.

It is doubtful if the double appearance of the same account in Matthew proves the written character of the material.[3] Such doublets are indeed present in Matthew and imply that one and the same account could be available in two versions, one from Mark and one from the Q material.[4] But this feature could appear also if one of the two versions was carried by oral media. It might be a means to implant an episode or saying by repetition.

As it seems, Matthew found the living voice of his teacher partly enclosed in the signs of written media. Seen by themselves, such media might in the long run make the tradition impersonal. They objectify it and remove a portion of learning and internalization from the immediate chain of personal confrontation.[5] The written character of Mark and some of the Q material might in a certain sense have effected an alienation of the Jesus tradition among the transmitters. The relation to the living voice of Jesus was complicated by abstract notions emerging from an objectifying written text.

Oral tradition and transmission, which relate more directly to the situation of the transmitters,[6] may be a more suitable means to carry and convey traditions that are of vital importance for the present and the future.[7] Orality is empathetic and participatory rather than objectively distanced.[8] In a setting fostering a keen interest in the teaching, the life and the status of Je-

---

Lehrer.

[1]   FINNEGAN, *Literacy,* 117–120, illustrates the potential feedback from written sources into oral forms among people in the Pacific during the 19th cent. and more recently.

[2]   Cf. ANDERSEN, Oral Tradition, 44.

[3]   *Contra* KÜMMEL, *Einleitung,* 40. Cf. correctly R.H. STEIN, *Synoptic Problem,* 107f.

[4]   Cf. e.g. Matt 5:32/Luke 16:18 with Matt 19:9/Mark 10:11f; Matt 10:38(f)/Luke 14:27 with Matt 16:24f/Mark 8:34f/Luke 9:23f; Matt 12:38(39)–40/Luke 11:29f with Matt 16:1–2a, 4/Mark 8:11f; Matt 13:12/Mark 4:25/Luke 8:18b with Matt 25:29/Luke 19:26. Further examples are listed by HAWKINS, *Horae Synopticae,* 82–99.

[5]   Cf. GÜTTGEMANNS, *Offene Fragen,* 137–143, 255.

[6]   KELBER, *The Oral and the Written Gospel,* 24, speaks of "the law of *social identification*" and contraposes this to verbatim memorization. But VANSINA, *Oral Tradition,* 120–123, points out in his discussion of "homeostasis"—the congruence between a society and its traditions—that the presence of archaisms, for instance, shows that there is no total congruence between the content and the concerns of the present. ONG, *Orality and Literacy,* 47, realizes that archaisms do survive, but only, he claims, through their current use.

[7]   In describing the characteristics of orality, LORD, *Oral Tradition* 2:1 (1987) 63, states: "Oral traditional literature tends to make the songs and stories from the past serve the goals of the present for the sake of the future."

[8]   ONG, *Orality and Literacy,* 45f.

sus, the teacher, we expect factors preventing the Jesus tradition from its total literarization to be inherent in the transmission process. These factors come to the surface in the existence of special oral traditions and in the re-oralization of the written traditions.

3.2.2. The Oral Traditions

If we substract from Matthew the material shared with Mark and Luke, a large number of unparallelled verses and pericopes remain.[1] It is extremely difficult to determine which of these come from a pre-Matthean tradition and constitute the so-called M material. S.H. Brooks, who provides the most extended attempt to identify and isolate the traditional character of most of the unparallelled material, uses four criteria: synoptic comparison, style, vocabulary and content.[2] We should, however, be aware that these criteria allow only for a limited degree of certainty. The criteria of style and content depend to a large extent upon the interpreter's own view of what constitutes logical sequence and coherence or disjunctions. If we believe that oral media carried the M material and that the written account which now contains this material is a written narrative infused with oral features,[3] the search for an exact logical consistency becomes even more difficult. And the other two criteria are insufficient by themselves.

Brooks first identifies fourteen M-sayings (Matt 5:19; Matt 5:21f; Matt 5:23f; Matt 5:27f; Matt 5:33–35, 37a, b; Matt 5:36; Matt 6:1–6, 16–18; Matt 6:7f; Matt 10:5b–6; Matt 10:23b; Matt 23:2f, 5; Matt 23:8–10; Matt 23:15; Matt 23:16–22, 24).[4] On the basis of the ideologies and life settings of these sayings, he also isolates and analyses five further unparallelled sayings as traditional units (7:6; 12:36f; 18:18; 18:19f; 19:12).[5] Scholars vary in assigning different parts of the unparallelled material to tradition. My own discussion below favours a view on the antithetical construction in the Antitheses and on 10:23b, and to some degree also on 18:18,[6] different from the one proposed by Brooks. Additional M material is probably present in the narrative meshalim, which Brooks does not treat, especially in 13:24–30, 44–50; 18:23–35; 20:1–16; 21:28–32; 25:1–13, 31–46. It is not possible to discuss each item separately here. But if we accept, with some caution and modification, Brooks' identification of the M-sayings, we will have a picture sufficiently clear for the present purposes.

---

[1] Cf. e.g. the table given by DAVIES/ALLISON, *Matthew* I, 121–124.
[2] *Matthew's Community*, 17–19.
[3] See below pp. 347f.
[4] *Matthew's Community*, 25–71. The reference to 23:33 in chart 2 (*ibid.*, 161) is probably a mistake.
[5] *Matthew's Community*, 87–110.
[6] See below pp. 357, 359f, 391–395. Cf. also the comments on 5:19 below p. 353.

The old view was that the M material existed in mainly written form.[1] But modern scholars point to its oral character. Both Brooks and H.-T. Wrege, who have given the most recent and detailed studies of the special material, conceive mainly oral media.[2] If we compare the M material with how Matthew incorporates Mark (and the Q material), we do not find much indication of written means to transmit the M material. Matthew gives no evidence in this case that he uses a coherent and unified tradition. With the possible exception of some narrative meshalim,[3] the M material appears in the Matthean framework as individual sayings scattered out at various places. There are no large blocks exhibiting a specific order. If there are no clear traces of written media, we must assume an oral media unaffected by developed literary conceptions.

Wrege's discussion implies that the Matthean community used oral media because the transmitting members were largely illiterate.[4] Without taking account of studies with other emphases, Wrege echos the long-standing influence of the early form-critical view on synoptic tradition and transmission.[5] For the problem at hand, this view not only raises the question why the highly educated rabbis later preferred—at least theoretically—oral tradition and transmission, but also makes us wonder about the actual role of the transmitter most evident to us, the author of the narrative. We gained a different impression in the previous chapters of my study. Matthew, I argued, regarded himself as one of the pupils and scribes aiming to learn and understand in the school of Jesus. This suggested a more specific setting of transmission than the illiterate community. In the present chapter, I also ventured the hypothesis that the narrative meshalim were in the hands of certain specialists in the community. And in spite of the fact that Matthew seems to incorporate M-sayings at separate places, there is evidence that the transmission was not totally uncontrolled. Certain items exhibit thematic similarities:[6] related concepts of eschatological judgement are present in 5:19; 5:21f; 12:36f; the reproach against those who perform acts of piety in order to be seen by others appears in 6:1–6, 16–18; 23:2f, 5. Such thematic connections may of course occur in material transmitted by illiterate

---

1 Cf. STREETER, *The Four Gospels*, 150, 223–270, 512; E. HIRSCH, *Frühgeschichte des Evangeliums* II, 332–338; KILPATRICK, *Origins*, 24f, 28, 31f, 35f; MANSON, *Sayings of Jesus*, 21–26 (first published in 1937).

2 S.H. BROOKS, *Matthew's Community*, 111–113; WREGE, *Sondergut*, 9f.

3 The considerations above pp. 323f may suggest that some basic texts of the narrative meshalim were carefully memorized.

4 *Sondergut*, 9f.—WREGE, *ibid.*, 10, concludes: "Unser form- und traditionsgeschichtlicher Ansatz bedeutet damit, daß die unliterarische Gemeinde, die wir als Trägerin der Überlieferungsprozesse annehmen dürfen bzw. müssen, eine Instanz auch gegenüber der literarischen Redaktionsarbeit des Evangelisten (Mt) bleibt."

5 For a positive assessment of the form-critical view on literacy and orality, cf. STRECKER, Schriftlichkeit oder Mündlichkeit, 159–172.

6 Cf. S.H. BROOKS, *Matthew's Community*, 74–83, 99, 109.

groups. But what is even more significant is that also sayings which, taken by themselves, are difficult to reconcile apparently belonged to the M material:[1] 23:3 seems to affirm the teaching authority of certain synagogue leaders, while 23:8–10 refuses to accept any other didactic authority but God and Jesus, and while 23:15; 23:16–22, 24 suggest that the opponents are blind guides offering erroneous interpretation; 5:33–35, 37 forbid swearing in any form, while 23:16–22 presupposes that there is a proper way of swearing. Although the tensions between the separate sayings may reflect different stages during the history of the Matthean community, they must eventually have emerged as part of the tradition which was at the evangelist's disposal at one and the same time. J. Vansina speaks of "the known tendency of the mind in memory to construct a coherent discourse."[2] The untrained memory tends to level the contradictions. This tendency makes likely that tensions and irregularities should have been eliminated, had the transmission been without any control whatsoever from qualified transmitters. Perhaps they kept such sayings separate, until the evangelist tried to resolve the tensions by placing them within a narrativized account. It is clear, in any event, that the transmitters were not illiterates. They were educated and capable persons. In accordance with the broad scepticism towards the written word in antiquity,[3] the transmitters used oral media of transmission out of choice, not because they were unable to write. They *preferred* not to fix the tradition in writing.

This is not without significance. As a member of the community, Matthew regarded the M material as his "own" tradition. It gives us therefore information "from the inside."[4] Its transmission reflects the situation of the community to a larger extent than Mark and the Q material, which were originally shaped externally to the experiences of the Matthean community. In addition, the M material contained sayings of his venerated teacher. When we view the tradition in the context of its social and existential relevance for the community, its total literarization becomes inconceivable and its remaining oral character becomes understandable. *Through the oral means of transmission, the tradition with which Matthew was most closely associated remained a living text in which he continuously heard and internalized the voice of Jesus, his only teacher.*

3.2.3. The Re-oralization of Traditions

If Matthew preferred to transmit his "own" tradition with oral media, it is conceivable that he adopted also the written traditions through a process

---

[1] Cf. S.H. BROOKS, *Matthew's Community,* 83f, 110.
[2] *Oral Tradition,* 171.
[3] See above pp. 164f and the literature referred to there.
[4] Cf. VANSINA, *Oral Tradition,* 197–199.

containing a certain oral hermeneutic. The attitude to a written text indeed varies in different cultures. Even literate cultures accord different degrees of respect to what is written down.[1] But written texts, especially those regarded as authoritative, often continue to have an oral dimension.[2] The immediate effect of the writing down of a tradition is the transition from sounds recomposed by a storyteller to sounds read/heard from a manuscript, not necessarily from sound to silence.[3] Usually an important tradition does not die out after it has been recorded in writing.[4] The writing may affect it in certain ways.[5] But it continues to be told and may at a later time once again be recorded.[6]

M.A. Mills, a scholar of folklore, speaks of the process of re-oralization. She thinks of scripture's perpetual return to oral currency, "called for by the very nature of scripture as a peculiarly authoritative kind of text, as words to live by in the profoundest sense."[7] Re-oralization generates, according to Mills, scripture's interpretations in context and takes place in small groups that are negotiating for shared meaning and cohesion. There is evidence that Matthew's use of the written tradition in the framework of his narrative reflects a similar process of re-oralization.[8]

In spite of the broad and basic adherence to the written traditions, Matthew also shows a significant amount of creativity. Table two above shows not only that Matthew adhered to Mark, but also that he felt free to *leave* the Markan context and insert other material. The Sermon on the Mount is the clearest example, but there are also several non-Markan pericopes at other places. In addition, Matthew sometimes *omitted* Markan material: his narrative does not contain the episodes about the healing of the man with an unclean spirit (Mark 1:23–28), the deaf mute (Mark 7:32–36) and the blind man at Bethsaida (Mark 8:22–26);[9] we do not find the episodes about an exorcist (Mark 9:38–40) and a poor widow's offering (Mark 12:41–44); the narrative mashal about the growing seed (Mark 4:26–29) is also missing.

---

[1] FINNEGAN, *Literacy,* 81.

[2] This is the main focus in the study by GRAHAM, *Beyond the Written Word.*

[3] BOOMERSHINE, *Semeia* 39 (1987) 61; BALCH, *Forum* 7:3–4 (1993) 192.

[4] Cf. e.g. VANSINA, *Oral Tradition,* 31.

[5] KELBER, *The Oral and the Written Gospel,* 217f, speaks in such cases of "secondary orality" as distinguished from "primary orality," which he detects on the presynoptic stage of transmission. Cf. also ONG, *Orality and Literacy,* 11, 136f. I find it difficult to accept the notion that any presynoptic unit constituted primary orality, if this is taken to mean that such units were totally untouched by writing.

[6] ONG, *Semeia* 39 (1987) 9, states: "Putting an utterance into script can only interrupt discourse, string it out indefinitely in time and space. But not 'fix' it."

[7] Folkloristic Concern, 232.

[8] In a subsequent section, I will study some of the creative interpretation of the Markan pericopes and the Q material visible in *individual* Matthean pericopes. Here I will focus on the incorporation of the traditions in the Matthean framework.

[9] Mark 8:22–26 may however have influenced Matt 9:27–31.

Some of these pericopes are lacking also in Luke.[1] But it is still legitimate to assume that Matthew felt free to omit certain units present in his version of Mark.

If we focus on Matt 1–13, there are especially two features suggesting that the Markan material was deeply embedded in the mind of Matthew. First, Matthew sometimes *changed the order* of the Markan material. Table two shows, for instance, that after leaving the Markan context at Mark 1:39 to insert the Sermon on the Mount, at Matt 7:28f Matthew returned to Mark 1:22. And after using Mark 1:40–45, he went back to Mark 1:29ff, then forward to Mark 4:35ff, and only subsequently continued with Mark 2:3ff. And similarly, after using Mark 2:18–22, he turned to several other verses and pericopes occurring at various places later in the Markan account. Not until 12:1ff did he return to Mark 2:23ff. The parable chapter also exhibits some rearrangements. Second, Matthew sometimes *foreshadowed* material which is present later in the Markan account and which Matthew himself subsequently would use more explicitly. This is not only the case when one of the doublets depends on a similar account in the Q material,[2] but also when two Matthean passages—one of which is given in brackets in table two—correspond to one Markan parallel. For instance, Matt 9:27–31; 10:17f, 21f do not have Lukan parallels at the same place in the narrative, but they foreshadow the fuller use of the Markan material in Matt 20:29–34; 24:9, 10, 13. Separate verses may have a similar foreshadowing function. 5:29, 30; 9:36 also lack clear Lukan parallels, but they recur in the use of the Markan tradition in 18:9; 18:8; 14:14.

These two features are explainable only if the Markan account as a whole was actively present to Matthew.[3] The technique of foreshadowing by repetition is an oral feature preparing the listener for what is to be expected.[4] And a purely literary approach to the written text would require too complicated a technique of cross-references and cross-checking to account for the change of order. As F.G. Kenyon pointed out long ago,[5] there were normally no visible signs of where various parts of a composition written on a scroll began or ended at this time.[6] The matter was further complicated through the need to roll and re-roll the scroll. Once a passage in a scroll was located, there would be no way to refer to it by paragraph or page. The in-

---

[1] So Mark 4:26–29; 7:32–36; 8:22–26.

[2] Cf. above p. 338 n. 4.

[3] In addition to these two features emerging from the structural framework, there is a certain terminological and theological dependence on Mark. See U. LUZ, *Matthäus* I, 56–58.

[4] See LOHR, *CBQ* 23 (1961) 411, and the literature referred to there.

[5] *Books and Readers,* 66f, 113.

[6] As RIESNER, Jesus as Teacher and Preacher, 207 n. 5, points out, it is an overstatement to say that ancient texts had no visual aids at all. And later, through the centuries, certain divisions emerged in different MSS. Cf. METZGER, *Text,* 21–31.

timate knowledge of the writing that was required in order to locate a passage in a scroll actually obviated the need to identify it exactly. And we have yet no clear evidence that Mark was originally written on anything else than a common scroll.[1] Therefore, the very physical nature of written texts makes it likely that people quoted from memory rather than located the passage in a writing.[2] In addition, we should not exclude the possibility that the school of the Matthean community had secretaries and that Matthew himself composed his narrative by dictating orally.[3]

A certain creativity existed also within the broad and basic adherence to the Q material.[4] In the midst of verbal agreement, there are also examples exhibiting no significant degree of exactness. Items no. 52, 55, 60, 68, which in table three appear within brackets, even show such striking disagreements that it is difficult to determine if the items actually belonged to the Q material shared by Matthew and Luke or not.[5] But we may also mention, for instance, parts of items no. 7, 36, 48, 57, 58. It is evident that for Matthew the written Q material was open to a rather flexible adoptation.

The creativity is also in this case due to the active presence of the written material in the mind of Matthew. We may recall two factors pointing in this direction. First, if with virtually all scholars we assume that Luke mostly represents the order of the Q material more faithfully than Matthew, several Matthean *transpositions* are evident. The right column of table three shows sufficient irregularities to suggest the existence of deliberate transpositions, though of course the original order of some items is uncertain. Within certain individual items, such as no. 4, 9, 23, 33, 36, 37, the order of various parts of sayings is also different in Matthew than in Luke. Second, it happened occasionally that Matthew *doubled* one and the same item in the Q material and used it on two independent occasions. This is evident in item no. 14 of table three, and perhaps also in no. 30. Since it was difficult to locate passages in a writing exactly, these features are difficult to account for by referring to several scannings of a document, even if the document

---

[1] But cf. the circumstantial considerations by C.H. ROBERTS, *JTS* 40 (1939) 253–257. Roberts has repeated his view on this matter in several later studies.

[2] For similar observations, see FULLER, Classics and the Gospel, 187f; ONG, *Orality and Literacy,* 119; ACHTEMEIER, *JBL* 109 (1990) 27; ANDERSEN, Oral Tradition, 44.

[3] For the importance of the secretary in the Greco-Roman environment, see RICHARDS, *Secretary,* 14–127, 199f. His treatment of the Pauline material (*ibid.,* 128–198, 201) is, however, more hypothetical. Cf. the critique by LINDEMANN, *TLZ* 117 (1992) 915–917.

[4] I cannot discuss here separately whether Matthew and Luke had somewhat different versions of the Q material. This is indeed possible in cases with no evident redactional interest behind the differences. For further discussion, see SATO, *Q und Prophetie,* 47–62.

[5] For a critical account of the differences between various Matthean and Lukan Q passages, cf. LINTON, Q-Problem, 43–59.

would have existed in the form of a codex.[1]
The creative use of the written traditions resulted ultimately in a self-contained narrative. I cannot reherse all the various suggestions made for a basic principle guiding the structure of Matthew as a whole.[2] But even the most prominent alternatives fail to convince as structural patterns governing the narrative in its totality.

There are three main alternatives. B.W. Bacon's influential proposal was published already in 1918.[3] His fivefold structure has the advantage of being based on the recurrent formula καὶ ἐγένετο ὅτε ἐτέλεσεν ὁ Ἰησοῦς (7:28; 11:1; 13:53; 19:1; 26:1).[4] By itself, the formula probably concludes the previous speeches.[5] Within the flow of the narrative, it also leads the readers/hearers on to the next phase of the story.[6] The structural function is there, irrespective of Bacon's suggestion concerning the allusions to the Pentateuch. But the proposal also contains considerable limitations. It leaves Matt 1–2 and 26–28 outside of the basic scheme and it does not explain sufficiently well the function of material that appears between the speeches. The five occurrences of the formula point to one structural pattern, but not to a basic pattern governing the total structure of Matthew.[7]

The second alternative, associated especially with C.H. Lohr,[8] also takes the spee-

---

1 SATO, *Q und Prophetie*, 64f, ventures the hypothesis that the Q material was written on a codex to which pages could be easily added. This is possible, but difficult to prove. Clear evidence of a pre-Christian codex is still missing. Cf. the recent appendix by METZGER, *Text*, 260f (with lit.).

2 For literature and surveys of the discussion, see SENIOR, *Matthew*, 20–27; STANTON, *ANRW* II 25:3 (1985) 1903–1906; D.R. BAUER, *Structure*, 21–55; DAVIES/ALLISON, *Matthew* I, 58–72; FRANCE, *Matthew: Evangelist and Teacher*; 141–153; U. LUZ, *Matthäus* I, 15–28; SAND, *Matthäus-Evangelium*, 39–42. In addition to the literature mentioned there, cf. also HELLHOLM, *SEÅ* 51–52 (1986–87) 80–89; KINGSBURY, *Matthew: Structure, Christology, Kingdom*, ix–xx.

3 *The Expositor* 15 (1918) 56–66. Cf. also *idem, JBL* 47 (1928) 208; *idem, Studies*, xv, 81f.

4 KEEGAN, *CBQ* 44 (1982) 415–430, claims the same formalistic function of the introductory passages (4:25–5:2; 9:36f; 13:1–3; 18:1–3; 24:3f) of the speeches. For criticism, see FRANCE, *Matthew: Evangelist and Teacher*, 142f.

5 Cf. KINGSBURY, *Matthew: Structure, Christology, Kingdom*, 6; HELLHOLM, *SEÅ* 51–52 (1986–87) 88f.

6 Already BACON, *The Expositor* 15 (1918) 65, understood the formula—he calls it "colophon"—as a link to the following narrative. So also more recently e.g. GOODING, *RB* 85 (1978) 229–331; WILKENS, *NTS* 31 (1985) 24; GNILKA, *Matthäusevangelium* I, 283; SCHENK, *Sprache des Matthäus*, 440; SYREENI, *Sermon on the Mount*, 81f; D.R. BAUER, *Structure*, 33, 129; FRANCE, *Matthew: Evangelist and Teacher*, 145; KINGSBURY, *Matthew: Structure, Christology, Kingdom*, 6 (though only when the formula itself is regarded as connected with the primary clause it modifies); U. LUZ, *Matthäus* I, 19.

7 For further criticism, see W.D. DAVIES, *Setting of the Sermon on the Mount*, 14–25; H.B. GREEN, *SE* 4 (1968) 48–50; D.R. BAUER, *Structure*, 27–35; KINGSBURY, *Matthew: Structure, Christology, Kingdom*, xiv, 5–7.

8 *CBQ* 23 (1961) 427–430. Cf. somewhat earlier FENTON, *SE* 1 (1959) 179. Later scholars have used and developed Lohr's proposal in different ways. Cf. e.g. GAECHTER, *Kunst*, 13; H.B. GREEN, *SE* 4 (1968) 54–59; P.F. ELLIS, *Matthew*, 10–13; GOODING, *RB* 85 (1978) 227–238; COMBRINK, *Neot* 16 (1982) 16–19; *idem, TynBul* 34 (1983) 70–87.—RIESNER, *TBei* 9 (1978) 172–182, tries to show that Jesus' spee-

ches seriously. In distinction to Bacon's proposal, this alternative tries to account for the relation of the speeches to each other and to the narrative material through a chiastic outline of the whole narrative. Lohr places Matt 13 in the middle of the narrative and sees correspondences between Matt 1–4 and 26–28 (narratives), Matt 5–7 and 23–25 (speeches), Matt 8–9 and 19–22 (narratives), Matt 10 and 18 (speeches) and Matt 11–12 and 14–17 (narratives). This structure carries credibility by giving the fivefold formula its structural importance and by relating both the longest (Matt 5–7 and 23–25) and the shortest (Matt 10 and 18) speeches to each other. Matt 10 and 18 also show similarities through the almost equal length of the two speeches.[1] But it is more difficult to evaluate the structure in relation to motifs occurring at different places in the narrative. For instance, the central importance of Matt 13 is not evident from a thematic point of view.[2] It is possible that Lohr discovered one of the structures used by Matthew, but the proposal does not cover the totality of the narrative.[3]

The third major proposal, advocated especially by J.D. Kingsbury and his student D.R. Bauer, also has the advantage of being based on an existent formula, ἀπὸ τότε ἤρξατο ὁ Ἰησοῦς (4:17; 16:21).[4] This formula divides the narrative into three parts (1:1–4:16; 4:17–16:20; 16:21–28:20). But it is questionable if we can regard the formulas "as veritable superscriptions for whole sections of the Gospel."[5] Also 1:1 is given this function. It is possible to question if 1:1 is a superscription to 1:2–4:16.[6] In particular, we should notice that ἀπὸ τότε, despite the asyndetic construction,[7] on both occasions relates to past events, to Jesus' settlement in Capernaum after the arrest of John the Baptist (4:12f) and to Peter's declaration at Caesarea Philippi (16:13–20).[8] The formula does not function as a superscription to what follows only. In addition, certain motifs occur in all the different parts and distort therefore the neat structure from a thematical point of view.[9] We may also ask why these particular formulas, and

---

ches exhibit a chiastic structure.

[1]   U. LUZ, *Matthäus* I, 17.

[2]   In the structure proposed by H.B. GREEN, *SE* 4 (1968) 58, Matt 11 forms the centre. In the alternative of GOODING, *RB* 85 (1978) 235f, 11:1–13:52 takes the central position.

[3]   For further criticism, see D.R. BAUER, *Structure*, 36–40.

[4]   D.R. BAUER, *Structure, passim,* esp. 73–108; KINGSBURY, *Matthew: Structure, Christology, Kingdom,* 7–37. Kingsbury builds on STONEHOUSE, *Witness of Matthew and Mark,* 129–131; LOHMEYER, *Matthäus,* 1, 64, 264; KRENTZ, *JBL* 83 (1964) 409–414. Cf. also already HAWKINS, *Horae Synopticae,* 168; ALLEN, *Matthew,* 35, 180; MCNEILE, *Matthew,* 44f, 244.

[5]   KINGSBURY, *Matthew: Structure, Christology, Kingdom,* 9.

[6]   Cf. e.g. U. LUZ, *Matthäus* I, arguing that it refers to Matt 1; DORMEYER, Mt 1,1 als Überschrift, 1361–1363, arguing that it refers to Matthew as a whole.

[7]   KINGSBURY, *Matthew: Structure, Christology, Kingdom,* xvi n. 26, xx, defends his position by referring primarily to the fact that ἀπὸ τότε is asyndetic in 4:17; 16:21. But this is not sufficient. As an example that the asyndeton does not prevent a substantial connection with what comes previously, we may refer to the discussion concerning the relation between 16:18 and 16:19 above pp. 249f.

[8]   Cf. NEIRYNCK, *ETL* 64 (1988) 21–59; HOWELL, *Inclusive Story,* 129; ALLISON, Matthew: Structure, 1203.

[9]   KINGSBURY, *Matthew as Story,* 40; idem, *Matthew: Structure, Christology, Kingdom,* xii, now acknowledges that the three parts are not to be treated as separate blocks of material and that the formula merely introduces a new phase in the ministry of Jesus. Cf. also somewhat earlier *idem, JSNT* 21 (1984) 4; *idem, JSNT* 25 (1985) 75f; *idem, Matthew,* 29f. Already STONEHOUSE, *Witness of Matthew and Mark,* 129f, gave

not, for instance, the ones proposed by Bacon, are to be placed at the centre of the structure.

Matthew's narrative seems to be structurally mixed. Several scholars doubt that Matthew structured the totality of his narrative according to one basic principle.[1] It is indeed evident that he worked with structural elements within individual units of the narrative.[2] The formulas καὶ ἐγένετο ὅτε ἐτέλεσεν ὁ Ἰησοῦς (7:28; 11:1; 13:53; 19:1; 26:1) and ἀπὸ τότε ἤρξατο ὁ Ἰησοῦς (4:17; 16:21) are the most evident examples. There are also other formulaic features which might correspond to each other.[3] But they do not appear as macro-structural principles for the narrative in its totality. There are obviously various structural patterns within Matthew.[4]

It is possible that the lack of a formal symmetry of perfectly balanced sections further reflects an oral hermeneutic imposed on the written traditions. Oral cultures are more interested in events, in actions and happenings,[5] than in exact stylistic structures and in what something "is" as such. E.A. Havelock brought attention to this already thirty years ago.[6] Plato's critique of the Homeric poets representing the oral mind-set of the time directs itself towards their "opinion" (δόξα) expressed in a tribal encyclopedia of pluralised and visually concrete happenings instead of in abstract thoughts integrated into systems of cause and effect. The poets located the doings and happenings in episodes. They gave, according to Havelock's reading of Plato, the episodes their narrative association and relevance by placing them within a narrative situation which, in turn, was located "in the context of a great and compendious story."[7] Oral cultures narrativize their own existence and environment.[8]

The narrativizing tendency is present also in Matthew. It may serve as an

---

attention to this.

[1]   Cf. e.g. GUNDRY, *Matthew,* 10f; SENIOR, *Matthew,* 25f; FRANCE, *Matthew,* 57; STANTON, *ANRW* II 25:3 (1985) 1905; DAVIES/ALLISON, *Matthew* I, 61; DOYLE, *RB* 95 (1988) 37; GNILKA, *Matthäusevangelium* II, 523; FRANCE, *Matthew: Evangelist and Teacher,* 147f; U. LUZ, *Matthäus* I, 16.

[2]   U. LUZ, *Matthäus* I, 19–23, summarizes 9 such elements. Cf. already LOHR, *CBQ* 23 (1961) 405–427, 430–434. See further below pp. 369–378.

[3]   Cf. e.g. 4:23; 9:35 (καὶ περιῆγεν ... διδάσκων ἐν ταῖς συναγωγαῖς αὐτῶν καὶ κηρύσσων τὸ εὐαγγέλιον τῆς βασιλείας καὶ θεραπεύων πᾶσαν νόσον καὶ πᾶσαν μαλακίαν; 5:17; 10:34 (μὴ νομίσητε ὅτι ἦλθον); 11:25; 12:1; 14:1 (ἐν ἐκείνῳ τῷ καιρῷ). Cf. further the examples given by HAWKINS, *Horae Synopticae,* 168f. Mention should also be made of the passion predictions (16:21; 17:22f; 20:17–19), with the uniform reference to the resurrection on the third day (τῇ τρίτῃ ἡμέρᾳ ἐγερθήσεται [ἐγερθῆναι 16:21]). For the passion predictions, see BAYER, *Jesus' Predictions,* 182–190.

[4]   SYREENI, *Sermon on the Mount,* 114, speaks of "rival structuring principles."

[5]   Cf. the definition of narrative events above p. 206.

[6]   *Preface to Plato,* 165–193. HAVELOCK, *Muse,* 1–18, gives a survey of his subsequent studies of the oral-literate problem in Greek antiquity.

[7]   *Preface to Plato,* 176.

[8]   Cf. HAVELOCK, *Muse,* 76; ONG, *Oral Tradition* 2:1 (1987) 378.

explanation of the mixed structures.[1] The various formulas are then controlable features of how Matthew intended the flow of the story. The development does not emerge out of a meta-theoretical system, but from indications in the narrative itself.[2] Even the chiastic patterns may help the readers/hearers to relate later parts of the narrative to earlier parts.[3] To be sure, the impact of literacy was present in Matthew's environment. His narrative certainly contains elements reflecting the literacy of its author. It is, after all, a written narrative. And narratives occur both in primary oral cultures and in highly literate societies.[4] But Matthew maintained an "oral sensibility."[5] He did not extract information from the traditions in order to produce a collection of important ideas. Instead he narrativized his situation by telling another story about Jesus' history. He was interested in the teaching as part of the life-story of a specific teacher. He maintained a framework which gave the sayings a narrative situation. In using the traditions, he ultimately created another story with its own internal development and movement, its narrative.

Matthew's treatment of the written traditions therefore reflects a process of re-oralization in various ways.[6] The written form of the Markan narrative and the Q material did not cause Matthew to regard the Jesus tradition as entirely fixed and stereotyped. He never used the written traditions as sources in the strict sense.[7] They were not merely read and reproduced passively. They were actively heard and recomposed. We may indeed say that the Markan account and the Q material were to Matthew "words to live

---

[1]   Cf. SENIOR, *Matthew,* 26f; FRANCE, *Matthew: Evangelist and Teacher,* 149–153; U. LUZ, *Matthäus* I, 24–28.

[2]   Cf. GOODING, *RB* 85 (1978) 227; COMBRINK, *TynBul* 34 (1983) 69f; KINGSBURY, *JSNT* 25 (1985) 62; U. LUZ, *Matthäus* I, 17.

[3]   COMBRINK, *TynBul* 34 (1983) 70–87, tries to correlate the chiastic means (the signifier) with the narrative message of the story (the signified). Cf. also *idem, Neot* 16 (1982) 10, 19.

[4]   ONG, *Orality and Literacy,* 133, 138–155.—KELBER, *Semeia* 39 (1987) 119, calls narrative "the most thoroughly textualized piece." I find this to be an exaggeration. Although the extended and linearly plotted narration about the career of a historical person may reflect a high degree of literacy, the narrative form itself is not necessarily, as far as I can see, a sign of literacy.

[5]   I have borrowed this expression from CROSSAN, *In Fragments,* 37–40, whose concern is "the mechanics of a *writer* for whom *orality* is still quite dominant" (*ibid.,* 39).

[6]   LORD, Gospels, 58–91, believes that the sequences and verbal correspondences between the gospel narratives are best explained by a process of oral traditional literary composition, without dependence on written tradition. Lord's discussion, however, does not include the possibility of scripture's perpetual return to oral currency. As TALBERT, Response, 95–99, points out, the types of evidence cited by Lord may also be present in written traditions. Cf. also HENAUT, *Oral Tradition,* 108–113.

[7]   ANDERSEN, Oral Tradition, 51, states: "In a largely oral culture you do not simply 'check' tradition by consulting the written text, for the written text is not yet considered as a 'source'." Cf. already LORD, *Singer of Tales,* 100f.

by in the profoundest sense."[1] They were not present as external sources of reference merely, but as living traditions which he had actively internalized. They contained the precious words of the teacher whose teaching, life and person he deeply cherished. Although the written traditions originated externally to Matthew's own social and existential situation, he incorporated them into a narrativized account as he and his community were seeking for meaning and internal cohesion. *The setting and the motives of transmission correlated with a preference for oral traditions and with a process that continuously re-oralized the written traditions.*[2]

4. The Preservation and Elaboration of Traditions

As a final step, I will try to see how the setting determined by the authority of Jesus as teacher and the person-oriented motives of transmission correlated with the process of preserving and elaborating traditions. Again, Matthew does not provide explicit evidence of this process. The setting of transmission in a school of trained specialists suggests that the transmission was an act separated from the use of the traditions in the community. And the keen interest in Jesus' teaching as rooted in his past history implies a procedure where preservation and elaboration are distinguishable.[3] The Jesus tradition was important also independently of the practical activities fostering an "updating" of the tradition. I will therefore discuss the preservation and the elaboration in separate sections. But due to the character of the material, *I will look primarily for aims and intentions in the present text rather than for hypothetical procedures at earlier stages in the transmission process.*

It is impossible to give an exhaustive account and treat all the Jesus-sayings. I will concentrate on some sayings and small collections of sayings and see how the process of preservation and elaboration relates to the setting and motives of transmission in these cases. Many scholars have already noticed that Matthew enhances Jesus as teacher by presenting long units of several sayings, speeches. This needs no further demonstration. I will pay attention to other features. First, I will study how the aim to preserve the Jesus tradition occurs in sayings which are often seen as the result of a high degree of creativity, *the alleged prophetic oracles.* They are particularly useful as a test case, because *if there are visible intentions of preserving the tradition even in the alleged prophetic oracles, it is legitimate to assume that*

---

[1]   MILLS, Folkloristic Concern, 232.

[2]   KELBER, *The Oral and the Written Gospel*, 93, acknowledges the ongoing existence of synoptic orality, in spite of his emphasis on Mark's disruption of the oral currency on the pre-synoptic level. Cf. also *idem, Semeia* 39 (1987) 101.

[3]   See above pp. 254–261, 306.

a similar attitude pertained to further spectra of the transmitted material.
As a second step, I will look at the elaboration resulting in a *structural significance* of the Jesus-sayings. I will concentrate on structural patterns
which raise what Jesus says above the normal flow of the story. Third, I
will study the elaboration aiming to give the Jesus-sayings a pronounced *argumentative character*. The focus will be on sayings containing a quotation
from the OT.

4.1. Preservation within Creativity

I mentioned above that there was probably no entirely free incorporation
and integration of traditions from other persons into the Jesus tradition.[1] It
is time to substantiate this claim. Matthew did live in a sociocultural situation of transmission where some integration of foreign traditions seems to
have existed. This was the case especially in certain prophetic circles in ancient Israel.[2] In chapter three I tried to show that the prophetic disciples not
only interpreted the tradition from their own master, but also integrated influences from other prophets into the tradition of the prophet they themselves adhered to. The settings and the motives of transmission effected both
an interpretative development and an integrative concentration of the tradition.[3] Did Matthew then differ from this practice?

The problem of whether some of the material appearing on the lips of Jesus in the gospel narratives had its origin in words uttered by Christian prophets has occupied the attention of scholars for a long time. Already the
early form critics differed somewhat in their answers to the problem.[4] R.
Bultmann thought that Christian prophets often formulated utterances of
the spirit and sayings of the risen Lord.[5] Since all the words of Jesus essentially served as a vehicle for the voice of the risen Lord, the early communities incorporated prophetic oracles into the dominical tradition without
any concern at any stage of the transmission to keep the two separated. M.
Dibelius claimed that there were regulatory words from the historical Jesus
and inspirational words infused by the spirit of the Lord.[6] The early communities used the two within one and the same paraenetic activity. The inspirational words functioned on the same level as the regulatory words,

---

[1]   See above p. 319.

[2]   We may also recall how the Qumranites retrospectively ascribed precepts to the
Teacher—the Mosaic prophet. See above pp. 188–193, 195.

[3]   See above pp. 176–188, 195.

[4]   Cf. my remarks in the introduction above pp. 15–17, 24.

[5]   *Geschichte der synoptischen Tradition,* 40 n. 2, 134f, 160, 176, 393. Cf. also
idem, Ergänzungsheft, 51f.

[6]   *Formgeschichte,* 239–265, 279–287. Dibelius speaks only rarely of *prophetic*
speech in the Christian communities.

since they were all said "in the Lord."[1] But Dibelius also recognized the early Christian interest in collecting genuine Jesus-sayings. Besides the levelling of the words in the paraenetic activity, there was an awareness that some words came from Jesus himself and as such were particularly important.[2]

Despite the extended criticism that Bultmann and his followers—especially E. Käsemann in his analysis of prophetic "sentences of holy law"[3]—received on these matters,[4] the discussion continues. In recent years, M.E. Boring has repeatedly tried to sharpen the issue and bring it to a further level of clarification.[5] His aim is to trace the Jesus-sayings which originated when the Christian prophets delivered their messages directly from the risen Jesus to the Christian community or, as representatives of the community, to the general public. The question at hand for the present inquiry is how this creativity related to the preserved tradition in the Matthean community.[6] Did Matthew allow new and independent oracles from Christian prophets in his community to enter into the tradition as Jesus-sayings placed in a pre-Easter context?

4.1.1. The Material

To make text work possible, Boring sets up certain analytical criteria.[7] The

---

[1]   Cf. DIBELIUS, *Formgeschichte,* 242: "Man wird vielmehr daran zu erinnern haben, daß alle Sprüche der christlichen Paränese als vom Geist oder vom Herrn gewirkt galten, so daß sie alle, wenn auch nicht als Mahnungen des Herrn, so doch als Mahnungen 'im Herrn' erschienen."

[2]   Cf. DIBELIUS, *Formgeschichte,* 243: "Wie sich im Urchristentum von Anfang an neben enthusiastischen auch nomistische Gedanken gezeigt haben, so steht neben dem pneumatischen Interesse, für das alle christliche Paränese den einen göttlichen Ursprung hat, die Wertschätzung der T r a d i t i o n , der A u t h e n t i e und der A u t o r i t ä t."

[3]   *New Testament Questions,* 66–81.—Related to this form is the "eschatological correlative." R.A. EDWARDS, *ZNW* 60 (1969) 9–20, claims that this form first occurred in four (Luke 11:30/Matt 12:40; Luke 17:24/Matt 24:27; Luke 17:26/Matt 24:37; Luke 17:28, 30/Matt 24:38f) of the six son of man sayings in Q and was used in the celebration of the eucharist. D. SCHMIDT, *JBL* 96 (1977) 517–522, argues that the form was not a creation of the early Church but adopted by the Christian prophets from the "prophetic correlative" found in the LXX. But none of these correlatives is prophetic by definition. See AUNE, *Prophecy,* 168f.

[4]   Cf. the mainly negative assessments of Bultmann's view by NEUGEBAUER, *ZNW* 53 (1962) 218–228; DUNN, *NTS* 24 (1978) 175–198; HILL, *New Testament Prophecy,* 160–174; AUNE, *Prophecy,* 233–240; RIESNER, *Lehrer,* 8–11. For criticism of Käsemann's definition and prophetic location of "sentences of holy law," see BERGER, *NTS* 17 (1970–71) 10–40; *idem, TZ* 28 (1972) 305–330. See further excursus 14 below.— The dissertation by C. FORBES, *Prophecy and Inspired Speech in Early Christianity and Its Hellenistic Environment.* Macquarie University 1987, was not available to me.

[5]   See most recently *Continuing Voice.*

[6]   For an assessment of the prophetic oracles in a broader perspective, see excursus 14 below.

[7]   *Continuing Voice,* 155–186, 189f. Cf. already *idem, JBL* 91 (1972) 501–521.

particular *forms* and *items of content* characterizing prophetic speech must be present. This would suggest that a prophet is the author of the saying. But since also Jesus himself could have uttered prophetic sayings, it must also be probable that the sayings existed *independently* of their present narrative context and that they are *secondary*. This would indicate that they were formulated by a person other than Jesus and that they have been projected from a post-Easter to a pre-Easter context.

Boring has defined the texts which might imply that prophets in the Matthean community creatively used or authored prophetic oracles. Some oracles were inherited from the tradition as already integrated within a pre-Easter context. But according to Boring,[1] 5:3–12, 18, 19; 6:14f; 7:2, 20–23; 10:5b–6, 17–22, 23; 12:33–35; 13:35; 16:17–19; 17:20; 18:18, 19f; 19:12, 23b; 22:3; 23:1–39 might disclose this kind of prophetic activity in the Matthean community itself.[2] He mentions also 28:18b–20, but this utterance is still located in a post-Easter context and therefore not relevant here. Boring is himself sceptical about ascribing the possible, though often vague, prophetic characteristics of 5:19; 6:14f; 7:2; 10:5b–6, 17–22; 16:17–19; 18:19f to persons in the Matthean community. I will leave them out of consideration. He also recognizes that the prophetic features in 5:3–12, 18; 12:33–35; 13:35; 17:20; 19:12, 23b; 22:3; 23:1–39 do not depend on the incorporation of entirely new and independent oracles. These instances merely represent prophetic amplifications of already existing Jesus-sayings. 5:3–12, 18 still deserve some attention since, in Boring's view, they reflect the use of forms that are typically prophetic. A discussion of them may illustrate to what extent and how prophetic interests actually influenced the use of the already existing tradition. 7:20–23; 10:23; 18:18 remain as possible reflections of how new and independent prophetic oracles were integrated into the Jesus-tradition and put within a pre-Easter context by prophets in the Matthean community or persons active in the Matthean stream of tradition.

4.1.2. Matthew 5:3–12; 5:18

5:3–12 is in its present form the result of work on the tradition. Typical Matthean vocabulary appears.[3] Among the beatitudes without parallel in Luke (5:5, 7–10), 5:10 probably reflects Matthean work.[4] The work creates

---

[1]   *Continuing Voice*, 247–255. The arguments are presented more fully in *idem, Sayings*, 204–216.

[2]   BORING, *Sayings*, 212, discusses also 10:24, 27, 40–42; 11:28–30. But in the more recent study, *Continuing Voice*, he does not mention these passages.

[3]   Cf. δικαιοσύνη (5:6, 10), ἡ βασιλεία τῶν οὐρανῶν (5:3, 10).

[4]   So most scholars. Cf. e.g. WALTER, *SE* 4 (1968) 247; STRECKER, *NTS* 17 (1970–71) 267; FRANKEMÖLLE, *BZ* 15 (1971) 56f; GUELICH, *JBL* 95 (1976) 430f; *idem, Sermon on the Mount*, 93; TUCKETT, *NovT* 25 (1983) 201f; DAVIES/ALLISON,

a neat structure with two pairs of four beatitudes in the third person (5:3–6, 7–10), each pair concluded with a reference to δικαιοσύνη and each containing approximately thirty-six words,[1] and with a π-alliteration in the first pair (πτωχοί, πενθοῦντες, πραεῖς, πεινῶντες).[2] The ninth beatitude consisting of thirty-four or thirty-five words appears in the second person and links with the following pericope.

Boring finds several prophetic features in the text, though he acknowledges the problem of giving them an exact tradition-historical location.[3] However, some of the features carry no evident prophetic marks. The phrases from Scripture placed on Jesus' lips in 5:5, 8 are not prophetic at all. They are taken from the Psalms.[4] The "sentence of holy law" in 5:7 is likewise an insufficient indication. K. Berger has shown that this kind of pronouncements are at home also in wisdom circles.[5] As a Matthean example, we may refer to the alleged "sentence of holy law" in 5:19. Even if this would be a saying that originated in the post-Easter situation of the Matthean community,[6] which is far from certain,[7] the form and the items of content give no secure evidence for a prophetic influence. The content of this pronouncement implies instead that an interest to secure the right teaching influenced the Matthean formulation of the saying—we may leave the question of origin open. To be sure, Berger does not consider the fact that prophets could use sapiential forms.[8] But we could also say the reverse: wisdom teachers could use prophetic forms.[9] The interchangeability of different life settings for one and the same form suggests that this criterion is too uncertain in order to be used for confining the origin or elaboration of a saying to a particular group of people.[10] Boring also fails to mention that the first eight beatitudes appear in the common third person form, which

---

Matthew I, 434, 459; U. LUZ, *Matthäus* I, 200, 214.

[1] Cf. SCHNIEWIND, *Matthäus*, 40; FRANKEMÖLLE, *BZ* 15 (1971) 55; DUPONT, *Béatitudes* III, 309; MCELENEY, *CBQ* 43 (1981) 13; U. LUZ, *Matthäus* I, 199f.

[2] C. MICHAELIS, *NovT* 10 (1968) 148–161. For a similar, but fivefold, π-alliteration in Heb 1:1, see D.A. BLACK, *WTJ* 49 (1987) 189; ÜBELACKER, *Hebräerbrief* I, 88.

[3] *Sayings*, 206; *idem, Continuing Voice*, 249.

[4] Cf. SATO, *Q und Prophetie*, 263.

[5] BERGER, *NTS* 17 (1970–71) 10–40; *idem, TZ* 28 (1972) 305–330. Berger argues that the "sentences" are wisdom instructions used in the initial catechetical activity of the community. As it seems, Berger's hypothesis was not entirely new. Cf. SCHWEIZER, *NTS* 16 (1969–70) 226f n. 3, referring to an unpublished paper by G.-C. Kähler.

[6] HEUBÜLT, *ZNW* 71 (1980) 144; GUNDRY, *Matthew*, 81f, think that the verse stems from Matthew's own redaction.

[7] SCHÜRMANN, *Untersuchungen*, 126, states: "Die Forschung ist sich einig in dem Urteil, daß Mt 5,19 dem Matthäus schon *überkommenes Überlieferungsgut* darstellt." Some would even trace it back to Jesus himself. So e.g. BANKS, *JBL* 93 (1974) 238–240; RIESNER, *Lehrer*, 456–460.

[8] Cf. SATO, *Q und Prophetie*, 266; BORING, *Continuing Voice*, 162.

[9] Cf. e.g. above p. 83.

[10] Cf. DUNN, *NTS* 24 (1978) 182.

perhaps is less original than the second person form,[1] though this is uncertain.[2] M. Sato notices that this weakens the prophetic force and character of the beatitudes.[3]

What remains are features reflecting the use of the preserved tradition. Prophetic motifs are present in 5:10, 11f. Of special importance is the motif of persecution.[4] The Matthean term διώκειν appears in all three verses.[5] 5:12 relates it to the prophets "before you" (τοὺς πρὸ ὑμῶν). And this motif depends on the tradition. 5:11f builds on a tradition reflected also in Luke 6:22f, where the motif of persecution is present without the use of διώκειν.[6] Further, it is difficult to assume that 5:10 ever existed as an independent saying. It brings nothing new beyond what was already present in the tradition. 5:10a draws on 5:11 and 5:10b on 5:3b,[7] in both cases on beatitudes with clear roots in the tradition. The similarities with 1 Pet 3:14 might even imply that the Matthean work on 5:10 proceeded from a traditional kernel. The prophetic motif was therefore not new, and it did not, as far as we can tell, exist independently of its present context. If prophets were at work, their activity did not consist in the formulation of entirely new characteristics added to sayings. They depended upon the preserved tradition.

In 5:18, Boring assumes,[8] the Matthean community has associated a prophetic saying from Q more closely with prophetic forms. The circumstances behind 5:18 are indeed extremely difficult—if not impossible—to ascertain. However, the prophetic features in the present text are not always evident. Although the introductory formula ἀμὴν γὰρ λέγω ὑμῖν might be

---

[1] So e.g. WALTER, SE 4 (1968) 250–253; SCHWEIZER, NTS 19 (1972–73) 124 n. 1; MCELENEY, CBQ 43 (1981) 11; GUNDRY, Matthew, 67f; BROER, Seligpreisungen, 12, 17–19, 29f, 32–38; U. LUZ, Matthäus I, 201. For a different view, cf. the extensive discussion by DUPONT, Béatitudes I, 272–298, who is followed by e.g. KIEFFER, Weisheit und Segen, 35.—PUECH, RB 98 (1991) 87–106, argues that the Matthean version is older because the number of beatitudes (8+1) corresponds to a standard literary form found in Sir 14:20–27 and, perhaps, 4Q525 frg. 2. But for critique, cf. VIVIANO, BARev 18:6 (1992) 66; idem, SEÅ 58 (1993) 80–84.

[2] GUELICH, JBL 95 (1976) 415; TUCKETT, NovT 25 (1983) 197; DAVIES/ALLISON, Matthew I, 445f, leave the issue open.

[3] SATO, Q und Prophetie, 263, ascribes the third person format to QMt and concludes: "Hier liegt kein prophetisches Stück mehr vor, sondern ein endzeitlich-weisheitlicher Lehrtext."

[4] BORING, Sayings, 206, mentions also ἀγαλλιᾶσθε, which in view of Luke 1:47; 10:21; Rev 19:7 has overtones of the prophetic exaltation of the spirit. But this seems to be a remote point.

[5] STECK, Israel, 23, 25, believes διώκειν to be pre-Matthean. But see TUCKETT, NovT 25 (1983) 203 n. 46.

[6] It is not necessary here to decide when the motif of persecution first entered into the tradition. It seems that the general perspective on the Q material as either sapiential or prophetic is decisive. Cf. the different proposals of KLOPPENBORG, Formation of Q, 173, 190, and SATO, Q und Prophetie, 258–260.

[7] Cf. WALTER, SE 4 (1968) 247; STRECKER, NTS 17 (1970–71) 267; FRANKEMÖLLE, BZ 15 (1971) 56.

[8] Sayings, 207; idem, Continuing Voice, 249.

an addition,[1] it constitutes no unequivocal evidence of the prophetic origin
and character of the saying. V. Hasler's hypothesis that this formula originated with the early Christian prophets in the Hellenistic church is unlikely.[2] Since there are only three possible indications of a pre-Christian use of
the non-responsorial ἀμήν,[3] the proposal fails to explain from where the
prophets took the formula, were it not already present in the Jesus tradition,[4] at least in some version.[5] Moreover, it is not certain that only the
early Christian prophets adopted the formula. It is hardly an equivalent to
the OT messenger formula.[6] The introductory ἀμήν-formula grounds the
authority in the speaker himself, not in God. In the NT, and with two exceptions also in the NT apocrypha,[7] it always occurs on Jesus' lips—not a
Christian prophet's—and is carried by his own intrinsic authority.

The remaining prophetic feature depends also in this case on the preserved tradition. The declaration that something will not take place until
something else (of an eschatological nature) happens probably reflects
prophetic influence. The formula οὐ μὴ ... ἕως (ἄν)/μέχρις οὖ often appears
in sayings which explicitly or implicitly relate the present situation to decisive events of the end-time,[8] and this might be characteristic of prophetic

---

1   The formula is not present in Luke 6:17. Moreover, ἀμὴν λέγω appears more often in Matthew than in the other synoptics, altogether 31 times (including 18:19) as compared to 13 times in Mark and 6 times in Luke. The formula with γάρ occurs only in Matt
10:23; 13:17; 17:20.

2   *Amen,* 168–187.

3   BERGER, *Amen-Worte,* 4–6, brings attention to rec. A of T. Abr. 8, 20 (James'
ed. 85 line 19, 102 line 2). He defends the non-Christian character of these instances in
ZNW 63 (1972) 47–50. But cf. G.-C. KÄHLER, *TLZ* 97 (1972) 201; Joachim JERE-
MIAS, *ZNW* 64 (1973) 123.—STRUGNELL, *HTR* 67 (1974) 177–182; BIETENHARD,
NIDNTT I, 98, bring attention to a Hebrew letter written with ink on an ostracon from
the 7th cent. B.C.E., published by NAVEH, *IEJ* 10 (1960) 129–136, pl. 17. The term אמן
appears on line 11. But it is not certain that this use is non-responsorial. Cf. BERGER,
Amen-Worte, 2f; Joachim JEREMIAS, *ibid.,* 122; CHILTON, *ZNW* 69 (1978) 205.

4   This argument speaks against the assumption that the formula orginated in an apocalyptic context where the introductory ἀμήν was part of a legitimation formula for eschatological asseverations, as is the thesis of BERGER, *Amen-Worte; idem, ZNW* 63 (1972)
45–75. Berger gives a certain justification for his view when he points to the replacement
of ἦ μήν in Gen 22:17 (LXX) with ἀμήν in rec. A of T. Abr. 8 (James' ed. 85 line 19).
The question is of course if the use in T. Abr. 8 is pre-Christian. Cf. the previous note.

5   CHILTON, *ZNW* 69 (1978) 203–211, proposes that Jesus addressed his hearers
with "in truth" (Aram. בקושטא), which was translated into Greek as ἀμήν. But this hypothesis is not unproblematic. Cf. the critique by RIESNER, *Lehrer,* 381f.

6   *Contra* HASLER, *Amen,* 174–180; BERGER, *Amen-Worte,* 124–130. For critique
of Hasler and Berger on this point, see SATO, *Q und Prophetie,* 245f. Cf. also AUNE,
Prophecy, 164.

7   Act. Pt. et Andr. 5 (LIPSIUS/BONNET [eds.], *Acta* I, 120 line 9); Act. Thom. 158
(LIPSIUS/BONNET [eds.], *Acta* II, 269 line 7).

8   Cf. Matt 10:23; Mark 9:1/Matt 16:28/Luke 9:27; Matt 23:39/Luke 13:35; Mark
13:30/Matt 24:34/Luke 21:32; Mark 14:25/Matt 26:29/Luke 22:16, 18.—The formula is
of course present also in sayings which do not concern eschatology. Cf. Matt 5:26/Luke
12:59; John 13:38.

diction.[1] But even if this formula is an addition to the tradition, which is not certain,[2] we find no evidence of a complete saying originating as a new and independent oracle from a prophet in the Matthean community. The prophets only adopted a traditional saying to their own diction.

5:3–12, 18 exemplify the prophets' use of the tradition. The prophetic influence is not as strong as it may seem on first sight. And when such an influence is present, it does not emerge as the result of a creativity relying exclusively on charismatic inspiration. Prophetic items of content and prophetic forms are here *interpretative* measures shaping and actualizing the *preserved* tradition.

4.1.3. Matthew 7:20–23; 10:23; 18:18

The next step is to discuss the passages which Boring regards as new and independent additions to the Jesus tradition. 7:20–23 reflects, according to Boring, the activity of a Christian prophet in the Matthean community.[3] A prophet has taken up a traditional saying and reformulated it as a word of the risen Lord to the contemporary situation. The reformulation is in Boring's view more than an incidental influence on the way things get said in the Matthean community.

A first modification of this hypothesis concerns Boring's isolation of the saying. 7:20 belongs to the previous unit. Together with 7:16a it forms an inclusio to 7:16b–19. Matthean diction is visible in 7:21.[4] And its parallel in Luke 6:46 does not appear together with the parallel to 7:22f in Luke 13:25–27.[5] There is only evidence, therefore, that 7:22f formed a unit in the tradition. The eschatological orientation, the concern with false prophecy and the authoritative tone of judgement in 7:22f suggest prophetic influences in the formulation of a traditional saying recorded also in Luke 13:25–27.[6]

The second modification concerns the claim that the saying was uttered as a word of the risen Lord. It did not float around entirely freely in the tradi-

---

[1]   PEABODY, *JBL* 97 (1978) 391–409; CRAWFORD, *JBL* 101 (1982) 225–244; KLOPPENBORG, *Formation of Q*, 153; SATO, *Q und Prophetie*, 159, 243. Cf. also BERGER, *Amen-Worte*, 73f.

[2]   Cf. e.g. CRAWFORD, *JBL* 101 (1982) 232f.

[3]   *Sayings*, 208; *idem, Continuing Voice*, 250.

[4]   See U. LUZ, *Matthäus* I, 402 n. 7.

[5]   The resemblance with Matt 7:21 in Justin, Apol. I 16:9; 2 Clem. 4:2; Gos. Naz. frg. 6 (Greek text in STROKER, *Extracanonical Sayings*, 71), probably depends on the synoptics. See W.-D. KÖHLER, *Rezeption des Matthäusevangeliums*, 181 n. 3; 132–134; 298. For P. Egerton 2 frg. 2^r (Greek text in STROKER, *Extracanonical Sayings*, 16), cf. similarly in HENNECKE/SCHNEEMELCHER (eds.), *Apokryphen* I, 83.

[6]   BORING, *Sayings*, 208, mentions also the allusion to Jer 14:14 in Matt 7:22 and to Ps 6:8 (should be Ps 6:9 according to both MT and LXX) in Matt 7:23. It is possible, but far from evident, that such re-presentation of Scripture reflects prophetic influence.

tion. M. Sato believes that Luke 13:23f, 25–27, 28f, 34f reflect the order within the Q material.[1] There is in these cases a common sequence in the material which Luke shares with Matthew.[2] If Sato is correct, 7:22f was located within a series of Jesus-sayings already in the tradition. It is of course possible that a Christian prophet might loosen the saying from its context and use it as an isolated utterance. But such an assumption is a mere conjecture. The evidence available suggests that the prophet used a saying that was preserved precisely as something which the earthly Jesus had said.

In the discussion about prophetic influences behind the missionary speech, Boring focuses on 10:23 specifically.[3] In his view, the saying originated as a pronouncement of a Christian prophet in the Matthean stream of tradition. The life setting was a commissioning service. Since there was a clear tradition that a missionary should stand firm in the face of opposition, the call to flee shows, according to Boring, that belief in the spirit even could legitimize actual breaks with the tradition.

Prophetic influence is indeed visible in 10:23. The form relating the present situation to decisive events of the end-time is emphatically present (οὐ μὴ ... ἕως [ἄν]).[4] There are also signs that the saying, while exhibiting several Matthean features,[5] comes from the tradition.[6] The decisive evidence is not the (awkward) language used[7] but the implication of 10:23b. The mention of Israelite cities as unexplored objects of mission fits better at a time earlier than the second half of the first century C.E.[8] And it is difficult to believe that 10:23a and 10:23b ever existed independently of each other.[9] 10:23a is in itself a torso and the statement in 10:23b, that the disciples will not complete the cities of Israel, presupposes something, most likely the reference to the city and the call to flee in 10:23a.[10]

However, it is difficult to ascertain that 10:23 originated with a prophet

---

1   *Q und Prophetie*, 42f. Cf. also KLOPPENBORG, *Formation of Q*, 223–237.
2   See items 48–51 in table 3 above. I differ only in relating Luke 13:24, not 13:23f, to Matt 7:13f.
3   *Sayings*, 208–212; idem, *Continuing Voice*, 250–252.
4   Cf. SATO, *Q und Prophetie*, 217.
5   Cf. e.g. DAVIES/ALLISON, *Matthew* II, 188.
6   *Contra* FRANKEMÖLLE, *Jahwebund*, 130–133; GUNDRY, *Matthew*, 194f; GNILKA, *Matthäusevangelium* I, 374f.
7   The presence of ταύτῃ and the definite article in front of ἑτέραν is often regarded as a sign of an earlier (Aramaic) tradition. But there is no close connection here to the city mentioned in 10:15. And τῇ πόλει ταύτῃ ... τὴν ἑτέραν, which is the original reading, correspond to each other in the sense that "this city" stands over "the next (city)." See GUNDRY, *Matthew*, 195; GNILKA, *Matthäusevangelium* I, 374f n. 14.
8   BARTNICKI, *TZ* 43 (1987) 316f, argues that the mission to Israel implies also mission to non-Jews. In view of 10:5b–6, this is unlikely.
9   *Contra* DUPONT, *NovT* 2 (1958) 230–238; KÜMMEL, Naherwartung, 41f; HARE, *Jewish Persecution*, 110f; GRÄSSER, *Parusieverzögerung*, 137; SABOURIN, *BTB* 7 (1977) 5. —MCDERMOTT, *BZ* 28 (1984) 236–240, regards 10:23a as traditional and 10:23b as (probably) redactional.
10   BARTNICKI, *TZ* 43 (1987) 315.

in the Matthean stream of tradition and was transmitted as an independent saying. Its origin is simply impossible to determine. It is not satisfying merely to claim that it is "notoriously difficult" to fit 10:23 into the pre-Easter ministry of Jesus.[1] V. Hampel is a recent representative of a number of scholars who are quite certain that such a setting is in fact conceivable.[2] Concerning the transmission, H. Schürmann suggests that 10:23 followed in Q the unit recorded in Matt 10:19/Luke 12:11f, which Matthew supplemented with Mark 13:9, 11–13.[3] The similarities between the introductions in Matt 10:19/Luke 12:11 and in Matt 10:23 are indeed striking. Others point to the possibility that 10:23 appeared in Q's missionary speech, reflected in Luke 10:2–16.[4] The various opinions of scholars depend in this case on the fact that there is simply not enough evidence.[5] This calls for some caution before claiming that 10:23 originated and circulated as an independent saying. The analytical criteria for establishing the existence of a new and independent oracle cannot be used with sufficient clarity and coherence in this case.

It is also unlikely that 10:23 represents a break with the tradition. The emphasis is not on escaping from persecution, as Boring says. W.G. Kümmel and E. Grässer see rightly that 10:23b concerns primarily the continued mission of the disciples.[6] This does not imply that 10:23b is unconnected with the call to flee in 10:23a, as Kümmel and Grässer continue to argue. On the contrary, fleeing is a way to carry the mission further. The Matthean γάρ in the ἀμήν-clause suggests that the disciples should flee to the next town *because* of the urgency to missionize Israel.[7] Comparison of 10:22f with 24:13f confirms the emphasis on mission.[8] 10:22b and 24:13 contain the identical promise that the one who endures to the end will be saved (ὁ δὲ ὑπομείνας εἰς τέλος οὗτος σωθήσεται). 24:14 continues by stating that the gospel will be preached to the whole world before the end comes. The focus is clearly on the continued mission, though in a world-wide perspective. 10:23 centres on the mission to Israel before the end comes. The task of completing the cities of Israel is so great that it cannot be ac-

---

[1] BORING, *Sayings,* 210; idem, *Continuing Voice,* 250.

[2] *TZ* 45 (1989) 20–27. Hampel lists other scholars with the same opinion (*ibid.,* 24 n. 70). Both U. LUZ, *Matthäus* II, 107f, 113f, and DAVIES/ALLISON, *Matthew* II, 189f, recognize the possibility that the saying goes back to Jesus.

[3] *Untersuchungen,* 150–156.

[4] GEIST, *Menschensohn,* 228–230; U. LUZ, *Matthäus* II, 106 n. 8; DAVIES/ALLISON, *Matthew* II, 188.

[5] Cf. the conclusion by KÜNZI, *Naherwartungslogion,* 180: "Ein *Beweis* dafür, daß Mt 10,23 überarbeitet oder später gebildet wäre, ist bis jetzt nicht erbracht."

[6] KÜMMEL, Naherwartung, 43; GRÄSSER, *Parusieverzögerung,* 137.

[7] WEAVER, *Missionary Discourse,* 100.

[8] There might have been a close connection between the two verses in the tradition. The parallel to Matt 24:9–14 in Mark 13:9–13 shows several similarities with Matt 10:17–22.

complished before the eschaton,[1] but its urgency demands that the disciples respond to persecution by fleeing from one city to the next.[2] This understanding is against the tradition.[3]

If my observations are correct, the prophetic influence on 10:23 cannot be ascribed to a prophet uttering a new and independent saying. It is at least as probable that the prophetic features are the result of an activity which faithfully adhered to the intentions in the preserved tradition.

The third instance of interest is 18:18. Boring believes that this verse originated as a prophetic declaration.[4] It was later combined with the less prophetic tradition reflected in 16:17–19, which Matthew related to the Markan account about Peter's confession.

There are two objections to this hypothesis. The first concerns the criteria for arguing that 18:18 is prophetic at all. They consist of the ἀμήν-formula and the legal sounding declaration expressed in an antithetical parallelism similar to "sentences of holy law." But as we have seen, the criteria building on the presence of an ἀμήν-formula and "sentences of holy law" are ambiguous. And legal declarations and antithetical parallelisms were certainly not used in prophetic circles only. Boring mentions also that John 20:23 reflects a prophetic use of the saying. But C.H. Dodd claimed that John knew only a synoptic-like tradition in mainly oral form. 20:23 represents, in Dodd's view, a tradition which is merely akin to the Matthean tradition and which John has followed independently.[5] If Dodd was correct,[6] John's use says nothing about the origin and character of the saying in the Matthean stream of tradition. There are no certain criteria for determining the prophetic character of the saying.

Second, it is far from certain that 18:18 is earlier than 16:19.[7] To be sure, such arguments as the ones claiming that the attribution of authority to an indvidual goes before the attribution to a group or that 16:16 is better

---

[1]   I cannot here discuss separately what the coming of the son of man refers to exactly. It must suffice to say that it does not function as an exact chronological fixation in the Matthean context. Cf. SAND, *Matthäus*, 225: "Mt hat das konsequent eschatologische Menschsohnwort nicht zeitlich (...) sondern endzeitlich verstanden."

[2]   The term τελεῖν can mean "to complete," not only "to finish" as in 7:28; 11:1; 13:53; 19:1; 26:1—in 10:23 this would take the sense "to go through" (cf. e.g. NRSV).

[3]   In spite of his emphasis on persecution, BAMMEL, *ST* 15 (1961) 92 n. 8, adds that the present context of 10:23 implies the theme of mission.

[4]   *Sayings,* 213f; idem, *Continuing Voice,* 252f.

[5]   *Historical Tradition,* 349. Cf. similarly BEASLEY-MURRAY, *John,* 383.

[6]   For a recent elaboration of Dodd's study, see DUNN, John and the Oral Gospel Tradition, 351–379.

[7]   Several scholars claim that 16:19 formed the basis of 18:18. So e.g. G. KLEIN, *ZTK* 58 (1961) 326f; TRILLING, *Israel,* 157f; W.G. THOMPSON, *Matthew's Advice,* 193f; STRECKER, *Weg der Gerechtigkeit,* 223; BULTMANN, *Geschichte der synoptischen Tradition,* 150f; BORNKAMM, "Bind" and "Loose," 94; SCHNACKENBURG, *Matthäusevangelium* II, 172f; GNILKA, *Matthäusevangelium* II, 55f; DAVIES/ALLISON, *Matthew* II, 639f.

anchored in the context are too general in order to carry much weight. But the use of οὐρανοί/οὐρανός in 16:19 and 18:18 seems to be significant. 16:19 uses the plural; 18:18 the singular. Matthew elsewhere uses both, mostly the plural. The distinction between the singular and the plural is perhaps more significant than commonly assumed.[1] In any event, when Matthew juxtaposes heaven and earth, he always uses the singular,[2] except in 16:19.[3] It probably reflects Matthean work. The mention of heaven and earth together is an important feature in Matthew.[4] Only in three cases is the juxtaposition present in the parallels.[5] The parallels to 6:10, 19f in Luke 11:2; 12:33 do not mention heaven and earth together. 5:34f; 28:18 are special material. It is easier, therefore, to assume a change from the plural in 16:19 to the singular in 18:18 than the reverse. The plural in 16:19 is in this perspective an isolated occurrence in Matthew. And it cannot be explained as harmonization with the plural in 16:17, 19a.[6] Matthew elsewhere maintains the singular in contexts using the plural.[7] It indicates rather that 16:19 is the earlier version. Boring admits that 16:19 is not strongly prophetic. If 16:19 is the more original version, the tradition in 18:18 did not originate as a prophetic declaration. And if prophetic features are present in 18:18, which as we saw is questionable, they emerged through the use of an existing tradition.

The evidence available implies that the prophetic influences in the Matthean community manifested themselves as *interpretative* activities. As E. Schweizer puts it, "the true prophet is the interpreter of the commissions of Jesus."[8] Jesus-sayings from the past remained the basis of any contemporizing address to the community.[9] It is indeed possible that the prophets did utter new and independent oracles. But Matthew did apparently not allow them to enter into the Jesus tradition as pre-Easter Jesus-sayings. *There was no entirely free incorporation and integration of new and independent oracles into the Jesus tradition.* Within the creativity, there was the aim to preserve.

---

1   So TORM, *ZNW* 33 (1934) 48–50.
2   5:18, 34f; 6:10, 19f; 11:25; 18:18; 24:35; 28:18.
3   TRILLING, *Israel*, 157f n. 59; W.G. THOMPSON, *Matthew's Advice*, 189, 193f.
4   SCHNEIDER, "Im Himmel – auf Erden," 288f, 292–297; SYREENI, *JSNT* 40 (1990) 3–13.
5   Matt 5:18/Luke 16:17; Matt 11:25/Luke 10:21 (but not in P[45]); Matt 24:35/Mark 13:31/Luke 21:33.
6   *Contra* GNILKA, *Matthäusevangelium* II, 55.
7   Cf. e.g. 5:18 with 5:16, 19, 20 or 6:10 with 6:9, 14 or 24:35 with 24:36.
8   *NTS* 16 (1969–70) 228.—STANTON, *Gospel*, 345, states: "The expansions ... are not the work of a Christian prophet, but of an 'exegete'." But this implies an unnecessary dichotomy between prophet and exegete.
9   Cf. for earlier layers in the Jesus tradition, J. WANKE, *"Bezugs- und Kommentarworte,"* 114.

4.1.4. The Criteria for Preservation

Matthew's aim to preserve—even protect—the Jesus tradition implies the existence of criteria which controlled the incorporation of additional material.[1] J.D.G. Dunn stresses the early Christians' need to test prophetic oracles.[2] He lists three criteria for the testing: the criterion of past revelation, the criterion of present conduct and the criterion of community benefit. The third is an extension of the second.

The criterion of present conduct is most evident in Matthew. Jesus warns specifically against false prophets in 7:15–23. He even points to persons who, it seems, prophecied in the name of the Lord (7:22). Whatever their exact identity,[3] there is no reason to minimize their impact in the Matthean community.[4] The reference to false prophets is present only in Matthew.[5] And Jesus states that a tree can be known only by the fruit it produces (ποιεῖν).[6] There is a strong emphasis on the correlation between words and deeds.[7]

The criterion of right conduct implies some kind of standard according to which the behaviour is judged. The special material in 24:11f shows that false prophecy results in lawlessness.[8] And lawlessness is lack of love, both for God and for fellow-men—the emphasis is here on the latter.

It is therefore not improbable that Matthew and his circle of transmitters tested the prophetic oracles on the basis of the correlation with the love command. Jesus ascribes a fundamental and non-questionable status to the command to love in two pericopes. When the Matthean Jesus quotes the OT, he usually relates the quotation to an elaborated argumentation.[9] But in two pericopes, the quotations appear as entirely sufficient in themselves.

In 22:34–40 Jesus quotes Deut 6:5 and Lev 19:18. A comparison with Mark 12:28–34/Luke 10:25–28 shows that Matthew has sharpened the principal and exegetical character of the issue at stake. The stated aim to test (πειράζειν) the wisdom of Jesus, the absence of a reference to Deut 6:4, with

---

[1] Already EASTON, *Gospel,* 118, spoke about the corporate "censorship" of the Christian community.

[2] *NTS* 24 (1978) 175–198.

[3] G. BARTH, Law, 73–75, identifies them with antinomians. So also COTHENET, Les prophètes chrétiens, 300.—HILL, *Bib* 57 (1976) 340–348, thinks of two separate groups, Pharisaic teachers from the outside (7:15–20) and charismatic prophets from within the community (7:21–23). But cf. the criticism by Hill's own student CHARETTE, *Recompense,* 124f n. 3.—DAVIES/ALLISON, *Matthew* I, 701; U. LUZ, *Matthäus* I, 403, list other proposals.

[4] *Contra* STRECKER, *Weg der Gerechtigkeit,* 137f n. 4.

[5] Cf. the parallels in Luke 6:43f, 46; 13:25–27.

[6] Cf. 3:10; 12:33; 13:23, though the use of the image is different in each case.

[7] See above p. 325.

[8] It is probable that this text reflects the situation of the Matthean community. See U. LUZ, *Matthäus* I, 403 n. 22.

[9] See below pp. 378–396.

the resulting—probably intentional[1]—focus on the actual commandments to love, and perhaps the mention of a νομικός,[2] a specialist in legal matters, give the impression of a sharply formulated discussion of much importance. These differences are all to some extent in agreement with Luke 10:25–28,[3] and it is not certain, therefore, that they reflect Matthew's own work with the tradition.[4] But Matthew maintains them. And only in Matt 22:36 does the questioner ask about the greatest commandment in the Torah, not merely about the first commandment of all, as in Mark 12:28, and not merely about the practice recommended in order to inherit eternal life, as in Luke 10:25. And only in Matt 22:40 does Jesus add that the writings of the prophets—not only the Law—depend on the double love command.[5] A legal and exegetical issue of high principal value is at stake.

Matthew puts all the emphasis upon Jesus' response containing the OT quotations. Mark 12:32–34 follows up the quotations by an account about the questioner's reaction, by another Jesus-saying and by a concluding comment from the narrator. Luke 10:25–28 puts the OT quotation on the lips of the questioner himself. The Lukan Jesus merely affirms the quotation. In striking contrast, Matthew places the quotations on Jesus' own lips and ends the unit without further comments. The Matthean Jesus adds only brief explanatory remarks. Jesus, the normative character of the story, is the one who quotes the OT, which carries all the necessary force to answer the issue at stake. The quotation of the double love command is a response to an exegetical issue and presents itself the hermeneutical programme according to which the Law and the prophets—Scripture as a whole—should be understood.[6]

It is likely, therefore, that the double love command served as the main criterion for testing new oracles, both in regard to the continuity with past revelation—the command is taken from the OT and present in Mark 12:28–34 as a dominical saying—and in regard to conduct. This accords with the standard implied in 7:15–23 and 24:11f.

Love for God is implicitly the concern of the quotations in 4:4, 7, 10. They belong to the pericope about the testing of Jesus (4:1–11). Within the three scenes appearing with increased intensity in 4:1–4, 5–7, 8–10, the quotations constantly occur as the second part of a dialogue between Satan and Jesus. It is probable that they were present already in the tradition re-

---

1 BANKS, *Jesus and the Law,* 168.
2 The term is textcritically uncertain.
3 Other agreements are listed by e.g. VOUGA, *Jésus et la loi,* 135.
4 Different explanations are given by BORNKAMM, *Geschichte und Glaube* III, 44 (a common dependence on an earlier version of Mark); BURCHARD, Liebesgebot, 42–51 (a common dependence on a tradition reflected also in Mark); FULLER, Doppelgebot, 317–322 (a common dependence on a source [Q] independent of Mark).
5 Cf. BERGER, *Gesetzesauslegung,* 230.
6 See further GERHARDSSON, Hermeneutic Program, 129–150.

flected also in Luke 4:1–13.[1] The Matthean account contains essential principles. It functions to focalize the fundamental perspective according to which Jesus' earthly ministry develops in the subsequent narrative.[2]

Jesus quotes the OT isolated from an elaborated argument also here. He replies to the testing merely with quotations from the Torah. In 4:4 he quotes from Deut 8:3, in 4:7 from Deut 6:16 and in 4:10 from Deut 6:13. Matthew does not expand or rearrange the tradition in order to give the quotations a more argumentative function. Only the brief command ὕπαγε σατανᾶ (4:10) appears as a distinctive Matthean feature outside of the quotations.[3] The OT speaks for itself.[4]

4:1–11 and 22:34–40 contain the most evident connections with the Shemaᶜ in Matthew. In 22:34–40 the relation comes to the surface in the quotation of Deut 6:5. In 4:1–11 all the quotations are taken from Deut 6–8, passages in close proximity to the Shemaᶜ text in Deut 6:4f. The three testings seem to follow—in the order they appear in Matthew—the rabbinic interpretation of the threefold command to love God with all your heart, with all your soul and with all your might.[5] This means, according to the rabbis, that you should love God with both your inclinations, even if God takes your life and with your whole property.[6] Jesus loves God by allowing the word of God and not the evil inclination to reign his heart, by acknowledging God alone to decide over his life and by renouncing all the properties of this world for the service of God. Also other texts in Matthew show, as we have seen, signs of connections with the Shemaᶜ. But 4:1–11 and 22:34–40 are the only two in which the confession guides Jesus' actual quotation from the OT.

Thus, Jesus' use of the OT in 4:1–11 and 22:34–40 depends on the essential and non-questionable status of the Shemaᶜ. Jesus does not relate the quotation to an elaborated argument in these passages. As it seems, *the essential criterion controling the incorporation of additional material into the Jesus tradition was the first part of the Shemaᶜ—solely or as combined with Lev 19:18.* The confession was fundamental and served as the criterion of past revelation, recorded in the Torah itself. And since it contains commandments for proper behaviour, it was also the standard of conduct and com-

---

1   WILKENS, *NTS* 28 (1982) 479–489, contends that Matthew created the pericope merely on the basis of Mark 1:12f and that Luke 4:1–13 depends on the Matthean version. Besides neglecting the general dependence on tradition which Matthew exhibits, Wilkens also fails to account properly for the non-Matthean features, and in particular for the fact that γέγραπται used in 4:4, 6, 7, 10 elsewhere always is in harmony with one or both of the other synoptics (Matt 11:10/Luke 7:27 [cf. Mark 1:2]; Matt 21:13/Mark 11:17/Luke 19:46; Matt 26:31/Mark 14:27).

2   See GERHARDSSON, *ST* 27 (1973) 73–106.

3   Cf. also 16:23.

4   Cf. GERHARDSSON, *EvT* 42 (1982) 121.

5   See GERHARDSSON, *Testing of God's Son,* 71–79.

6   Cf. m. Ber. 9:5; Sifre on Deut 6:5 and above pp. 300–302.

munity benefit.

The criterion of past revelation consisted, in the end, of the preserved Jesus tradition as a whole, a vital ingredient of which was the Shemaᶜ. Matthew pictures, as we saw in the previous chapter, the tradition as located in Jesus' past history as teacher. Jesus himself is not primarily a prophet in Matthew.[1] While the portrayal of the disciples integrates the model of the prophet (5:12; 10:41; 23:34), the crowd's conception of John the Baptist as a prophet in 14:5; 21:26 has already been evaluated as insufficient (11:9). The first time προφήτης appears in reference to Jesus (13:57), it does not carry the definite article. The saying is merely a common aphoristic mashal,[2] which Jesus perhaps uses in order to conform to the situation of his audience. Subsequently, the term reflects the conception only of persons outside of the group of Jesus' followers (16:14; 21:11, 46). The last impression conveyed by the related verb is thoroughly negative (26:68).[3] The criterion of past revelation did not reside in a prophet. The decisive revelation comes through the words and deeds of a specific teacher in the past.

This adherence to past tradition accords with the dominant person-oriented motives of transmission. The Jesus of history was the only legitimate teacher with the only legitimate teaching. The motives of transmission centred not *only* on the teaching and not *only* on the life or status of the teacher. *If only the teaching in itself had been decisive, we would expect some important sayings to be either anonymous or ascribed to various persons in Matthew.* We find this in the rabbinic literature.[4] It would not have been important to identify constantly the utterances in reference to Jesus' name. *If only the life or the status of the teacher had been of importance, it is likely that new sayings from other individuals, such as Christian prophets, would have been incorporated and integrated into the Jesus tradition as pre-Easter Jesus-sayings.* But teacher and teaching belonged closely together. It must have been important to transmit not only teaching in general, but what Matthew and his circle of transmitters preserved as Jesus' own teaching.[5]

---

[1] KINGSBURY, *Matthew: Structure, Christology, Kingdom,* 88f. This is admitted by BORING, *Continuing Voice,* 72, 255f.

[2] For references to the use of similar, though not identical, expressions, cf. U. LUZ, *Matthäus* II, 385 n. 16.—Even SAND, *Gesetz,* 142f, acknowledges that 13:57 is not to be used as an argument for regarding Jesus as a prophet in Matthew.

[3] KNOWLES, *Jeremiah in Matthew's Gospel,* 152–157, 160, does not pay sufficient attention to the form of 13:57 and to what characters that are said to regard Jesus as a prophet in 16:14; 21:11, 46; 26:68. In my opinion, this neglect causes Knowles to overestimate the importance of Jesus as a prophet for Matthew himself.

[4] See above pp. 138f.

[5] U. LUZ, *ZNW* 84 (1993) 174, comes to the conclusion that Matthew shows no awareness of the problem of fictional additions to the tradition since the evangelist belonged to a community integrating them into its living, oral transmission. This may be the impression we gain when focusing only on the additions which did enter into Matthew. But I differ from Luz in considering the transmission itself as a more conscious act separate from other activities and with the aim of protecting the tradition from additions which

The presence of the risen Lord in the activities of the community did not, as Bultmann believed, effect a total levelling of the distinction between pre- and post-Easter sayings. Against the early form-critics, J. Roloff rightly stressed that even the episodes about Jesus exhibited historicizing tendencies throughout the transmission process.[1] Matthew showed a similar attitude both in the story he wrote and in his actual transmission work. In spite of the belief in the risen Lord, he regarded Jesus and his teaching as firmly anchored within a historical situation of the past. This constituted a decisive criterion which controlled the transmission and protected the tradition from entirely foreign influences.[2] *The prophetic address remained in the Jesus tradition an interpreted and actualized report of the teaching which Jesus had given once and for all.* Within the creativity, there was the aim to preserve.[3]

Excursus 14: *Prophetic Oracles in Early Christianity?*

Boring rightly rejects the influential criticism which F. Neugebauer put forward against Bultmann's hypothesis concerning prophetic oracles in early Christianity. Neugebauer claimed that prophetic material was always handed down under the name of its own author.[4] This fails to convince.[5] The prophetical books in the OT do carry the name of a prophet. But a study of their growth shows that prophetic disciples attributed their own elaborations to a prophetic master. I have called this "secondary attribution."[6] The material was not handed down under the name of its *own* author. And the Qumran community recorded the teaching of the Righteous Teacher, who was considered to be an authoritative prophet, without explicit authorial identification at all.[7] Similar practices may occasionally have occurred in early Christianity.[8] By the same token, the distinction between the genres "gospel"—if we can speak of such a

---

were, so to say, too "fictional."

1   ROLOFF, *Kerygma*, 270, states his thesis concisely: "Unsere Untersuchung hat zu dem Ergebnis geführt, daß historisierende Motive innerhalb des von uns überschaubaren Gestaltungs- und Tradierungsprozesses der Jesusgeschichten von den Anfängen an eine weit größere Rolle gespielt haben, als vielfach angenommen worden ist."

2   Cf. TRILLING, *KD* 23 (1977) 103: "Matthäus wird offenkundig von einem sicheren Empfinden für authentisch Jesuanisches geleitet, wenn er Akzente setzt, interpretiert, ja kritisch Stellung nimmt."

3   Cf. SCHWEIZER, *NTS* 16 (1969–70) 217: "In modern terms: Matthew is definitely sceptical about a kerygma-theology, in which the Gospel would be totally identified with the preaching after Easter without being safeguarded by a strict faithfulness to Jesus' own teaching."

4   *ZNW* 53 (1962) 221f.

5   Cf. SATO, *Q und Prophetie*, 7; BORING, *Continuing Voice*, 30f.

6   See above pp. 140–148.

7   See above pp. 148–153.

8   AUNE, *Prophecy*, 415 n. 9, mentions the following examples: Acts 13:2; Rom 11:25f; 1 Cor 15:51f; 1 Thess 4:15ff; 1 Tim 4:1ff; Jude 17f (cf. 2 Pet 3:2–4); Eusebius, Hist. Eccl. III 5:3. However, the prophetic origin is sometimes difficult to prove.—RIESNER, *Lehrer*, 9f, apparently using a statement of NEUGEBAUER, *ZNW* 53 (1962) 224, claims that the prophet's name is not missing in Acts 10:19; 11:12, 28; 13:2; 21:4, 11. But the name is present only in 11:28; 21:10f.

genre at all—and "apocalypse" does not automatically affect the pre-synoptic stage of transmission. Neugebauer argues that the anonymity of the former genre and the claim of (pseudonymous) authorship of the latter made it natural that named prophetic oracles entered into apocalyptic writings without diffusion into the gospel narratives.[1] Bultmann's reference to Rev 3:20; 16:15 therefore neglects, according to Neugebauer, the difference in genre.[2] But this objection is valid only at a stage when the Jesus tradition appears in the full form of a gospel narrative, not before.[3]

A broad spectrum of ancient literature makes evident that sayings of various persons were occasionally transmitted under the name of another historical individual. We have noticed the presence of this phenomenon in ancient Israel and ancient Judaism.[4] It also appears in the Greek-Hellenistic world. As is well known, already Plato sometimes attributes his own views to Socrates.[5] D.E. Aune points to two other examples in which historical individuals are attributed utterances originating after their death. One is the ode to Persephone which according to a local Theban legend preserved in Pausanias, Description of Greece IX 23:4, was ascribed to the poet Pindar (c. 518–438 B.C.E.). The other is an oracle which according to Philostratus, Vit. Ap. 8:31, was ascribed to Apollonius of Tyana of the first century C.E.[6] Similar phenomena appear in early Christianity. Most evident is the fact that Paul is stated as the author of the Pastorals. The Christian teaching that Paul delivered constituted the named tradition through which these three letters achieved their identity and authority.[7] The letters served as substitutions whereby Paul's apostolic presence was apparently extended in view of his own delay and absence (1 Tim 3:14f; 4:13). These examples indeed differ from the situation where a resurrected person directly communicates sayings which are incorporated into the story of his life as a historical individual. The named individuals are all dead in these examples. But they do suggest a process in which sayings of various kinds were retrospectively identified as utterances from another person than the one from whom they actually originated.

If it was possible to ascribe utterances to dead persons, we must acknowledge the possibility that a person held be risen from the dead could be the object of similar attributions. But this is not to say that prophetic oracles originating within the Christian communities were incorporated and integrated into the context of the earthly Jesus' ministry without any distinction. The separation of pre-Easter and post-Easter sayings was not necessarily blurred. On the contrary, *because* the early Christians believed that Jesus had been raised from the dead, the possibility existed that the oracles remained identified as sayings of the *risen* Jesus. Of course, this could not happen in cases where the historical individual was not the object of a resurrection belief.

The instances in which prophets explicitly speak with the voice of Jesus confirm this.[8] In Acts 21:10f Agabus, the prophet, introduces his oracles with a kind of mes-

---

1   *ZNW* 53 (1962) 224–226.
2   Cf. BULTMANN, *Geschichte der synoptischen Tradition,* 134.
3   To be sure, in his criticism of Neugebauer on this point, BORING, *Continuing Voice,* 28, perhaps underestimates the narrative elements which, without being bound to the gospel genre, might have been present already at a pre-synoptic stage.
4   See above pp. 138f, 140–148, 173–188.
5   Cf. e.g. STREETER, *The Four Gospels,* 370; RYDBECK, Prometheus, 94.
6   AUNE, *Prophecy,* 235f.
7   MEADE, *Pseudonymity,* 118–139.
8   HAWTHORNE, Christian Prophets, 127f, uses Hebrews, textual variants and John as evidence of prophetic speech. But this is to beg the question at stake.

senger formula identifying the saying as an utterance of the holy spirit.[1] The spirit is in Acts the speaking agent also of other oracles using the first person form in reference to Jesus (10:19f; 13:2). And there is no reason to separate a saying of the spirit from a saying of the risen Christ.[2] Acts 16:6f uses τὸ ἅγιον πνεῦμα and τὸ πνεῦμα Ἰησοῦ interchangeably.[3] The book of Revelation, which is a prophecy to some extent (1:3; 22:18),[4] uses the voice of Jesus to address the present and future situation (1:8, 11, 17–20; 2:1–3:22; 16:15; 22:7, 12f, 16, 20).[5] But these utterances are constantly attributed to the exalted Lord.[6] In the letters to the seven churches, they are identified as sayings of the spririt (2:7, 11, 17, 29; 3:6, 13, 22). The texts show clearly that it is the spirit or the risen Christ—not the earthly Jesus—that speaks through the prophets.

A somewhat different picture emerges from the second century and onwards. According to Origen (c. 185–254 C.E.), Cels. 7:9, Celsus claimed that there were many Christian prophets who, although of no name, assumed the motions and gestures of inspired persons and spoke, each for himself, in the first person as God (ὁ θεός), God's son (θεοῦ παῖς) or divine spirit (πνεῦμα θεῖον). The distinction between pre-Easter and post-Easter sayings was not always maintained.[7] Nevertheless, we find no large number of entirely new synoptic-like sayings in the later Christian literature. The sayings proclaiming the gospel of salvation were apparently already thoroughly collected and presented in the canonical gospel narratives.[8] Certain second century texts show also that there remained an awareness of the distinction between pre- and post-Easter sayings. To prove his case, Bultmann himself refers to Odes Sol. 42:6.[9] In this early Christian hymn-book from Syria,[10] the inspired singer repeatedly, and without explicit remarks, shifts from his own diction to the voice of Jesus in the form of first person utterances (8:8–19; 10:4–6; 17:6–16; 22:1–12; 28:9–20; 31:6–13; 36:3–8; 41:8–10; 42:3–20).[11] 42:6 gives the programmatic legitimation for this shift.[12] It is all the more noteworthy that on this occasion a reference to Jesus' resurrection precedes the declaration that Jesus will speak by the mouths of others, presumably prophets:[13]

---

1   Cf. also Acts 11:28.

2   *Contra* BORING, *JBL* 91 (1972) 508.

3   Cf. e.g. BRUCE, *Acts,* 327: "Since His ascension it is by His Spirit that Jesus communicates with His people."

4   Cf. e.g. ULFGARD, *Feast and Future,* 13 (with lit.).—HILL, *New Testament Prophecy,* 169f, claims that Revelation is atypical of early Christian prophecy. But for criticism of this view, see AUNE, *Prophecy,* 416 n. 13.

5   BORING, *NovT* 34 (1992) 334–359, argues that Revelation as a whole represents the voice of Jesus implicitly.

6   Cf. DUNN, *NTS* 24 (1978) 180; HILL, *New Testament Prophecy,* 168.

7   Cf. e.g. the 2nd cent. Apocalypse of Peter, in which revelatory material is set within the earthly ministry of Jesus.

8   Joachim JEREMIAS, *Jesusworte,* 111f; HOFIUS, *TRE* 2 (1978) 109; *idem,* "Unbekannte Jesusworte," 382.

9   *Geschichte der synoptischen Tradition,* 135 n. 1.

10   The Odes are not merely, with HILL, *New Testament Prophecy,* 164; RIESNER, *Lehrer,* 9, to be regarded as gnostic material irrelevant for the study of the NT. Already R. ABRAMOWSKI, *ZNW* 35 (1936) 45, 62–64, pointed out several non-gnostic elements. For a more recent treatment, see AUNE, *NTS* 28 (1982) 435–460.

11   These units are marked out separately in CHARLESWORTH (ed.), *Odes.* The identification of some units is uncertain. Cf. the cautious comment by BESKOW/HIDAL, *Salomos Oden,* 79f.

12   AUNE, *NTS* 28 (1982) 439, 444.

13   HILL, *New Testament Prophecy,* 164, follows the old assumption that the state-

"Then I arose and am with them, and I will speak by their mouth." This is not an isolated occurrence. Boring refers to Hermas and rightly detects the voice of the risen Christ.[1] But when the old lady speaks to Hermas with the "I" of Jesus, her revelation takes the voice of the risen and exalted one who stands before the Father (Herm. Vis. III 9:10).[2] G.F. Hawthorne mentions also Melito of Sardis.[3] But again, when Melito brings out a long series of "I am" sayings, it is the voice of the Lord who had already "clothed himself with man," "suffered," "been bound," "been judged," "been buried" and who "arose from the dead" that utters the cry (On Pascha 100–103). Other texts could be mentioned. According to O. Hofius, the real agrapha—i.e. sayings ascribed to the earthly Jesus and not recorded in the oldest version of the canonical gospel narratives—that can be compared with sayings in the synoptic gospel narratives are very few,[4] and the ones existing hardly originated as prophetic oracles.[5]

Two negative implications emerge. First, *early Christianity did not easily shift the authorial identification of sayings from a Christian prophet to Jesus*. This observation is in harmony with the distinction that Paul makes between what he himself says and what the Lord says (1 Cor 7:10–40; 9:14; 11:23; 15:3; 1 Thess 4:15). Paul may have considered his apostolic commission as a call to preach in prophetic terms.[6] But regardless of whether the sayings of the Lord in all cases actually go back on a dominical tradition or not,[7] it is evident that Paul is anxious to keep sayings ascribed to himself and sayings ascribed to the Lord separate. The explicit evidence from the NT identifies Jesus as the speaking subject of prophetic oracles *already from the beginning*. No text shows clearly that oracles became related to Jesus only subsequently.

Second, *the normal procedure in early Christianity was not to project post-Easter sayings into the pre-Easter ministry of Jesus*. In the NT, as often also in later texts, the explicit prophetic oracles appear on the lips of the *risen* Christ. The evidence suggests that they also remained sayings of the risen Christ. There are no episodal comments implying a projection back into Jesus' earthly ministry. The book of Revelation shows that as late as at the end of the first century C.E., prophetic utterances continued to be identified as utterances of the risen Christ.

---

ment refers to believers in general. But see AUNE, *Prophecy,* 416 n. 13.

[1]   *Continuing Voice,* 161.

[2]   Especially Herm. Mand. 11 illustrates Hermas' interest in prophecy. See REILING, *Hermas,* though Reiling does not believe that Hermas was himself a Christian prophet (*ibid.,* 155–170).

[3]   Christian Prophets, 129.—HAWTHORNE, *ibid.,* 128f, brings attention also to the Didache as the teaching of the Lord and to Justin Martyr's use of Jesus-sayings. But in addition to the questionable authenticity of the subtitle of the Didache, we should note that the teaching does not—with some apparent exceptions (8:2; 9:5)—appear on the lips of Jesus. Cf. RORDORF, Jesus Tradition, 412f. And as already FASCHER, *ΠΡΟΦΗΤΗΣ,* 213, pointed out, Justin regards the Christian prophets as interpreters (ἐξηγηταί). Cf. Dial. 68:6. With the possible exception of Apol. I 61:4; Dial. 35:3; 47:5, Justin usually quotes or harmonizes sayings from the synoptic narratives themselves. Cf. KOESTER, *Christian Gospels,* 360–402.

[4]   HOFIUS, *TRE* 2 (1978) 108; *idem,* "Unbekannte Jesusworte," 371–379, counts 9, of which only 4 seem to be entirely independent creations.

[5]   HOFIUS, "Unbekannte Jesusworte," 380f.

[6]   Cf. the basic thesis of SANDNES, *Paul.*

[7]   Cf. e.g. HARTMAN, *Prophecy,* 181–190; DUNGAN, *Sayings.*

4.2. Structural Elaboration of Traditions

The next step of my inquiry is to relate the setting and the motives of trans-mission to the elaboration of traditions. The aim to preserve the tradition did not exclude elaboration. It put certain limits and shows that elaboration was a conscious act of maintaining the tradition by actualizing it.

I am interested only in features revealing careful attempts to enhance in-dividual Jesus-sayings or small collections of Jesus-sayings. There are two broad tendencies: the *structural* and the *argumentative* elaboration. The first has to do with the creation of structures in individual text-units. Al-though Matthew did not mould his story into a formal symmetry of exact sections, he disclosed a structural aim within certain units of his narrative. This may sometimes be due merely to his fondness of stylistic features.[1] But he often used the style for a certain communicative purpose. The structural elaboration is also, as we will see, a means to put emphasis on what Jesus says.

4.2.1. Structures within Pericopes

Two structural features within whole pericopes aim to increase the impor-tance of the Jesus-sayings. Through probable elaboration of the tradition, *Matthew located the Jesus-sayings either towards the climatic end or at the centre of sequences and text-units.*[2]

In the vast majority of cases, the Jesus-sayings appear at the end of the pericope. This is a natural narrative device which was not new with Matt-hew. But Matthew strengthened it. It is perhaps most evident in Matthew's tendency to sharpen the *sequential division* of a pericope, with the result that the Jesus-sayings occur at or towards the climatic end of a sequence.[3]

A few brief examples suffice to illustrate this practice. In 9:2–8 Matthew uses καὶ ἰδού (9:2, 3) to create two sequences (9:2, 3–8). The division is not as clear in Mark 2:3–12.[4] In this way, the saying in 9:2c appears at the end of a sequence. In 9:9–13 Matthew also separates two sequences (9:9, 10–

---

[1] I am not certain that FILSON, *JBL* 75 (1956) 230, is correct to ascribe "broken pat-terns" in Matthew to the evangelist's "dominant interest in topical arrangement of ma-terial." Matthew's general way of working on the tradition by means of structural elabo-ration testifies against this.

[2] Matthew places sayings also at the beginning of a pericope. Cf. e.g. 15:32. But these instances are exceptions and usually not the result of work with the tradition. And if the unit to which 15:32 belongs is defined as 15:29–38 instead of 15:32–38, a different pattern emerges. See below pp. 376f.

[3] In some cases the sequential division is present already in the tradition. Cf. e.g. Matt 4:3f, 5–7, 8–10 with Luke 4:3f, 5–8, 9–12, though the order of the second and third sequence is different; Matt 8:19f, 21f with Luke 9:57f, 59f; Matt 15:1–9, 10f, 12–20 with Mark 7:1–7, 14f, 17–23; Matt 17:14–18, 19f with Mark 9:14–27, 28f.

[4] It is possible that καὶ ἰδού in Matt 9:2/Luke 5:18 was present in the tradition.

13). The unit does not, as Mark 2:13–17, explicitly relate the house of the second sequence to the person called for discipleship in the first sequence. Jesus' command in 9:9b follows therefore towards the end of a rather independent sequence. In 9:18–26 Matthew distinguishes three sequences (9:18f, 20–22, 23–26). The text does not, as Mark 5:35, connect the second and the third sequence. The Jesus-saying in 9:22 occurs, therefore, towards the end of a self-contained sequence focusing on the interaction between Jesus and the woman.[1] In 15:21–28 Matthew again creates three sequences (15:22–23a, 23b–24, 25–28) after an initial comment (15:21). The second sequence is not present in Mark 7:24–30, which contains only one comprehensive scene. In the Matthean account, the first sequence ends with the narrator's comment about Jesus' silence and the second with a restrictive Jesus-saying. After the inclusion of a saying from the tradition (Matt 15:26/Mark 7:27), the third sequence brings the decisive Jesus-saying towards the end.[2] In 21:12–17 Matthew forms two sequences (21:12f, 14–16) with a concluding comment (21:17). Mark 11:15–17 gives only the first sequence. Both Matthean sequences contain an authoritative Jesus-saying at the end. In 26:36–46 Matthew distinguishes four sequences (26:37f, 39–41, 42f, 44–46) after an initial comment and Jesus-saying (26:36). The second, third and fourth sequence contain each the pattern of Jesus going away from the disciples, praying and returning. The sequential division is visible also in Mark 14:32–42. But by adding ἐκ δευτέρου (26:42) and ἐκ τρίτου (26:44), which probably is the original reading, Matthew sharpens the division. The first, second and fourth sequence ends with a Jesus-saying. The same tendency is visible also in 26:47–56. The repeated ἰδού (...) εἷς τῶν marks the beginning of two sequences (26:47–50, 51–56). This strengthens the division present in Mark 14:43–52. Matthew further adds a Jesus-saying towards the end of the first sequence (26:50) and abbreviates the episodal remarks after the final saying in the second sequence. In this way, both sequences contain an authoritative Jesus-saying towards the end.[3]

Matthew also worked with the centre of pericopes. Signs of this work emerges from *numerical* considerations.[4] Perhaps Matthew wanted to stress the importance of discipleship in 4:18–22 by placing ἠκολούθησαν of 4:20 in the middle of the unit. There are fourty-four words before and after this term.[5] It is the first time ἀκολουθεῖν occurs in the narrative. Matthew repeats it in 4:22, instead of using ἀπέρχεσθαι present in Mark 1:20. The term

---

[1] Cf. TRUMMER, *Die blutende Frau*, 89.

[2] Cf. below p. 377.

[3] Luke also adds a Jesus-saying (22:48) and ends the second unit with a Jesus-saying (22:52b–53). But the sequential division is not as clear as in Matthew.

[4] For numerical patterns in Matthew, see SMIT SIBINGA, Eine literarische Technik, 99–105; *idem, ST* 29 (1975) 71–79. Cf. also GERHARDSSON, *Mighty Acts*, 40f, 53, 78; SCHEDL, *Christologie*, 75f; U. LUZ, *Matthäus* I, 20, *passim*.

[5] I follow the reading in the 26th edition of Nestle-Aland.

is important in Matthew.[1] Further, in 9:27–31 the emphatic ναί of the two blind men (9:28) constitutes the middle term. If we include αὐτῷ in 9:27, we find thirty-seven words before and after ναί. It is an important expression of belief in the miraculous power of Jesus, the son of David. We have also seen that the doublet in 20:29–34 places the prayer of the blind men (20:31b) at the centre and that the mention of the resurrection in 28:5b–6 appears as in the middle of 28:1–10.[2]

It also happens that Jesus-sayings, or vital parts of them, form the centre of pericopes.[3] We already noticed that ὁ Ἰησοῦς εἶπεν αὐτῷ and the following saying occurs in the middle of 16:13–20.[4] The structural centre corresponds with the importance of the statement. We may mention four further examples. First, the expression πληρῶσαι πᾶσαν δικαιοσύνην in 3:15 constitutes the centre of 3:13–17. Provided we accept Ἰωάννης in 3:14 and αὐτῷ, τό, τοῦ and καί in 3:16 as original, there are forty-eight words before and after the expression. We do not find this pattern in the parallels (Mark 1:9–11/Luke 3:21f). And no doubt, the theme of fulfilling all righteousness as presented in 3:15 is vitally important in Matthew,[5] no matter how we interpret it.[6] Second, the statement θέλω, καθαρίσθητι in 8:3a appears in the middle of 8:1–4. There are thirty words before and after the brief saying.[7] The saying is present also in the tradition (Mark 1:41), but it does not form the centre of the unit there.[8] In Matthew it is an important expression of Jesus' will and ability to cleanse. Matthew takes over the Markan way of preparing and following up the Jesus-saying (Mark 1:40, 42). The request of the leper prepares the use of both θέλειν and καθαρίζειν (8:2), and the narrator tells about the result of Jesus' performative words by using καθαρίζειν again (8:3b). Matthew elsewhere maintains the Q tradition that the cleansing of the lepers is an aspect of Jesus' total ministry (Matt 11:5/Luke 7:22). The Matthean Jesus expects also his disciples to cleanse the lepers (10:8). Third, the whole Jesus-saying in 12:11f, including the introduction ὁ δὲ εἶπεν αὐτοῖς, occurs almost at the centre of 12:9–14. There are twenty-six words before and twenty-seven words after the say-

---

1 See KINGSBURY, *JBL* 97 (1978) 56–73.

2 See above pp. 265f, 318.

3 For the central position of some dialogues, see above p. 239 n. 8 and below p. 376f. For the central position of (parts of) an OT quotation, see below pp. 380, 389.

4 See above pp. 278f.

5 U. LUZ, *Matthäus* I, 153, states: "Auf den Einwand des Täufers antwortet Jesus mit einem Satz, der ein zentrales Anliegen matthäischer Theologie enthält."

6 EISSFELDT, *ZNW* 61 (1970) 210–213, lists the interpretation of various scholars. For more recent discussion, see PRZYBYLSKI, *Righteousness,* 91–94; GIESEN, *Christliches Handeln,* 21–41; POPKES, *ZNW* 80 (1989) 1–23; HAGNER, Righteousness, 115–118; WOUTERS, *"... wer den Willen meines Vaters tut,"* 214–217.

7 I follow the reading in the 26th edition of Nestle-Aland.

8 Luke also takes it over in 5:13, but he does not place it at the structural centre.

ing.[1] This pattern is not present in the parallels (Mark 3:1–6/Luke 6:6–11). The structural position accords with the importance of the saying. "To do good on the sabbath" (τοῖς σάββασιν καλῶς ποιεῖν) relates to the dominating Matthean themes of mercy and love.[2] Fourth, Matthew combines the sequential division of 26:36–46 with a numerical structure. 26:40f is at the centre of the pericope. If we accept οὖ in 26:36 and τό in 26:45, there are seventy-nine words before and after 26:40f. If we further isolate these two central verses, the important term γρηγορῆσαι in 26:40 appears at the centre. There are in 26:40f eighteen words before and after γρηγορῆσαι.[3] The parallels exhibit no such pattern (Mark 14:32–42/Luke 22:39–46). The term is important. 26:36–46 uses it both before (26:38) and after (26:41) its occurrence in 26:40. Already 24:36–44, 25:1–13 stress the need for watchfulness. And the immediate context of 26:36–46 relates indirectly to the theme of watchfulness. In 26:31 Jesus foretells that all the disciples will be deserters, and in 26:56 the narrator concludes that all the disciples deserted Jesus and fled. They were not watchful.

We cannot be entirely sure that the numerical patterns always reflect a *deliberate* means to elaborate the traditions. They are not consistently worked out in Matthew as a whole. They may occasionally be accidental. But the patterns are there, and in comparison with the other synoptics they do appear—in these instances at least—as peculiar to Matthew.[4]

4.2.2. Structures within Episodal Comments

The second structural elaboration enhancing the words of Jesus concerns the episodal comments which usually surround a saying. There are two related aspects of this kind of elaboration. They concern the *generalizing* and the *focalizing* work on the episodal comments.

Matthew often relates the episodal comment and the Jesus-saying to each other. We have already noticed the close connection between Jesus' verbal teaching and the narrator's episodal comments.[5] Jesus' words are difficult to understand apart from their episodal location, because Jesus himself is the ultimate centre of the entire tradition. Matthew sometimes uses structural strategies to strengthen the connection. Most evident are the catchwords between the episodal comment, which occasionally includes a saying of another character, and the Jesus-saying. Matthew agrees with one or both of the parallels in using such catch-words in for instance 4:18f (ἁλεεῖς); 8:2f

---

[1]   I follow the reading in the 26th edition of Nestle-Aland. I cannot find alternative readings which are original and even out the number of words here.

[2]   See U. LUZ, *Matthäus* II, 239f.

[3]   The numerical pattern of the whole pericope is thus 79+18+1+18+79=195.

[4]   I have counted the words only. It is possible also to count syllables. But this seems even more difficult and hypothetical to me.

[5]   See above pp. 264–266.

(θέλειν ... καθαρίζειν); 9:14f (νηστεύειν); 9:21f (σῷζειν); 12:46, 48–50 (μήτηρ, ἀδελφοί); 13:54, 57 (πατρίς); 20:17f (ἀναβαίνειν εἰς Ἰεροσόλυμα). He is alone to use the technique in, for instance, 8:19, 22 (ἀκολουθεῖν);[1] 11:20f (αἱ δυνάμεις αἱ γενόμεναι, μετανοεῖν); 12:1, 3 (πεινᾶν); 12:10f (ἄνθρωπος); 17:6f (φοβεῖσθαι). Further examples could be mentioned. They represent a prominent structural signal for the integration of Jesus-sayings into certain episodal settings. *Matthew did not conceive the Jesus-sayings as isolated units without episodal situation.*

Of course, this narrativizing tendency does not mean that the Jesus-sayings are entirely subordinated to the episodes. *Matthew also generalizes the Jesus-sayings beyond the flow of the narrative and the episodal context of individual passages.* We can assume that Jesus' words carry no special relevance beyond the immediate situation in which they occur on a few occasions only.[2] As a matter of course, the generalizing tendency is most evident in the long speeches. Matt 5–7, 10, 13, 18 and 23–25 rarely give the individual sayings any further episodal context than the general one of the whole speech. And when they do, as Matt 13, the episodal comments increase the importance of Jesus' words.

We also find the same tendency in cases where Matthew presents the sayings separately or in smaller units. Two procedures exemplify the generalizing tendency. First, Matthew often keeps the episodal comment *unspecified*. Apart from the long speeches, we see this most clearly in 11:20–24, 25–30. The Jesus-saying in 11:21–24 comes from the Q material.[3] Matthew probably relocated the saying from its place in Q's missionary speech,[4] which is the setting of Luke 10:12–15.[5] A remark in 11:20 precedes the saying. It is probably a Matthean creation shaped on the basis of the words in the traditional saying itself (αἱ δυνάμεις αἱ γενόμεναι, μετανοεῖν).[6] The episodal comment is abrupt and unspecified, aiming only towards the saying. In 11:25–30 Matthew combines two separate sayings with only a brief introductory comment. 11:25–27 is Q material.[7] 11:28–30 is special material. Matthew does not give another remark to introduce the second saying. Instead he creates one comprehensive saying which relates only vaguely to the unspecified situation depicted in 11:25a.

Second, Matthew sometimes generalizes the *addressee(s)* of the Jesus-

---

1　Cf. also the following comment in 8:23.
2　Cf. 8:7, 32; 12:13; 14:18, 29; 15:34; 20:21, 32.
3　Cf. Luke 10:12–15.
4　URO, *Sheep Among the Wolves,* 83–85.
5　Cf. also Matt 10:15.
6　COMBER, *CBQ* 39 (1977) 497–504, claims that 11:20 functions as a title which Matthew develops in the following saying. This might be the intention Matthew wanted to convey to the readers/hearers. But in his own work of composing the narrative, Matthew developed 11:20 on the basis of a traditional saying.
7　Cf. Luke 10:21f.

sayings. 8:10 may serve as an illustration. Although 8:5–9 describes Jesus' conversation with a centurion, 8:10 pictures Jesus as speaking to "those who followed" (τοῖς ἀκολουθοῦσιν)—even without the reference that Jesus spoke to those who followed "him" (αὐτῷ), added in some variant readings. This harks back all the way to 8:1 and passes by the situational comment in 8:5. Luke 7:9 defines the addressee more clearly. Jesus there turns to the crowd following him. The Lukan verse also relates to the previous conversation by mentioning that Jesus spoke upon hearing "these things" (ταῦ-τα)—i.e. what the centurion just said—and that Jesus was amazed at the centurion. Matt 8:10 says only that Jesus was amazed when he heard. It is difficult to know which version of the passage is earlier,[1] and we cannot be absolutely sure that Luke 7:9a is closer to Q than Matt 8:10a.[2] But the abbreviated Matthean form is in harmony with Matthew's habit of sometimes shortening the episodal elements of the tradition. As it thus seems, Matthew allows Jesus' authoritative voice to stand out as an address to a broader audience than the centurion only.[3]

The generalizing pattern in the episodal comments thus leads us to the abbreviating structures resulting in a focalization on the Jesus-sayings. J.C. Hawkins noticed long ago that Matthew tends to abbreviate, by condensation or omission, the episodal features of the tradition.[4] Hawkins gave attention to 8:1–4; 8:18, 23–27; 8:28–34; 9:1–8, 18–26; 14:13–21; 17:14–21; 20:29–34; 26:17–19, with parallels in both Mark and Luke,[5] further to 13:54–58; 14:3–5, 6–12, 34–36; 21:18–20, with parallels only in Mark, and to 8:5–10, 13; 11:2–6, with parallels only in Luke. H.J. Held brought the observation a step further by showing that the abbreviation of the tradition is a Matthean means of interpretation, especially in the miracle stories.[6] According to Held, the shortening in 8:2–4, 14f, 16f, 28–34; 9:2–8 effects a focus on christology, in 9:18–26, 27–31 on faith and in 14:15–21; 15:32–38; 17:14–20 on discipleship. In several of the passages brought out by Hawkins and Held, the abbreviated episodal features do not relate to a significant Jesus-saying.[7] The technique is not used only to enhance what Jesus

---

[1]   WEGNER, *Hauptmann*, 7–16, surveys several different theories concerning the relationship between Matt 8:5–10, 13 and Luke 7:1–10.

[2]   WEGNER, *Hauptmann*, 209–212, thinks that the abbreviated form of Matt 8:10a is closer to Q than Luke 7:9a. But he builds exclusively on what he considers to be typically Matthean and Lukan words or expressions, without considering broader tendencies in the work the tradition.

[3]   So GUNDRY, *Matthew*, 144. Cf. also DAVIES/ALLISON, *Matthew* II, 24.

[4]   *Horae Synopticae*, 158–160.

[5]   Luke also shortens Mark—though not always, sometimes his accounts are longer—but, with one exception (Luke 9:37–43a/Mark 9:14–29/Matt 17:14–20), never as much as Matthew does.

[6]   Miracle Stories, 168–192, 213–215, 223–225.

[7]   Cf. 8:14f, 16f, 28–34; 14:3–5, 6–12, 34–36; 20:29–34. In 9:27–31 Matthew focuses on the confession of the blind men in 9:28. See above p. 371. And the abbreviation

says. But—if we follow my own demarcation of the units—in such passages as 8:2–4; 8:5–10, 13; 8:23–27; 9:2–8, 18–26; 11:2–6; 14:13–21; 15:29–38; 17:14–20; 21:18–20; 26:17–19, *the abbreviation of the episodal comments effects a focalization on the Jesus-saying,* which is sometimes placed in a dialogue with other characters.[1]

Let me add some further examples. In 15:1f Matthew shortens the episodal comment of Mark 7:1–5 and gives the following Jesus-saying immediately;[2] in 17:22f Matthew frames the Jesus-saying with much briefer and unspecified episodal remarks than in both Mark 9:30–32 and Luke 9:43b–45; in 19:21 Matthew omits the comment that Jesus looked at and loved the rich man (Mark 10:21);[3] in 20:17 Matthew leaves out the reference that Jesus walked ahead and that those who followed were amazed and feared (Mark 10:32);[4] in 26:39a Matthew does not mention the remark about what Jesus prayed (Mark 14:35) but reserves this for the Jesus-saying in 26:39b;[5] in 26:59–61 Matthew abbreviates the episode about the false testimonies (Mark 14:55–59) and goes on more directly to the dialogue between Jesus and the high priest in 26:62–64.[6] The abbreviation by means of condensation or omission relates in all these cases to an important Jesus-saying. It happens also that Matthew leaves out unnecessary episodal comments completely and presents the Jesus-saying in one sequence.[7] There is in these cases a tendency to reduce the episodal comments to what is necessary only for the narrative flow of the story and to focalize the Jesus-sayings themselves.

4.2.3. Structures between Sayings

The third structural elaboration aimed to increase the importance of Jesus' words concerns the relation between different sayings in one and the same pericope. This relation appears in two ways. Matthew may connect a Jesus-saying with *utterances of other characters* or with *other Jesus-sayings* in the same pericope.

We noticed in chapter four that several of the units characterizing Jesus as διδάσκαλος carry the characteristics of a responsive chreia.[8] What Jesus says as teacher occurs in a dialogical situation. Matthew does not only pre-

---

in 13:54–58 is probably not due to a concentration on the Jesus-saying itself.

1 See below pp. 376f.

2 Luke 11:37f is also shorter than Mark 7:1–5.

3 Luke 18:22 also omits the Markan comment, but it adds the rather superfluous ἀκούσας δέ.

4 This is omitted also in Luke 18:31.

5 This is omitted also in Luke 22:41.

6 Luke 22:66f has no reference to false testimonies.

7 Cf. Matt 12:3–8/Mark 2:25–28/Luke 6:3–5; Matt 16:24–28/Mark 8:34–9:1 (Luke 9:23–27 also presents the Jesus-saying in one sequence); Matt 19:23f/Mark 10:23–25 (Luke 18:24f also presents the Jesus-saying in one sequence).

8 See above pp. 214f.

sent the teaching in long speeches and with general or focalized episodal features. It does of course happen that Matthew diminishes the dialogical character of a situation.[1] But the reverse is more common. There is a general tendency to *sharpen the dialogical situation* depicted in the tradition.

I have selected three examples. First, in 19:3–12 Matthew forms three sequences (19:3–6, 7–9, 10–12). Each sequence contains a question—by the Pharisees or the disciples—and an authoritative answer by Jesus. These dialogical sequences are not present in Mark 10:2–12, which does not have the third sequence at all. Second, in 19:16–22 Matthew again creates three sequences (19:16f, 18f, 20f) before the concluding remark (19:22). And again, each sequence exhibits the same pattern of question and answer. Mark 10:17–22/Luke 18:18–23 contains this sequence only twice. Third, in 22:41–46 Matthew sharpens the pattern of a question by Jesus (22:42a), an answer by the opponents (22:42b) and an authoritative final question by Jesus (22:43–45). Mark 12:35–37a/Luke 20:41–44 contains no dialogue at all. And while the parallels report that Jesus had silenced the opponents before he raised the question about David's son (Mark 12:34b/Luke 20:40), Matthew reserves this until also the issue about David's son has been discussed in the form of a dialogue (22:46). In cases of this kind, Matthew purposely relates the Jesus-sayings to utterances from other characters.

The dialogue is sometimes even the vital centre of a text-unit. This seems to be the case especially when Jesus dialogues with his disciples. We saw in the previous chapter that the dialogue between Jesus and the disciples forms the centre of 8:23–27.[2] There are other examples, like the two feeding accounts. The conversation with the disciples in 14:16f appears at the midpoint of 14:13–21. There are sixty-five words before and after the dialogue.[3] The interaction between Jesus and the disciples is not at the centre of Mark 6:32–44/Luke 9:10b–17 in the same sharp way. Further, the dialogue between Jesus and the disciples in 15:32f is at the centre of 15:29–38. The isolation of the unit is here somewhat uncertain. The summary in 15:29–31 should probably be included. It provides the general situation of the feeding account and corresponds in this way to 14:13f, which gives a briefer but similar episodal framework to the account about the feeding of the five thousand.[4] 15:39 might, however, fall outside of the unit and relate to the following. It corresponds to 14:23.[5] And 14:23 starts a new unit.[6] As in

---

[1] Cf. Matt 16:5–12/Mark 8:14–21; Matt 24:1f/Mark 13:1f/Luke 21:5f.

[2] See above p. 239 n. 8.

[3] I follow the reading in the 26th edition of Nestle-Aland. It is not necessary to decide if Ἰησοῦς is original or not in 14:16.

[4] Both 14:13 and 15:29 depict how Jesus moves away from a place (ἐκεῖθεν), and both 14:14 and 15:30 speak of how Jesus cured (ἐθεράπευσεν) the crowd(s).

[5] Cf. the use of καὶ ἀπολύσας τοὺς ὄχλους ἀνέβη εἰς τὸ ὄρος in 14:23 and καὶ ἀπολύσας τοὺς ὄχλους ἐνέβη εἰς τὸ πλοῖον in 15:39.

[6] 14:22 may be a "transition verse."

14:13, 15, the narrator says in 14:23 that Jesus is by himself (κατ' ἰδίαν) and that it was evening (ὀψίας δὲ γενομένης). If we accept 15:29–38 as a unit, we will find sixty-six words before προσκαλεσάμενος in 15:32 and sixty-six words after τοσοῦτον in 15:33,[1] leaving a central dialogue with fourty-six words.[2] The dialogue is not in the exact middle of Mark 7:31–8:9. While the speeches and the general or focalizing episodal comments enhance the Jesus-sayings by lifting them beyond the specific situations, *the dialogues show that the force of certain sayings depends on the dialectic of an interaction.*

Several pericopes also contain more than one Jesus-saying. While it happens that Matthew reduces the number of sayings to one,[3] he often also maintains several utterances. In certain cases, there is even a tendency to elaborate the tradition by *placing the different sayings in such a relation to each other that one of the sayings stands out as the most important one.*

I have selected three examples which point to different ways of relating the Jesus-sayings. In 15:21–28 the *narrator's introductions* to the sayings are of significance. We have already noticed the threefold sequential arrangement created by Matthew. The Matthean narrator builds up the expectation through his introductions to what Jesus says and his comments on what Jesus does not say. The narrator first states merely ὁ δὲ οὐκ ἀπεκρίθη αὐτῇ λόγον (15:23); he then twice introduces the two negative sayings with the brief ὁ δὲ ἀποκριθεὶς εἶπεν (15:24, 26); and he finally prepares the positive and decisive exclamation with the longer τότε ἀποκριθεὶς ὁ Ἰησοῦς εἶπεν αὐτῇ (15:28). The Markan narrator says only καὶ εἶπεν αὐτῇ (7:29). In distinction to the previous comments in Matthew, this last one starts with the emphatic τότε, mentions Jesus by name and shows with αὐτῇ explicitly that Jesus now speaks to the persistent woman. 16:5–12, the second example, relates two Jesus-sayings by means of an *inclusio*. The decisive expression of the unit is προσέχετε (δὲ) ἀπὸ τῆς ζύμης τῶν φαρισαίων καὶ σαδδουκαίων uttered by Jesus. Matthew creates the utterance from a saying in Mark 8:15. But in his own account, Matthew uses it twice, in the first saying (16:6) and at the end of the second saying (16:11b), thus forming an inclusio with only a comment by the disciples and questions posed by Jesus in between. 19:16–22 shows, as the third example, that also the *content* of various Jesus-sayings in a pericope relate to each other in such a way that the last one stands out as the most important one. We already noticed the threefold dialogical character of the unit. After a remark about who is good

---

1   The reason why ὁ δὲ Ἰησοῦς in 15:32 is not included in the central part might be that at προσκαλεσάμενος Matthew starts adhering more closely to Mark than previously in the unit.

2   I follow the reading in the 26th edition of Nestle-Aland.

3   Cf. Matt 8:23–27/Mark 4:35–41/Luke 8:22–25; Matt 8:28–9:1/Mark 5:1–20/Luke 8:26–39; Matt 20:29–34/Mark 10:46–52/Luke 18:35–43 (cf. also Matt 9:27–31).

(19:17a), Jesus refers in the first two sequences merely to the command-ments already known to and practised by the young man (19:17b–19). The last saying adds another aspect to what is required for attaining eternal life. In 19:21 Matthew indicates the importance of the saying by shifting ἕν σε ὑστερεῖ in Mark 10:21 to εἰ θέλεις τέλειος εἶναι.[1] This is a substantial deve-lopment in content when compared with the previous sayings, the first one of which starts with the similar but less radical εἰ δὲ θέλεις εἰς τὴν ζωὴν εἰσ-ελθεῖν (19:17).[2] Through this shift, the importance of discipleship as per-fection comes to the fore. Matthew thus relates the Jesus-sayings to each other through elaboration of the narrator's introductions, through inclusio and through the content of the sayings. He creates a strong emphasis on cer-tain words of Jesus.

4.3. Argumentative Elaboration of Traditions

There are numerous argumentative features in Matthew. I will study only the argumentation related to sayings in which Jesus quotes the OT explicit-ly. The OT is an obvious authority in Matthew. The Jesus tradition arose and developed within a cultural matrix accepting and building on the OT as normative revelation. The OT exhibited constantly its authoritative in-fluence.[3] But with Jesus and his teaching another authority entered into the situation. We have already seen that the Matthean Jesus quotes the OT with-out further comments only in 4:1–11; 22:34–40. In spite of its authoritative status, Jesus is usually not content with merely quoting the OT. It is of in-terest to see how the two—the OT and Jesus' own words—relate to each other in the argumentation concerned with particular issues in Matthew. How did Matthew elaborate the argumentation in the Jesus-sayings con-taining a quotation from the OT? If Jesus' own authority remained funda-mental and decisive even in these cases, it is of course likely that it was vital in the argumentative development of other parts of the Jesus tradition as well.[4]

---

[1]   Luke 18:22 has ἔτι ἕν σοι λείπει.

[2]   The two steps introduced in this manner do not imply two levels of morality. See G. BARTH, Law, 95–99. Nor is it evident that it implies two ways to God for Jews, one for the ordinary Jews and one for the Jewish Christians, as argued by HARRINGTON, The Rich Young Man, 1425–1432. In 5:48 Jesus speaks of perfection in quite absolute terms as a requirement for all who are to be sons of the heavenly Father (cf. 5:45), not merely as a superior level (for Jewish Christians) contrasted to a minimum standard (for ordinary Jews).

[3]   See my remarks already in the introduction p. 21.

[4]   I have not made extensive use of rhetorical tools to analyze the arguments. Such a study requires, in my estimation, a deeper comparison with rhetorical handbooks and other rhetorical texts than was possible here. Thus, for instance, I have used the term "elaboration" throughout this study without limiting it to denote only a rhetorical elabora-tion exercise (ἐργασία). For an application of progymnastic rhetoric, especially the elabo-ration of the chreia, on the gospel tradition, see MACK/ROBBINS, *Patterns of Persuasion*.

4.3.1. The Material

Matthew's use of the OT has been the object of several lengthy studies.[1] I will concentrate on what I call the "OT sayings," i.e. *the sayings in which Jesus himself quotes the OT explicitly.* There are many sayings alluding to the OT in Matthew.[2] On some occasions, the allusions amount to actual quotations.[3] But on other occasions, they are embedded within Jesus' own figure of speech or expression, sometimes to the extent that an appreciation of their communicative function requires a deep involvement in the cultural situation of the language.[4] For my purposes, the allusions are of little interest. They do not identify the traditions by reference to anything else than Jesus himself. Jesus remains here the sole authority. It is sufficient to concentrate on instances in which the context or the actual Jesus-saying itself show clearly that Jesus refers to another authority than himself, the OT.

The Matthean Jesus quotes the OT explicitly twenty-five times. With two exceptions (22:37, 39), he shows that he is about to quote the OT by identifying the quotation in some way: nine times he defines it as a word spoken by God (5:21, 27, 31, 33, 38, 43; 15:4; 19:4f; 22:31); three times he refers to the name of the presumed author, Isaiah (13:14; 15:7) or David (22:43); on seven occasions he refers to the OT as a written and anonymous body of scriptures by using γέγραπται (4:4, 7, 10; 11:10; 21:13; 26:31)[5] or ἐν ταῖς γραφαῖς (21:42); twice he uses τί ἐστιν (9:13; 12:7), once τό (19:18) and once ὅτι (21:16). I have already treated the use of the OT in 4:4, 7, 10; 22:37, 39. Jesus here relies entirely on the OT. We may also exclude 21:13. The quotation is in this case not a vital part of an argumentative elaboration. There remains nineteen instances. They fall into three groups.

21:13 belongs to the first of the two scenes in 21:12f, 14–17, which together constitute the Matthean account about the cleansing of the temple. In comparison with Mark 11:17, the most evident differences in the quotation of Isa 56:7 and Jer 7:11 are the Matthean form of a statement instead of a question and the absence of any reference to the Gentiles. But it is difficult to ascertain that these variations actually are the result of work on the tradition. The same differences appear also in Luke 19:46, which in addition exhibits other minor agreements with Matt 21:13 against Mark 11:17.[6] And the

---

[1] For an overview of the most important contributions, see STANTON, *ANRW* II 25:3 (1985) 1930–1934. Cf. also the recent study by KNOWLES, *Jeremiah in Matthew's Gospel,* arguing that the use of Jeremiah contributes to a christocentric Deuteronomistic perspective in Matthew. Also CHARETTE, *Recompense,* 168, considers his study as dealing primarily with Matthew's use and understanding of the OT.

[2] For discussion of several allusions both inside and outside of the Jesus-sayings, see GUNDRY, *Use of the Old Testament,* 28–66, 69–89, 127–147.

[3] Cf. e.g. 10:35f; 12:40; 18:16; 21:33; 23:39; 26:64; 27:46.

[4] Cf. HARTMAN, Scriptural Exegesis, 135.

[5] Cf. also 26:24.

[6] Cf. the absence of ἐδίδασκεν and the presence of ὑμεῖς δὲ αὐτὸν ποιεῖτε/ἐποιήσατε instead of ὑμεῖς δὲ πεποιήκατε.

quotation is not used in a discussion with a stated thesis. It is used to defend an action. The most significant work on the tradition is here instead the subsequent addition of 21:14–17, with the quotation from Ps 8:3. This expansion is sufficient to give the whole pericope of 21:12–17 an argumentative pattern. I will treat it below.

4.3.2. Argumentation within Quotations from the Tradition

The first and largest group consists of sayings which contained the OT quotation already in the tradition. This is the case in 11:10; 15:4, 8f, 19:4f, 18f; 21:42; 22:32, 44; 26:31. The argumentative elaboration here manifests itself as expansions and/or rearrangements of the sayings and their episodal settings.

The quotation in 11:10 belongs to 11:7–15. With some minor changes, 11:7–11 is taken over from a tradition recorded also in Luke 7:24–28.[1] Of the remaining verses, 11:14f appears as an independent addition with no synoptic parallel. While 11:12f is similar to Luke 16:16, the presence of Matthean diction—and perhaps also the different contextual location—implies that its occurrence here is the result of work on the tradition.[2]

The Matthean expansion of the tradition results in a significant structure and argument, in which the quotation from Exod 23:20 and Mal 3:1 plays an important role.[3] The saying concerns the identity of John the Baptist. The expansion makes the words ὃς κατασκευάσει τὴν ὁδόν σου ἔμπροσθέν σου—the first six words belong to the quotation—occur at the very centre of the pericope.[4] The discussion about John's identity is focused on his function to prepare the way before Jesus. The argumentation of the saying confirms this structural pattern. In 11:7b–9 Jesus presents the first part of the argumentation by stating a number of questions.[5] Only the last one is given an affirmative answer.[6] The οὗτός ἐστιν in 11:10 shows that the OT quotation defines the identity of John. And the stress is, as we saw, on his function to prepare the way before Jesus. The second part of the saying (11:11–15), which contains the Matthean expansion, forms an argumentation developing the definition given in the quotation. 11:11f first gives two theses connected with δέ. 11:13f then supports the theses with two rationales con-

---

[1] For the quotation itself, cf. also Mark 1:2.—It is not necessary to determine the character of Q at this point. Cf. the discussion about commentary words by J. WANKE, *"Bezugs- und Kommentarworte,"* 31–35; KLOPPENBORG, *Formation of Q,* 108–110; ERNST, *Johannes der Täufer,* 61–63.

[2] *Contra* ERNST, *Johannes der Täufer,* 63–66, 169. Concerning the presence of 11:12f in Q, see the cautious remarks by U. LUZ, *Matthäus* II, 172f.

[3] For the form of the quotation, see GUNDRY, *Use of the Old Testament,* 11f.

[4] In the text accepted by the 26th edition of Nestle-Aland, there are 65 words before and after this phrase.

[5] The proposition in 11:8c serves merely to imply a negative answer to the previous question.

[6] Cf. THEISSEN, *Lokalkolorit und Zeitgeschichte,* 36.

nected with a simple καί and introduced with γάρ. The second rationale forms the climax. The αὐτός ἐστιν points back to the definition previously given in the OT quotation. But this time the text goes on to define John as the coming Elijah in explicit terms.[1] Although it is uncertain how prominent the expectation about Elijah as the forerunner of the Messiah was in the first century C.E.,[2] this definition harks back implicitly to John's function of preparing the way for Jesus. As it therefore appears, the OT is not independent of Jesus' own words. The quotation, with its emphasis on John's function to prepare the way before Jesus, has been the basis for an expansion of a traditional Jesus-saying into a more elaborated argumentation about John's identity.

The two quotations in 15:4, 8f are part of 15:1–20. In distinction to Mark 7:23, Matt 15:20b concludes the unit by explicitly referring back to the issue initially brought up in 15:2. The unit consists of four sequences (15:1–9, 10f, 12–14, 15–20). Among the differences from Mark 7:1–23,[3] the absence of an explanation to the practice of the Jews (Mark 7:3f), the rearrangement of the OT quotations in the first sequence and the addition of the statements concerning the plant not planted by the Father and the blind guides in the third (Matt 15:13f) are most evident.[4]

The different order of the OT quotations is held together by an implicit drive to produce a more argumentative presentation of the Jesus-saying in the first sequence. The rearrangement of the quotations to appear in the order of first referring to Exod 20:12/Deut 5:16 and Exod 21:17 and subsequently to Isa 29:13 has the effect of proving the latter. The issue is stated in 15:2 and concerns the breaking of the tradition of the elders. Instead of explaining the Jewish practice, the Matthean version immediately counters the initial question of the Pharisees and scribes. Picking up the very words used by the opponents (διὰ τί ... παραβαίνειν), Jesus at once poses a counterquestion. He subsequently justifies (γάρ) the thesis implicit in the question, that the opponents themselves transgress God's commandment, with a critical discussion of the Jewish embellishment of Exod 20:12/Deut 5:16 and Exod 21:17. The quotation from Isa 29:13 follows only after Jesus has established that the opponents make void the word of God for the sake of their traditions. Instead of being an introduction to Jesus' attack, Isa 29:13 forms the concluding climax of the first sequence. Jesus' opposition to the Jewish leaders and vice versa is in this way put in sharper relief and the is-

---

[1] Cf. ERNST, *Johannes der Täufer,* 170; WEBB, *John the Baptizer,* 57, 59.

[2] Cf. esp. Mal 3:23f; Sir 48:10; Mark 9:11–13/Matt 17:10–12; Justin, Dial. 49:1; b. ʿErub. 43a–b (bar.). These and other references are critically evaluated by FAIERSTEIN, *JBL* 100 (1981) 75–86. Cf. also the more positive evaluation of the evidence by ALLISON, *JBL* 103 (1984) 256–258, and the affirmation of Faierstein's assessment by FITZMYER, *JBL* 104 (1985) 295f.

[3] For the most important differences, see U. LUZ, *Matthäus* II, 416f.

[4] It is possible that 15:14 partly builds on Q material. Cf. Luke 6:39.

sue is argued more consistently than in Mark.

The Matthean addition to Mark in 15:13f is in harmony with this emphasis and builds on the first sequence. Just as the commandment/word of God—not merely of Moses, as in Mark 7:10—is not to be set aside by the tradition of the elders, so every plant that the heavenly Father has not planted will be uprooted; and just as the opponents teach merely human precepts according to Isa 29:13, so they are also blind guides. By rearrangement and expansion, Matthew thus moulds the OT quotations into an elaborated argumentation.

The two quotations in 19:4f belong to 19:3–12 consisting of three dialogical sequences—two with the Pharisees and one with the disciples (19:3–6, 7–9, 10–12).[1] In comparison with Mark 10:2–12,[2] the main differences are the rearrangement of the quotations and the addition of the special material in 19:10–12.[3]

The rearrangement develops the argumentation in the first sequence. The Pharisees state the issue (19:3). It concerns not only—as in Mark—the right of a man to divorce his wife, but his right to divorce her for any cause (κατὰ πᾶσαν αἰτίαν). Instead of referring the Pharisees to what Moses commanded and correcting their use of Deut 24:1, the Matthean Jesus immediately proves his case by means of a quotation from Gen 1:27 and 2:24 as the word of the Creator. Then, in 19:6, he draws the conclusions marked by ὥστε and οὖν.

The second sequence brings forth an authoritative Jesus-saying which elaborates the argumentation of the previous sequence.[4] Jesus first refers back to the quotations and then embellishes them with his own authoritative statement. Just as he in 19:4 introduces the proof from the OT by referring to how it was ἀπ᾽ ἀρχῆς, so in 19:8 he gives a similar reference (ἀπ᾽ ἀρχῆς δὲ οὐ γέγονεν οὕτως) before the decisive λέγω δὲ ὑμῖν statement.

The special material in the third sequence also elaborates the argumentation of the first sequence. Through the term αἰτία, the disciples' statement in 19:10 makes a connection back to the initial issue in 19:3. In the following response, Jesus refers to τὸν λόγον (τοῦτον).[5] Since he uses γάρ—not ὅτι *recitativum*—as a connection to the next phrase in 19:12, τὸν λόγον

---

[1]   See above p. 376.

[2]   For 19:9, cf. also Matt 5:32; Luke 16:18.

[3]   S.H. BROOKS, *Matthew's Community,* 107–109, considers 19:12 as traditional. If Justin, Apol. I 15:4, is independent of Matthew, as BLINZLER, Justinus, 45–55; GNIL-KA, *Matthäusevangelium* II, 151, believe, 19:11 might also be pre-Matthean. But Justin might here depend on Matthew. So BELLINZONI, *Sayings,* 60f; SAND, *Reich Gottes,* 24, 53; MASSAUX, *Influence de l'Évangile de Saint Matthieu,* 470; W.-D. KÖHLER, *Rezeption des Matthäusevangeliums,* 230, 560. In view of the absence of any parallel to 19:10–12 in Mark and Luke, the occurrence of all the three verses within the present context is probably Matthean.

[4]   The strong emphasis indicated by λέγω δὲ ὑμῖν is not present in Mark 10:11.

[5]   It is not necessary to decide whether τοῦτον is secondary or not.

(τοῦτον) must refer back to a previous word,[1] most likely to the one in 19:9.[2] Perhaps it focuses on the implication of 19:9 that forbids remarriage. The word cannot be grasped by everyone, because the gift of not marrying (again) has been given only to some—the "eunuchs." The emphasis on not remarrying is in harmony with the first sequence. As we just noticed, 19:8 introduces the authoritative statement in 19:9 in a manner which reveals the connection to the previous proof from the OT. It seems that also the third sequence develops the quotations. Matthew, it seems, created a pattern in which Jesus first presents an argumentation with proof from the OT and a concluding thesis, and then elaborates the proofs in authoritative sayings, one of which comes from the Markan tradition and one of which comes from elsewhere (Matthew's own hand or another tradition).

The quotations in 19:18f belong to 19:16–22, which contains three dialogical sequences (19:16f, 18f, 20f) and a concluding remark (19:22).[3] They relate also to the following teaching given to the disciples in 19:23–30. The whole unit is framed by the issue concerning having or inheriting eternal life (19:16, 29). There are in comparison with Mark and Luke especially three small differences which reveal the attempt to elaborate Jesus' use of the OT.

First, while both the Markan and the Lukan Jesus present the quotation from Exod 20:12–16/Deut 5:16–20 as prohibitive aorist subjunctives, the Matthean Jesus uses future indicatives preceded by τό. Since the order of the various items mentioned in the quotation agrees with the MT also in Matthew,[4] the change into future indicatives is only partially explained as adherence to the LXX.[5] Through this change, the prohibitions appear more as principles in an argumentation than as directives about an action.

Second, the Matthean Jesus adds a reference to Lev 19:18, "a great maxim in the Torah" (כלל נדול בחורה) according R. Akiba (y. Ned. 41c; Sifra on 19:18; Gen. Rab. 24:7). The addition of this reference raises the quotation in Matt 19:18f to a fundamental level. Lev 19:18 is in Matt 22:39 one of the two principles on which the Law and the prophets depend.[6] It appears as an essential ingredient in the hermeneutical programme according to which the Matthean Jesus interprets and applies the OT.

Third, the first and the last sequence of 19:16–22 correspond to each other through εἰ (δὲ) θέλεις,[7] which we do not find in Mark and Luke. The exhortation to keep the commandments follows after the first occurrence of

---

1 *Contra* GNILKA, *Matthäusevangelium* II, 155.
2 Cf. SAND, *Reich Gottes,* 53f.
3 See above p. 376.
4 The presence of μὴ ἀποστερήσῃς in Mark 10:19 is textcritically uncertain. It is missing in both Matthew and Luke.
5 GUNDRY, *Use of the Old Testament,* 19.
6 See above pp. 361f. Cf. also 5:43–48.
7 Cf. above p. 378.

the expression; Jesus' exhortation about the further requirement follows after the second occurrence. The correspondence between the first and third sequence results in the impression that the Matthean Jesus elaborates the OT.

The quotation in 21:42 belongs to 21:40–43(–44),[1] which constitutes the concluding application of the narrative mashal concerning the wicked tenants in 21:33–39. In comparison with Mark 12:9–11/Luke 20:15b–18, Matt 21:40–43(–44) exhibits two specific features which sharpen the argumentative function of the OT.

First, as a result of changes in the tradition,[2] the Matthean version presents a dialogue in which the opponents provide the answer to a question posed by Jesus. The dialogue does not appear in Mark, and in Luke Jesus gives himself the answer, to which the people react merely with a brief μὴ γένοιτο (Luke 20:16). The dialogical form in Matthew creates the expectation of an argumentation.

Second, while Jesus quotes Ps 118:22f with identical words in both Mark and Matthew,[3] the Matthean Jesus adds a statement of his own in 21:43.[4] Its location, and perhaps even creation,[5] is Matthean. Jesus alludes in his own statement to the previous response by the opponents with the catch-word καρποί and makes a connection to the quotation with διὰ τοῦτο.[6] In this way, Jesus develops polemically the suggestion made by the opponents and adheres to Ps 118:22f as the basic proof of his own statement.

The quotation in 22:32 occurs towards the end of 22:23–33, which exhibits two parts (22:23–28, 29–33). In comparison with Mark 12:24–

---

[1] It is not impossible that 21:44 is original. Cf. METZGER, *Textual Commentary*, 58; SNODGRASS, *Wicked Tenants*, 66–68.

[2] SNODGRASS, *Wicked Tenants*, 61, argues that the dialogue is earlier since the parable "is much more effective if the hearers pronounce their own judgment in keeping with the classic parable form," which Snodgrass exemplifies by reference to 2 Sam 12:1f. But there are no evident reasons for assuming that the narrative meshalim developed from more to less effective forms, and it is difficult to ascertain that 2 Sam 12:1f—even if the saying of David himself in 12:5f is taken into account—represents the classical form of a narrative mashal.

[3] The quotation is shorter in Luke 20:17.

[4] Matt 21:44—if original—might be from the tradition. Cf. Luke 20:18.

[5] SNODGRASS, *Wicked Tenants*, 68–71, argues that 21:43, 44 existed together already in the double tradition. In particular, the use of ἡ βασιλεία τοῦ θεοῦ instead of ἡ βασιλεία τῶν οὐρανῶν may reflect influence from the tradition. But it is not impossible that the use of ἡ βασιλεία τοῦ θεοῦ in 21:43 is due to its occurrence in 21:31. Cf. also 12:28; 319:24 and the discussion by PAMMENT, *NTS* 27 (1981) 211–232; WOUTERS, *"... wer den Willen meines Vaters tut,"* 88–103; THOMAS, *NTS* 39 (1993) 136–146, all three recognizing that the use of ἡ βασιλεία τοῦ θεοῦ instead of ἡ βασιλεία τῶν οὐρανῶν is not insignificant in Matthew, though they draw different conclusions from this observation.

[6] TILLING, *Israel*, 60, stresses that the connection made by means of διὰ τοῦτο refers to the whole mashal about the wicked tenants. But as already ZAHN, *Matthäus*, 629f, indicated, there is also—and perhaps primarily—an argumentative relation between the quotation itself and 21:43.

27/Luke 20:34–39, the Matthean Jesus produces a clearer argumentation in the second part of the unit.

Jesus first states the thesis that the Sadducees go astray because they know neither the Scriptures nor the power of God (22:29). The Matthean Jesus gives his thesis in the form of a clear proposition, not a question like in Mark 12:24.[1] The following two rationales are linked to the previous with γάρ (22:30) and connected with each other by means of δέ (22:31). The first provides the explanation why the Sadducees go astray in the specific issue about remarriage after the resurrection. The second, containing the quotation from Exod 3:6, addresses the more general issue about why the Sadducees do not know the Scriptures and the power of God in their view of the resurrection. In 22:31 Jesus refers to the resurrection (ἡ ἀνάστασις) of the dead instead of using the verb (ἐγείρεσθαι) present in Mark 12:26/Luke 20:37. This is congruent with the terminology taken over from the tradition earlier in the pericope (22:23, 28, 30). The quotation becomes more explicitly directed towards the general issue at stake. What the Sadducees say about the resurrection is contrasted by what God says.[2] The Matthean Jesus also introduces the OT quotation as a word from God addressed directly to the present generation (τὸ ῥηθὲν ὑμῖν). In Mark 12:26/Luke 20:37 the quotation remains something that God said (εἶπεν) or Moses disclosed (ἐμήνυσεν) in the past. The change in the Matthean version intensifies the argumentative force of the quotation.[3] Taken together, the rationales explain why the Sadducees go astray in the specific and in the general issue. Again, an OT saying appears as a vital part in an argumentative elaboration of the Jesus tradition.

The quotation in 22:44 appears within 22:41–46. Matthew puts it in the form of a dialogue.[4] In comparison with the parallels in Mark 12:35–37a/Luke 20:41–44, Matt 22:42–45 shows specific characteristics pointing to a more elaborated argumentative situation and function of the OT saying.

The dialogical form makes the issue appear more fundamental and principal. The question does not concern, as in Mark and Luke, how the Jewish representatives can say that the Messiah is the son of David. It is more precise and deals with whose son the Messiah is (22:42, 45). The readers/hearers consequently expect the Jesus-saying to bring a conclusive argumentation into the dialogue. Although the Matthean Jesus puts his words in the form of a question (22:43–45), there are in comparison with Mark and Luke at least two differences implying a more argumentative situation and function of the quotation.

First, Jesus actualizes and vitalizes the OT quotation more clearly in

---

1   The Lukan Jesus does not say that the Sadducees go astray (πλανᾶν).
2   Cf. PATTE, *Matthew*, 311.
3   Cf. GUNDRY, *Matthew*, 446; SAND, *Matthäus*, 445.
4   See above p. 376.

Matthew than in the parallels. The Markan Jesus introduces the quotation as something which David said (εἶπεν) in the holy spirit; the Lukan Jesus introduces it as something which David says in the book of Psalms (λέγει ἐν βίβλῳ ψαλμῶν). In Matthew David calls (καλεῖ) the Messiah lord, speaking (λέγων) the words of Ps 110:1 in the spirit. This change makes the quotation more immediately applicable to the present situation.

Second, the Matthean version makes the link to the issue under discussion more explicit by means of a twofold οὖν (22:43, 45). While we cannot exclude the possibility that there might have been some connecting words in the tradition,[1] the parallel occurrence of οὖν is present in Matthew only. It increases the logical connection in the saying. The first οὖν picks up the answer which the Pharisees give on Jesus' question about whose son the Messiah is. The second indicates that Jesus forms a final question on the basis of his quotation. The second question contains therefore a concluding proposition implicitly.[2] Jesus does not claim that the opinion of the Pharisees is wrong. The double occurrence of οὖν instead strengthens the impression that the Pharisees have to reconcile their answer with the proof from the OT. If the Pharisees admit that the Messiah is the son of David, they must, because of Ps 110:1, also recognize him as son of a higher dignity.[3] Otherwise they do not understand the OT.[4] The force of this argumentation is indicated in the final comment (22:46),[5] which only Matthew places after the Jesus-saying.[6] Through the implicit argumentation from the OT, Jesus has conclusively silenced the listeners. Matthew gives the OT saying an increased argumentative situation and force.

The quotation in 26:31 is part of 26:31–35. The pericope exhibits two dialogical sequences. In 26:31–33 the dialogue centres on the threefold σκανδαλίζεσθαι, and in 26:34f on the twofold ἀπαρνεῖσθαι. Only the first Jesus-saying shows an elaborated argumentative character. This is provided by the quotation from the OT. In comparison with Mark 14:27f, the saying in Matt 26:31f displays especially two distinctive features sharpening the argumentative function of the quotation.

First, the Matthean version introduces the quotation with γέγραπται γάρ instead of the Markan ὅτι γέγραπται. This is in harmony with Matthew's normal way to signal the rationale for a previous command, statement or

---

[1] Cf. the presence of γάρ and οὖν in Luke 20:42, 44.

[2] HELD, *Miracle Stories*, 236 n. 4, remarks in this connection that "here no answer is nevertheless an answer."

[3] WREDE, *Vorträge*, 174; GIBBS, *NTS* 10 (1963–64) 461; SUHL, *ZNW* 59 (1968) 61; KINGSBURY, *Matthew: Structure, Christology, Kingdom*, 101f.

[4] Cf. U. LUZ, *Christologie*, 225: "Von ihrer Position her können sie also ihre eigene Bibel nicht mehr verstehen."

[5] Cf. GIBBS, *NTS* 10 (1963-64) 461; SUHL, *ZNW* 59 (1968) 79f; BURGER, *Davidssohn*, 89f, though Burger emphasizes Jesus' use of κύριος on the cost of the statement that the issue actually concerns the sonship of the Messiah.

[6] Cf. Mark 12:34b/Luke 22:40.

question.[1] In this case, Jesus justifies a thesis with the OT.

Second, within the quotation of Zech 13:7 itself, the Matthean version changes the chiastic pattern in Mark and advances διασκορπισθήσονται.[2] In this way, a future indicative verb starts both parts of the quotation. The change is not due to harmonization with the LXX only.[3] Since the verbs point to future happenings, it has also the effect of strengthening the previous thesis by emphasizing the predictive character of its rationale. The work on the tradition reflected in 26:31 elaborates therefore Jesus' argumentative use of the OT.

To summarize and conclude, several OT sayings in Matthew belong to a tradition which has been the object of expansion and/or rearrangement. In 11:10; 15:4, 8f; 19:4f, 18f; 21:42; 22:32, 44; 26:31 the OT sayings are part of a reasoning which is more deductive than the tradition. The OT quotation itself may serve different functions in the argumentation, mostly of course as a proof. But it never stands alone, separated from Jesus' own words. Matthew achieves this deductive logic by working on the setting of the quotation, on the quotation itself or on both together. The expansion consists of additions to the setting and/or the actual quotation. The rearrangement manifests itself through the different order of words and phrases in the setting and/or actual quotation. The two means of working on the tradition—expansion and rearrangement—often occur within one and the same unit. At the end, *Jesus emerges as a person using the OT as authoritative Scripture but still developing its logical function and force. He incorporates it within his own elaborated argumentation in the story.*

4.3.3. Argumentation within Matthean Quotations

The second manner of elaborating argumentative patterns was to add an OT quotation to an already existing Jesus-saying. This procedure is reflected in 9:13; 12:7; 13:14f; 21:16. I will here bring a further aspect into the analysis. I will not study the logic of the argumentation *in* the story only. It is of special interest to see how the logic in the story relates to the personal authority of Jesus that emerges *out of* the story.[4] In other words, does the readers'/hearers' recognition of Jesus' argumentation with the OT depend on their previous recognition of Jesus himself, or does the logic of the argumentation suffice in itself to convince the readers/hearers?

9:11 states the issue of the scene depicted in 9:10–13 in the form of a question. It concerns Jesus' table fellowship with tax collectors and sinners.

---

1 R.A. EDWARDS, *CBQ* 52 (1990) 649.
2 Matthew also adds τῆς ποίμνης.
3 Cf. GUNDRY, *Use of the Old Testament*, 25–28.
4 MACK/ROBBINS, *Patterns of Persuasion*, 128, 132, 137f, 141, make a distinction between the rhetoric "in" the story and "of" the story.

The quotation in 9:13 is part of Jesus' response. In Mark 2:17/Luke 5:31f Jesus answers merely by means of an aphoristic mashal functioning as the general premise of the conclusion. This way of arguing is insufficient in Matthew. By including the command to learn Hos 6:6,[1] the Matthean Jesus forms a thesis based on an authority recognized, though not correctly understood,[2] by the opponents.

The thesis depends on the Matthean story about Jesus. Matthew presents a rationale (γάρ) for the preceding command to learn the OT. It concerns Jesus' vocation and action and implies that the quotation is ultimately christological.[3] This use of the γάρ-clause is according to R.A. Edwards ideological: it "reveals the assumptions of the speaker ... after the command, statement, or question has been spoken."[4] In this case, the argumentation in the saying is connected with the argument arising out of the whole story. The recognition of the thesis based on the OT depends on the recognition of Jesus' vocation and action.

The case of 12:1–8 is clearly stated in 12:2. In contrast to the inquiring question in Mark 2:24/Luke 6:2, the Pharisees make an accusation concerning what is lawful to do on the sabbath. The reference to the example of David is insufficient as a response in Matthew.[5] Without interrupting the Jesus-saying with another introductory formula,[6] the Matthean version holds together the response and elaborates the argumentation by adding an analogy from the Torah (12:5), a comparison between lesser and greater (12:6) and a quotation of Hos 6:6 (12:7).[7] The first and the last of these base their force on the OT, with the quotation developed into an implicit thesis.

A self-referential statement in the form of a rationale (γάρ) follows the quotation also here. It points to the assumption of the speaker. If the Pharisees had acknowledged Jesus as lord over the sabbath, they would have realized that the disciples are guiltless in view of Hos 6:6.[8] In addition, 12:1–8 as a whole illustrates in what way Jesus' yoke and burden are easy and light (11:30). The aim to establish the guiltless status of the disciples by reference to the OT depends then at the end on Jesus' intrinsic authority emerging out of the story.[9]

The case of 13:10–17 is clearly formulated in 13:10. While Mark

---

[1] For arguments against the assumption that the quotation was part of the tradition, see HILL, *NTS* 24 (1978) 107f.

[2] Cf. HILL, *NTS* 24 (1978) 111.

[3] Cf. above p. 272.

[4] *CBQ* 52 (1990) 646.

[5] DAUBE, *New Testament*, 67–71.

[6] Cf. καὶ ἔλεγεν αὐτοῖς in Mark 2:27/Luke 6:5.—It is not certain that the following Jesus-saying in Mark 2:27 was part of the tradition available to Matthew. It is missing also in Luke.

[7] MACK/ROBBINS, *Patterns of Persuasion*, 132–139.

[8] Cf. VERSEPUT, *Rejection*, 169–172.

[9] Cf. MACK/ROBBINS, *Patterns of Persuasion*, 137f.

4:10/Luke 8:9 points merely to an interest in the narrative meshalim, Matthew sharpens the issue to concern why Jesus speaks in such a way to the crowd(s). The answer consists of three segments (13:11f, 13–15, 16f). The first presents a thesis (ὅτι) consisting in the opposition between what is given to the disciples and not given to the crowd(s), with the subsequent rationale (γάρ) in the form of an aphoristic mashal. The second refers to the issue and presents an explanatory thesis (ὅτι) consisting in the opposition between seeing and not seeing, hearing and neither hearing nor understanding. The OT quotation is not brought in as a rationale. The introductory formula does not in this case contain γάρ, ἵνα or ὅπως, as we find elsewhere in Matthew.[1] Jesus instead states the fulfilment of Isa 6:9f as a consequence (καί) affirming—not actually proving—the thesis. The OT is for the disciples more relevant as an affirmation of already held convictions than as a proof. Through the location of ὑμῶν δέ at the beginning of the third segment,[2] the thesis that the eyes and the ears of the disciples are blessed appears in implicit contrast to the eyes and ears of the crowd(s) and functions therefore as a further answer to the initial question. The rationale (γάρ) consists of an authoritative ἀμήν-saying providing the background of Jesus' thesis.[3]

The quotation is a vital part in an attempt to elaborate the argumentation in the Jesus-saying. The first and third segment are constructed out of individual elements located at separate places in Mark and/or Luke. The almost complete quotation of Isa 6:9f probably reflects Matthew's work on the tradition.[4] The two other synoptics allude to Isa 6:9f without introducing it as a quotation (Mark 4:12/Luke 8:10). Matt 13:13 maintains the allusion, with the important change of ἵνα into ὅτι. But the Matthean Jesus also adds the actual quotation. This is congruent with the sharpened issue initially raised by the disciples. The response receives in this way an affirmation through a decisive reference to the authoritative word of God.

The quotation is deliberately connected with the broader account about the sower and its interpretation. This is indicated by the location of 13:14f at the almost exact centre of 13:3–23.[5] The mashal about the sower concerns the hearers of the word and is fundamental to the six narrative meshalim in 13:24–30, 31f, 33, 44, 45f, 47f.[6] Hearing and understanding are also the concern of 13:14f. The quotation therefore depends on Jesus' broader activity as a "mashalist." Isa 6:9f functions as an affirmation *because* the

---

1   Cf. 1:22; 2:5, 15, 23; 3:3; 4:14; 8:17; 12:17; 13:35; 21:4.
2   Cf. the emphatic ὑμῖν δέδοται γνῶναι in 13:11.
3   Cf. R.A. EDWARDS, *CBQ* 52 (1990) 647, classifying this occurrence of γάρ within clauses that provide the "plot background."
4   U. LUZ, *Matthäus* II, 301f.
5   In the text accepted by the 26th edition of Nestle-Aland, there are 162 words before and 164 words after 13:14f.
6   GERHARDSSON, *NTS* 14 (1967–68) 165–193; *idem, NTS* 19 (1972–73) 16–37.

Matthean Jesus now speaks in narrative meshalim to crowd(s) showing no signs of understanding. Jesus' activity puts the Scripture into the right perspective. The full force of the quotation depends essentially on the broad perspective of the story about Jesus.

The Matthean account of the cleansing of the temple exhibits two scenes, which both contain an OT saying. The scene in 21:12f appears also in the two other synoptics (Mark 11:15–17/Luke 19:45f). With the exception of the narrator's comment in 21:17,[1] the second scene in 21:14–17, including the quotation of Ps 8:3,[2] seems to be an addition to the tradition.[3] It is also more argumentative. It depicts the quotation as an answer to an issue explicitly brought out by the high priests and scribes. The case concerns the children's cry. If the high priests and the scribes had really read Ps 8:3, they would have realized that the children's cry was acknowledged by God. The tradition is expanded through the creation of a new argumentation in which Jesus resolves the matter by reference to the OT.

The argumentative force of the OT depends on basic intentions emerging out of the whole story. Already in 11:25 Jesus praises his Father for the revelation he has given to the infants but not to the wise and intelligent ones. Within the whole gospel tradition, Jesus uses νήπιοι to refer to the children only in this utterance—and its parallel (Luke 10:21)—and the quotation in 21:16. The children are further acknowledged later in the narrative. In answering the question concerning who is greatest in the kingdom of heaven, Jesus brings forth a child as the example to follow (18:1–4). And later he takes a step further by presenting the children as models for those to whom the kingdom belongs (19:14). The high priests and the scribes had of course read Ps 8:3. But they fail to interpret it in the light of Jesus' mission. Ps 8:3 justifies the children's praise *because* Jesus elsewhere acknowledges them. The presentation of Jesus emerging out of the story constitutes the condition under which his argumentation by means of the OT in the story gains its force.

We have seen that Matthew inserts an OT quotation into an utterance of Jesus in 9:13; 12:7; 13:14f; 21:16. *There emerges a significant interaction between deductive and inductive logic of argumentation.* On one hand, Jesus teaches by means of more deductive logic than in the tradition. The OT sayings contain deductive reasoning as the result of elaborative work with

---

[1] Cf. Mark 11:11b.

[2] The close adherence to the LXX is not an indication that the quotation is taken from the tradition. Cf. STENDAHL, *School of Matthew*, 134f; ROTHFUCHS, *Erfüllungszitate*, 24.

[3] It is questionable if e.g. E. KLOSTERMANN, *Matthäusevangelium*, 167; BULTMANN, *Geschichte der synoptischen Tradition*, 34; SCHWEIZER, *Matthäus*, 266, are correct to assume that Luke 19:39f reflects the tradition on which Matt 21:15f builds. The opponents' identity and the utterance are totally different in the two versions. Cf. BURGER, *Davidssohn*, 86f; GNILKA, *Matthäusevangelium* II, 207.

the available material. It was not sufficient to present a teacher who merely stated his declarations. He argues his point. On the other hand, the OT sayings remain dependent on Jesus' intrinsic authority emerging out of the whole story. The logos relies on the ethos, to speak in rhetorical terms. The deductive argumentation made by reference to the OT depends on the total flow of the narrative and relates to the depiction of Jesus' own authority. This shows that *the elaborative argumentation is not the result of a diminished view of Jesus' teaching authority. On the contrary, the readers'/hearers' recognition of the argumentation in the story relies ultimately on their recognition of the Jesus image emerging out of the whole story.*

4.3.4. Argumentation within the Antitheses

The third manner of elaborating certain argumentative patterns was to create an antithetical construction in which the OT relates to certain authoritative words of Jesus. In the Antitheses Jesus quotes (5:21, 27, 38, 43), paraphrases (5:31) and summarizes (5:33) passages from the OT. All six introduce the reference to the OT with ἐρρέθη—a divine passive.

The amount of Matthean elaboration in the antithetical formula itself has been estimated variously. The influential view of R. Bultmann was that Matthew took over the first, the second and the fourth construction and himself created the third, the fifth and the sixth.[1] Bultmann claimed that the counterdemand of the primary formulas could never have been transmitted isolated from the thesis, that the secondary Antitheses have synoptic parallels which do not exhibit the antithetical form and that while the counterdemands of the primary formulas transcend the prohibitions in the theses, the ones of the secondary formulas instead contradict the demands—once the concession (5:31)—in the theses. G. Strecker finds it necessary to revise Bultmann's arguments.[2] None of them is sufficient, according to Strecker. While he arrives at the same conclusion as Bultmann, he puts more emphasis on Matthew's use of the Decalogue in the primary Antitheses, on Matthew's fondness of number three, on wordstatistics and on Matthew's conservative attitude to the tradition. In his view, Matthew received the primary formulas from Q[Mt].

There are other opinions, apart from this majority view.[3] On one hand, H.-T. Wrege and his teacher Joachim Jeremias ascribe all six formulas to the tradition.[4] The Matthean Jesus elsewhere fulfils rather than abrogates

---

[1]   *Geschichte der synoptischen Tradition,* 142–144.

[2]   *ZNW* 69 (1978) 36–72.

[3]   Many scholars agree that some Antitheses come from the tradition and some from Matthew, but they differ from Bultmann and Strecker concerning which ones. Cf. the scholars mentioned by BERNER, *Bergpredigt,* 209f n. 79; STRECKER, *ZNW* 69 (1978) 40 n. 7. In addition, cf. GUELICH, *NTS* 22 (1975–76) 444–457.

[4]   WREGE, *Überlieferungsgeschichte,* 2f, 56f, 66–94, esp. 82, 93; Joachim JERE-

the Law, and for this reason it is unlikely that Matthew should have created any of the formulas. Matthew took them over from certain law-free churches, which had collected them as separate units in the oral tradition. On the other hand, there is a trend to ascribe all six constructions to Matthew himself. I. Broer and M.J. Suggs, in particular, advocate this proposal.[1] They argue that the antithetical construction as well as the emphatic ἐγώ of Jesus are present in other instances where the creative activity of Matthew is visible.

While it is evident that Matthew adhered to the tradition when he created the Antitheses as a whole, the absence of an antithetical argumentation in the parallel material is a decisive factor speaking against a pre-Matthean origin of the construction. The reference to the ἀλλά-construction in Luke 6:27 does not suffice. J. Dupont shows that the construction with πλήν ... ἀλλά followed by λέγω ὑμῖν (6:24, 27) is Lukan.[2] This raises the possibility that the construction is of Matthean origin.[3] To the observations already made by Broer and Suggs, it is possible to add some statistical reflections.

The use of ἐρρέθη is significant. It is the only common element in the introductory formula of all six theses. Different forms of λέγειν are present approximately twohundred and eighty-nine times in Matthew. The aorist passive occurs nineteen times. The indicative is not found outside of the Antitheses, but the passive participial of the aorist, which is not used in Mark and Luke, appears in thirteen Matthean formulations (1:22; 2:15, 17, 23; 3:3; 4:14; 8:17; 12:17; 13:35; 21:4; 22:31; 24:15; 27:9). Since the most vital element of the introductory formula is characteristic of Matthew's own diction, it is certainly possible that the whole antithetical argumentation is his creation.

The introductory formula of the counterdemands centres on ἐγώ ... λέγω. Matthew uses ἐγώ in its nominative form[4] approximately twenty-eight times.[5] The pronoun appears in a self-referential statement by Jesus sixteen times.[6] In addition, Matthew uses κἀγώ approximately nine times.[7] Six of

---

MIAS, *Neutestamentliche Theologie,* 240f;

[1]   BROER, *BZ* 19 (1975) 50–63; SUGGS, Antitheses, 433–444. Cf. also BROER, *Freiheit vom Gesetz,* 102–107.

[2]   *Béatitudes* I, 189–191. Dupont does not, however, reject entirely all resemblances between Matthew and Luke. Cf. further SUGGS, Antitheses, 439–441; GUELICH, *NTS* 22 (1976) 450 n. 4.

[3]   In addition to the synoptic parallels, we may also mention Jas 5:12 as related to Matt 5:33–37. Jas 5:12 exhibits no antithetical format. HARTIN, *James,* 190f, considers the Matthean form to be more developed and later than the one in James.

[4]   In addition, ἐμοῦ, μου, ἐμοί, μοι, ἐμέ and με occur. Altogether the pronoun appears 221 times, including the use in variant readings of some MSS.

[5]   Mark has 16 and Luke 20 or 21 (counting also 11:20) occurrences of ἐγώ.

[6]   5:22, 28, 32, 34, 39, 44; 8:7; 10:16; 12:27, 28; 14:27; 20:22; 21:27; 23:34; 26:39; 28:20.

[7]   Mark does not give any instance of the crasis, provided κἀγώ in some MSS of 11:29a is secondary; Luke has 5.

these instances occur within self-referential statements by Jesus.[1] The Matthean Jesus thus uses ἐγώ in reference to himself on twenty-two occasions. Mark contains nine or ten occasions;[2] Luke has twelve or thirteen.

Six of the self-referential instances are part of Matthew's special material.[3] In the nine instances belonging to the double tradition, Matthew alone uses the term seven or eight times.[4] It is absent only once or twice in Matthew when present in the parallel Lukan passage.[5] In the five instances belonging to the triple tradition, Matthew is twice entirely alone to use the pronoun.[6] Mark and Luke never agree against Matthew to use ἐγώ.[7] In two instances belonging to passages which Matthew shares with Mark only, the pronoun is present in both synoptics.[8] But on five or six other occasions, Mark has the pronoun where it is absent in the parallel Matthean passage.[9]

What is significant is that Matthew has a self-referential ἐγώ used by Jesus more often than any of the other two synoptics, that Matthew has an additional ἐγώ in seven or eight cases of passages parallelled in Luke, while the opposite is true only once or twice, and that Mark and Luke never agree against Matthew to use ἐγώ. In the passages where the term appears in Luke but not in Matthew, its presence is probably due to Lukan work on the tradition.[10] And the absence of the term in passages taken over from Mark is never due to omission of the term only. It is always the result of the omission of a whole phrase[11] or of a change in the grammatical construction.[12]

In the majority of cases where only Matthew uses the term in the double and triple tradition, ἐγώ is a Matthean addition. This is quite evident in 5:32;

---

1   10:32, 33; 11:28; 16:18; 21:24 (*bis*). In 18:33 κἀγώ is part of a narrative meshalim given by Jesus.

2   In Mark 14:58 Jesus is quoted by someone else.

3   5:22, 28, 34; 11:28; 16:18; 28:20.

4   Matt 5:39/Luke 6:29; Matt 5:44/Luke 6:27; Matt 8:7/Luke 7:6; Matt 10:16/Luke 10:3 (with some MSS of Luke 10:3 including ἐγώ); Matt 10:32/Luke 12:8; Matt 10:33/Luke 12:9; Matt 23:34/Luke 11:49. If ἐγώ is secondary in Luke 11:20, Matt 12:28 is also to be counted here.

5   Matt 7:7/Luke 11:9. Cf. also Matt 19:28/Luke 22:29.

6   Matt 5:32/Mark 10:11/Luke 16:18; Matt 21:24b/Mark 11:29b/Luke 20:3 (with some MSS of Mark 11:29b reading ἐγώ λέγω instead of ἐρῶ). Matt 5:32 does not, strictly speaking, belong to the triple tradition, because Mark 10:11 has its actual parallel in Matt 19:9. But the saying is at least attested in all three gospels. Cf. tables 2 and 3 above.

7   In Matt 21:24a/Mark 11:29a/Luke 20:3, Matthew and Luke agree against Mark in having κἀγώ, if the Markan text is original. In Matt 26:39/Mark 14:36/Luke 22:42, Matthew and Mark agree against Luke.

8   Matt 14:27/Mark 6:50; Matt 20:22/Mark 10:38.

9   Matt 20:22f/Mark 10:38f (with some MSS of Matt 20:22f including two of the three "missing" instances of ἐγώ); Matt 26:61/Mark 14:58 (though Jesus is only quoted here); Matt 26:64/Mark 14:62. Cf. also Matt 17:18/Mark 9:25, where the whole Jesus-saying is absent in Matthew.

10   For discussion of the pronoun in Luke, see HOWARD, *Ego,* 174–183.

11   Matt 17:18/Mark 9:25; Matt 20:22f/Mark 10:38f; Matt 26:64/Mark 14:62 (cf. Matt 14:27).

12   Matt 26:61/Mark 14:58.

21:24b. It is more difficult to determine the issue in passages with a parallel only in Luke, but its presence is probably the result of Matthean addition to the tradition in the majority of the seven or eight instances.

The ἐγώ in 5:39, 44 is probably Matthean. We have seen that even Bultmann and his followers admit that Matthew created the fifth and the sixth antithetical construction.

It is possible that the ἐγώ of Jesus in 8:7 is caused by the implication that Jesus would enter the house of a Gentile.[1] This would accord well with the Matthean emphasis in 15:21–28, where Jesus' initial reservation towards the Canaanite woman in 15:23f is an addition to Mark 7:24–30. The Lukan parallel gives no indication that the term was present in the tradition.

The occurrence in 10:16 is to be judged together with the use of the term in 23:34. Both verses contain ἐγὼ ἀποστέλλω. Most scholars regard the ἐγώ in 23:34 as Matthean.[2] Since Luke exhibits no specific interest in wisdom speculations, it is unlikely that he would have altered an original ἐγώ into ἡ σοφία τοῦ θεοῦ in 11:49.[3] Matthew also includes ἐγώ in front of ἀποστέλλω in the OT quotation in 11:10, probably depending on the LXX.[4] The parallel in Luke 7:27 does not have the pronoun; nor does Mark 1:2. In fact, 10:16; 11:10; 23:34 are the only Matthean instances in which ἀπο-στέλλω is used in this form by Jesus, and in each case the verb is preceded by ἐγώ. Since the pronoun was probably added by Matthew in 11:10; 23:34, it is likely that the same was the case in 10:16.

H. Geist argues convincingly that κἀγώ is Matthean in 10:32, 33.[5] To be sure, Matthew normally maintains the expression ὁ υἱὸς τοῦ ἀνθρώπου when it is present in the tradition.[6] This is the case even in his use of Mark 8:38, which is related to Matt 10:32f/Luke 12:8f, in 16:27. But it is probable that the presence of ἐν ἐμοί in Matt 10:32a/Luke 12:8a caused Matthew to use κἀγώ also in the second half of the verse, thus avoiding the awkward change from the first to the third person. As a negative parallel, Matthew then forms 10:33 in a similar style.

As it appears, only five of the twenty-two relevant occurrences of the pronoun come from the tradition.[7] At least nine have been inserted by Matthew.[8] Another six appear in Matthew's special material. Jesus' self-referential ἐγώ sometimes also exhibits a certain emphasis outside of the Antitheses.[9] 8:7; 10:16; 11:28; 23:34; 28:20—all instances in which the pronoun

---

[1]   So e.g. DAHL, *Matteusevangeliet* I, 112; GNILKA, *Matthäusevangelium* I, 301.

[2]   GARLAND, *Matthew 23,* 172 n. 34, presents a list of scholars for and against this assumption.

[3]   SUGGS, *Wisdom,* 14, 135.

[4]   The LXX of Exod 23:20 and Mal 3:1 contains the pronoun.

[5]   *Menschensohn,* 294–300.

[6]   Cf. COLPE, *TDNT* VIII, 442 n. 297.

[7]   Matt 12:27/Luke 11:19; Matt 14:27/Mark 6:50; Matt 20:22/Mark 10:38; Matt 21:27/Mark 11:33/Luke 20:8; Matt 26:39/Mark 14:36.

[8]   In two cases—Matt 12:28/Luke 11:20; Matt 21:24a/Mark 11:29a/Luke 20:3—we may leave the issue open.

[9]   *Contra* STRECKER, *ZNW* 69 (1978) 45.—GNILKA, *Matthäusevangelium* I, 152, agrees with Strecker that the emphatic ἐγώ is not present outside of the Antitheses. Still, in commenting on 10:16 he states: "Den Aspekt des Schutzes wird das im griechischen Text vorangestellte '*ich* sende euch' nahebringen wollen" (*ibid.,* 376). Earlier he calls this a "verstärkendes ἐγώ" added to the tradition by Matthew (*ibid.,* 373).

is peculiar to Matthew—use ἐγώ without any immediately corresponding subject causing the pronoun. These data indicate that Matthew had a special interest in creating patterns stressing the ἐγώ of Jesus.[1]

Matthew also discloses an interest in other parts of the counterdemand. Although the narrative does not employ the whole phrase ἐγὼ δὲ λέγω ὑμῖν elsewhere, it uses related expressions to set Jesus-sayings apart from what other characters say. 16:18 follows up Simon Peter's previous confession by a Jesus-saying containing κἀγὼ δέ σοι λέγω; 21:27 agrees with Mark 11:33/Luke 20:8 to use ἐγὼ λέγω ὑμῖν in a negative response to the opponents. There are also relevant expressions without ἐγώ. Matthew employs λέγω ὑμῖν in authoritative Jesus-sayings approximately fifty-two times. This is more often than in Mark and Luke together.[2] The exact expression λέγω δὲ ὑμῖν is present on seven occasions outside of the Antitheses. Four of them are peculiar to Matthew.[3] This expression alludes in 19:9 to the counterdemand of the third Antithesis (5:32), though without the antithetical format. We may also note the authoritative ἀμήν-sayings appearing thirty or thirty-one times in Matthew.[4] Although Matthew sometimes gives the Markan ἀμήν-sayings without the introductory ἀμήν,[5] it is also often taken over from the tradition,[6] added to the Markan tradition[7] and used in material with only vague or no parallels.[8]

Together with the observations made by Broer and Suggs, these data suggest that Matthew did himself form the antithetical pattern in 5:21–48. If no trace of the antithetical construction is present in the parallel material and if most of the individual words and expressions occur in one form or the other elsewhere in the narrative, with the most vital words exhibiting distinctively Matthean features, it is probable that Matthew was indeed the one mainly responsible for the present antithetical format.

In the antithetical construction itself, Jesus asserts his views on the basis

---

[1] An inquiry into the use of other forms of ἐγώ would probably confirm my conclusion. Cf. e.g. 11:28–30.

[2] Mark uses λέγω ὑμῖν 11 times; Luke 35.

[3] 8:11; 12:6, 36; 19:9. Cf. also Matt 6:29/Luke 12:27; Matt 17:12/Mark 9:13; Matt 26:29/Mark 14:25.

[4] The presence of ἀμήν in 18:19 is textcritically uncertain.

[5] Matt 12:31/Mark 3:28; Matt 12:39; 16:4/Mark 8:12; Matt 26:29/Mark 14:25. But we should notice that Luke never agrees with Mark in using ἀμήν in these cases. Mark 12:43 does not have a Matthean parallel.

[6] Matt 10:42/Mark 9:41; Matt 16:28/Mark 9:1; Matt 19:28/Mark10:29; Matt 21:21/Mark 11:23; Matt 24:34/Mark 13:30; Matt 26:13/Mark 14:9; Matt 26:21/Mark 14:18; Matt 26:34/Mark 14:30.

[7] Matt 19:23/Mark 10:23; Matt 24:2/Mark 13:2. Luke 18:24; 21:6 do not have ἀμήν.—It is also often peculiar to Matthew in the double tradition. Cf. Matt 5:26/Luke 12:59; Matt 8:10/Luke 7:9; Matt 10:15/Luke 10:12; Matt 11:11/Luke 7:28; Matt 13:17/Luke 10:24; Matt 17:20/Luke 17:6; Matt 18:13/Luke 15:5; Matt 23:36/Luke 11:51; Matt 24:47/Luke 12:44.

[8] 5:18; 6:2, 5, 16; 10:23; 18:3, 18 (19); 21:31; 25:12, 40, 45.

of his authoritative ἐγώ.[1] True, some Antitheses contain deductive patterns of argumentation after the initial formula.[2] Jesus does continue to argue his case sometimes. But in the antithetical construction itself, the OT does not function as a proposition or a proof in an extended line of reasoning. It serves the depiction of the customary hearing of God's word, which Jesus deepens by means of his own authoritative declarations. When Matthew formed his own argumentative pattern, the ethos of Jesus was very much at the centre. *The antithetical form makes the argumentation entirely dependent upon Jesus' intrinsic authority.* The ultimate basis and force of the argumentation depended on Jesus as a teacher with irrefutable authority.[3]

Matthew's own work with the tradition reflects the transmission. It implies that the Jesus tradition did not develop from more to less inductive logic only. What Jesus said in the tradition might often have been in need of supporting argumentation. But *the argumentative elaboration of the tradition did not go only in one direction. There was an interchange between deductive and inductive logic in Jesus' use of the OT, where the latter remained fundamental.* The essential motives of transmission centred on a person whose authoritative status as the only normative teacher had already been accepted and validated by Matthew and his circle of transmitters. The logical reasoning would at the end not be recognized by persons who had not already accepted Jesus himself. Teacher and teaching were inseparable. The argumentative elaboration in the story therefore remained bound to the authority of Jesus emerging out of the story. *By combining the two aspects of the elaboration, Matthew created a teacher whose use and interpretation of the OT no one in the community could question any further.*[4]

5. Summary and Conclusions

This chapter tried to answer if and how Matthew's transmission of the Jesus tradition was similar and dissimilar to the patterns described in chapter three. These patterns concerned the personal specificity in the transmission process. It was necessary to study the three areas where the specificity was especially evident in the sociocultural situation: the identification of traditions, the means of transmission and the preservation and elaboration of traditions.

1. There is a unique identification of utterances as Jesus-sayings in Matthew. As a deliberate means to identify a saying, Matthew strengthens the named attribution of sayings to Jesus through his work on the tradition. His

---

[1]   See above pp. 294–296.
[2]   KENNEDY, *New Testament Interpretation,* 56f.
[3]   Cf. MACK, *Rhetoric,* 98.
[4]   Cf. the conclusion by MACK/ROBBINS, *Patterns of Persuasion,* 207f.

consistent use of Ἰησοῦς to introduce the sayings functions to concentrate all important utterances to one specific person who had lived within a certain historical situation of the past. Sayings of other characters are important only as they relate to Jesus. These features reflect the personal specificity in the transmission. *Because the one named Jesus was the only normative teacher, it was important to isolate the Jesus tradition from foreign influences and to treat all other sayings as subordinated to what Jesus had said and done.*

2. Matthew's narrative reveals the means of transmission indirectly. The story of the narrative indicates how Matthew conceptualized the means of transmission. It conveys an emphasis on appropriating Jesus' teaching in word and deed through active hearing and practice. This reflects the verbal and behavioural means of transmission among the transmitters in the community. *The integrated means of transmission, where the words of the tradition are continuous with the rest of life, emerges naturally in a context influenced by orality and person-oriented motives of transmission.*

Matthew's actual use of the main verbal traditions conforms to the authorial conceptions of transmission reflected in the story. The written character of Mark and the Q material did not make the voice of Jesus impersonal. The oral media of the M material show that the Matthean transmitters preferred to transmit traditions of social and existential importance orally. Through a process of re-oralization, the written traditions were accordingly also incorporated as living words into Matthew's narrativized account. *The setting and the motives of transmission effected a careful work with an oral hermeneutic which secured the social and existential importance of the traditions.*

3. The same correlation also applies to the process of preserving and elaborating traditions. The aim to preserve the tradition accords with the increased identification of Jesus-sayings. Foreign material originating with early Christian prophets in the Matthean community did not enter into the body of pre-Easter Jesus-sayings to any larger extent. A decisive criterion manifested in right conduct was the past revelation, a vital part of which was the interpreted Shemaᶜ. The transmission was controlled by what was preserved as past tradition. *Within a setting where transmission is a specific act motivated by a special interest in the teaching as integrated within the past history of Jesus, the aim to preserve and protect the Jesus tradition remained essential.*

Preservation is not opposed to elaboration. The structural and argumentative elaboration of traditions also show signs of a correlation with the specific setting and motives of transmission. Matthew tends to enhance the Jesus-sayings by locating them at the end or at the centre of a pericope, by generalizing or focalizing the episodal comments, by placing the sayings within dialogues and by relating the sayings to each other in a significant manner. What Jesus says is of uttermost importance within the narrative flow of a story. Moreover, a study of sayings in which Jesus quotes the OT explicitly shows that Matthew tends to increase the argumentative force of the Jesus-sayings: he takes over such quotations from the tradition and elaborates the argumentation of the sayings in the story; he adds new quotations into sayings which both develop the argumentation in the story and build on Jesus' authoritative status emerging out of the story; he creates a new antithetical pattern in which Jesus asserts his own declarations on the basis of his own ethos. *The setting determined by Jesus' own didactic authority and by person-oriented motives of transmission fostered an elaboration that enhanced the Jesus-sayings and increased the irrefutable status of Jesus' teaching.*

A correlation between the setting and the motives of transmission on one hand, and the process of transmission on the other, did therefore exist in the three broad areas of transmission worked out in chapter three. Matthew was also in this sense part of a cultural field in ancient Israel and ancient Judaism. But just as the cumulative presence of all three motives of transmission in the school of Matthew's community levelled the phenomenological variety in the sociocultural situation, some areas of Matthew's transmission work exhibited *unique* features. Most evident is the identification of traditions. The rabbinic literature also identifies the tradition by reference to the name of a teacher. But we do not find the same unique focus on *one* name with a specially emphatic connotation. This also led to the aim of preserving the Jesus tradition by isolating it. The prophetic circles in ancient Israel concentrated the tradition by integrating influences from other prophets. Matthew concentrates it mainly by *protecting* it from the sayings of others. These factors are inconceivable without the special setting and the cumulative force of the motives of transmission. Certainly, there are also features which are not specifically unique. The oral hermeneutic imposed on the tradition containing the words of the teaching master reflects what we found also in certain prophetic circles in ancient Israel and at Qumran. Although it has not been possible here to put the structural and argumentative elaboration of the tradition in an exact comparative perspective, we cannot exclude the possibility that such features are present also elsewhere in writings from ancient Israel and ancient Judaism—and indeed from the Greco-Roman world. But *the constant focus on Jesus and the protection of the Jesus tradition remain unique within Matthew's sociocultural situation of transmission.* G. Kittel's old statement, to which I referred at the beginning of my study,[1] still holds true as far as Matthew is concerned. For Matthew, Jesus was indeed the *only* teacher!

---

[1]   See the introduction pp. 14f.

Concluding Remarks

Each of the previous chapters contained a summarizing and concluding section at the end. There is no need to repeat here what has already been said. It is only necessary to make some general and final remarks relating more clearly to the issues mentioned in the introduction to the whole study and indicate some areas in need of further study.

Ignatius' and Clement's interest in Jesus as the only teacher did not build on a random phenomenon merely. They struck, perhaps without knowing it themselves, on one of the central features in early Christian transmission of what Jesus said and did. The modern studies by G. Kittel, R. Bultmann, M. Dibelius, B. Gerhardsson and R. Riesner have one thing in common: the insistence that an appreciation of the constant focus on Jesus in the gospel narratives is essential for a fuller understanding of the tradition and transmission in the young Christian communities.

My study was placed within a scholarly discussion which—to simplify somewhat—stressed either the common settings and practical motives of transmission (Bultmann, Dibelius) or the separate settings and non-practical motives of transmission (Gerhardsson, Riesner). In both cases the assumption was of course that the settings and the motives interacted with the actual transmission process. Was the focus on Jesus the result of a transmission fostered mainly by various activities and needs in the communities? Or was it the focus on Jesus that caused and guided the transmission? The two options are by no means exclusive of each other. The focus on Jesus may certainly have been strengthened through certain activities and needs without being caused by them. It is a matter of emphases and priorities, but important ones. They affect decisively our view of the transmission. Without denying the existence of practical considerations and influences in the young Christian communities, I tried to account for the aspects unrelated to the common activities and needs, and to see how these aspects correlated with the actual transmission process.

Matthew conceptualized the focus on Jesus in his notion about Jesus as the only teacher. Jesus' statement "for one is your teacher" (εἷς γάρ ἐστιν ὑμῶν ὁ διδάσκαλος) in 23:8 carries a significance which goes far beyond its immediate context. The notion is an important feature in Matthew's whole narrative and an index to realities—conceptions and practices—in his community. The previous chapters have shown that it related to broad and essential aspects of Matthew's understanding of Jesus' active ministry and was a vital force in his transmission of the Jesus tradition. By studying it from different perspectives, *we detected reflections of a separate setting exhibiting non-practical motives of transmission which correlated with the way the Jesus tradition was actually preserved and elaborated.* This is, in my judgement, the main general result of the present study. The conception of Jesus as the only teacher defined the setting of transmission as the school of Jesus. The transmitters, including Matthew in particular, regarded themselves as pupils of no one else but Jesus. This setting was probably separate from the rest of the activities in the community. The transmitters of this school transmitted because they cherished Jesus' teaching, life and person for their own sake. They were not left only to immediate considerations about the present and the future activities and needs of the community. Their personal involvement in the content of the tradition—the "inner" tradition—effected a transmission which in various ways enhanced Jesus to an exclusive status of authority.

The main result has several important corollaries. Let me mention three of them. One concerns the reliability of the transmission in the Matthean community. This issue is not only a modern quest caused by our own standards of historical accuracy. Matthew's persistent interest in always relying on the past tradition in his controlled treatment of the Jesus tradition implies that he himself was a transmitter conscious of the distinctions as well as interactions between preservation and elaboration. A separate setting of transmission may point to a technical awareness of how to transmit the material, but it does not say much about why it should be transmitted. The presence of additional factors is necessary. If the setting was also identified as the school of Jesus and exhibited an interest in Jesus' teaching as intimately linked with his life and person, *we have all the essentials for assuming the existence of transmitters highly able and motivated to preserve the tradition faithfully also within their own and the community's creative elaborations.* Chapter six showed that such an assumption holds true even at a close inspection of the actual material.

This leads to another important corollary. Although I have emphasized the non-practical motives of transmission, I have also stressed the importance of placing the transmission within the broad context of the transmitters' social and existential situation. The transmission was not entirely passive, unaffected by the transmitters' environment and convictions. The discussion of the oral and written means of transmission paid special attention to this, but it was fundamental to the whole approach of this study. *Any study of the technical matters of transmission must go hand in hand with a serious appreciation of the transmitters themselves.* This means that the Christian transmitters did not merely register the tradition for preservation passively. They were real persons affected by the tradition; it concerned, and had to concern, their present situation deeply. But by the same token, this does not mean that the transmitters were entirely oriented towards the needs of their community. Such a misunderstanding has sometimes led to the simplified assumption that the transmitters preserved only traditions that were immediately relevant for themselves and their community, and adapted them freely to the present situation. There is an important distinction, in my view, between a present need and a vital belief coloured by the past tradition. We have seen that the transmitters' situation in no way resulted in a total indifference to the past tradition. On the contrary, their personal involvement in the Jesus tradition correlated closely with—even promoted—a careful and controlled transmission process. This study has tried to avoid both extremes, pointing to the intricate interaction between preservation and elaboration in the Matthean transmission of the Jesus tradition.

Another corollary concerns the sociocultural situation of transmission. Comparison is, it seems, implicit in most forms of historical research. I have worked on the assumption that each phenomenon of transmission must be seen within a field of cultural continuity relating to the past and to the future. The main result of the study emanated, to a large extent, on the basis of related phenomena of transmission in ancient Israel and ancient Judaism—before and after Matthew. There were both similarities and contrasts, but the result was anchored in Matthew's own cultural matrix of transmission. As an outcome of this approach, *some phenomenological patterns of transmission in various corners of the ancient Israelite and Jewish culture have emerged.* I tried to keep the material broad enough to allow the postulation of some general patterns, and at the same time I tried to be detailed enough to allow some firm conclusions. This investigation— and even more my own experiences in making the research—has shown that historical phenomena are open to adequate historical explanations only when we avoid isolating them from the comparative perspective gained from other material of relevance. While the sociocultural reconstruction was aimed primarily for a study of the Matthean transmission of the Jesus tradition, its general character may have repercussions for other studies dealing with the same problems in other material related to ancient Israel and ancient Judaism.

Finally we then arrive at areas and material in need of further investigation. The most evident limitation of the present study is of course that it deals primarily with the narrative of one gospel only. The various conclusions and the result with its corollaries concern first of all Matthew's narrative, not Mark's, not Luke's and indeed not John's. This limitation avoids a common criticism against assuming a rather controlled transmission process, namely the differences between the gospel narratives themselves. Even if the present study indicates that this criticism neglects much of the elaboration and variety that such an assumption actually allows for, a full response would have to analyze the gospel tradition as represented in each gospel narrative and at each definable stage of the pre-synoptic transmission. It would then be of analytical value to put questions similar to the ones put in this study to all the material, though it is possible that the comparative model would need to be enriched and that the answers would be somewhat different.

This brings us to the comparative material. It would be desirable sometimes to go into further depth in studying each item in each piece of material from ancient Israel and ancient Judaism, always asking the same basic questions. And an account of the Greco-Roman material would indeed be helpful in order to see what patterns exist there and how they merge with or differ from what we found in the first part of this study. The relationship between the Pauline literature and the post-Pauline tradition should also belong to this broadened perspective.

There are of course numerous individual issues in Matthew which need to be addressed more thoroughly. We could ask if there were forms and genres particularly suitable to express and communicate the person-oriented motives of transmission, especially the didactic-biographical motives; we could study each separate Jesus-saying and ask about its significance in relation to the episodal context and the argument of the whole story, constantly with an eye on the transmission process. More could be mentioned.

Other scholars are today working in these areas from different perspectives and with a different set of material and questions. Where our interests merge, there may be fruitful discussions in the common search for a fuller understanding of tradition and transmission in early Christianity. The present study hopes to have shown that one way to seek is to follow the traces of Jesus, the only teacher.

Abbreviations

I have used the abbreviations listed in *Journal of Biblical Literature* 107 (1988) 579–596. For the sources not listed there, I have used *Theological Dictionary of the New Testament*. Vol. 1. Grand Rapids 1964, xvi–xl, and J.A. Fitzmyer, *The Dead Sea Scrolls*. Major Publications and Tools for Study. SBLRBS 20. Atlanta ³1990, 3–53, addendum. In addition, the following abbreviations occur:

AAA	Acta Academiae Aboensis
AARSU	Annales Academiae Regiae Scientiarum Upsaliensis
AASF.DHL	Annales Academiae Scientiarum Fennicae. Dissertationes Humanarum Litterarum
AAWG.PH	Abhandlungen der Akademie der Wissenschaften. Philologisch-historische Klasse
ABD	The Anchor Bible Dictionary
ABLSOT	The Albert Bates Lord Studies on Oral Tradition
ACJD	Abhandlungen zum christlich-jüdischen Dialog
ACNT	Augsburg Commentary on the New Testament
AdB	Autour de Bible
AnGreg	Analecta Gregoriana
ANTZ	Arbeiten zur neutestamentlichen Theologie und Zeitgeschichte
AramB	The Aramaic Bible
ASLG	Auctoritate Societatis Litterarum Gottingensis
ATRSup	*Anglican Theological Review. Supplementary Series*
AUU.HR	Acta universitatis Upsaliensis. Historia Religionum
BAB	Beck's Archäologische Bibliothek
BdM	Bibliothèque de *Muséon*
BEATAJ	Beiträge zur Eforschung des Alten Testaments und des antiken Judentums
BEFAR	Bibliothèque des écoles françaises d'Athènes et de Rome
BÉHÉ.SR	Bibliothèque de l'école des hautes études. Sciences religieuses
BeO	Biblica et Orientalia
BH	Bibliothèque Historique
BibK	Bibel-Kommentar
BibKar A	Bibliotheca Karaitica. Series A
BibTod	*Bible Today*
BibTS	Biblisch-Theologische Studien
BISNELC	Bar-Ilan Studies in Near Eastern Languages and Culture
BS	The Biblical Seminar
BSGRT	Bibliotheca Scriptorum Graecorum et Romanorum Teubneriana
BTH	Bibliothèque de théologie historique
BU	Biblische Untersuchungen
CBW	Cities in the Biblical World
CD	*La Ciudad de Dios*
CCWJCW	Cambridge Commentaries on Writings of the Jewish & Christian World 200 BC to AD 200
CLS	Clavis Linguarum Semiticarum
CNI	*Christian News from Israel*
CRHPR	Cahiers de la revue d'histoire et de philosophie religieuses
CSHJ	Chicago Studies in the History of Judaism
CTS.RR	College Theology Society. Resources in Religion
DAWB.SSA	Deutsche Akademie der Wissenschaften zu Berlin. Schriften der Sektion für Altertumswissenschaft
EAEHL	*Encyclopedia of Archaeological Excavations in the Holy Land*
EH	Europäische Hochschulschriften
EUS	European University Studies
F&F	Foundations & Facets
FAT	Forschungen zum Alten Testament

FS	Festschrift
GBS.NT	Guides to Biblical Scholarship. New Testament Series
GFC	Garland Folklore Casebooks
Gos. Naz.	Gospel of the Nazaraeans
HB	Herderbücherei
HSCL	Harvard Studies in Comparative Literature
Inv.	De Inventione
JBQ	*Jewish Bible Quarterly* (=*Dor le Dor*)
JC	Judaica et Christiana
JCP.NS	Jews' College Publications. New Series
JSPSup	Journal for the Study of the Pseudepigrapha. Supplement Series
KatBl	*Katechetische Blätter*
KBANT	Kommentare und Beiträge zum Alten und Neuen Testament
KNT	Kommentar till Nya testamentet
KomNT	Kommentar zum Neuen Testament
LEC	Library of Early Christianity
LTPM	Louvain Theological & Pastoral Monographs
LumVit	*Lumen Vitae*
MBT	Münsterische Beiträge zur Theologie
MD	*Maison Dieu*
MdB	Le monde de la Bible
MThA	Münsterische Theologische Abhandlungen
MTL	Marshall's Theological Library
MTS	Marburger Theologische Studien
NABPR.BS	National Association of Baptist Professors of Religion. Bibliographic Series
NGS	New Gospel Studies
NIDNTT	*The New International Dictionary of New Testament Theology*
NRSV	New Revised Standard Version
NTM	New Testament Message
OCT	Oxford Centre Textbooks
OECT	Oxford Early Christian Texts
OTM	Oxford Theological Monographs
PP	Päpste und Papsttum
PsVTGr	Pseudepigrapha Veteris Testamenti Graece
PTS	Patristische Texte und Studien
QM	Qumranica Mogilanensia
11QT	Temple Scroll from Qumran Cave 11
SAC	Studies in Antiquity and Christianity
SAOC	Studies in Ancient Oriental Civilization
SBEC	Studies in the Bible and Early Christianity
SCL	Studies in Classical Literature
ScrMin	Scripta Minora
SEG	*Supplementum Epigraphicum Graecum*
SFSHJ	South Florida Studies in the History of Judaism
SGFWJ	Schriften (herausgegeben von) der Gesellschaft zur Förderung der Wissenschaft des Judentums
SH	Studia Hellenistica
SHR	Studies in the History of Religions
SKK.NT	Stuttgarter Kleiner Kommentar. Neues Testament
SMU	Studia Missionalia Upsaliensia
SNTU	Studien zum Neuen Testament und seiner Umwelt
SNVAO.HF	Skrifter utgitt av det norske videnskaps-akademi i Oslo. Historisk-filosofisk klasse
SPHomSer	Scholars Press Homage Series
SPS	Sacra Pagina Series
SSAC	Sussidi allo studio delle antichità cristiane
StudDel	Studia Delitzschiana
SubBib	Subsidia Biblica

SVS	Sammlung gemeinverständlicher Vorträge und Schriften aus dem Gebiet der Theologie und Religionsgeschichte
TA	Theologische Arbeiten
TAB	Texte und Arbeiten zur Bibel
TH	Théologie historique
THAT	*Theologisches Handwörterbuch zum Alten Testament*
TheolDiss	Theologische Dissertationen
TI	Theological Inquiries
TNTC	Tyndale New Testament Commentaries
TSAJ	Texte und Studien zum Antiken Judentum
TSJTSA	Texts and Studies of the Jewish Theological Seminary of America
TTK	*Tidskrift for Teologi og Kirke*
TUMSR	Trinity University Monograph Series in Religion
UNDCSJCA	University of Notre Dame Center for the Study of Judaism and Christianity in Antiquity
UrbT	Urban-Taschenbücher
VGSup	Supplements to Vigiliae Christianae
WdF	Wege der Forschung
YJS	Yale Judaic Studies
ZWB	Zürcher Werkkommentare zur Bibel.

Bibliography

1. Primary Sources and Translations

a) *The Bible with Apocrypha and Pseudepigrapha:*

Biblia Hebraica Stuttgartensia. Editio funditus renovata. Eds., K. Elliger – W. Rudolph. Stuttgart 1967/77.
Septuaginta. Ed., A. Rahlfs. Stuttgart 1935.
Septuaginta. Vetus Testamentum Graecum. Auctoritate Academiae Scientiarum Gottingensis or Auctoritate Societatis Litterarum Gottingensis (=ASLG) editum. Göttingen 1931ff (not complete).
The Fourth Book of Ezra. The Latin Version Edited from the MSS. TextsS 3:2. Ed., R.L. Bensly. Cambridge 1895.
Ecclesiastico. Testo ebraico con apparato critico e versioni greca, latina e sirica. Pubblicazioni del seminario di semistica 1. Ed., F. Vattioni. Napoli 1968.
L'ecclésiastique ou la sagesse de Jésus, fils de Sira. Vols. 1–2. BÉHÉ.SR 10:1–2. Ed., I. Lévi. Paris 1898, 1901.
Sapientia Iesu Filii Sirach. ASLG 12:2. Ed., J. Ziegler. Göttingen 1965.
The Hebrew Text of the Book of Ecclesiasticus. SSS 3. Ed., I. Lévi. Leiden 1904.
Die Weisheit des Jesus Sirach. Hebräisch und Deutsch mit einem hebräischen Glossar. Ed., Rudolf Smend. Berlin 1906.
Apocalypsis Henochi Graece. PsVTGr 3 (pp. 1–44). Ed., M. Black. Leiden 1970.
The Ethiopic Book of Enoch. A New Edition in the Light of the Aramaic Dead Sea Fragments. Ed., M.A. Knibb in consultation with E. Ullendorff. Vols. 1–2. Oxford 1978.
Fragmenta Pseudepigraphorum quae supersunt Graeca. Collected by A.-M. Denis. PsVTGr 3 (pp. 45–238). Leiden 1970.
Paraleipomena Jeremiou. SBLTT 1. Eds., R.A. Kraft – A.-E. Purintun. Missoula 1972.
The Testaments of the Twelve Patriarchs. A Critical Edition of the Greek Text. PsVTGr 1:2. Ed., M. de Jonge. Leiden 1978.
The Testament of Abraham. The Greek Text now first edited with an Introduction and Notes. TextsS 2:2 (pp. 1–130). Ed., M.R. James. Cambridge 1892.
The Greek New Testament. Eds., K. Aland – M. Black – C.M. Martini – B.M. Metzger – A. Wikgren. London ³1975.
Novum Testamentum Graece. Eds., K. Aland – M. Black – C.M. Martini – B.M. Metzger – A. Wikgren. Stuttgart 1979.
Acta Apostolorum Apocrypha. Partis alterius. Vols. 1–2. Eds., R.A. Lipsius – M. Bonnet. Leipzig 1898, 1903.
The Odes of Solomon. SBLTT 13. Ed., J.H. Charlesworth. Chico 1977.
The Testament of Solomon. Edited from Manuscripts at Mount Athos, Bologna, Holkham Hall, Jerusalem, London, Milan, Paris and Vienna. UNT 9. Ed., C.C. McCown. Leipzig 1922.

The Holy Bible containing the Old and New Testaments. New Revised Standard Version (=NRSV). Nashville 1990.
The Apocrypha and Pseudepigrapha of the Old Testament in English (=APOT). Vols. 1–2. Ed., R.H. Charles. Oxford 1913.
The Old Testament Pseudepigrapha. Vols. 1–2. Ed., J.H. Charlesworth. London 1983, 1985.
The Apocryphal Old Testament. Ed., H.F.D. Sparks. Oxford 1984.

Box, G.H. – Oesterley, W.O.E., The Book of Sirach, *APOT* 1 (1913) 268–517.

Georgi, D., Weisheit Salomos, *JSHRZ* 3:4 (1980) 391–478.

Sauer, G., Jesus Sirach (Ben Sira), *JSHRZ* 3:5 (1981) 483–644.

Neutestamentliche Apokryphen in deutscher Übersetzung. Vols. 1–2. Eds., E. Hennecke – W. Schneemelcher. Tübingen ⁵1987, ⁵1989.

James, M.R., *The Apocryphal New Testament*. Oxford 1924.

Beskow P. – Hidal, S., *Salomos Oden*. Den äldsta kristna sångboken översatt och kommenterad. Stockholm 1980.

b) *Dead Sea Scrolls:*

The Books of Enoch. Aramaic Fragments of Qumrân Cave 4. Ed., J.T. Milik. Oxford 1976.

Discoveries in the Judean Desert (=*DJD*). Vol. 1: Qumran Cave I. Eds., D. Barthélemy – J.T. Milik. Oxford 1955.

-, Vol. 2: Les Grottes de Murabbaʿât. Eds., P. Benoit – J.T. Milik – R. de Vaux. Oxford 1961.

-, Vol. 3: Les "petites grottes" de Qumrân. Eds., M. Baillet – J.T. Milik – R. de Vaux. Oxford 1962.

-, Vol. 4: The Psalms Scroll of Qumrân Cave 11. Ed., J.A. Sanders. Oxford 1965.

-, Vol. 5: Qumrân Cave 4, I (4Q158–4Q186). Ed., J.M. Allegro. Oxford 1968.

-, Vol. 6: Qumrân grotte 4, II Archéologie, Teffilin, Mezuzot et Targums (4Q128–4Q157). Eds., R. de Vaux – J.T. Milik. Oxford 1977.

-, Vol. 7: Qumrân grotte 4, III (4Q482–4Q520). Ed., M. Baillet. Oxford 1982.

-, Vol. 8: The Greek Minor Prophets Scroll from Naḥal Ḥever (8ḤevXIIgr). Ed., E. Tov. Oxford 1990.

Documents of Jewish Sectaries. Vol. 1. Ed., S. Schechter. Cambridge 1910.

The Essenes according to the Classical Sources. OCT 1. Eds., G. Vermes – M.D. Goodman. Sheffield 1989.

The Genesis Apocryphon of Qumran Cave 1. A Commentary. BeO 18A. Ed., J.A. Fitzmyer. Rome ²1971.

A Manual of Palestinian Aramaic Texts (Second Century B.C.–Second Century A.D.). BeO 34. Eds., J.A. Fitzmyer – D.J. Harrington. Rome 1978.

The Dead Sea Psalms Scroll. Ed., J.A. Sanders. Ithaca 1967.

The Dead Sea Scrolls Uncovered. The First Complete Translation and Interpretation of 50 Key Documents Withheld for Over 35 Years. Eds., R.H. Eisenman – M. Wise. Shaftesbury 1992.

The Temple Scroll. Vols. 1–3 with suppl. Ed., Y. Yadin. Jerusalem 1977–1983.

Die Texte aus Qumran. Hebräisch und Deutsch. Ed., E. Lohse. München ²1971.

Aramaic Texts from Qumran with Translations and Annotations. Vol. 1. SSS 4. Eds., B. Jongeling – C.J. Labuschagne – A.S. van der Woude. Leiden 1976.

Baillet, M., Un recueil liturgique de Qumrân, grotte 4: "Les Paroles des Luminaires," *RB* 68 (1961) 195–250.

Jonge, M. de – Woude, A.S. van der, 11Q Melchizedek and the New Testament, *NTS* 12 (1965–66) 301–326.

Milik, J.T., Review of P. Wernberg-Møller, *The Manual of Discipline*. Leiden 1957, *RB* 67 (1960) 410–416.

Puech, É., 4Q525 et les péricopes des Béatitudes en Ben Sira et Matthieu, *RB* 98 (1991) 80–106.

Woude, A.S. van der, Melchisedek als himmlische Erlösergestalt in den neugefundenen eschatologischen Midraschim aus Qumran Höhle XI, *OTS* 14 (1965) 354–373.

Carmignac, J. – Guilbert, P., *Les Textes de Qumrân*. Traduits et annotés. AdB. Paris 1961.

Carmignac, J. – Cothenet, É. – Lignée, H., *Les Textes de Qumrân*. Traduits et annotés. AdB. Paris 1963.

Charles, R.E., Fragments of a Zadokite Work, *APOT* 2 (1913) 799–834.

Maier, J., *The Temple Scroll*. An Introduction, Translation & Commentary. JSOTSup 34. Sheffield 1985.

Vermes, G., *The Dead Sea Scrolls in English*. Sheffield ³1987.

Wernberg-Møller, P., *The Manual of Discipline*. Translated and Annotated with an Introduction. STDJ 1. Leiden 1957.

c) *Jewish-Hellenistic Literature:*

Aristae ad Philocratem Epistula. BSGRT. Ed., P. Wendland. Leipzig 1900.

Philo. Vols. 1–10. LCL. Transl., F.H. Colson – G.H. Whitaker – R. Marcus. London 1929–1962.

Pseudo-Philon, *Les Antiquités Bibliques*. Vols. 1–2. SC 229, 230. Eds., D.J. Harrington – C. Perrot – P.-M. Bogaert. Paris 1976.

Josephus. Vols. 1–9. LCL. Transl., H.S.J. Thackeray – R. Marcus – A. Wikgren – L.H. Feldman. London 1926–1965.

Philo, *Questiones et Solutiones in Genesin et Exodum*. Vols. 1–2. LCL. Transl., R. Marcus. London 1953.

d) *Rabbinic Literature and Targumim:*

Mishnayoth. Printed Hebrew Text, Introduction, English Translation, Introduction, Notes, Supplement, Appendix, Indexes, Addenda, Corrigenda. Vols. 1–7. Ed., P. Blackman. Gateshead ²1983.

Tosephta. Based on the Erfurt and Vienna Codices. Ed., M.S. Zuckermandel. With Supplement to the Tosephta by S. Liebermann. Jerusalem 1970 (=1937).

Der babylonische Talmud mit Einschluss der Vollständigen Mišnah. Vols. 1–9. Ed., L. Goldschmidt. Berlin 1897–1935.

... תלמוד ירושלמי. Jerusalem 1969 (=Krotoshin 1866).

Aboth de Rabbi Nathan. Ed., S. Schechter. Corrected edition. Hildesheim 1979 (orig. Wien 1887).

Masechet Derech Eretz Zutta. Ed., D. Sperber. Jerusalem ²1982.

Mekilta de-Rabbi Ishmael. Vols. 1–3. Ed., J.Z. Lauterbach. Philadelphia 1933–1935.

... ספרא דבי רב. Ed., I.H. Weiß. New York 1947 (=Wien 1862).

Siphre d' be Rab. Fasciculus primus: Siphre ad Numeros adjecto Siphra zutta. Corpus Tannaiticum III 3:1. Ed., H.S. Horovitz. Jerusalem 1966 (=Leipzig 1917).

Siphre ad Deuteronomium. Corpus Tannaiticum III 3:2. Ed., L. Finkelstein. New York 1969 (=Berlin 1939).

... מדרש תנאים. Ed., D. Hoffmann. Jerusalem 1984 (=Berlin 1908–1909).

... מדרש רבה על חמשה חמשי תורה וחמש מגלות. Jerusalem 1961 (=Wilna 1887).

Pesikta de Rav Kahana. According to an Oxford Manuscript. Ed., B. Mandelbaum. New York ²1987.

... מדרש פסיקתא רבתי. Ed., M. Friedmann. Tel Aviv 1963 (=Wien 1880).

... מדרש תנחומא. Ed., S. Buber. Jerusalem 1964 (=Wilna 1885).

... מדרש תהלים. Ed., S. Buber. Jerusalem 1966 (=Wilna 1891).

Midrash Seder Olam. A Photostatic Reproduction of Ber Ratner's Edition of the Text,

Notes and Introduction. With a prefatory scholarly survey ... by S.K. Mirsky. New York 1966.

The Bible in Aramaic. Vols. 1–4a. Ed., A. Sperber. Leiden 1959–1968.

The Fragment-Targums of the Pentateuch According to their Extant Sources. Vol. 1. AnBib 76. Ed., M.L. Klein. Rome 1980.

Neophyti 1. Targum Palestinese MS de la Biblioteca Vaticana. Vols. 1–5. Textos y estudios 7–11. Ed., A. Díez Macho. Madrid 1968–1978.

Targum Pseudo-Jonathan of the Pentateuch. Text and Concordance. Ed., E.G. Clarke with collaboration by W.E. Aufrecht, J.C. Hurd, and F. Spitzer. Hoboken 1984.

Danby, H., *The Mishnah*. Translated from the Hebrew with Introduction and Brief Explanatory Notes. Oxford 1933.

Neusner, J. *et al., The Tosefta*. Translated from the Hebrew. Vols. 1–6. New York 1977–1986.

The Babylonian Talmud. Vols. 1–17. Ed., I. Epstein. London 1961.

Neusner, J., *The Talmud of the Land of Israel*. A Preliminary Translation and Explanation. Chicago Studies in the History of Judaism. Chicago 1982ff (not complete).

Übersetzung des Talmud Yerushalmi. Eds., M. Hengel – (J. Neusner – H.P. Rüger –) P. Schäfer. Tübingen 1976ff (not complete).

The Minor Tractates of the Talmud. Vols. 1–2. Ed., A. Cohen. London [2]1971.

Neusner, J., *Sifra*. An Analytical Translation. Vols. 1–3. BJS 138–140. Atlanta 1988.

Kuhn, K.G., *Tannaitische Midrashim: Sifre zu Numeri*. Rabbinische Texte 2 Lieferung 1–12. Stuttgart 1933–1959.

Hammer, R., *Sifre*. A Tannaitic Commentary on the Book of Deuteronomy. Translated from the Hebrew with Introduction and Notes. YJS 24. New Haven 1986.

Midrash Rabbah. Translated into English with Notes, Glossary and Indices. Vols. 1–9. Eds., H. Freedman – M. Simon. London [3]1983.

Braude W.G. – Kapstein, I.J., *Pěsiḵta dě-Raḇ Kahǎna*. R. Kahana's Compilation of Discourses for Sabbaths and Festal Days. Philadelphia 1975.

Braude, W.G., *Pesikta Rabbati*. Discourses for Feasts, Fasts, and Special Sabbaths. Vols. 1–2. YJS 18. New Haven 1968.

Bietenhard, H., *Midrasch Tanḥuma B*. R. Tanḥuma über die Tora, genannt Midrasch Jelammedenu. Vols. 1–2. JC 5–6. Bern 1980, 1982.

Braude, W.G., *The Midrash on Psalms*. Vols. 1–2. YJS 13. New Haven 1959.

McNamara, M., *Targum Neofiti 1: Genesis*. Translated, with Apparatus and Notes. AramB 1a. Edinburgh 1992.

Maher, M., *Targum Pseudo-Jonathan: Genesis*. Translated, with Introduction and Notes. AramB 1b. Edinburgh 1992.

Grossfeld, B., *The Targum Onqelos to Genesis*. Translated, with a Critical Introduction, Apparatus, and Notes. AramB 6. Wilmington 1988.

–, *The Targum Onqelos to Leviticus and The Targum Onqelos to Numbers*. Translated, with Apparatus, and Notes. AramB 7. Wilmington 1988.

–, *The Targum Onqelos to Deuteronomy*. Translated, with Apparatus, and Notes. AramB 9. Wilmington 1988.

Klein, M.L., *The Fragment-Targums of the Pentateuch* According to their Extant Sources. Vol. 2. AnBib 76. Rome 1980.

Harrington, D.J. – Saldarini, A.J., *Targum Jonathan of the Former Prophets*. Introduction, Translation and Notes. AramB 10. Wilmington 1987.

Chilton, B.D., *The Isaiah Targum*. Introduction, Translation, Apparatus and Notes. AramB 11. Wilmington 1987.

Cathcart K.J. – Gordon, R.P., *The Targum of the Minor Prophets*. Translated, with a Critical Introduction, Apparatus, and Notes. AramB 14. Wilmington 1989.

e) *Early Christian Literature:*

Die ältesten Apologeten. Texte mit kurzen Einleitungen. Ed., E.J. Goodspeed. Göttingen 1914.
The Apostolic Fathers. Vols. 1–2. LCL. Transl., K. Lake. London 1912, 1913.
Die Apostolischen Väter. Griechisch-deutsche Parallelausgabe auf der Grundlage der Ausgaben von F.X. Funk, K. Bihlmeyer und M. Whittaker. Transl., A. Lindemann – H. Paulsen. Tübingen 1992.
Clemens Alexandrinus, *Protrepticus und Paedagogus*. GCS 12. Ed., O. Stählin. Leipzig ²1936.
–, *Stromata*. Buch I–VI. GCS 52. Eds., O Stählin – L. Früchtel. Berlin ³1960.
–, *Stromata*. Buch VII–VIII. GCS 17. Ed., O. Stählin. Leipzig 1909.
Eusèbe de Césarée, *La Préparation Évangelique*. Livres 8–10. Introduction, traduction et notes. SC 369. Eds., G. Schroeder – É. des Places. Paris 1991.
Eusebius, *The Ecclesiastical History*. Vols. 1–2. LCL. Transl. K. Lake – J.E.L. Oulton. London 1926, 1932.
Hippolytus, *Refutatio Omnium Haeresium*. PTS 25. Ed., M. Marcovich. Berlin 1086.
Melito of Sardis, *On Pascha* and Fragments. OECT. Ed., S.G. Hall. Oxford 1979.
Origen, *Contre Celse*. Livres 7–8. Introduction, texte critique, traduction et notes. SC 150. Ed., M. Borret. Paris 1969.

f) *Greco-Roman Literature:*

Die Fragmente der Vorsokratiker. Griechisch und Deutsch. Vols. 1–2. Eds., H. Diels – W. Krantz. Hildesheim ⁶1992 (=1951, 1952).
Rhetores Graeci. Vol. 2. Ed., E. Spengel. Leipzig 1854.
Aeschylus. Vols. 1–2. LCL. Transl., H. Weir Smyth. London 1922, 1926.
Aristotle, *The "Art" of Rhetoric*. LCL. Transl., J.H. Freese. London 1926.
Cicero, *De Inventione*. LCL 2 (pp. 2–345). Transl., H.M. Hubbell. London 1949.
–, *Orator*. LCL. Transl., H.M. Hubbell. London 1939.
–, *De Oratore*. Books 1–2. LCL. Transl., E.W. Sutton – H. Rackham. London 1942.
Dionysius of Halicarnassus, *The Critical Essays*. Vols. 1–2. LCL. Transl., S. Usher. London 1974, 1985.
Epictetus. Vols. 1–2. LCL. Transl., W.A. Oldfather. London 1925, 1928.
Euripides. Vols. 1–4. LCL. Transl., A.S. Way. London 1912.
Hesiod, *The Homeric Hymns and Homerica*. LCL. Transl., H.G. Evelyn-White. London 1914.
Lucian, *Hermotimus*. LCL 6 (pp. 260–415). Transl., K. Kilburn. London 1959.
Lysias. LCL. Transl., W.R.M. Lamb. London 1930.
Pausanias, *Description of Greece*. Vols. 1–4. LCL. Transl., W.H.S. Jones – H.A. Ormerod. London 1918–1935.
Philodemus of Gadara, *De ira liber*. BSGRT. Ed., C. Wilke. Leipzig 1914.
–, Περὶ παρρησίας. BSGRT. Ed., A. Olivieri. Leipzig 1914.
Philostratus, *The Life of Appolonius of Tyana*. Vols. 1–2. LCL. Transl., F.C. Conybeare. London 1912.
Plato, *The Apology*. LCL 1 (pp. 68–145). Transl., H.N. Fowler. London 1914.
–, *Menexenus*. LCL 9 (pp. 332–381). Transl., R.G. Bury. London 1929.
Plutarch, *Lives*. Vols. 1–11. LCL. Transl., B. Perrin. London 1914–1926.

-, *Moralia*. Vols. 1–16. LCL. Transl., F.C. Babbitt *et al.* London 1926–1969.
Quintillian, *Institutio Oratoria*. Vols. 1–4. LCL. Transl., H.E. Butler. London 1920–1922.
Thucydides, *History of the Pelloponesian War*. Vols. 1–4. LCL. Transl., C.F. Smith. London 1919–1923.

g) *Inscriptions and Papyri:*

Corpus Inscriptionum Iudaicarum (=*CII*). Recueil des inscriptions juives qui vont du IIIe siècle avant Jésus-Christ au VIIe siècle de notre ère. Vol. 2. SSAC 3. Ed., J.-P. Frey. Roma 1952.
The Oxyrhynchus Papyri. Vol. 6 (no. 930 pp. 295–296). Eds., B.P. Grenfell – A.S. Hunt. London 1908.
-, Vol. 18 (no. 2190 pp. 145–149). Eds., E. Lobel – C.H. Roberts – E.P. Wegener. London 1941.
Supplementum Epigraphicum Graecum (=*SEG*). Vol. 23. Ed., A.G. Woodhead. Lugundi Batavorum 1968.
Avigad, N., Baruch the Scribe and Jerahmeel the King's Son, *IEJ* 28 (1978) 52–56.
Naveh, J., A Hebrew Letter from the Seventh Century B.C., *IEJ* 10 (1960) 129–139.

h) *Text Collections:*

The Chreia in Ancient Rhetoric. Vol 1: The *Progymnasmata*. SBLTT 27, Graeco-Roman Religion Series 9. Eds., R.F. Hock – E.N. O'Neil. Atlanta 1986.
Narrative Parallels to the New Testament. SBLRBS 22. Ed., F. Martin. Atlanta 1988.
Ancient Quotes & Anecdotes. From Crib to Crypt. F&F: Reference Series. Ed., V.K. Robbins. Sonoma 1989.
Stroker, W.D., *Extracanonical Sayings of Jesus*. SBLRBS 18. Atlanta 1989.

2. Reference Works

Aland, K. (ed.), *Synopsis Quattuor Evangeliorum*. Locis parallelis evangeliorum apocryphorum et patrum adhibitis. Stuttgart [13]1985.
Aland, K. (ed.), *Vollständige Konkordanz zum griechischen Neuen Testament*. Unter Zugrundelegung aller kritischen Textausgaben und des Textus Receptus. Vols. 1–2. Berlin 1978–1983.
Allenbach, J. – Benoît, A. *et al.* (eds.), *Biblia Patristica*. Index des citations et allusions bibliques dans la littérature patristique. Vols. 1–4, suppl. Paris 1975–1987.
Barthélemy, D. – Rickenbacher, O. (eds.), *Konkordanz zum hebräischen Sirach,* mit syrisch-hebräischem Index. Göttingen 1973.
Bauer, W., *Griechisch-deutsches Wörterbuch* zu den Schriften des Neuen Testaments und der frühchristlichen Literatur. Eds., K. Aland – B. Aland. Berlin [6]1988.
Blass, F. – Debrunner, A., *A Greek Grammar of the New Testament* and Other Early Christian Literature. Transl. and rev., R.W. Funk. Chicago 1961.
Blass, F. – Debrunner, A., *Grammatik des neutestamentlichen Griechisch*. Rev., F. Rehkopf. Göttingen [14]1975.
Blomqvist, J. – Jastrup, P.O., *Grekisk grammatik*. Copenhagen 1991.
Boismard, M.-E. – Lamouille, A., *Synopsis Graeca Quattuor Evangeliorum*. Leuven 1986.
Charlesworth, J.H. *et al., Graphic Concordance to the Dead Sea Scrolls*. Tübingen 1991.
Crossan, J.D., *Sayings Parallels*. A Workbook for the Jesus Tradition. F&F: NT. Phila-

delphia 1986.

Dalman, G.H., *Aramäisch-neuhebräisches Handwörterbuch zu Targum, Talmud und Midrasch*. Mit Lexikon der Abbreviaturen von G.H. Händler und einem Verzeichnis der Mischna-Abschnitte. Hildesheim ³1967.

Edwards, R.A., *A Concordance to Q*. SBLSBS 7. Chico 1975.

Eisenman, R.H. – Robinson, J.M., *A Facsimile Edition of the Dead Sea Scrolls*. Prepared with an Introduction and Index. Vols. 1–2. Washington 1991.

Fitzmyer, J.A., *An Introductory Bibliography for the Study of Scripture*. SubBib 3. Rome ³1990.

-, *The Dead Sea Scrolls*. Major Publications and Tools for Study. SBLRBS 20. Atlanta ³1990.

Forestell, J.T., *Targumic Traditions and the New Testament*. An Annotated Bibliography with a New Testament Index. SBLAS 4. Chico 1979.

Garland, D.E., *One Hundred Years of Study on the Passion Narratives*. NABPR.BS 3. Macon 1989.

Gesenius, W., *Hebräisches und aramäisches Handwörterbuch über das Alte Testament*. Vol. 1. Eds., U. Rüterswörden – R. Meyer – H. Donner. Berlin ¹⁸1987.

Gesenius, W. – Kautzsch, E., *Gesenius' Hebrew Grammar*. Oxford ²1910.

Hatch, E. – Redpath, H.A., *A Concordance to the Septuagint* and the other Greek Versions of the Old Testament (including the Apocryphal Books). Oxford 1897.

Hawkins, J.C., *Horae Synopticae*. Contributions to the Study of the Synoptic Problem. Oxford ²1909.

Hoffmann, E.G. – Siebenthal, H. von, *Griechische Grammatik zum Neuen Testament*. Riehen 1985.

Jastrow, M., *A Dictionary of the Targumim, the Talmud Babli and Yerushalmi, and the Midrashic Literature*. Vols. 1–2. London 1886, 1903.

Kiessling, E. (ed.), *Wörterbuch der griechischen Papyrusurkunden* mit Einschluß der griechischen Inschriften, Aufschriften, Ostraka, Mumienschilder usw. aus Ägypten. Vol. 4, suppl. 1. Marburg 1944–1971 (vol. 4), Amsterdam 1969–1971 (suppl. 1).

Köhler (Koehler), L. – Baumgartner, W., *Lexicon in Veteris Testamenti libros*. Leiden ²1958.

-, *Hebräisches und aramäisches Lexikon zum Alten Testament*. Vols. 1–4. Leiden ³1967ff (not complete).

Kuhn, K.G. (ed.), *Konkordanz zu den Qumrantexten*. Göttingen 1960.

-, *et al.*, Nachträge zur "Konkordanz zu den Qumrantexten," *RevQ* 4 (1963) 163–234.

Levias, C., *A Grammar of the Aramaic Idiom Contained in the Babylonian Talmud*. Cincinnati 1900.

Liddell, H.G. – Scott, R., *A Greek-English Lexicon*. A New Edition Revised and Augmented throughout by H.S. Jones *et al.*, suppl. ed., E.A. Barber. Oxford ⁹1940, 1968 (suppl.).

Lisowsky, G., *Konkordanz zum hebräischen Alten Testament*. Stuttgart ²1958.

Longstaff, T.R.W. – Thomas, P.A. (eds.), *The Synoptic Problem*. A Bibliography, 1716–1988. NGS 4. Macon 1988.

Mandelkern, S., *Veteris Testamenti Concordantiae hebraicae atque chaldaicae*. Jerusalem ⁹1971.

Margolis, M.L., *A Manual of the Aramaic Language of the Babylonian Talmud*. CLS 3. München 1910.

Mayer, G., *Index Philoneus*. Berlin 1974.

Metzger, B.M., *A Textual Commentary on the Greek New Testament*. London 1971.

Morgenthaler, R., *Statistik des neutestamentlichen Wortschatzes*. Zürich ³1982.

-, *Statistik des neutestamentlichen Wortschatzes*. Beiheft zur 3. Auflage. Zürich 1982.

Moulton, J.H., *A Grammar of New Testament Greek*. Vol. 1. Edinburgh [3]1908.

Orchard, J.B. (ed.), *A Synopsis of the Four Gospels* in Greek. Arranged According to the Two-Gospel Hypothesis. Edinburgh 1983.

Preisgke, F., *Wörterbuch der griechischen Papyrusurkunden* mit Einschluß der griechischen Inschriften Aufschriften Ostraka Mumienschilder usw. aus Ägypten. Vols. 1–3. Ed., E. Kießling. Berlin 1925–1931.

Rengstorf, K.H. (ed.), *A Complete Concordance to Flavius Josephus*. Vols. 1–4, suppl. 1 by A. Schalit. Leiden 1968 (suppl.), 1973–1983.

Smend, Rudolf, *Griechisch-Syrisch-Hebräischer Index zur Weisheit des Jesus Sirach*. Berlin 1907.

Wagner, G. (ed.), *An Exegetical Bibliography of the New Testament*. Matthew and Mark. Macon 1983.

Wal, A. van der, *Amos*. A Classified Bibliography. Amsterdam [3]1986.

Waltke, B.K. – O'Connor, M., *An Introduction to Biblical Hebrew Syntax*. Winona Lake 1990.

Zerwick, M., *Biblical Greek*. SPBI 114. Rome 1963.

3. Secondary Literature

Aalen, S., *Die Begriffe 'Licht' und 'Finsternis'* im Alten Testament, im Spätjudentum und im Rabbinismus. SNVAO II HF 1951:1. Oslo 1951.

-, Visdomsforestillingen og Jesu kristologiske selvbevisshet, *SEÅ* 37–38 (1972–73) 35–46.

-, *Kristologien i de synoptiske evangelier*. Oslo [3]1979.

Abel, E.L., The Psychology of Memory and Rumor Transmission and Their Bearing on Theories of Oral Transmission in Early Christianity, *JR* 51 (1971) 270–281.

Aberbach, M., Educational Institutions and Problems During the Talmudic Age, *HUCA* 37 (1966) 107–120.

-, The Relations Between Master and Disciple in the Talmudic Age, in: H.J. Zimmels *et al.* (eds.), *Essays presented to Chief Rabbi I. Brodie on the Occasion of His Seventieth Birthday*. JCP.NS 3. London 1967, 1–24.

-, The Change from a Standing to a Sitting Posture by Students after the Death of Rabban Gamaliel, in: H.Z. Dimitrovsky (ed.), *Exploring the Talmud*. Vol 1. New York 1976, 277–283.

Abrahams, I., *Studies in Pharisaism and the Gospels*. Vols. 1–2. Cambridge 1917, 1924.

Abramowski, L., Die "Erinnerungen der Apostel" bei Justinus, in: P. Stuhlmacher (ed.), *Das Evangelium und die Evangelien*. Vorträge vom Tübinger Symposium 1982. WUNT 28. Tübingen 1983, 341–353.

Abramowski, R., Der Christus der Salomooden, *ZNW* 35 (1936) 44–69.

Abrams, M.H., *A Glossary of Literary Terms*. Fort Worth [5]1988.

Achtemeier, P.J., *Omne Verbum Sonat:* The New Testament and the Oral Environment of Late Western Antiquity, *JBL* 109 (1990) 3–27.

Ackroyd, P.R., The Vitality of the Word of God in the Old Testament. A Contribution to the Study of the Transmission and Exposition of Old Testament Material, *ASTI* 1 (1962) 7–23.

-, Apocalyptic in its Social Setting. Review of P.D. Hanson, *The Dawn of Apocalyptic*. Philadelphia 1975, *Int* 30 (1976) 412–415.

-, A Judgment Narrative between Kings and Chronicles? An Approach to Amos 7:9–17, in: G.W. Coats *et al.* (eds.), *Canon and Authority*. Essays in Old Testament Religion and Theology. Philadelphia 1977, 71–87.

–, Isaiah I–XII: Presentation of a Prophet, in: J.A. Emerton (ed.), *Congress Volume Göttingen 1977.* VTSup 29. Leiden 1978, 16–48.

–, Isaiah 36–39: Structure and Function, in: W.C. Delsman *et al.* (eds.), *Von Kanaan bis Kerala.* FS J.P.M. van der Ploeg. Neukirchen-Vluyn 1982, 3–21.

Ahlström, G.W., Oral and Written Transmission. Some Considerations, *HTR* 59 (1966) 69–81.

–, The House of Wisdom, *SEÅ* 44 (1979) 74–76.

Albeck, C., *Einführung in die Mischna.* SJ 6. Berlin 1971.

Albertz, R., Das Deuterojesaja-Buch als Fortschreibung der Jesaja-Prophetie, in: E. Blum *et al.* (eds.), *Die Hebräische Bibel und ihre zweifache Nachgeschichte.* FS R. Rendtorff. Neukirchen-Vluyn 1990, 241–256.

Albright, W.F. – Mann, C.S., *Matthew.* Introduction, Translation, and Notes. AB 26. Garden City 1971.

Alexander, L., The Living Voice: Scepticism towards the Written Word in Early Christian and in Graeco-Roman Texts, in: D.J.A. Clines *et al.* (eds.), *The Bible in three dimensions.* Essays in celebration of forty years of Biblical Studies in the University of Sheffield. JSOTSup 87. Sheffield 1990, 221–247.

Alexander, P.S., Rabbinic Biography and the Biography of Jesus: A Survey of the Evidence, in: C.M. Tuckett (ed.), *Synoptic Studies.* The Ampleforth Conferences of 1982 and 1983. JSNTSup 7. Sheffield 1984, 19–50.

–, Quid Athenis et Hierosolymis? Rabbinic Midrash and Hermeneutics in the Graeco-Roman World, in: P.R. Davies *et al.* (eds.), *A Tribute to Geza Vermes.* Essays on Jewish and Christian Literature and History. JSOTSup 100. Sheffield 1990, 101–124.

–, Orality in Pharisaic-rabbinic Judaism at the Turn of the Eras?, in: H. Wansbrough (ed.), *Jesus and the Oral Gospel Tradition.* JSNTSup 64. Sheffield 1991, 159–184.

Allen, W.C., *A Critical and Exegetical Commentary on the Gospel according to S. Matthew.* ICC. Edinburgh 1907.

Allison, D.C., Jr, The Authorship of 1 QS III,13–IV,14, *RevQ* 10 (1980) 257–268.

–, "Elijah Must Come First," *JBL* 103 (1984) 256–258.

–, Jesus and Moses (Mt 5:1–2), *ExpTim* 98 (1987) 203–205.

–, Two Notes on a Key Text: Matthew 11:25–30, *JTS* 39 (1988) 477–485.

–, Matthew: Structure, Biographical Impulse, and the *Imitatio Christi,* in: F. Van Segbroeck *et al.* (eds.), *The Four Gospels 1992.* FS F. Neirynck. BETL 100. Leuven 1992, 1203–1221.

Alon, G., *Jews, Judaism and the Classical World.* Studies in Jewish History in the Times of the Second Temple and Talmud. Jerusalem 1977.

Andersen, F.I. – Freedman, D.N., *Hosea.* A New Translation with Introduction and Commentary. AB 24. Garden City 1980.

Andersen, Ø., Oral Tradition, in: H. Wansbrough (ed.), *Jesus and the Oral Gospel Tradition.* JSNTSup 64. Sheffield 1991, 17–58.

Applebaum, S., Review of K. Bringmann, *Hellenistische Reform und Religionsverfolgung in Judäa.* Göttingen 1983, *Gnomon* 57 (1985) 191–193.

Arens, E., *The ἦλθον-Sayings in the Synoptic Tradition.* A Historico-Critical Investigation. OBO 10. Fribourg 1976.

Arvedson, T., *Das Mysterium Christi.* Eine Studie zu Mt 11.25–30. Uppsala 1937.

Attridge, H.W., Historiography, in: M.E. Stone (ed.), *Jewish Writings of the Second Temple Period.* Apocrypha, Pseudepigrapha, Qumran Sectarian Writings, Philo, Josephus. CRINT II 2. Assen 1984, 157–184.

Auld, A.G., *Amos.* OTG. Sheffield 1986.

Aune, D.E., The Odes of Solomon and Early Christian Prophecy, *NTS* 28 (1982) 435–460.

-, *Prophecy in Early Christianity and the Ancient Mediterranean World*. Grand Rapids 1983.

-, *The New Testament in Its Literary Environment*. LEC 8. Philadelphia 1987.

-, Prolegomena to the Study of Oral Tradition in the Hellenistic World, in: H. Wansbrough (ed.), *Jesus and the Oral Gospel Tradition*. JSNTSup 64. Sheffield 1991, 59–106.

Avigad, N., The Seal of Seraiah (Son of) Neriah (Hebrew with English summary), *ErIsr* 14 (1978) 86–87.

-, *Hebrew Bullae from the Time of Jeremiah*. Remnants of a Burnt Archive. Jerusalem 1986.

-, The Contribution of Hebrew Seals to an Understanding of Israelite Religion and Society, in: P.D. Miller, Jr *et al.* (eds.), *Ancient Israelite Religion*. FS F.M. Cross. Philadelphia 1987, 195–209.

-, Hebrew Seals and Sealings and Their Significance for Biblical Research, in: J.A. Emerton (ed.), *Congress Volume Jerusalem 1986*. VTSup 40. Leiden 1988, 7–16.

Baasland, E., Jesu minste bud? Eksegetiske bemerkninger til Matteus 5,19(f), *TTK* 1 (1983) 1–12.

Bacher, W., *Die Agada der Tannaiten*. Vols. 1–2. Straßburg ²1903, 1890.

-, *Die exegetische Terminologie der jüdischen Traditionsliteratur*. Vols. 1–2. Leipzig 1899, 1905.

-, D'une nouvelle explication de l'expression וְאִיתְּמָא, *REJ* 54 (1907) 273–275.

-, *Tradition und Tradenten in den Schulen Palästinas und Babyloniens*. Studien und Materialien zur Entstehungsgeschichte des Talmuds. SGFWJ. Leipzig 1914.

Bachmann, M., *Jerusalem und der Tempel*. Die geographisch-theologischen Elemente in der lukanischen Sicht des jüdischen Kultzentrums. BWANT 109. Stuttgart 1980.

Bacon, B.W., The "Five Books" of Matthew against the Jews, *The Expositor* 15 (1918) 56–66.

-, Jesus and the Law. A Study of the First 'Book' of Matthew (Mt. 3–7), *JBL* 47 (1928) 203–231.

-, *Studies in Matthew*. London 1930.

Balch, D.L., The Canon. Adaptable and Stable, Oral and Written. Critical Questions for Kelber and Riesner, *Forum* 7:3–4 (1993) 183–205.

Balogh, J., "Voces Paginarum". Beiträge zur Geschichte des lauten Lesens und Schreibens, *Philologus* 82 (1927) 84–109, 202–240.

Baltzer, D., *Ezechiel und Deuterojesaja*. Berührungen in der Heilserwartung der beiden großen Exilspropheten. BZAW 121. Berlin 1971.

Baltzer, K., *Die Biographie der Propheten*. Neukirchen-Vluyn 1975.

Bamberger, B.J., Revelations of Torah After Sinai. An Aggadic Study, *HUCA* 16 (1941) 97–113.

Bammel, E., Matthäus 10,23, *ST* 15 (1961) 79–92.

-, *Jesu Nachfolger*. Nachfolgeüberlieferungen in der Zeit des frühen Christentums. StudDel 3:1. Heidelberg 1988.

Banks, R., Matthew's Understanding of the Law: Authenticity and Interpretation in Matthew 5:17–20, *JBL* 93 (1974) 226–242.

-, *Jesus and the Law in the Synoptic Tradition*. SNTSMS 28. Cambridge 1975.

Barbour, R.S., Uncomfortable Words. VIII Status and Titles, *ExpTim* 82 (1970–71) 137–142.

Bardtke, H., Qumrān und seine Probleme. Teil II. Die Kupferrollen, *TRu* 33 (1968) 185–236.

Bar-Ilan, M., Writing in Ancient Israel and Early Judaism. Part Two: Scribes and Books in the Late Second Commonwealth and Rabbinic Period, in: M.J. Mulder (ed.), *Miqra*.

Reading, Translation and Interpretation of the Hebrew Bible in Ancient Judaism and Early Christianity. CRINT II 1. Assen 1988, 21–38.

Barrett, C.K., School, Conventicle, and Church in the New Testament, in: K. Aland *et al.* (eds.), *Wissenschaft und Kirche*. FS E. Lohse. TAB 4. Bielefeld 1989, 96–110.

Barth, G., Auseinandersetzungen um die Kirchenzucht im Umkreis des Matthäusevangeliums, *ZNW* 69 (1978) 158–177.

-, Bergpredigt. I: Im Neuen Testament, *TRE* 5 (1980) 603–618.

-, Matthew's Understanding of the Law, in: G. Bornkamm *et al.*, *Tradition and Interpretation in Matthew*. London ²1982, 58–164.

Barth, H., *Die Jesaja-Worte in der Josiazeit*. Israel und Assur als Thema einer produktiven Neuinterpretation der Jesajaüberlieferung. WMANT 48. Neukirchen-Vluyn 1977.

Bartholomew, G.L., Feed My Lambs: John 21:15–19 as Oral Gospel, *Semeia* 39 (1987) 69–96.

Bartnicki, R., Das Trostwort an die Jünger in Mt 10,23, *TZ* 43 (1987) 311–319.

Basser, H.W., The Rabbinic Citations in Wacholder's the Dawn of Qumran, *RevQ* 11 (1984) 549–560.

-, Derrett's "Binding" Reopened, *JBL* 104 (1985) 297–300.

-, Marcus's "Gates": A Response, *CBQ* 52 (1990) 307–308.

Bauer, D.R., *The Structure of Matthew's Gospel*. A Study in Literary Design. JSNTSup 31. Sheffield 1988.

Bauer, W. – Paulsen, H., *Die Briefe des Ignatius von Antiochia und der Polykarpbrief*. HNT 18:2. Tübingen ²1985.

Baumann, A., Urrolle und Fasttag. Zur Rekonstruktion der Urrolle des Jeremiabuches nach den Angaben in Jer 36, *ZAW* 80 (1968) 350–373.

Baumbach, G., Die Mission im Matthäus-Evangelium, *TLZ* 92 (1967) 889–893.

Baumgarten, A.I., The Pharisaic *Paradosis*, *HTR* 80 (1987) 63–77.

Baumgarten, J.M., 1QSa 1.11—Age of Testimony or Responsibility?, *JQR* 49 (1958–59) 157–160.

-, The Unwritten Law in the Pre-Rabbinic Period, *JSJ* 3 (1972) 7–29.

-, The Heavenly Tribunal and the Personification of Ṣedeq in Jewish Apocalyptic, *ANRW* II 19:1 (1979) 219–239.

-, Recent Qumran Discoveries and Halakhah in the Hellenistic-Roman Period, in: S. Talmon (ed.), *Jewish Civilization in the Hellenistic-Roman Period*. JSPSup 10. Sheffield 1991, 147–158.

Baumgartner, W., Die literarischen Gattungen in der Weisheit des Jesus Sirach, *ZAW* 34 (1914) 161–198.

Bayer, H.F., *Jesus' Predictions of Vindication and Resurrection*. The provenance, meaning and correlation of the Synoptic predictions. WUNT 2:20. Tübingen 1986.

Beall, T.S., *Josephus' Description of the Essenes Illustrated by the Dead Sea Scrolls*. SNTSMS 58. Cambridge 1988.

Beare, F.W., The Mission of the Disciples and the Mission Charge: Matthew 10 and Parallels, *JBL* 89 (1970) 1–13.

-, *The Gospel according to Matthew*. A Commentary. Oxford 1981.

-, Jesus as Teacher and Thaumaturge: the Matthean Portrait, *SE* 7 (TU 126) (1982) 31–39.

Beasley-Murray, G.R., *John*. WBC 36. Waco 1987.

Becker, H.-J., *Auf der Kathedra des Mose*. Rabbinisch-theologisches Denken und anti-rabbinische Polemik in Matthäus 23,1–12. ANTZ 4. Berlin 1990.

Becker, Joachim, Erwägungen zur ezechielischen Frage, in: L. Ruppert *et al.* (eds.), *Künder des Wortes*. Beiträge zur Theologie der Propheten. FS J. Schreiner. Würzburg 1982, 137–149.

-, Ez 8–11 als einheitliche Komposition in einem pseudepigraphischen Ezechielbuch, in: J. Lust (ed.), *Ezekiel and His Book*. Textual and Literary Criticism and their Interrelation. BETL 74. Leuven 1986, 136–150.

Becker, Jürgen, *Das Heil Gottes*. Heils- und Sündenbegriffe in den Qumrantexten und im Neuen Testament. SUNT 3. Göttingen 1964.

Begg, C.T., A Bible Mystery: The Absence of Jeremiah in the Deuteronomistic History, *IBS* 7 (1985) 139–164.

-, The Non-Mention of Ezekiel in Deuteronomistic History, the Book of Jeremiah and the Chronistic History, in: J. Lust (ed.), *Ezekiel and His Book*. Textual and Literary Criticism and their Interrelation. BETL 74. Leuven 1986, 340–343.

-, Ben Sirach's Non-mention of Ezra, *BN* 42 (1988) 14–18.

-, Review of H.-J. Stipp, *Elischa – Propheten – Gottesmänner*. St. Ottilien 1987, *CBQ* 51 (1989) 352–353.

Behm, J., καρδία, *TDNT* 3 (1965) 608–613.

Bellinzoni, A.J., *The Sayings of Jesus in the Writings of Justin Martyr*. NovTSup 17. Leiden 1967.

Berger, K., *Die Amen-Worte Jesu*. Eine Untersuchung zum Problem der Legitimation in apokalyptischer Rede. BZNW 39. Berlin 1970.

-, Zu den sogenannten Sätzen heiligen Rechts, *NTS* 17 (1970–71) 10–40.

-, *Die Gesetzesauslegung Jesu*. Ihr historischer Hintergrund im Judentum und im Alten Testament. WMANT 40. Neukirchen-Vluyn 1972.

-, Zur Geschichte der Einleitungsformel "Amen, ich sage euch," *ZNW* 63 (1972) 45–75.

-, Die sog. "Sätze heiligen Rechts" im N.T., *TZ* 28 (1972) 305–330.

-, Die königlichen Messiastraditionen des Neuen Testaments, *NTS* 20 (1973–74) 1–44.

-, *Formgeschichte des Neuen Testaments*. Heidelberg 1984.

Bergquist, J.L., Prophetic Legitimation in Jeremiah, *VT* 39 (1989) 129–139.

Berlin, A., On the Meaning of *rb*, *JBL* 100 (1981) 90–93.

Berner, U., *Die Bergpredigt*. Rezeption und Auslegung im 20. Jahrhundert. GTA 12. Göttingen 1979.

Berridge, J.M., Jeremia und die Prophetie des Amos, *TZ* 35 (1979) 321–341.

Bertram, G., μωρός κτλ., *TDNT* 4 (1967) 832–847.

Betz, H.D., *Nachfolge und Nachahmung Jesu Christi im Neuen Testament*. BHT 37. Tübingen 1967.

-, *Essays on the Sermon on the Mount*. Philadelphia 1985.

-, The Problem of Christology in the Sermon on the Mount, in: T.W. Jennings, Jr (ed.), *Text and Logos*. The Humanistic Interpretation of the New Testament. SPHomSer. Atlanta 1990, 191–209.

Betz, O., *Offenbarung und Schriftforschung in der Qumransekte*. WUNT 6. Tübingen 1960.

-, Rechtfertigung in Qumran, in: J. Friedrich *et al.* (eds.), *Rechtfertigung*. FS E. Käsemann. Tübingen 1976, 17–36.

-, Jesus and the Temple Scroll, in: J.H. Charlesworth (ed.), *Jesus and the Dead Sea Scrolls*. AB Reference Library. New York 1993, 75–103.

Betz, O. – Riesner, R., *Jesus, Qumran und der Vatikan*. Klarstellungen. Gießen ²1993.

Beuken, W.A.M., *Haggai – Sacharja 1–8*. Studien zur Überlieferungsgeschichte der frühnachexilischen Prophetie. SSN 10. Assen 1967.

Beyer, K., *Semitische Syntax im Neuen Testament*. Vol. 1. SUNT 1. Göttingen 1962.

Beyerlin, W., *Reflexe der Amosvisionen im Jeremiabuch*. OBO 93. Fribourg 1989.

Bi(c)kerman(n), É.(J.), *Der Gott der Makkabäer*. Untersuchungen über Sinn und Ursprung der makkabäischen Erhebung. Berlin 1937.

-, La chaîne de la tradition pharisienne, *RB* 59 (1952) 44–54.

-, *The Jews in the Greek Age.* Cambridge MA 1988.

Bietenhard, H., ἀμήν, *NIDNTT* 1 (²1980) 97–99.

Bilde, P., *Flavius Josephus between Jerusalem and Rome.* His Life, his Works, and their Importance. JSPSup 2. Sheffield 1988.

Birkeland, H., *Zum hebräischen Traditionswesen.* Die Komposition der prophetischen Bücher des Alten Testaments. ANVAO. HF 1938:1. Oslo 1938.

Bjørndalen, A.J., Erwägungen zur Zukunft der Amazja und Israels nach der Überlieferung Amos 7,10–17, in: R. Albertz *et al.* (eds.), *Werden und Wirken des Alten Testaments.* FS C. Westermann. Göttingen 1980, 236–251.

Black, D.A., Hebrews 1:1–4: A Study in Discourse Analysis, *WTJ* 49 (1987) 175–194.

Black, M., Theological Conceptions in the Dead Sea Scrolls, *SEÅ* 18–19 (1953–54) 72–97.

-, *An Aramaic Approach to the Gospels and Acts.* Oxford ³1967.

Blair, E.P., *Jesus in the Gospel of Matthew.* Nashville 1960.

Blank, J., Neutestamentliche Petrus-Typologie und Petrusamt, *Concilium* 9 (1973) 173–179.

-, Lernprozesse im Jüngerkreis Jesu, *TQ* 158 (1978) 163–177.

Blenkinsopp, J., *A History of Prophecy in Israel.* Philadelphia 1983.

Blinzler, J., Justinus Apol. I, 15,4 und Matthäus 19,11–12, in: A. Descamps *et al.* (eds.), *Mélanges Bibliques.* FS B. Rigaux. Gembloux 1970, 45–55.

Blomberg, C.L., New Testament genre criticism for the 1990s, *Themelios* 15 (1990) 40–49.

Blomqvist, J., Apokryfer och pseudepigrafer, in: *"God och nyttig läsning."* Om Gamla Testamentets Apokryfer. Stockholm 1988, 175–214.

Bocheński, J.M., *Was ist Autorität?* Einführung in die Logik der Autorität. HB 439. Freiburg 1974.

Bockmuehl, M.N.A., *Revelation and Mystery* in Ancient Judaism and Pauline Christianity. WUNT 2:36. Tübingen 1990.

-, A Slain Messiah in 4Q Serekh Milchamah (4Q285)?, *TynBul* 43:1 (1992) 155–169.

Boehmer, J., "Jahwes Lehrlinge" im Buch Jesaja, *ARW* 33 (1936) 171–175.

Bohren, R., *Das Problem der Kirchenzucht im Neuen Testament.* Zürich 1952.

Boman, T., *Die Jesus-Überlieferung im Lichte der neueren Volkskunde.* Göttingen 1967.

Bonnard, P., Matthieu, éducateur du peuple chrétien, in: A. Descamps *et al.* (eds.), *Mélanges Bibliques.* FS B. Rigaux. Gembloux 1970, 1–7.

Bonnard, P.-E., *Le Second Isaïe, son disciple et leurs éditeurs.* Isaïe 40–66. Ébib. Paris 1972.

Bonsirven, J., *Le Judaïsme Palestinien* au temps de Jésus-Christ. Sa théologie. BTH. Vols. 1–2. Paris 1934, 1935.

Boogaart, T.A., *Reflections on Restoration.* A Study of Prophecies in Micah and Isaiah about the Restoration of Northern Israel. Groningen 1981.

Boomershine, T.E., Peter's Denial as Polemic or Confession: The Implications of Media Criticism for Biblical Hermeneutics, *Semeia* 39 (1987) 47–68.

Borgen, P., "At the Age of Twenty" in 1QSa, *RevQ* 3 (1961) 267–277.

Boring, M.E., How May We Identify Oracles of Christian Prophets in the Synoptic Tradition? Mark 3:28–29 as a Test Case, *JBL* 91 (1972) 501–521.

-, *Sayings of the Risen Jesus.* Christian Prophecy in the Synoptic Tradition. Cambridge 1982.

-, *The Continuing Voice of Jesus.* Christian Prophecy and the Gospel Tradition. Louisville 1991.

-, The Voice of Jesus in the Apocalypse of John, *NovT* 34 (1992) 334–359.

Bornkamm, G., *Geschichte und Glaube.* Gesammelte Aufsätze. Vol. 3. BEvT 48. München 1968.

-, End-Expectation and Church in Matthew, in: G. Bornkamm *et al., Tradition and Interpretation in Matthew*. London ²1982, 15–57.

-, The Stilling of the Storm in Matthew, in: G. Bornkamm *et al., ibid.*, 52–57.

-, The Authority to "Bind" and "Loose" in the Church in Matthew's Gospel: The Problem of Sources in Matthew's Gospel, in: G. Stanton (ed.), *The Interpretation of Matthew*. IRT 3. Philadelphia 1983, 85–97.

Boström, L., *The God of the Sages*. The Portrayal of God in the Book of Proverbs. ConBOT 29. Stockholm 1990.

Botterweck, G.J., Zur Authentizität des Buches Amos, *BZ* 2 (1958) 176–189.

Boyce, M., The Poetry of the *Damascus Document* and its Bearing on the Origin of the Qumran Sect, *RevQ* 14 (1990) 615–628.

Brändle, F., Jesucristo, único maestro y sabiduría de Dios en Mateo, *RevistEspir* 43 (1984) 187–209.

Braun, H., *Qumran und das Neue Testament*. Vols. 1–2. Tübingen 1966.

Braun, W., Were the New Testament Herodians Essenes? A Critique of an Hypothesis, *RevQ* 14 (1989) 75–88.

Bregman, M., Another Reference to "A Teacher of Righteousness" in Midrashic Literature, *RevQ* 10 (1979) 97–100.

Bright, J., *Jeremiah*. A New Translation with Introduction and Commentary. AB 21. Garden City 1965.

-, *A History of Israel*. Philadelphia ³1981.

-, The Date of the Prose Sermons of Jeremiah, in: L.G. Perdue *et al.* (eds.), *A Prophet to the Nations*. Essays in Jeremiah Studies. Winona Lake 1984, 193–212.

Bringmann, K., *Hellenistische Reform und Religionsverfolgung in Judäa*. Eine Untersuchung zur jüdisch-hellenistischen Geschichte (175–163 v. Chr.). AAWG.PH 3:132. Göttingen 1983.

Broer, I., Die Antithesen und der Evangelist Mattäus. Versuch, eine alte These zu revidieren, *BZ* 19 (1975) 50–63.

-, *Freiheit vom Gesetz und Radikalisierung des Gesetzes*. Ein Beitrag zur Theologie des Evangelisten Matthäus. SBS 98. Stuttgart 1980.

-, *Die Seligpreisungen der Bergpredigt*. Studien zu ihrer Überlieferung und Interpretation. BBB 61. Bonn 1986.

Brooke, G.(J.), Qumran Pesher: Towards the Redefinition of a Genre, *RevQ* 10 (1981) 483–503.

-, *Exegesis at Qumran*. 4QFlorilegium in its Jewish Context. JSOTSup 29. Sheffield 1985.

-, Introduction, in: G.J. Brooke (ed.), *Temple Scroll Studies*. Papers presented at the International Symposium on the Temple Scroll, Manchester, December 1987. JSPSup 7. Sheffield 1989, 13–19.

Brooks, O.S., Sr, Matthew XXVIII 16–20 and the Design of the First Gospel, *JSNT* 10 (1981) 2–18.

Brooks, S.H., *Matthew's Community*. The evidence of his special sayings material. JSNTSup 16. Sheffield 1987.

Brown, J.P., An Early Revision of the Gospel of Mark, *JBL* 78 (1959) 215–227.

Brown, R.E., *The Gospel according to John*. Introduction, Translation and Notes. AB 29, 29a. New York ²1966.

-, *The Birth of the Messiah*. A commentary on the infancy narratives in Matthew and Luke. London 1977.

Brown, R.E. – Donfried, K.P. – Reumann, J. (eds.), *Peter in the New Testament*. A Collaborative Assessment by Protestant and Roman Scholars. Minneapolis 1973.

Brown, S., The Two-fold Representation of the Mission in Matthew's Gospel, *ST* 31 (1977) 21–32.

-, The Mission to Israel in Matthew's Central Section (Mt 9 35–11 1), *ZNW* 69 (1978) 73–90.

-, The Matthean Community and the Gentile Mission, *NovT* 22 (1980) 193–221.

-, Universalism and Particularism in Matthew's Gospel: A Jungian Approach, in: D.J. Lull (ed.), *Society of Biblical Literature 1989 Seminar Papers*. SBLSP 28. Atlanta 1989, 388–399.

Brownlee, W.H., The Wicked Priest, the Man of Lies, and the Righteous Teacher—the Problem of Identity, *JQR* 73 (1982) 1–37.

-, *Ezekiel 1–19*. WBC 28. Waco 1986.

Bruce, F.F., *Commentary on the Book of the Acts*. The English Text with Introduction, Exposition and Notes. NICNT. Grand Rapids 1981 (=1954).

-, Holy Spirit in the Qumran Texts, *ALUOS* 6 (1969) 49–55.

Brueggemann, W., Unity and Dynamic in the Isaiah Tradition, *JSOT* 29 (1984) 89–107.

Buchanan, G.W., The Priestly Teacher of Righteousness, *RevQ* 6 (1969) 553–558.

-, The Office of Teacher of Righteousness, *RevQ* 9 (1977) 241–243.

Büchler, A., Learning and Teaching in the Open Air in Palestine, *JQR* 4 (1913–14) 485–491.

Büchsel, F., δέω (λύω), *TDNT* 2 (1964) 60–61.

Bultmann, R., *Die Geschichte der synoptischen Tradition*. FRLANT 29. Göttingen 9̂1979.

-, *Die Geschichte der synoptischen Tradition*. Ergänzungsheft. Bearb. von G. Theissen – P. Vielhauer. Göttingen 5̂1979.

Burchard, C., Das doppelte Liebesgebot in der frühen christlichen Überlieferung, in: E. Lohse *et al.* (eds.), *Der Ruf Jesu und die Antwort der Gemeinde*. FS Joachim Jeremias. Göttingen 1970, 39–62.

-, Review of S. Szyszman, *Le Karaïsme*. Lausanne 1980, *RevQ* 11 (1983) 279–285.

Burger, C., *Jesus als Davidssohn*. Eine traditionsgeschichtliche Untersuchung. FRLANT 98. Göttingen 1970.

-, Jesu Taten nach Matthäus 8 und 9, *ZTK* 70 (1973) 272–287.

Burgmann, H., Das umstrittene Intersacerdotium in Jerusalem 159–152 v. Chr., *JSJ* 11 (1980) 135–176.

-, Review of B.E. Thiering, *Redating the Teacher of Righteousness*. Sydney 1979, *RevQ* 10 (1980) 314–317.

-, Wer war der "Lehrer der Gerechtigkeit?," *RevQ* 10 (1981) 553–578.

Burnett, F.W., *The Testament of Jesus-Sophia*. A Redaction-Critical Study of the Eschatological Discourse in Matthew. Lanham 1981.

-, Characterization and Christology in Matthew: Jesus in the Gospel of Matthew, in: D.J. Lull (ed.), *Society of Biblical Literature 1989 Seminar Papers*. SBLSP 28. Atlanta 1989, 588–603.

Burridge, R.A., *What are the Gospels?* A Comparison with Graeco-Roman Biography. SNTSMS 70. Cambridge 1992.

Butterworth, M., *Structure and the Book of Zechariah*. JSOTSup 130. Sheffield 1992.

Byrskog, S., *Nya testamentet och forskningen*. Några aktuella tendenser inom de nytestamentliga exegetiken. Religio 39. Lund 1992.

-, Review of H. Wansbrough (ed.), *Jesus and the Oral Gospel Tradition*. Sheffield 1991, *STK* 69 (1993) 85–87.

Callaway, P.(R.), Source Criticism of the Temple Scroll: The Purity Laws, *RevQ* 12 (1986) 213–222.

-, *The History of the Qumran Community*. An Investigation. JSPSup 3. Sheffield 1988.

-, The Temple Scroll and the Canonization of Jewish Law, *RevQ* 13 (1988) 239–250.

-, Qumran Origins: From the *Doresh* to the *Moreh*, *RevQ* 14 (1990) 637–650.

Camp, L., *Hiskija und Hiskijabild*. Analyse und Interpretation von 2 Kön 18–20. MThA 9. Altenberge 1990.

Campbell, K.M., The New Jerusalem in Matthew 5.14, *SJT* 31 (1978) 335–363.

Campenhausen, H. von, *Kirchliches Amt und geistliche Vollmacht* in den ersten drei Jahrhunderten. BHT 14. Tübingen ²1963.

Cancik, H., Bios und Logos. Formengeschichtliche Untersuchungen zu Lukians 'Demonax', in: H. Cancik (ed.), *Markus-Philologie*. Historische, literargeschichtliche und stilistische Untersuchungen zum zweiten Evangelium. WUNT 33. Tübingen 1984, 115–130.

Caragounis, C.C., *The Son of Man*. Vision and Interpretation. WUNT 38. Tübingen 1986.

-, *Peter and the Rock*. BZNW 58. Berlin 1990.

Carlston, C.E., Betz on the Sermon on the Mount—A Critique, *CBQ* 50 (1988) 47–57.

Carmignac, J., Le document de Qumrân sur Melkisédeq, *RevQ* 7 (1970) 343–378.

-, Qui était le Docteur de Justice?, *RevQ* 10 (1980) 235–246.

-, Précisions, *RevQ* 10 (1981) 585–586.

-, Die Theologie des Leidens in den Hymnen von Qumran, in: K.E. Grözinger *et al.* (eds.), *Qumran*. WdF 410. Darmstadt 1981, 312–340.

Carr, D.M., What Can We Say about the Tradition History of Isaiah? A Response to Christopher Seitz's *Zion's Final Destiny,* in: E.H. Lovering, Jr (ed.), *Society of Biblical Literature 1992 Seminar Papers*. SBLSPS 31. Atlanta 1992, 583–597.

Carroll, R.P., The Elijah-Elisha Sagas: Some Remarks on Prophetic Succession in Ancient Israel, *VT* 19 (1969) 400–415.

-, *When Prophecy Failed*. Reactions and responses to failure in the Old Testament prophetic traditions. London 1979.

-, Twilight of Prophecy of Dawn of Apocalyptic, *JSOT* 14 (1979) 3–35.

-, *From Chaos to Covenant*. Uses of Prophecy in the Book of Jeremiah. London 1981.

-, *Jeremiah*. A Commentary. OTL. London 1986.

Carter, W., Kernels and Narrative Blocks: The Structure of Matthew's Gospel, *CBQ* 54 (1992) 463–481.

-, The Crowds in Matthew's Gospel, *CBQ* 55 (1993) 54–67.

Casey, M., The Jackals and the Son of Man (Matt. 8.20 // Luke 9.58), *JSNT* 23 (1985) 3–22.

Cazelles, H., מָשַׁח, *TWAT* 5 (1986) 28–46.

Chajes, Z.H., *The Student's Guide Through the Talmud*. New York ²1960.

Charette, B., *The Theme of Recompense in Matthew's Gospel*. JSNTSup 79. Sheffield 1992.

-, 'To Proclaim Liberty to the Captives'. Matthew 11.28–30 in the Light of OT Prophetic Expectation, *NTS* 38 (1992) 290–297.

Charlesworth, J.H., From Jewish Messianology to Christian Christology. Some Caveats and Perspectives, in: J. Neusner *et al.* (eds.), *Judaisms and Their Messiahs at the Turn of the Christian Era*. Cambridge 1987, 225–264.

-, Foreword: Qumran Scrolls and a Critical Consensus, in: J.H. Charlesworth (ed.), *Jesus and the Dead Sea Scrolls*. AB Reference Library. New York 1993, xxxi–xxxvi.

Chatman, S., *Story and Discourse*. Narrative Structure in Fiction and Film. Ithaca 1978.

Childs, B.S., *Memory and Tradition in Israel*. SBT 37. London 1962.

-, *Isaiah and the Assyrian Crisis*. SBT 2:3. London 1967.

-, *Introduction to the Old Testament as Scripture*. Philadelphia 1979.

Chilton, B., "Amen": an Approach through Syriac Gospels, *ZNW* 69 (1978) 203–211.

-, Targumic Transmission and Dominical Tradition, in: R.T. France *et al.* (eds.), *Gospel Perspectives*. Vol. 1. Sheffield 1980, 21–45.

-, *The Glory of Israel*. The Theology and Provenience of the Isaiah Targum. JSOTSup 23. Sheffield 1983.

-, *Profiles of a Rabbi*. Synoptic Opportunities in Reading About Jesus. BJS 177. Atlanta 1989.

Christ, F., *Jesus Sophia*. Die Sophia-Christologie bei den Synoptikern. ATANT 57. Zürich 1970.

Civil, M., Education (Mesopotamia), *ABD* 2 (1992) 301–305.

Clark, M.L., *Higher education in the ancient world*. London 1971.

Claudel, G., *La confession de Pierre*. Trajectoire d'une péricope évangélique. Ébib nouvelle série 10. Paris 1988.

-, Review of C.C. Caragounis, *Peter and the Rock*. Berlin 1990, *Bib* 71 (1990) 570–576.

Clements, R.E., *Prophecy and Tradition*. Oxford 1975.

-, *Isaiah and the Deliverance of Jerusalem*. A Study of the Interpretation of Prophecy in the Old Testament. JSOTSup 13. Sheffield 1980.

-, *Isaiah 1–39*. NCB. London 1980.

-, The Prophecies of Isaiah and the Fall of Jerusalem in 587 B.C., *VT* 30 (1980) 421–436.

-, The Ezekiel tradition: prophecy in a time of crisis, in R. Coggins *et al.* (eds.), *Israel's Prophetic Tradition*. FS P.R. Ackroyd. Cambridge 1982, 119–136.

-, The Unity of the Book of Isaiah, *Int* 36 (1982) 117–129.

-, *A Century of Old Testament Study*. Cambridge ²1983.

-, Beyond Tradition-History. Deutero-Isaianic Development of First Isaiah's Themes, *JSOT* 31 (1985) 95–113.

-, The Chronology of Redaction in Ezekiel 1–24, in: J. Lust (ed.), *Ezekiel and His Book*. Textual and Literary Criticism and their Interrelation. BETL 74. Leuven 1986, 283–294.

-, The Prophet and his Editors, in: D.J.A. Clines *et al.* (eds.), *The Bible in three dimensions*. Essays in celebration of forty years of Biblical Studies in the University of Sheffield. JSOTSup 87. Sheffield 1990, 203–220.

Clifford, R.J., The Unity of the Book of Isaiah and Its Cosmogonic Language, *CBQ* 55 (1993) 1–17.

Cody, A., *A History of Old Testament Priesthood*. AnBib 35. Rome 1969.

Cohen, S.J.D., Epigraphical Rabbis, *JQR* 72 (1981) 1–17.

-, Patriarchs and Scholarchs, *PAAJR* 48 (1981) 57–85.

Collins, J.J., The Origin of the Qumran Community: A Review of the Evidence, in: M.P. Horgan *et al.* (eds.), *To Touch the Text*. FS J.A. Fitzmyer. New York 1989, 159–178.

-, The Sage in the Apocalyptic and Pseudepigraphic Literature, in: J.G. Gammie *et al.* (eds.), *The Sage in Israel and the Ancient Near East*. Winona Lake 1990, 343–354.

Collins, R.F., Matthew's ἐντολαί. Towards an Understanding of the Commandments in the First Gospel, in: F. Van Segbroeck *et al.* (eds.), *The Four Gospels 1992*. FS F. Neirynck. BETL 100. Leuven 1992, 1325–1348.

Collins, T., *The Mantle of Elijah*. The Redaction Criticism of the Prophetical Books. BS 20. Sheffield 1993.

Colpe, C., ὁ υἱὸς τοῦ ἀνθρώπου, *TDNT* 8 (1972) 400–477.

Colunga, A., "A nadie llaméis padre sobre la tierra, porque uno sólo es vuestro padre, el que está en los cielos" (Mt., 23,9), in: R.M. Díaz (ed.), *Miscellanea Biblica B. Ubach*. Scripta et documenta 1. Montisserrati 1953, 333–347.

Comber, J.A., The Composition and Literary Characteristics of Matt 11:20–24, *CBQ* 39 (1977) 497–504.

-, The Verb *Therapeuō* in Matthew's Gospel, *JBL* 97 (1978) 431–434.

Combrink, H.J.B., The Macrostructure of the Gospel of Matthew, *Neot* 16 (1982) 1–20.

-, The Structure of the Gospel of Matthew as Narrative, *TynBul* 34 (1983) 61–90.

Conybeare, F.C., Christian Demonology. III., *JQR* 9 (1896–97) 444–470.

Conzelmann, H., Paulus und die Weisheit, *NTS* 12 (1965–66) 231–244.

-, συνίημι κτλ., *TDNT* 7 (1971) 888–896.

-, φῶς κτλ., *TDNT* 9 (1974) 310–358.

-, Die Schule des Paulus, in: C. Andersen *et al.* (eds.), *Theologia crucis – signum crucis.* FS E. Dinkler. Tübingen 1979, 85–96.

Cook, M.J., *Mark's Treatment of the Jewish Leaders.* NovTSup 51. Leiden 1978.

Cope, O.L., *Matthew, A Scribe Trained for the Kingdom of Heaven.* CBQMS 5. Washington 1976.

Cothenet, É., Les prophètes chrétiens dans l'Évangile selon saint Matthieu, in: M. Didier (ed.), *L'Évangile selon Matthieu.* Rédaction et théologie. BETL 29. Gembloux 1972, 281–308.

Coulot, C., *Jésus et le disciple.* Étude sur l'autorité messianique de Jésus. Ébib 8. Paris 1987.

Crawford, B.S., Near Expectation in the Sayings of Jesus, *JBL* 101 (1982) 225–244.

Crenshaw, J.L., Wisdom and Authority: Sapiential Rhetoric and its Warrants, in: J.A. Emerton (ed.), *Congress Volume Vienna 1980.* VTSup 32. Leiden 1981, 10–29.

-, Review of A. Lemaire, *Les écoles et la formation de la Bible dans l'ancien Israël.* Fribourg 1981, *JBL* 103 (1984) 630–632.

-, Education in Ancient Israel, *JBL* 104 (1985) 601–615.

Crook, M.B., A Suggested Occasion for Isaiah 9 2–7 and 11 1–9, *JBL* 68 (1949) 213–224.

Crosby, M.H., *House of Disciples.* Church, Economics, and Justice in Matthew. Maryknoll 1988.

Cross, F.M., Jr, *The Ancient Library of Qumran & Modern Biblical Studies.* Grand Rapids ²1961.

Crossan, J.D., *In Fragments.* The Aphorisms of Jesus. San Francisco 1983.

Culley, R.C., Oral Tradition and Biblical Studies, in: J.M. Foley (ed.), *Oral-Formulaic Theory.* A Folklore Casebook. GFC 5. New York 1990, 189–225.

Cullmann, O., *Petrus. Jünger – Apostel – Märtyrer.* Das historische und das theologische Petrusproblem. Zürich 1952.

-, Πέτρος, Κηφᾶς, *TDNT* 6 (1968) 100–112.

Culpepper, R.A., *The Johannine School.* An Evaluation of the Johannine-School Hypothesis based on an Investigation of the Nature of Ancient Schools. SBLDS 26. Missoula 1975.

-, *Anatomy of the Fourth Gospel.* A Study in Literary Design. F&F: NT. Philadelphia 1983.

Dahl, N.A., *Matteusevangeliet.* Vols. 1–2. Oslo 1965 (vol. 2), ²1973 (vol. 1).

Dalman, G., *Jesus-Jeschua.* Die drei Sprachen Jesu. Jesus in der Synagoge, auf dem Berge, beim Passahmahl, am Kreuz. Leipzig 1922.

-, *Die Worte Jesu* mit Berücksichtigung des nachkanonischen jüdischen Schrifttums und der aramäischen Sprachen. Leipzig ²1930.

-, *Arbeit und Sitte in Palästina.* Vols. 1–7. Gütersloh 1928–1942.

Daube, D., Public Pronouncement and Private Explanation in the Gospels, *ExpTim* 57 (1945–46) 175–177.

-, Rabbinic Methods of Interpretation and Hellenistic Rhetoric, *HUCA* 22 (1949) 239–

262.

-, *The New Testament and Rabbinic Judaism*. London 1956.

-, Responsibilities of Master and Disciples in the Gospels, *NTS* 19 (1972–73) 1–15.

Davidson, M.J., *Angels at Qumran*. A Comparative Study of 1 Enoch 1–36, 72–108 and Sectarian Writings from Qumran. JSPSup 11. Sheffield 1992.

Davies, E.W., *Prophecy and Ethics*. Isaiah and the Ethical Traditions of Israel. JSOTSup 16. Sheffield 1981.

Davies, M., *Matthew*. Readings: A New Biblical Commentary. Sheffield 1993.

Davies, P.R., *Qumran*. CBW. Guildford 1982.

-, *The Damascus Covenant*. An Interpretation of the "Damascus Document." JSOTSup 25. Sheffield 1983.

-, Eschatology at Qumran, *JBL* 104 (1985) 39–55.

-, Qumran Beginnings, in: K.H. Richards (ed.), *Society of Biblical Literature 1986 Seminar Papers*. SBLSP 25. Atlanta 1986, 361–368.

-, *Behind the Essenes*. History and Ideology in the Dead Sea Sect. BJS 94. Atlanta 1987.

-, The Teacher of Righteousness and the "End of Days," *RevQ* 13 (1988) 313–317.

-, The Temple Scroll and the Damascus Document, in: G.J. Brooke (ed.), *Temple Scroll Studies*. Papers presented at the International Symposium on the Temple Scroll Manchester, December 1987. JSPSup 7. Sheffield 1989, 201–210.

-, The Birthplace of the Essenes: Where is "Damascus?," *RevQ* 14 (1990) 503–519.

-, Halakhah at Qumran, in: P.R. Davies *et al.* (eds.), *A Tribute to Geza Vermes*. Essays on Jewish and Christian Literature and History. JSOTSup 100. Sheffield 1990, 37–50.

-, Communities at Qumran and the Case of the Missing 'Teacher', *RevQ* 15 (1991) 275–286.

Davies, W.D., 'Knowledge' in the Dead Sea Scrolls and Matthew 11:25–30, *HTR* 46 (1953) 112–139.

-, *The Setting of the Sermon on the Mount*. Cambridge 1964.

-, The Jewish Sources of Matthew's Messianism, in: J.H. Charlesworth (ed.), *The Messiah*. Developments in Earliest Judaism and Christianity. The First Princeton Symposium on Judaism and Christian Origins. Minneapolis 1992, 494–511.

Davies, W.D. – Allison, D.C., Jr, *The Gospel according to Saint Matthew*. Vols. 1–2. ICC. Edinburgh 1988, 1991 (not complete).

Davis, E.F., *Swallowing the Scroll*. Textuality and the Dynamics of Discourse in Ezekiel's Prophecy. JSOTSup 78. Sheffield 1989.

Davis, J.A., *Wisdom and Spirit*. An Investigation of 1 Corinthians 1.18–3.20 against the Background of Jewish Sapiential Traditions in the Greco-Roman Period. Lanham 1984.

Dearman, J.A., My Servants the Scribes: Composition and Context in Jeremiah 36, *JBL* 109 (1990) 403–421.

Déaut, R. le, Traditions targumiques dans le corpus paulinien? (Hebr 11,4 et 12,24, Gal 4,29–30, II Cor 3,16), *Bib* 42 (1961) 28–48.

Dechent, H., Der "Gerechte" – eine Bezeichnung für den Messias, *TSK* 100 (1927–28) 439–443.

Deissler, A., Das "Echo" der Hosea-Verkündigung im Jeremiabuch, in: L. Ruppert *et al.* (eds.), *Künder des Wortes*. Beiträge zur Theologie der Propheten. FS J. Schreiner. Würzburg 1982, 61–75.

Deissmann, A., The Name 'Jesus', in: G.K.A. Bell *et al.* (eds.), *Mysterium Christi*. Christological Studies by British and German Theologians. London 1930, 1–27.

Delcor, M., Contribution à l'étude de la législation des sectaires de Damas et de Qumrân,

RB 61 (1954) 533–553, *RB* 62 (1955) 60–75.

-, The Melchizedek Figure from Genesis to the Qumran Texts and the Epistle to the Hebrews, *JSJ* 2 (1971) 115–135.

-, Qumrân. Littérature essénienne, *DBSup* 9 (1979) 828–960.

Dell, A., Matthäus 16,17–19, *ZNW* 15 (1914) 1–49.

Delorme, J., *Gymnasion*. Étude sur les monuments consacrés à l'éducation en Grèce (des origines à l'Empire romain). BEFAR 196. Paris 1960.

Demsky, A., Education in the Biblical Period, *EncJud* 6 (1971) 381–398.

-, On the Extent of Literacy in Ancient Israel, in: J. Amitai (ed.), *Biblical Archaeology Today*. Proceedings of the International Congress of Biblical Archaeology, Jerusalem, April 1984. Jerusalem 1985, 349–353.

-, Writing in Ancient Israel and Early Judaism. Part One: The Biblical Period, in: M.J. Mulder (ed.), *Miqra*. Reading, Translation and Interpretation of the Hebrew Bible in Ancient Judaism and Early Christianity. CRINT II 1. Assen 1988, 2–20.

Denis, A.-M., *Les thèmes de connaissance dans le Document de Damas*. SH 15. Louvain 1967.

Derrett, J.D.M., Mt 23,8–10 a Midrash on Is 54,13 and Jer 31,33–34, *Bib* 62 (1981) 372–386.

-, Binding and Loosing (Matt 16:19; 18:18; John 20:23), *JBL* 102 (1983) 112–117.

Deutsch, C., The Sirach 51 Acrostic: Confession and Exhortation, *ZAW* 94 (1982) 400–409.

-, *Hidden Wisdom and the Easy Yoke*. Wisdom, Torah and Discipleship in Matthew 11.25–30. JSNTSup 18. Sheffield 1987.

-, Wisdom in Matthew: Transformation of a Symbol, *NovT* 32 (1990) 13–47.

DeVries, S.J., *1 Kings*. WBC 12. Waco 1985.

Dewey, J., Oral Methods of Structuring Narrative in Mark, *Int* 43 (1989) 32–44.

DeWitt, N.W., *Epicuros and His Philosophy*. Minneapolis 1954.

Dibelius, M., *Die Formgeschichte des Evangeliums*. Tübingen ²1933.

Dietrich, E.L., Das religiös-emphatische Ich-Wort bei den jüdischen Apokalyptikern, Weisheitslehrern und Rabbinen, *ZRGG* 4 (1952) 289–311.

Dietrich, W., *Jesaja und die Politik*. BEvT 74. München 1976.

Díez Macho, A., The recently discovered Palestinian targum: its antiquity and relationship with the other targums, in: *Congress Volume Oxford 1959*. VTSup 7. Leiden 1960, 222–245.

Dihle, A., Die Evangelien und die griechische Biographie, in: P. Stuhlmacher (ed.), *Das Evangelium und die Evangelien*. Vorträge vom Tübinger Symposium 1982. WUNT 28. Tübingen 1983, 383–411.

Dillistone, F.W., Wisdom, Word, and Spirit. Revelation in the Wisdom Literature, *Int* 2 (1948) 275–287.

Dillon, J.T., The Effectiveness of Jesus as Teacher, *LumVit* 36 (1981) 135–162.

Dimant, D., Qumran Sectarian Literature, in: M.E. Stone (ed.), *Jewish Writings of the Second Temple Period*. Apocrypha, Pseudepigrapha, Qumran Sectarian Writings, Philo, Josephus. CRINT II 2. Assen 1984, 483–550.

Dobschütz, E. von, Matthew as Rabbi and Catechist, in: G. Stanton (ed.), *The Interpretation of Matthew*. IRT 3. Philadelphia 1983, 19–29.

Dodd, C.H., Jesus as Teacher and Prophet, in: G.K.A. Bell *et al.* (eds.), *Mysterium Christi*. Christological Studies by British and German Theologians. London 1930, 51–66.

-, *The Apostolic Preaching* and its Developments. London ²1944.

-, *Historical Tradition in the Fourth Gospel*. Cambridge 1963.

Dohmen, C., Zur Gründung der Gemeinde von Qumran (1QS VIII–IX), *RevQ* 11 (1982)

81–96.

Dombkowski Hopkins, D., The Qumran Community and 1Q Hodayot: A Reassessment, *RevQ* 10 (1981) 323–364.

Dombrowski, B.W., היחד in 1QS and τὸ κοινόν. An Instance of Early Greek and Jewish Synthesis, *HTR* 59 (1966) 293–307.

Donaldson, J., The Title Rabbi in the Gospels—Some Reflections on the Evidence of the Synoptics, *JQR* 63 (1972–73) 287–291.

Donaldson, T.L., *Jesus on the Mountain.* A Study in Matthean Theology. JSNTSup 8. Sheffield 1985.

Donner, H., *Geschichte des Volkes Israel und seiner Nachbarn in Grundzügen.* Vols. 1–2. GAT 4. Göttingen 1984, 1986.

Doran, R., Jason's Gymnasion, in: H.W. Attridge *et al.* (eds.), *Of Scribes and Scrolls.* Studies on the Hebrew Bible, Intertestamental Judaism, and Christian Origins. FS J. Strugnell. CTS.RR 5. Lanham 1990, 99–109.

Dormeyer, D., Evangelium als literarische Gattung und als theologischer Begriff. Tendenzen und Aufgaben der Evangelienforschung im 20. Jahrhundert, mit einer Untersuchung des Markusevangeliums in seinem Verhältnis zur antiken Biographie. Erster Teil: Evangelium als literarische Gattung, *ANRW* II 25:2 (1984) 1545–1634.

-, *Evangelium als literarische und theologische Gattung.* ErFor 263. Darmstadt 1989.

-, Mt 1,1 als Überschrift zur Gattung und Christologie des Matthäus-Evangeliums, in: F. Van Segbroeck *et al.* (eds.), *The Four Gospels 1992.* FS F. Neirynck. BETL 100. Leuven 1992, 1361–1383.

Downing, F.G., Contemporary Analogies to the Gospels and Acts: 'Genres' or 'Motifs'?, in: C.M. Tuckett (ed.), *Synoptic Studies.* The Ampleforth Conferences of 1982 and 1983. JSNTSup 7. Sheffield 1984, 51–65.

-, The Social Contexts of Jesus the Teacher: Construction or Reconstruction, *NTS* 33 (1987) 439–451.

Doyle, B.R., Matthew's Intention as Discerned by His Structure, *RB* 95 (1988) 34–54.

Driver, G.R., 'Another Little Drink'—Isaiah 28:1–22, in: P.R. Ackroyd *et al.* (eds.), *Words and Meanings.* FS D.W. Thomas. Cambridge 1968, 47–67.

-, Myths of Qumran, *ALUOS* 6 (1969) 23–48.

Dürr, L., *Das Erziehungswesen im Alten Testament und im antiken Orient.* MVAG 36:2. Leipzig 1932.

Duhm, B., *Das Buch Jesaia.* HKAT 3:1. Göttingen 1892.

-, *Das Buch Jeremia.* HKAT 11. Tübingen 1901.

Duling, D.C., Solomon, Exorcism, and the Son of David, *HTR* 68 (1975) 235–252.

-, The Therapeutic Son of David: An Element in Matthew's Christological Apologetic, *NTS* 24 (1978) 392–410.

-, Binding and Loosing: Matthew 16:19; Matthew 18:18; John 20:23, *Forum* 3:4 (1987) 3–31.

-, Matthew's Plurisignificant "Son of David" in Social Science Perspective: Kinship, Kingship, Magic and Miracle, *BTB* 22 (1992) 99–116.

Dungan, D.L. *The Sayings of Jesus in the Churches of Paul.* The Use of the Synoptic Tradition in the Regulation of Early Church Life. Oxford 1971.

Dunn, J.D.G., Prophetic 'I'-Sayings and the Jesus Tradition: The Importance of Testing Prophetic Utterances within Early Christianity, *NTS* 24 (1978) 175–198.

-, *Christology in the Making.* A New Testament Inquiry into the Origins of the Doctrine of the Incarnation. London [2]1989.

-, John and the Oral Gospel Tradition, in: H. Wansbrough (ed.), *Jesus and the Oral Gospel Tradition.* JSNTSup 64. Sheffield 1991, 351–379.

-, Matthew's Awareness of Markan Redaction, in: F. Van Segbroeck *et al.* (eds.), *The*

Four Gospels 1992. FS F. Neirynck. BETL 100. Leuven 1992, 1349–1359.

Dupont, J., "Vous n'aurez pas achevé les villes d'Israël avant que le Fils de l'homme ne vienne" (Mat. X 23), *NovT* 2 (1958) 228–244.

–, Nova et vetera (Mt 13,52), in: *L'Évangile hier et aujourd'hui*. FS F.-J. Leenhardt. Genève 1968, 55–63.

–, *Les Béatitudes*. Vols. 1–3. Ébib. Paris ²1969–1973.

–, Le point de vue de Matthieu dans le chapitre des paraboles, in: M. Didier (ed.), *L'Évangile selon Matthieu*. Rédaction et théologie. BETL 29. Gembloux 1972, 221–259.

Dupont-Sommer, A., *The Dead Sea Scrolls*. A Preliminary Survey. Oxford 1952.

–, *Les écrits esséniens découverts près de la Mer Morte*. BH. Paris 1959.

Easton, B.S., *The Gospel Before the Gospels*. London 1928.

Eaton, J.(H.), The Origin of the Book of Isaiah, *VT* 9 (1959) 138–157.

–, The Isaiah tradition, in: R. Coggins *et al.* (eds.), *Israel's Prophetic Tradition*. FS P.R. Ackroyd. Cambridge 1982, 58–76.

Eco, U., *The Role of the Reader*. Explorations in the semiotics of texts. London 1981.

Edwards, J.R., The Use of προσέρχεσθαι in the Gospel of Matthew, *JBL* 106 (1987) 65–74.

Edwards, R.A., The Eschatological Correlative as a *Gattung* in the New Testament, *ZNW* 60 (1969) 9–20.

–, *The Sign of Jonah* in the Theology of the Evangelists and Q. SBT 2:18. London 1971.

–, *Matthew's Story of Jesus*. Philadelphia 1985.

–, Uncertain Faith: Matthew's Portrait of the Disciples, in: F.F. Segovia (ed.), *Discipleship in the New Testament*. Philadelphia 1985, 47–61.

–, Narrative Implications of *Gar* in Matthew, *CBQ* 52 (1990) 636–655.

–, Characterization of the Disciples as a Feature of Matthew's Narrative, in: F. Van Segbroeck *et al.* (eds.), *The Four Gospels 1992*. FS F. Neirynck. BETL 100. Leuven 1992, 1305–1323.

Ehrhardt, A., Jewish and Christian Ordination, *JEH* 5 (1954) 125–138.

Eichrodt, W., *Ezekiel*. A Commentary. OTL. London 1970.

Eisenman, R.H., *James the Just in the Habakkuk Pesher*. SPB 35. Leiden 1986.

Eissfeldt, O., Der Anlaß zur Entdeckung der Höhle und ihr ähnliche Vorgänge aus älterer Zeit, *TLZ* 74 (1949) 597–600.

–, *The Old Testament*. An Introduction. Oxford 1966.

–, Πληρῶσαι πᾶσαν δικαιοσύνην in Matthäus 3 15, *ZNW* 61 (1970) 209–215.

Elliger, K., *Die Einheit des Tritojesaia* (Jesaia 56–66). BWANT 9. Stuttgart 1928.

–, Der Prophet Tritojesaja, *ZAW* 49 (1931) 112–141.

–, *Deuterojesaja in seinem Verhältnis zu Tritojesaja*. BWANT 11. Stuttgart 1933.

–, *Deuterojesaja*. 1. Teilband: Jesaja 40,1–45,7. BKAT 6:1. Neukirchen-Vluyn 1978.

Ellis, E.E., Paul and His Co-Workers, *NTS* 17 (1970–71) 437–452.

Ellis, P.F., *Matthew: His Mind and His Message*. Collegeville 1974.

Ellison, H.L., ῥαββί, *NIDNTT* 3 (1978) 115–116.

Elon, M., Takkanot, *EncJud* 15 (1971) 712–728.

Emerton, J.A., Binding and Loosing—Forgiving and Retaining, *JTS* 13 (1962) 325–331.

Emmerson, G.I., *Hosea*. An Israelite Prophet in Judean Perspective. JSOTSup 28. Sheffield 1984.

Engberg-Pedersen, T., Erfaring og åbenbaring i Siraks Bog, in: T. Engberg-Pedersen *et al.* (eds.), *Tradition og nybrud*. Jødedommen i hellenistisk tid. Forum for bibelsk eksegese 2. København 1990, 93–122.

Engnell, I., *Gamla Testamentet*. En traditionshistorisk inledning. Vol. 1. Stockholm 1945.

-, Profetia och tradition. Några synpunkter på ett gammaltestamentligt centralproblem, *SEÅ* 12 (1948) 94–123.

-, *The Call of Isaiah.* An Exegetical and Comparative Study. UUÅ 1949:4. Uppsala 1949.

-, Amos bok, *SBU* 1 (²1962) 66–67.

-, Hesekiels bok, *SBU* 1 (²1962) 946–951.

-, Hoseas bok, *SBU* 1 (²1962) 983–987.

-, Jeremias bok, *SBU* 1 (²1962) 1098–1106.

-, Jesajas bok, *SBU* 1 (²1962) 1143–1147.

-, Lärjungar. 1. GT, *SBU* 1 (²1962) 1557–1558.

-, *Critical Essays on the Old Testament.* London 1970.

Erlandsson, S., *Jesaja.* Angered 1983.

Ernst, J., *Johannes der Täufer.* Interpretation – Geschichte – Wirkungsgeschichte. BZNW 53. Berlin 1989.

Eslinger, L., Inner-Biblical Exegesis and Inner-Biblical Allusion: The Question of Category, *VT* 42 (1992) 47–58.

Evans, C.A., The Genesis Apocryphon and the Rewritten Bible, *RevQ* 13 (1988) 153–165.

Fabry, H.-J., יַחַד, *TWAT* 3 (1982) 595–603.

Faierstein, M.M., Why Do the Scribes Say That Elijah Must Come First?, *JBL* 100 (1981) 75–86.

Falk, Z.W., Binding and Loosing, *JJS* 25 (1974) 92–100.

Fanning, B.M., *Verbal Aspect in New Testament Greek.* OTM. Oxford 1990.

Fascher, E., *Die formgeschichtliche Methode.* Eine Darstellung und Kritik. Zugleich ein Beitrag zur Geschichte des synoptischen Problems. BZNW 2. Gießen 1924.

-, ΠΡΟΦΗΤΗΣ. Eine sprach- und religionsgeschichtliche Untersuchung. Gießen 1927.

-, Jesus der Lehrer. Ein Beitrag zur Frage nach dem "Quellenort der Kirchenidee," *TLZ* 79 (1954) 325–342.

-, Der Logos-Christos als göttlicher Lehrer bei Clemens von Alexandrien, in: *Studien zum Neuen Testament und zur Patristik.* FS E. Klostermann. TU 77. Berlin 1961, 193–207.

Feldman, L.H., Hengel's *Judaism and Hellenism* in Retrospect, *JBL* 96 (1977) 371–382.

- How Much Hellenism in Jewish Palestine?, *HUCA* 57 (1986) 83–111.

-, Josephus's Portrait of Joshua, *HTR* 82 (1989) 351–376.

-, Review of M. Hengel – C. Markschies, *The 'Hellenization' of Judea in the First Century after Christ.* London 1989, *JSJ* 22 (1991) 142–144.

Fenton, J.C., Inclusio and Chiasmus in Matthew, *SE* 1 (TU 73) (1959) 174–179.

Ferguson, E., Jewish and Christian Ordination, *HTR* 56 (1963) 13–19.

Festinger, L., *A Theory of Cognitive Dissonance.* Evanston 1957.

Fey, R., *Amos und Jesaja.* Abhängigkeit und Eigenständigkeit des Jesaja. WMANT 12. Neukirchen-Vluyn 1963.

Fichtner, J., Jesaja unter den Weisen, *TLZ* 74 (1949) 75–80.

Filson, F.V., Broken Patterns in the Gospel of Matthew, *JBL* 75 (1956) 227–231.

Finnegan, R., *Oral Poetry.* Its nature, significance and social context. Cambridge 1977.

-, *Literacy and Orality.* Studies in the Technology of Communication. Oxford 1988.

-, What is Oral Literature Anyway? Comments in the Light of Some African and Other Comparative Material, in: J.M. Foley (ed.), *Oral-Formulaic Theory.* A Folklore Casebook. GFC 5. New York 1990, 243–282.

Fischel, H.A., Studies in Cynicism and the Ancient Near East: The Transformation of a *Chria,* in: J. Neusner (ed.), *Religions in Antiquity.* Essays in Memory of E.R. Goodenough. SHR 14. Leiden 1968, 372–411.

-, *Rabbinic Literature and Greco-Roman Philosophy.* A Study of Epicurea and Rhetorica in Early Midrashic Writings. SPB 21. Leiden 1973.

Fishbane, M., *Biblical Interpretation in Ancient Israel.* Oxford 1985.

-, Use, Authority and Interpretation of Mikra at Qumran, in: M.J. Mulder (ed.), *Miqra.* Reading, Translation and Interpretation of the Hebrew Bible in Ancient Judaism and Early Christianity. CRINT II 1. Assen 1988, 339–377.

-, From Scribalism to Rabbinism: Perspectives on the Emergence of Classical Judaism, in: J.G. Gammie *et al.* (eds.), *The Sage in Israel and the Ancient Near East.* Winona Lake 1990, 439–456.

Fisher, L.R., Can This Be the Son of David?, in: F.T. Trotter (ed.), *Jesus and the Historian.* FS E.C. Colwell. Philadelphia 1968, 82–97.

Fitzmyer, J.A., *Essays on the Semitic Background of the New Testament.* SBLSBS 5. Missoula 1971.

-, *A Wandering Aramean.* Collected Aramaic Essays. SBLMS 25. Missoula 1979.

-, More About Elijah Coming First, *JBL* 104 (1985) 295–296.

Flender, H., Lehren und Verkündigung in den synoptischen Evangelien, *EvT* 25 (1965) 701–714.

Flusser, D., The Apocryphal Book of *Ascensio Isaiae* and the Dead Sea Sect, *BIES* 17 (1952) 28–47.

-, Two Notes on the Midrash on 2 Sam. VII, *IEJ* 19 (1959) 99–109.

-, Melchizedek and the Son of Man, *CNI* 17 (1966) 23–29.

Foerster, W., ἐξουσία, *TDNT* 2 (1964) 562–574.

-, Ἰησοῦς, *TDNT* 3 (1965) 284–293.

Fohrer, G., Tradition und Interpretation im Alten Testament, *ZAW* 73 (1961) 1–30.

-, *Studien zur alttestamentlichen Prophetie (1949–1965).* BZAW 99. Berlin 1967.

-, *Elia.* ATANT 53. Zürich ²1968.

-, *Introduction to the Old Testament.* London 1970.

Foley, J.M., *The Theory of Oral Composition.* History and Methodology. Bloomington 1988.

Forkman, G., *The Limits of the Religious Community.* Expulsion from the Religious Community within the Qumran Sect, within Rabbinic Judaism, and within Primitive Christianity. ConBNT 5. Lund 1972.

Fornberg, T., *Jewish-Christian Dialogue and Biblical Exegesis.* SMU 47. Uppsala 1988.

-, Review of H.D. Betz, *Essays on the Sermon on the Mount.* Philadelphia 1985, *SEÅ* 53 (1988) 123–124.

-, *Matteusevangeliet 1:1–13:52.* KNT 1A. Uppsala 1989.

Forster, E.M., *Aspects of the Novel.* London 1927.

Fraade, S.D., The Early Rabbinic Sage, in: J.G. Gammie *et al.* (eds.), *The Sage in Israel and the Ancient Near East.* Winona Lake 1990, 417–436.

France, R.T., Mark and the Teaching of Jesus, in: R.T. France *et al.* (eds.), *Gospel Perspectives.* Vol. 1. Sheffield 1980, 101–136.

-, Jewish Historiography, Midrash, and the Gospels, in: R.T. France *et al.* (eds.), *Gospel Perspectives.* Vol 3. Sheffield 1983, 99–127.

-, *The Gospel according to Matthew.* An Introduction and Commentary. TNTC. Leichester 1985.

-, *Matthew: Evangelist and Teacher.* Exeter 1989.

Frankemölle, H., Die Makarismen (Mt 5,1–12; Lk 6,20–23). Motive und Umfang der redaktionellen Komposition, *BZ* 15 (1971) 52–75.

-, *Jahwebund und Kirche Christi.* Studien zur Form- und Traditionsgeschichte des "Evangeliums" nach Matthäus. NTAbh Neue Folge 10. Münster 1974.

–, Evangelist und Gemeinde. Eine methodenkritische Besinnung (mit Beispielen aus dem Matthäusevangelium), *Bib* 60 (1979) 153–190.

–, Zur Theologie der Mission im Matthäusevangelium, in: K. Kertelge (ed.), *Mission im Neuen Testament*. QD 93. Freiburg 1982, 93–129.

Friedrich, G., κηρύσσω, *TDNT* 3 (1965) 697–714.

Friedrich, J.(H.), *Gott im Bruder?* Eine methodenkritische Untersuchung von Redaktion, Überlieferung und Traditionen in Mt 25,31–46. CThM 7. Stuttgart 1977.

–, Wortstatistik als Methode am Beispiel der Frage einer Sonderquelle im Matthäus-evangelium, *ZNW* 76 (1985) 29–42.

Frövig, D.A., *Das Selbstbewusstsein Jesu als Lehrer und Wundertäter nach Markus und der sogenannten Redequelle untersucht*. Ein Beitrag zur Frage nach der Messianität Jesu. Leipzig 1918.

Fuller, R.H., Das Doppelgebot der Liebe. Ein Testfall für die Echtheitskriterien der Worte Jesu, in: G. Strecker (ed.), *Jesus Christus in Historie und Theologie*. FS H. Conzelmann. Tübingen 1975, 317–329.

–, Classics and the Gospels: The Seminar, in: W.O. Walker, Jr (ed.), *The Relationships Among the Gospels*. An Interdisciplinary Dialogue. TUMSR 5. San Antonio 1978, 173–192.

Funk, R.W., *The Poetics of Biblical Narrative*. F&F: Literary Facets. Sonoma 1988.

Gaechter, P., *Die literarische Kunst im Matthäus-Evangelium*. SBS 7. Stuttgart 1965.

Gärtner, B., The Habakkuk Commentary (DSH) and the Gospel of Matthew, *ST* 8 (1954) 1–24.

Gammie, J.G., The Sage in Sirach, in: J.G. Gammie *et al.* (eds.), *The Sage in Israel and the Ancient Near East*. Winona Lake 1990, 355–372.

Gammie, J.G. – Perdue, L.G. (eds.), *The Sage in Israel and the Ancient Near East*. Winona Lake 1990.

Gandz, S., The Rōbeh רוֹבֶה or the Official Memorizer of the Palestinian Schools, *PAAJR* 7 (1935–36) 5–12.

García Martínez, F., Review of J.H. Charlesworth, *The Discovery of a Dead Sea Scroll (4Q Therapeia)*. Texas 1985, *JSJ* 17 (1986) 242–244.

García Martínez, F. – Woude, A.S. van der, A "Groningen" Hypothesis of Qumran Origins and Early History, *RevQ* 14 (1990) 521–541.

Garland, D.E., *The Intention of Matthew 23*. NovTSup 52. Leiden 1979.

Gaston, L., The Messiah of Israel As Teacher of the Gentiles. The Setting of Matthew's Christology, *Int* 29 (1975) 24–40.

Gatzweiler, K., Les récits de miracles dans l'Évangile selon saint Matthieu, in: M. Didier (ed.), *L'Évangile selon Matthieu*. Rédaction et théologie. BETL 29. Gembloux 1972, 209–220.

Geist, H., *Menschensohn und Gemeinde*. Eine redaktionskritische Untersuchung zur Menschensohnprädikation im Matthäusevangelium. FB 57. Würzburg 1986.

Genette, G., *Narrative Discourse*. An Essay in Method. Ithaca 1980.

–, *Narrative Discourse Revisited*. Ithaca 1988.

Gerhardsson, B., Review of A.H.J. Gunneweg, *Mündliche und schriftliche Tradition der vorexilischen Prophetenbücher*. Göttingen 1959, *SEÅ* 25 (1960) 175–181.

–, Nycklamakten enligt Skriften, in: E. Segelberg (ed.), *Himmelrikets nycklar*. Predikningar och föredrag hållna vid Kyrklig Förnyelses Kyrkodagar kring Bikten och Själa-vården i Upsala 1962. Saltsjöbaden 1963, 41–74.

–, *Memory and Manuscript*. Oral Tradition and Written Transmission in Rabbinic Judaism and Early Christianity. ASNU 22. Lund ²1964.

–, *Tradition and Transmission in Early Christianity*. ConNT 20. Lund 1964.

–, *The Testing of God's Son* (Matt 4:1–11 & par). An Analysis of an Early Christian

Midrash. ConBNT 2. Lund 1966.

-, The Parable of the Sower and its Interpretation, *NTS* 14 (1967–68) 165–193.

-, Jésus livré et abandonné d'après la passion selon saint Matthieu, *RB* 76 (1969) 206–227.

-, Monoteism och högkristologi i Matteusevangeliet, *SEÅ* 37–38 (1972–73) 125–144.

-, The Seven Parables in Matthew XIII, *NTS* 19 (1972–73) 16–37.

-, Gottes Sohn als Diener Gottes. Messias, Agape und Himmelsherrschaft nach dem Matthäusevangelium, *ST* 27 (1973) 73–106.

-, Sacrificial Service and Atonement in the Gospel of Matthew, in: R.J. Banks (ed.), *Reconciliation and Hope*. FS L.L. Morris. Exeter 1974, 25–35.

-, The Hermeneutic Program in Matthew 22:37–40, in: R. Hamerton-Kelly *et al.* (eds.), *Jews, Greeks and Christians*. Religious Cultures in Late Antiquity. FS W.D. Davies. Leiden 1976, 129–150.

-, *The Mighty Acts of Jesus according to Matthew*. ScrMin 1978–79:5. Lund 1979.

-, *The Origins of the Gospel Traditions*. London 1979.

-, Review of M.D. Goulder, *Midrash and Lection in Matthew*. London 1974, *SEÅ* 45 (1988) 147–149.

-, *The Ethos of the Bible*. Philadelphia 1981.

-, Confession and Denial Before Men: Observations on Matt. 26:57–27:2, *JSNT* 13 (1981) 46–66.

-, "An ihren Früchten sollt ihr sie erkennen." Die Legitimitätsfrage in der matthäischen Christologie, *EvT* 42 (1982) 113–126.

-, Der Weg der Evangelientradition, in: P. Stuhlmacher (ed.), *Das Evangelium und die Evangelien*. Vorträge vom Tübinger Symposium 1982. WUNT 28. Tübingen 1983, 78–102.

-, The Narrative Meshalim in the Synoptic Gospels. A Comparison with the Narrative Meshalim in the Old Testament, *NTS* 34 (1988) 339–363.

-, The Narrative Meshalim in the Old Testament Books and in the Synoptic Gospels, in: M.P. Horgan *et al.* (eds.), *To Touch the Text*. FS J.A. Fitzmyer. New York 1989, 289–304.

-, The Gospel Tradition, in: D.L. Dungan (ed.), *The Interrelations of the Gospels*. A Symposium led by M.-É. Boismard – W.R. Farmer – F. Neirynck, Jerusalem 1984. BETL 95. Leuven 1990, 497–545.

-, If We Do Not Cut the Parables Out of Their Frames, *NTS* 37 (1991) 321–335.

-, Illuminating the Kingdom: Narrative Meshalim in the Synoptic Gospels, in: H. Wansbrough (ed.), *Jesus and the Oral Gospel Tradition*. JSNTSup 64. Sheffield 1991, 266–309.

-, The Shemaᶜ in Early Christianity, in: F. Van Segbroeck *et al.* (eds.), *The Four Gospels 1992*. FS F. Neirynck. BETL 100. Leuven 1992, 275–293.

Gese, H., Komposition bei Amos, in: J.A. Emerton (ed.), *Congress Volume Vienna 1980*. VTSup 32. Leiden 1981, 74–95.

Gevaryahu, H.M.I., Biblical Colophons: A Source for the "Biography" of Authors, Texts and Books, in: G.W. Anderson *et al.* (eds.), *Congress Volume Edinburgh 1974*. VTSup 28. Leiden 1975, 42–59.

-, Privathäuser als Versammlungsstätten von Meister und Jüngern, *ASTI* 12 (1983) 5–12.

-, The School of Isaiah. Biography and Transmission in the Book of Isaiah, *JBQ* 18 (1989–90) 62–68.

Gibbs, J.M., Purpose and Pattern in Matthew's Use of the Title 'Son of David', *NTS* 10 (1963–64) 446–464.

-, The Son of God as the Torah Incarnate in Matthew, *SE* 4 (TU 102) (1968) 38–46.

Giesen, H., *Christliches Handeln*. Eine redaktionskritische Untersuchung zum δικαιο-σύνη-Begriff im Matthäus-Evangelium. EH 23:181. Frankfurt am Main 1982.

-, Jesu Krankenheilungen im Verständnis des Matthäusevangeliums, in: L. Schenke (ed.), *Studien zum Matthäusevangelium*. FS W. Pesch. SBS. Stuttgart 1988, 79–106.

Gilat, Y.D., Eliezer ben Hyrcanus, *EncJud* 6 (1971) 619–623.

-, *R. Eliezer ben Hyrcanus*. A Scholar Outcast. BISNELC. Ramat-Gan 1984.

Gilbert, M., Wisdom Literature, in: M.E. Stone (ed.), *Jewish Writings of the Second Temple Period*. Apocrypha, Pseudepigrapha, Qumran Sectarian Writings, Philo, Josephus. CRINT II 2. Assen 1984, 283–324.

-, The Book of Ben Sira: Implications for Jewish and Christian Traditions, in: S. Talmon (ed.), *Jewish Civilization in the Hellenistic-Roman Period*. JSPSup 10. Sheffield 1991, 81–91.

Ginzberg, L., *Eine unbekannte jüdische Sekte*. Hildesheim 1972 (=New York 1922).

Gitay, Y., Deutero-Isaiah: Oral or Written, *JBL* 99 (1980) 185–197.

Glasson, T.F., An Early Revision of the Gospel of Mark, *JBL* 85 (1966) 231–233.

Glombitza, O., Die Titel διδάσκαλος und ἐπιστάτης für Jesus bei Lukas, *ZNW* 49 (1958) 275–278.

Glucker, J., *Antiochus and the Late Academy*. Hypomnemata 56. Göttingen 1978.

Gnilka, J., *Die Verstockung Israels*. Isaias 6,9–10 in der Theologie der Synoptiker. SANT 3. München 1961.

-, Zur Theologie des Hörens nach den Aussagen des Neuen Testaments, *BibLeb* 2 (1961) 71–81.

-, Das Verstockungsproblem nach Matthäus 13,13–15, in: W.P. Eckert *et al.* (eds.), *Antijudaismus im Neuen Testament?* Exegetische und systematische Beiträge. ACJD 2. München 1967, 119–134.

-, *Der Kolosserbrief*. HTKNT 10:1. Freiburg 1980.

-, *Das Matthäusevangelium*. Vols. 1–2. HTKNT 1:1–2. Freiburg 1986, 1988.

Görg, M., שׁבע, *TWAT* 3 (1982) 1012–1032.

-, Jesaja als Kinderlehrer? Beobachtungen zur Sprache und Semantik in Jes 28,10 (13), *BN* 29 (1985) 12–16.

Goia, F., *La comunità di Qumrân*. Proposte educative. Rome 1979.

Goldblatt, H., The Rabbis of the Babylonian Talmud: A Statistical Analysis, in: J. Neusner *et al.* (eds.), *From Ancient Israel to Modern Judaism*. Intellect in Quest of Understanding. FS M. Fox. Vol. 2. BJS 173. Atlanta 1989, 81–89.

Goldenberg, R., The Deposition of Rabban Gamaliel II: an Examination of the Sources, *JJS* 23 (1972) 167–190.

-, The Problem of Originality in Talmudic Thought, in: J. Neusner *et al.* (eds.), *From Ancient Israel to Modern Judaism*. Intellect in Quest of Understanding. FS M. Fox. Vol. 2. BJS 173. Atlanta 1989, 19–27.

Goldin, J., Several Sidelights of a Torah Education in Tannaite and Early Amorical Times, in: J. Bergman *et al.* (eds.), *Ex orbe religionum*. FS G. Widengren. Leiden 1972, 176–191.

Goldschmidt, W., *Comparative Functionalism*. An Essay in Anthropological Theory. London 1966.

Goldstein, J.(A.), *I Maccabees*. A New Translation with Introduction and Commentary. AB 41. Garden City 1976.

-, Jewish Acceptance and Rejection of Hellenism, in: E.P. Sanders *et al.* (eds.), *Jewish and Christian Self-Definition*. Vol 2. London 1981, 64–87.

-, *II Maccabees*. A New Translation with Introduction and Commentary. AB 41a. Garden City 1983.

Golka, F.W., Die israelitische Weisheitsschule oder 'des Kaisers neue Kleider', *VT* 33

(1983) 257–270.

-, Die Königs- und Hofsprüche und der Ursprung der israelitischen Weisheit, *VT* 36 (1986) 13–36.

Good, D., The Verb ἀναχωρέω in Matthew's Gospel, *NovT* 32 (1990) 1–12.

Good, E.M., The Composition of Hosea, *SEÅ* 31 (1966) 21–63.

Goodblatt, D.M., *Rabbinic Instruction in Sasanian Babylonia*. SJLA 9. Leiden 1975.

Gooding, D.W., Structure littéraire de Matthieu, XIII,53 à XVIII,35, *RB* 85 (1978) 227–252.

Goodman, P., *The Structure of Literature*. Chicago 1954.

Goody, J., *The domestication of the savage mind*. Cambridge 1977.

Gordis, G.M., Prophetic Superscriptions and the Growth of a Canon, in: G.W. Coats *et al.* (eds.), *Canon and Authority*. Essays in Old Testament Religion and Theology. Philadelphia 1977, 56–70.

Gordis, R., The Composition and Structure of Amos, *HTR* 33 (1940) 239–251.

Goshen-Gottstein, M.H., "Sefer Hagu"—the End of a Puzzle, *VT* 8 (1958) 286–288.

Goulder, M.D., Review of M.J. Suggs, *Wisdom, Christology, and Law in Matthew's Gospel*. Cambridge MA 1970, *JTS* 22 (1971) 568–569.

-, *Midrash and Lection in Matthew*. The Speaker's Lectures in Biblical Studies 1969–71. London 1974.

Grässer, E., *Das Problem der Parusieverzögerung in den synoptischen Evangelien und in der Apostelgeschichte*. BZNW 22. Berlin ³1977.

Graham, W.A., *Beyond the Written Word*. Oral Aspects of Scripture in the History of Religion. Cambridge 1987.

Grams, R., The Temple Conflict Scene: A Rhetorical Analysis of Matthew 21–23, in: D.F. Watson (ed.), *Persuasive Artistery*. FS G.A. Kennedy. JSNTSup 50. Sheffield 1991, 41–65.

Grassi, J.A., *Teaching the Way*. Jesus, the Early Church and Today. Washington 1982.

-, Matthew as a Second Testament Deuteronomy, *BTB* 19 (1989) 23–29.

Gray, G.B., *A Critical and Exegetical Commentary on the Book of Isaiah*. Vol. 1. ICC. Edinburgh 1912.

Grayston, K., The Translation of Matthew 28.17, *JSNT* 21 (1984) 105–109.

Green, H B., The Structure of St Matthew's Gospel, *SE* 4 (TU 102) (1968) 47–59.

Green, W.S., Introduction, in: W.S. Green (ed.), *Persons and Institutions in Early Rabbinic Judaism*. BJS 3. Missoula 1977, 1–7.

-, What's in a Name?—The Problematic of Rabbinic "Biography," in: W.S. Green (ed.), *Approaches to Ancient Judaism:* Theory and Practice. BJS 1. Missoula 1978, 77–96.

-, Palestinian Holy Men: Charismatic Leadership and Rabbinic Tradition, *ANRW* II 19:2 (1979) 619–647.

Greenberg, M., *Ezekiel 1–20*. A New Translation with Introduction and Commentary. AB 22. Garden City 1983.

Greenfield, J.C., Review of J.H. Charlesworth, *The Discovery of a Dead Sea Scroll (4Q Therapeia)*. Texas 1985, *IEJ* 36 (1986) 118–119.

Greenspahn, F.E., Why Prophecy Ceased, *JBL* 108 (1989) 37–49.

Grimm, W., ἐπιστάτης, *EWNT* 2 (1981) 93–94.

Groß, K., *Die literarische Verwandtschaft Jeremias mit Hosea*. Leipzig 1930.

Guelich, R.A., *"Not to Annul the Law Rather to Fullfill the Law and the Prophets."* An Exegetical Study of Jesus and the Law in Matthew with Emphasis on 5:17–48. Hamburg 1967.

-, The Antitheses of Matthew V.21–48: Traditional and/or Redactional?, *NTS* 22 (1975–76) 444–457.

-, The Matthean Beatitudes: "Entrance-Requirements" or Eschatological Blessings?, *JBL*

95 (1976) 415–434.

-, *The Sermon on the Mount*. A Foundation for Unterstanding. Waco 1982.

-, The Gospel Genre, in: P. Stuhlmacher (ed.), *Das Evangelium und die Evangelien*. Vorträge vom Tübinger Symposium 1982. WUNT 28. Tübingen 1983, 183–219.

Güttgemanns, E., *Offene Fragen zur Formgeschichte des Evangeliums*. Eine methodologische Skizze der Grundlagenproblematik der Form- und Redaktionsgeschichte. BEvT 54. München 1970.

Gundry, R.H., The Narrative Framework of Matthew XVI 17–19. A Critique of Professor Cullmann's Hypothesis, *NovT* 7 (1964) 1–9.

-, *The Use of the Old Testament in St. Matthew's Gospel* with Special Reference to the Messianic Hope. NovTSup 18. Leiden 1967.

-, *Matthew*. A Commentary on His Literary and Theological Art. Grand Rapids 1982.

Gunkel, H., Elisha—The Successor of Elijah (2 Kings II.1–18), *ExpTim* 41 (1929–30) 182–186.

Gunneweg, A.H.J., *Mündliche und schriftliche Tradition der vorexilischen Prophetenbücher* als Problem der neueren Prophetenforschung. FRLANT 73. Göttingen 1959.

Guttmann, A., The Problem of the Anonymous Mishna. A Study in the History of the Halakah, *HUCA* 16 (1941) 137–155.

Haag, H., בֵּן, *TWAT* 1 (1973) 670–682.

-, *Der Gottesknecht bei Deuterojesaja*. ErFor 233. Darmstadt 1985.

Haenchen, E., Matthäus 23, in: J. Lange (ed.), *Das Matthäus-Evangelium*. WdF 525. Darmstadt 1980, 134–163.

Hagner, D., Righteousness in Matthew's Theology, in: M.J. Wilkins *et al.* (eds.), *Worship, Theology and Ministry in the Early Church*. FS R.P. Martin. Sheffield 1992, 101–120.

Hahn, F., *Das Verständnis der Mission im Neuen Testament*. WMANT 13. Neukirchen-Vluyn 1963.

-, *Christologische Hoheitstitel*. Ihre Geschichte im frühen Christentum. FRLANT 83. Göttingen [4]1974.

Haldar, A., *Associations of Cult Prophets Among the Ancient Semites*. Uppsala 1945.

Halperin, D.J., Crucifixion, the Nahum Pesher, and the Rabbinic Penalty of Strangulation, *JJS* 32 (1981) 32–46.

Hamerton-Kelly, R.G., *Pre-Existence, Wisdom, and the Son of Man*. A Study of the Idea of Pre-Existence in the New Testament. SNTSMS 21. Cambridge 1973.

Hampel, V., "Ihr werdet mit den Städten Israels nicht zu Ende kommen." Eine exegetische Studie über Matthäus 10,23, *TZ* 45 (1989) 1–31.

Hanson, A.T., Handauflegung I, *TRE* 14 (1985) 415–422.

Hanson, P.D., *The Dawn of Apocalyptic*. Philadelphia 1975.

Hanssen, O.C., *Handspåleggelsens funksjon ved kristen initiasjon i Apostlenes Gjerninger*. Lund 1987.

Haran, M., On the Diffusion of Literacy and Schools in Ancient Israel, in: J.A. Emerton (ed.), *Congress Volume Jerusalem 1986*. VTSup 40. Leiden 1988, 81–95.

Hardmeier, C., Die Propheten Micha und Jesaja im Spiegel von Jeremia XXVI und 2 Regum XVIII–XX. Zur Prophetie-Rezeption in der nach-joschijanischen Zeit, in: J.A. Emerton (ed.), *Congress Volume Leuven 1989*. VTSup 43. Leiden 1991, 172–189.

Hare, D.R.A., *The Theme of Jewish Persecution of Christians in the Gospel According to St Matthew*. SNTSMS 6. Cambridge 1967.

-, *The Son of Man Tradition*. Minneapolis 1990.

-, *Matthew*. Interpretation. Louville 1993.

Hare, D.R.A. – Harrington, D. J., "Make Disciples of All the Gentiles" (Mt 28:19), *CBQ* 37 (1975) 359–369.

Harrington, D.J., The Wisdom of the Scribe According to Ben Sira, in: J.J. Collins *et al.* (eds.), *Ideal Figures in Ancient Judaism*. Profiles and Paradigms. SBLSCS 12. Chico 1980, 181–188.

-, *The Gospel of Matthew*. SPS 1. Collegeville 1991.

-, The Rich Young Man in Mt 19,16–22: Another Way to God for Jews?, in: F. Van Segbroeck *et al.* (eds.), *The Four Gospels 1992*. FS F. Neirynck. BETL 100. Leuven 1992, 1425–1432.

Harris, W.V., *Ancient Literacy*. Cambridge MA 1989.

Hartin, P.J., *James and the Q Sayings of Jesus*. JSNTSup 47. Sheffield 1991.

Hartman, L., *Prophecy Interpreted*. The Formation of Some Jewish Apocalyptic Texts and of the Eschatological Discourse Mark 13 Par. ConBNT 1. Lund 1966.

-, Scriptural Exegesis in the Gospel of St. Matthew and the Problem of Communication, in: M. Didier (ed.), *L'Évangile selon Matthieu*. Rédaction et théologie. BETL 29. Gembloux 1972, 131–152.

-, Till frågan om evangeliernas litterära genre, *AARSU* 21 (1978) 5–22.

-, *Till Herrens Jesu namn*. Tro & Tanke 1993:4. Uppsala 1993.

Hartmann, T., רַב, *THAT* 2 (²1979) 715–726.

Hasler, V., *Amen*. Redaktionsgeschichtliche Untersuchung zur Einführungsformel der Herrenworte "Wahrlich ich sage euch." Zürich 1969.

Haspecker, J., *Gottesfurcht bei Jesus Sirach*. Ihre religiöse Struktur und ihre literarische und doktrinäre Bedeutung. AnBib 30. Rome 1967.

Havelock, E.A., *Preface to Plato*. Cambridge MA 1963.

-, *The Muse Learns to Write*. Reflections on Orality and Literacy from Antiquity to the Present. New Haven 1986.

Hawthorne, G.F., The Role of Christian Prophets in the Gospel Tradition, in: G.F. Hawthorne *et al.* (eds.), *Tradition and Interpretation in the New Testament*. FS E.E. Ellis. Grand Rapids 1987, 119–133.

Head, P.M., Christology and Textual Transmission: Reverential Alterations in the Synoptic Gospels, *NovT* 35 (1993) 105–129.

Heil, J.P., *The Death and Resurrection of Jesus*. A Narrative-Critical Reading of Matthew 26–28. Minneapolis 1991.

Held, H.J., Matthew as Interpreter of the Miracle Stories, in: G. Bornkamm *et al.*, *Tradition and Interpretation in Matthew*. London ²1982, 165–299.

Helderman, J., Melchisedeks Wirkung. Eine traditionsgeschichtliche Untersuchung eines Motivkomplexes in NHC IX, 1,1–27,10 (*Melchisedek*), in: J.-M., Sevrin (ed.), *The New Tesament in Early Christianity*. BETL 86. Leuven 1989, 335–362.

Hellholm, D., En textgrammatisk konstruktion i Matteusevangeliet, *SEÅ* 51–52 (1986–87) 80–89.

Henderson, I.A., *Didache* and Orality in Synoptic Comparison, *JBL* 111 (1992) 283–306.

Hengel, M., Die Synagogeninschrift von Stobi, *ZNW* 57 (1966) 145–183.

-, *Judaism and Hellenism*. Studies in their Encounter in Palestine during the Early Hellenistic Period. Vols. 1–2. London 1974.

-, Review of T. Middendorp, *Die Stellung Jesu Ben Siras zwischen Judentum und Hellenismus*. Leiden 1972, *JSJ* 5 (1974) 83–87.

-, Qumrān und der Hellenismus, in: M. Delcor (ed.), *Qumrān. Sa piété, sa théologie et son milieu*. BETL 46. Leuven 1978, 333–372.

-, Jesus als messianischer Lehrer der Weisheit und die Anfänge der Christologie, in: *Sagesse et religion*. Colloque de Strasbourg (octobre 1976). Paris 1979, 148–188.

-, *Jews, Greeks and Barbarians*. Aspects of the Hellenization of Judaism in the Pre-Christian Period. London 1980.

-, *The Charismatic Leader and His Followers*. SNTW. Edinburgh 1981.

-, *Studies in the Gospel of Mark*. London 1985.

Hengel, M. – Markschies, C., *The 'Hellenization' of Judea in the First Century after Christ*. London 1989.

Hentschel, G., *Die Elijaerzählungen*. Zum Verhältnis von historischem Geschehen und geschichtlicher Erfahrung. ETS 33. Leipzig 1977.

Hermisson, H.-J., *Studien zur israelitischen Spruchweisheit*. WMANT 28. Neukirchen-Vluyn 1968.

-, Voreiliger Abschied von den Gottesknechtsliedern, *TRu* 49 (1984) 209–222.

Hernaut, B.W., *Oral Tradition and the Gospels*. The Problem of Mark 4. JSNTSup 82. Sheffield 1993.

Herner, S., Erziehung und Unterricht in Israel, in: C. Adler *et al.* (eds.), *Oriental Studies dedicated to P. Haupt*. Baltimore 1926, 58–66.

Herrmann, S., *Die prophetischen Heilserwartungen im Alten Testament*. Ursprung und Gestaltwandel. BWANT 85. Stuttgart 1965.

-, Jeremia – der Prophet und die Verfasser des Buches Jeremia, in: P.-M. Bogaert (ed.), *Le livre de Jérémie*. Le prophète et son milieu, les oracles et leur transmission. BETL 54. Leuven 1981, 197–214.

-, Jeremia/Jeremiabuch, *TRE* 16 (1987) 568–586.

Herzberg, H.W., Die Nachgeschichte alttestamentlicher Texte innerhalb des Alten Testaments, in: P. Volz *et al.* (eds.), *Werden und Wesen des Alten Testaments*. Vorträge gehalten auf der internationalen Tagung alttestamentlicher Forscher zu Göttingen vom 4–10 September 1935. BZAW 66. Berlin 1936, 110–121.

Heubült, C., Mt 5 17-20. Ein Beitrag zur Theologie des Evangelisten Matthäus, *ZNW* 71 (1980) 143–149.

Hiers, R.H., "Binding" and "Loosing": The Matthean Authorizations, *JBL* 104 (1985) 233–250.

Hill, D., Δίκαιοι as a Quasi-Technical Term, *NTS* 11 (1964–65) 296–302.

-, *The Gospel of Matthew*. NCB. London 1972.

-, False Prophets and Charismatics: Structure and Interpretation in Matthew 7,15–23, *Bib* 57 (1976) 327–348.

-, Christian Prophets as Teachers or Instructors in the Church, in: J. Panagopoulos (ed.), *Prophetic Vocation in the New Testament and Today*. NovTSup 45. Leiden 1977, 108–130.

-, On the Use and Meaning of Hosea VI.6 in Matthew's Gospel, *NTS* 24 (1978) 107–119.

-, *New Testament Prophecy*. MTL. London 1979.

-, Son and Servant: An Essay on Matthean Christology, *JSNT* 6 (1980) 2–16.

-, The Figure of Jesus in Matthew's Story: A Response to Professor Kingsbury's Literary-Critical Probe, *JSNT* 21 (1984) 37–52.

Hillyer, N., Ἡρῳδιανοί, *NIDNTT* 3 (1978) 441–443.

Hirsch, E., *Frühgeschichte des Evangeliums*. Vol. 2. Tübingen 1941.

Hirsch, E.D., Jr, *Validity in Interpretation*. New Haven 1967.

Hobbs, T.R., *2 Kings*. WBC 13. Waco 1985.

Höffken, P., Notizen zum Textcharakter von Jesaja 7,1–17, *TZ* 36 (1980) 321–337.

Høgenhaven, J., *Gott und Volk bei Jesaja*. Eine Untersuchung zur biblischen Theologie. ATDan 24. Leiden 1988.

Hoenig, S.B., On the Age of Mature Responsibility in 1QSa, *JQR* 48 (1957–58) 371–375.

-, The Age of Twenty in Rabbinic Tradition and 1QSa, *JQR* 49 (1958–59) 209–214.

Hoet, R., *"Omnes autem vos fratres estis."* Etude du concept ecclésiologique des "frères" selon Mt 23,8–12. AnGreg 232. Rome 1982.

Hoffmann, P., Der Petrus-Primat im Matthäusevangelium, in: J. Lange (ed.), *Das Matthäus-Evangelium*. WdF 525. Darmstadt 1980, 415–440.

Hofius, O., Agrapha, *TRE* 2 (1978) 103–110.

-, "Unbekannte Jesusworte," in: P. Stuhlmacher (ed.), *Das Evangelium und die Evangelien*. Vorträge vom Tübinger Symposium 1982. WUNT 28. Tübingen 1983, 355–382.

Hoh, J., Der christliche γραμματεύς, *BZ* 17 (1926) 256–269.

Holladay, W.L., Prototype and Copies: A New Approach to the Poetry-Prose Problem in the Book of Jeremiah, *JBL* 79 (1960) 351–367.

-, The Identification of the Two Scrolls of Jeremiah, *VT* 30 (1980) 452–467.

-, A Fresh Look at "Source B" and "Source C" in Jeremiah, in: L.G. Perdue *et al.* (eds.), *A Prophet to the Nations*. Essays in Jeremiah Studies. Winona Lake 1984, 213–228.

-, *Jeremiah*. Vols. 1–2. Hermeneia. Philadelphia 1986 (vol. 1), Minneapolis 1989 (vol. 2).

Holmberg, B., *Paul and Power*. The Structure of Authority in the Primitive Church as Reflected in the Pauline Epistles. ConBNT 11. Lund 1978.

Holm-Nielsen, S., *Hodayot*. Psalms from Qumran. ATDan 2. Aarhus 1960.

-, "Ich" in den Hodajoth und die Qumrängemeinde, in: H. Bardtke (ed.), *Qumrān-Probleme*. Vorträge des leipziger Symposions über Qumrān-Probleme von 9. bis 14. Oktober 1961. DAWB.SSA 42. Berlin 1963, 217–229.

Honeyman, A.M., Notes on a Teacher and a Book, *JJS* 4 (1953) 131–132.

Horst, J., οὖς, *TDNT* 5 (1967) 543–558.

Hossfeldt, F., *Untersuchungen zu Komposition und Theologie des Ezechielbuches*. FB 20. Würzburg 1977.

Howard, V.P., *Das Ego Jesu in den synoptischen Evangelien*. Untersuchungen zum Sprachgebrauch Jesu. MTS 14. Marburg 1975.

Howell, D.B., *Matthew's Inclusive Story*. A Study in the Narrative Rhetoric of the First Gospel. JSNTSup 42. Sheffield 1990.

Howie, C.G., *The Date and Composition of Ezekiel*. JBLMS 4. Philadelphia 1950.

Hruby, K., La notion d'ordination dans la tradition juive, *MD* 102 (1970) 30–56.

Hubbard, B.J., *The Matthean Redaction of a Primitive Apostolic Commissioning:* An Exegesis of Matthew 28:16–20. SBLDS 19. Missoula 1974.

Hübner, H., *Das Gesetz in der synoptischen Tradition*. Studien zur These einer progressiven Qumranisierung und Judaisierung innerhalb der synoptischen Tradition. Göttingen ²1986.

Hultgård, A., *L'eschatologie des Testaments des Douze Patriarches*. Vol. 1. AUU.HR 6. Uppsala 1977.

Hultkrantz, Å., *Metodvägar inom den jämförande religionsforskningen*. Stockholm 1973.

Hummel, R., *Die Auseinandersetzung zwischen Kirche und Judentum im Matthäusevangelium*. BEvT 33. München 1966.

Hyatt, J.P., Jeremiah and Deuteronomy, in: L.G. Perdue *et al.* (eds.), *A Prophet to the Nations*. Essays in Jeremiah Studies. Winona Lake 1984, 113–127.

-, The Deuteronomic Edition of Jeremiah, in: L.G. Perdue *et al.* (eds.), *A Prophet to the Nations*. Essays in Jeremiah Studies. Winona Lake 1984, 247–267.

Imschoot, P. van, Sagesse et esprit dans l'Ancient Testament, *RB* 47 (1938) 23–49.

Irvine, S.A., *Isaiah, Ahaz, and the Syro-Ephraimitic Crisis* (SBLDS 123). Atlanta 1990.

-, The Isaianic *Denkschrift*: Reconsidering an Old Hypothesis, *ZAW* 104 (1992) 216–231.

Ittmann, N., *Die Konfessionen Jeremias*. Ihre Bedeutung für die Verkündigung des Propheten. WMANT 54. Neukirchen-Vluyn 1981.

Jacob, E., Wisdom and Religion in Sirach, in: J.G. Gammie *et al.* (eds.), *Israelite Wisdom*. FS S. Terrien. Missoula 1978, 247–260.

Jacobs, L., Halakhah le-Moshe mi-Sinai, *EncJud* 7 (1971) 1167.

Jaeger, W., *Paideia*. Die Formung des griechischen Menschen. Vols. 1–3. Berlin 1934–1947.

Jamieson-Drake, D.W., *Scribes and Schools in Monarchic Judah*. A Socio-Archeological Approach. JSOTSup 109, SWBA 9. Sheffield 1991.

Jaubert, A., "Le pays de Damas," *RB* 65 (1958) 214–248.

Jenni, E., למד, *THAT* 1 (³1978) 872–875.

Jensen, J., *The Use of tôrâ by Isaiah*. His Debate with the Wisdom Tradition. CBQMS 3. Washington 1973.

Jeppesen, K., Herrens lidende tjener i historien og traditions-historien, in: K. Jeppesen *et al.* (eds.), *Texter & Tolkningar*. Ti studier i Det gamle Testamente. Århus 1986, 113–126.

Jeppesen, K. – Otzen, B. (eds.), *The Productions of Time*. Tradition History in Old Testament Scholarship. Sheffield 1984.

Jepsen, A., Die Nebiah in Jes 8 3, *ZAW* 72 (1960) 267–268.

Jeremias, G., *Der Lehrer der Gerechtigkeit*. SUNT 2. Göttingen 1963.

Jeremias, Joachim, Zur Hypothese einer schriftlichen Logienquelle Q, *ZNW* 29 (1930) 147–149.

-, *Unbekannte Jesusworte*. Unter Mitwirkung von O. Hofius. Gütersloh ³1963.

-, Ἠλ(ε)ίας, *TDNT* 2 (1964) 928–941.

-, κλείς, *TDNT* 3 (1965) 744–753.

-, *Abba. Studien zur neutestamentlichen Theologie und Zeitgeschichte*. Göttingen 1966.

-, Μωυσῆς, *TDNT* 4 (1967) 848–873.

-, *Jerusalem in the Time of Jesus*. An Investigation into Economic and Social Conditions during the New Testament Period. London 1969.

-, *Neutestamentliche Theologie*. Erster Teil: Die Verkündigung Jesu. Gütersloh 1971.

-, Zum nicht-responsorischen Amen, *ZNW* 64 (1973) 122–123.

Jeremias, Jörg, נבִיא, *THAT* 2 (²1979) 7–26.

-, *Der Prophet Hosea*. ATD 24:1. Göttingen 1983.

Johnson, M.D., Reflections on a Wisdom Approach to Matthew's Christology, *CBQ* 36 (1974) 44–64.

Jones, A., *The Gospel According to St Matthew*. A Text and Commentary for Students. London 1965.

Jones, D., The Traditio of the Oracles of Isaiah of Jerusalem, *ZAW* 67 (1955) 226–246.

Jonge, M. de, χρίω κτλ., *TDNT* 9 (1974) 509–517.

-, The Main Issues in the Study of the Testaments of the Twelve Patriarchs, *NTS* 26 (1980) 508–524.

Joüon, P., Qu'étaient les 'Fils des Prophètes' (Bᵉné hannᵉbî'îm)?, *RSR* 16 (1926) 307–312.

Kähler, C., Zur Form- und Traditionsgeschichte von Matth. XVI.17–19, *NTS* 23 (1976–77) 36–58.

Kähler, G.-C., Review of K. Berger, *Die Amen-Worte Jesu*. Berlin 1970, *TLZ* 97 (1972) 200–202.

Käsemann, E., *New Testament Questions of Today*. NTL. London 1969.

Kaiser, O., *Introduction to the Old Testament*. A Presentation of its Results and Problems. London 1975.

-, Gottesgewißheit und Weltbewußtsein in der frühhellenistischen jüdischen Weisheit, in: T. Rendtorff (ed.), *Glaube und Toleranz*. Das theologische Erbe der Aufklärung. Gütersloh 1982, 76–88.

-, Judentum und Hellenismus. Ein Beitrag zur Frage nach dem hellenistischen Einfluß auf Kohelet und Jesus Sirach, *VF* 27 (1982) 68–86.

-, *Isaiah 1–12*. A Commentary. OTL. London ²1983.

-, Jesaja/Jesajabuch, *TRE* 16 (1987) 636–658.

Kampling, R., Jesus von Nazaret – Lehrer und Exorzist, *BZ* 30 (1986) 237–248.

Kane, J.P., The Ossuary Inscriptions of Jerusalem, *JSS* 23 (1978) 268–282.

Kapelrud, A.S., לָמַד, *TWAT* 4 (1983) 576–582.

-, The Traditio-historical Study of the Prophets, in: K. Jeppesen *et al.* (eds.), *The Productions of Time*. Tradition History in Old Testament Scholarship. Sheffield 1984, 53–66.

Kapera, Z.J., A Review of East European Studies on the Temple Scroll, in: G.J. Brooke (ed.), *Temple Scroll Studies*. Papers presented at the International Symposium on the Temple Scroll, Manchester, December 1987. JSPSup 7. Sheffield 1989, 275–286.

-, A Preliminary Subject Bibliography of 4QMMT: 1956–1991, in: Z.J. Kapera (ed.), *Qumran Cave IV and MMT*. Special Report. Kraków 1991, 75–80.

Karrer, M., Der lehrende Jesus. Neutestamentliche Erwägungen, *ZNW* 83 (1992) 1–20.

Keck, L.E., Toward the Renewal of New Testament Christology, *NTS* 32 (1986) 362–377.

Keegan, T.J., Introductory Formulae for Matthean Discourses, *CBQ* 44 (1982) 415–430.

Kelber, W.H., *The Oral and the Written Gospel*. The Hermeneutics of Speaking and Writing in the Synoptic Tradition, Mark, Paul and Q. Philadelphia 1983.

-, Biblical Hermeneutics and the Ancient Art of Communication: A Response, *Semeia* 39 (1987) 97–105.

-, Narrative as Interpretation and Interpretation of Narrative: Hermeneutical Reflections on the Gospels, *Semeia* 39 (1987) 107–133.

Kennedy, G.A., *New Testament Interpretation through Rhetorical Criticism*. Chapel Hill 1984.

Kenyon, F.G., *Books and Readers in Ancient Greece and Rome*. Oxford 1932.

Kessler, M., The Significance of Jer 36, *ZAW* 81 (1969) 381–383.

Keyes, C.F., Charisma: From Social Life to Sacred Biography, in: M.A. Williams (ed.), *Charisma and Sacred Biograpy*. JAAR Thematic Studies 48:3, 4. Missoula 1982, 1–22.

Kieffer, R., Weisheit und Segen als Grundmotive der Seligpreisungen bei Mattäus und Lukas, in: E. Fuchs (ed.), *Theologie aus dem Norden*. SNTU A:2. Linz 1976, 29–43.

-, "Mer-än"-kristologin hos synoptikerna, *SEÅ* 44 (1979) 134–147.

Kilpatrick, G.D., *The Origins of the Gospel According to St. Matthew*. Oxford 1946.

Kilunen, J., Der nachfolgewillige Schriftgelehrte. Matthäus 8.19–20 im Verständnis des Evangelisten, *NTS* 37 (1991) 268–279.

Kingsbury, J.D., *The Parables of Jesus in Matthew 13*. A Study in Redaction-Criticism. London 1969.

-, Observations on the "Miracle Chapters" of Matthew 8–9, *CBQ* 40 (1978) 559–573.

-, The Verb *Akolouthein* ("to follow") as an Index of Matthew's View of his Community, *JBL* 97 (1978) 56–73.

-, The Figure of Peter in Matthew's Gospel as a Theological Problem, *JBL* 98 (1979) 67–83.

-, The Figure of Jesus in Matthew's Story: A Literary-Critical Probe, *JSNT* 21 (1984) 3–36.

-, The Figure of Jesus in Matthew's Story. A Rejoinder to David Hill, *JSNT* 25 (1985) 61–81.

-, *Matthew*. Proclamation Commentaries. Philadelphia ²1986.

-, The Developing Conflict Between Jesus and the Jewish Leaders in Matthew's Gospel: A Literary-Critical Study, *CBQ* 49 (1987) 57–73.

-, *Matthew as Story*. Philadelphia ²1988.

-, On Following Jesus: The 'Eager' Scribe and the 'Reluctant' Disciple (Matthew 8.18–22), *NTS* 34 (1988) 45–59.

-, Reflections on 'the Reader' of Matthew's Gospel, *NTS* 34 (1988) 442–460.

-, *Matthew: Structure, Christology, Kingdom*. Minneapolis ²1989.

-, Conclusion: Analysis of a Conversation, in: D.L. Balch (ed.), *Social History of the Matthean Community*. Cross-disciplinary Approaches. Minneapolis 1991, 259–269.

-, The Plot of Matthew's Story, *Int* 46 (1992) 347–356.

Kirkpatrick, P.G., *The Old Testament and Folklore Study*. JSOTSup 62. Sheffield 1988.

Kirschner, R., Imitatio Rabbini, *JSJ* 17 (1986) 70–79.

Kitchen, K.A., Egypt and Israel during the First Millenium B.C., in: J.A. Emerton (ed.), *Congress Volume Jerusalem 1986*. VTSup 40. Leiden 1988, 107–123.

Kittel, B.P., *The Hymns of Qumran*. Translation and Commentary. SBLDS 50. Chico 1981.

Kittel, G., *Die Probleme des palästinischen Spätjudentums und das Urchristentum*. BWANT 1. Stuttgart 1926.

-, ἀκολουθέω κτλ., *TDNT* 1 (1964) 210–216.

-, ἀκούω, *TDNT* 1 (1964) 216–221.

Kjær-Hansen, K., *Studier i navnet Jesus*. Aarhus 1982.

Kjær Nielsen, H., *Heilung und Verkündigung*. Das Verständnis der Heilung und ihres Verhältnisses zur Verkündigung bei Jesus und in der ältesten Kirche. ATDan 22. Leiden 1987.

Klauck, H.-J., *Judas – ein Jünger des Herrn*. QD 3. Freiburg 1987.

Klein, G., Die Verleugnung des Petrus. Eine traditionsgeschichtliche Untersuchung, *ZTK* 58 (1961) 285–328.

Klein, H., Das Glaubensverständnis im Matthäusevangelium, in: F. Hahn *et al.* (eds.), *Glaube im Neuen Testament*. FS H. Binder. BibTS 7. Neukirchen-Vluyn 1982, 29–42.

Kleinknecht, K.T., *Der leidende Gerechtfertigte*. Die alttestamentlich-jüdische Tradition vom 'leidenden Gerechten' und ihre Rezeption bei Paulus. WUNT 2:13. Tübingen ²1988.

Kloppenborg, J.S., *The Formation of Q*. Trajectories in Ancient Wisdom Collections. SAC. Philadelphia 1987.

Klostermann, A., *Schulwesen im alten Israel*. Leipzig 1908.

Klostermann, E., *Das Matthäusevangelium*. HNT 4. Tübingen ²1927.

Knibb, M.A., *The Qumran Community*. CCWJCW 2. Cambridge 1987.

-, The Teacher of Righteousness—A Messianic Title?, in: P.R. Davies *et al.* (eds.), *A Tribute to Geza Vermes*. Essays on Jewish and Christian Literature and History. JSOTSup 100. Sheffield 1990, 51–65.

Knierim, R., Criticism of Literary Features, Form, Tradition, and Redaction, in: D.A. Knight *et al.* (eds.), *The Hebrew Bible and its Modern Interpreters*. SBLBMI 1. Philadelphia 1985, 123–165.

Knight, D.A., *Rediscovering the Traditions of Israel*. The Development of the Traditio-Historical Research of the Old Testament, with Special Consideration of Scandinavian Contributions. SBLDS 9. Missoula 1973.

-, Tradition History, *ABD* 6 (1992) 633–638.

Knight, G.A.F., *Servant Theology*. A Commentary on the Book of Isaiah 40–55. ITC. Edinburgh 1984.

Knowles, M., *Jeremiah in Matthew's Gospel*. The Rejected-Prophet Motif in Matthaean

Redaction. JSNTSup 68. Sheffield 1993.

Kobelski, P. J., *Melchizedek and Melchireša'*. CBQMS 10. Washington 1981.

Koch, K., *Was ist Formgeschichte?* Methoden der Bibelexegese. Neukirchen-Vluyn ³1974.

-, צדק, *THAT* 2 (²1979) 507–530.

-, *The Prophets*. Vols. 1–2. London 1982, 1983

Koch, K. *et al., Amos*. Untersucht mit den Methoden einer strukturalen Formgeschichte. Vol. 1. AOAT 30. Neukirchen-Vluyn 1976.

Köhler (Koehler), L., *Das formgeschichtliche Problem des Neuen Testamentes*. SVS 127. Tübingen 1927.

-, Lautes Lesen, *ZAW* 32 (1912) 240.

Köhler, W.-D., *Die Rezeption des Matthäusevangeliums in der Zeit vor Irenäus*. WUNT 2:24. Tübingen 1987.

Kölichen, J.-C. von, Der "Lehrer der Gerechtigkeit" und Hos 10:12 in einer rabbinischen Handschrift des Mittelalters, *ZAW* 74 (1962) 324–327.

Koenen, K., *Ethik und Eschatologie im Tritojesajabuch*. Eine literarkritische und redaktionskritische Studie. WMANT 62. Neukirchen-Vluyn 1990.

Koester, H., *Ancient Christian Gospels*. Their History and Development. London 1990.

Koffmahn, E., Rechtsstellung und hierarchische Struktur des יחד von Qumran. Eine juristische Person und eine religiöse Gemeinschaft nach dem mosaischen Gesetz, *Bib* 42 (1961) 433–442.

-, Die staatsrechtliche Stellung der essenischen Vereinigungen in der griechisch-römischen Periode, *Bib* 44 (1963) 46–61.

Kohler, K., Abba, Father. Title of Spiritual Leader and Saint, *JQR* 13 (1901) 567–580.

Kook, A.I., The Sage is More Important Than the Prophet, *Judaism* 21 (1972) 311–312.

Kosch, D., *Die eschatologische Tora des Menschensohnes*. Untersuchungen zur Rezeption der Stellung Jesu zur Tora in Q. NTOA 12. Fribourg 1989.

Koskenniemi, E., *Apollonios von Tyana in der neutestamentlichen Exegese*. Forschungsbericht und Weiterführung der Diskussion. Åbo 1992.

Kraemer, D., On the Reliability of Attributions in the Babylonian Talmud, *HUCA* 60 (1989) 175–190.

Kratz, R.G., *Kyros in Deuterojesaja-Buch*. Redaktionsgeschichtliche Untersuchungen zur Entstehung und Theologie von Jes 40–55. FAT 1. Tübingen 1991.

Krauss, S., *Talmudische Archäologie*. SGFWJ. Vols. 1–3. Leipzig 1910–1912.

-, Outdoor Teaching in Talmudic Times, *JJS* 1 (1948–49) 82–84.

Kremers, H., Leidensgemeinschaft mit Gott im Alten Testament. Eine Untersuchung der "biographischen" Berichte im Jeremiabuch, *EvT* 13 (1953) 122–140.

Krentz, E., The Extent of Matthew's Prologue. Toward the Structure of the First Gospel, *JBL* 83 (1964) 409–414.

Kretzer, A., *Die Herrschaft der Himmel und die Söhne des Reiches*. Eine redaktionsgeschichtliche Untersuchung zum Basileiabegriff und Basileiaverständnis im Matthäusevangelium. SBM 10. Stuttgart 1971.

Kruse, C.G., Community Functionaries in the Rule of the Community and the Damascus Document: A Test of Chronological Relationships, *RevQ* 10 (1981) 543–551.

Küchler, M., *Frühjüdische Weisheitstraditionen*. Zum Fortgang weisheitlichen Denkens im Bereich des frühjüdischen Jahweglaubens. OBO 26. Fribourg 1979.

Kümmel, W.G., Die Naherwartung in der Verkündigung Jesu, in: E. Dinkler (ed.), *Zeit und Geschichte*. FS R. Bultmann. Tübingen 1964, 31–46.

-, Die Weherufe über die Schriftgelehrten und Pharisäer (Matthäus 23,13–36), in: W.P. Eckert *et al.* (eds.), *Antijudaismus im Neuen Testament?* Exegetische und systematische Beiträge. ACJD 2. München 1967, 135–147.

-, *Einleitung in das Neue Testament.* Heidelberg [21]1983.

Künzel, G., *Studien zum Gemeindeverständnis des Matthäus-Evangeliums.* CThM 10. Stuttgart 1978.

Künzi, M., *Das Naherwartungslogion Matthäus 10,23.* Geschichte seiner Auslegung. BGBE 9. Tübingen 1970.

Kuhn, H.-W., *Enderwartung und gegenwärtiges Heil.* Untersuchungen zu den Gemeindeliedern von Qumran mit einem Anhang über Eschatologie und Gegenwart in der Verkündigung Jesu. SUNT 4. Göttingen 1966.

Kuhn, K.G., The Two Messiahs of Aaron and Israel, in: K. Stendahl (ed.), *The Scrolls and the New Testament.* New York 1957, 54–64.

Kuhn, P., *Offenbarungsstimmen im Antiken Judentum.* Untersuchungen zur Bat Qol und verwandten Phänomenen. TSAJ 20. Tübingen 1989.

Kvalbein, H., *Jesus og de fattige.* Jesu syn på de fattige og hans bruk av ord for "fattig." Oslo 1981.

-, *Fortolkning til Matteusevangeliet.* Vols. 1–2. Bibelverket. Oslo 1989, 1990.

Laato, A., *Who is Immanuel?* The Rise and the Foundering of Isaiah's Messianic Expectations. Åbo 1988.

-, *The Servant of YHWH and Cyrus.* A Reinterpretation of the Exilic Messianic Programme in Isaiah 50–55. ConBOT 35. Stockholm 1992.

Lachs, S.T., *A Rabbinic Commentary on the New Testament.* The Gospels of Matthew, Mark, and Luke. Hoboken 1987.

Lambrecht, J., *Out of the Treasure.* The Parables in the Gospel of Matthew. LTPM 10. Louvain 1992.

Lang, B., *Die weisheitliche Lehrrede.* Eine Untersuchung von Sprüche 1–7. SBS 54. Stuttgart 1972.

-, Schule und Unterricht im alten Israel, in: M. Gilbert (ed.), *La Sagesse de l'Ancien Testament.* BETL 51. Leuven 1979, 186–201.

-, *Ezechiel.* Der Prophet und sein Buch. ErFor 153. Darmstadt 1981.

-, *Monotheism and the Prophetic Minority.* An Essay in Biblical History and Sociology. SWBA 1. Sheffield 1983.

-, *Wisdom and the Book of Proverbs.* A Hebrew Goddess Redefined. New York 1986.

-, Street Theater, Raising the Dead, and the Zoroastrian Connection in Ezekiel's Prophecy, in: J. Lust (ed.), *Ezekiel and His Book.* Textual and Literary Criticism and their Interrelation. BETL 74. Leuven 1986, 297–316.

Lange, J., *Das Erscheinen des Auferstandenen im Evangelium nach Matthäus.* Eine traditions- und redaktionsgeschichtliche Untersuchung zu Mt 28,16–20. FB 11. Würzburg 1973.

Laperrousaz, E.-M., Les "ordonnances premières" et les "ordonnances dernières" dans les manuscrits de la Mer Morte, in: A. Caqout *et al.* (eds.), *Hommages à A. Dupont-Sommer.* Paris 1971, 405–419.

-, Critères internes de datation des manuscrits de la Mer Morte: "Ordonnances premières" et "ordonnances dernières," *RevQ* 13 (1988) 453–464.

-, A propos du Maître de Justice et du temple de Jérusalem: Deux problèmes de nombre, *RevQ* 15 (1991) 265–274.

Lapide, P., *Die Bergpredigt – Utopie oder Programm?* Mainz [4]1984.

Lapin, H., Rabbi, *ABD* 5 (1992) 600–602.

Larsson, E., *Christus als Vorbild.* Eine Untersuchung zu den paulinischen Tauf- und Eikontexten. ASNU 23. Uppsala 1962.

-, Paulus och den hellenistiska församlingsteologin. Ett blad i den vetenskapliga dogmbildningens historia, *SEÅ* 28–29 (1963–64) 81–110.

Latham, J.E., *The Religious Symbolism of Salt.* TH 64. Paris 1982.

Lausberg, H., *Elemente der literarischen Rhetorik*. Eine Einführung für Studierende der klassischen, romanischen, englischen und deutschen Philologie. München ⁹1987.

-, *Handbuch der literarischen Rhetorik*. Eine Grundlegung der Literaturwissenschaft. Stuttgart ³1990.

Lee, T.R., *Studies in the Form of Sirach 44–50*. SBLDS 75. Atlanta 1986.

Leeuwen, (R.)C. van, עד, *THAT* 2 (²1979) 209–221.

-, The Sage in the Prophetic Literature, in: J.G. Gammie *et al.* (eds.), *The Sage in Israel and the Ancient Near East*. Winona Lake 1990, 295–306.

Légasse, S., Scribes et disciples de Jésus, *RB* 68 (1961) 321–345, 481–506.

-, L'"antijudaïsme" dans l'Évangile selon Matthieu, in: M. Didier (ed.), *L'Évangile selon Matthieu*. Rédaction et théologie. BETL 29. Gembloux 1972, 417–428.

Lehmann, M.R., 11QPsᵃ and Ben Sira, *RevQ* 11 (1983) 239–251.

Leivestad, R., An Interpretation of Matt 11 19, *JBL* 71 (1952) 179–181.

-, Das Dogma von der prophetenlosen Zeit, *NTS* 19 (1972–73) 288–299.

Lella, A.A. di, *The Hebrew Text of Sirach*. A Text-Critical and Historical Study. SCL 1. The Hague 1966.

-, Conservative and Progressive Theology: Sirach and Wisdom, *CBQ* 28 (1966) 139–154.

-, Sirach 51:1–12: Poetic Structure and Analysis of Ben Sira's Psalm, *CBQ* 48 (1986) 395–407.

Lemaire, A., *Les écoles et la formation de la Bible dans l'ancien Israël*. OBO 39. Fribourg 1981.

-, Sagesse et écoles, *VT* 34 (1984) 270–281.

-, L'enseignement essénien et l'école de Qumrân, in: A. Caqout *et al.* (eds.), *Hellenica et Judaica*. FS V. Nikiprowetzky. Louvain 1986, 191–203.

-, Vers l'histoire de la rédaction des Livres des Rois, *ZAW* 98 (1986) 221–236.

-, The Sage in School and Temple, in: J.G. Gammie *et al.* (eds.), *The Sage in Israel and the Ancient Near East*. Winona Lake 1990, 165–181.

-, Education (Israel), *ABD* 2 (1992) 305–312.

Lenhardt, P., Voies de la continuité juive. Aspects de la relation maître-disciple d'après la littérature rabbinique ancienne, *RSR* 66 (1978) 489–516.

Lescow, T., Jesajas Denkschrift aus der Zeit des syrisch-ephraimitischen Krieges, *ZAW* 85 (1973) 315–331.

Lesky, A., Homeros. IX. Die Hymnen, *PWSup* 11 (1968) 824–831.

Levin, C., *Die Verheißung des neuen Bundes* in ihrem theologiegeschichtlichen Zusammenhang ausgelegt. FRLANT 137. Göttingen 1985.

Levine, A.-J., *The Social and Ethnic Dimensions of Matthean Salvation History*. "Go nowhere among the Gentiles ..." (Matt. 10:5b). SBEC 14. Lewiston 1988.

Levison, J.R., Did the Spirit Inspire Rhetoric? An Exploration of George Kennedy's Definition of Early Christian Rhetoric, in: D.F. Watson (ed.), *Persuasive Artistery*. FS G.A. Kennedy. JSNTSup 50. Sheffield 1991, 25–40.

Lewy, H., Aristotle and the Jewish Sage According to Clearchus of Soli, *HTR* 31 (1938) 205–235.

Lieberman, S., *Hellenism in Jewish Palestine*. Studies in the Literary Transmission, Beliefs and Manners of Palestine in the I Century B.C.E.–IV Century C.E. TSJTSA 18. New York 1950.

Lightstone, J.N., *Yosé the Galilean*. I. Traditions in Mishnah-Tosefta. SJLA 31. Leiden 1979.

-, Yosé the Galilean in Mishnah-Tosefta and the History of Early Rabbinic Judaism, *JJS* 31 (1980) 37–45.

Lignée, H., La place du livre des Jubilés et du Rouleau du Temple dans l'histoire du mouvement Essénien. Ces deux ouvrages ont-ils été écrits par le Maître de Justice?, *RevQ* 13 (1988) 331–345.

Lim, T.H., The Wicked Priest of the Groningen Hypothesis, *JBL* 112 (1993) 415–425

Limbeck, M., *Matthäus-Evangelium*. SKK.NT 1. Stuttgart ²1988.

Lincoln, A.T., Matthew—A Story for Teachers?, in: D.J.A. Clines *et al.* (eds.), *The Bible in three dimensions*. Essays in celebration of forty years of Biblical Studies in the University of Sheffield. JSOTSup 87. Sheffield 1990, 103–125.

Lindblom, J., *Jesu missions- och dopbefallning*. Matt. 28:18–20. Tillika en studie över det kristna dopets ursprung. Stockholm 1919.

-, *Prophecy in Ancient Israel*. Oxford 1962.

Lindemann, A., Review of E.R. Richards, *The Secretary in the Letters of Paul*. Tübingen 1991, *TLZ* 117 (1992) 915–917.

Linton, O., The Demand for a Sign from Heaven (Mk 8,11–12 and Parallels), *ST* 19 (1965) 112–129.

-, The Q-Problem Reconsidered, in: D.E. Aune (ed.), *Studies in New Testament and Early Christian Literature*. FS A.P. Wikgren. NovTSup 33. Leiden 1972, 43–59.

Lipiński, E., Royal and State Scribes in Ancient Judaism, in: J.A. Emerton (ed.), *Congress Volume Jerusalem 1986*. VTSup 40. Leiden 1988, 157–164.

Lips, H. von, *Glaube – Gemeinde – Amt*. Zum Verständnis der Ordination in den Pastoralbriefen. FRLANT 122. Göttingen 1979.

-, *Weisheitliche Traditionen im Neuen Testament*. WMANT 64. Neukirchen-Vluyn 1990.

Lipscomb, W.L. – Sanders, J.A., Wisdom at Qumran, in: J.G. Gammie *et al.* (eds.), *Israelite Wisdom*. FS S. Terrien. Missoula 1978, 277–285.

Liver, J., The "Sons of Zadok the Priests" in the Dead Sea Sect, *RevQ* 6 (1967) 3–30.

Liwak, R., *Überlieferungsgeschichtliche Probleme des Ezechielbuches*. Eine Studie zu postezechielischen Interpretationen und Komposition. Bochum 1976.

Ljungman, H., *Das Gesetz erfüllen*. Matth. 5,17ff. und 3,15 untersucht. LUÅ N.F. I 50:6. Lund 1954.

Loader, W.R.G., Son of David, Blindness, Possession, and Duality in Matthew, *CBQ* 44 (1982) 570–585.

Löhr, M., *Bildung aus dem Glauben*. Beiträge zum Verständnis der Lehrreden des Buches Jesus Sirach. Bonn 1975.

Lövestam, E., Davids-son-kristologin hos synoptikerna, *SEÅ* 37–38 (1972–73) 196–210.

Lohfink, G., *Wem gilt die Bergpredigt?* Beiträge zu einer christlichen Ethik. Freiburg 1988.

Lohfink, N., Glauben lernen in Israel, *KatBl* 108 (1983) 84–99.

-, Gottesvolk als Lerngemeinschaft. Zur Kirchenwirklichkeit im Buch Deuteronomium, *BK* 39 (1984) 90–100.

Lohfink, N. – Bergman, J., אֶחָד, *TWAT* I (1973) 210–218.

Lohmeyer, E., *Das Evangelium des Matthäus*. Für den Druck erarbeitet und herausgeben von W. Schmauch. MeyerK. Göttingen ³1962.

Lohr, C.H., Oral Techniques in the Gospel of Matthew, *CBQ* 23 (1961) 403–435.

Lohse, E., *Die Ordination im Spätjudentum und im Neuen Testament*. Göttingen 1951.

-, ῥαββί, ῥαββουνί, *TDNT* 6 (1968) 961–965.

-, "Ich aber sage euch," in: E. Lohse *et al.* (eds.), *Der Ruf Jesu und die Antwort der Gemeinde*. FS Joachim Jeremias. Göttingen 1970, 189–203.

Long, B.O., Prophetic Authority as Social Reality, in: G.W. Coats *et al.* (eds.), *Canon and Authority*. Essays in Old Testament Religion and Theology. Philadelphia 1977, 3–20.

Lord, A.B., *The Singer of Tales*. HSCL 24. Cambridge MA 1960.

-, The Gospels as Oral Traditional Literature, in: W.O. Walker, Jr (ed.), *The Relationships Among the Gospels*. An Interdisciplinary Dialogue. TUMSR 5. San Antonio 1978, 33–91.

-, Memory, Fixity, and Genre in Oral Traditional Poetries, in: J.M. Foley (ed.), *Oral Traditional Literature*. FS A.B. Lord. Columbus 1981, 451–461.

-, Characteristics of Orality, *Oral Transmission* 2:1 (1987) 54–72.

Ludwig, J., *Die Primatworte Mt 16,18.19 in der altkirchlichen Exegese*. NTAbh 19:4. Münster 1952.

Lührmann, D., Ein Weisheitspsalm aus Qumran (11QPs[a] XVIII), *ZAW* 80 (1968) 87–98.

-, Rechtfertigung und Versöhnung. Zur Geschichte der paulinischen Tradition, *ZTK* 67 (1970) 437–452.

Lundbom, J.R., Baruch, Seraiah, and Expanded Colophons in the Book of Jeremiah, *JSOT* 36 (1986) 89–114.

Luria, S., Zur Quelle von Mt 8 19, *ZNW* 25 (1926) 282–286.

Lust, J., "Gathering and Return" in Jeremiah and Ezekiel, in: P.-M. Bogaert (ed.), *Le livre de Jérémie*. Le prophète et son milieu, les oracles et leur transmission. BETL 54. Leuven 1981, 119–142.

Luz, M., A Description of the Greek Cynic in the Jerusalem Talmud, *JSJ* 20 (1989) 49–60.

Luz, U., Die Erfüllung des Gesetzes bei Matthäus (Mt 5,17–20), *ZTK* 75 (1978) 398–435.

-, The Disciples in the Gospel according to Matthew, in: G. Stanton (ed.), *The Interpretation of Matthew*. IRT 3. Philadelphia 1983, 98–128.

-, Geschichte/Geschichtsschreibung/Geschichtsphilosophie IV. Neues Testament, *TRE* 12 (1984) 595–604.

-, Die Wundergeschichten von Mt 8–9, in: G.F. Hawthorne *et al.* (eds.), *Tradition and Interpretation in the New Testament*. FS E.E. Ellis. Grand Rapids 1987, 149–161.

-, *Das Evangelium nach Matthäus*. Vols. 1–2. EKKNT 1:1–2. Zürich [2]1989 (vol. 1), 1990 (vol. 2) (not complete).

-, Das Primatwort Matthäus 16.17–19 aus wirkungsgeschichtlicher Sicht, *NTS* 37 (1991) 415–433.

-, Eine thetische Skizze der Matthäischen Christologie, in: C. Breytenbach *et al.* (eds.), *Anfänge der Christologie*. FS F. Hahn. Göttingen 1991, 221–235.

-, The Son of Man in Matthew: Heavenly Judge or Human Christ, *JSNT* 48 (1992) 3–21.

-, Review of D.B. Howell, *Matthew's Inclusive Story*. Sheffield 1990, *TLZ* 117 (1992) 189–191.

-, Fiktivität und Traditionstreue im Matthäusevangelium im Lichte griechischer Literatur, *ZNW* 84 (1993) 153–177.

Maass, F., "Tritojesaja?," in: F. Maass (ed.), *Das ferne und nahe Wort*. FS L. Rost. BZAW 105. Berlin 1967, 153–163.

Maccoby, H., *Judas Iscariot and the Myth of Jewish Evil*. London 1992.

Mack, B.L., *Wisdom and the Hebrew Epic*. Ben Sira's Hymn in Praise of the Fathers. CSHJ. Chicago 1985.

-, Sirach (Ecclesiasticus), in: B.W. Anderson (ed.), *The Books of the Bible*. Vol. 2. New York 1989, 65–86.

-, *Rhetoric and the New Testament*. GBS.NT. Minneapolis 1990.

Mack, B.L. – Murphy, R.E., Wisdom Literature, in: R.A. Kraft *et al.* (eds.), *Early Judaism and its Modern Interpreters*. SBLMI 2. Philadelphia 1986, 371–410.

Mack, B.L. – Robbins, V.K., *Patterns of Persuasion in the Gospels*. F&F: Literary Facets. Sonoma 1989.

Maier, G., *Mensch und freier Wille*. Nach den jüdischen Religionsparteien zwischen Ben Sira und Paulus. WUNT 12. Tübingen 1971.

–, Die jüdischen Lehrer bei Josephus. Einige Beobachtungen, in: O. Betz *et al.* (eds.), *Josephus-Studien*. Untersuchungen zu Josephus, dem antiken Judentum und dem Neuen Testament. FS O. Michel. Göttingen 1974, 260–270.

–, *Matthäus-Evangelium*. Vols. 1–2. BibK Edition C: C 30, B 2. Stuttgart 1979, 1980.

Maier, J., *Geschichte der jüdischen Religion*. Von der Zeit Alexanders des Grossen bis zur Aufklärung mit einem Ausblick auf das 19./20 Jahrhundert. Berlin 1972.

–, Zum Begriff יחד in den Texten von Qumran, in: K.E. Grözinger *et al.* (eds.), *Qumran*. WdF 410. Darmstadt 1981, 225–248.

–, Von Eleazar bis Zadok: CD V,2–5, *RevQ* 15 (1991) 231–241.

Malherbe, A.J., Self-Definition among Epicureans and Cynics, in: B.F. Meyer *et al.* (eds.), *Jewish and Christian Self-Definition*. Vol. 3. London 1982, 46–59.

Malina, B.J., *The New Testament World*. Insights from cultural anthropology. Atlanta 1981.

–, *Christian Origins and Cultural Anthropology:* Practical Models for Biblical Interpretation. Atlanta 1986.

Malina, B.J. – Neyrey, J.H., *Calling Jesus Names*. The Social Value of Labels in Matthew. F&F: Social Facets. Sonoma 1988.

Malina, B.J. – Rohrbaugh, R.L., *Social Science Commentary on the Synoptic Gospels*. Minneapolis 1992.

Mallau, H.H., Baruch/Baruchschriften, *TRE* 5 (1980) 269–276.

Manson, T.W., Review of Joachim Jeremias, *Die Gleichnisse Jesu*. Göttingen [2]1952, *NTS* 1 (1954–55) 57–62.

–, *The Sayings of Jesus*. As Recorded in the Gospels according to St. Matthew and St. Luke arranged with Introduction and Commentary. Grand Rapids 1979.

Marböck, J., *Weisheit im Wandel*. Untersuchungen zur Weisheitstheologie bei Ben Sira. BBB 37. Bonn 1971.

–, Gesetz und Weisheit. Zum Verständnis des Gesetzes bei Jesus Ben Sira, *BZ* 20 (1976) 1–21.

–, Sir 38,24–39,11: Der schriftgelehrte Weise. Ein Beitrag zu Gestalt und Werk Ben Siras, in: M. Gilbert (ed.), *La Sagesse de l'Ancien Testament*. BETL 51. Leuven 1979, 293–316.

Marcus, J., The Gates of Hades and the Keys of the Kingdom (Matt 16:18–19), *CBQ* 50 (1988) 443–455.

Marquet, C., Ne vous faites pas appeler 'maître'. Matthieu 23,8–12, *Christus* 30 (1983) 88–102.

Marrou, H.I., *A History of Education in Antiquity*. London 1956.

Marshall, H., Palestinian and Hellenistic Christianity: Some Critical Comments, *NTS* 19 (1972–73) 271–287.

Martin, M., *The Scribal Character of the Dead Sea Scrolls*. Vols. 1–2. BdM 44–45. Louvain 1958.

Mason, R.A., The Relation of Zech 9–14 to Proto-Zechariah, *ZAW* 88 (1976) 227–239.

–, The Purpose of the "Editorial Framework" of the Book of Haggai, *VT* 27 (1977) 413–421.

Massaux, É., *Influence de l'Évangile de Saint Matthieu* sur la littérature chrétienne avant Saint Irénée. BETL 75. Leuven [2]1986.

Matera, F.J., *Passion Narratives and Gospel Theologies*. Interpreting the Synoptics Through Their Passion Stories. TI. New York 1986.

-, The Plot of Matthew's Gospel, *CBQ* 49 (1987) 233–253.

Matheus, F., *Singt dem Herrn ein neues Lied.* Die Hymnen Deuterojesajas. SBS 141. Stuttgart 1990.

May, H.G., Towards an Objective Approach to the Book of Jeremiah: The Biographer, *JBL* 61 (1942) 139–155.

Mays, J.L., *Amos.* A Commentary. OTL. London 1969.

-, *Hosea.* A Commentary. OTL. London 1969.

McCarter, P.K., Jr, *1 Samuel.* A New Translation with Introduction, Notes & Commentary. AB 8. Garden City 1980.

McConnell, R.S., *Law and Prophecy in Matthew's Gospel.* The Authority and Use of the Old Testament in the Gospel of St. Matthew. TheolDiss 2. Basel 1969.

McDermott, J.M., Mt. 10:23 in Context, *BZ* 28 (1984) 230–240.

McEleney, N.J., The Beatitudes of the Sermon on the Mount/Plain, *CBQ* 43 (1981) 1–13.

McKane, W., *Prophets and Wise Men.* SBT 44. London 1965.

-, Relations Between Poetry and Prose in the Book of Jeremiah with Special Reference to Jeremiah III 6–11 and XII 14–17, in: L.G. Perdue *et al.* (eds.), *A Prophet to the Nations.* Essays in Jeremiah Studies. Winona Lake 1984, 269–284.

-, *A Critical and Exegetical Commentary on Jeremiah.* Vol. 1. ICC. Edinburgh 1986 (not complete).

McKay, J.W., Man's Love for God in Deuteronomy and the Father/Teacher – Son/Pupil Relationship, *VT* 22 (1972) 426–435.

McKenzie, J.L., *Second Isaiah.* Introduction, Translation and Notes. AB 20. Garden City 1968.

McKenzie, S.L., *The Trouble with Kings.* The Composition of the Books of Kings in the Deuteronomistic History. VTSup 42. Leiden 1991.

McNamara, M., *The New Testament and the Palestinian Targum to the Pentateuch.* AnBib 27. Rome 1966.

McNeile, A.H., *The Gospel According to St. Matthew.* The Greek Text with Introduction, Notes, and Indices. Thornapple Commentaries. London 1915.

Meade, D.G., *Pseudonymity and Canon.* An Investigation into the Relationship of Authorship and Authority in Jewish and Earliest Christian Tradition. WUNT 39. Tübingen 1986.

Meeks, W.A., *The Prophet-King.* Moses Traditions and the Johannine Christology. NovTSup 14. Leiden 1967.

-, Moses as God and King, in: J. Neusner (ed.), *Religions in Antiquity.* Essays in Memory of E.R. Goodenough. SHR 14. Leiden 1968, 354–371.

Meier, J.P., Salvation-History in Matthew: In Search of a Starting Point, *CBQ* 37 (1975) 203–215.

-, *Law and History in Matthew's Gospel.* A Redactional Study of Mt. 5:17–48. AnBib 71. Rome 1976.

-, Nations or Gentiles in Matthew 28:19?, *CBQ* 39 (1977) 94–102.

-, *The Vision of Matthew.* Christ, Church, and Morality in the First Gospel. TI. New York 1979.

-, *Matthew.* NTM 3. Wilmington 1980.

-, John the Baptist in Matthew's Gospel, *JBL* 99 (1980) 383–405.

-, Review of C.C. Caragounis, *Peter and the Rock.* Berlin 1990, *CBQ* 53 (1991) 492–493.

Melugin, R.F., *The Formation of Isaiah 40–55.* BZAW 141. Berlin 1976.

Ménard, J.E., Le traité de Melchisédek de Nag Hammadi, *RevScRel* 64 (1990) 235–243.

Mendecki, N., Ezechielische Redaktion des Buches Jeremia?, *BZ* 35 (1991) 242–247.

Mensching, G., *Soziologie der Religion*. Bonn 1947.

Menzies, R.P., *The Development of Early Christian Pneumatology* with special reference to Luke-Acts. JSNTSup 54. Sheffield 1991.

Merendino, R.P., *Der Erste und der Letzte*. Eine Untersuchung von Jes 40–48. VTSup 31. Leiden 1981.

-, Allein und einzig Gottes prophetisches Wort: Israels Erbe und Auftrag für alle Zukunft (Jesaja 50,4–9a.10), *ZAW* 97 (1985) 344–366.

Mettinger, T.N.D., *Solomonic State Officials*. A Study of the Civil Government Officials of the Israelite Monarchy. ConBOT 5. Lund 1971.

-, *A Farewell to the Servant Songs*. A Critical Examination of an Exegetical Axiom. ScrMin 1982–83:3. Lund 1983.

Metzger, B.M., The Furniture in the Scriptorium at Qumran, *RevQ* 1 (1959) 509–515.

-, *The Text of the New Testament*. Its Transmission, Corruption, and Restoration. Oxford [3]1992.

Meye, R.P., Messianic Secret and Messianic Didache in Mark's Gospel, in: F. Christ (ed.), *Oikonomia*. Heilsgeschichte als Thema der Theologie. FS O. Cullmann. Hamburg 1967, 57–68.

-, *Jesus and the Twelve*. Discipleship and Revelation in Mark's Gospel. Grand Rapids 1968.

Meyer, B.F., *The Aims of Jesus*. London 1979.

Meyer, R., Melchisedek von Jerusalem und Moresedek von Qumran, in: P.A.H. de Boer (ed.), *Volume du Congrès Genèva 1965*. VTSup 15. Leiden 1966, 228–239.

-, προφήτης κτλ., *TDNT* 6 (1968) 812–828.

Michaelis, C., Die Π-Alliteration der Subjektsworte der ersten 4 Seligpreisungen in Mt. V 3–6 und ihre Bedeutung für den Aufbau der Seligpreisungen bei Mt., Lk. und in Q, *NovT* 10 (1968) 148–161.

Michaelis, W., ὁδηγός, -έω, *TDNT* 5 (1967) 97–102.

Michaels, J.R., Christian Prophecy and Matthew 23:8–12. A Test Exegesis, in: G. MacRae (ed.), *Society of Biblical Literature 1976 Seminar Papers*. SBLSP 10. Missoula 1976, 305–312.

Michel, A., *Le Maître de Justice* d'après les documents de la Mer Morte, la littérature apocryphe et rabbinique. Avignon 1954.

Michel, D., Zur Eigenart Tritojesajas, *TViat* 10 (1965–66) 213–230.

-, Deuterojesaja, *TRE* 8 (1981) 510–530.

Michel, O., "Diese Kleinen" – eine Jüngerbezeichnung Jesu, *TSK* 108 (1937–38) 401–415.

-, The Conclusion of Matthew's Gospel. A Contribution to the History of the Easter Message, in: G. Stanton (ed.), *The Interpretation of Matthew*. IRT 3. London 1983, 30–41.

Middendorp, T., *Die Stellung Jesu Ben Siras zwischen Judentum und Hellenismus*. Leiden 1972.

Milik, J.T., Le travail d'édition des manuscrits de Qumran. La Grotte 4 de Qumran (4Q), *RB* 63 (1956) 60–62.

-, *Ten Years of Discovery in the Wilderness of Judaea*. SBT 26. London 1959.

-, *Milkî-ṣedeq et Milkî-reša'* dans les anciens écrits juifs et chrétiens, *JJS* 23 (1972) 95–144.

Millard, A.R., An Assessment of the Evidence for Writing in Ancient Israel, in: J. Amitai (ed.), *Biblical Archaeology Today*. Proceedings of the International Congress of Biblical Archaeology, Jerusalem, April 1984. Jerusalem 1985, 301–312.

Miller, J.M., The Elisha Cycle and the Accounts of the Omride Wars, *JBL* 85 (1966) 441–454.

Miller, J.W., *Das Verhältnis Jeremias und Hesekiels sprachlich und theologisch unter-sucht*, mit besonderer Berücksichtigung der Prosareden Jeremias. Assen 1955.

Miller, M.P., The Function of Isa 61 1–2 in 11Q Melchizedek, *JBL* 88 (1969) 467–469.

Mills, M.A., Domains of Folkloristic Concern: The Interpretation of Scriptures, in: S. Niditch (ed.), *Text and Tradition*. The Hebrew Bible and Folklore. SBLSS. Atlanta 1990, 231–241.

Minear, P.S., The Disciples and the Crowds in the Gospel of Matthew, *ATRSup* 3 (1974) 28–44.

-, *Matthew: The Teacher's Gospel*. London 1984.

Mohrlang, R., *Matthew and Paul*. A comparison of ethical perspectives. SNTSMS 48. Cambridge 1984.

Moiser, J., The Structure of Matthew 8–9: A Suggestion, *ZNW* 76 (1985) 117–118.

Mommer, P., *Samuel*. Geschichte und Überlieferung. WMANT 65. Neukirchen-Vluyn 1991.

Moor, J.C. de, Lexical Remarks Concerning *yaḥad* and *yaḥadw, VT* 7 (1957) 350–355.

Moore, G.F., *Judaism in the First Centuries of the Christian Era*. The Age of the Tannaim. Vols. 1–3. Cambridge MA 1927–1930.

Morawe, G., *Aufbau und Abgrenzung der Loblieder von Qumrân*. Studien zur gattungs-geschichtlichen Einordnung der Hodajôth. TA 16. Berlin 1961.

-, Vergleich des Aufbaus der Danklieder und hymnischen Bekenntnislieder (1QH) von Qumran mit dem Aufbau der Psalmen im Alten Testament und im Spätjudentum, *RevQ* 4 (1963) 323–356.

Morris, L., The Gospels and the Jewish Lectionaries, in: R.T. France *et al.* (eds.), *Gospel Perspectives*. Vol 3. Sheffield 1983, 129–156.

Mowery, R.L., Subtle Differences: The Matthean "Son of God" References, *NovT* 32 (1990) 193–200.

Mowinckel, S., *Zur Komposition des Buches Jeremia*. VidS II HF 1913:5. Kristiania 1914.

-, *Profeten Jesaja*. En bibelstudiebok. Oslo 1925.

-, *Jesaja-disiplene*. Profetien fra Jesaja til Jeremia. Oslo 1926.

-, Die Komposition des deuterojesajanischen Buches, *ZAW* 49 (1931) 87–112, 242–260.

-, Die Komposition des Jesajabuches Kap. 1–39, *AcOr* 11 (1933) 267–292.

-, *Prophecy and Tradition*. The Prophetic Books in the Light of the Study of the Growth and History of the Tradition. ANVAO. HF 1946:3. Oslo 1946.

-, The Hebrew Equivalent of Taxo in Ass. Mos. IX, in: G.W. Anderson *et al.* (eds.), *Congress Volume Copenhagen 1953*. VTSup 1. Leiden 1953, 88–96.

-, *He That Cometh*. Oxford 1956.

Müller, M., *Der Ausdruck "Menschensohn" in den Evangelien*. Voraussetzungen und Bedeutung. ATDan 17. Leiden 1984.

Müller, P., *Anfänge der Paulusschule*. Dargestellt am zweiten Thessalonicherbrief und am Kolosserbrief. ATANT 74. Zürich 1988.

Müller, P.-G., *Der Traditionsprozeß im Neuen Testament*. Kommunikationsanalytische Studien zur Versprachlichung des Jesusphänomens. Freiburg 1982.

Muilenburg, J., Form Criticism and Beyond, *JBL* 88 (1969) 1–18.

-, Baruch the Scribe, in: L.G. Perdue *et al.* (eds.), *A Prophet to the Nations*. Essays in Jeremiah Studies. Winona Lake 1984, 229–245.

Mundle, W., πέτρα, *NIDNTT* 3 (1978) 381–385.

Muraoka, T., Sir. 51,13–30: An Erotic Hymn to Wisdom, *JSJ* 10 (1979) 166–178.

Murphy-O'Connor, J., La genèse littéraire de la règle de la communauté, *RB* 76 (1969) 528–549.

-, An Essene Missionary Document? CD II,14–VI,1, *RB* 77 (1970) 201–229.

-, A Literary Analysis of Damascus Document XIX,33–XX,34, *RB* 79 (1972) 544–564.

-, The Essenes and their History, *RB* 81 (1974) 215–244.

-, Demetrius I and the Teacher of Righteousness (I Macc., X,25–45), *RB* 83 (1976) 400–420.

-, Judah the Essene and the Teacher of Righteousness, *RevQ* 10 (1981) 579–585.

-, The Damascus Document Revisited, in: K.H. Richards (ed.), *Society of Biblical Literature 1986 Seminar Papers*. SBLSP 25. Atlanta 1986, 369–383.

Mussner, F., Die Beschränkung auf einen einzigen Lehrer. Zu einer wenig beachteten *differentia specifica* zwischen Judentum und Christentum, in: G. Müller (ed.), *Israel hat dennoch Gott zum Trost*. FS S. Ben-Chorin. Trier 1978, 33–43.

-, *Tractate on the Jews*. The Significance of Judaism for Christian Faith. London 1984.

-, Rückfrage nach Jesus. Bericht über neue Wege und Methoden, *TBer* 13 (1985) 165–182.

-, *Die Kraft der Wurzel*. Judentum – Jesus – Kirche. Freiburg ²1987.

-, Die Stellung zum Judentum in der "Redenquelle" und in ihrer Verarbeitung bei Matthäus, in: L. Schenke (ed.), *Studien zum Matthäusevangelium*. FS W. Pesch. SBS. Stuttgart 1988, 209–225.

Nauck, W., Salt as a Metaphor in Instructions for Discipleship, *ST* 6 (1952) 165–178.

Naveh, J., A Medical Document or a Writing Exercise? The So-called 4Q Therapeia, *IEJ* 36 (1986) 52–55.

Neirynck, F., Les Femmes au Tombeau: Étude de la rédaction Matthéenne (Matt. XXVIII.1–10), *NTS* 15 (1968–69) 168–190.

-, 'Από τότε ἤρξατο and the Structure of Matthew, *ETL* 64 (1988) 21–59.

Nelson, M.D., *The Syriac Version of the Wisdom of Ben Sira Compared to the Greek and Hebrew Materials*. SBLDS 107. Atlanta 1988.

Nepper-Christensen, P., *Das Matthäusevangelium*. Ein judenchristliches Evangelium? ATDan 1. Aarhus 1958.

-, *Matthæusevangeliet*. En kommentar. Århus 1988.

Neugebauer, F., Geistsprüche und Jesuslogien, *ZNW* 53 (1962) 218–228.

Neusner, J., *Development of a Legend*. Studies on the Traditions Concerning Yoḥanan ben Zakkai. SPB 16. Leiden 1970.

-, *The Rabbinic Traditions About the Pharisees Before 70*. Vols. 1–3. Leiden 1971.

-, *Eliezer ben Hyrcanus*. The Tradition and the Man. Vols. 1–2. SJLA 3–4. Leiden 1973.

-, The Traditions Concerning Yoḥanan ben Zakkai: Reconsiderations, *JJS* 24 (1973) 65–73.

-, Exegesis and the Written Law, *JSJ* 5 (1974) 176–178.

-, The Present State of Rabbinic Biography, in: G. Nahon et al. (eds.), *Hommage à G. Vajda*. Études d'histoire et de pensée juives. Louvain 1980, 85–91.

-, *From Mishnah to Scripture*. The Problem of the Unattributed Saying With Special Reference to the Division of Purities. BJS 67. Chico 1984.

-, *In Search of Talmudic Biography*. The Problem of the Attributed Saying. BJS 70. Chico 1984.

-, *The Memorized Torah*. The Mnemonic System of the Torah. BJS 96. Chico 1985.

-, *Oral Tradition in Judaism*. The Case of the Mishnah. ABLSOT 1. New York 1987.

-, Did the Talmud's Authorship Utilize Prior "Sources?" A Response to Halivini's *Sources and Traditions*, in: J. Neusner et al. (eds.), *From Ancient Israel to Modern Judaism*. Intellect in Quest of Understanding. FS M. Fox. Vol. 2. BJS 173. Atlanta 1989, 53–79.

Newman, J., *Semikhah* (Ordination). A Study of its Origin, History and Function in

Rabbinic Literature. Manchester 1950.

Newsom, C.A., The Sage in the Literature of Qumran: The Functions of the *Maśkîl*, in: J.G. Gammie *et al.* (eds.), *The Sage in Israel and the Ancient Near East*. Winona Lake 1990, 373–382.

Neymeyr, U., *Die christlichen Lehrer im zweiten Jahrhundert*. Ihre Lehrtätigkeit, ihr Selbstverständnis und ihre Geschichte. VGSup 4. Leiden 1989.

Neyrey, J.H., The Thematic Use of Isaiah 42,1–4 in Matthew 12, *Bib* 63 (1982) 457–473.

Nicholson, E.W., *Preaching to the Exiles*. A Study of the Prose Tradition in the Book of Jeremiah. Oxford 1970.

Nickelsburg, G.W.E., *Jewish Literature Between the Bible and the Mishnah*. A Historical and Literary Introduction. London 1981.

-, Enoch, Levi, and Peter: Recipients of Revelation in Upper Galilee, *JBL* 100 (1981) 575–600.

Niditch, S (ed.), *Text and Tradition*. The Hebrew Bible and Folklore. SBLSS. Atlanta 1990.

Niehr, H., סֹפֵר, *TWAT* 5 (1986) 921–929.

Nielsen, E., *Oral Tradition*. A Modern Problem in Old Testament Introduction. SBT 11. London 1954.

Nielsen, I., Undervisningens fysiske rammer, in: C.G. Tortzen *et al.* (eds.), *Den hellenistiske skole*. Hellenismestudier 8. Aarhus 1993, 74–86.

Nilsson, M.P., *Die hellenistische Schule*. München 1955.

Nissinen, M., *Prophetie, Redaktion und Fortschreibung im Hoseabuch*. Studien zum Werdegang eines Prophetenbuches im Lichte von Hos 4 und 11. AOAT 231. Neukirchen-Vluyn 1991.

Normann, F., *Christos Didaskalos*. Die Vorstellung von Christus als Lehrer in der christlichen Literatur des ersten und zweiten Jahrhunderts. MBT 32. Münster 1967.

North, C.R., Living Issues in Biblical Scholarship. The Place of Oral Tradition in the Growth of the Old Testament, *ExpTim* 61 (1949–50) 292–296.

-, The "Former Things" and the "New Things" in Deutero-Isaiah, in: H.H. Rowley (ed.), *Studies in Old Testament Prophecy*. FS T.H. Robinson. Edinburgh 1950, 111–126.

-, *The Suffering Servant in Deutero-Isaiah*. An Historical and Critical Study. Oxford ²1956.

Nyberg, H.S., Das textkritische Problem des Alten Testaments am Hoseabuche demonstriert, *ZAW* 52 (1934) 241–254.

-, *Studien zum Hoseabuche*. Zugleich ein Beitrag zur Klärung des Problems der alttestamentlichen Textkritik. UUÅ 1935:6. Uppsala 1935.

Oberlinner, L., "... sie zweifelten aber" (Mt 28,17b). Eine Anmerkung zur matthäischen Ekklesiologie, in: L. Oberlinner *et al.* (eds.), *Salz der Erde – Licht der Welt*. Exegetische Studien zum Matthäusevangelium. FS A. Vögtle. Stuttgart 1991, 375–400.

Obrist, F., *Echtheitsfragen und Deutung der Primatsstelle Mt 16,18f. in der deutschen protestantischen Theologie der letzten dreissig Jahre*. NTAbh 21:3–4. Münster 1961.

Oepke, A., ἐπιστάτης, *TDNT* 2 (1964) 622–623.

Östborn, G., *Tōrā in the Old Testament*. A Semantic Study. Lund 1945.

Ogawa, A., *L'histoire de Jésus chez Matthieu*. La signification de l'histoire pour la théologie matthéenne. EH 23:116. Frankfurt am Main 1979.

Ollrog, W.-H., *Paulus und seine Mitarbeiter*. Untersuchungen zu Theorie und Praxis der paulinischen Mission. WMANT 50. Neukirchen-Vluyn 1979.

Olsson, B., *Structure and Meaning in the Fourth Gospel*. A Text-Linguistic analysis of John 2:1–11 and 4:1–42. ConBNT 6. Lund 1974

Olyan, S.M., Ben Sira's Relationship to the Priesthood, *HTR* 80 (1987) 261–286.

Ong, W.J., *Orality and Literacy*. The Technologizing of the Word. London 1982.

–, Orality-Literacy Studies and the Unity of the Human Race, *Oral Tradition* 2:1 (1987) 371–382.

–, Text as Interpretation: Mark and After, *Semeia* 39 (1987) 7–26.

Orton, D.E., *The Understanding Scribe*. Matthew and the Apocalyptic Ideal. JSNTSup 25. Sheffield 1989.

Oswalt, J.N., *The Book of Isaiah*. Chapters 1–39. NICOT. Grand Rapids 1986.

Overman, J.A., *Matthew's Gospel and Formative Judaism*. The Social World of the Matthean Community. Minneapolis 1990.

Pamment, M., The Kingdom of Heaven According to the First Gospel, *NTS* 27 (1981) 211–232.

–, The Son of Man in the First Gospel, *NTS* 29 (1983) 116–129.

Parsons, M.C., *The Departure of Jesus in Luke-Acts*. The Ascension Narratives in Context. JSNTSup 21. Sheffield 1987.

–, Reading a Beginning/Beginning a Reading: Tracing Literary Theory in Narrative Openings, *Semeia* 52 (1990) 11–31.

Parzen, H., The *Ruaḥ HaḲodesh* in Tannaitic Literature, *JQR* 20 (1929–30) 51–76.

Patte, D., *Early Jewish Hermeneutic in Palestine*. SBLDS 22. Missoula 1975.

–, *The Gospel According to Matthew*. A Structural Commentary on Matthew's Faith. Philadelphia 1987.

–, Prolegomena to a Study of the Disciples in Matthew. Paper presented at the SNTS Conference at Cambridge 1988, 1–54.

Paul, S., Literary and Ideological Echoes of Jeremiah in Deutero-Isaiah, in: P. Peli (ed.), *Proceedings of the Fifth World Congress of Jewish Studies*. Jerusalem, 3–11 August 1969. Vol. 1. WUJS. Jerusalem 1972, 102–120.

Pauritsch, K., *Die neue Gemeinde: Gott sammelt Ausgestossene und Arme (Jesaia 56–66)*. Die Botschaft des Tritojesaia-Buches literar-, form-, gattungskritisch und redaktionsgeschichtlich untersucht. AnBib 47. Rome 1971.

Pautrel, R., Ben Sira et le stoïcisme, *RSR* 51 (1963) 535–549.

Payne, P.B., Midrash and History in the Gospels with Special Reference to R.H. Gundry's *Matthew*, in: R.T. France *et al.* (eds.), *Gospel Perspectives*. Vol 3. Sheffield 1983, 177–215.

Peabody, D., A Pre-Markan Prophetic Sayings Tradition and the Synoptic Problem, *JBL* 97 (1978) 391–409.

Pearson, B.A., Hellenistic-Jewish Wisdom Speculation and Paul, in: R.L. Wilken (ed.), *Aspects of Wisdom in Judaism and Early Christianity*. UNDCSJCA 1. Notre Dame 1975, 43–66.

Pedley, K.G., The Library at Qumran, *RevQ* 2 (1959) 21–41.

Perkins, P., *Jesus as Teacher*. Cambridge 1990.

Perls, A., Das Plagium, *MGWJ* 58 (1914) 305–322.

Pesce, M., Discepolato gesuano e discepolato rabbinico. Problemi e prospettive della comparazione, *ANRW* II 25:1 (1982) 351–389.

Pesch, R., *Simon-Petrus*. Geschichte und geschichtliche Bedeutung des ersten Jüngers Jesu Christi. PP 15. Stuttgart 1980.

Pesch, W., *Matthäus der Seelsorger*. Das neue Verständnis der Evangelien dargestellt am Beispiel von Matthäus 18. SBS 2. Stuttgart 1966.

Péter, R., L'imposition des mains dans l'Ancien Testament, *VT* 27 (1977) 48–55.

Petersen, D.L., *Late Israelite Prophecy*. Studies in Deutero-Prophetic Literature and in Chronicles. SBLMS 23. Missoula 1977.

–, *The Roles of Israel's Prophets*. JSOTSup 17. Sheffield 1981.

Petzke, G., *Die Traditionen über Apollonius von Tyana und das Neue Testament*. SCHNT 1. Leiden 1970.

Pfeifer, G., Die Ausweisung eines lästigen Ausländers. Amos 7 10–17, *ZAW* 96 (1984) 112–118.

–, Das Ja des Amos, *VT* 39 (1989) 497–503.

–, Über den Unterschied zwischen Schriftstellern des zwanzigsten Jahrhunderts nach und des ersten Jahrtausends vor Christus. Zur Entstehung des Amosbuches, *VT* 41 (1991) 123–127.

Phillips, A., The Ecstatics' Father, in: P.R. Ackroyd *et al.* (eds.), *Words and Meanings*. FS D.W. Thomas. Cambridge 1968, 183–194.

Philonenko, M., Le Maître de justice et la Sagesse de Salomon, *TZ* 14 (1958) 81–88.

–, *Les interpolations chrétiennes des Testaments des Douze Patriarches et les manuscrits du Qoumrân*. CRHPR 35. Paris 1960.

–, Un titre messianique de Bar Kokheba, *TZ* 17 (1961) 434–435.

Pilch, J.J., Teacher for a troubled Church: Matthew's Jesus, *BibTod* 25 (1987) 23–28.

Ploeg, J. van der, Le rôle de la tradition orale dans la transmission du texte de l'ancien testament, *RB* 54 (1947) 5–41.

Plöger, O., *Theokratie und Eschatologie*. WMANT 2. Neukirchen-Vluyn 1959.

Plümacher, E., Eine Thukydidesreminiszenz in der Apostelgeschichte (Act 20,33–35 – Thuk. II 97,3f), *ZNW* 83 (1992) 270–275.

Pohlmann, K.-F., *Ezechielstudien*. Zur Redaktionsgeschichte des Buches und zur Frage nach den ältesten Texten. BZAW 202. Berlin 1992.

Polag, A., *Die Christologie der Logienquelle*. WMANT 45. Neukirchen-Vluyn 1977.

Popkes, W., Die Gerechtigkeitstradition im Matthäus-Evangelium, *ZNW* 80 (1989) 1–23.

Porter, J.R., The origins of prophecy in Israel, in: R. Coggins *et al.* (eds.), *Israel's Prophetic Tradition*. FS P.R. Ackroyd. Cambridge 1982, 12–31.

Pouilly, J., L'Évolution de la Législation Pénale dans la Communauté de Qumrân, *RB* 82 (1975) 522–551.

–, *La Règle de la Communauté de Qumrân*. Son évolution littéraire. CahRB 17. Paris 1976.

Powell, M.A., *What Is Narrative Criticism?* GBS.NT. Minneapolis 1990.

–, The Plot and Subplots of Matthew's Gospel, *NTS* 38 (1992) 187–204.

Pregeant, R., The Wisdom Passages in Matthew's Story, in: D.J. Lull (ed.), *Society of Biblical Literature 1990 Seminar Papers*. SBLSP 29. Atlanta 1990, 469–493.

Preuß, H.D., *Einführung in die alttestamentliche Weisheitsliteratur*. UrbT 383. Stuttgart 1987.

–, Zum deuteronomistischen Geschichtswerk, *TRu* 58 (1993) 229–264.

Przybylski, B., *Righteousness in Matthew and his world of thought*. SNTSMS 41. Cambridge 1980.

Puech, É., Les écoles dans l'Israël préexilique: données épigraphiques, in: J.A. Emerton (ed.), *Congress Volume Jerusalem 1986*. VTSup 40. Leiden 1988, 189–203.

Puskas, C.B., *An Introduction to the New Testament*. Peabody 1989.

Qimron, E. – Strugnell, J., An Unpublished Halakhic Letter from Qumran, in: J. Amitai (ed.), *Biblical Archaeology Today*. Proceedings of the International Congress of Biblical Archaeology, Jerusalem, April 1984. Jerusalem 1985, 400–407.

Quesnel, M., *Jésus-Christ selon saint Matthieu*. Synthèse théologique. Paris 1991.

Rabinowitz, I., The Guides of Righteousness, *VT* 8 (1958) 391–404.

–, The Qumran Author's *spr hhgw/y*, *JNES* 20 (1961) 109–114.

–, The Qumran Hebrew Original of Ben Sira's Concluding Acrostic on Wisdom, *HUCA* 42 (1971) 173–184.

Rabinowitz, L.I., Rabbi, Rabbinate, *EncJud* 13 (1971) 1445.

Rad, G. von, Die Stadt auf dem Berge, *EvT* 8 (1948–49) 439–447.

–, *Wisdom in Israel.* London 1972.

–, *Old Testament Theology.* Vols. 1–2. London 1975.

Radday, Y.T. – Wickmann, D., The Unity of Zechariah Examined in the Light of Statistical Linguistics, *ZAW* 87 (1975) 30–55.

Raitt, T.M., *A Theology of Exile.* Judgment/Deliverance in Jeremiah and Ezekiel. Philadelphia 1977.

Redditt, P.L., Israel's Sheppherds: Hope and Pessimism in Zechariah 9–14, *CBQ* 51 (1989) 631–642.

Reeves, J.C., The Meaning of *Moreh Ṣedeq* in the Light of 11QTorah, *RevQ* 13 (1988) 287–298.

Reiling, J., *Hermas and Christian Prophecy.* A Study of the Eleventh Mandate. NovTSup 37. Leiden 1973.

Reisch, E., Διδάσκαλος, *PW* 5 (1905) 401–406.

Reiser, M., *Syntax und Stil des Markusevangeliums* im Licht der hellenistischen Volksliteratur. WUNT 2:11. Tübingen 1983.

Reiser, W., Eschatologische Gottessprüche in den Elisa-Legenden, *TZ* 9 (1953) 321–338.

Renaud, B., L'alliance éternelle d'Éz 16:59–63 et l'alliance nouvelle de Jér 31:31–34, in: J. Lust (ed.), *Ezekiel and His Book.* Textual and Literary Criticism and their Interrelation. BETL 74. Leuven 1986, 335–339.

Rendtorff, R., Erwägungen zur Frühgeschichte des Prophetentums in Israel, *ZTK* 59 (1962) 145–167.

–, προφήτης κτλ., *TDNT* 6 (1968) 796–812.

–, Zur Komposition des Buches Jesaja, *VT* 34 (1984) 295–320.

–, *The Old Testament.* An Introduction. London 1985.

–, Between Historical Criticism and Holistic Interpretation: New Trends in Old Testament Exegesis, in: J.A. Emerton (ed.), *Congress Volume Jerusalem 1986.* VTSup 40. Leiden 1988, 298–303.

–, Jesaja 6 im Rahmen der Komposition des Jesajabuches, in: J. Vermeylen (ed.), *The Book of Isaiah – Le Livre d'Isaïe.* Les oracles et leurs relectures. Unité et complexité de l'ouvrage. BETL 81. Leuven 1989, 73–82.

Rengstorf, K.H., διδάσκω κτλ., *TDNT* 2 (1964) 135–165.

–, μανθάνω κτλ., *TDNT* 4 (1967) 390–461.

Reventlow, H.G., Das Ende der sog. "Denkschrift" Jesajas, *BN* 38–39 (1987) 62–67.

Richards, R.E., *The Secretary in the Letters of Paul.* WUNT 2:42. Tübingen 1991.

Richter, A., Hauptlinien in Deuterojesaja-Forschung von 1964–1979, in: C. Westermann, *Sprache und Struktur der Prophetie Deuterojesajas.* CThM 11. Stuttgart ²1981, 89–131.

Rickenbacher, O., *Weisheitsperikopen bei Ben Sira.* OBO 1. Fribourg 1973.

Riesener, I., *Der Stamm עבד im Alten Testament.* Eine Wortuntersuchung unter Berücksichtigung neuerer sprachwissenschaftlicher Methoden. BZAW 149. Berlin 1979.

Riesenfeld, H., The Gospel Tradition and its Beginnings, *SE* 1 (TU 73) (1959) 43–65.

Riesner, R., Der Aufbau der Reden im Matthäus-Evangelium, *TBei* 9 (1978) 172–182.

–, Jüdische Elementarbildung und Evangelienüberlieferung, in: R.T. France *et al.* (eds.), *Gospel Perspectives.* Vol. 1. Sheffield 1980, 209–223.

–, *Jesus als Lehrer.* Eine Untersuchung zum Ursprung der Evangelien-Überlieferung. WUNT 2:7.Tübingen ³1988.

–, Jesus as Teacher and Preacher, in: H. Wansbrough (ed.), *Jesus and the Oral Gospel Tradition.* JSNTSup 64. Sheffield 1991, 185–210.

-, Review of D. Wenham, *The Rediscovery of Jesus' Eschatological Discourse*. Sheffield 1984, *TZ* 46 (1990) 82–83.

-, Teacher, in: J.B. Green *et al.* (eds.), *Dictionary of Jesus and the Gospels*. Downers Grove 1992, 807–811.

Rießler, P., Unterricht im A.T., *TQ* 91 (1909) 606–607.

Rietzschel, C., *Das Problem der Urrolle*. Ein Beitrag zur Redaktionsgeschichte des Jeremiabuches. Gütersloh 1966.

Rignell, L.G., Das Orakel "Maher-salal Has bas." Jesaja 8, *ST* 10 (1956) 40–52.

Ringgren, H., Oral and Written Transmission in the O.T., *ST* 3 (1949) 34–59.

-, Literarkritik, Formgeschichte, Überlieferungsgeschichte, *TLZ* 91 (1966) 641–650.

-, אָב, *TWAT* 1 (1973) 1–19.

Robbins, V.K., The Chreia, in: D.E. Aune (ed.), *Greco-Roman Literature and the New Testament*. SBLSBS 21. Atlanta 1988, 1–23.

-, *Jesus the Teacher*. A Socio-Rhetorical Interpretation of Mark. With a New Introduction. Minneapolis ²1992.

Roberts, C.H., The Ancient Book and the Ending of St Mark, *JTS* 40 (1939) 253–257.

Roberts, J.J.M., Isaiah in Old Testament Theology, *Int* 36 (1982) 130–143.

Robinson, B.P., Peter and His Successors: Tradition and Redaction in Matthew 16.17–19, *JSNT* 21 (1984) 85–104.

Robinson, J.M., Jesus as Sophos and Sophia: Wisdom Tradition and the Gospels, in: R.L. Wilken (ed.), *Aspects of Wisdom in Judaism and Early Christianity*. UND-CSJCA 1. Notre Dame 1975, 1–16.

-, The Sayings Gospel Q, in: F. Van Segbroeck *et al.* (eds.), *The Four Gospels 1992*. FS F. Neirynck. BETL 100. Leuven 1992, 361–388.

Römheld, D., *Wege der Weisheit*. Die Lehren Amenemopes und Proverbien 22,17–24,22. BZAW 184. Berlin 1989.

Rofé, A., The Classification of the Prophetical Stories, *JBL* 89 (1970) 427–440.

-, *The Prophetical Stories*. The Narratives about the Prophets in the Hebrew Bible. Their Literary Types and History. Jerusalem 1988.

Roloff, J., *Das Kerygma und der irdische Jesus*. Historische Motive in den Jesus-Erzählungen der Evangelien. Göttingen ²1973.

-, *Die Kirche im Neuen Testament*. NTD Ergänzungsreihe 10. Göttingen 1993.

Romaniuk, C., Le thème de la Sagesse dans les documents de Qumrân, *RevQ* 9 (1978) 429–435.

Rordorf, W., Does the Didache Contain Jesus Tradition Independently of the Synoptic Gospels?, in: H. Wansbrough (ed.), *Jesus and the Oral Gospel Tradition*. JSNTSup 64. Sheffield 1991, 394–423.

Rosenberg, B.A., The Complexity of Oral Tradition, *Oral Tradition* 2:1 (1987) 73–90.

Rosmarin, A., *Moses im Lichte der Agada*. New York 1932.

Rost, L., Gruppenbildungen im Alten Testament, *TLZ* 80 (1955) 1–8.

Roth, C., The Teacher of Righteousness and the Prophecy of Joel, *VT* 13 (1963) 91–95.

-, Minhagim Books, *EncJud* 12 (1971) 26–31.

Rothfuchs, W., *Die Erfüllungszitate des Matthäus-Evangeliums*. Eine biblisch-theologische Untersuchung. BWANT 88. Stuttgart 1969.

Rothkoff, A., Moses, *EncJud* 12 (1971) 393–398.

-, Semikhah, *EncJud* 14 (1971) 1140–1142.

Rowley, H.H., 4QpNahum and the Teacher of Righteousness, *JBL* 75 (1956) 188–193.

Rudolph, W., *Hosea*. KAT 13:1. Gütersloh 1966.

-, *Jeremia*. HAT 1:12. Tübingen ³1968.

-, *Joel – Amos – Obadja – Jona*. Mit einer Zeittafel von A. Jepsen. KAT 13:2. Gütersloh 1971.

Rüger, H.P., *Text und Textform im hebräischen Sirach.* Untersuchungen zur Textgeschichte und Textkritik der hebräischen Sirachfragmente aus der Kairoer Geniza. BZAW 112. Berlin 1970.

-, Oral Tradition in the Old Testament, in: H. Wansbrough (ed.), *Jesus and the Oral Gospel Tradition.* JSNTSup 64. Sheffield 1991, 107–120.

Ruppert, L., *Der leidende Gerechte.* Eine motivgeschichtliche Untersuchung zum Alten Testament und zwischentestamentlichen Judentum. FB 5. Würzburg 1972.

-, Beobachtungen zur Literar- und Kompositionskritik von Hosea 1–3, in: L. Ruppert *et al.* (eds.), *Künder des Wortes.* Beiträge zur Theologie der Propheten. FS J. Schreiner. Würzburg 1982, 163–182.

Ruprecht, E., Die ursprüngliche Komposition der Hiskia-Jesaja-Erzählungen und ihre Umstrukturierung duch den Verfasser des deuteronomistischen Geschichtswerkes, *ZTK* 87 (1990) 33–66.

Rydbeck, L., Från Prometheus härstammar allt som mänskligheten kan: om den antika, grekiska kulturens inriktning mot det förflutna, in: *Människan i samspel.* FS A. Werner. Lund 1990, 89–107.

Rylaarsdam, J.C., *Revelation in Jewish Wisdom Literature.* Chicago 1946.

Sabourin, L., "You Will Not Have Gone Through All the Towns of Israel, Before the Son of Man Comes" (Mat 10:23b), *BTB* 7 (1977) 5–11.

Safrai, S., Elementary Education, its Religious and Social Significance in the Talmudic Period, in: H.H. Ben-Sasson *et al.* (eds.), *Jewish Society Through the Ages.* London 1971, 148–169.

-, Tales of the Sages in the Palestinian Tradition and the Babylonian Talmud, *ScrHier* 22 (1971) 209–232.

-, Education and the Study of the Torah, in: S. Safrai *et al.* (eds.), *The Jewish People in the First Century.* Historical Geography, Political History, Social, Cultural and Religious Life and Institutions. CRINT I 2. Assen 1976, 945–970.

-, Oral Tora, in: S. Safrai (ed.), *The Literature of the Sages.* Vol. 1. CRINT II 3:1. Assen 1987, 35–119.

-, Halakha, in: S. Safrai (ed.), *The Literature of the Sages.* Vol. 1. CRINT II 3:1. Assen 1987, 121–209.

Saggin, L., Magister vester unus est, Christus (Mt 23,10), *VD* 30 (1952) 205–213.

Saito, T., *Die Mosevorstellungen im Neuen Testament.* EH 23:100. Bern 1977.

Salas, A., El tema de la "Montaña" en el primer evangelio. ¿Precisión geográfica o motivación teológica?, *CD* 188 (1975) 3–17.

Saldarini, A.J., Johanan ben Zakkai's Escape from Jerusalem. Origin and Development of a Rabbinic Story, *JSJ* 6 (1975) 189–204.

-, "Form Criticism" of Rabbinic Literature, *JBL* 96 (1977) 257–274.

-, Reconstructions of Rabbinic Judaism, in: R.A. Kraft *et al.* (eds.), *Early Judaism and its Modern Interpreters.* SBLBMI 2. Philadelphia 1986, 437–477.

-, *Pharisees, Scribes and Sadducees in Palestinian Society.* A Sociological Approach. Wilmington 1988.

Sand, A., *Das Gesetz und die Propheten.* Untersuchungen zur Theologie des Evangeliums nach Matthäus. BU 11. Regensburg 1974.

-, Propheten, Weise und Schriftkundige in der Gemeinde des Matthäusevangeliums, in: J. Hainz (ed.), *Kirche im Werden.* Studien zum Thema Amt und Gemeinde im Neuen Testament. Paderborn 1976, 167–184.

-, *Reich Gottes und Eheverzicht im Evangelium nach Matthäus.* SBS 109. Stuttgart 1983.

-, *Das Evangelium nach Matthäus.* RNT. Regensburg 1986.

-, *Das Matthäus-Evangelium.* ErFor 275. Darmstadt 1991.

-, Review of C.C. Caragounis, *Peter and the Rock.* Berlin 1990, *TRev* 88 (1992) 29–30.

Sandelin, K.-G., *Wisdom as Nourisher.* A Study of an Old Testament Theme, its Development within Early Judaism and its Impact on Early Christianity. AAA. Ser. A 64:3. Åbo 1986.

Sanders, E.P., *The Tendencies of the Synoptic Tradition.* SNTSMS 9. Cambridge 1969.

-, *Paul and Palestinian Judaism.* A Comparison of Patterns of Religion. London 1977.

-, *Jewish Law from Jesus to the Mishnah.* Five Studies. London 1990.

Sanders, E P. – Davies, M., *Studying the Synoptic Gospels.* London 1989.

Sanders, J.T., *Ben Sira and Demotic Wisdom.* SBLMS 28. Chico 1983.

Sandnes, K.O., *Paul—One of the Prophets?* A Contribution to the Apostle's Self-Understanding. WUNT 2:43. Tübingen 1991.

Sato, M., *Q und Prophetie.* Studien zur Gattungs- und Traditionsgeschichte der Quelle Q. WUNT 2:29. Tübingen 1988.

Sauer, G., אזר, *THAT* 1 (³1978) 104–107.

Sawyer, J.F.A., Daughter of Zion and Servant of the Lord in Isaiah: A Comparison, *JSOT* 44 (1989) 89–107.

Schäfer, P., *Die Vorstellung vom heiligen Geist in der rabbinischen Literatur.* SANT 28. München 1972.

-, *Studien zur Geschichte und Theologie des rabbinischen Judentums.* AGJU 15. Leiden 1978.

-, Die Flucht Johanan b. Zakkais aus Jerusalem und die Gründung des 'Lehrhauses' in Jabne, *ANRW* II 19:2 (1979) 43–101.

-, Research into Rabbinic Literature: An Attempt to Define the *Status Quaestionis, JJS* 37 (1986) 139–152.

Schäfer-Lichtenberger, C., 'Josua' und 'Elischa' – eine biblische Argumentation zur Begründung der Autorität und Legitimität des Nachfolgers, *ZAW* 101 (1989) 198–222.

Schawe, E., *Gott als Lehrer im Alten Testament.* Eine semantisch-theologische Studie. Fribourg 1979.

Schechter, S., The Rabbinical Concept of Holiness, *JQR* 10 (1897–98) 1–12.

-, Some Rabbinic Parallels to the New Testament, *JQR* 12 (1899–1900) 415–433.

Schedl, C., *Rufer des Heils in heilloser Zeit.* Der Prophet Jesajah Kapitel I–XII logotechnisch und bibeltheologisch erklärt. Paderborn 1973.

-, *Zur Christologie der Evangelien.* Wien 1984.

Schenk, W., Das "Matthäusevangelium" als Petrusevangelium, *BZ* 27 (1983) 58–80.

-, *Die Sprache des Matthäus.* Die Text-Konstituenten in ihren makro- und mikrostrukturellen Relationen. Göttingen 1987.

Schiffman, L.H., *The Halakhah at Qumran.* SJLA 16. Leiden 1975.

-, *Sectarian Law in the Dead Sea Scrolls.* Courts, Testimony and the Penal Code. BJS 33. Chico 1983.

-, *The Eschatological Community of the Dead Sea Scrolls.* A Study of the Rule of the Congregation. SBLMS 38. Atlanta 1989.

-, *Miqsat maʿaśeh ha-torah* and the Temple Scroll, *RevQ* 14 (1990) 435–457.

-, Messianic Figures and Ideas in the Qumran Scrolls, in: J.H. Charlesworth (ed.), *The Messiah.* Developments in Earliest Judaism and Christianity. The First Princeton Symposium on Judaism and Christian Origins. Minneapolis 1992, 116–129.

Schildenberger, J., Die Bedeutung von Sir 48,24f. für die Verfasserfrage von Is 40–66, in: H. Junker *et al.* (eds.), *Alttestamentliche Studien.* FS F. Nötscher. BBB 1. Bonn 1950, 188–204.

Schimanowski, G., *Weisheit und Messias.* Die jüdischen Voraussetzungen der urchristlichen Präexistenzchristologie. WUNT 2:17. Tübingen 1985.

Schlatter, A., *Der Evangelist Matthäus. Seine Sprache, sein Ziel, seine Selbständigkeit.* Stuttgart ³1948.

Schlott, A., *Schrift und Schreiber im Alten Ägypten.* BAB. München 1989.

Schmauch, W., *Orte der Offenbarung und der Offenbarungsort im Neuen Testament.* Göttingen 1956.

Schmidt, D., The LXX *Gattung* "Prophetic Correlative," *JBL* 96 (1977) 517–522.

Schmidt, K.L., *Der Rahmen der Geschichte Jesu.* Literarkritische Untersuchungen zur ältesten Jesusüberlieferung. Berlin 1919.

Schmidt, W.H., Die deuteronomistische Redaktion des Amosbuches, *ZAW* 77 (1965) 168–193.

Schmithals, W., *Einleitung in die drei ersten Evangelien.* Berlin 1985.

Schmitt, A., *Entrückung – Aufnahme – Himmelfahrt.* Untersuchungen zu einem Vorstellungsbereich im Alten Testament. FB 10. Würzburg 1973.

Schmitt, H.-C., *Elisa.* Traditionsgeschichtliche Untersuchungen zur vorklassischen nordisraelitischen Prophetie. Gütersloh 1972.

–, Prophetie und Tradition. Beobachtungen zur Frühgeschichte des israelitischen Nabitums, *ZTK* 74 (1977) 255–272.

–, Prophetie und Schultheologie im Deuterojesajabuch. Beobachtungen zur Redaktionsgeschichte von Jes 40–55, *ZAW* 91 (1979) 43–61.

Schnabel, E.J., *Law and Wisdom from Ben Sira to Paul.* A Tradition Historical Enquiry into the Relation of Law, Wisdom, and Ethics. WUNT 2:16. Tübingen 1985.

Schnackenburg, R., Die Erwartung des "Propheten" nach dem Neuen Testament und den Qumran-Texten, *SE* 1 (TU 73) (1959) 622–639.

–, Petrus im Matthäusevangelium, in: *À cause de l'évangile.* Études sur les Synoptiques et les Actes. FS J. Dupont. LD 123. Paris 1985, 107–125.

–, *Matthäusevangelium.* Vols. 1–2. Die neue EB 1:1–2. Würzburg 1985, 1987.

–, "Jeder Schriftgelehrte, der ein Jünger des Himmelreiches geworden ist" (Mt 13,52), in: K. Aland *et al.* (eds.), *Wissenschaft und Kirche.* FS E. Lohse. TAB 4. Bielefeld 1989, 57–69.

–, "Siehe da mein Knecht, den ich erwählt habe ..." (Mt 12,18). Zur Heiltätigkeit Jesu im Matthäusevangelium, in: L. Oberlinner *et al.* (eds.), *Salz der Erde – Licht der Welt.* Exegetische Studien zum Matthäusevangelium. FS A. Vögtle. Stuttgart 1991, 203–222.

Schneider, G., ῥαββί κτλ., *EWNT* 3 (1983) 493–495.

–, "Im Himmel – auf Erden," eine Perspektive matthäischer Theologie, in: L. Schenke (ed.), *Studien zum Matthäusevangelium.* FS W. Pesch. SBS. Stuttgart 1988, 283–297.

Schniewind, J., *Das Evangelium nach Matthäus.* NTD 2. Göttingen ⁹1960.

Schoedel, W.R., *Ignatius of Antioch.* A Commentary of the Letters of Ignatius of Antioch. Hermeneia. Philadelphia 1985.

Schöllgen, G., Wandernde oder seßhafte Lehrer in der Didache?, *BN* 52 (1990) 19–26.

Scholtissek, K., *Die Vollmacht Jesu.* Traditions- und redaktionsgeschichtliche Analysen zu einem Leitmotiv markinischer Christologie. NTAbh Neue Folge 25. Münster 1992.

Schoors, A., *I Am God Your Saviour.* A Form-Critical Study of the Main Genres in Is. XL–LV. VTSup 24. Leiden 1973.

Schottroff, W., *'Gedenken' im Alten Orient und im Alten Testament.* WMANT 15. Neukirchen-Vluyn 1964.

Schreiner, J., Das Buch jesajanischer Schule, in: J. Schreiner (ed.), *Wort und Botschaft.* Eine theologische und kritische Einführung in die Probleme des Alten Testaments. Würzburg 1967, 143–162.

Schrenk, G., δίκαιος, *TDNT* 2 (1964) 182–191.

-, πατήρ, *TDNT* 5 (1967) 974–1014.

Schubert, K., Testamentum Juda 24 im Lichte der Texte von Chirbet Qumran, *WZKM* 53 (1957) 227–236.

-, Die Messiaslehre in den Texten von Chirbet Qumran, in: K.E. Grötzinger *et al.* (eds.), *Qumran.* WdF 410. Darmstadt 1981, 341–364.

Schubert, M., *Schöpfungstheologie bei Kohelet.* BEATAJ 15. Frankfurt am Main 1989.

Schürer, E., *The History of the Jewish People in the Age of Jesus Christ (175 B.C.– A.D. 135).* A New English Version Revised and Edited by G. Vermes *et al.* Vols. 1– 3. Edinburgh 1973–1987.

Schürmann, H., *Traditionsgeschichtliche Untersuchungen zu den synoptischen Evangelien.* KBANT. Düsseldorf 1968.

-, Lehrende in den neutestamentlichen Schriften. Ihre Angewiesenheit auf andere geistliche Gaben und ihre Verwiesenheit an andere geistliche Dienste, in: W. Baier *et al.* (eds.), *Weisheit Gottes – Weisheit der Welt.* FS J. Ratzinger. Vol. 1. St. Ottilien 1987, 419–440.

Schult, H., עמש, *THAT* 2 (²1979) 974–982.

Schulz, A., *Nachfolgen und Nachahmen.* Studien über das Verhältnis der neutestamentlichen Jüngerschaft zur urchristlichen Vorbildethik. SANT 6. München 1962.

Schulz, P., *Der Autoritätsanspruch des Lehrers der Gerechtigkeit in Qumran.* Meisenheim am Glan 1974.

Schwartz, D.R., On Two Aspects of a Priestly View of Descent at Qumran, in: L.H. Schiffman (ed.), *Archaeology and History in the Dead Sea Scrolls.* The New York University Conference in Memory of Y. Yadin. JSPSup 8. Sheffield 1990, 157–179.

Schweitzer, F.M., The Teacher of Righteousness, in: Z.J. Kapera (ed.), *Mogilany 1989.* Papers on the Dead Sea Scrolls offered in memory of J. Carmignic. Vol. 2. QM 3. Kraków 1991, 53–97.

Schweizer, E., *Church Order in the New Testament.* SBT 32. London 1961.

-, Observance of the Law and Charismatic Activity in Matthew, *NTS* 16 (1969–70) 213– 230.

-, Formgeschichtliches zu den Seligpreisungen Jesu, *NTS* 19 (1972–73) 121–126.

-, *Das Evangelium nach Matthäus.* NTD 2. Göttingen ³1981.

-, Matthew's Church, in: G. Stanton (ed.), *The Interpretation of Matthew.* IRT 3. London 1983, 129–155.

Scott, B.B., *Hear Then the Parable.* A Commentary on the Parables of Jesus. Minneapolis 1989.

-, The Birth of the Reader, *Semeia* 52 (1990) 83–102.

Segal, M.H., The Habakkuk "Commentary" and the Damascus Fragments, *JBL* 70 (1951) 131–147.

Segbroeck, F. Van, Jésus rejeté par sa patrie (Mt 13,54–58), *Bib* 49 (1968) 167–198.

Seidelin, P., Der ʿEbed Jahwe und die Messiasgestalt im Jesajatargum, *ZAW* 35 (1936) 194–231.

Seifrid, M.A., *Justification by Faith.* The Origin and Development of a Central Pauline Theme. NovTSup 68. Leiden 1992.

Seitz, C.R., Isaiah 1–66: Making Sense of the Whole, in: C.R. Seitz (ed.), *Reading and Preaching the Book of Isaiah.* Philadelphia 1988, 105–126.

-, *Theology in Conflict.* Reactions to the Exile in the Book of Jeremiah. BZAW 176. Berlin 1989.

-, Mose als Prophet. Redaktionsthemen und Gesamtstruktur des Jeremiabuches, *BZ* 34 (1990) 234–245.

-, *Zion's Final Destiny.* The Development of the Book of Isaiah. A Reassessment of Isaiah 36–39. Minneapolis 1991.

Sekine, S., *Die Tritojesajanische Sammlung (56–66) redaktionsgeschichtlich untersucht.* BZAW 175. Berlin 1989.

Sekki, A.E., *The Meaning of Ruaḥ at Qumran.* SBLDS 110. Atlanta 1989.

Sellers, O.R., A Possible Old Testament Reference to the Teacher of Righteousness, *IEJ* 5 (1955) 93–95.

Sellin, G., "Gattung" und "Sitz im Leben" auf dem Hintergrund der Problematik von Mündlichkeit und Schriftlichkeit synoptischer Erzählungen, *EvT* 50 (1990) 311–331.

Senior, D.(P.), *The Passion Narrative According to Matthew.* A Redactional Study. BETL 39. Leuven 1975.

-, *What Are They Saying About Matthew?* New York 1983.

Shanks, H., Is the Title "Rabbi" Anachronistic in the Gospels, *JQR* 53 (1962–63) 337–345.

-, Origins of the Title "Rabbi," *JQR* 59 (1968–69) 152–157.

-, Jeremiah's Scribe and Confidant Speaks from a Hoard of Clay Bullae, *BARev* 13:5 (1987) 58–65.

-, Blood on the Floor at New York Dead Sea Scroll Conference. Qumran Scriptorium Reinterpreted as a Dining Room, *BARev* 19:2 (1993) 63–68.

-, The Qumran Settlement. Monastery, Villa or Fortress?, *BARev* 19:3 (1993) 62–65.

Sheppard, G.T., Wisdom and Torah: The Interpretation of Deuteronomy Underlying Sirach 24:23, in: G.A. Tuttle (ed.), *Biblical and Near Eastern Studies.* FS W.S. LaSor. Grand Rapids 1978, 166–176.

Sheridan, M., Disciples and Discipleship in Matthew and Luke, *BTB* 3 (1973) 235–255.

Shiloh, Y., *Excavations at the City of David.* I. 1978–1982. Interim Report of the First Five Seasons. Qedem 19. Jerusalem 1984.

-, The City of David: 1978–1983, in: J. Amitai (ed.), *Biblical Archaeology Today.* Proceedings of the International Congress of Biblical Archaeology, Jerusalem, April 1984. Jerusalem 1985, 451–462.

-, A Group of Hebrew Bullae from the City of David, *IEJ* 36 (1986) 16–38.

Shiloh, Y. – Tarler, D., Bullae from the City of David. A Hoard of Seal Impressions from the Israelite Period, *BA* 49 (1986) 196–209.

Shils, E., *Tradition.* London 1981.

Shimoff, S.R., Hellenization among the Rabbis: Some Evidence from Early Aggadot Concerning David and Solomon, *JSJ* 18 (1987) 168–187.

Shuler, P.L., *A Genre for the Gospels.* The Biographical Character of Matthew. Philadelphia 1982.

-, The Genre(s) of the Gospels, in: D.L. Dungan (ed.), *The Interrelations of the Gospels.* A Symposium led by M.-É. Boismard – W.R. Farmer – F. Neirynck, Jerusalem 1984. BETL 95. Leuven 1990, 459–483, 495–496.

Shupak, N., The 'Sitz im Leben' of the Book of Proverbs in the Light of a Comparison of Biblical and Egyptian Wisdom Literature, *RB* 94 (1987) 98–119.

Siegel, J.P., Two Further Medieval References to the Teacher of Righteousness, *RevQ* 9 (1978) 437–440.

Sievers, J., *The Hasmoneans and Their Supporters.* From Mattathias to the Death of John Hyrcanus I. SFSHJ 06. Atlanta 1990.

Sigal, P., *The Halakah of Jesus of Nazareth according to the Gospel of Matthew.* Lanham 1986.

Silberman, N.A., Ossuary, *BARev* 17:3 (1991) 73–74.

Simian-Yofre, H., Wächter, Lehrer oder Interpret? Zum theologischen Hintergrund von Ez 33,7–9, in: L. Ruppert et al. (eds.), *Künder des Wortes.* Beiträge zur Theologie der Propheten. FS J. Schreiner. Würzburg 1982, 151–162.

Sjöberg, E., πνεῦμα, πνευματικός, *TDNT* 6 (1968) 375–389.

Skehan, P.W., The Acrostic Poem in Sirach 51:13–30, *HTR* 64 (1971) 387–400.

Skehan, P.W. – Lella, A.A. di, *The Wisdom of Ben Sira*. AB 39. Garden City 1987.

Slusser, M., Reading Silently in Antiquity, *JBL* 111 (1992) 499.

Smelik, K.A.D., *Converting the Past*. Studies in Ancient Israelite and Moabite Historiography. OTS 28. Leiden 1992.

Smend, Rudolf, *Die Weisheit des Jesus Sirach erklärt*. Berlin 1906.

Smend, Rudolf, Der biblische und der historische Elia, in: G.W. Anderson *et al.* (eds.), *Congress Volume Edinburgh 1974*. VTSup 28. Leiden 1975, 167–184.

–, *Die Entstehung des Alten Testaments*. TW 1. Stuttgart 1978.

Smit Sibinga, J., Eine literarische Technik im Matthäusevangelium: in: M. Didier (ed.), *L'Évangile selon Matthieu*. Rédaction et théologie. BETL 29. Gembloux 1972, 99–105.

–, The Structure of the Apocalyptic Discourse, Matthew 24 and 25, *ST* 29 (1975) 71–79.

Smith, M., *Tannaitic Parallels to the Gospels*. SBLMS 6. Philadelphia 1951.

–, A Comparison of Early Christian and Early Rabbinic Tradition, *JBL* 82 (1963) 169–176.

–, *Palestinian Parties and Politics that Shaped the Old Testament*. London [2]1987.

Smith, R.H., *Matthew*. ACNT. Minneapolis 1989.

Smith, T.V., *Petrine Controversies in Early Christianity*. WUNT 2:15. Tübingen 1985.

Snaith, J.G., *Ecclesiasticus* or the Wisdom of Jesus Son of Sirach. CBC. Cambridge 1974.

Snodgrass, K., *The Parable of the Wicked Tenants*. An Inquiry into Parable Interpretation. WUNT 27. Tübingen 1983.

Soares Prabhu, G.M., *The Formula Quotations in the Infancy Narrative of Matthew*. An Enquiry into the Tradition History of Mt 1–2. AnBib 63. Rome 1976.

Soggin, J.A., *Joshua*. A Commentary. OTL. London 1979.

Sperber, D., *A Commentary on Derech Eretz Zuta*. Chapters Five to Eight. Ramat-Gan 1990.

Spicq, C., Une allusion au Docteur de Justice dans Matthieu, XXIII,10?, *RB* 66 (1959) 387–396.

–, *Notes de lexicographie néo-testamentaire*. Vols. 1–2, suppl. OBO 22:1–3. Fribourg 1978, 1982.

Stacey, D., *Prophetic Drama in the Old Testament*. London 1990.

Stadelmann, H., *Ben Sira als Schriftgelehrter*. Eine Untersuchung zum Berufsbild des vor-makkabäischen Sôfēr unter Berücksichtigung seines Verhältnisses zu Priester-, Propheten- und Weisheitslehrertum. WUNT 2:6. Tübingen 1980.

Stanton, G.(N), *Jesus of Nazareth in New Testament Preaching*. SNTSMS 27. Cambridge 1974.

–, Matthew as a Creative Interpreter of the Sayings of Jesus, in: P. Stuhlmacher (ed.), *Das Evangelium und die Evangelien*. Vorträge vom Tübinger Symposium 1982. WUNT 28. Tübingen 1983, 273–287.

–, The Origin and Purpose of Matthew's Gospel. Matthean Scholarship from 1945 to 1980, *ANRW* II 25:3 (1985) 1889–1951.

–, The Origin and Purpose of Matthew's Sermon on the Mount, in: G.F. Hawthorne *et al.* (eds.), *Tradition and Interpretation in the New Testament*. FS E.E. Ellis. Grand Rapids 1987, 181–192.

–, *A Gospel for a New People*. Studies in Matthew. Edinburgh 1992.

–, Matthew: βίβλος, εὐαγγέλιον, or βίος?, in: F. Van Segbroeck *et al.* (eds.), *The Four Gospels 1992*. FS F. Neirynck. BETL 100. Leuven 1992, 1187–1201.

Starcky, J., Les quatre étapes du messianisme à Qumrân, *RB* 70 (1963) 481–505.

–, Les Maîtres de Justice et la chronologie de Qumrân, in: M. Delcor (ed.), *Qumrān*. Sa piété, sa théologie et son milieu. BETL 46. Leuven 1978, 249–256.

Steck, H.O., *Israel und das Gewaltsame Geschick der Propheten*. Untersuchungen zur Überlieferung des deuteronomistischen Geschichtsbildes im Alten Testament, Spätjudentum und Urchristentum. WMANT 23. Neukirchen-Vluyn 1967.

-, *Überlieferung und Zeitgeschichte in den Elia-Erzählungen*. WMANT 26. Neukirchen-Vluyn 1968.

-, Das Problem theologischer Strömungen in nachexilischer Zeit, *EvT* 28 (1968) 445–458.

-, *Bereitete Heimkehr*. Jesaja 35 als redaktionelle Brücke zwischen dem Ersten und dem Zweiten Jesaja. SBS 121. Stuttgart 1985.

-, *Der Abschluß der Prophetie im Alten Testament*. Ein Versuch zur Frage der Vorgeschichte des Kanons. BibTS 17. Neukirchen-Vluyn 1991.

-, *Studien zu Tritojesaja*. BZAW 203. Berlin 1991.

Stegemann, H., *Die Entstehung der Qumrangemeinde*. Bonn 1971.

-, Die "Mitte der Schrift" aus der Sicht der Gemeinde von Qumran, in: M. Klopfenstein *et al.* (eds.), *Mitte der Schrift?* Ein jüdisch-christliches Gespräch. Texte des Berner Symposions von 6.–12. Januar 1985. JC 2. Bern 1987, 149–184.

-, The Origins of the Temple Scroll, in: J.A. Emerton (ed.), *Congress Volume Jerusalem 1986*. VTSup 40. Leiden 1988, 235–256.

-, Das Gesetzeskorpus der "Damaskusschrift" (CD IX–XVI), *RevQ* 14 (1990) 409–434.

-, The 'Teacher of Righteousness' and Jesus: Two Types of Religious Leadership in Judaism at the Turn of the Era, in: S. Talmon (ed.), *Jewish Civilization in the Hellenistic-Roman Period*. JSPSup 10. Sheffield 1991, 196–213.

-, Is the Temple Scroll a Sixth Book of the Torah—Lost for 2,500 Years?, in: H. Shanks (ed.), *Understanding the Dead Sea Scrolls*. New York 1992, 126–136.

Stein, R.H., The "Redaktionsgeschichtlich" Investigation of a Markan Seam (Mc 1 21f.), *ZNW* 61 (1970) 70–94.

-, *The Synoptic Problem*. An Introduction. Grand Rapids 1987.

-, Matthew—Luke Agreements Against Mark: Insight from John, *CBQ* 54 (1992) 482–502.

Stein, S., The Influence of Symposia Literature on the Literary Form of the Pesaḥ Haggadah, *JJS* 8 (1957) 13–44.

Stemberger, G., *Das klassische Judentum*. Kultur und Geschichte der rabbinischen Zeit (70 n. Chr. bis 1040 n. Chr). München 1979.

-, *Der Talmud*. Einführung – Texte – Erläuterungen. München 1982.

-, *Pharisäer, Sadduzäer, Essener*. SBS 144. Stuttgart 1991.

Stendahl, K., Kerygma und Kerygmatisch. Von zweideutigen Ausdrücken der Predigt der Urkirche – und unserer, *TLZ* 77 (1952) 715–720.

-, *The School of Matthew* and its Use of the Old Testament. ASNU 20. Lund ²1968.

Stern, D., *Parables in Midrash*. Narrative and Exegesis in Rabbinic Literature. Cambridge MA 1991.

Sternberg, M., *Expositional Modes and Temporal Ordering in Fiction*. Baltimore 1978.

Stipp, E.-J., *Elischa – Propheten – Gottesmänner*. Die Kompositionsgeschichte des Elischazyklus und verwandter Texte, rekonstruiert auf der Basis von Text- und Literarkritik zu 1 Kön 20.22 und 2 Kön 2–7. ATAT 24. St. Ottilien 1987.

Stock, A., Is Matthew's Presentation of Peter Ironic?, *BTB* 17 (1987) 64–69.

Stoebe, H.J., Noch einmal zu Amos VII 10–17, *VT* 39 (1989) 341–354.

Stone, M.E., Ideal Figures and Social Context: Priest and Sage in the Early Second Temple Age, in: P.D. Miller, Jr *et al.* (eds.), *Ancient Israelite Religion*. FS F.M. Cross. Philadelphia 1987, 575–586.

Stonehouse, N.B., *The Witness of Matthew and Mark to Christ*. Philadelphia 1944.

Strack, H.L. – Billerbeck, P., *Kommentar zum Neuen Testament aus Talmud und Midrasch*. Vols. 1–4. Vols. 5–6 ed. by Joachim Jeremias. München 1924–1928, 1956, 1961.

Strack, H.L. – Stemberger, G., *Introduction to the Talmud and Midrash*. Edinburgh 1991.

Strecker, G., Die Makarismen der Bergpredigt, *NTS* 17 (1970–71) 255–275.

-, *Der Weg der Gerechtigkeit*. Untersuchung zur Theologie des Matthäus. FRLANT 82. Göttingen ³1971.

-, Die Antithesen der Bergpredigt (Mt 5 21–48 par), *ZNW* 69 (1978) 36–72.

-, Review of M.J. Suggs, *Wisdom, Christology, and Law in Matthew's Gospel.* Cambridge MA 1970, *TLZ* 98 (1973) 519–522.

-, The Concept of History in Matthew, in: G. Stanton (ed.), *The Interpretation of Matthew*. IRT 3. Philadelphia 1983, 67–84.

-, *The Sermon on the Mount*. An Exegetical Commentary. Edinburgh 1988.

-, Schriftlichkeit oder Mündlichkeit der synoptischen Tradition? Anmerkungen zur formgeschichtlichen Problematik, in: F. Van Segbroeck *et al.* (eds.), *The Four Gospels 1992*. FS F. Neirynck. BETL 100. Leuven 1992, 159–172.

Streeter, B.H., *The Four Gospels*. A Study of Origins. Treating of the Manuscript Tradition, Sources, Authorship, & Dates. London 1926.

Strugnell, J., "Amen, I Say Unto You" in the Sayings of Jesus and in Early Christian Literature, *HTR* 67 (1974) 177–182.

-, The Qumran Scrolls: A Report on Work in Progress, in: S. Talmon (ed.), *Jewish Civilization in the Hellenistic-Roman Period*. JSPSup 10. Sheffield 1991, 94–106.

Stuart, D., *Hosea – Jonah*. WBC 31. Waco 1987.

Stuhlmacher, P., *Gerechtigkeit Gottes bei Paulus*. FRLANT 87. Göttingen ²1966.

-, *Das paulinische Evangelium*. I. Vorgeschichte. FRLANT 95. Göttingen 1968.

-, Das paulinische Evangelium, in: P. Stuhlmacher (ed.), *Das Evangelium und die Evangelien*. Vorträge vom Tübinger Symposium 1982. WUNT 28. Tübingen 1983, 157–182.

-, The Genre(s) of the Gospels, in: D.L. Dungan (ed.), *The Interrelations of the Gospels*. A Symposium led by M.-É. Boismard – W.R. Farmer – F. Neirynck, Jerusalem 1984. BETL 95. Leuven 1990, 484–494.

-, Das Christusbild der Paulus-Schule – eine Skizze, in: J.D.G. Dunn (ed.), *Jews and Christians*. The Parting of the Ways A.D. 70 to 135. The Second Durham-Tübingen Research Symposium on Earliest Christianity and Judaism (Durham, September, 1989). WUNT 66. Tübingen 1992, 159–175.

Sturdy, J.V.M., The authorship of the "prose sermons" of Jeremiah, in: J.A. Emerton (ed.), *Prophecy*. FS G. Fohrer. BZAW 150. Berlin 1980, 143–150.

Suggs, M.J., *Wisdom, Christology, and Law in Matthew's Gospel*. Cambridge MA 1970.

-, The Antitheses as Redactional Products, in: G. Strecker (ed.), *Jesus Christus in Historie und Theologie*. FS H. Conzelmann. Tübingen 1975, 433–444.

Suhl, A., Der Davidssohn im Matthäus-Evangelium, *ZNW* 59 (1968) 57–81.

Sutcliffe, E.F., *The Monks of Qumran* as Depicted in the Dead Sea Scrolls. London 1960.

Swanepoel, M.G., Ezekiel 16: Abandoned Child, Bride Adorned or Unfaithful Wife?, in: P.R. Davies *et al.* (eds.), *Among the Prophets*. Language, Image and Structure in the Prophetic Writings. JSOTSup 144. Sheffield 1993, 84–104.

Sweeney, M.A., *Isaiah 1–4 and the Post-Exilic Understanding of the Isaianic Tradition*. BZAW 171. Berlin 1988.

Syreeni, K., *The Making of the Sermon on the Mount*. A procedural analysis of Matt-

hew's redactoral activity. Vol. 1. AASF.DHL 44. Helsinki 1987.
-, Between Heaven and Earth: On the Structure of Matthew's Symbolic Universe, *JSNT* 40 (1990) 3–13.
Szyszman, S., *Le Karaïsme*. Ses doctrines et son histoire. BibKar A:1. Lausanne 1980.
Tabor, J.D., A Pierced or Piercing Messiah?—The Verdict Is Still Out, *BARev* 18:6 (1992) 58–59.
Tagawa, K., People and Community in the Gospel of Matthew, *NTS* 16 (1969–70) 149–162.
Talbert, C.H., *What Is a Gospel?* The Genre of the Canonical Gospels. Philadelphia 1977.
-, Oral and Independent or Literary and Interdependent? A Response to Albert B. Lord, in: W.O. Walker, Jr (ed.), *The Relationships Among the Gospels*. An Interdisciplinary Dialogue. TUMSR 5. San Antonio 1978, 93–102.
Talmon, S., The "Comparative Method" in Biblical Interpretation—Principles and Problems, in: J.A. Emerton (ed.), *Congress Volume Göttingen 1977*. VTSup 29. Leiden 1978, 320–356.
-, Heiliges Schrifttum und Kanonische Bücher aus jüdischer Sicht – Überlegungen zur Ausbildung der Grösse "Die Schrift" im Judentum, in: M. Klopfenstein *et al.* (eds.), *Mitte der Schrift?* Ein jüdisch-christliches Gespräch. Texte des Berner Symposions von 6.–12. Januar 1985. JC 2. Bern 1987, 45–79.
-, The Emergence of Jewish Sectarianism in the Early Second Temple Period, in: P.D. Miller, Jr *et al.* (eds.), *Ancient Israelite Religion*. FS F.M. Cross. Philadelphia 1987, 587–616.
-, *The World of Qumran from Within*. Collected Studies. Jerusalem 1989.
-, Oral Tradition and Written Transmission, or the Heard and the Seen Word in Judaism of the Second Temple Period, in: H. Wansbrough (ed.), *Jesus and the Oral Gospel Tradition*. JSNTSup 64. Sheffield 1991, 121–158.
-, The Concepts of *Māšîaḥ* and Messianism in Early Judaism, in: J.H. Charlesworth (ed.), *The Messiah*. Developments in Earliest Judaism and Christianity. The First Princeton Symposium on Judaism and Christian Origins. Minneapolis 1992, 79–115.
Taylor, V., *The Formation of the Gospel Tradition*. London 1933.
-, *The Names of Jesus*. London 1954.
-, *New Testament Essays*. London 1970.
Tcherikover, V., *Hellenistic Civilization and the Jews*. Philadelphia 1959.
Teeple, H.M., *The Mosaic Eschatological Prophet*. JBLMS 10. Philadelphia 1957.
-, The Oral Tradition That Never Existed, *JBL* 89 (1970) 56–68.
Teicher, J.L., The Dead Sea Scrolls—Documents of the Jewish-Christian Sect of Ebionites, *JJS* 2 (1951) 64–99.
-, Jesus in the Habakkuk Scroll, *JJS* 3 (1952) 53–55.
Terrien, S., Amos and Wisdom, in: J.L. Crehshaw (ed.), *Studies in Ancient Israelite Wisdom*. New York 1976, 448–455.
Theißen, G., *Urchristliche Wundergeschichten*. Ein Beitrag zur formgeschichtlichen Erforschung der synoptischen Evangelien. SNT 8. Gütersloh 1974.
-, *Lokalkolorit und Zeitgeschichte in den Evangelien*. Ein Beitrag zur Geschichte der synoptischen Tradition. NTOA 8. Fribourg 1989.
Thiel, W., *Die deuteronomistische Redaktion von Jeremia 1–25*. WMANT 41. Neukirchen-Vluyn 1973.
-, *Die deuteronomistische Redaktion von Jeremia 26–45*. Mit einer Gesamtbeurteilung der deuteronomistischen Redaktion des Buches Jeremia. WMANT 52. Neukirchen-Vluyn 1981.
-, Deuteronomistische Redaktionsarbeit in den Elia-Erzählungen, in: J.A. Emerton (ed.),

Congress Volume Leuven 1989. VTSup 43. Leiden 1991, 148–171.

-, Review of D.W. Jamieson-Drake, *Scribes and Schools in Monarchic Judah.* Sheffield 1991, *TLZ* 12 (1991) 898–900.

Thiering, B.E., *Redating the Teacher of Righteousness.* Sydney 1979.

Thomas, J.C., The Kingdom of God in the Gospel According to Matthew, *NTS* 39 (1993) 136–146.

Thompson, J.A., *The Book of Jeremiah.* NICOT. Grand Rapids 1980.

Thompson, W.G., *Matthew's Advice to a Divided Community.* Mt. 17,22–18,35. AnBib 44. Rome 1970.

-, Review of M.J. Suggs, *Wisdom, Christology, and Law in Matthew's Gospel.* Cambridge MA 1970, *CBQ* 33 (1971) 145–146.

-, Reflections on the Composition of Mt 8:1–9:34, *CBQ* 33 (1971) 365–388.

-, *Matthew's Story.* Good News for Uncertain Times. New York 1989.

Thyen, H., *Studien zur Sündenvergebung* im Neuen Testament und seinen alttestamentlichen und jüdischen Voraussetzungen. FRLANT 96. Göttingen 1970.

Tiede, D.L., *The Charismatic Figure as Miracle Worker.* SBLDS 1. Missoula 1972.

Tilborg, S. van, *The Jewish Leaders in Matthew.* Leiden 1972.

-, Matthew 27.3–10: an Intertextual Reading, in: S. Draisma (ed.), *Intertextuality in Biblical Writings.* FS B. van Iersel. Kampen 1989, 159–174.

Torm, F., Der Pluralis οὐρανοί, *ZNW* 33 (1934) 48–50.

Tortzen, C.G., Hvordan lærte oldtidens børn at læse og skrive?, in: C.G. Tortzen *et al.* (eds.), *Den hellenistiske skole.* Hellenismestudier 8. Aarhus 1993, 7–38.

Townsend, J.T., Matthew XXIII.9, *JTS* 12 (1961) 56–59.

Trever, J.C., The Book of Daniel and the Origin of the Qumran Community, *BA* 48 (1985) 89–102.

-, The Qumran Teacher—Another Candidate?, in: C.A. Evans *et al.* (eds.), *Early Jewish and Christian Exegesis.* Studies in Memory of W.H. Brownlee. SPHomSer 10. Atlanta 1987, 101–121.

Trilling, W., *Das wahre Israel.* Studien zur Theologie des Matthäus-Evangeliums. SANT 10. München ³1964.

-, Die Wahrheit von Jesus-Worten in der Interpretation neutestamentlicher Autoren, *KD* 23 (1977) 93–112.

Trummer, P., *Die blutende Frau.* Wunderheilung im Neuen Testament. Freiburg 1991.

Tucker, G.M., Prophetic Authenticity. A Form-Critical Study of Amos 7:10–17, *Int* 27 (1973) 423–434.

-, Prophecy and the Prophetic Literature, in: D.A. Knight *et al.* (eds.), *The Hebrew Bible and its Modern Interpreters.* SBLBMI 1. Philadelphia 1985, 325–368.

Tuckett, C.M., The Beatitudes: A Source-Critical Study, *NovT* 25 (1983) 193–207.

Übelacker, W.G., *Der Hebräerbrief als Appell.* I. Untersuchungen zu *exordium, narratio* und *postscriptum* (Hebr 1–2 und 13,22–25). ConBNT 21. Stockholm 1989.

Ulfgard, H., *Feast and Future.* Revelation 7:9–17 and the Feast of Tabernacles. ConBNT 22. Stockholm 1989.

Unterman, J., *From Repentance to Redemption.* Jeremiah's Thought in Transition. JSOTSup 54. Sheffield 1987.

Urbach, E. E., The Talmudic Sage—Character and Authority, in: H.H. Ben-Sasson *et al.* (eds.), *Jewish Society Through the Ages.* London 1971, 116–147.

The Sages. Their Concepts and Beliefs. Cambridge MA ²1979.

Urman, D., Jewish Inscriptions from Dabbura in the Golan, *IEJ* 22 (1972) 16–23.

-, Golan, *EAEHL* 2 (1976) 453–467.

Uro, R., *Sheep Among the Wolves.* A Study on the Mission Instructions of Q. AASF.DHL 47. Helsinki 1987.

Uspensky, B., *A Poetics of Composition*. The Structure of the Artistic Text and Typology of a Compositional Form. Berkeley 1973.

Vanderkam, J.C., Zadok and the *spr htwrh hhtwm* in Dam. Doc. V,2–5, *RevQ* 11 (1984) 561–570.

Vansina, J., *Oral Tradition as History*. London 1985.

Vaux, R. de, Fouilles au Khirbet Qumrân. Rapport préliminaire sur la deuxième campagne, *RB* 61 (1954) 206–236.

-, *Ancient Israel*. Its Life and Institutions. London ²1965.

-, *Archaeology and the Dead Sea Scrolls*. The Schweich Lectures of the British Academy 1959. London 1973.

Vermes, G., *Scripture and Tradition in Judaism*. Haggadic Studies. SPB 4. Leiden ²1973.

-, *Jesus the Jew*. A historian's reading of the Gospels. London 1973.

-, *Post-Biblical Jewish Studies*. SJLA 8. Leiden 1975.

-, The Essenes and History, *JJS* 32 (1981) 18–31.

-, The Oxford Forum for Qumran Research Seminar on the Rule of War from Cave 4 (2Q285), *JJS* 43 (1992) 85–90.

Vermeylen, J., *Du prophète Isaïe à l'apocalyptique*. Isaïe, I–XXXV, miroir d'un demi-millénaire d'expérience religieuse en Israël. Vols. 1–2. Ébib 13, 29. Paris 1977, 1978.

-, Le Proto-Isaïe et la sagesse d'Israel, in: M. Gilbert (ed.), *La Sagesse de l'Ancien Testament*. BETL 51. Leuven 1979, 39–58.

-, L'unité du livre d'Isaïe, in: J. Vermeylen (ed.), *The Book of Isaiah – Le Livre d'Isaïe*. Les oracles et leurs relectures. Unité et complexité de l'ouvrage. BETL 81. Leuven 1989, 11–53.

Verseput, D.J., *The Rejection of the Humble Messianic King*. A Study of the Composition of Matthew 11–12. EUS. Frankfurt am Main 1986.

-, The Role and Meaning of the 'Son of God' Title in Matthew's Gospel, *NTS* 33 (1987) 532–556.

-, The Faith of the Reader and the Narrative of Matthew 13.53–16.20, *JSNT* 46 (1992) 3–24.

Viberg, Å., *Symbols of Law*. A Contextual Analysis of Legal Symbolic Acts in the Old Testament. ConBOT 34. Stockholm 1992.

Vieweger, D., Die Arbeit des jeremianischen Schülerkreises am Jeremiabuch und deren Rezeption in der literarischen Überlieferung der Prophetenschrift Ezechiels, *BZ* 32 (1988) 15–34.

Vincent, J.J., Didactic Kerygma in the Synoptic Gospels, *SJT* 10 (1957) 262–273.

-, Did Jesus Teach His Disciples to Learn by Heart?, *SE* 3 (TU 88) (1964) 105–118.

Vinson, R.B., A Comparative Study of the Use of Enthymemes in the Synoptic Gospels, in: D.F. Watson (ed.), *Persuasive Artistery*. FS G.A. Kennedy. JSNTSup 50. Sheffield 1991, 119–141.

Viviano, B.T., *Study as Worship*. Aboth and the New Testament. SJLA 26. Leiden 1978.

-, Rabbouni and Mark 9:5, *RB* 97 (1990) 207–218.

-, Social World and Community Leadership: The Case of Matthew 23.1–12, 34, *JSNT* 39 (1990) 3–21.

-, Beatitudes Found Among Dead Sea Scrolls, *BARev* 18:6 (1992) 53–55, 66.

-, Eight Beatitudes at Qumran and in Matthew? A New Publication from Cave Four, *SEÅ* 58 (1993) 71–84.

Vögtle, A., Messiasbekenntnis und Petrusverheißung. Zur Komposition Mt 16,13–23 Par., *BZ* 1 (1957) 252–272, *BZ* 2 (1958) 85–103.

-, Das christologische und ekklesiologische Anliegen von Mt. 28,18–20, *SE* 2 (TU 87)

(1964) 266–294.

Vogler, W., *Judas Iskarioth*. Untersuchungen zu Tradition und Redaktion von Texten des Neuen Testaments und außerkanonischer Schriften. TA 42. Berlin 1983.

Volz, P., *Die Eschatologie der jüdischen Gemeinde* im neutestamentlichen Zeitalter nach den Quellen der rabbinischen, apokalyptischen und apokryphen Literatur. Tübingen 1934.

Vorster, W., Intertextuality and Redaktionsgeschichte, in: S. Draisma (ed.), *Intertextuality in Biblical Writings*. FS B. van Iersel. Kampen 1989, 15–26.

Vouga, F., *Jésus et la loi* selon la tradition synoptique. MdB. Genève 1988.

Vries, B. de, Baraita, Beraitot, *EncJud* 4 (1971) 189–193.

Wach, J., *Meister und Jünger*. Zwei religionssoziologische Betrachtungen. Leipzig 1924.

-, *Sociology of Religion*. Chicago 1944.

-, Master and Disciple: Two Religio-Sociological Studies, *JQ* 42 (1962) 1–21.

Wacholder, B.Z., *The Dawn of Qumran*. The Sectarian Torah and the Teacher of Righteousness. HUCM 8. Cincinnati 1983.

-, The "Sealed" Torah versus the "Revealed" Torah: An Exegesis of Damascus Covenant V,1–6 and Jeremiah 32,10–14, *RevQ* 12 (1986) 351–368.

-, Does Qumran Record the Death of the *Moreh?* The Meaning of *he'aseph* in Damascus Covenant XIX,35, XX,14, *RevQ* 13 (1988) 323–330.

-, The Ancient Judaeo-Aramaic Literature (500–164 BCE). A Classification of Pre-Qumranic Texts, in: L.H. Schiffman (ed), *Archaeology and History in the Dead Sea Scrolls*. The New York University Conference in Memory of Y. Yadin. JSPSup 8. Sheffield 1990, 257–281.

Wagner, S., יָרָה, *TWAT* 3 (1982) 909–930.

Wainwright, E.M., *Towards a Feminist Critical Reading of the Gospel according to Matthew*. BZNW 60. Berlin 1991.

Walker, R., *Die Heilsgeschichte im ersten Evangelium*. FRLANT 91. Göttingen 1967.

Wallendorff, P., מורה הצדק. *Rättfärdighetens lärare*. En exegetisk undersökning. Helsingfors 1964.

Walter, N., Die Bearbeitung der Seligpreisungen durch Matthäus, *SE* 4 (TU 102) (1968) 246–258.

Wanke, G., *Untersuchungen zur sogenannten Baruchschrift*. BZAW 122. Berlin 1971.

Wanke, J., *"Bezugs- und Kommentarworte" in den synoptischen Evangelien*. Beobachtungen zur Interpretationsgeschichte der Herrenworte in der vorevangelischen Überlieferung. ETS 44. Leipzig 1981.

Wansbrough, H. (ed.), *Jesus and the Oral Gospel Tradition*. JSNTSup 64. Sheffield 1991.

Watson, D.F., *Invention, Arrangement, and Style*. Rhetorical Criticism of Jude and 2 Peter. SBLDS 104. Atlanta 1988.

-, Review of B.L. Mack, *Rhetoric and the New Testament*. Minneapolis 1990, *Bib* 72 (1991) 116–119.

Watts, J.D.W., *Isaiah*. Vols. 1–2. WBC 24, 25. Waco 1985, 1987.

Weaver, D.J., *Matthew's Missionary Discourse*. A Literary Critical Analysis. JSNTSup 38. Sheffield 1990.

Webb, R.L., *John the Baptizer and Prophet*. A Socio-Historical Study. JSNTSup 62. Sheffield 1991.

Weber, M., *Wirtschaft und Gesellschaft*. Grundriss der verstehenden Soziologie. Tübingen ⁵1976.

Weder, H., *Die "Rede der Reden."* Eine Auslegung der Bergpredigt heute. Zürich ²1987.

-, "But I say to you ..." Concerning the Foundations of Jesus' Interpretation of the Law in the "Sermon on the Mount," in: T.W. Jennings, Jr (ed.), *Text and Logos*. The Humanistic Interpretation of the New Testament. SPHomSer. Atlanta 1990, 211–228.

Wegner, U., *Der Hauptmann von Kafarnaum* (Mt 7,28a; 8,5–10.13 par Lk 7,1–10). Ein Beitrag zur Q-Forschung. WUNT 2:14. Tübingen 1985.

Weinfeld, M., *Deuteronomy and the Deuteronomic School*. Oxford 1972.

-, *The Organizational Pattern and the Penal Code of the Qumran Sect*. A Comparison with Guilds and Religious Associations of the Hellenistic-Roman Period. NTOA 2. Fribourg 1986.

Weingreen, J., *From Bible to Mishna*. The continuity of tradition. Manchester 1976.

Weippert, H., *Die Prosareden des Jeremiabuches*. BZAW 132. Berlin 1973.

-, Das deuteronomistische Geschichtswerk. Sein Ziel und Ende in der neueren Forschung, *TRu* 50 (1985) 213–249.

Weiss, H.-F., διδάσκω κτλ., *EWNT* 1 (1980) 764–769.

Weiss, W., *"Eine neue Lehre in Vollmacht."* Die Streit- und Schulgespräche des Markus-Evangeliums. BZNW 52. Berlin 1989.

Wellhausen, J., *Das Evangelium Matthaei*. Berlin 1904.

Wenham, D., *The Rediscovery of Jesus' Eschatological Discourse*. Gospel Perspectives 4. Sheffield 1984.

Werlitz, J., *Studien zur literarkritischen Methode*. Gericht und Heil in Jesaja 7,1–17 und 29,1–8. BZNW 204. Berlin 1992.

Wernberg-Møller, P., צדק, צדיק and צדוק in the Zadokite Fragments (CDC), the Manual of Discipline (DSD) and the Habakkuk-Commentary (DSH), *VT* 3 (1953) 310–315.

-, Some Passages in the "Zadokite" Fragments and their Parallels in the Manual of Discipline, *JSS* 1 (1956) 110–128.

-, The Nature of the *Yaḥad* according to the Manual of Discipline and Related Documents, *ALUOS* 6 (1969) 56–81.

Werner, W., Vom Prophetenwort zur Prophetentheologie. Ein redaktionskritischer Versuch zu Jes 6,1–8,18, *BZ* 29 (1985) 1–30.

-, *Eschatologische Texte in Jesaja 1–39*. Messias, heiliger Rest, Völker. FB 46. Würzburg [2]1986.

Westerholm, S., *Jesus and Scribal Authority*. ConBNT 10. Lund 1978.

Westermann, C., *Isaiah 40–66*. A Commentary. OTL. London 1969.

-, שרת, *THAT* 2 ([2]1979) 1019–1022.

Wevers, J.W., *Ezekiel*. NCB. London 1969.

Whitley, C.F., The Language and Exegesis of Isaiah 8 16–23, *ZAW* 90 (1978) 28–43.

Whybray, R.N., *The Intellectual Tradition in the Old Testament*. BZAW 135. Berlin 1974.

-, *Isaiah 40–66*. NCB. London 1975.

-, Prophecy and Wisdom, in: R. Coggins *et al*. (eds.), *Israel's Prophetic Tradition*. FS P.R. Ackroyd. Cambridge 1982, 181–199.

-, *The Second Isaiah*. OTG. Sheffield 1983.

-, The social world of the wisdom writers, in: R.E. Clements (ed.), *The World of Ancient Israel*. Sociological, Anthropological and Political Perspectives. Cambridge 1989, 227–250.

-, The Sage in the Israelite Royal Court, in: J.G. Gammie *et al*. (eds.), *The Sage in Israel and the Ancient Near East*. Winona Lake 1990, 133–139.

Widengren, G., *Literary and Psychological Aspects of the Hebrew Prophets*. UUÅ 1948:10. Uppsala 1948.

Wieder, N., The "Law-Interpreter" of the Sect of the Dead Sea Scrolls: The Second Moses, *JJS* 4 (1953) 158–175.

Wiefel, W., Vätersprüche und Herrenworte. Ein Beitrag zur Frage der Bewahrung mündlicher Traditionssätze, *NovT* 11 (1969) 105–120.

Wieser, F.E., *Die Abrahmvorstellungen im Neuen Testament*. EH 23:317. Bern 1987.

Wilcox, M., Peter and the Rock: A Fresh Look at Matthew XVI.17–19, *NTS* 22 (1975–76) 73–88.

Wildberger, H., Die Rede Ratsake vor Jerusalem, *TZ* 35 (1979) 35–47.

-, *Jesaja*. Vols. 1–3. BKAT 10:1–3. Neukirchen-Vluyn 1972–1982.

Wilkens, W., Die Redaktion des Gleichniskapitels Mark. 4 durch Matth., *TZ* 20 (1964) 305–327.

-, Die Versuchung Jesu nach Matthäus, *NTS* 28 (1982) 479–489.

-, Die Komposition des Matthäus-Evangeliums, *NTS* 31 (1985) 24–38.

Wilkins, M.J., *The Concept of Disciple in Matthew's Gospel* As Reflected in the Use of the Term Μαθητής. NovTSup 59. Leiden 1988.

Willi-Plein, I., *Vorformen der Schriftexegese innerhalb des Alten Testaments*. Untersuchungen zum literarischen Werden der auf Amos, Hosea und Micha zurückgehenden Bücher im hebräischen Zwölfprophetenbuch. BZAW 123. Berlin 1971.

-, *Prophetie am Ende*. Untersuchungen zu Sacharja 9–14. BBB 42. Köln 1974.

Williams, J.G., The Prophetic "Father." A Brief Explanation of the Term "Sons of the Prophets," *JBL* 85 (1966) 344–348.

Wilson, R.R., *Prophecy and Society in Ancient Israel*. Philadelphia 1980.

-, The Community of the Second Isaiah, in: R. Seitz (ed.), *Reading and Preaching the Book of Isaiah*. Philadelphia 1988, 53–70.

Winter, B.W., The Messiah as the Tutor: The Meaning of καθηγητής in Matthew 23:10, *TynBul* 42 (1991) 152–157.

Winton Thomas, D., The Dead Sea Scrolls: What May We Believe?, *ALUOS* 6 (1969) 7–20.

Wise, M.O., *A Critical Study of the Temple Scroll from Qumran Cave 11*. SAOC 49. Chicago 1990.

-, The Teacher of Righteousness and the High Priest of the Intersacerdotium: Two Approaches, *RevQ* 14 (1990) 587–613.

Wolff, H.W., Hoseas geistige Heimat, *TLZ* 81 (1956) 83–94.

-, *Frieden ohne Ende*. Eine Auslegung von Jes. 7,1–7 und 9,1–6. BibS(N) 35. Neukirchen-Vluyn 1962.

-, *Amos' geistige Heimat*. WMANT 18. Neukirchen-Vluyn 1964.

-, *Hosea*. A Commentary on the Book of the Prophet Hosea. Hermeneia. Philadelphia 1974.

-, *Joel and Amos*. A Commentary on the Books of the Prophets Joel and Amos. Hermeneia. Philadelphia 1977.

-, Haggai/Haggaibuch, *TRE* 14 (1985) 355–360.

-, *Dodekapropheton 6. Haggai*. BKAT 14:6. Neukirchen-Vluyn 1986.

-, *Studien zur Prophetie*. Probleme und Erträge. TBü 76. München 1987.

Wong, K.-C., *Interkulturelle Theologie und multikulturelle Gemeinde im Matthäusevangelium*. Zum Verhältnis von Juden- und Heidenchristen im ersten Evangelium. NTOA 22. Fribourg 1992.

Woude, A.S. van der, *Die messianischen Vorstellungen der Gemeinde von Qumrân*. Assen 1957.

-, χρίω κτλ., *TDNT* 9 (1974) 517–520.

-, Three classical prophets: Amos, Hosea and Micah, in: R. Coggins *et al.* (eds.), *Israel's Prophetic Tradition*. FS P.R. Ackroyd. Cambridge 1982, 32–57.

-, Wicked Priest or Wicked Priests? Reflections on the Identification of the Wicked Priest in the Habakkuk Commentary, *JJS* 33 (1982) 349–359.

-, The Dead Sea Scrolls: Some Issues, *SEÅ* 57 (1992) 86–101.

-, Fünfzehn Jahre Qumranforschung (1974–1988), *TRu* 54 (1989) 221–261, *TRu* 55

(1990) 245–307, *TRu* 57 (1992) 1–57, 225–253.

Wouters, A., *"... wer den Willen meines Vaters tut."* Eine Untersuchung zum Verständnis vom Handeln im Matthäusevangelium. BU 23. Regensburg 1992.

Wrede, W., *Vorträge und Studien.* Tübingen 1907.

Wrege, H.-T., *Die Überlieferungsgeschichte der Bergpredigt.* WUNT 9. Tübingen 1968.

-, *Das Sondergut des Matthäus-Evangeliums.* ZWB. Zürich 1991.

Wright, B.G., *No Small Difference.* Sirach's Relationship to Its Hebrew Parent Text. SBLSCS 26. Atlanta 1989.

Wright, D.P., The Gesture of Hand Placement in the Hebrew Bible and in Hittite Literature, *JAOS* 106 (1986) 433–446.

-, *The Disposal of Impurity.* Elimination Rites in the Bible and in Hittite and Mesopotamian Literature. SBLDS 101. Atlanta 1987.

Wright, D.P. – Milgrom, J. – Fabry, H.-J., סמך, *TWAT* 5 (1986) 880–889.

Würthwein, E., *Die Bücher der Könige.* Vol. 2. ATD 11:2. Göttingen 1984.

Wuellner, W.H., *The Meaning of "Fishers of Men."* NTL. Philadelphia 1967.

Yadin, Y., A Note on Melchizedek and Qumran, *IEJ* 15 (1965) 152–154.

-, *The Temple Scroll.* The Hidden Law of the Dead Sea Sect. London 1985.

Yee, G.A., *Composition and Tradition in the Book of Hosea.* A Redaction Critical Investigation. SBLDS 102. Atlanta 1987.

Zahn, T., *Das Evangelium des Matthäus.* KomNT 1. Leipzig ³1910.

Zeitlin, S., A Reply, *JQR* 53 (1962–63) 345–349.

-, The Title Rabbi in the Gospels is Anachronistic, *JQR* 59 (1968–69) 158–160.

Zeller, D., Jesus als vollmächtiger Lehrer (Mt 5–7) und der hellenistische Gesetzgeber, in: L. Schenke (ed.), *Studien zum Matthäusevangelium.* FS W. Pesch. SBS. Stuttgart 1988, 299–317.

Zias, J. – Charlesworth, J.H., Crucifixion: Archaeology, Jesus, and the Dead Sea Scrolls, in: J.H. Charlesworth (ed.), *Jesus and the Dead Sea Scrolls.* AB Reference Library. New York 1993, 273–289.

Ziesler, J.A., *The Meaning of Righteousness in Paul.* A Linguistic and Theological Enquiry. SNTSMS 20. Cambridge 1972.

Zimmerli, W., Zur Struktur der alttestamentlichen Weisheit, *ZAW* 51 (1933) 177–204.

-, *Gottes Offenbarung.* Gesammelte Aufsätze zum Alten Testament. TBü 19. München 1963.

-, *Studien zur alttestamentlichen Theologie und Prophetie.* Gesammelte Aufsätze. Vol. 2. TBü 51. München 1974.

-, Prophetic Proclamation and Reinterpretation, in: D.A. Knight (ed.), *Tradition and Theology in the Old Testament.* Philadelphia 1977, 69–100.

-, Vom Prophetenwort zum Prophetenbuch, *TLZ* 104 (1979) 481–496.

-, Das Phänomen der "Fortschreibung" im Buche Ezechiel, in: J.A. Emerton (ed.), *Prophecy.* FS G. Fohrer. BZAW 150. Berlin 1980, 174–191.

-, *Grundriß der alttestamentlichen Theologie.* TW 3. Stuttgart ⁴1982.

-, Ezechiel/Ezechielbuch, *TRE* 10 (1982) 766–781.

-, *Ezekiel.* A Commentary on the Book of the Prophet Ezekiel. Vols. 1–2. Hermeneia. Philadelphia 1979, 1983.

Zimmermann, A.F., *Die urchristlichen Lehrer.* Studien zum Tradentenkreis der διδάσκαλοι im frühen Urchristentum. WUNT 2:12. Tübingen ²1988.

Zobel, K., *Prophetie und Deuteronomium.* Die Rezeption prophetischer Theologie durch das Deuteronomium. BZAW 199. Berlin 1992.

Zuck, R.B., Hebrew Words for "Teach," *BSac* 121 (1964) 228–235.

Zumstein, J., *La relation du maître et du disciple dans le bas-judaïsme palestinien et dans l'évangile selon Matthieu.* Mémoire de l'Institut des sciences bibliques de l'Université de Lausanne. Lausanne 1971.

-, *La condition du croyant dans l'évangile selon Matthieu.* OBO 16. Fribourg 1977.

Indices